Psychiatric Mental Health Nursing

Second Edition

Psychiatric Mental Health Nursing

Second Edition

Katherine M. Fortinash, MSN, RNCS, CNS
Certified Clinical Specialist
Adult Psychiatric Mental Health Nursing;
Clinical Nurse Specialist/Senior Systems Specialist
Sharp Mesa Vista Hospital
Sharp Behavioral Health Services
San Diego, California;
Consultant
San Diego, California

Patricia A. Holoday-Worret, MSN, RNCS, CNS
Certified Clinical Specialist
Adult Psychiatric Mental Health Nursing;
Professor, Psychiatric Mental Health Nursing
Palomar College
San Marcos, California;
Consultant
San Diego, California

M Mosby

St. Louis Baltimore Boston Carlsbad Chicago Minneapolis New York Philadelphia Portland
London Milan Sydney Tokyo Toronto

www.mosby.com

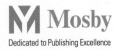
Mosby
Dedicated to Publishing Excellence

Editor-in-Chief: Sally Schrefer
Editor: Jeanne Allison
Developmental Editor: Jeff Downing
Project Manager: John Rogers
Senior Production Editor: Cheryl A. Abbott
Designer: Kathi Gosche

Mosby, Inc.
A Harcourt Health Sciences Company
11830 Westline Industrial Drive
St. Louis, Missouri 63146

Printed in the United States

International Standard Book Number 0-3230-0648-5

99 00 01 02 03 CL/KPT 9 8 7 6 5 4 3 2 1

CONTRIBUTORS

Donna C. Aguilera, RN, PhD, FAAN, FIAEP
Disaster Mental Health Services, American Red Cross
Private Practice and Consultant
Beverly Hills and Sherman Oaks, California

Merry A. Armstrong, DNSc, ARNP
Assistant Professor
Intercollegiate Center for Nursing Education
Washington State University
Spokane, Washington

Margaret T. Barker, RN, MSW, LCSW
Psychiatric Social Worker
Private Practice
La Mesa, California

Anne Clarkin-Watts, MSW, LCSW
Private Practice
San Diego, California

Phillip R. Deming, MA, MDiv, Chaplain
Pastoral Care and Education, Sharp HealthCare
Behavioral Health Services
San Diego, California

Carmel Bitondo Dyer, MD
Assistant Professor of Medicine
Director of Geriatrics Program
Baylor College of Medicine
Houston, Texas

Marjorie Lee Ferguson, MN, RNCS, FNP
Clinical Nurse Specialist
Child and Adolescent Psychiatric Mental Health
 Nursing
Family Nurse Practitioner
San Diego, California

Mary S. Gleason, MSN, RNCS
Director of Clinical Services; Geriatric Program
Harris County Hospital District
Baylor College of Medicine
Houston, Texas

Ruth N. Grendell, DNSc, RN
Professor
Point Loma Nazarene University
San Diego, California

Bonnie Hagerty, RN, PhD, CS
Associate Professor
School of Nursing
University of Michigan
Ann Arbor, Michigan

Linda Hollinger-Smith, RN, PhD
Assistant Dean, Academic Systems
Director of Nursing, Rush Primary Care Institute
Rush–Presbyterian–St. Luke's Medical Center
Chicago, Illinois

Charles Kemp, RN, CRNH
Lecturer
School of Nursing
Baylor University
Dallas, Texas

Joyce Laben, RN, MSN, JD, CS, FAAN
Professor of Nursing Emerita
Vanderbilt University
Nashville, Tennessee

Richard C. Lucas, MD, JD
Adolescent Unit Director
Charter Behavioral Health Systems;
Assistant Clinical Professor of Psychiatry
University of California, San Diego
San Diego, California

Shelly F. Lurie, MS, RN, CS-P
Faculty Associate
School of Nursing
The Johns Hopkins University;
Nurse Psychotherapist
Private Practice
Baltimore, Maryland

Pamela E. Marcus, RN, MSCS-P
Nurse Psychotherapist
Private Practice
Upper Malboro, Maryland

Susan Fertig McDonald, RN, MSN, CNS
Clinical Nurse Specialist
San Diego VA Health Care System
San Diego, California

Monica Molloy, MSN, RNC
Clinical Nurse Specialist
Division of Psychiatric Nursing
Department of Psychiatry and Behavioral Sciences
Medical University of South Carolina
Charleston, South Carolina

Diane Podsedly Oran, MN, RN, CS
Director of Crisis Response
Counseling Services, Inc.
Portland, Maine

Kathleen Pace-Murphy, PhD, RNCS
Regional Health Care Service–Medical
G.D. Searle and Company;
Clinical Assistant Professor
Baylor College of Medicine;
Department of Medicine
Assistant Professor
Texas Tech University
School of Nursing
Houston, Texas

Terry Patterson, MN, RN, CNS, ARNP
Instructor
Intercollegiate Center for Nursing Education
Washington State University, Eastern Washington
    University, and Whitworth College
Spokane, Washington

Barbara A. Redding, RN, EdD
Professor
College of Nursing
University of South Florida
Tampa, Florida

Nan Rich, RN, CS, PMHNP, PhD(c)
Doctoral Candidate
University of California, San Francisco;
Eastmoreland Hospital, Portland
Nursing Home Consultation Service
Portland, Oregon

Ona Z. Riggin, EdD, ARNP
Distinguished Service Professor
Chair, Graduate Program
College of Nursing
University of South Florida
Tampa, Florida

Alwilda Scholler-Joquish, MN, MS, PhD, RN, CS
Assistant Professor
School of Nursing
Texas Tech Health Sciences Center
Lubbock, Texas

Jay Sherr, PharmD, BCPP
Clinical Assistant Professor
School of Pharmacy
Research Assistant Professor
Maryland Psychiatric Research Center
School of Medicine
University of Maryland, Baltimore
Catonsville, Maryland

Kathryn Thomas, PhD, RN, CS-P, FAACS
Associate Professor
Villa Julie College
Private Practice
Baltimore, Maryland

James Turnbull, MD, FRCP(c)
Medical Director, Outpatient Services
Frontier Health, Inc.;
Clinical Professor
Department of Family Medicine and Psychiatry
Quillen College of Medicine
East Tennessee State University
Kingsport, Tennessee

Joan C. Urbancic, PhD, MSN, RN, CS
Professor
McAuley School of Nursing
University of Detroit Mercy
Detroit, Michigan

Gwen van Servellen, RN, PhD, FAAN
Professor
School of Nursing
University of California, Los Angeles
Los Angeles, California

Kathleen M. Walker, RN, MS, CS
Psychiatric Clinical Nurse Specialist
University of Tennessee at Knoxville, College of Nursing
Johnson City, Tennessee

Mary Magenheimer Webster, MS, CS
Psychiatric Nurse Liaison
Spokane, Washington

William R. Whetstone, RN, PhD
Professor and Assistant Chair
Division of Nursing
California State University, Dominguez Hills
Carson, California

Theresa Williams-Hessling, MA, MFCC, ATR
Art Therapist and Marriage, Family, and Child Counselor
Private Practice
San Diego, California

REVIEWERS

For those who struggle with mental disorders every day on their journey toward mental health and for the students, nurses, and caregivers whose lives they touch. Our wish is that this text brings knowledge, wisdom, and hope.

PREFACE

Psychiatric Mental Health Nursing, now in its second edition, is prepared to meet the health care challenges of the new millenium. As research continues to expand in the areas of psychobiology and psychopharmacology, nurses continue to integrate the current plethora of biologic information with the caring concepts of the psychosocial models. Newer, more effective, and less toxic medications present new hope for clients and families experiencing the effects of mental disorders. This presents new challenges for nurses, who must prepare themselves to educate clients, families, and community about current trends in treatment modalities, with a sense of cautious optimism. The implication of psychiatric nursing is that these findings must be incorporated into all areas of the discipline. This is especially true for psychopharmacology "to ensure safe and effective care of people with mental illness and the advancement of the specialty" (ANA, 1994).

The health care delivery system continues to be influenced by the revolutionary changes in the industry, most specifically, managed care organizations. The shift of clients with mental disorders from inpatient treatment to alternative, less costly care options, such as partial hospital programs, outpatient clinics, and community agencies, continues to challenge nurses and other health care disciplines. Although inpatient psychiatric care is available for individuals whose illness demands it, the typical lengths of stay in acute care settings continue to be dramatically reduced.

Along with extraordinary changes in psychobiology, the next century promises to infuse the health care delivery system with dramatic information about the cultural and spiritual aspects of clients with mental disorders and their families. Mental health facilities are calling on hospital chaplains and other clergy to assist clients and families in addressing their spiritual concerns within a nondenominational context. These spiritual therapists are part of the professional, interdisciplinary health care team and provide a much-needed service to those in need of spiritual care. Another challenge for nurses and other health care disciplines in keeping with current, dynamic cultural changes is that of cultural awareness. Although nurses have always addressed the cultural and spiritual needs of their clients, current mandates from specific managed care organizations are requiring further knowledge and education in these critical areas in several states across the country.

Now, as in the past, psychiatric mental health nurses are called on to blend their broad base of scientific knowledge and interpersonal skills to meet the traditional and current challenges of providing effective quality care. Whatever changes await psychiatric nursing in the new millenium, one thing remains constant: student nurses, new graduates, and seasoned practitioners alike will meet the challenges, as always, with energy, enthusiasm, and concern for their clients.

APPROACH AND INTENDED USE

This second edition of *Psychiatric Mental Health Nursing* continues to stress the challenges and discoveries of the biologic revolution as health care delivery moves into the twenty-first century. Integration of the client's biologic psychosocial needs remains the focus of nursing care, with additional emphasis on cultural and spiritual areas of concern. Nurses and associated professionals continue to focus on attaining, maintaining, and promoting the client's integrity and dignity while meeting those needs. This text illustrates a balanced nursing and medical approach, with strong emphasis on DSM-IV guidelines and related treatments. Although psychiatric nursing is thoroughly discussed as it relates to various well-regarded theorists, the text does not advocate any one specific nursing framework. This timely, state-of-the-art text is primarily intended to help students and practicing psychiatric nurses deliver professional nursing care for clients and their families, regardless of time, place, or circumstances.

The nursing process, a time-proven, six-step problem-solving method, is featured as a distinct section in relevant chapters. Interesting case studies depicting "real-life" situations followed by a series of questions are interspersed throughout the various stages of the nursing process section to stimulate student learning and critical thinking. This section also includes comprehensive nursing care plans that begin with a case study, followed by relevant DSM-IV and NANDA diagnoses. Client outcomes are identified, interventions with rationales are presented, and an evaluative statement is provided.

The major organizing structures for the disorders chapters include both the diagnoses of the North American Nursing Diagnosis Association (NANDA, 1999) and the American Psychiatric Association (APA) *Diagnostic and Statistical Manual of Mental Disorders,* fourth edition (APA, 1994). We strongly believe in the practicality and effectiveness of the collaborative efforts of nursing and medicine whenever possible. We contend that the use of current NANDA terminology most accurately describes the therapeutic services and contributions of nurses and also reflects contemporary nursing actions and responses. Application and use of refined diagnostic labels are essential to the evolution of the language and discipline of nursing.

STRUCTURE AND ORGANIZATION

Part One, Introduction to Psychiatric Mental Health Nursing, presents concepts and issues fundamental to psychiatric mental health nursing. The reader is introduced to concepts that not only define nursing as an art and a science but also reveal the substantive changes and trends that currently shape and challenge traditional professional nursing roles in the area of mental health. Typical student experiences and concerns specific to the role of psychiatric nursing are uniquely presented in the forms of clinical rewards, challenges, and solutions. This information will be very helpful for students as they enter and interact in the psychiatric setting. Theoretic perspectives that provide the framework for mental and emotional disorders are thoroughly explored with clear, specific examples of each therapeutic modality. A comprehensive chapter on psychobiology is presented, which thoroughly explores the biologic components and their role in mental and emotional disorders. Clear, concise examples are depicted with vivid full-color illustrations of biologic effects on brain chemistry. Legal and ethical issues specific to clients with mental disorders are described. Patients' rights related to mental illness are carefully defined, and relevant case law is cited. Cultural issues are discussed, offering a cross-section of the various cultures. Explanation of how cultural beliefs affect clients' attitudes toward health care and care-giving practices is provided, with emphasis on mental health and mental disorders.

Part Two, Dynamics of Nursing Practice, discusses the two essential components of the nursing role. The chapter on the nursing process presents the foundations of critical thinking, intuitive skills, and problem-solving approaches used by nurses as they practice their discipline in a variety of clinical and community settings. Several helpful assessment and interview tools are featured, including a treatment plan, a standardized care plan, and a clinical pathway. Each phase of the nursing process is carefully explained with examples provided. Nursing Outcomes Classification (NOC) and Nursing Interventions Classification (NIC) and their relationship to NANDA are explored. The second chapter of this unit discusses the most valuable tool of the psychiatric nurse—that of communication—with emphasis on the essential components of the therapeutic nurse-client relationship.

Part Three, Developmental Aspects Across the Life Span, analyzes the stages of growth and development in separate chapters about childhood and adolescence, adulthood, and the elderly. Critical tasks that need to be met or mastered for clients to move forward developmentally are discussed from a variety of theoretic perspectives.

Part Four, Psychiatric Disorders, focuses on 10 major disorders generated by DSM-IV criteria. Each disorder is presented in terms of a brief description, history, etiology, epidemiology, and prognosis. The nursing process is presented as a separate section at the end of each chapter, with discussion of each nursing process step. A detailed nursing care plan is presented in this section, beginning with a case study, followed by DSM-IV multiaxial diagnoses and relevant nursing diagnoses. Client outcomes are identified based on the nursing diagnosis statement, inter-

ventions and their rationales are presented, and an evaluation statement is noted. Collaboration between nursing and medicine is evident throughout the nursing process section, most notably in columns depicting a side-by-side listing of DSM-IV and typical NANDA diagnoses and in the multiaxial diagnostic segments preceding the nursing care plans.

Part Five, Therapeutic Modalities, emphasizes the five major therapeutic modalities used to treat clients in the psychiatric setting. The chapter on interactive therapies presents discussion of the different theoretic concepts in the form of practical examples and scenarios typically found in a mental health facility. The chapter on psychopharmacology offers a thorough description of medications typically used to treat mental illness, as well as their therapeutic and nontherapeutic effects, recommended dosages, nursing implications, and other critical information. Forty perforated, detachable drug cards in the back of the book accompany this chapter for the learner's convenience. Crisis intervention is discussed, tracing the historical development of this modality and describing its major components. A separate chapter is devoted to activity therapies, such as occupational, recreational, art, music, and dance therapies, emphasizing the text's interdisciplinary focus. Special consideration is given to the nurse's role in each therapeutic task, function, or activity.

Part Six, Contemporary Issues, describes a variety of timely issues and concerns experienced by clients in different settings and treated by psychiatric nurses. Such important topics as surviving violence, suicide, grief and loss, AIDS, psychologic aspects of physiologic illness, and persons with chronic mental illness are discussed in this unit. An in-depth chapter exploring nursing care in the community and home-based treatment settings follows. The text concludes with a state-of-the-art chapter on spirituality and its relevance and importance in the mental health setting.

DESIGN AND KEY FEATURES

Bright and vivid full-color design permeates this text to promote visual appeal, emphasize and distinguish key pedagogic features, and graphically portray illustrations of critical psychiatric nursing concepts for students in the new millenium. Numerous full-color brain scans and drawings of psychobiologic concepts are presented in relevant chapters throughout the text. Many boxes, tables, and other figures summarize and highlight important information.

Each chapter has several standard features that make critical information more accessible for learning:

- **Objectives,** placed at the beginning of the chapter, emphasize the most important concepts.
- **Key Terms** with definitions are presented at the beginning of the chapter and are highlighted throughout the chapter in bold type.

- A **Summary of Key Concepts** concludes each chapter, summarizing the most significant ideas to be remembered.

Other important key features are highlighted by a unique design and included in relevant chapters.

- A detailed **Nursing Care Plan** is presented as part of the nursing process section. It begins with a case study, followed by DSM-IV multiaxial diagnoses and relevant nursing diagnoses. Client outcomes based on the nursing diagnoses statements are identified, interventions with rationales are presented, and an evaluative statement concludes the care plan.
- **Case Study** boxes with critical thinking components integrate critical thinking questions or statements following realistic case studies to foster students' problem-solving skills and application of the concepts presented. Different steps of the nursing process are featured throughout these case studies to help students in areas such as assessment, diagnosis, and outcomes.
- **Nursing Care in the Community** boxes discuss community perspectives on particular disorders and issues.
- **Clinical Alert** boxes throughout the text highlight critical information relevant to clinical practice.
- **DSM-IV Criteria** boxes present the DSM-IV criteria for particular disorders.
- **Collaborative Diagnoses** boxes present DSM-IV and NANDA diagnoses relevant for a certain disorder.
- **Client & Family Teaching Guidelines** provide education for both the client and the family on various concerns for a particular disorder.
- **Clinical Symptoms** boxes summarize the symptoms that indicate a certain disorder.
- **Additional Treatment Modalities** boxes summarize various modalities and interventions that are used in conjunction with nursing interventions in the treatment of a particular disorder.
- **Understanding & Applying Research** boxes summarize a research study related to a disorder and its application to nursing interventions.
- **Nursing Assessment Questions** boxes present questions that should be included in the assessment of a particular disorder.
- Forty perforated **drug cards** containing essential information about the most common and important psychiatric medications are in the back of the book. These cards can be torn out and easily used for reference in clinical settings.
- **Clinical pathways,** for various disorders and from different institutions, are presented to demonstrate the importance and usefulness of this interdisciplinary tool in the treatment of mental disorders.
- A **Glossary** in the back provides concise updated definitions of the commonly used nomenclature found throughout the book.

TEACHING-LEARNING PACKAGE
A complete ancillary package to enhance teaching and learning is provided for this text.

Instructor's Resource Manual and Test Bank
The *Instructor's Resource Manual and Test Bank* to accompany *Psychiatric Mental Health Nursing* includes many features that will supplement and enhance teaching and learning from the textbook. Critical thinking exercises, enrichment activities, and multimedia resources are provided for each text chapter. Strategies for teaching psychiatric nursing and suggested course outlines for courses of varying lengths are presented. Student worksheets for each chapter are included. The text bank has approximately 700 questions in NCLEX format and provides the applicable nursing process step, cognitive level of each question, and answer rationale.

Mosby's Psychiatric Nursing Transparency Acetates, Second Edition
The second edition of Mosby's *Psychiatric Nursing Transparency Acetates* contains 48 two-color and full-color transparencies, covering many topics in psychiatric nursing. These transparencies provide a visual learning experience to reinforce knowledge and understanding.

Computerized Test Bank
The computerized version of the test bank is available in IBM and Macintosh versions. It comes with an instruction manual and allows users to edit, add, delete, or select questions on the computer.

TERMINOLOGY AND LANGUAGE
We have made every effort to remove evidence of sexism from this text. Whenever possible, we have attempted to use plural nouns and pronouns in place of the singular *his* or *her*. We recognize the contribution of both men and women to the nursing profession. However, clarity sometimes has dictated the use of *she* for nurse and *he* for client.

We have chosen to use the term *client* instead of *patient* because we view individuals receiving treatment as significant participants in the reciprocal process of treatment. We also recognize that *family* can refer not only to blood relatives but friends and significant others. However, the term *family* is generally used for simplicity.

ACKNOWLEDGMENTS
We would like to thank the following individuals who provided valuable assistance to us in so many ways.

- Elizabeth Campbell Atkinson, OTR, Program Director, Alpine Special Treatment Center, Alpine, California (San Diego area), for writing the Behavior Therapy section of Chapter 3, Theoretic Perspectives.

- Kathy Susan Sweet, LPT, Patient Access Representative, Sharp Memorial Hospital and Sharp Mary Birch Hospital, San Diego, California, for her library research.

The authors want to thank Jeff Downing, Developmental Editor; Jeanne Allison, Editor; Cheryl Abbott, Senior Production Editor; John Rogers, Project Manager; and all those at Mosby who helped with this challenging project.

We wish to pay a special tribute to the late Dr. George G. Glenner, past co-contributor, for his landmark research on Alzheimer's disease; to Joy Glenner, CEO/President of the George G. Glenner Alzheimer's Family Centers, San Diego, California; and to Geraldine I. Strachan, RN, MSNEd, Dr. Glenner's former colleague and co-contributor. Their work with clients and families who are affected by Alzheimer's disease and other related cognitive disorders have provided a legacy for the work to continue and enduring hope for a cure.

We also wish to remember the late Vincent R. Pieranunzi, MSN, RN, PhD, whose initial contributions to the chapters on *Cultural Issues* and *Disorders of Childhood and Adolescence* greatly enhanced this text.

We want to thank Marjorie F. Bendik, RN, DNSc, for her past contributions in Chapter 14, *The Schizophrenias*.

We are proud to launch this new edition of our textbook and invite psychiatric nursing students and nurses at all levels to meet the challenges presented and to apply the concepts in clinical practice. As we approach the new millennium and meet the dynamic forces influencing health care and health care delivery, the time-honored role of psychiatric nursing holds steady in the twenty-first century. It is our hope that the content described in this textbook will serve as an anchor amid the inevitable turbulence of change. We wish you well in your professional journey and feel confident that you will successfully meet these challenges while experiencing the joy and wonder of psychiatric nursing.

Kathi Fortinash and Pat Holoday-Worret

BRIEF CONTENTS

CONTENTS

Introduction to Psychiatric Mental Health Nursing

Ntesie
Ashanti, West Africa

This symbol, signifying wisdom, knowledge, and prudence, is derived from the Ashanti people of Ghana, West Africa. A literal translation of the symbol is "What I hear, I keep . . . I consider and keep what I learn." The Ashanti often stamp cloth with many symbols in graphic patterns that represent and convey their ideals, proverbs, history, and beliefs. The chapters in Part One discuss fundamental concepts of psychiatric nursing for the readers to "learn and keep" throughout their endeavors in this field.

CHAPTER 1

Foundations of Psychiatric Mental Health Nursing

Patricia A. Holoday-Worret

OBJECTIVES

- Define and describe psychiatric mental health nursing.

- Distinguish between a therapeutic and a social relationship.

- Explain the four stages of the nurse-client relationship.

- Identify the American Nurses Association Standards of Care.

- Describe protective defenses.

- Compare and contrast mental health with mental disorder.

- Discuss the roles of several members of the mental health team.

- Identify significant trends in health care and their effects on psychiatric nursing.

Psychiatric mental health nursing exists because there is a definable need for that discipline of nursing. Psychiatric mental health nurses assist clients (individuals, families, community) to achieve and maintain mental health, and they treat clients when mental disorders or life crises disrupt progress and function.

DESCRIPTION OF PSYCHIATRIC MENTAL HEALTH NURSING

Psychiatric mental health nursing is a specialty within the nursing profession that focuses primarily on the use of therapeutic interpersonal interactions and biologic and interpersonal interventions with clients. Professional mandates include the promotion of mental health, the prevention and treatment of mental disorders, and rehabilitation after disorders occur. Psychiatric nursing is one of four core mental health practice areas designated since 1946 by the National Mental Health Act to serve in this capacity. The other practice areas include psychiatry, psychology, and social work (Redick, 1994).

PREPARATION FOR PSYCHIATRIC MENTAL HEALTH NURSING

Effective client care in any psychiatric setting requires extensive knowledge and comprehension of both mental health and mental disorders. This knowledge and understanding are derived from two main sources: education and experience.

EDUCATION

Formal education of psychiatric nurses is governed and overseen by state boards of registered nursing and is influenced by national psychiatric nurses associations (see Appendix C). Theory-based knowledge is necessary to generate relevant, logical critical thinking about client con-

Autodiagnosis
Examination of one's own thoughts, feelings, perceptions, and attitudes about a particular client.

Content The topics or subjects covered during conversation.

Epigenesis
Developmental concept developed by Erikson: genetics and environmental experiences, which begin with conception and continue throughout life and determine the person's personality and the mentally healthy or destructive responses to the world.

Incidence
The frequency of occurrences of a specific disorder within a designated period (number of new cases).

Nomenclature
Names or terms making up a set or a system.

Objectivity
Remaining free from bias, prejudice, and personal identification in an interaction with another person and being able to process information based on facts.

Prevalence The number of existing cases of a specific disorder in a normal population at a given time.

Primary prevention
Prevention efforts that focus on reduction of the incidence of mental disorders within the community; directed toward occurrence of mental health problems, with emphasis on health promotion and prevention of disorders.

Process A series of progressive and interdependent steps toward a goal.

Protective defenses Automatic or learned psychologic processes that keep the threat of internal and external stressors and dangers out of awareness.

Secondary prevention
Prevention efforts directed toward reducing the prevalence of mental disorders through early identification of problems and early treatment of those problems; occurs after the problem arises and aims to shorten the course or duration of the episode.

Stereotype
A simplified, standardized conception or image that is invested with special meaning and held in common by members of a group.

Stigma A mark of disgrace or defect.

Subjectivity Emphasizing one's own words, attitudes, and opinions in an interaction with another person.

Tertiary prevention Prevention efforts that have the dual focus of reducing residual effects of the disorder and rehabilitating the individual.

Therapeutic alliance The relationship between therapist and client; it is the vehicle used to assist the client in working toward wellness.

ditions and situations and to form problem-solving skills that will assist clients on their journey toward mental health. This education has its basis in several disciplines and is derived from areas that include the following:

Physical sciences
Natural sciences
Behavioral sciences
Humanities
The art and science of nursing

EXPERIENCE

Education is necessary, but experience must be the companion to affect successful interventions in psychiatric nursing. Nurses who practice in any psychiatric setting unanimously agree that a solid education is essential, but there is no substitute for experience. Learned skills are honed only through exposure to challenging situations that involve opportunities to choose and practice appropriate, effective interventions with clients. Although mental disorders are identifiable by specific, academically defined criteria, it takes time and practice to recognize the myriad of ways that disorders may be manifested. The uniqueness of each human being affects symptom portrayal and can affect the caregiver's interpretation, unless sufficient experience is the guide. Nurses in the psychiatric setting are aware that contact with many different clients and situations is necessary to forge competence and confidence.

PRACTICE STANDARDS
PURPOSE

A profession has the task of developing standards of practice that serve as a model for conduct and a gauge by which it measures performance and competence. Standards also communicate values, priorities, and patterns of excellence.

Standards of nursing practice are also guidelines that direct provision of care for clients during promotion and maintenance of health, prevention of illness and injury, and restoration of health.

Standards of care and practice for psychiatric mental health nurses were developed by the American Nurses Association (ANA) (1994b) and continue to describe nursing functions. They follow the steps of the nursing process and provide a framework within which psychiatric mental health nursing is implemented and evaluated.

AMERICAN NURSES ASSOCIATION STANDARDS OF PSYCHIATRIC MENTAL HEALTH CLINICAL NURSING PRACTICE: STANDARDS OF CARE*

Standard I
Assessment
The psychiatric mental health nurse collects client health data.

During the nurse's interview with the client or other reliable reporters, relevant information is obtained that enables the nurse to make decisions about the client's situation and to begin to formulate a plan of care. In the interview process, the nurse utilizes multiple skills of observation, communication, and assessment techniques and then records the review. When data collection is completed, the nurse prioritizes the information.

Standard II
Diagnosis
The psychiatric mental health nurse analyzes the assessment data in determining diagnoses.

Through synthesis and analysis of the collected data, the nurse determines patterns of client responses that represent needs, problems, or actual/potential psychiatric disorders. Nursing diagnoses are derived using the accepted classification of the North American Nursing Diagnosis Association (NANDA). Nursing diagnoses will also be closely associated with the client's psychiatric diagnosis when applicable.

Standard III
Outcome Identification
The psychiatric mental health nurse identifies expected outcomes individualized to the client.

The nurse and client together determine the ultimate goals (expected outcomes) for the client's health that can be expected from health care. The goals are identified and documented. Expected outcomes are realistic, attainable, measurable, and client focused. They not only provide a target for the client to reach but also provide a basis of information to measure health status and progress or lack of progress.

Standard IV
Planning
The psychiatric mental health nurse develops a plan of care that prescribes interventions to attain expected outcomes.

An individualized, prioritized plan of care is developed by the nurse in collaboration with the client and significant others and is used to guide interventions to ulti-

*From American Nurses Association: *A statement on psychiatric-mental health clinical nursing practice and standards of psychiatric-mental health clinical nursing practice,* Washington, DC, 1994b, The Association.

mately achieve the client's expected outcomes. The care plan is utilized by all health team members and is modified as changes occur in the client's health status or progress.

Standard V
Implementation
The psychiatric mental health nurse implements the interventions identified in the plan of care.

Psychiatric mental health nurses practice according to their level of educational preparation and certification. Nurses select interventions according to client need, their own level of practice, and in keeping with the care plan that has been established for the client.

Basic Practice Level

At the basic level of practice, nurses may intervene in the following ways.

Counseling
The psychiatric mental health nurse uses counseling interventions to assist clients in improving or regaining their previous coping abilities, in fostering mental health, and in preventing mental illness and disability.

Counseling is described by the ANA as including interviewing and communication techniques, problem solving, crisis intervention, stress management, and behavior modifications.

Milieu Therapy
The psychiatric mental health nurse provides, structures, and maintains a therapeutic environment in collaboration with the client and other health care providers.

The environment is used as a therapeutic tool to modify behaviors, teach skills, and encourage communication between the client and others. The nurse in milieu therapy provides structure and support and promotes growth through role modeling and opportunities for interactions.

Self-Care Activities
The psychiatric mental health nurse structures interventions around the client's activities of daily living to foster self-care and mental and physical well-being.

A primary concept in psychiatric mental health nursing is to encourage independence within a client's ability and capacity. In keeping with this principle, clients are urged to take responsibility for their care, and in turn they experience increased self-esteem, along with improved function and health.

Psychobiologic Interventions
The psychiatric mental health nurse uses knowledge of psychobiologic interventions and applies clinical skills to restore the client's health and prevent further disability.

Nursing interventions with clients in a psychiatric setting frequently include the use of medications, so nurses have responsibility for thorough knowledge, preparation, and experience in this area. Other psychologic interventions also require nurses' participation, observation, and teaching skills.

Health Teaching
The psychiatric mental health nurse, through health teaching, assists clients in achieving satisfying, productive, and healthy patterns of living.

Nurses teach multiple topics to clients in the psychiatric setting, offering feedback for learning and opportunities for the practice of skills.

Case Management
The psychiatric mental health nurse provides case management to coordinate comprehensive health services and ensure continuity of care.

Nurses participate in client care and comprehensively oversee the care provided by other members of the health team or agencies when appropriate.

Health Promotion and Health Maintenance
The psychiatric mental health nurse employs strategies and interventions to promote and maintain mental health and prevent mental illness.

Aside from secondary psychiatric nursing interventions employed after clients' problems have been identified, the nurse at this level also engages in promotion of mental health and prevention of mental disorder.

Advanced Practice Level

The following interventions may be employed only by clinical specialists who are certified in advanced psychiatric mental health nursing.

Psychotherapy
The certified specialist in psychiatric mental health nursing uses individual, group, and family psychotherapy; child psychotherapy; and other therapeutic treatments to assist clients in fostering mental health, preventing mental illness and disability, and improving or regaining previous health status and functional abilities.

The psychiatric mental health nurse clinical specialist uses a wide range of knowledge to intervene with clients. The nurse and client agree to a contract and work within its parameters. The nurse at this level is autonomous in therapeutic modalities but collaborates appropriately when warranted.

Prescription of Pharmacologic Agents
The certified specialist prescribes pharmacologic agents in accordance with the state nursing practice act to treat symptoms of psychiatric illness and improve functional health status.

The nurse at this level, in accordance with government

regulation and state nursing practice acts and with full knowledge of psychopharmacologic agents, prescribes medications and manages the client's regimen.

Consultation

The certified specialist provides consultation to health care providers and others to influence the plans of care for clients and to enhance the abilities of others to provide psychiatric and mental health care and effect change in systems.

The nurse clinical specialist at this level provides consultation regarding changes in agencies or systems when necessary.

Evaluation

The psychiatric mental health nurse evaluates the client's progress in attaining expected outcomes.

Evaluation of client health status and progress is done at this level.

The standards of client care provide a frame-work for psychiatric mental health nursing practice and evaluation. These criteria help nurses clearly define role responsibilities and outcomes for which they are accountable during the process of caring for clients in any psychiatric setting.

The scope of practice for psychiatric mental health nursing is also based on knowledge of and compliance with standards of professional performance. Some of these standards are directly related to client care (quality of care, ethics, performance evaluation, collaboration, use of appropriate resources); others are directed beyond that performance level but still address the professional role (research, advanced education, specialty certification, advanced practice, continuing education, memberships in organizations) (ANA, 1994b).

ADDITIONAL PERFORMANCE STANDARDS

The ANA Standards of Care previously mentioned describe two levels of nursing practice within the specialty of psychiatric mental health nursing (the generalist and the clinical specialist) and discuss criteria that determine the nurse's responsibility and accountability at each level. Other standards also govern nursing performance and are listed as follows:

Professional standards of practice
Professional code of nursing
Specialty certification
State-registered nurses license (RN)
State nursing practice act
Educational level of the RN
Personal competence
Policies and procedures of individual facility
Position description in work setting (clearly defined)

In addition to these standards, nurses also choose to practice in one or more of the following subspecialty areas:

Clinical
Educational
Administration
Research

MENTAL HEALTH AND MENTAL DISORDER

Psychiatric mental health nurses are required to have thorough knowledge and understanding of both mental health and mental disorder. The terms *mental health* and *mental disorder* are complex and defy simplistic operational definitions. A discussion of these concepts follows.

MENTAL HEALTH

Mental health consists of multiple and varied components, and many are unmeasurable by scientific standards. For this reason, a concise, encompassing definition of mental health does not exist, although several definitions appear in the literature. This emphasizes the fact that human beings are not simply defined or described or predictable. Each individual brings his or her own uniqueness to the world and interacts with it in a way that is unlike any other person.

No two people have the same experience. Two children born into the same home and of the same parents may have entirely different life experiences. Two people witnessing the same event may have similar but different perceptions. Individual responses are considered healthy or disordered as measured by psychiatric, psychologic, and sociocultural standards.

Physical health is more easily defined because of specific parameters rooted in physical science (anatomy, physiology, chemistry, microbiology). These parameters can be measured by exacting diagnostics (e.g., laboratory tests, pathology examinations, radiology, nuclear medicine). More precise definitions of physical health can be derived based on the presence or absence of specific anatomic or physiologic components. It is frequently more difficult to identify mental disorders because of the lack of definitive, tangible, low-cost diagnostic methods.

Often mental health has been presented through linear paradigms that depict the components of mental health ranging from optimal mental wellness to extreme mental disorder. The one-dimensional presentation in Figure 1-1 does not incorporate or consider all of the components that make up mental health or that may malfunction to constitute mental disorder. Figure 1-2 shows a more representative illustration of mental health and mental disorder.

Several components of mental health appear in Box 1-1. To be mentally healthy, one need not demonstrate or exhibit all of the characteristics that appear in this box. As stated previously, some symptoms of dysfunction are likely to appear in even the healthiest individuals; conversely, healthy components can be found in persons with serious mental disorder.

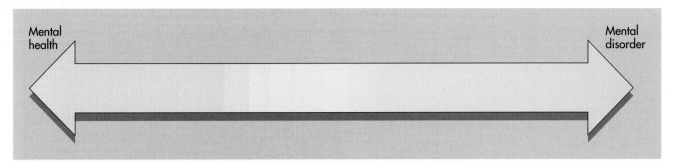

Figure 1-1   One-dimensional presentation of mental health and mental disorder.

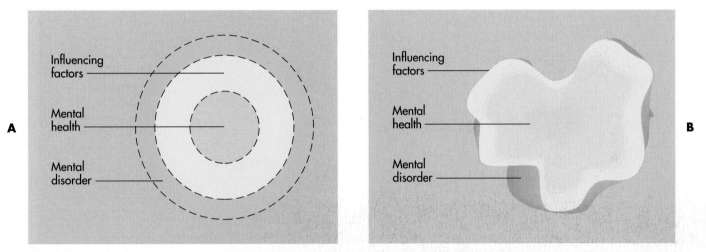

Figure 1-2   **A,** Mental health is the core; influencing internal and external factors surround the core; mental disorder is the outer layer. Dividing each component are broken lines that represent the dynamic states of each component that change continually across the life span, depending on the individual's intrapersonal characteristics, interpersonal relationships, and environmental events and circumstances. **B,** Representation of how this may occur in one instance—in its dynamic state.

Factors that contribute to and influence mental health or mental disorder are also numerous and varied (Box 1-2) and can be broadly categorized as intrapersonal, interpersonal, or environmental.

Every infant comes into the world with certain inborn responses. The child is not a blank slate, or *tabula rasa* (Kaplan and Sadock, 1994). Recent research demonstrates that the newborn is endowed with these responses and interacts with the environment to produce behaviors that uniquely define the child.

The concept of **epigenesis,** described first by Erikson (1963), considers several factors that influence development and ultimately shape the individual. Erikson wrote that genetics and environmental experiences, which begin with conception (pregnancy, intrauterine development, childbirth) and continue throughout life, determine the person's personality and his or her mentally healthy or de-

structive responses to the world. In addition, the individual must have the capacity to successfully structure experience at every stage of development and contend with and negotiate the given environment to maintain health.

Theory pertaining to origins of mental health has been contemplated and shaped by a few influential thinkers and expanded by many of their followers. The question still remains concerning the degree to which the potential toward health or disorder is present at conception or is modified by effects of the environment (i.e., nature versus nurture).

At present, the pendulum has swung back toward biologic elements as causal factors of mental health or disorder. Psychiatric nurses need to stay informed of the latest developments, and not lose sight of the psychologic, sociologic, behavioral, cultural, and spiritual factors that may also influence their clients' health.

Box 1-1 Components of Mental Health

Presence of anatomic and physiologic components necessary to function in the world
Absence of signs and symptoms of mental disorder
Freedom from excessive mental and emotional disability and pain
Ability to
Perceive self, others, and events correctly
Recognize own strengths, weaknesses, capabilities, and limitations
Separate fantasy from reality
Think clearly
    Problem solve
    Use good judgment
    Reason logically
    Reach insightful conclusions
Negotiate each developmental stage
Attain and maintain positive self-system
    Self-concept
    Self-image
    Self-esteem
Accept self and others as uniquely different but humanly similar
Appreciate life
Find beauty, joy, and goodness in self, others and environment
Be creative
Be optimistic but realistic
Use talents to fullest
Involve self in purposeful, meaningful life work
Engage in play
Develop and demonstrate appropriate sense of humor
Express emotions

Exhibit congruent behaviors
Accept responsibility for actions
Control impulses and behavior
Be accountable for own behaviors
Respect societal rules and sanctions
Learn from experiences
Maintain wholesome values and belief system
Cope with internal and external stressors in constructive and adaptive ways
Return to usual or higher function after crises
Delay gratification
Function independently
Maintain reasonable expectations concerning self and others
Adapt to social environment
Relate to others
    Form relationships
    Maintain close, meaningful, loving, adaptive relationships
    Work and play well with others
    Be intimate, appropriately and selectively
    Respond to others in need
    Feel and exhibit compassion and empathy toward others
    Demonstrate culturally and socially acceptable interpersonal interactions
    Manage interpersonal conflict constructively
    Give and receive gracefully
    Learn from and teach others
    Function interdependently
Seek self-actualization
Attain self-defined spirituality

Box 1-2 Influencing Factors for Mental Health or Disorder

Inherited factors
    Predisposition
    Capacities
    Limitations
Pregnancy environment and experience (from conception to birth)
Psychoneuroimmunologic factors
Biochemical influences
Hormonal influences
Family
    Composition
    Birth position
    Bonding
    Members' mental health
Developmental events
    Completion of clearly defined stages
    Resolution of developmental crises
Culture
Subculture
Values
Belief systems
Perception of self

Cognitive abilities
    Capacity
    Volition
Personality traits and states
Goals, aspirations
World view
Internal stressors
External stressors
Support systems
    Choice
    Availability
Negative influences
    Internal/external
    Mental disorders
    Crime
    Drugs
    Psychosocial stressors
    Poverty
Demographic factors
Geographic location
Health practices and beliefs
Spirituality/religion

Protective Defenses

Most healthy individuals want to and strive to feel good about themselves and their goals, accomplishments, and relationships. They want to be content with the world as they know it. It must be noted that healthy individuals also strive to avoid anxiety, distress, discomfort, and pain.

Mature adults, however, realize that some negative aspects of life, such as excessive responsibilities, disappointment, loss, embarrassment, nonfulfillment, and rejection, are inevitable and intrinsically woven into the very fabric of life. All individuals, in an attempt to maintain contentment, employ a variety of methods in an effort to accomplish feeling good while avoiding pain. Some of the methods are automatic responses, whereas other responses are purposeful and planned techniques or are strategies that are learned.

Automatic responses were first described in detail by Freud, who named them defense mechanisms, and were thought to be mostly unconscious. This concept was soon challenged by other schools of psychology that disagreed with, or added to, Freud's concepts. Positive theories were presented to demonstrate that consciously planned strategies and methods, coupled with skill rehearsal and practice, could dramatically reduce dysfunction for some individuals, thus giving control to the individual. It was believed by many therapists that automatic defense mechanisms were used by clients as a way to contend with stress and manage anxiety but that most individuals could also learn purposefully planned and appropriate strategies or methods for overcoming some psychologic difficulties and life crises.

The concept of **protective defenses,** or ways that clients manage the negative aspects of life, is still being examined and considered by nursing, psychiatry, psychology, and social work when formulating interdisciplinary treatment plans. Both automatic mechanisms and planned strategies that are employed by clients need to be understood and considered during client care. Both types of defenses, automatic responses (Box 1-3) and consciously employed strategies (Box 1-4), are presented in this text.

MENTAL DISORDER

It seems logical that deviations in the factors that influence mental health or disorder (see Box 1-2) would define mental disorder. It remains a term, however, that is not easily defined. In its most recent discussions of the term *mental disorder,* the American Psychiatric Association (APA) states that it "implies a distinction between mental and physical disorders that is a reductionistic anachronism of mind/body dualism" (APA, 1994). In other words, the word *mental* does not adequately include the many varied aspects of mental disorders.

Like the concept of mental health, the concept of mental disorder encompasses far too many components and situations to be covered in one operational definition. Mental disorders are well described in the *Diagnostic and*

Statistical Manual of Mental Disorders, fourth edition (DSM-IV), but definition remains imperfect. With that qualifier, the APA (1994) defines mental disorder as

. . . clinically significant behavioral or psychological syndrome or pattern that occurs in an individual and is associated with present distress (e.g., a painful symptom) or disability (i.e., impairment in one or more important areas of functioning) or with a significantly increased risk of suffering death, pain, disability, or an important loss of freedom.

Research and Epidemiology Relating to Mental Disorders

Two significant psychiatric epidemiologic studies have revealed startling results about mental disorders. The first landmark survey is the Epidemiologic Catchment Area (ECA) study (Robins and Regier, 1991), and the second is the National Comorbidity Survey (NCS) (Maxman and Ward, 1995). Although the surveys were conducted at separate times and with different but large sample sizes, the findings are similar and conclude that one third to one half of all adults in the United States will have a mental disorder in their lifetime.

In the ECA survey, researchers from the National Institute of Mental Health (NIMH) interviewed almost 20,000 adults in multiple sites to establish the 1-year and lifetime prevalence of 30 mental disorders (Robins and Regier, 1991). Researchers from the NCS interviewed 8098 adults regarding 17 of the most commonly occurring disorders (Kessler et al, 1994). The ECA and NCS concluded that mental disorders affected approximately 20% to 30% of adults in the United States during the year preceding the interviews and 32% to 50% throughout their lives (Maxman and Ward, 1995). Table 1-1 presents mental disorders in order of their prevalence.

The ECA survey stated that most clients with mental disorders were more likely to be treated by general practitioners, internists, psychologists, nurses, and social workers (nonpsychiatrists). Both studies clarified the need for health care professionals in all fields to be aware of psychopathology (Maxman and Ward, 1995).

Nursing implication. Nurses are aware that healthy individuals may employ many defenses during stressful situations throughout their life span. Recovery and healthful adaptation after stressful times can be measured by the following criteria:

- Maintenance of reality orientation
- Restoration of equilibrium
- Continued involvement in purposeful work
- Evidence of continued cognitive and emotional growth
- Ability to problem solve
- Continued involvement in nurturing and interdependent interpersonal/social network

Box 1-3   Defense Mechanisms and Strategies

Repression: The active unconscious process of keeping out or ejecting from the consciousness ideas or impulses that are unacceptable to the person.
Example: An adult male who was sexually abused as a child has no recollection of the events.

Denial: Refusal to perceive or face unpleasant reality as it actually exists.
Example: Nonacceptance of a fatal diagnosis, such as AIDS.

Rationalization: Use of a contrived, socially acceptable and logical explanation to justify unpleasant material and to keep it out of consciousness.
Example: A high-school graduate who does not get accepted to a prestigious military academy says he could never tolerate the regimentation anyway.

Projection: Attributing one's own unacceptable motives or characteristics to another person or group.
Example: A paranoid person uses projection frequently in always seeing "the others" as hostile.

Displacement: The discharge of pent-up feelings (frequently hostility) onto something or someone else in the environment that is less threatening than the original source of the feelings.
Example: After her boss berates her publicly, a woman comes home and starts an argument with her neighbor over parking rights.

Reaction formation: Prevention of awareness or expression of unacceptable desires by adoption of opposite behaviors in an exaggerated way.
Example: A woman who does not want her child before it is born becomes overly protective after the birth, refusing to leave the child's side.

Intellectualization: The overuse of abstract thinking or generalizations to control or minimize painful feelings
Example: A man who faces a pending divorce engages in lengthy and lofty discourse about divorce statistics and process during a support group but never talks about his own fears and feelings.

Undoing: Atonement for or attempt to dissipate unacceptable acts or wishes.
Examples: 1) A man has an affair with another woman, then buys his wife a new car. 2) A professional berates her colleague and causes her to lose her job, then offers to help take care of the colleague's child.

Compensation: Counterbalance for deficiencies in one area by excelling in another area.
Example: A young man who fails at sports studies hard and becomes valedictorian of his graduating class.

Identification: Incorporation of the image of an emulated person, then acting, thinking, and feeling like that person (unconscious mental mimicry).
Example: Gang members dress exactly like their leader and steal from neighbors as the leader does.

Introjection: Treating something outside the self as if it is actually inside the self.
Example: A child who fears dragons "becomes" a dragon in serious play, thus assimilating the fearful experience.

Sublimation: Modification of an instinctual but socially unacceptable impulse into a constructive acceptable behavior.

Examples: 1) An aggressive young man becomes a star hockey player. 2) A woman with strong sexual urges becomes a sculptor.

Regression: Returning to an earlier level of adaptation
Examples: 1) An adolescent who is under stress curls up on his bed with a stuffed teddy bear, sucks his thumb, and does not speak. 2) An adult client admitted to the psychiatric unit with a diagnosis of psychosis is found smearing feces on the wall.

Suppression: The conscious inhibition of an impulse, idea, or affect. The person has full awareness of the behavior.
Example: A man on his way to give a major speech is told by his wife that she is divorcing him. He decides not to think about it until his speech is over, and puts it out of his mind so he can complete his task.

Humor: Emphasis on ironic or amusing components of a crisis, conflict, or stressor.
Example: Two people leave a room after being strongly disciplined by their boss and burst into laughter, which they had restrained. They jokingly discuss the only thing each focused on—a large piece of the boss's hair that stuck straight up in the air and bobbed up and down as he paced around the room and crowed at them.

Splitting: Compartmentalization of opposite-affect states and failure to integrate positive and negative aspects of self or others, resulting in polarized images of self and others as all good or all bad.
Example: A client on a psychiatric unit tells Nurse A that she is "the kindest, smartest, most well-prepared nurse on the unit." She tells Nurse B, who sets limits on the client's behavior, that she is "stupid and insensitive, and it's a miracle she ever got an RN license."

Self-Observation: Reflection on one's own behavior, thoughts, and feelings, followed by appropriate response.

Self-Assertion: Expression of thoughts and feelings in direct ways that are not manipulative or intimidating.

Altruism: Devotion of self to serving others as a way to manage conflict and stress; differs from reaction formation in that it is gratifying but not self-sacrificing.
Example: Some nuns, priests, rabbis, ministers, nurses, physicians, firefighters, and paramedics, to name a few, often serve people for unselfish reasons and gain satisfaction through giving.

Affiliation: Turning to others for support and help when stressed or conflicted, without attempting to make others responsible for taking care of the person.
Example: A woman is widowed and moves across the country to be near her family of origin and friends from her past.

Anticipation: Anticipating consequences of events yet to come and thinking of options, solutions, and alternatives; also can include experiencing the feelings associated with these thoughts (a "mental rehearsal" of future events).
Example: A hard-working attorney, called to interview for partnership in a law firm, spends the rest of the day rehearsing and experiencing the event.

Box 1-3   Defense Mechanisms and Strategies—cont'd

Help-Rejecting Complaining: Repeated requests for help, suggestions, or advice that is then rejected; request disguises covert feelings of reproach or hostility for others; complaints may be about problems of life or physical or psychologic symptoms.
Example: A woman constantly calls her grown and married children to complain about her physical pains and loneliness but constantly refuses to take any helpful steps they suggest to alleviate her situation.
Passive Aggression: Expression of aggression toward others in indirect and nonassertive ways; covert hostility and resentment masked by overt compliance.
Example: A girl who is jealous because her best friend dated a boy she wanted to date agrees to meet her friend for lunch and then arrives an hour late, apologizing profusely and begging forgiveness.
Omnipotence: Feeling or acting superior to others or as if one has special abilities or power.
Example: An inept and underachieving son of a dynamic business tycoon struts around his own plush but token office and treats others condescendingly.

Isolation of Affect: Separation of feelings from thoughts and ideas that are originally associated with them.
Example: A woman describes in full detail the traumatic event of watching her friend get hit by a truck and killed but displays no emotion.
Fantasy: Gratification of frustrated desires, achievements, and relationships by substituting them with daydreams and imagery.
Example: An unpopular high-school senior is left out of social events but spends her spare time imagining herself dressing for and going to the senior prom with the class football hero.
Acting Out: The use of actions versus reflection or true experiencing of feelings to deal with stress and conflict.
Example: A student learns he or she has failed a course, then smashes a window in the classroom, leaves, and drinks six beers.

Box 1-4   Conscious Measures as Defenses

Exercising
Calling a friend
Talking to a parent or significant other
Going to a movie
Crying
Eating
Dancing
Reading
Volunteering time
Writing in a journal
Sleeping
Practicing relaxation techniques
Going to the theater
Attending church or community meetings
Writing letters to friends, family, or others
Getting involved in purposeful work

Table 1-1   Prevalence Rates of Mental Disorders

Rank	Disorder	Percentage of Adult Americans Affected
First	Anxiety disorders	14.4-17.2
Second	Substance abuse disorders	8.8-11.3
Third	Mood disorders	4.3-11.3
Fourth	Cognitive impairment disorder	5.9
Fifth	Schizophrenia	0.5-1

Modified from Maxman J, Ward N: *Essential psychopathology and its treatment*, New York, 1995, WW Norton.

Problems may arise in the following situations: when the individual's internal and/or external stressors are greater than the capacity to contend with them; when the individual's perception is that the obstacle cannot be overcome; or when the individual uses one or more defenses exclusively, especially those that distort reality.

When the nurse recognizes the client's use of defenses, it is possible to accept them as part of the individual's attempts to contend with the situation or to intervene if the defenses are inhibiting development or are interfering with reality orientation. The nurse's action depends on level of education and clinical experience.

An inexperienced psychiatric mental health nurse will generally not confront or attempt to remove the client's protective defenses. Instead, the focus is one of support and assistance in identifying the client's positive characteristics and in the development of strengths through the establishment and maintenance of the nurse-client relationship.

The experienced nurse will move beyond these limits

to challenge defenses in the interest of the client's cognitive and emotional growth. Through insight, the client is guided toward subsequent behavioral changes that are practiced in the safety of the relationship, then generalized in the client's life outside of therapy.

Psychobiology

Epidemiologic studies have been instrumental in the current paradigm shift that caused the NIMH to name the 1990s the *Decade of the Brain.* Epidemiologic investigation and studies are "based on the assumption that human disease has causal and preventive factors" (Betemps and Ragiel, 1994), which are identified through systematic assessment of populations that manifest symptoms that can be classified. Epidemiology employs the scientific measures of *prevalence* and *incidence.*

Prevalence refers to the number of cases of a specific disorder in a normal population at a given time. **Incidence** refers to the frequency of occurrences of a specific disorder within a designated time (number of new cases).

Before World War II, the biologic model greatly influenced epidemiology. During World War II, however, it was determined that stress was a major cause of psychiatric disorders. These findings led to an emphasis on social influences, thus changing the study of etiology and epidemiology relating to mental disorders in the United States (Grob, 1992; Klerman, 1990). The development of sociologic and psychologic frameworks of psychiatry during this time dramatically turned the focus of intervention from biology toward social psychologic aspects of mental disorders.

In the 1970s, the focus of intervention began to turn back toward biologic causes of psychiatric disorders. The greatest momentum for this shift came from the Epidemiologic Catchment Area survey begun by the NIMH (Klerman, 1986). Basic goals of the ECA program include the following:

> Estimate rates of prevalence and incidence of specific mental disorders
> Estimate rates of mental health services use
> Study factors influencing the development and continuance of disorders
> Study factors influencing use of services (Eaton, 1984)

The ECA surveys created a shift in research that once again focused on biologic causes of mental disorders. From the mid-1980s to the present, there has been an explosion of research in this area. More has been learned about psychiatric disorders in the last 10 years than at any other time in history. Biologic research findings appear throughout this textbook.

Stigma of Mental Disorders

Mental disorders are presented in the DSM-IV (APA, 1994), where it states that the manual is a classification of disorders and not a classification of people. The meaning of that statement is significant for psychiatric mental health nurses who act as client advocates for the reduction of **stereotyping,** judgmentalism, disrespectful labeling, and the **stigma** that has been associated with mental disorders. Instead of referring to a person by a diagnosis, the nurse refers to the person who has a diagnosis.

Example 1

Correct: "Admitted a 19-year-old male for suicide threats, resulting from several days' use of crystal methamphetamine. Put him in the quiet area, on close watch precautions."

Incorrect: "Admited a crystal meth addict who is threatening to kill himself. Put him with the alcoholic in Room 25."

Example 2

Correct: "A family has been added to my cases. The father has a diagnosis of bipolar disorder, manic phase. His daughter has out-of-control behavior, which is due to alcoholism."

Incorrect: "They've added a manic to my caseload. His daughter is an alcoholic and lives with him. They fight constantly."

Nurses specializing in psychiatric mental health are continually faced with situations in which they need to keep reminding themselves, and perhaps each other, that client behaviors and responses are a product of the disorder. *The client is not the disorder.* Respect for the individual, regardless of the condition or the situation, should remain constant. Limits may have to be set on behavior, but the client needs to maintain dignity, which is facilitated by being treated respectfully by the nurse.

In addition to immediate practice, nurses have the opportunity to reduce stigma by educating the general population about causes and treatments of mental disorders and the needs of mental health clients. Stigmatizing and stereotyping continue to hover over persons with mental disorder and their families and are fueled by ignorance and fear. Stigma increases the problems faced by psychiatric clients, and these problems will increase only as the trend of present-day funding reroutes essential monies away from their care. Because of economic reallocation, homelessness will increase, and the issues surrounding it will become more difficult. Some problems faced by those with mental disorders include the following:

> Homelessness
> Housing discrimination
> Unstable living conditions
> Job discrimination
> Diminished self-esteem

Inappropriate or inadequate treatment
Inability to seek treatment
Alienation, isolation
Loss of entitlements

With enlightenment and advocacy, these individuals can obtain the following:

Access to education
Job opportunities
Health insurance coverage
Adequate treatment
Adequate housing
Research
Appropriate personal and human contact

People with mental disorders (psychiatric diagnoses) are feared or perceived as dangerous, violent, and aggressive, and are blamed for their illness. In fact, they are more likely to be passive, withdrawn, and isolated. (The major mental disorders are described in Part Four of this text.) Nurses can be instrumental in modifying or significantly changing the public's attitude regarding mental disorders and the client's experience of rejection to one of acceptance.

PSYCHIATRIC DIAGNOSES

Psychiatric diagnoses are precise descriptions and classifications of mental disorders. They are necessary and important for several reasons, such as communication, treatment, prognosis, and funding.

Communication

Each psychiatric diagnosis represents a specific set of symptoms or a syndrome. The criteria for each disorder enable mental health care providers to communicate with each other without having to explain symptoms when discussing the diagnoses. Staff should bear in mind that each client will present a unique expression of the disorder.

Educating individuals about psychiatric disorders is effective because the psychiatric classification of disorders is clearly defined and therefore can be communicated to learners in an organized way.

Treatment

Staff members are prepared to begin symptom-specific treatment based on a client's diagnosis. They know that the approaches (biologic and interpersonal) will vary, depending on the diagnosis. For example, preparation of the staff and the psychiatric setting will be different for a client reported with a diagnosis of paranoid schizophrenia with acutely psychotic symptoms and aggressive behavior toward others than will preparation for a client with a diagnosis of major depression and severely withdrawn behavior.

Prognosis

Some psychiatric diagnoses have more favorable prognoses than do others. Mental health care providers remain hopeful and convey that hope to clients. However, they are aware that a goal of treatment may be to return a client to a level of function experienced before an acute exacerbation of a chronic disorder, without expecting a cure of the disorder. The prognosis for some adjustment disorders, for example, is more favorable than the prognosis for one of the schizophrenias that has a chronic course.

Funding

It is a well-established fact that money is required to pay for services delivered during the care of clients, regardless of the psychiatric setting. Whether the source is private or public, certain criteria must be met to receive payment, and the client's diagnosis is a major factor.

On a larger scale, research monies are targeted for investigation of designated diagnoses. Research may be carried out in the private sector (e.g., drug companies) or public sector (e.g., government mental health agencies).

DIAGNOSTIC NOMENCLATURES
DSM

A **nomenclature** of psychiatric diagnoses developed by the American Psychiatric Association is widely accepted in the United States as the official diagnostic criteria in clinical, research, and educational settings. The diagnoses are published in the *Diagnostic and Statistical Manual of Mental Disorders*, fourth edition (DSM-IV). See Appendix A for the complete listing of DSM-IV diagnoses.

NANDA

Nursing has formed its own nomenclature of nursing diagnoses. Many of the current diagnoses published by the North American Nursing Diagnosis Association (NANDA) are applicable in the psychiatric setting. The NANDA nursing classification is relatively young, but with each conference and publication, new diagnoses are evolving for psychiatric clients.

The nursing process.   The nursing **process** is a scientific, problem-solving method that assists nurses in total client care. This important process consists of six steps: assessment, diagnosis, outcome identification, planning, implementation, and evaluation. Chapter 7 is devoted to a thorough description and explanation of the nursing process as it relates to psychiatric nursing.

COLLABORATIVE DIAGNOSES

In the interest of establishing itself as a separate science, nursing has passed through a time when it attempted to use its own classification apart from medical diagnoses. Textbooks for psychiatric nurses were sometimes written with chapter headings directed at client behaviors rather than psychiatric diagnoses. It was more difficult for students first exposed to psychiatry to associate the psychiatric (admitting) diagnosis of a mental disorder with the nursing diagnosis and subsequent combined treatment. It seems clear that a coexistence of medical and nursing diagnoses is essential for the ultimate collaborative, interdisciplinary care of clients. Only through this synergy will clients' needs be fully met. Clinical pathways are utilized in many psychiatric settings as interdisciplinary tools during client treatment. Several sample clinical pathways appear in Chapter 7.

THE NURSING ROLE

Traditionally, psychiatric nurses have focused on psychosocial aspects of the client (individual, group, family, community) as the client conducted life and managed or failed to manage the challenges, tasks, demands, and problems of life. In this endeavor, psychiatric nurses have been concerned primarily with the client's perceptual, mental, emotional, and behavioral responses to internal and external stressors and crises. In addition, they assessed factors that enhanced or inhibited the client's ability and capacity to cope with these challenges and with real or perceived threats to stability. At the heart of psychiatric nurses' interactions was the interpersonal relationship (therapeutic alliance), which still remains the emphasis of treatment. Even though many other biologic and scientific factors have major influence, the nurse-client interaction is the catalyst for client participation and progression toward wellness.

Psychiatric nursing has changed considerably over time. Actual formalization of this specialty did not begin until the mid-1950s. Nursing texts before this were often vague and ambiguous when describing interpersonal nurse-client interactions. They offered little information about specific nursing interventions or rationale for those interventions. Although most authors agreed that the nurse-client relationship was a key to client wellness, examples of successful interactions with clients were not clearly defined to help nurses learn how to be effective therapeutic communicators.

After the National Mental Health Act was passed in 1946, the nursing profession responded to a mandate calling for an increase of activity in mental health nursing. Several graduate programs in psychiatric nursing were begun, and produced the nursing leaders who "set the stage in the 1950s for the importance of the one-to-one nurse-

---

Box 1-5   Essential Characteristics of a Successful Therapist

Empathy Considered by many to be the most important element of a therapeutic relationship and necessary for client to feel understood; encompasses placing self in client's internal perception without losing objectivity or identity.

Warmth Being wholly and intently attentive to the interaction, which results in client feeling accepted and significant; conveyance of warmth also means nonpossessive caring and avoiding emotional entanglements while maintaining boundaries.

Genuineness Verbal and nonverbal messages are entirely congruent with way nurse feels; honest, sincere, open; "real" responses; does not imply "tell all"; requires discriminating responses.

Respect Unconditional positive regard for client's uniqueness regardless of his or her present life situation; valuing the client and conveying recognition of client's human worth; does not mean allowing or condoning inappropriate behaviors.

Concreteness Involves use of specific, realistic terminology rather than vague, abstract jargon or concepts; assists client to speak concretely; clearly fosters self-understanding; helps in problem solving and formulating plans and alternatives.

Immediacy Interactions and communication focus on interpersonal relationship as it exists; client relationship with the nurse is a "snapshot" of problems experienced in other relationships and needs to be addressed.

Confrontation Constructive confrontation is necessary for client behavioral changes. If the client remains unaware of problems or if problems go unaddressed, he or she will continue to conduct life in the same self-defeating patterns and will avoid getting well. The nurse discusses discrepancies and incongruities. Timing is important. The nurse avoids outbursts that may occur for the sake of relief of the nurse's frustration.

Self-Disclosure Nurse volunteers personal information (ideas, feelings, experiences) only when relevant to the client's concerns and interests (client is the focus); nurse redirects conversation back to client problems, situations, or events; nurse assists clients in recognizing that problems being experienced are not unique—that client is not alone and that others will support client through difficult times; nurse models success in problem solving.

patient relationship" (Lego, 1995). Significance of the therapeutic alliance has never diminished. Following is a description of the art and science of the nurse-client relationship.

THE NURSE-CLIENT RELATIONSHIP
The Art

The art of caring is embodied in the therapeutic nurse-client relationship, which is the basis for psychiatric mental health nursing. The relationship, often referred to as a *therapeutic alliance*, is used as a therapeutic vehicle to effect change, promote growth, and heal mental and emotional wounds. It has been identified as one of the most crucial components of the entire health care delivery process (Lego, 1995; Peplau, 1952; Ruben, 1990; Thompson, 1990) and has a primary purpose of optimal well-being of the client (Bernstein and Bernstein, 1985).

Hildegard Peplau, a pioneer in psychiatric nursing, first described the nurse's relationship with the client in her text, *Interpersonal Relations in Nursing* (1952). Thereafter, Peplau and other psychiatric nurse practitioners and authors continued to develop and refine nursing theory that described and interpreted the relationship. Even though significant changes occurred between 1974 and 1994 in the care of people with actual and potential mental disorders, "the one-to-one relationship remained a core modality in psychiatric mental health nursing practice" (Beeber, 1995).

The art of a therapeutic relationship includes essential characteristics of the nurse that facilitate client participation in his or her own care toward the ultimate purpose of wellness. These essential characteristics of a successful therapist were first identified nearly 30 years ago by Carkhoff (Carkhoff, 1969; Carkhoff and Traux, 1967) and have become classic, core conditions for facilitative interpersonal relationships. The characteristics are empathy, warmth, genuineness, respect, concreteness, immediacy, confrontation, and self-disclosure, which are described in Box 1-5.

Concept of helping.   A major objective for nurses is client participation in his or her own care within the client's capacity. The ultimate goal is eventual client self-sufficiency, which is achieved through self-searching and self-help. Nurses facilitate this growth process by understanding that concept before undertaking the role of care provider in the psychiatric setting.

The helping process is complex. It is not unique to health care providers but is practiced by all caring and concerned individuals. Many motives exist for the act of helping. It is imperative that psychiatric nurses, who work with an exceptionally vulnerable population, assess their own interests in helping and become aware of their personal needs and reasons for serving others. Some reasons cited by Brammer (1993) include the following:

- *Desire to contribute to society.* A feeling of wanting to give back to the world describes this altruistic urge to make things better than they are. By contributing to society, the person feels more worthwhile. Beginning to help in tangible, concrete ways versus grandiose ways is recommended.

- *Need to protect others.* Helping may take the form of protecting the individual. Sometimes, rescuing others from consequences of their own decisions and behaviors is counterproductive (e.g., a family member's codependent protective behavior toward a person with alcoholism). Objective assessment of the client's condition and situation is necessary to know when protection for health and safety's sake is legitimate and when it fosters dependence or encourages, rather than eliminates, maladaptive behavior.

- *Need for love.* If when helping others the focus is on the helper's own need for love and attention, the result becomes counterproductive. Awareness of the need to be needed is important, because a consequence of serving others to the exclusion of getting one's own needs met leads inevitably to disappointment and burnout, resulting in decreased capacity and ability to help others. Clients must not be the source of this love.

- *Need for control or power.* Clients often see helpers as more powerful because of their presumed knowledge, coupled with the client's sense of vulnerability during both acute and chronic dysfunction or disorder. When helpers are aware of this need to influence others or to gain prestige and praise, they can act to correct their motive for helping and focus on the client's needs. Gratitude and praise are then received appropriately.

- *Need for personal satisfaction.* Balanced, healthy individuals who work in helping professions often describe personal satisfaction from working with and watching individuals overcome adversity, achieve goals, and experience growth. To know that the helper facilitated these changes is rewarding and often brings great satisfaction to the helper.

- *Need for personal insight.* While working with clients who have personal problems, a helper may use the relationship to solve his or her own problems. Awareness of this vicarious learning is important as constant reminder to focus on clients and their issues. Many helpers who have worked through their own similar problems become effective therapists and are able to offer empathy and insight to their clients who move toward change and growth.

Above are some reasons why helpers enter the psychotherapeutic arena. Many motives are unconscious and can be brought to awareness through a process of **autodiagnosis:** examination of one's own thoughts, feelings, perceptions, and attitudes about a particular client. Motives can also be discovered through continual education and supervision by effective instructors, mentors, or professional peers, who will assist the helper in confronting areas that may be problematic.

Outcomes of helping.   Helping is a process that aims to assist another person as follows:

Help himself or herself
Choose a direction in life
Find purpose for existing
Solve problems
Survive crises
Share life with others in work, play, and love

Helping is not about doing "to" or "for" another when the person can function autonomously or with guidance and assistance. Only when the client takes responsibility for life through independence (within his or her own ability, age, stage of development, life situation) can that person experience the freedom to grow. The helper's task is awareness of self, awareness of client needs, and utilization of skills to set the client free, with tools to forge his or her own life.

The Science

The term *science* is broadly used to describe the systematic operationalization of the nurse-client relationship. The essential characteristics mentioned earlier, plus the desire to help people in the psychiatric setting, are just the prerequisites of psychiatric mental health nursing. The nurse also needs to know how to help. This requires learning tangible skills that are used in conjunction with the helping characteristics previously described—skills that are put into action in the form of specific interventions directed at identified client needs and problems.

Only four decades ago, nurses' interventions with clients in psychiatric settings were focused primarily on keeping them safe, carrying out medical orders, and helping them (by whatever nursing means were available) to be comfortable. Care was largely custodial. Nursing textbooks lacked specific instructions for effective, meaningful interactions to benefit clients and were often vague, ambiguous, abstract, and general regarding nursing interventions. At present, instructions are clear and specific regarding nursing activities with psychiatric clients.

The nurse-client interpersonal relationship involves the integration of many components to be successful. In addition to previously defined characteristics and the willingness or desire to help people solve their problems, the nurse also must have knowledge of content that includes but is not limited to the following:

Principles of the nurse-client relationship
Nursing scope of practice
Mental health and mental disorder
Psychiatric diagnoses
    DSM
    NANDA
Nursing process
Therapeutic treatment modalities
Current epidemiology and research
Prevention of disorders (levels)
Roles of the mental health team
Trends and issues regarding the future

Principles of the nurse-client relationship.   The therapeutic interpersonal relationship that develops between the nurse and the client is a vehicle for effecting client change and growth. The following are principles and guidelines for developing and maintaining the relationship:

The relationship is therapeutic rather than social.
The focus remains on the client's issues rather than on the nurse's or other issues.
The relationship is purposeful and goal directed.
It is objective versus subjective in quality.
It is time limited versus open ended.

Box 1-6 **Signs of Unhealthy Boundaries**	
Going against personal values or rights to please another	Allowing someone to take as much as they can from you
Not noticing when someone displays inappropriate boundaries	Letting others direct your life
Not noticing when someone invades your boundaries	Letting others describe your reality
Talking at an intimate level on the first meeting	Letting others define you
Falling in love with a new acquaintance	Believing others can anticipate your needs
Falling in love with anyone who reaches out	Expecting others to fill your needs automatically
Being overwhelmed by (preoccupied with) a person	Falling apart so someone will take care of you
Acting on first sexual impulse	Self-abuse
Being sexual for your partner, not yourself	Sexual and physical abuse
Accepting food, gifts, touch, or sex that you do not want	Food abuse
Touching a person without asking	Loaning money you do not have
Taking as much as you can for the sake of getting	Flirting; sending mixed messages
Giving as much as you can for the sake of giving	Telling all

Therapeutic versus social.   A therapeutic relationship is formed to help clients solve problems, make decisions, achieve growth, learn coping strategies, let go of unwanted behaviors, reinforce self-worth, and examine relationships. The meetings between nurse and client are not for mutual satisfaction. Although the nurse can be friendly with the client, the nurse is not there to be the client's friend. Because boundaries define us and our roles and are important in any relationship, especially in a therapeutic relationship, trying to be a client's friend blurs boundaries and confuses roles. The nurse helps the client increase awareness of boundaries and practice boundary-setting (Box 1-6).

Some social conversation is usual at the beginning of meetings and may help to establish or maintain rapport. Occasionally during meetings, superficial or social conversation may briefly reappear, but the majority of conversation is focused and therapeutic. Table 1-2 compares therapeutic with social interactions.

Client focus.   Frequently during a session, a client redirects the focus away from self by changing the subject, talking about the weather, or focusing on the nurse (nurse's appearance, personal problems, problems in the milieu), or other issues. The nurse recognizes this as a divergent tactic that is probably a form of resistance. The nurse then confronts the behavior in a matter-of-fact way and refocuses the client. Clients do this for one or more of several reasons: resistance to discussing anxiety-producing material, boredom, repetition of material previously discussed with other therapists, or inability to stay cognitively focused because of a mental disorder.

Goal direction.   The primary purpose of a therapeutic relationship is helping clients to meet adaptive goals. Together the client and nurse determine problematic issues and collaboratively decide what the client needs and is able to achieve. Once goals are established, the nurse and client agree to work toward those goals and put intentions into action and modify strategies when necessary until the identified goals are achieved. The activities involved are usually many and varied, but each activity is purposefully planned with the client's goals in mind.

Objective versus subjective.   Nurses can be therapeutic only if they remain objective. **Objectivity** refers to remaining free from bias, prejudice, and personal identification in interaction with the client and being able to process information based on facts. **Subjectivity,** on the other hand, refers to emphasis on one's own feelings, attitudes, and opinions when interacting with the client. When nurses act subjectively in relation to the client's problems or situations, they lose effectiveness in the relationship. By stepping back, the nurse can see things realistically rather than becoming overly and personally involved with the client's issues.

This, of course, does not imply that the nurse withdraws from feeling or constructs barriers to protect himself or herself by intellectualizing or avoiding responses. With knowledge, awareness, and practice, the nurse can be both objective and fully attentive to clients' situations and needs.

An example of objectivity versus subjectivity is the nurse's ability to remain empathic instead of becoming sympathetic when interacting with a client, even though the nurse may have experienced a similar, painful situation. For instance, consider a nurse who has lost a child in an accident and then encounters a client who is depressed and grieving the recent death of his or her own child. The nurse demonstrates objectivity by allowing and facilitating the client's full expression of thoughts and feelings and then responding in a warm, empathic way that remains client centered. This approach helps the client relieve pent-up feelings in a normal grieving process, allows him or her to feel understood, and helps the client to process and organize thoughts directed toward solving problems.

An example of nontherapeutic subjectivity is a nurse in the same situation who hears the client's expression of feelings and responds with excessive self-disclosure about his or her own similar experience. This approach represents a loss of therapeutic boundaries by identifying with

Table 1-2	**Therapeutic Versus Social Interactions**
Therapeutic	**Social**
Offer client therapeutic assistance	Give and receive friendship equally
Focus on client's needs	Meet both person's needs
Discuss client's perception, thoughts, feelings, and behaviors	Share mutual ideas and experiences
Actively listen and use therapeutic communication, skills, and techniques	Give opinions and advice
Encourage client to choose subject for discussion	Randomly discuss topics at will or whim
Encourage client to problem solve toward independence	Insist on helping as a friend; tolerate dependence
Keep no secrets that may harm client	Promise to keep secrets at any cost
Set goals with client	Goals of relationship not important
Remain objective	Become subjectively involved
Maintain healthy boundaries	Accept blurred boundaries
Evaluate interactions with client	Avoid relational evaluations

the client's problem—becoming enmeshed in the situation by personalizing it. The client's response will most likely be negative. The client will probably stop sharing information because he or she feels unimportant and negated, or because he or she worries that the nurse is fragile or inept and cannot even manage his or her own problems.

Time-limited interactions.   Before the relationship is established, the nurse sets necessary parameters of the relationship by agreeing with the client on the days and times when they will meet and on the numbers of times meetings will take place. Such structure helps the client realize that this relationship has limits and is not open ended (i.e., the client cannot see the nurse whenever he or she wants and for as long as he or she wants).

The principle of time-limited interaction is important for several reasons. Sometimes clients have not learned during formative relationships that limits are important for all relationships and that without limits problems are inevitable. When participants define the amount of time they are willing and able to give, then anxiety-provoking guesswork is eliminated and individuals can decide how to make appropriate use of the time they have together. Also, all relationships have inevitable endings. Much grief is avoided if both the nurse and the client are certain of the parameters of their relationship and enforce them together. The relationship is a microcosm of the client's relationships outside of their meetings and serves as a model for the client to successfully begin and appropriately let go of subsequent relationships.

Stages of the nurse-client relationship.   Every relationship between the nurse and the client is unique because of the qualities each participant brings to the interaction process and because of the human chemistry that develops between them. There are, however, definitive phases that relationships undergo. The astute nurse identifies these phases as they occur to more effectively facilitate the client's progress.

Preorientation phase.   During this initial phase before the nurse and the client ever meet, the nurse must accomplish several tasks. The first is to gather data about the client, his or her condition, and present situation. Information is taken from all available sources (client's chart; staff report; physician's report; input from family or other reliable sources, such as police and ambulance attendants).

From the information gathered, the nurse engages in a period of autodiagnosis regarding his or her thoughts, feelings, perceptions, and attitudes about this particular client. Judgmentalism, biases, or stereotyping may arise that can influence the pending contact in a nontherapeutic way. For example, if the nurse learns information that reminds him or her of a loved one or of a despised or feared person, the nurse's response to the client could be subjective and ineffective if the facts are not closely examined.

Consider Nurse A, whose father was dependent on alcohol and verbally abused her mother when he drank.

What are some possible responses Nurse A may demonstrate in the following situations if she does not engage in autodiagnosis?

A male client is admitted to the unit because of inebriation and wife abuse.

A matronly female is admitted to the unit with major depression. Her husband drinks and abuses her.

Nurse A's conscious efforts to examine each situation and put it in an objective perspective are important if judgmentalism and stereotyping are to be avoided.

Orientation phase.   Following nurse-client introduction, the relationship begins to grow. During this stage, participants become acquainted, build trust and rapport, and demonstrate acceptance of the process that will take place when the client begins to work on important issues.

The contract.   A contract is established in the orientation phase of the relationship. The contract may be formal or informal, written or verbal. Nurses most frequently use verbal, informal contracts with clients in acute care settings in which the client and nurse are more continually together. It may be necessary for the nurse to write a more specific, formalized contract for clients who are seen outside of an acute care setting.

The contract may be succinct and still be effective and efficient. For example, the nurse on an inpatient unit may say to the client: "I will be your contact person while you are in the (facility). I work Monday through Friday from 8 AM to 4 PM. Because of your schedule on this unit, it seems that the best time for us to meet is 9 AM. Is that a good time for you?" If the client agrees, the contract is established.

In a community setting (home care, partial-day treatment program, halfway house), the nurse would probably write a contract for the client, specifying dates, days, and times of meetings, and phone numbers where the nurse can be reached if the client has questions between appointments. Some contracts clearly define client behaviors expected to occur between meetings and goals to be reached.

Regardless of the type of contract, the nurse explains the purpose of the meetings, what may be expected during the meetings, and roles of both nurse and client. Together, they determine long-term goals and short-term objectives for reaching those goals.

Dependability is imperative and nurses must keep all appointments with clients. Even at times when circumstances prevent this, the nurse contacts the client to explain the situation and sets a new meeting time. Client dependability is also expected and conveyed.

During the orientation stage, client strengths, limitations, and problem areas are identified by both the client and the nurse. Outcome criteria are established, and a plan of care is formulated. Client's responses to this phase vary widely.

Working phase. The orientation phase ends and the working phase begins when the client takes responsibility for his or her own behavior change. This means committing to working on issues and concerns that have caused disruptions in the client's life.

Prioritizing clients' needs helps determine those problems that will require immediate attention and promotes an organized way to manage the problems. A general principle is that safety and health problems supersede any others. For example, it is always determined first that clients are free from danger to self or others and that physical needs are met before traditional therapy begins. Then behaviors that are socially unacceptable are modified (e.g., hostile remarks, swearing, isolation, poor hygiene). The nurse assists the client to change problematic behaviors in a safe environment in which the client can practice new skills and behaviors.

As nurses gain experience, they are better able to recognize when their clients are in the working phase. Sometimes clients tell their "story" but do not do the work to change. Seasoned nurses are able to separate the provocative content from actual process and growth.

Termination phase. In this stage the relationship comes to a close. Termination begins in the orientation phase when the nurse states meeting times with the client. This lets the client know that the relationship is about to begin, but that it also has parameters and will end. It avoids confusion on the part of the client, who occasionally is unable or unwilling to recognize the boundaries of the relationship and wants to contact the nurse outside of the facility or after the client has been discharged. The nurse does not continue relationships after the client leaves treatment.

Termination generally occurs when the client has improved and has been discharged, but it may also occur if the client or nurse is transferred. When termination is anticipated, the nurse employs strategies to prepare for the event. Ending treatment may sometimes be traumatic for clients who have come to value the relationship and the help. Some methods that the nurse may use when preparing for termination include the following:

Reducing the amount of time spent with the client in each session and increasing the amount of time between sessions, as the condition improves.

Beginning to work on preparation for the client's post-discharge situation (plans for future) rather than focusing on new or past problems.

Having the client identify changes he or she has made toward growth; sharing perceptions of the client's growth.

Helping the client express feelings about ending the relationship; telling the client if the relationship has been pleasant.

When nurses recognize relationship stages and are aware of the strategies and responses during each stage, the course of the therapeutic process runs more smoothly. The nurse is not caught off guard or shocked when responses are other than anticipated. When nurses are unaware of potential client responses, they may take responsibility for what seems like failure or may even abandon the relationship because it is unrewarding or unfulfilling. When the nurse is aware of responses that may occur, however, he or she is prepared to use strategies that facilitate client growth.

ROLES OF THE MENTAL HEALTH TEAM

Nurses play a major role in all aspects of mental health care (e.g., prevention, treatment, rehabilitation) and work collaboratively with other disciplines.

Clients involved in mental health care are usually treated by an interdisciplinary team of care providers. The roles of mental health team members vary widely, but each role exists primarily to assist the client in achieving and maintaining optimum wellness.

The healthy client-member relationship works toward eventual client independence within his or her capacity. Team members provide the tools that clients use to shape their lives and the relationship within which the client practices learned behaviors. Although health team members cooperatively formulate goals and objectives for clients within the system, each role differs with respect to the following:

Philosophy
Conceptual bases
Theoretic frameworks
Preparatory education
Purpose
Methods of intervention

Roles of the mental health team appear in Box 1-7.

TREATMENT

Clients who require treatment enter the mental health system in one of several ways. They may voluntarily seek intervention themselves in any number of psychiatric settings (therapists office, community clinic, acute care hospital setting). Clients may also be brought into the system by family, friends, service agencies, ambulance, or law enforcement agencies and for many reasons. The following are reasons that necessitate intervention and treatment.

Symptoms are painful or intolerable.
  Example: A mother of four is unable to leave her house each day until she compulsively cleans the entire house.
Symptoms are unmanageable by the client or significant others.

Box 1-7   Roles of the Mental Health Team

Psychiatric Nurse

Nurses have the most widely focused position description of any of the member roles. This depends on their license and certification mandates, the policies of the psychiatric facility or care setting, and their experience. They interact with clients in individual and group settings; manage client care; administer and monitor medications; assist with numerous psychiatric and physical treatments; participate in interdisciplinary team meetings; teach clients and families; take responsibility for client records; act as a client advocate; interact with clients' significant others; and assess and intervene with clients' psychiatric, biologic, psychosocial, cultural, and spiritual problems.

Licensed vocational nurses provide direct client support. Registered nurses have expanded roles of unit management and decision making in addition to client interaction. Master's- and doctoral-prepared nurses act as clinical specialists in individual, group, and family therapy, with expanded roles within psychiatric settings, or they act autonomously in private practice.

In some states clinical nurse specialists prescribe medications and manage client caseloads. A master's or doctoral degree is required to teach nursing education. Graduate nurses frequently conduct psychiatric research or act as administrators of psychiatric settings.

Psychiatric Social Worker

This graduate-level position allows members to work with clients on an individual basis, conduct group therapy sessions, work with clients' families, and act as liaisons with the community to place clients after discharge. They emphasize intervention with the client in the social environment in which he or she will live.

Psychiatric Technician

The licensed psychiatric technician has direct client contact in a psychiatric setting and usually reports to the registered nurse. Technicians are trained to observe and record symptoms and intervene under supervision. In some states they can administer medications under the supervision of a registered nurse.

Mental Health Worker

Some facilities call this position mental health counselor. It is an unlicensed position in which the member acts only under the supervision of an RN in assisting clients with activities of daily living, maintaining the schedule, and providing general support. Some mental health workers have minimal education in psychiatry; others may work in this position while accruing hours toward master's or doctoral degrees. They do not administer medications.

Psychiatrist

A psychiatrist is a licensed medical physician who specializes in psychiatry. Responsibilities include admitting clients into acute care settings, prescribing and monitoring psychopharmacologic agents, administering electroshock therapy, conducting individual and family therapy, and participating in interdisciplinary team meetings that focus on his or her clients.

Psychologist

A psychologist is a licensed individual with a doctoral degree in psychology. There are several different psychology tracks. Preparation is for assessment and treatment of psychologic and psychosocial problems of individuals, families, or groups (including industrial, educational, environmental). Psychologists do not prescribe or administer medications. Many psychologists administer psychometric tests that aid in the diagnosis of disorders.

Marriage, Family, Child Counselor

These are licensed individuals who frequently work in private practice. They are prepared to work with individuals, couples, families, and groups, and emphasize the interpersonal aspects of achieving and maintaining relationships.

Case Managers

This position is continuously redefined. Nurses are qualified for this position because of their diverse education. Case managers facilitate delivery of individualized, coordinated care in cost-effective ways. Managed care and case management are not interchangeable concepts. *Managed care* refers to a system of cost-containment programs that are utilized to direct, control, and approve access to services and costs within the health care delivery system. *Case management* is a process in the managed care strategy (Mullahy, 1995). Case managers need to know the various types of hospitalization and outpatient care settings, the coverage offered by different payers (insurance companies, health maintenance organizations, preferred provider organizations), and the impact of federal and state legislation. Case managers serve as a connection between agencies to provide the most favorable outcomes for the client.

Example: The client refuses to take medications that control disruptive symptoms associated with chronic schizophrenia.

Daily function is disrupted as a result of the disorder.

Example: A husband is so depressed, he cannot get up to go to work or complete daily household duties and family responsibilities.

Life crises occur because of symptoms.

Example: An adolescent is admitted to the hospital after trying to commit suicide.

Crimes are committed as a result of the disorder.

Example: A single mother of two toddlers is jailed because of using and selling street drugs.

Psychiatric mental health nurses are frequently involved in the care of clients with mental disorders, in various settings.

THERAPEUTIC TREATMENT MODALITIES

A virtual revolution in mental health care has occurred in the past few years in which traditional inpatient hospitalization has been replaced with an entire range of care options. These optional care modalities may offer cost-effective, creative, client-focused alternatives to traditional treatment. Nurses' awareness of these shifts in treatment methods will ensure optimum client care.

Multiple methods may be used during intervention with clients in any psychiatric setting that include, but are not limited to, inpatient hospital or treatment center, outpatient day treatment program, clinic, home, community center, crisis center, place of employment, or school. The choice of methods for intervening with clients' needs and problems is influenced by several factors, including the following:

The client's presenting problems
The client's knowledge about treatment methods
The client's ability to make treatment choices
The therapist's theoretic background, training, and philosophy
Type of setting
Available resources

Approaches vary widely among the scores of available therapies, and it is not an uncommon practice to incorporate several methods (eclectic approach) during treatment. Generally, clients admitted to an acute care psychiatric setting will receive both interactive and biologic types of therapy. Any range of methods may be employed in community settings.

Interactive therapies include all of those in which the client has interpersonal contact with one or more therapists and includes interaction with other clients. Biologic therapies include use of medications, electroshock therapy, and, more rarely, psychosurgery. Interactive therapies most often used regardless of the theoretic framework, or conceptual model on which they are based, take the form of one-to-one therapy, group therapy, and adjunctive therapies. Box 1-8 lists therapeutic treatment modalities that may be offered in traditional and nontraditional settings. A description of therapies is presented in Part Five.

CHANGES IN TREATMENT

Historically, when individuals had serious, unremitting mental disorders that resulted in the inability to function in society, they were sent to live in institutions. These were either state-funded hospitals where persons with mental disorders would probably remain for the duration of their lives, or these were private facilities if their families could

Box 1-8	Therapeutic Treatment Modalities

Psychotherapy
Crisis intervention
Milieu therapy
Support, psychosocial
　　Caregiver support
Therapeutic processes
　　Transference (psychology)
　　Countertransference (psychology)
Transactional analysis
Reality therapy
Validation therapy
Symbolism (psychology)
　　Metaphor
Socioenvironmental therapy
　　Client passes
　　Group psychotherapy
Psychodrama
Role playing
Support groups
Residential care
Family therapy
Marital therapy
Behavior modification
　　Assertiveness training
　　Behavior contracting
　　Behavior therapy
　　Cognitive therapy
　　Biofeedback
　　Relaxation techniques
　　　　Distraction
　　　　Guided imagery
　　　　Meditation
Biofeedback
Hypnosis
Art therapy
Play therapy
Pet therapy
Music therapy
Dance therapy
Bibliotherapy
Guided imagery
Substance dependence program
Rehabilitation, psychosocial

and would pay for them. Some events occurred that dramatically changed the face of history relating to the treatment of people with mental disorders. The move out of institutions and into the community for treatment was primarily influenced by the following events.

The impetus for deinstitutionalization came from several sources. One was the 1949 government grant awards through the National Mental Health Act for community treatment of clients with mental disorders. A second source was the use of antipsychotic medications that began in the 1950s and provided more complete relief to clients plagued by life-hampering psychotic symptoms. Because of medications, clients were able to leave mental institutions and, in many cases, function in society once again. Third was the Mental Health Centers Act of 1963, which called for development of comprehensive community mental health programs across the nation.

Prevention of Mental Disorders

In response to the mandate to treat clients in the community setting, Gerald Caplan proposed a model for preventive care of persons with mental disorders in his textbook, *Principles of Preventive Psychiatry* (1964). The model is still widely accepted, quoted, and utilized. Although originally written for psychiatry, the model has been adopted by many other disciplines. Psychiatric nurses use the effective principles in providing care for their clients, and the model is a primary focus for community health nurses because of its adaptability to biologic, psychologic, or social problems and needs.

The model proposes three levels of prevention of illness and disorder: *primary prevention, secondary prevention,* and *tertiary prevention.* Some subsequent theorists state that there are actually four levels, because the primary level includes two steps: promotion and prevention (Clark, 1992; Leavell, 1965).

Box 1-9   Examples of Prevention Levels

Primary Prevention
- Teach stress reduction and stress management techniques to any population
- Present seminar for school-age children and parents on drug actions and effects
- Teach parenting skills and normal child development expectations to pregnant couples
- Lead a group that cleans cluttered grounds of a troubled tenement lot to begin a garden

Secondary Prevention
- Treat individuals in any psychiatric setting (inpatient, home, clinic, day treatment), after diagnosis has been identified, by any approved method of therapy (interactive or biologic medications)
- Refer clients who demonstrate symptoms to other appropriate mental health care providers (psychometric testing, medication consultation, family therapy)

Tertiary Prevention
- Provide family support and education to assist in early identification of symptoms that may occur in the future
- Engage couple in therapy to learn new ways to relate to each other in their marriage
- Provide ongoing outpatient therapy group that meets for mutual support of members, education, and assessment of progress

---

Levels of prevention.   Primary prevention focuses on reduction of the incidence of mental disorders within the community. It is directed toward occurrence of mental health problems, with emphasis on health promotion and prevention of disorders. Nursing interventions may concentrate on the client, the environment, or both. For example, the nurse may help the client to learn about and cope with life stressors or strive to diminish the numbers of stressors in the community.

Secondary prevention is directed toward reducing the prevalence of mental disorders through early identification of problems and early treatment of those problems. This stage occurs after the problem arises and aims to shorten the course or duration of the episode.

Tertiary prevention has the dual focus of reducing residual effects of the disorder and rehabilitating the individual who experienced the mental disorder. Examples of primary, secondary, and tertiary prevention appear in Box 1-9.

Psychiatric nurses who are familiar with this model will benefit as nursing practice continues to move out into the community. As funding becomes more constricted, a primary mission is to increase intervention at the primary prevention level. An even more important reason for primary prevention is to assist clients in avoiding pitfalls whenever possible through increased awareness and education.

THE FUTURE
PROVISION OF CARE

Without exception, the contemporary dominant issue in mental health is managed care. Managed care is composed of a system of providers that regulates and dictates how health care is delivered and financed. The outcomes of managed care for clients and families with mental disorders and other disorders are conservatively reported to be ineffective. Open, honest reports state that managed care, especially for the persistently severe, chronic population of mentally disordered clients, is nothing short of disastrous. The National Alliance for Mental Illness reported dramatic underservice of that population as long ago as 1997 (NAMI, 1997).

During the decade of the 1980s there was an "unprecedented boom in psychiatric care" (Mohr, 1998). It was abundant. Psychiatric care facilities grew in numbers during this golden era. As we are poised to enter the next century, clients with mental disorders are consistently denied access to care or are undertreated if care is provided because of the constraints that limit funding for services. Clients' conditions and situations no longer dictate intervention and treatment; however, availability of funds does, and funds are controlled by cost-effective managed care organizations.

Clients, especially those with chronic, persistent, and severe mental disorders, are frequently encountered in home care or other community settings or are admitted to acute care facilities, where the time to intervene, treat, and monitor treatment effects is greatly limited under the present dictums. Because of lack of funding, clients are often discharged before they are ready to leave. They frequently reenter the system within a short period and are unable to function because of persistent symptoms of their undertreated disorder. This phenomenon is commonly referred to as *the revolving door syndrome.*

The above precedent has changed the way that nurses practice. To effectively serve the consumer, nurses must accomplish a lot in a short time. In these turbulent times, nurses must be flexible. They have historically demonstrated an awareness that opportunity is the companion of change. With that in mind, nurses must seek the opportunity for providing thorough care, in every challenge, whether these are limited client contacts or clients prematurely discharged as a result of funding restrictions.

Other opportunities exist that focus on the psychiatric nurse. With the decided advantage of having the ability to monitor medical and medication needs of clients, and in the interest of cost-effectiveness, nurses can compete for positions that may expand their roles. In addition, nurses who stay abreast of trends through their active involvement in nursing, political, and consumer interest organizations become aware of current issues and may participate in discussions and decision-making processes, thereby offering constructive solutions to some of the salient problems that plague the health care field.

OTHER ADVANCES
In addition to the economic and political factors that influence the future of psychiatric mental health nursing, other factors require consideration.

Psychobiology
The decade of the 1990s was named by Congress as "the Decade of the Brain." More has been learned about mental disorders and treatment in the past decade than was learned in all the years before that time. Neurobiology is a favorite topic in the explosion of information that surrounds psychiatric mental health. Great strides have been made in this area to determine causes for some disorders, and successful treatment cannot be far behind. Psychobiology is a necessary topic to be incorporated into nursing education.

Medical Technology
In this text, readers will discover the impact that expanding technology has had on psychiatry. Modern brain imaging techniques such as MRI, PET, and CAT scans have revolutionized diagnosis of mental disorders. Brain surgery done by stereotactic methods may become even more sophisticated in the future. Research in circadian rhythms and their influence on mental disorders is well documented.

Constant discovery of new psychopharmacologic agents is certain to alter the future treatment of disorders. Clients might be able to automatically monitor their own medication levels and replenish them before minor symptoms become extreme disorders. For example, anxiety levels may be monitored by unobtrusively connected mechanisms that will signal an individual to perform his or her own therapy before a full-blown panic attack occurs.

CRITICAL THINKING
One of nursing's finest tools is the ability to critically think through situations and content to arrive at solutions and decisions that are based in logic and fact. Critical thinking is an acquired skill that evolves with knowledge, experience, intent, and practice. It is the responsibility of every psychiatric nurse to learn these skills. Some nursing disciplines may be less challenging because they offer the nurse more predictable structure and prepared formulas for working with clients. Psychiatric nursing has structured principles but requires the nurse to continually apply critical thinking because of the dynamic nature of clients and the unique manifestations of mental disorders.

A definition of critical thinking is the use of cognitive skills and strategies that is purposeful, reasoned, and goal directed and that increases the probability of a desirable outcome in decision making and problem solving.

The following elements are necessary when learning critical thinking:

An attitude toward recognizing when a critical thinking skill is needed and a willingness to apply it (openmindedness, awareness of psychologic blocks and biases)

Readiness and ability to learn the skills of critical thinking

Practice of structure-training exercises designed to facilitate transfer of information across contexts

Teaching and application of self-monitoring skills so that critical thinking can be examined and feedback can be given

The use of critical thinking in the psychiatric setting will enable the nurse to interact and communicate with clients more effectively, suspend judgments, convey information to peers that is based in fact, and problem solve with a focus on the client's objectives.

Summary of Key Concepts

1. Psychiatric mental health nursing is a specialty within nursing and is recognized as one of the four core mental health practice areas.
2. The therapeutic nurse-client relationship is the basis of psychiatric mental health nursing.
3. The client's needs are the focus of a therapeutic relationship.
4. The four stages of the nurse-client relationship are preorientation, orientation, working, and termination.
5. The ANA Standards of Care follow the steps of the nursing process and provide a framework within which psychiatric mental health nursing can be implemented and evaluated.
6. There is no one definition for mental health. Mental health is influenced by numerous and varied factors.
7. Protective defenses are the psychologic processes used to protect the person from internal and external stressors and dangers.
8. Traditional mental health care in an inpatient setting is significantly decreasing as delivery systems in the community and the home become more prevalent.
9. The most effective mental health care will be delivered through a team approach, which applies the expertise of multiple mental health disciplines.
10. Psychobiologic research supports a biologic basis for many mental disorders, with significant implications for psychiatric mental health nursing.
11. Expanding scientific technology is an important influence for the future of psychiatric mental health nursing.
12. Critical thinking is a necessary skill for psychiatric mental health nurses.

REFERENCES

American Journal of Nursing: Health care reform (video), 32nd biennial convention of Sigma Theta Tau, Alan Trench/Helene Fuld Trust, 1993.

American Nurses Association: *Psychiatric mental health nursing.* Psychopharmacology project, Washington, DC, 1994a, The Association.

American Nurses Association: *A statement on public mental health clinical nursing practice and standards of public mental health nursing practice,* Washington, DC, 1994b, The Association.

American Nurses Association: *Standards of clinical nursing practice,* Kansas City, Mo, 1991, The Association.

American Psychiatric Association: *Diagnostic and statistical manual of mental disorders,* ed 4, Washington, DC, 1994, The Association.

Beeber LS: The one-to-one relationship in nursing practice: the next generation. In Anderson CA, editor: *Psychiatric nursing 1974 to 1994: a report on the state of the art,* St. Louis, 1995, Mosby.

Bernstein L, Bernstein R: *Interviewing: a guide for health professions,* Norwalk, Conn, 1985, Appleton Century Crofts.

Betemps E, Ragiel C: Psychiatric epidemiology: facts and myths on mental health and illness, *J Nursing* 32:23, 1994.

Brammer L: *The helping relationship: process and skills,* Boston, 1993, Allyn & Bacon.

Calabria M, Macrae J: *Suggestions for thought by Florence Nightingale,* Philadelphia, 1994, University of Pennsylvania Press.

Caplan G: *Principles of preventive psychiatry,* New York, 1964, Basic Books.

Carkhoff R: *Helping and human realities,* New York, 1969, Holt, Rinehart, & Winston.

Carkhoff R, Traux C: *Toward effective counseling and psychotherapy,* Chicago, 1967, Aldine Publishing.

Clark MJ: *Nursing in the community,* Norwalk, Conn, 1992, Appleton & Lange.

Eaton W et al: The design of the epidemiologic catchment area surveys, *Arch of Gen Psychiatry* 41:942, 1984.

Erikson E: *Childhood in society,* ed 2, New York, 1963, WW Norton.

Grob G: *From asylum to community,* Princeton, 1991, Princeton University Press.

Grob GN: Mental health policy in America, *Health Affairs* Fall:7, 1992.

Huffman K, Vernoy M, Williams B: *Psychology in action,* ed 2, New York, 1995, John Wiley & Sons.

Kaplan H, Sadock B: *Synopsis of psychiatry,* ed 6, Baltimore, 1994, Williams & Wilkins.

Kessler RC et al: Lifetime and 12 month prevalence of DSM-IV psychiatric disorders in the United States, *Arch of Gen Psychiatry* 51:8, 1994.

Klerman GL: The National Institute of Mental Health Epidemiology Catchment Area (NIMH-ECA) Program, *Soc Psychiatry Psychiatr Epidemiol* 21:159, 1986.

Klerman GL: Paradigm shifts in U.S. epidemiology since World War II, *Soc Psychiatry Psychiatr Epidemiol* 25:27, 1990.

Kraus JB: *Health care reform: essential mental health services,* Washington DC, 1993, American Nurses Publishing.

Leavell HR et al: *Preventive medicine for the doctor in his community,* ed 3, New York, 1965, McGraw-Hill.

Lego S: The one-to-one nurse-patient relationship. In Anderson CA, editor: *Psychiatric nursing 1974 to*

1994: a report on the state of the art, St. Louis, 1995, Mosby.

Maxman J, Ward N: *Essential psychopathology and its treatment*, New York, 1995, WW Norton.

Mohr W: Managed care and mental health services: how we got to where we are, *J Am Psychiatr Nurses Assoc* 4:5, 1998.

Monderscheid R, Sonnenschein M, editors: *Mental health in the United States, 1996*, Department of Health and Human Services Publication, Washington, DC, 1996, U.S. Government Printing Office.

Mullahy C: *The case manager's handbook*, Gaithersburg, Md, 1995, Aspen Publications.

North American Nursing Diagnosis Association: *Nursing diagnoses: definitions and classification*, Philadelphia, 1996, The Association.

National Alliance of Mentally Ill: Millions with serious brain disorders at risk for managed care, *NAMI Advocate* 19(2), 1997.

National Alliance of Mentally Ill: Overcoming depression in an era of managed care, *NAMI Advocate* 20(2), 1998.

O'Toole A, Loonis M: Revision of the phenomena of concern for psychiatric mental health nursing, *Arch Psychiatric Nurs* 3:5, 1989.

Peplau H: *Interpersonal relations in nursing*, New York, 1952, CP Putnam.

Redick R et al: Expansion and evolution of mental health care in the United States, *Center for Mental Health Services Publications No. 210*, 1994.

Robins L, Regier D, editors: *Psychiatric disorders in America: the epidemiological catchment area study*, New York, 1991, Free Press.

Ruben BD: The health caregiver-patient relationship: pathology, etiology, treatment. In Ray EB, Donohan L, editors: *Communication and health: systems and applications*, Hillsdale, NJ, 1990, Lawrence Earlbaum.

Thompson TL: Patient health care: issues in communication. In Ray EB, Donohan L, editors: *Communication and health: systems and applications*, Hillsdale, NJ, 1990, Lawrence Earlbaum.

Tommasini N: Private insurance coverage for treatment of mental illness, *Arch Psychiatric Nurs*, vol 1, 1994.

U.S. Department of Health and Human Services: *Healthy People 2000: national health promotion and disease prevention objectives*, Boston, 1992, Jones & Bartlet.

CHAPTER 2

Clinical Experiences: Rewards, Challenges, and Solutions

Patricia A. Holoday-Worret

OBJECTIVES

- Discuss reasons for nurses' fears of entering the psychiatric setting.

- Explain direction and intention in the psychiatric setting.

- Describe the importance of focusing on client strengths.

- Discuss the clinical priorities of nursing diagnoses and nursing interventions.

- Tell why it is important to think and observe for fluctuating symptoms rather than static behavior patterns and responses (more or less versus all or none).

- Explain the importance of avoiding evaluative responses when communicating with clients.

- Explain why it is better to simply observe client behavior than to draw inferences about it.

- Discuss reasons for stating observations versus making inferences and for presenting alternatives versus solutions.

- Discuss the importance of managing frustration with client noncompliance and nonparticipation.

Nurses select psychiatric mental health nursing as their career for several reasons. Two primary reasons are that nurses derive strong satisfaction from interpersonal interactions with their clients (individuals, groups, families, community) and that nurses believe that their clients will derive positive outcomes as a result of these interactions. Caring for clients in the psychiatric setting brings many **rewards** and **challenges**.

REWARDS

In addition to satisfaction gained from working with clients in the specialty of psychiatric mental health nursing, many other rewards are voiced when nurses are asked to share their personal experiences in a clinical setting. Some comments of nurses follow:

"There is no such thing as boredom in this field of nursing."

"To assist one person back from wanting to die, into choosing life again, makes my own life worthwhile."

"No two days are ever the same, because of the dynamic nature of the human mind and clients' behaviors."

"In all my nursing experience, I have come to think there is no greater pain than the kind that these clients endure, so I consider that helping them to meet their needs is a profound privilege."

"When I see the reaction of a client who suddenly has that "ah ha" experience (gains insight), I feel as if I were handed a gift."

"Working with a family and watching them come back together and heal after the disruption caused by a member's disorder is an enriching event for any nurse fortunate enough to observe it."

"I use such a wide scope of my nursing background (education, knowledge, and skills) in psychiatric mental health nursing. It is much more than tending only to people's minds and emotions!"

Nurses in multiple psychiatric settings expressed the last comment. When one is caring for clients in this specialty, more is necessary and required than knowledge and skill with psychiatric disorders. Clients within the psychiatric mental health system often have many other problems in addition to mental and emotional ones. These may include physical, cultural, spiritual, and social disorders and dysfunctions as well. Nurses are able to intervene in the client's behalf in all areas.

For instance, clients with mental disorders are frequently unable or unwilling to notify the nurse when they have physical problems because the disorder may include symptoms of a lack of awareness, inability to correctly interpret internal stimuli, or inability to process information, among other reasons. The nurse needs to be alert in recognizing when physical symptoms are a problem even if clients do not voice them, as in the following clinical situation:

Nancy was admitted to the psychiatric setting with a diagnosis of psychosis of an unspecified type. She was incoherent and exhibited bizarre delusions and hallucinations; among other statements, she kept repeating, "I have knives sticking into me when I go to the bathroom." Staff members were unable to decipher this comment, but Donna, the charge nurse, had a urine culture ordered. It revealed that Nancy had a very severe urinary tract infection, requiring antibiotic therapy.

In this instance, if the nurse had focused only on the client's psychiatric symptoms and narrowly interpreted the client's comment, she may have missed the opportunity to prevent the client from experiencing more serious complications. The nurse was aware that psychiatric nursing includes drawing from knowledge and using skills from each discipline in nursing.

CHALLENGES AND SOLUTIONS

The rewards of psychiatric mental health nursing are many, but it is also realistic to recognize challenges that nurses may encounter when they begin working in the psychiatric setting. Some of these challenges are

KEY TERMS

Challenge A demand to engage that may be inviting, stimulating, or difficult.

Frustration The state one experiences when plans or expectations are negated or thwarted.

Indifference Lack of interest or concern about a person or activity.

Inference A conclusion or opinion about a topic, activity, or person.

Neutrality Equal support of all sides of a matter.

Preconceive Form an idea, image, or feeling before actual contact with an object or person.

Reward Something given or received in return for service or merit.

Self-doubt Uncertainty or distrust of one's own ability, talent, or worth.

Solution An explanation, answer, or clarification.

Stereotype Form an oversimplified, standardized opinion of a person or object; often done before receiving adequate information.

Table 2-1	Suggested Solutions to Key Challenges of Working in the Psychiatric Mental Health Nursing Setting
Challenges	**Solutions**
Allay fear and anxiety by avoiding stereotyping people with mental disorders.	Learn and understand formal psychiatric diagnoses (DSM-IV). Select safe units on which to begin interactions. Become familiar with unit policies and role expectations. Interact with clients.
Address self-doubt about performance inadequacy and concern about one's own stability or mental health.	Learn the principles of psychiatric mental health nursing. Learn and use therapeutic communication techniques. Make yourself available to clients to gain experience. Practice communication skills. Review content about personal boundaries. Seek supervision or counseling. Maintain a positive cognitive set. Practice positive affirmations.
Become action oriented through direction and intention.	Prepare daily objectives that are client focused. Validate objectives with the client, the staff, and the client's treatment plan. Meet objectives by participating with intent. Involve the client in meeting objectives.
Focus on client strengths.	Identify strengths with the client. Focus on strengths. Provide positive feedback to the client regarding strengths. Encourage activities and behaviors that will increase and reinforce those strengths.
Prioritize nursing diagnoses and nursing interventions.	Attend to safety and health issues first by ensuring client safety and prevention of self-harm or harm to others.
Think in terms of more or less versus all or none.	Keep the client-expected outcomes hopeful but realistic. Avoid predicting client progress. Be prepared for and accept an unpredictable course toward wellness. Avoid absolute "black and white" thinking.
Avoid evaluative statements and responses when communicating with clients.	Focus on behaviors, not on the person. Be neutral but not indifferent. Avoid evaluative statements. Use statements of recognition.
Make observations instead of inferences.	Respond through observation instead of inference. Validate interpretations with the client to reach mutual conclusions. Explore difficult conclusions with the client.
Offer alternatives rather than solutions.	Help the client express concerns and problems. Allow expression of feelings. Help the client problem solve toward solutions. Avoid giving advice. Offer multiple alternatives or options only when the client is unable to do so. Facilitate choices.
Avoid frustration with clients.	Include the client in the plan of care. Teach and monitor skills that support growth. Work collaboratively with the client.

included here for the purpose of helping nurses to increase their awareness of the challenges that may arise when they start to interact with clients who have mental disorders. This content will also help nurses to prepare to meet these challenges with either **solutions** presented here or with solutions that the nurse may have in mind. Neither the challenges nor the solutions are intended to be conclusive; rather, they may provide the basis for thoughtful discussion with peers and/or instructors about events that occur in the clinical setting and the nurse's responses to them.

In any event, actual challenges will undoubtedly prove to be thought provoking and stimulating, will provide growth, and in most instances will be interesting. The diligence required by the nurse to meet challenges will also be accompanied by many rewards. Key challenges and some solutions are presented in Table 2-1.

CHALLENGE: FEAR OF ENTERING THE PSYCHIATRIC SETTING

New experiences usually include some measure of anxiety that is actually a healthy response, alerting the individual to prepare for new information and change. Very often, however, when nurses first enter a psychiatric setting, the expectation for rewards may be overshadowed by fear. Many sources may be attributed to the generation of fear concerning this arena, but two salient reasons are **preconceived** stereotypes and **self-doubt** about performance or one's own stability.

PRECONCEIVED STEREOTYPES

To **stereotype** is to form an oversimplified, standardized opinion of a person or group of people, and this is often done without adequate information. Unfortunately, the general public often stereotypes people with mental disorders as "insane," "out of control," and "dangerous." Films and books reinforce this unrealistic image and add to the fear. The beginning nurse, without experience, prepares to feel unsafe in these imagined circumstances.

Solutions to this challenge include:
Learn and understand the formal psychiatric diagnoses (DSM-IV).
Select safe units on which to begin interactions.
Become familiar with unit policies and role expectations (agency and nursing program).
Interact with clients.

An understanding of mental disorders, coupled with an opportunity to interact with individuals who have the disorders, will quickly dispel stereotypes. Only a small percentage of people with mental disorders are dangerous toward others, and they will usually not be placed directly with other clients on units that are managed effectively.

The nurse will soon begin to see clients as humans with problems who are to be helped, not feared.

Unit safety, a paramount issue, is the responsibility of the facility and staff. The nurse has a personal obligation to be thoroughly oriented to each unit and familiar with policies, procedures, and role expectations. Nurses with little experience will not be assigned to units where clients are potentially dangerous, unless the units are monitored by teaching staff who assume responsibility for safety. Well-operated units are usually safe.

Of course, the nurse does not provoke a situation that results in disruption. If disruption does occur, the beginning nurse should get experienced assistance immediately and assist in ushering uninvolved clients away from the area, both for the clients' protection and to prevent escalation of anxiety.

SELF-DOUBT

Self-doubt comes from several sources. In conjunction with the nurse's role in the psychiatric setting, two main sources of self-doubt are beliefs about performance inadequacy and concern about one's own stability or mental health.

Beliefs About Performance Inadequacy

Fear of performance inadequacy is a fear experienced by novice nurses who tend to believe that they will not know what to say or do to help clients with their problems. "I don't know what to say to them" is a frequent remark when nurses have had little exposure to or experience with clients in this setting. They hear interactions between clients and more experienced staff members, who frequently seem to find the perfect words for the clients. But they must remember that this seemingly simple process of communication is both an art and a science. The science or skills can be learned, and most communicators become artful with practice!

Solutions to this challenge include:
Learn principles of psychiatric mental health nursing.
Learn and use therapeutic communication techniques.
Make yourself available to clients to gain experience.
Practice communication skills.

Nurses just starting in psychiatry have the responsibility of learning correct therapeutic communication techniques and practicing them in order to become skillful communicators. Chapter 8 further discusses some techniques.

Nurses need to be realistic about their performance expectations. They are not expected to be seasoned therapists during early encounters with clients. With opportunity, time, and attention toward becoming skillful, they will ultimately succeed. Response selection, correctness, and timing will continue to improve. As a result, both nurses and clients will benefit.

Precise words are not nearly as important as the capacity to convey a sense of caring to the client. Mistakes in communication inevitably will occur. However, these will be overlooked and forgiven if the client senses that the nurse has genuine empathy and a willingness to assist the client on his or her journey to wellness.

Concern About One's Own Mental Health

Some psychiatric mental health nurses fear that their own stability or mental health is inadequate for this type of nursing or is compromised by being in the setting. The nurse who has difficulty maintaining personal boundaries may not feel emotionally strong enough to tolerate the depth of human problems in a psychiatric facility. This can be especially true if the nurse has had serious mental or emotional dysfunction in the past or is currently experiencing overwhelming personal life stressors.

Newcomers sometimes say, "I worry that this could happen to me" or "My problems seem greater than some of theirs—why are they in the hospital and I'm not?" Undoubtedly, the reader has also heard of what is commonly called the "medical or nursing student's syndrome," meaning that the student believes he or she experiences symptoms of every disorder studied! Nurses sometimes fail to give themselves credit for their capacity to function in times of psychosocial stressors.

<u>Solutions</u> to this challenge include:
Review content about personal boundaries.
Seek supervision or counseling.
Maintain a positive cognitive set.
Practice positive affirmations.

Maintaining personal boundaries is essential in a therapeutic relationship. The nurse can then be empathic about the client's situation without becoming so personally involved that he or she loses objectivity and effectiveness. This topic is also covered more thoroughly in Chapters 1 and 8. The nurse with healthy boundaries and a healthy ego is prepared to maintain personal mental health.

It is important to discuss concerns about one's own mental health. Relief may come when the topic is addressed during a student or staff conference and the nurse learns that worry is not unique and that solutions are available. Deep concern requires conferring with an instructor or counselor who will objectively assess the problem and advise the nurse whether further counseling will be helpful.

Self-defeating thoughts can become self-fulfilling prophecies if repeated often enough. When the nurse continually focuses on worry, fear, or inadequacy, then successful role performance becomes difficult or impossible. Thinking positive thoughts constitutes possessing a positive cognitive set. This is a positive outlook toward the world and others, and the belief that success is possible and that one can achieve what one believes (but one should be realistic about goals).

In conjunction with conscious efforts to maintain a positive cognitive set, the nurse can practice positive affirmations, which are self-confirming and self-supporting messages that reinforce confidence and enhance performance. They can be self-fulfilling prophecies toward success. Examples of positive affirmations are the following:

"I am able to study, learn, and practice this new and challenging content."
"Every day, I become more proficient in nurse-client interactions."
"I am as good at interviewing clients as I am supposed to be at this time."
"I use therapeutic communication techniques."
"I am relaxed and more capable each day."
"Instructors and staff are here to assist me."
"The client heals self, and I facilitate that progress within my capacity; that capacity grows each day."

Once again—and it cannot be said too often—fears will decrease and confidence will increase with greater knowledge, time, experience, and the resulting successful interpersonal interactions.

CHALLENGE: DIRECTION AND INTENTION

Entering any unfamiliar environment that requires performance is a challenge. The nurse who enters the psychiatric setting is there primarily to help clients achieve the following:

Increase awareness of personal and relational issues that impair mental health and impede growth.
Discuss difficult issues during therapeutic interactions.
Engage in the problem-solving process.
Share thoughts and feelings.
Identify positive aspects of self and life.
Accept self and others.
Learn new skills for building competence and improving relationships.

To assist the client in these areas, the nurse must first have a plan in mind (direction) and be ready to engage, based on sound principles (intention). When nurses fail to become active participants in the nurse-client relationship, both the client and the nurse fall short of meeting potential objectives, goals, and needs. Being action oriented means moving beyond observing and assessing to becoming an actual facilitator. This does not imply that the nurse takes charge and does things to or for the client. It does imply, however, that the client and the nurse work together to formulate a personal plan of care and then collaboratively implement the plan.

Objectives and goals are met only when there is a purposeful plan that provides direction and the plan is put into action by intention. Sometimes nurses write exquisite client-focused objectives but fail to refer to or follow the plan in order to meet the objectives. Unless the plan is kept in mind, they revert to merely assessing, observing, and recording, rather than interacting with a purpose.

Solutions to this challenge include:
Prepare daily objectives that are client focused.
Validate objectives with the client, the staff, and the client's treatment plan.
Meet objectives by participating with intent.
Involve the client in meeting objectives.

CHALLENGE: FOCUS ON CLIENT STRENGTHS

Some psychiatric mental health nurses who are just beginning a nursing rotation or career have a tendency to focus mainly on the client's disorders instead of on their healthy aspects and strengths. Psychiatric disorders often seem dramatic and fascinating, so it is easy to understand why the nurse's attention is directed toward dysfunction instead of health. In addition, there is a great deal to learn about psychiatric disorders, so energy gets channeled into learning and applying information about disorders and dysfunction versus strengths.

Solutions to this challenge include:
Identify strengths *with* the client.
Focus on strengths.
Provide positive feedback to the client regarding strengths.
Encourage activities and behaviors that will increase and reinforce those strengths.

The nurse's contact time with a client will be spent helping him or her overcome problems that stem from the disorders. But, more important, the nurse will also help the client build strengths, increase competence, and accentuate and reinforce reasons for living (Figure 2-1). With the treatment plan in mind, the nurse provides activities and encourages participation that will foster mental and emotional health and growth.

For several reasons, it may not be possible for some clients to identify their strengths directly after admission to the facility. For example, a psychotic state, severe depression, substance intoxication, or low self-esteem could all interfere with this process. However, as soon as these symptoms diminish, the nurse again focuses on the client's strengths. Some techniques for accomplishing focus on strengths include:

Ask the client's opinion about personal strengths and attributes.
Ask the client his or her reasons for getting well.

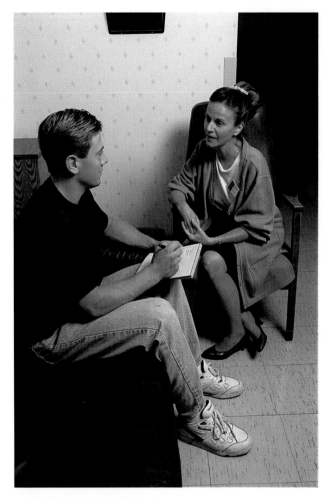

Figure 2-1 An interaction between a psychiatric nurse and an adolescent client. The nurse and the adolescent are discussing his strengths while he makes a list to keep for personal reference and reflection. (Copyright Cathy Lander-Goldberg, Lander Photographics.)

Allow time for the client to process thoughts—they may not come easily.
Suggest that the client write a list of his or her strengths if he or she is unable to verbalize them.
If the client is unable to think of strengths, ask what a spouse, child, friend, member of the clergy, or significant other would say about the client.
Have staff members share observations about the client's strengths.

Staff members can also chart clients' strengths along with other progress to inform members of the mental health team of important areas for focus. This ensures continuity of care and additional potential for reinforcement.

NOTE: Clients who are grandiose, or have an exaggerated view of themselves, will probably have little difficulty telling about their real and imagined strengths and attributes. The nurse will be prepared to accept the client's behavior within appropriate limits and use therapeutic techniques to help him or her to stay in touch with reality.

CHALLENGE: ESTABLISHING CLINICAL PRIORITIES

Prioritization of both nursing diagnoses and nursing interventions is essential to meet the client's needs in a timely manner. Prioritization means that the nurse follows several steps:

Obtain all necessary data.
Organize and sort information.
Attend to client problems and needs in order of significance:
1. Safety/health
2. Intrapersonal issues
3. Interpersonal issues

NURSING DIAGNOSIS PRIORITY

When a client is admitted for psychiatric problems, the admission information may clearly state which problems are more urgent than others. However, often the admitting information is incomplete and the nurse must interview the client and significant others to determine prioritization of nursing diagnoses.

A major principle of psychiatric nursing is that safety and health issues are addressed first, as in the following clinical situation:

A 23-year-old female client was admitted to the unit following a suicide attempt. She had been severely depressed for several weeks, was currently abusing multiple substances, and had been treated at age 16 for anorexia nervosa. She lost 15 pounds during the month before admission.

Each problem is of major importance, but the primary concern and first priority are to sustain and maintain the client's life. The following clinical situation concerns a holistic priority:

A 63-year-old male client was admitted to the acute care psychiatric facility by the police, who were called because the client was shouting loudly and incoherently in his apartment and had barricaded his door. He had been grieving his wife's recent death, so the landlord became concerned about his behavior and sought help from the police. On admission, the experienced nurse assessed the client during an interview. Amidst his incoherence, he stated that his "wife gave him his insulin because she loved him." The nurse asked the laboratory to do his blood work, STAT. The client's psychiatric symptoms were actually from an insulin reaction, and the nurse's awareness kept him from becoming more disordered.

In this instance the experienced psychiatric nurse was aware that medical problems can often affect a client's responses and behaviors. A common problem that can exist in psychiatric settings is the tendency to concentrate solely on psychiatric and communication problems and issues and ignore or forget medical and other aspects that include physical, cultural, spiritual, and psychosocial components. Nursing is a holistic practice and requires assessment of all aspects of the client, regardless of the type of unit to which the client is admitted.

Solutions to such challenges include:
List all client problems and needs, after thorough assessment.
Convert client problems to nursing diagnoses.
Prioritize nursing diagnoses.
Practice prioritization of both the diagnosis and the interventions.

Following an intake history, the nurse must determine an order of importance for every problem identified during assessment. In the psychiatric setting it is easy to miss medical and other problems because psychiatric and communication problems and needs are often so outstanding. A helpful exercise when beginning psychiatric nursing is to develop hypothetical clinical situations containing multiple client problems and to practice prioritizing.

NURSING INTERVENTION PRIORITY

Prioritizing interventions within each nursing diagnosis is also necessary. For instance, consider a care plan that includes the priority nursing diagnosis of violence, risk for: self-directed. The nurse is aware that a necessary nursing intervention is to establish a relationship in which the client can express thoughts and feelings about suicide and reasons for living. However, this intervention, even though important and at the heart of psychiatric nursing, is secondary to ensuring client safety and prevention of self-harm.

Solutions to such challenges include:
Consider the client's unique manifestations of the nursing diagnosis.
Prioritize nursing interventions under each nursing diagnosis.

CHALLENGE: MORE OR LESS VERSUS ALL OR NONE

Unlike most physical sciences that are predictable and exact, psychiatry can sometimes seem elusive to the beginning nurse. The definition, description, and categorization of psychiatric diagnoses in the *Diagnostic and Statistical Manual of Mental Disorders,* fourth edition (DSM-IV), appear exact. However, because of the complex nature of human beings, symptoms of the same name are manifested and expressed in unique ways by each client.

The nurse may initially think in absolutes, seeing symptoms as being totally present or totally absent (i.e., *all or none*). In reality, the client's symptoms may change slightly or dramatically over hours or days (i.e., *more or less*). Because psychiatric symptoms cannot always be measured by laboratory values, charts, and graphs, they are sometimes overlooked or missed completely by beginning nurses. Subtle changes may be clues that more dramatic changes are coming, so increases or decreases in symptoms need to be carefully noted, as in the following clinical situation:

Charlotte was admitted to the psychiatric acute care unit because she was jogging down the center of a busy two-way traffic boulevard and taunting motorists. She was wearing multiple layers of brightly colored clothes, high heels, and excessive jewelry. On admission she shouted out about the indignity of having to be in this facility against her will, which she termed a violation of her "personal, important rights." She was diagnosed with bipolar disorder, manic type.

After several days of quiet surroundings, consistent unit routines, staff interventions, and medication (which she had stopped taking before admission), she calmed. Staff reports and charting stated that she seemed ready to return home.

Just before discharge, however, her contact staff person noted that she began to change her clothes every few hours and that the content of her conversation centered on "very important" things she was planning to accomplish when she got home. The staff member asked her if she had been taking her medication. Charlotte admitted she had been putting it in the toilet because she was getting too "normal" to get her plans accomplished. Discharge was postponed.

<u>Solutions</u> to this challenge include:
Keep clients' expected outcomes hopeful but realistic.
Avoid predicting client progress.
Be prepared for and accept an unpredictable course toward wellness.
Avoid absolute "black and white" thinking.

Symptoms are dynamic and are more like shades of gray than black and white. So the nurse should observe for fluctuation of symptoms rather than static, set patterns of behaviors and responses.

A client who is paranoid, for instance, may demonstrate mistrust by being loud and accusatory on admission. He may then quiet down but remain guarded, suspicious, and controlled on subsequent days. The symptom of paranoia is the same, but the manifestations change, depending on the client's internal stimuli, the unit environment, the present situation or events, and the client's personality style.

Another point is to write care plans reflecting realistic appraisal of the client's symptoms, as seen in the following partial nursing care plan. Note that the correct realistic expectations indicate symptom reduction (more or less) rather than total absence (all or none).

Nursing Diagnosis: Thought processes, altered, related to impaired ability to process internal and external stimuli and related to stressful current family and work situation; manifested by guarded and suspicious behavior and statements that other clients are stealing his clothes and that staff want to harm him.

Expected Outcomes:

Correct	*Incorrect*
Client will demonstrate decreased delusions of persecution within 1 week.	Paranoid delusions will be absent in 1 week.

In some cases it is unrealistic to expect complete absence of symptoms. Interdisciplinary treatment plans aim at symptom reduction within reasonable time limits, with concurrent expectations that clients will achieve these objectives with assistance. Symptom "cure" is an unreasonable expectation for some clients.

CHALLENGE: EVALUATIVE RESPONSES

A general principle in psychiatric nursing states that when communicating with clients the nurse will avoid using evaluative statements and responses that indicate approval or disapproval (e.g., "good or bad," "right or wrong") about the client's appearance, progress, or behavior. A more effective response from the nurse is neutral recognition. Consider the following clinical situation:

Mrs. H., a 72-year-old woman, was hospitalized following the death of her spouse of 53 years. Although she had been suffering from major depression and chronic low self-esteem for several decades, he had remained loyal and loving. After admission, Mrs. H. wore dark, drab clothing every day and cared for her hygiene only after constant encouragement from staff. After several days, she showered and came to breakfast wearing a pink printed dress. Jane, a nurse with little experience, was assigned to the unit. She said, "Oh, Mrs. H., you look so pretty in that pink dress. It's so much better than all those dark clothes you've been wearing." Mrs. H. lowered her head and returned to her room. She refused breakfast, lunch, and activities, saying she didn't feel well. She came to dinner in her dark, drab clothing.

Withdrawn or depressed people reject praise because it is the opposite of their own present negative self-image. Praise conflicts with the client's mind-set of "I'm ugly," "I'm worthless," "I deserve nothing." The client either fails to hear the praise, or the praise is discredited. Disapproval only serves to reinforce pathology, so it, too, needs to be avoided.

On the other hand, nurses sometimes learn to avoid direct approval or disapproval but mistakenly substitute indifference. Neutrality and indifference are not the same. **Indifference** manifests as disconnected, unconcerned, aloof separation from the client's needs and situation; it is the antithesis of psychiatric nursing. Nurses can still provide a necessary warm human experience and environment by maintaining **neutrality**—interaction with the client that shows respect and acceptance but not excessive approval or disapproval. Showing indifference toward a client who is mentally or emotionally compromised is like having the person take an ice cold shower in the dead of winter. It is certain to snuff out any spark of remaining spirit or hope.

<u>Solutions</u> to showing appropriate evaluative responses include:
Focus on behaviors, not on the person.
Be neutral but not indifferent.
Avoid evaluative statements.
Use statements of recognition.

Of course, limits may need to be appropriately set on self-defeating behaviors. When doing the latter, the nurse will comment on behaviors while avoiding statements about the person's worth. Compare the nurse's comments to the client in the following two examples:

> *Correct:* "During group yesterday, it was agreed that each client would be ready to go on the field trip by 8 AM. Because you are refusing to dress, the trip is behind schedule. The bus will leave in 15 minutes." *(Comment on behavior)*
> *Incorrect:* "You are so slow and undependable. Everyone is on the bus and thinks you're terrible for holding up the field trip." *(Comment on the person's worth)*

Neutral statements recognize the person's behavior. Recall Mrs. H. and the pink dress. Appropriate neutral statements to her would be, "I see you showered before breakfast, Mrs. H." and "You're wearing a pink printed dress today." These statements, which imply neither approval nor disapproval, offer recognition and may elicit responses from the client that promote further insight into her problems. Evaluative statements, on the other hand, close communication and the client either withdraws from the interaction or becomes defensive.

The following are two other examples of neutral statements:

> "You decided to join the group today, Tom. Seats are not assigned, so sit anywhere you wish."
> "I notice you received all your points yesterday for attending school and the scheduled activities, Amber."

Evaluative statements are discouraged for other reasons as well. If staff praises the client too soon, he or she may fear support will be withdrawn. Even though he or she is rehearsing new behaviors, the client may still feel vulnerable and revert to old behaviors to regain imagined loss of support. Or, a client may believe he or she is acceptable only if he or she looks or behaves in the specified evaluative way. If the client cannot comply with the evaluation, he or she may feel even more unworthy.

Some psychiatric nurses may disagree with this practice and freely offer praise for positive behavior. This practice has merit when it is clear that the client is ready to receive praise. Each case is unique, but the nurse has a responsibility to understand the client and the situation before choosing responses.

CHALLENGE: INFERENCES VERSUS OBSERVATIONS

It is sometimes difficult for the nurse who is new to the psychiatric setting to avoid inferences about a client's behavior. An **inference** is an interpretation of behavior that is made by finding motive and forming conclusions without having all of the information. When inferences are made, the nurse interprets the client's behavior, decides on a reason, assigns a motive, and forms a conclusion. There is great potential for error and unfairness in this process.

Some dangers in drawing inferences are that the nurse is operating from his or her own experience and frame of reference that may have little or no connection to the client's actual behavior. In addition, when the nurse makes an inference and forms a conclusion, the client is robbed of the opportunity to problem solve and share thoughts and ideas about important issues. A false conclusion may also misdirect treatment objectives.

Interpreting client behaviors and making inferences is not always negative, and seasoned nurses do it frequently. The difference is that experienced nurses take additional steps before final conclusions are reached.

<u>Solutions</u> to this challenge include:
Respond through observation instead of inference.
Validate interpretations with the client to reach mutual conclusions.
Explore conclusions with the client.

To avoid making inferences, the nurse operates from an understanding of the importance of obtaining a client's viewpoint about situations and events that affect his or her own life instead of forming a personal opinion. Also, the nurse draws conclusions by responding to client behaviors without interpreting them. This means that the nurse simply observes behaviors. For example:

> "I saw your wife leave, Jim, and now you're crying."
> "Yesterday you sat alone, Tommy, but today the other children joined you."

"Marsha, what you just said got a major reaction from the group."

Notice that the nurse does not offer any conclusions to these obviously significant situations. It may be difficult for the nurse to relinquish giving his or her concluding opinion, but it is a necessary, rewarding tactic.

The client will usually respond to the nurse's statement, and then communication, reasoning, and problem solving can begin. The more experienced nurse will continue beyond observation to interpretation. The critical difference is that the nurse immediately validates the interpretation with the client, and a mutual conclusion is formed or at least brought to awareness for future discussion. Here is an example of the entire four-step process.

1. "I saw your wife leave, Jim, and now you're crying." *(Observation)*
2. "You said earlier that she was coming in today to discuss a divorce." *(Interpretation)*
3. "Is that the reason you're feeling sad now?" *(Validation)*
4. "This might be a good time for us to discuss your relationship." *(Offer to explore the issue)*

Notice that the nurse is not guessing but rather is reasoning based on past information. Also, the client now has an opportunity to validate. The last important step is the nurse's willingness to be available to the client for processing this event through therapeutic communication.

CHALLENGE: ALTERNATIVES VERSUS SOLUTIONS

Nurses may feel inadequate before beginning to work in the psychiatric setting because they worry that they do not have answers for the clients' problems. Clients, not nurses, however, are responsible for their choices.

Solutions to this challenge include:
Help the client express concerns and problems.
Allow expression of feelings.
Help the client problem solve toward solutions.
Avoid giving advice.
Offer multiple alternatives or options only when the client is unable to do so.
Facilitate choices.

The nurse engages in therapeutic communication with the client, facilitating expression of thoughts and feelings. When the client is able to hear his or her own words, the problem-solving process has begun and the client starts to reach his or her own solutions.

It is important for the nurse to avoid giving advice. The client probably does not want the nurse's opinion as much as he or she wants the nurse to stay engaged while the client talks; there is a relief in expressing problems openly to a willing listener. If the client asks, "What would you do?" or "What do you think I should do?" the nurse can reply, "I think it is more important for you to decide what works best for you. Let's talk about your ideas."

Another reason to avoid offering advice and solutions is that doing so negates the client. He or she feels less worthwhile and maybe even infantilized, as if a parent were dictating how the client should conduct his or her life. Also, the nurse's solutions may not fit the client's lifestyle or self-image.

If the client for any reason (depression, cognitive impairment or deficit, state of crisis) is unable to come up with answers, the nurse can then offer alternatives or options. This means offering assistance and giving some prompting without providing answers or advising. For example:

"Some things that have worked for other people in similar situations are . . . [name several options]. Do any of these seem reasonable for you?"
"Have you considered . . . [give several choices]?"
"What are some of the options you have for placement when you're discharged? Some that come to mind are . . . [give several realistic and appropriate choices]."

The nurse may need to be more definitive in helping the client when the client sees no solutions. For example: "You said you are a workaholic and can't relax since you got your own business. What leisure activities have you enjoyed in the past? Which of those would you enjoy now if you had the time? What did you like most about [golfing, fishing]? Who do you trust to run the business while you take vacations? Since the business is open Monday through Friday, when could you find time to [golf, fish]?"

Most clients know the solutions they need and only require assistance to bring these solutions to their awareness.

CHALLENGE: FRUSTRATION WITH CLIENTS

To frustrate means to nullify, defeat, make worthless, or negate plans or directions of another person. **Frustration** is a difficult state to experience, tolerate, or, sometimes, let go. It arises when efforts or plans fail to materialize according to expectations. Frustration may prevail in health care, especially when the caregiver is new at his or her field, and nurses in the psychiatric setting are no exception in this matter.

Prepared with carefully studied and learned theory, and ready to apply the theory through utilization of skills based on principles, the nurse enters the arena of psychiatric mental health to care for clients with mental disorders who are probably also undergoing life crises as a result. Plans are carefully made to interact with the client and intervene in current problems and needs fulfillment. Assessment is made of the client and the events and situations surrounding the client. Problems and needs are identified, and a plan directed at solutions is formulated, with the intent of carrying out the plan and evaluating the progress.

The nurse may use one or more of the planned interventions with success. It is not uncommon, however, in this setting for clients to not cooperate with the best-made plans. Frustration can occur when the client has different plans or refuses to engage in the nurse's plan because of one or more reasons. In addition to frustration, the nurse may experience loss of confidence, embarrassment, rejection, anger, and/or thoughts of failure. These can be exaggerated responses toward the noncompliant client and with time should be modified or eliminated, because they are usually unproductive.

Solutions: When frustration occurs in an exaggerated way, the nurse must step back, put the situation into realistic perspective, and review some basic principles of psychiatric mental health nursing. This may involve validating and discussing the situation with appropriate staff, the instructor, and peers.

The nurse may have lost contact with the fact that client plans and interventions must be:
Client focused versus nurse focused and require client input.
Goal directed (client's goals versus nurse's goals). If the nurse ignores the client's needs or objectives when making the plan, the goals will usually fail to materialize.
Objective versus subjective in approach. The nurse must keep appropriate perspective and boundaries regarding the client and the problems.

A reaction to frustration for some beginning nurses is to abandon the plan, and in extreme cases, abandon the client. When the nurse has insight into the need of all individuals to have some control over their lives (even though limited in many cases because of symptoms), the nurse will begin to come closer to working *with* the client, rather than *on* the client. When clients believe they have had sufficient input into their plan of care, cooperation usually increases relative to the client's capacity to engage. The nurse needs to collaborate with the client on a mutually formulated plan of care.

Some specific client-focused objectives for the nurse to follow are:

Maintain awareness of the client's capability and capacity to engage in his or her own care.
Include the client in the plan of care.
Assist the client toward understanding positive aspects of self-help.
Encourage the client to engage in behaviors directed toward eliminating problems and maintaining health and well-being.
Teach client skills that will assist in making change possible.
Praise attempts to improve.
Continually evaluate progress and reassess changes.

The nurse will benefit from incorporating personal goals toward meeting the client's needs. These include:

Remain acceptant of the client's need to maintain some control over his or her own life.
Refrain from the need to complete your own agenda.
Refrain from abandoning the client if frustration arises (look for alternatives).
Remain objectively involved with problems.
Lighten up. Use appropriate humor and relaxation techniques when needed to diffuse tension.
Review principles frequently.
Get supervision (staff, instructor) to validate your own and the client's progress.

Summary of Key Concepts

1. Students may fear entering the psychiatric setting because of predetermined stereotypes of danger and self-doubt.
2. Students can remain realistic about their performance expectations.
3. Nurses need stable mental health themselves before they attempt to stabilize clients.
4. An action-oriented nurse will meet the client's treatment goals.
5. Focusing on client strengths fosters emotional and mental health and growth.
6. The priority intervention is to ensure client safety and prevent harm.
7. Comments to clients should focus on behavior, rather than personal worth.
8. Relating observations rather than inferences leaves the conclusions to the client.
9. Offering alternative problem-solving techniques gives control to the client and builds self-esteem, while providing the solution suggests that the client is incapable of handling the situation.

REFERENCES

Fortinash K, Holoday-Worret P: *Psychiatric nursing care plans*, ed 2, St. Louis, 1995, Mosby.

Holoday-Worret P: Accumulated clinical anecdotal notes (unpublished).

Peplau H: *Interpersonal relations in nursing*, New York, 1982, Putnam.

Theoretic Perspectives

Mary Magenheimer Webster

OBJECTIVES

- Discuss the basic concepts and application of each theory presented.

- Compare and contrast the various theoretic approaches to treatment.

- Describe the core concepts of rational emotive therapy (RET) and Alderian therapy and compare with Beck's newer cognitive therapy.

- Evaluate the appropriateness of the various therapies to specific client needs and symptoms.

- Apply the various theories to actual clinical practice situations.

- Develop a nursing care plan using one or more of the theories presented.

Alter ego A function of the therapist to reflect back the client's attitudes and feelings without including the client's negative connotations.

Cognitive triad Pattern of thinking noted in people with depression and characterized by (1) a negative self-assessment, (2) a negative view of the present, and (3) a negative view of the future.

Ego The organizing part of the personality that is in contact with reality and acts as a mediator between the id and reality to find an acceptable satisfaction of needs.

Ego state A coherent set of feelings developed by the child's organization of similar life experiences and accompanied by a related set of coherent and observable behavior patterns. There are three ego states defined in transactional analysis: parent, adult, and child.

Faulty information processing Fixed and rigid patterns of thinking that block the contextual aspects of a situation and are characteristic of people with depression.

Figure-background formation The concept that an organism's foremost need or specific interest will define the reality of the moment; component of Gestalt theory.

Final goal The unconscious goal of an ideal situation or perfection, which motivates an individual in present actions and influences the approach toward life, according to Adlerian theory.

Id The part of the personality that holds the instincts, primitive impulses, and all that is inherited, present at birth, and fixed in a person's psychic constitution.

Inferiority feelings Normal feelings that arise when individuals become aware of their imperfections, which motivate them to strive for mastery and competence, according to Adlerian theory.

Interactive context of behaviors The concept that behavior is shaped and reinforced by interaction with one's social system while the social system is being shaped and reinforced by the same interaction.

Libido The energy of the instincts held in the id.

Organismic self-regulation The concept that once the need is satisfied it will recede and allow the emergence of the next need.

Pleasure principle The goal of experiencing pleasure while avoiding pain. This principle represents the id's goal in the personality to satisfy a person's innate needs and instincts.

Reality principle The goal of postponing immediate gratification until a suitable object for this satisfaction is found. The ego is ruled by this principle.

Reframing A technique of changing the viewpoint of a situation and replacing it with another viewpoint that fits the facts equally well but changes the entire meaning.

Superego The part of the personality holding the internalization of the demands, prohibitions, and ideals of significant others (notably the parents). It is organized into two subsystems: the *conscience* (representing the demanding or forbidding aspects of the parents) and the *ego ideal* (representing the values thought to be morally good by the parents).

Unconditional positive regard The stance of the therapist modeling the unconditional acceptance of the client; based on the belief that the client is competent to direct himself or herself in a natural tendency to move forward toward integration.

The various theories of human behavior each have the common goal of producing frameworks that promote the understanding of the complexities of human behavior. They represent the theorists' attempts to organize and interpret data derived from human interactions and behaviors into a cohesive format from which one is better able to predict and interpret meanings and thus base effective interventions.

Theories are useful because they provide an organized way to view human behavior and, in so doing, suggest strategies to modify or change behavior. For example, if one views a disturbed behavior as resulting from intrapsychic conflicts, as in psychoanalytic theory, then it would follow that treatment would involve some type of exposure to the conflict, with the purpose of resolving that conflict. However, if one viewed the same behavior as stemming from an irrational thought or belief, as in the cognitive theories, then it would make sense that effective treatment would necessitate changing or altering the faulty belief system. The theory bases provide the framework for cohesive work and consistent treatment.

The difficulty, of course, lies in the multiple ways to view, organize, and interpret human behavior. The variety of theoretic perspectives represents the creativity and worldviews of their founders and reflects the cultural and social influences of their time. There is no dominant theory of human behavior, although all human behavior can be described by each theory. Either practitioners choose a theory that corresponds to their personal world-view and proceed to practice within that theory base, or they familiarize themselves with several theories and move fluidly within them, depending on the needs of their clients. Many therapists use an eclectic (varied) approach to treatment.

Therefore the beginning practitioner is wise to review the various theories and their unique applications. The beginner, as well as the seasoned practitioner, needs to consider the perspective of the theory, as well as its applicability in various practice settings.

The following are presented as an overview of various approaches and as an aid to the student in organizing and interpreting interactions and behaviors.

PSYCHOANALYTIC THEORY

Sigmund Freud (1856-1939) developed the first organized theory of personality (Figure 3-1). Before Freud, much of the thinking about personality development was based on vague philosophic approaches. Freud based his theory on clinical observations of the clients in his private practice and on his own subjective interpretations. Because of this subjective approach, the validity of his theory has been challenged. Nevertheless, Freud's theory of personality has formed the basis for psychoanalysis, which has been expanded and revised by subsequent theorists. Psychoanalytic theory has arguably been more popular in the United States than in other parts of the world.

THEORETIC OVERVIEW

Freud organized his theory of personality around three major themes: levels of consciousness, sexuality, and functions of the personality. Freud saw individuals as being driven by instinctual impulses and believed that the personality is organized to control these impulses to the individual's best advantage. At times, this control involves repression of certain impulses, thoughts, or experiences. Freud proposed that these repressed impulses continue to affect an individual's behavior throughout his or her lifetime, for good or ill, without the individual's awareness.

BASIC CONCEPTS
Levels of Consciousness

Freud's basic assumption was that all behavior is meaningful. The "little daily mistakes" of forgetting something, misplacing something, or misspeaking spring from a purposive desire that may or may not be known to the indi-

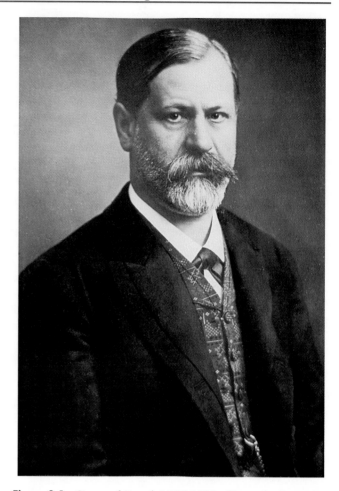

Figure 3-1   Sigmund Freud, 1856-1939. (From the Bettmann Archive.)

vidual (Freud, 1979). If it is unknown, it is said to spring from the unconscious. Freud proposed that people know only a small part of their inner life and nothing of many feelings and thoughts that occur outside their awareness (Freud, 1979).

Freud theorized that the unconscious is developed during the early years of life in the following way: a child is born into the world with a variety of physical needs such as hunger, thirst, and physical comfort. When these needs are met, the child experiences pleasure. The child's central purpose in life is the attainment of pleasure (Freud, 1979), and the child thoroughly enjoys all of the opportunities for attaining this pleasure, such as thumb sucking, elimination, and/or masturbation. However, around the age of 1 year, the child realizes that the mother, the primary caregiver and satisfier of needs, does not belong only to the child but is shared with other siblings and the father. A jealousy of the others follows, and at about the same time, more demands are placed on the child by these people. The child is asked to give up these pleasures and begin the process of becoming "civilized" via activities such as toilet training and ending thumb sucking.* The child eventually gives up these pleasures as a result of adult interventions that may be perceived as threats of disapproval, withdrawal, or the possibility of physical harm. Initially the child only pretends to take on the parental attitude, but gradually the child accepts the adult values as truth. For this acceptance to happen, the child must undergo a reversal of feelings associated with the previous physical pleasures. In doing this, the memory rejects the pleasurable experiences and also the whole period of life associated with those memories. That period of life is seen as "unworthy" and "repulsive" compared with the adult standard (Freud, 1979). This part of life is relegated to the unconscious, the level of consciousness that holds the "forgotten" or repressed thoughts, feelings, and memories. Freud theorized that this occurs in the first 5 years of life and would explain the absence of memories most people have about their very early childhood. This "forgotten" part of the self remains active, however, and shapes relationships and interactions.

Functions of the Personality and Levels of Consciousness

As the child continues to grow, other processes occur in the organization of the personality. Freud saw the personality as consisting of three parts or systems: the id, the ego, and the superego. Each part has its own function within the personality.

Id.   The **id** is the part of the personality that holds what is inherited, present at birth, and fixed in a person's psychic constitution. The id contains the *instincts*, the primitive forces existing behind the tensions of the id that make somatic (bodily) demands (e.g., hunger, touch, thirst, sexuality). There are multiple instincts. Freud saw these instincts as the "ultimate causes of all activity" (Freud, 1960). Freud identified two main and oppositional categories of instincts: the life instinct and the death instinct. The aim of the life instinct is to bind things together into greater and greater unities that it strives to preserve. The death instinct tends to undo connections and destroy things, with the ultimate goal of reducing living things to an inorganic state (Freud, 1960). Such is the nature of the id that conflicting instincts can exist together and exert influence on an individual's behavior. The id is characterized by a subjectivity toward experience and a lack of logic, time, or morality. The id's goal in the personality is to satisfy a person's innate needs and instincts. The goal of experiencing pleasure while avoiding pain is called the **pleasure principle.** When acting under the pleasure principle, a person will seek immediate gratification of needs.

Libido.   The id holds the individual's instincts and drives for pleasure, and these instincts provide energy for the personality. This energy is called the **libido,** the energy with which sexual instincts function in all phases of life (Freud, 1979). The id holds instincts and drives for pleasure, things the child repressed during the early years. Consequently, the id and its energy, the libido, are in the unconscious and exert their influences outside of a person's awareness. Freud considered the id to be the most important influence throughout one's life.

Ego.   The **ego** develops from the id to function as an intermediary between the id and external reality. Its function is to mediate between the instincts of the id and the constraints of environment to find an acceptable and efficient satisfaction of needs. The ego is the only part of the personality that is in contact with reality. It is ruled by the **reality principle,** which aims to postpone immediate gratification until a suitable object for this satisfaction is found. Thus the ego is logical, organized, and causal and participates in problem solving. The ego's external, self-preserving function includes perception (storing experiences), adaptation, flight (escape), and activity (an attempt to modify the world to its own advantage). The ego's internal self-preserving functions involve gaining control over the demands of the instincts by deciding whether to satisfy, postpone, or suppress the demands (Freud, 1960). The ego functions as the organizer of the personality and strives to achieve harmony between the reality of the external world, the id, and the superego. Often this challenge produces anxiety. The ego is the aspect of the personality that experiences anxiety, as a signal to the self to protect oneself from some perceived danger (Freud, 1960). Since the ego has memories that can be recalled, it is associated with a level of consciousness known as the preconscious. Preconscious material can move from the unconscious to the conscious but can also be obstructed by resistance (Freud, 1960). Consciousness is an awareness of an experience at the moment it occurs. It is the awareness of daily living. When the attention is taken away from an experience, that experience goes to the preconscious level, where it subsequently can be retrieved.

Superego.   The **superego** develops from the ego as an internalization of the demands, prohibitions, and ideals of significant others (notably the parents). In fact, the superego can be viewed as a prolonging of the parental influence (Freud, 1960). The superego consists of two subsystems reflective of the parental influence: conscience and the ego ideal. The *conscience* represents the demanding or forbidding aspects of the parents. It represents what the individual thinks the parents considered morally wrong. The *ego ideal* evolves from the individual's perception of what the parents thought was morally good and includes ideals of strength, power, beauty, and success. The individual submits to the standards of conscience and ego

---

The time frame of rearing a child in nineteenth-century Vienna was different from our contemporary world, but the process was the same.

ideal and therefore continues on in a relationship with the parents. This relationship is acted out in other relationships. The ego must intervene to reach a satisfactory level of interaction with the superego. Conflicts arise when an individual cannot live up to the standards of the superego. Shame and a lowered sense of self-worth occur if a person cannot meet his or her ego ideal, and failure to live up to perceived moral standards can cause guilt.

Sexuality.   The second theme woven through Freud's theory of personality is that of sexuality. Before Freud's work, sexuality was thought to exist as an influence only after puberty. One of Freud's greatest contributions was the recognition that sexuality operates from the beginning of a child's development and that it gradually changes form from one phase to the next (Freud, 1979). Freud hypothesized that the stages of sexual development are predetermined and that this development is fueled by the energy from the libido. During the child's development this energy becomes focused on specific body parts considered erogenous zones and causes tension in those parts. This tension is relieved by manipulation of the body part, and the tension relief is experienced as pleasure. Freud saw the erogenous zones as progressing from the mouth (the oral phase—birth to 18 months) to the anus (the anal phase—18 months to 3 years) to the penis (the phallic phase—3 years to 5 years) and later to the entire genital area (the genital phase—15 years).*

Freud saw each of these periods as having a task and concomitant development of defense mechanisms to allow for the task accomplishments.

Oral phase (birth to 18 months).   The oral phase is characterized by the need to suck, and the infant receives pleasure from the satisfaction of that need. The infant will suck his or her fist, toy, blanket, and so on, if the nipple is not available.

Anal phase (18 months to 3 years).   The anal phase is characterized by increasing awareness of the anal sphincter and the ability or inability to exert control over it. The child receives pleasure from being able to "produce" or expel from this body part during bowel movements.

Phallic phase (3 years to 5 years).   The phallic phase is arguably the most challenged aspect of Freud's theory. Freud proposed that during this phase the young boy will touch his penis to receive pleasure and imagine sexual activity with the primary female in his life, his mother. However, he fears retaliation from his father in the form of castration. This desire for the mother and the fear of the father's reprisal is called the Oedipus complex (based on the Greek story of Oedipus, who killed his father and married his mother). According to Anna Freud, this conflict is

so great that the boy flees to latency, which is marked by an absence of sexual interest (Freud, 1979).

According to Freud, girls undergo a different type of trauma at this stage of development. Girls try to be similar to boys but recognize the "inferiority of the clitoris" compared with the penis and in disappointment turn away from sexual life (Freud, 1979). This aspect of Freud's theory on female sexuality has been challenged by subsequent psychoanalysts as representing a male-dominated view of experience.

Genital phase (15+ years).   The genital phase is marked by sexual maturity and pleasure in heterosexual relations.

TECHNIQUES

The techniques of psychoanalysis flow from the premise that the conflicts causing disturbances are held in the unconscious and that it is possible to move this material from the unconscious to the preconscious and finally into consciousness. Once it is in one's conscious awareness, the individual can decide how to deal with it in a more adaptive manner. The two main means to access this unconscious material are through free association in the therapy session and dream analysis.

Free Association

During the therapy session, the individual is encouraged to relax and to speak whatever comes to mind without judging its appropriateness or relatedness. To facilitate this process, the client reclines on a couch or lounge chair while the therapist sits behind out of view, so as to avoid any eye contact that may impede the client's flow of thoughts. The psychoanalyst listens for themes and recurrent distortions in the material presented and assists in clarifying the material through various means. The analyst may make an *interpretation*, which proposes an underlying cause for a client's expressed feeling. As therapy progresses, the analyst will examine *transference issues*, in which the client's repressed feelings and past relationships are acted out in the current relationship with the therapist. The analyst will examine the *resistance* of the client to the work of therapy. The resistances are exhibited by avoidance (canceling appointments, failure to free-associate, or talking about trivia) or more active means (rejecting an interpretation or acting out of a need). Resistances exist around areas of conflict and are clues to the therapist of repressed material.

Dream Analysis

Freud viewed dreams as a means of access to the unconscious. Freud believed that every dream demands the satisfaction of some intrinsic need or the solution of a conflict. Furthermore, Freud proposed that dreams make broader use of memory and linguistic symbols, since the id has more liberty in dreams than in waking periods (Freud, 1960). Therefore dream analysis involves the client free-

---

Freud did not consider the latency period (5 to 12 years) or the prepubescent period (12 to 15 years). These were added later by his daughter, Anna Freud, as she continued the theory development.

CLINICAL APPLICATION
Psychoanalytic Theory

The client is a 42-year-old woman who is being treated for a depression of 6 months' duration. She was divorced and has been married to her second husband for 6 years. She has two children by her first marriage: a son who is 14 years old and a daughter who is 11 years old. She worked as a bank teller until the symptoms of the depression forced her to stop 4 months ago. Her parents are living in the same city, but she rarely sees them.

Peggy has experienced anhedonia (loss of pleasure in life), decreased appetite, anxiety, and insomnia punctuated by nightmares.

The interaction that follows occurs 4 months into the client's treatment with a psychoanalyst. Peggy has previously discussed a recurring dream she has of a young child crying out into the darkness. Instead of stars in the dark sky, there are only eyes. The more the child cries, the smaller the child becomes.

Peggy:	[Angry] You just sit there, like a nothing. I don't even know if you're listening to me.
Therapist:	[Silence]
Peggy:	Well, are you?

Therapist:	[Silence]
Peggy:	[With sadness] This is so typical. I talk and no one listens, even when I pay them to.
Therapist:	[Silence]
Peggy:	Why is it I'm so unnoticeable? Can't you notice me, you bastard?
Therapist:	[Silence]
Peggy:	[In small voice] I feel small.
Therapist:	[Silence]
Therapist:	This is the experience of your dream: of crying out to eyes that watch but do not take the action that you expect. Because no action or rescue comes, you feel insignificant and angry. It may be helpful for you to consider whom you expected to take action. Your projected anger at me suggests a true anger at your father.

Continuing this work, Peggy eventually uncovers her anger at her father for his absence during her upbringing, a pattern that continued with her husbands.

---

associating around a dream so that the analyst can determine the deep unconscious meanings and symbols involved.

ADLERIAN THERAPY

Alfred Adler (1870-1937) was a major contributor to the development of the psychodynamic model of therapy. His theory of personality development is rooted in the disciplines of psychotherapy, education, and anthropology. After an initial collaboration with Freud, Adler became dissatisfied with Freud's biologically determined approach and developed his Individual Psychology theory, which views human nature as being socially based. This approach to therapy focuses on the development and progression of a therapeutic relationship and presents a framework for understanding individuals within their social context.

THEORETIC OVERVIEW

Adler had an optimistic view of the nature of human beings. He saw them as being capable of living together cooperatively, working toward self-improvement and fulfillment, and contributing to the common welfare. Adler stressed the unity of personality. He believed that people could be understood as integrated and complete beings. This view emphasizes the purposeful nature of behavior, maintaining that the direction individuals are heading in is far more important than where they came from. People are seen as actors and creators of their lives and as being capable of developing unique lifestyles that are an expres-

sion of their goals. Individuals tend to create themselves rather than merely being shaped by their childhood experiences (Corey, 1991).

BASIC CONCEPTS
Phenomenologic Approach

The key point of Adlerian therapy is simply paying attention to the individual's way of understanding the world. Adler agreed with Freud that a person's personality is largely influenced by the first 6 years of life. Unlike Freud, however, Adler argued that it is not the events themselves that influence personality development but rather the individual's perception and interpretation of these events (Corey, 1991). Adler saw individuals as attributing meaning to these life experiences and thus creating a subjective reality to which they respond. This phenomenologic approach was first articulated by Adler and has been incorporated into many other forms of therapy, such as Gestalt, existential, and cognitive-behavioral.

Personality Development

Adler viewed personality development as a creative and active process. Unlike Freud, he believed that humans are motivated by social urges rather than sexual ones, with purposeful and goal-directed behavior and consciousness being at the center of the personality (Corey, 1991).

Adler proposed that personality development begins in infancy, and that humans gradually become aware of **inferiority feelings,** which arise when individuals become conscious of imperfections. "We cope with feelings of helplessness by striving for competence, mastery and perfection" (Corey, 1991). According to Adler, as soon as one experiences inferiority, one is motivated to strive for superiority. Adler maintained that the "goal of success pulled people toward mastery and enabled them to overcome obstacles" (Corey, 1991). Superiority, as viewed by Adler, refers to attaining a larger degree of one's potential versus being superior to others. One strives for competence in accordance with one's individual style.

Adler defined a **final goal** as an imagined ideal situation of perfection, completion, or overcoming of inferiority feelings. This is an unconscious goal. It is the movement toward this goal that guides one's actions in the present and influences one's approach to life. Adler referred to this unique approach as the *style of life* and saw it as the way individuals either approach or avoid the three tasks of life (work, love, and community).

Feeling of Community

One of Adler's most significant contributions was his acknowledgment of the individual's connection to society. Humans have a basic need to be accepted, to feel secure and worthwhile. *Gemeinschaftsgefühl*, or social interest, refers to an "individual's awareness of being part of the human community" and "one's attitude toward society, including striving for a better future for humanity" (Corey, 1991). Adler proposes that individuals are part of society and cannot be understood in isolation. Adler did not see a "fundamental conflict between self and society." He believed that the development of self and connectedness to the world are processes that influence one another in positive ways. "The greater one's personal development and the more one connects positively with others, the more one is able to learn and develop oneself" (Corey, 1991).

View of Pathology

Adler viewed psychologic disturbances as generally occurring in the presence of two conditions: an exaggerated inferiority feeling and an insufficient feeling of community. Under these conditions a person may experience or anticipate failure in a task that appears impossible and may become discouraged. Adler tended to use the term *discouraged* as opposed to terms such as *pathologic* or *sick*. When individuals are discouraged, they often resort to ways to relieve or mask, rather than overcome, their inferiority feelings. They attempt to bolster their feelings by "tricks," whereas they avoid actually confronting their seemingly impossible difficulties.

Discouraged people strive to protect their sense of self through *safeguarding devices*. Individuals can use safeguarding devices in attempts to excuse themselves from failure and/or depreciate others. Safeguarding devices include symptoms, depreciation, accusations, self-accusations, guilt, and various forms of distancing. Symptoms such as anxiety, phobias, and depression can all be used as excuses for avoiding life tasks and transferring responsibility to others. In this way individuals can use their symptoms to shield themselves from potential or actual failure in these tasks. Individuals may be able to do well in one or two tasks of life and have difficulties in only one (work, community, or love.)

Depreciation can be used to deflate the value of others, thereby achieving a sense of relative superiority. Accusations attribute the responsibility for a difficulty or failure to others in an attempt to relieve an individual of responsibility. Self-accusations can deter criticisms from others or elicit comforting assurances. Guilt may create a feeling of superiority over others and clear the way for continuing harmful actions.

TECHNIQUES

Adlerian counseling is described as a diplomatic, cooperative working relationship that establishes the feeling of equality (Stein, 1998). The work usually involves identifying, exploring, and modifying the unconscious final goal and the consistent patterns that support it. The goal is to assist the individual in becoming a more fully functioning person. During counseling the therapist provides information, teaching, guidance, and encouragement. Encouragement is believed to be the most powerful method available for changing a person's beliefs. It helps clients build self-confidence and stimulates courage. Courage is the willingness to act in ways that are consistent with social interest (Corey, 1991).

Adlerian therapy consists of either 12 steps or four stages. For the sake of clarity, the four stages are presented here. Within each stage, cognitive, emotional, and behavioral changes are encouraged. The four stages of Adlerian therapy are:

1. Establishing the therapeutic relationship
2. Exploring the client's psychologic dynamics
3. Encouraging the development of insight or self-understanding
4. Assisting the client in making new choices

Throughout these stages, Adlerian therapists adapt their approach to the uniqueness of the individual rather than adhering to specific techniques. The therapist always works within the phenomenologic framework. The stages are briefly summarized here.

Stage 1: Establishing the Relationship

The work of this stage is to establish a collaborative relationship and to help clients become more cooperative (as demonstrated by their ability to cooperate in therapy). One way to create a working therapeutic relationship is to help clients recognize their strengths and assets. The difficulties clients have struggled to overcome frequently provide the strengths used in therapy. During this stage the therapist's main techniques are listening, attending, empathizing, and demonstrating confidence in the client's ability to change. Once the client feels accepted and understood, he or she is more likely to focus on his or her goals for therapy. Adlerians use Socratic questioning (i.e., questions designed to reveal hidden ignorances or to elicit truths known to all) to clarify the client's goals and beliefs about self, others, and life. Mistaken ideas are identified and corrected to align with common sense. Often, symptoms provide an opportunity for this clarification. Symptoms may serve as excuses for avoiding something that the client is not doing. One way that the therapist can expose this is to ask the Socratic question: "If you did not have these symptoms, what would you do?" The client's answer is often quite revealing.

Stage 2: Exploring the Individual's Dynamics

The aim of this stage is to assist clients in understanding the style of life and how it affects their functioning in all life tasks (Corey, 1991). The therapist serves to broaden the client's perspective beyond the narrow viewpoint. Always working within the phenomenologic framework, the therapist explores the client's motives, beliefs, feelings, and goals. Adlerian therapists go beyond feelings to explore the beliefs underlying them. They then confront faulty beliefs in order to free the client from them (Corey, 1991).

During this stage the therapist engages in a lifestyle assessment that includes descriptions of the client's family of origin, their relationships with the client, and early childhood memories and the meaning they hold for the client. This assessment helps the client discover the logic and interpretations that form the basis for the client's subjective view of reality. The therapist also evaluates the client's functioning in the three tasks of life: work, community, and love. Clients are asked about their satisfaction and level of goal accomplishment in each area.

Stage 3: Encouraging Insight

In this stage the therapist challenges the client to develop insights into self-defeating behaviors and goals by making tentative hypotheses and interpretations. Adlerians do not see insight as being necessary for an individual to make a behavioral change but rather as an adjunct. Interpretations are designed to create awareness of one's unique logic and goals and how these affect current behavior. Since no one can truly know the inner world of another, interpretations are presented in the form of open-ended sharings to be explored in the session (e.g., "Could it be that . . .? or "It seems to me that . . .") (Corey, 1991). It is important that these interpretations reflect an empathy for the client that has been developed in the previous stages.

Stage 4: Helping With Reorientation

This final stage is action oriented and involves putting the insights into practice (Corey, 1991). The therapist and the client actively problem solve ways for the client to make

---

CLINICAL APPLICATION
Adlerian Therapy

Peggy has been seeing an Adlerian therapist for a few weeks and is currently exploring her dynamics (stage 2) as the therapist encourages insight (stage 3). As in other forms of therapy, the stages often overlap.

Peggy:	I'm just so incompetent in my life. I don't seem to be able to do anything right.
Therapist:	You seem discouraged to me, Peggy. I know this struggle has been with you awhile. Could it be that "not doing anything right" is almost a lifestyle for you?
Peggy:	It sure seems to be lately. But I guess I've always worried about it—all my life.
Therapist:	I wonder what that could be about.
Peggy:	I've always thought that if I did things "just right" my parents—well, everybody—would notice, and everything would be OK.
Therapist:	So, it sounds to me as if the goal of all this may be to get reassurance from others that you are acceptable. Does that fit for you?

---

changes in life that are consistent with the newly established goals. Often clients are encouraged to act as if they were already the person they wish they were. This serves to undermine self-limiting assumptions (Corey, 1991). Adlerian therapists use many techniques in this stage but always select ones that are appropriate to the client's goals and views.

TRANSACTIONAL ANALYSIS

Transactional analysis (TA) provides an easily understood framework for examining human communication and its problems. It provides a straightforward approach to analyzing and changing communication that can be easily understood by a variety of clients and students, and it has become a popular mode of therapy since it was introduced by Eric Berne in 1961. Basically, TA can be used to identify an individual's dysfunctional life stances through the analysis and correction of communication patterns, both internal (self-talk) and external (communication with others), as well as examining how this dysfunction is communicated over a lifetime.

THEORETIC OVERVIEW

Berne proposes that young children are constantly organizing their life experiences and that similar thoughts, actions, and feelings become organized into ego states. An **ego state** is defined as a coherent set of feelings accompanied by a related set of coherent behavior patterns that are observable (Berne, 1964). Berne defines three ego states of an individual: *parent*, *adult*, and *child*. Individuals move fluidly from one ego state to another, depending on which ego state is active at the moment. These ego states are recognizable to observers and are consistent over time.

Parent Ego State

The parent ego state reflects the attitudes, beliefs, and behavioral patterns of the parental figures. The parent ego state can be the supportive "good parent" (the *nurturing parent*) or the never-pleased "bad parent" (the *critical parent*). The function of the parent ego state is to set limits, protect, support, and teach. It functions to save time for the individual by making many decisions and responses automatic (Berne, 1964). When a person acts from this ego state, the behaviors, words, and decisions will be automatic and imitative of the parental figures.

Adult Ego State

The adult ego state allows the individual to objectively appraise the reality of a situation without self-criticism or conceit. The adult ego state functions as a rational data-processing system to assist the individual in problem solving and dealing effectively with the outside world. As the rational ego state, the adult ego state is called on to mediate conflicts between the automatic parent and the impulsive child. When a person is acting from the adult ego state, the behaviors and decisions represent a rational and informed response to the situation.

Child Ego State

The child ego state holds the spontaneous urges and impulses of an individual. The creative, playful, and intuitive impulses are associated with the *natural child* or *free child* ego state. The shamefulness, fearfulness, anxiety, and inhibitions that result when the natural child is thwarted in some manner by the controlling parental influence is called the *adapted child* ego state. The function of the child ego state is to experience feelings and to act spontaneously and intuitively. When a person acts from this ego state, decisions will be impulsive.

Life Stances

Berne proposes that a person is always acting from one ego state or another but perhaps not consciously. The cumulative effect of early life experiences causes the individual to develop a *life stance*. The life stance is basically the individual's assessment of personal self-worth compared with others. Berne has identified four life stances: (1) I'm OK, you're OK; (2) I'm OK, you're not OK; (3) I'm not OK, you're OK; and (4) I'm not OK, you're not OK. Berne's position is that the individual's basic stance is enacted in his or her communication with self and others. By analyzing the ineffective communication pattern, the therapist and client can identify both the sources of dysfunction and healthier alternatives. It is the goal of TA to help individuals recognize their various ego states and be able to function within the appropriate one by choice.

BASIC CONCEPTS
Communication Patterns

Since Berne envisions that individuals always speak from one of the three ego states, he uses the ego states to analyze communication. TA represents an individual with three distinct ego states as depicted in the following illustration:

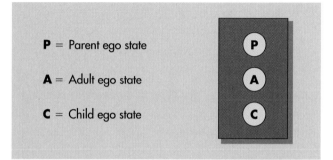

When analyzing communication from one person to another, Berne looks at transactions between the two individuals. A transaction is the smallest unit of interaction between two people and is represented by arrows designating the stimulus and the response. A transaction between two people is represented in the following illustration:

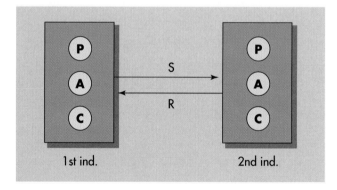

In this example, the first individual spoke from the adult ego state to the second individual's adult ego state, and the second individual responded from the adult ego state as well. This represents a *complementary* transaction or exchange. (A complementary exchange is also called a parallel exchange because the arrows are parallel to each other.) Complementary transactions are between role-appropriate ego states. The example above could be between two co-workers—two adults interacting with each other. The following illustration shows a complementary transaction between a mother and her child.

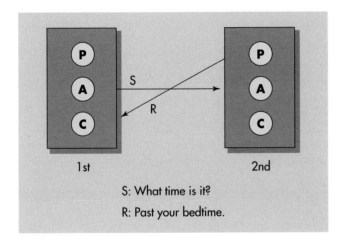

Berne proposes that communication is effective and functions if it is complementary (Berne, 1964) because it is experienced as being mutually satisfying and serves to further communication.

Differences arise when the transactions are not along complementary (or parallel) lines. This means that communication is not between role-appropriate ego states. The following illustration represents such a transaction and is known as a crossed transaction:

S: What time is it?

R: Past your bedtime.

In this case the first person initiated an adult-to-adult transaction. The second person, however, responded from the parent ego state, as if addressing a child. This is an example of a crossed transaction. Crossed transactions are experienced as dysfunctional and have the effect of stopping or inhibiting further communication. The most common form of a crossed transaction occurs when the stimulus is adult to adult but the response is either parent to child or child to parent (Berne, 1964).

Strokes

Strokes refer to the TA concepts of validation. All human beings attempt to validate their existence through words and/or touch. Transactions that result in increasing esteem are considered positive strokes. Those that produce negative feelings of belittlement are considered negative strokes. Conditional strokes are received for accomplishing something, whereas unconditional strokes are given just for being. Complementary communication tends to increase a person's self-validation because it is effective; crossed transactions are confusing and often discounting.

TECHNIQUES

The techniques of TA are actually the steps in the progression of therapy. This is designed to help individuals become aware of their interactive style as a reflection of their life stance and to assist them in choosing the most appropriate ego stances. The approach is educative and challenging. Therapy is divided into four sections: structural analysis, transactional analysis, game analysis, and script analysis. All are best accomplished in a group situation.

Structural Analysis

Structural analysis is the initial part of the therapy. It begins with the client identifying the problem or symptom to be relieved by the therapy. The client is then educated regarding the functions and purposes of various ego states. Work is done to assist the client in identifying the phenomena associated with his or her own ego state presentations and to clearly separate the various states. This is done through analyzing transactions with the therapist or through analyzing examples that the client brings to therapy.

The overall goal of structural analysis is to assist the client in functioning predominantly from the reality-testing ego state (i.e., the adult ego state) (Berne, 1972). However, to accomplish this, the therapist and client must identify the ego state that is carrying the symptoms with which the client presented (Berne, 1972). Consequently, the need exists to activate the adult ego state to rationally mediate between the more reactive and impulsive ego states. The goal of structural analysis is the mastery of internal conflicts through the diagnosis of ego states so that the adult ego state can maintain mastery of the personality in stressful situations. At the conclusion of structural analysis, the client may terminate or proceed to the next phase.

Transactional Analysis

Once clients are aware of their various ego states, they begin to examine when and how they are activated. The eventual goal of this phase is to establish the adult ego state in the executive role of the personality and actively choose when to release the child ego state or adult ego state and when to terminate their transactions (Berne, 1972). In group situations, clients learn how and when their parent or child ego state overrides their adult ego state and then learn to formulate adult responses.

One of the specific techniques the TA therapist uses throughout therapy, but especially at this stage, is inviting the client to be responsible for choosing more appropriate responses to situations. This involves changing inappropriate parent or child responses to the realm of the adult. As much as possible, these responses are framed in the positive. After analyzing transactions, the client may end therapy or proceed to look at how the various ego states affect larger segments of his or her interactions.

Game Analysis

Games are defined as a recurring set of transactions that have a concealed or ulterior motivation (Berne, 1972). Berne views games as having their origins in early childhood, when they are consciously initiated by the child. Over time, however, they become fixed in patterns, the origins are lost, and the ulterior nature is obscured (Berne, 1964). According to Berne, games are necessary and desirable because they provide structure for time. At question is whether the individual's games offer the best outcome for him or her (Berne, 1964).

Games employ ulterior transactions that are tied to the individual's life stance. An ulterior transaction involves the game player pretending to do one thing but really doing something else. Therefore all games will involve a con of some sort (Berne, 1972). Berne and others have defined many types of games, but all games have two characteristics: the ulterior quality and the "payoff" (Berne, 1964). Payoffs are the feelings that the game arouses within the individual.

Rather than examine the many games defined by Berne, one will be used to demonstrate game characteristics. A common game between spouses has been named "If It Weren't for You." As an example of this game, the wife complains that her husband restricts her social activities so that she never learned to dance. When she begins to change certain attitudes during her psychiatric treatment, her husband retreats from his previous stance and she is able to expand her social activities. She takes dancing lessons only to discover a horrible fear of dance floors! Her domineering husband was actually providing her a real service by preventing her from even becoming aware of her fears.

The transactional analysis of this game is illustrated as follows. The dotted lines represent the ulterior transaction.

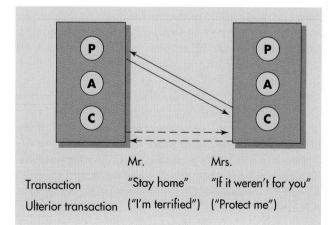

On the social level the game was a parent-child one with the husband as parent demanding that the wife stay home and care for the house. The wife responded as a child with "If it weren't for you."

On the ulterior level, the game is played between the child ego states, with the husband using his dominance to hide his child fear of desertion and the wife's child ego state seeking protection from fearful situations (Berne, 1964).

Script Analysis

Script theory holds that the child makes early decisions about self and begins to make a life plan based on that decision (Goulding and Goulding, 1979). This script is reflected in the predominance of one ego state over another, in the individual's transactions, and in the choice of games. Thus script analysis represents the final stage of therapy and focuses on the analysis of lifelong patterns. The script is seen as the adaptation of early childhood experiences that is played out through life by manipulating others to play the necessary roles (Berne, 1972). Scripts are analyzed by examining the material collected in and out of the group until the nature of the script becomes clear (Berne, 1972).

GESTALT THERAPY

Gestalt therapy was founded by Fred (Fritz) Perls, who began his career as a psychoanalyst. Over time, he became dissatisfied with some of Freud's beliefs. Specifically, Perls did not see intrapsychic conflicts as originating from conflicts with the id, ego, and superego, but rather from an individual's interactions with society. Gestalt therapy is considered a type of humanistic psychology.

THEORETIC OVERVIEW

Perls envisioned human beings as "organisms" (beings) with their own nature and also as being a part of nature. Organisms have emotions, impulses, intellect, and a history of experiences that all serve to direct and fulfill the organism in life. Perls theorized that society made demands on organisms (or individuals) to conform to certain standards of behavior. Perls theorized that as individuals comply with these "should" demands of society, they distance themselves from their own emotional experiences and, as a result, dissociate from being a part of nature (Stevens, 1975). The individual can no longer function at full capacity because of this alienation and separation from his or her nature. In fact, if allowed to continue, the individual may deteriorate in his or her functioning. In addition, this reliance on society for setting standards of behavior leaves the individual dependent on society for validation and support. To Perls, the result again is one of minimized functioning of the individual, because the individual cannot self-regulate but must rely on external factors that may be making inappropriate demands on him or her.

CLINICAL APPLICATION
Transactional Analysis

The client, Peggy, has been involved in an outpatient transactional analysis group to deal with the symptoms of her depression. She has so far identified her life stance as "I'm not OK, you're OK," and is currently working with other group members to learn more about the activation of ego states.

The group has been working for about 45 minutes, but Peggy has been silent.

Therapist:	Peggy, you've chosen to be quiet tonight.
Peggy:	I don't have much to offer. I learn a lot from listening to you.
Group member:	Do you mean you learn a lot from the therapist or from the group?
Peggy:	Well, the therapist, I guess. I mean, he is the expert and we are all just trying to learn from him.
Group member:	Sounds to me like you're coming from your child ego state. Big Daddy has all the

	answers for us poor kids.
Peggy:	Well, I do feel like I need help. I feel ashamed and scared and sad and I want someone to help me.
Therapist:	Perhaps that person is closer than you think. What would your last comment sound like, Peggy, if you were speaking from an adult ego state instead of a child one?
Peggy:	You mean, about being scared?
Therapist:	Yes.
Peggy:	Um, I'm having some uncomfortable feelings . . . that will probably pass in time when I choose to let them go . . . I'd like to figure out how to let them go.

In her last statement, Peggy identified the more rational, problem-solving response of the adult ego state.

BASIC CONCEPTS

Top Dog and Underdog

Perls created the terms *top dog* and *underdog* to represent this struggle. Top dog refers to the superego, the "shoulds" of life learned in society, and Perls notes that this is so strong a force that it is rarely understood. The underdog represents the id, the impulses and desires. The underdog is constantly working at evading the top dog, and the two are in constant strife, struggling for control. To a Gestaltist, cure represents the end of this control struggle between top dog and underdog, in that the struggle for supremacy is replaced by their natural acknowledgment and interaction (Stevens, 1975).

Figure-Background Formation

Another tenet of Gestalt therapy is that of **figure-background formation.** Basically, this means that reality is determined by the individual's specific interest and needs and that "whatever is the organism's foremost need, makes reality appear as it does" (Stevens, 1975). For clarification, consider the following situation: two people enter a restaurant. The first person is famished, having worked through the day, skipping both breakfast and lunch. The obvious need is hunger, and as the individual enters the restaurant, she notices the dessert tray by the entrance, the smells of cooking coming from the kitchen, and the food being eaten by other diners.

The second person enters the restaurant to use the telephone. Her car has broken down just outside, and she is late for a dinner meeting with a client. She needs to use the telephone to inform the client of her later arrival and to call a cab. She enters the restaurant and scans the lobby for a telephone. She is not particularly aware that this is a

restaurant; it just happened to be an open public building close to the spot of her car trouble.

In each example, reality was experienced differently, demonstrating the Gestaltist point of view that reality is determined by one's needs. Once the need is satisfied, it recedes and the next need emerges. Perls saw this as **organismic self-regulation** (Stevens, 1975).

However, if the need is not met, conflict ensues because Gestalt theory proposes that an organism cannot tolerate an unfinished situation. Gestalt therapy works to help an individual complete unfinished situations through helping the individual to differentiate the various aspects affecting any given moment or conflict and then to integrate them (Stevens, 1975).

Thus the emphasis in Gestalt therapy is always on the present moment, the "here and now," known as the *foreground*. Past events and experiences are useful in that they influence the present moment. Gestalt therapists illuminate their influence so as to allow the individual to integrate them.

TECHNIQUES

Chair Work

Perhaps the best-known Gestalt therapy technique is *chair work*. In this exercise, the client sits opposite an empty chair, which represents some aspect of the foreground. It may be a person, a physical sensation, or an emotion. The individual has a conversation with the empty chair, stating his or her concerns and point of view. At the conclusion of this statement, the therapist asks the individual to switch seats and roles and to make a reply to what has been said. (Thus a man may be speaking to his "empty-chair" father and then be asked to take the father's position, via the

CLINICAL APPLICATION
Gestalt Therapy

Peggy is in an outpatient group and is currently the focus of the work. She sits opposite an empty chair in the center of the group's circle. The therapist is standing behind her. She has just told the group that she felt sorry for her father, who had to work so hard all his life.

Therapist: Pretend your father is sitting in that chair. What would you like him to know?

Peggy: Hi, Dad. It's been a long time. You're looking good . . . I guess.

Therapist: [Silence]

Peggy: I really don't know what to say to you, Dad . . . except thank you for taking care of me

Therapist: [Silence]

Therapist: Can you remember a time he took care of you?

Peggy: No, I can't.

Therapist: Tell him.

Peggy: Dad, I don't know what to say to you, and I think that's a shame. I know you had to work hard to support us, but I work hard, too, and I still have more time for my kids than you did. What was the matter? Was it me?

Therapist: Switch chairs and answer your daughter.

Peggy: [As father] Hello, Peggy. I don't know what to say to you, either . . . I guess I never did. I always counted on your mother to do that. I tried to show you I loved you, but I guess I'm not good at showing it. Did I hurt you?

Therapist: Switch back.

Peggy: It's not anything big, Dad. It's just all those small little things that make me feel I'm not worth much if . . . if even my own father doesn't love me.

Therapist: [Silence]

Therapist: Switch chairs again.

Peggy: [As father] Well, Peggy, I do love you. I'm just lousy at showing it. You were always such a quiet little girl. I never knew what you were thinking. I don't know how girls think. Hell, I grew up with four brothers! But, Peggy, didn't you know I loved you?

Therapist: Switch back.

Peggy: I guess I did. I remember you carrying me back to my bed after I'd fall asleep watching TV with you. I always liked that.

Therapist: [Silence]

Peggy: I guess I was kind of in awe of you, Dad. I didn't know what to say to you, but I did not think that would be hard for you. You seemed to be able to handle anything. You always knew what to do, so I just guessed you'd know what to do with me, too.

The conversation goes on until both Peggy and the "father" feel it was completed.

---

chair, and respond to the son.) This switching back and forth is continued until the individual reaches some integration and the need recedes.

This technique illustrates the Gestalt approach of *differentiation* and *integration*. It allows the client to experience the many aspects of the moment. Indeed, "chair-workers" frequently remember sounds, lights, voice tones, colors, seasons, emotions, and interactions of others, along with their own self-expectations and reactions. This interplay adds to the texture and depth of the experience, which may have been flattened by the conflict of the unmet need. By becoming aware and accepting of the many aspects of the situation and by listening to them, the individual is in a position to integrate them. The individual does not need to bend only to "top dog," but will find a way to blend all of the acknowledged aspects of the situation. Perls has said that "true listening is understanding" (Stevens, 1975).

This aspect of Gestalt work is demonstrated again in dream work. To Perls a dream is a message that not only contains the kernels of an individual's life situation but also answers about how to change the nightmare of the situation. In Gestalt dream work the individual acts out the various aspects of the dream and listens to the message

of each aspect. The assumption is that each part of the dream is a projection of some aspect of the individual's life and consequently has a truth message that the individual finds difficult to hear or accept. By actually playing out the various parts of the dream while aware and in therapy, the individual is forced to identify with the various aspects of the dream and, in Gestalt terms, listen to it.

CLIENT-CENTERED THERAPY
THEORETIC OVERVIEW

Another form of humanistic psychology is client-centered therapy. It was developed in the 1940s by Carl Rogers, an American psychiatrist (Figure 3-2), who acknowledges his indebtedness to Gestalt psychology for its recognition of the wholeness and center relatedness of phenomena (Rogers, 1951). Rogers, too, extols the richness of experiences and the profound potential of human organisms to move forward. Indeed, it is this fundamental belief that the basic tendency of a human being is to move forward toward constructive change and integration that underlies client-centered (or Rogerian) therapy. The central hypothesis is that the individual has "sufficient capacity to deal constructively with all those aspects of his/her life that can

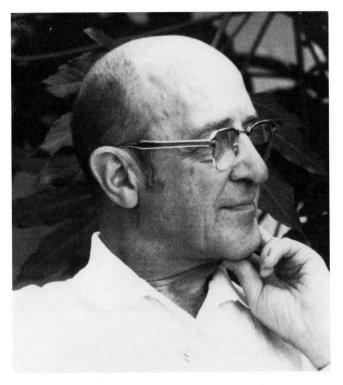

Figure 3-2 Carl Rogers, 1902-1987. (From the Bettmann Archive.)

potentially come into conscious awareness" (Rogers, 1951). The difficulty is that many aspects of the client's life or experiences are buried in shame, guilt, or denial. The individual's personality then works to continue to suppress thoughts or feelings that are not consistent with the individual's self-image. This suppression can cause difficulties in the individual's definition of self or in interpersonal relations. In addition, Rogers (1951) recognized that as society grew more and more diverse, it was less capable of supporting the individual in his or her definition of self. The goal of client-centered therapy is to bring these buried aspects of one's self to awareness, in full confidence that the individual will be able to accept these various parts, integrate them into an expanded self-concept, and live more fully and freely because energy is not being spent on suppression.

BASIC CONCEPTS

Rogers believed that within every human organism is "a whole person, distinctly organized" who can be approached directly in a therapy situation (Kovel, 1976). One of the basic tenets of client-centered therapy is the belief that at the core of the human organism is an organized self whose basic energy is moving forward toward integration of experiences. Another tenet at the core of this therapy is that interpersonal relationships are the basis for both health and neurosis, for it is in these aspects that the self is defined.

It therefore follows that a client-centered therapist would use the therapeutic relationship to support the growth of the client's inner self in its endeavors to comprehend, accept, and integrate those experiences that have been hidden from consciousness and prohibited from acceptance and integration. This is the core of Rogerian therapy.

TECHNIQUES

However simplistic the premise of client-centered therapy may sound, the practice of it is demanding on the therapist. It requires therapists to, as much as possible, totally accept the premise that an individual's natural tendency is to move forward toward integration. Therapists must be firmly grounded in this premise because all of their actions and words must flow from this basic premise in a consistent manner. Indeed, the only "technique" of client-centered therapy is to create a therapeutic relationship that is unconditionally accepting of and empathic to the client. This is called **unconditional positive regard.** That is, the therapist must demonstrate the belief that the client is competent to direct himself or herself (Rogers, 1951).

To demonstrate this belief, the therapist attempts to take on the client's frame of reference and perception of the world and relate it back to the client in an accepting and nonjudgmental way. The therapist does not attempt to change or challenge the client's thoughts or perceptions. In fact, just the opposite occurs. The therapist simply accepts and empathizes with what the client verbalized and relates it back without the negative connotation placed on it by the client. Rogers has described this tech-

---

CLINICAL APPLICATION
Client-Centered Therapy

Peggy is seeing a Rogerian therapist for treatment of her depression. She has been in individual therapy for about 6 weeks.

Therapist:	Come in, Peggy. I'm glad to see you.
Peggy:	Thanks, I'm glad to see you, too. It seems this is the only place I feel worth anything.
Therapist:	You can feel your worth here.
Peggy:	Yeah, everywhere else I feel like such a failure: as a wife, a mom, a daughter, even as a worker.
Therapist:	You carry a lot of roles and do a lot of things.
Peggy:	I guess I do and I worry about doing them right.
Therapist:	You're trying to do right by a lot of people.
Peggy:	Yeah, I am. It's hard, and I never know if what I'm doing is OK.
Therapist:	And yet, you keep doing your best.

The therapist demonstrates acceptance and positive regard for Peggy and encourages her to move toward self-reorganization.

| **Box 3-1** | **Client-Centered Therapist Technique** |

Allow the client to lead the therapy. The therapist does not suggest what should be discussed.

Attempt to accurately reflect the client's perception in a totally accepting and empathic manner.

Be completely nonjudgmental (knowing that the client's inner self is on a path toward development).

Reflect an attitude of wanting to help the client.

nique as functioning as an **alter ego** for the client's attitudes and feelings, which allows the client to see himself or herself "more clearly and to experience him/herself more significantly" (Rogers, 1951). The therapist is just as accepting and empathic toward the negative or contradictory aspects of an individual's presentation as of the more positive aspects. As the client experiences the safety of acceptance from the therapist, he or she is free to explore these newer or contradictory elements of his or her self with the same acceptance shown by the therapist. In this self-acceptance the client can accept and assimilate more experiences of the self in a broader way than before and move toward a reorganization of self that is more inclusive and comfortable because it is more consistently acceptable to the self (Box 3-1).

BEHAVIOR THERAPY

Behavior therapy involves attempting to modify an observable behavior. It differs from other therapies in that *the focus is on the behavior rather than the cause*. The behavior could be an emotional response, verbalization, or action.

THEORETIC OVERVIEW

One of the early theorists working with the concept of behaviors was Ivan Pavlov (1849-1936). Pavlov described the learned behavior he observed when a stimulus was present and when a response to that stimulus was given. He was well known for his studies with salivation of dogs. Pavlov first noted that dogs salivate when food is within their sight and that the salivation occurs even before the dog begins to eat. As an experiment, Pavlov would ring a bell and present food to the dog, and the dog would salivate. After repeating this sequence several times, the dog salivated with the ringing of the bell, whether or not the food was present. Pavlov called this *conditioned response* or *classical conditioning*.

Another theorist involved in early behaviorist work was B.F. Skinner (1904-1990). Skinner's belief was that virtually all behavior resulted from learned environmental experiences. He thought not only that human behavior is completely determined by one's history but also that one

learns from those experiences that have been repeatedly reinforced. This is known as *operant conditioning*.

Even though both of these theorists looked at behavior, Pavlov proved that the stimulus occurred before the behavior, and Skinner believed that the reinforcement should come after the behavior occurred. It is obvious, then, that Pavlov's theories of behavior were more experimentally driven, whereas Skinner took a more retrospective approach.

BASIC CONCEPTS

All therapies involve learning to some degree, but proponents of behavior therapy view client learning as the primary focus of their work. The behavioral therapist engages the client in an activity that is focused on learning about an unwanted or troubling behavior. By having the client focus on his or her problem behavior, it separates the problem or behavior from the client. The problem is something the client *has* rather than *is*. This process, in essence, allows the client to become a "scientist," and as such, the client is able to study the problem in an intellectual way rather than in an emotional way. Therefore there is some distance placed between the client and the problem behavior.

Once the problem behavior has become separate from the client and the client believes it is something he or she "has" rather than "is," the problem can more clearly be observed, dissected, and attacked. Because the problem is not part of the whole person, aggressive treatment will not interfere with the client-therapist relationship. The aggressive treatment will actually strengthen the therapeutic relationship because the therapist and client work together to diminish the problem.

The first goal of behavior therapy is to narrow the problem down to something tangible, clear-cut, and well defined. This allows the client to believe that the problem can be better controlled and removes the feelings of hopelessness and of being overwhelmed. Defining the problem therefore gives the client some relief from his or her symptoms.

TECHNIQUES
Systematic Desensitization

Systematic desensitization is a behavior therapy technique that was created by Joseph Wolpe for treatment of phobias. This treatment begins with a series of graded tasks to be performed by the client. The client is asked to perform an activity that is related to the phobia in some way but that is well within the client's ability. Because the task is easy for the client to accomplish, confidence is established and the client develops the feeling of anticipation and the desire to "get on with the treatment." At this stage the client usually wants to confront the phobia and do even more than what the therapist requires. As treatment progresses, the activities or tasks come closer to approaching the phobia. By the time the client is ready to deal with the phobia, it is generally at the client's insistence, since the therapist is still trying to restrain the client somewhat.

When it is time for the "real life" exposure, the exposure time should be 1 hour or more. This allows time for any feelings of fear, whether psychologic or physically manifested, to diminish naturally. Prolonged exposure allows the client to develop natural relaxation in spite of the phobic situation.

A common element of the task for the client is to keep a journal or log about the therapeutic experience. This enables the client to be the "scientist" and to record any reactions, feelings, and thoughts as they relate to the tasks of therapy. The process of keeping a journal also helps keep the problem narrow, clear-cut, and separate from the client. This method also helps keep physical symptoms distinct and accurate and reduces the likelihood that the client will exaggerate his or her reactions to the event at a later date.

Relaxation Training

Relaxation training is another technique of behavior therapy. There are a variety of relaxation techniques used to decrease anxiety or nervousness and to assist clients who experience sleep disorders.

One technique, known as *abdominal breathing*, can be used on its own or with other relaxation techniques. Abdominal breathing requires that the client breathe deeply by expanding the lower lungs and raising the abdomen and then exhaling. This technique encourages the body to relax and to slow down and thus promotes the feeling of calmness.

Progressive relaxation is another relaxation technique

in which there is systematic contracting and relaxing of different muscle groups. This allows the client to distinguish between the feeling of tension versus relaxation, which is the first step toward effective treatment.

Another technique is called *autogenics*. This technique uses self-talk to promote relaxation. For example, telling oneself "I can handle this," "I am calm," or "I am relaxed" can be helpful in ultimately achieving a relaxed state.

RATIONAL EMOTIVE THERAPY
THEORETIC OVERVIEW

Rational emotive therapy (RET) was developed by Albert Ellis during the 1960s and 1970s as he became disillusioned with the effectiveness of the psychoanalytic approach and yet found the behavioral approach to be limiting as well. Ellis views individuals as being able to actively and consciously choose their orientation toward themselves. His RET is designed to help individuals apply a scientific approach to their own situation to test the validity of their self-assumptions. In this way, Ellis views his approach as "humanistic" in that it encourages individuals to use their most human skill: to think about thinking (Ellis, 1973).

The goal of RET is to assist individuals in their unconditional self-acceptance, not in terms of performance or accomplishments, but only in terms of "being." Ellis points out that self-acceptance does not involve esteeming the self because esteeming implies rating or valuing oneself. In fact, he considers rating the self in any way to be "ridiculous." According to Ellis, the only aspects of a human being that can be rated are traits and performances, and these are distinctly separate from the self. The self is inherently valued. Yet Ellis sees many people choosing to base their self-worth on irrational philosophic premises about life and self. It is the goal of RET to empower individuals with the skills that scientifically challenge these irrational premises, so that they will behave differently (rationally) and enjoy life (Ellis, 1973). Although Ellis defines himself as a humanist, his groundbreaking work is the precursor to cognitive-behavioral therapy.

BASIC CONCEPTS

Ellis agrees with others that an individual must interpret data from the environment to make sense of it and respond to it. A basic premise of RET is that the way in which an individual interprets the data will affect his or her emotions and actions. For instance, if an individual interprets an argument with a significant other as "terrible" or "destructive," he or she may feel frightened and vulnerable. If, however, the individual views the argument as "clearing the air," he or she may feel validated and assertive. Ellis proposes that much of what individuals base their interpretation and behavior on are faulty assumptions learned so early that they are never questioned. These basic irrational ideas are listed in Box 3-2.

CLINICAL APPLICATION
Behavior Therapy

Peggy is working with a behavior therapist to deal with various aspects of her depression. Since she lost her job, she has noticed an increased fearfulness in her life, with old fears becoming more predominant. Especially troublesome is her fear of going to the grocery store.

In her first session she discussed experiencing physical sensations when she was in the store. She became dizzy and nauseated and experienced heart palpitations so often that she feared she would have a heart attack.

She and the therapist have defined the problem of their focus as "panicky/fearful feelings in grocery store."

The treatment begins with the therapist educating Peggy as to the physiologic basis of her symptoms. Her first assignment is to keep a journal of these feelings, noting their intensity and duration and the precipitating event. This begins the work of segmenting the problem and observing it in a scientific, nonemotional manner.

Box 3-2   **Basic Irrational Ideas According to Albert Ellis (RET)**

1. The idea that it is a dire necessity for an adult human to be loved or approved of by virtually every significant other person in his/her life
2. The idea that one should be thoroughly competent, adequate, and achieving in all possible respects, to consider oneself worthwhile
3. The idea that certain people are bad, wicked, or villainous, and that they should be severely blamed and punished for their villainy
4. The idea that it is awful and catastrophic when things are not the way one would like them to be
5. The idea that human unhappiness is externally caused, and that people have little or no ability to control their terrors and disturbances
6. The idea that it is easier to avoid, than to fail, life's difficulties and self-responsibilities
7. The idea that one's past history is an all-important determinant of one's present behavior, and that because something once strongly affected one's life, it should indefinitely affect it

From Ellis A: *Humanistic psychotherapy*, New York, 1973, McGraw-Hill.

ABCs

Ellis proposes that people upset themselves by holding onto and using these basic misassumptions. He demonstrates this interaction between thoughts and emotions with the ABCs of rational emotive therapy. *A* represents the action, activity, or agent (i.e., person) with whom the individual becomes upset. *B* represents the belief system activated by *A*. The belief can be rational or irrational. A rational belief *(rB)* can be supported by data, whereas an irrational belief *(iB)* cannot be supported by any evidence. Irrational beliefs frequently imply a demand for a certain outcome. These demands are frequently couched in phrases containing "should," "ought," or "must." *C* represents the consequence of belief and is either a rational consequence *(rC)* or an irrational consequence *(iC)*. Irrational consequences present as dysfunctional or self-defeating behaviors.

For an example of this ABC schema, consider a student who has received a low grade on an important examination. The grade represents the activating event. If the student evaluates this as a sign of poor performance in the course, this represents a rational belief because it is supported by the data. As a consequence, the student may ask the teacher for extra instruction, join a study group, or engage a tutor. This is a rational consequence to the rational belief and promotes a self-enhancing activity. If, however, the student responds with an irrational belief, the scenario will be different. Perhaps the student thinks, "This proves I'm incompetent and that I'll never make anything of my-

self. I ought to do better." As a consequence of this thinking, the student may become depressed, avoid interactions around the difficult subject, and eventually drop out of school. This represents an irrational consequence of an irrational belief.

To quickly identify the faulty assumptions and modify the consequent self-defeating behaviors, Ellis proposes that therapy include a combination of cognitive approaches and behavioral techniques but always within the structure of a therapeutic relationship that encourages the individual to express emotions. The therapist's stance is one of unconditional acceptance of the individual. This models the basic assumption that the self is totally acceptable, whereas traits or behaviors are to be evaluated. The RET therapist is active and directive, orientating the individual to the scientific method and its application in his or her situation.

TECHNIQUES

The therapy begins with an overview of RET. The therapist orients the individual to the premise that thoughts affect emotions, reactions, and behavior, and that many of one's thoughts are inaccurate. The therapist explains that much of the work will be examining the individual's thoughts and evaluating their accuracy, using the scientific method of testing hypotheses for validity.

The therapist then actively questions the individual to uncover the individual's basic stance toward self and the belief system that supports it. The RET therapist is direct, challenging, and often confrontive. The work is done through questioning rather than making interpretations or statements. The attempt is always to help the individual to become aware of and to challenge self-defeating thinking. RET therapists frequently ask, "How do you know that?" "What proof do you have to support that?" or "Are there other possible explanations?"

RET uses behavioral techniques to help undermine the cognitive aspect of self-defeating behavior. Once an individual is oriented to the therapy and has some recognition of that process, the therapist assigns "activity homework." These activities are designed to test some irrational belief held by the individual or to challenge the behavioral consequence of the irrational belief. The work should always focus on the symptom causing the most discomfort to the client. These activities are designed to proceed progressively and are unique to each individual. For example, Ellis has used role-playing to help individuals to become desensitized to rejection and has assigned progressive tasks to those who procrastinate. He has also assigned public-speaking engagements for shy individuals.

Through all of this, the therapist consistently points out that reality does not support the irrational belief held by the individual. For instance, the individual who is so afraid of rejection does not die or become a worthless person when rejected. The procrastinator does not have to write the world's greatest novel in order to be effective,

CLINICAL APPLICATION
Rational Emotive Therapy

Peggy is in the initial stages of RET and has been educated about the course of therapy, the ABCs, and the irrational ideas of life.

Peggy:	I'm so worthless.
Therapist:	Why do you say that?
Peggy:	I can't do anything.
Therapist:	What can't you do?
Peggy:	I can't be a good wife, or mother, or daughter. I even lost my job. I'm a failure in every aspect of my life.
Therapist:	Let's take them one by one. Which do you want to start with?
Peggy:	Uh, being a mom.
Therapist:	OK. What makes you think you're not a good mom?
Peggy:	I have no patience with the kids. I snap at them more than I used to . . . I don't do anything for them anymore. I used to make cookies or help them with their schoolwork.
Therapist:	Do you still fix dinner?
Peggy:	Sure, but the meals are not as good as they used to be.
Therapist:	Do you talk with the kids at all?
Peggy:	Of course! I keep up with their lives, but I'm not as involved as I should be.
Therapist:	So, you feed them and talk with them. Is that right?
Peggy:	That's right.
Therapist:	But you don't do all the things you think you should, like helping with schoolwork and making cookies. Is that right?
Peggy:	Yeah.
Therapist:	So, because you don't do at least two of the things you think you should, you've decided that you're a failure as a mom. Is that what you think?
Peggy:	Well, yes.
Therapist:	What do you think you're basing that on?
Peggy:	I guess one of those irrational ideas, that I have to be completely competent all the time and in all ways to be worthwhile.

The therapist continues to point out the irrational beliefs held by Peggy until she recognizes that reality does not support those beliefs.

and the shy person is able to speak publicly, albeit with some anxiety.

COGNITIVE THERAPY

Cognitive therapy was begun by Aaron Beck in the 1970s as an outgrowth of his interest in depression. Beck had accepted the Freudian hypothesis that depression represents hostility and that the client withdraws into himself or herself because of a need to suffer. As Beck studied the research, he found that people with depression consistently interpret their experiences in a negative way. As he reviewed this further, he developed a theory of depression and consequently a therapeutic approach based on identifying and counteracting an individual's negative thoughts (or cognitions). Beck acknowledges the contribution of the behavioral therapies in the development of cognitive therapy (especially evident in some of the techniques) (Beck et al, 1979). Beck, however, places much more importance on the internal (or mental) experiences of his clients than does behaviorism (Beck et al, 1979).

THEORETIC OVERVIEW

Beck holds, as do other theorists, that the way in which a person structures the world through thoughts and evaluations largely influences both affect and behaviors. The classic example of the glass filled with water to its midpoint serves to illustrate this point. If one observes the glass to be half empty, one may experience sadness stemming from the loss or fear that there may not be enough water. However, if one's reaction is that the glass is half full, one may be grateful that there is water at all or hopeful that there will be more.

BASIC CONCEPTS

Beck explored this concept with people who experienced depression and found a consistency in the way they structured their experiences. He organized this into a cognitive model of depression.

Cognitive Triad

The **cognitive triad** is Beck's term to identify three common characteristics in the thinking of people with depression. First, depressed people hold a very negative view of themselves, tending to see themselves as defective in some way (psychologically, morally, or physically). Because of these presumed defects, they tend to view themselves as worthless. Second, people with depression tend to evaluate ongoing life events in a negative way (e.g., the glass is *always* half empty). The person with depression tends to misinterpret available data so as to always result in a negative outcome (e.g., defeat, humiliation, rejection, or inadequacy). Third, the person with depression assumes that the future holds no promise and that the current difficulties will continue. He or she expects despair, frustration, and failure to persist (Figure 3-3).

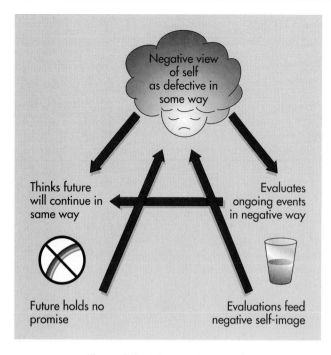

Figure 3-3 The cognitive triad.

The cognitive triad is basic to Beck's understanding of depression. He views all other symptoms of depression as connecting back to these cognitive patterns of negative self-image, negative interpretation of ongoing experiences, and negative view of the future.

Schemas
The term *schema* refers to an individual's organization of incoming data into meaningful patterns. Beck points out that although people tend to conceptualize situations in a variety of ways, an individual will be fairly consistent in interpreting similar sets of data. These schemas have been learned over time and represent attitudes or assumptions that have been formed on the basis of one's experiences. Schemas affect how an individual will cognitively structure experiences and consequently respond to them. Beck proposes that in a state of depression, dysfunctional schemas become prevalent and the data from a situation are distorted to fit the dysfunctional schema. The individual is no longer able to match an appropriate schema to a situation because the dysfunctional schema predominates over so much of the thinking. In effect, any stimulus will trigger the negative, dysfunctional schema. This would then explain why people with depression cannot "see" or respond to the many positive aspects of their lives.

Faulty Information Processing
The characteristics of a depressed person's thinking include **faulty information processing**. Beck calls depressed thinking "primitive" as opposed to more mature thinking. Primitive thinking is more absolute than relative, more

judgmental than flexible, and more invariable than variable. It is "black and white" thinking with the emphasis on black. Primitive thinking misses the context and variations of life and tends to be rigid and fixed. It locks the person with depression into a flat and unidimensional way of thinking, an "all or none" mentality whereby he or she views himself or herself and his or her actions as "all bad." Faulty patterns of processing information are the following:

- *Arbitrary inference:* Drawing a conclusion when evidence does not support it (e.g., deciding that one's boss is displeased with one's work because the boss did not greet one in the morning).
- *Selective abstraction:* Paying attention to only one detail of a situation, taking that detail out of context, and ascribing the meaning to the situation based on this singular detail. For example, a woman is explaining a plan to save enough money to go on a wonderful vacation to her depressed spouse. In the course of doing this, she mentions, "I've always wanted to go there." The depressed spouse then takes this one-sided comment out of context and decides that he has been a failure as a husband because he had not known this and therefore probably had never met her needs in any way.
- *Overgeneralization:* The practice of drawing a conclusion based on one incident and then applying it in general. For example, a person nervously spills a glass of water when talking with another person and concludes that he must be totally socially incompetent and unable to carry on even the simplest of conversations.
- *Magnification and minimization:* The inability to evaluate the importance or significance of an event to the point of creating a distortion. For example, a copy editor misses one minor misprint in a publication and berates herself for months for incompetence.
- *Personalization:* The tendency to assume that external events are related to one's self when there is no reason to make such a connection. For example, a mother makes cookies for her child's class and the next day a few of the children are ill. The mother assumes it is from her cookies, although she does not even know whether the ill children ate the cookies.
- *Absolute thinking:* The habit of defining experiences in one or two opposite categories (e.g., good or bad, perfect or flawed, healthy or sick, worthwhile or worthless).

In summary, the cognitive triad, the concept of schemas, and faulty information processing are the bases for Beck's cognitive therapy of depression. The techniques of cognitive therapy naturally flow from the theory base.

TECHNIQUES
The therapeutic approach in cognitive therapy is a combination of cognitive and behavioral techniques. The cognitive techniques help clients notice their own automatic

negative thoughts and the connection of those thoughts to moods and actions. The cognitive techniques also help individuals evaluate the presence or absence of evidence supporting the automatic thought, and to replace it with a more reality-based interpretation (similar to the scientific method approach of Ellis). The behavioral techniques are used to show individuals that they are capable of interrupting dysfunctional patterns.

Use of the Therapeutic Relationship

Beck repeatedly advises that the therapist must be well grounded in the theory before attempting the therapy. He warns that the techniques can seem "gimmicky" or contrived if they are not based on a solid understanding of the theory. In addition, he stresses the importance of a strong therapeutic relationship and interpersonal skills. It is not enough to simply perform the techniques; the interventions must be based on a sound understanding of the theory and presented within a strong therapeutic relationship of concern, acceptance, and empathy. Beck points out that the effectiveness of a therapeutic relationship depends greatly on the client's ability to experience and express feelings. Very often, people with depression do not think that they can honestly say how they feel and perceive a pressure to keep up a facade to hide the depth of their despair. This can lead them to think of themselves as dishonest and describe themselves as deceitful. It is only in an effective therapeutic relationship that they are able to act in an emotionally congruent manner. This helps to restore a sense of honesty and genuineness (Beck et al, 1979).

Although Beck proposes that all feelings are acceptable and open to discussion, he advises that the therapy time be structured so that the entire time is not used to express emotions. It is the work of therapy to explore the attitudes that cause the emotions, and this is a collaborative process.

The therapist begins by acknowledging the client's "personal paradigm." In this instance a paradigm is a person's model or view of the self. The client's paradigm is his or her particular presentation of the cognitive triad, schemas, and faulty information processing. The therapist has the client give examples of past and present events that confirm his or her negative ideas in an attempt to identify the underlying patterns of thoughts. The therapist makes no attempt to counteract or discount these beliefs. Rather, the cognitive therapist poses questions for the client's consideration. These questions are used to elicit what the client is thinking, as well as to plant the seed of other possibilities the client has ignored. Beck has found skillful questioning to be a useful device for identifying, considering, and correcting cognitions and beliefs (Beck et al, 1979).

Together, the therapist and client redefine the client's initial chief complaint into a target symptom that can be the focus of their work. A target symptom is defined as "any of the components of depressive disorder that involves suffering or functional disability" (Beck et al, 1979). Beck identifies five areas: affective symptoms; motivational symptoms (e.g., the desire to escape); cognitive difficulties; behavioral symptoms; and physiologic, or vegetative, symptoms. Selection of the target symptom is made by choosing the one that is most upsetting to the client and also amenable to therapy. The work is then to identify and correct the specific thinking that leads to these symptoms.

Reattribution Techniques

Perhaps the best-known specific cognitive techniques are reattribution techniques. These techniques are designed to assist the depressed individual who automatically assumes total blame or responsibility for anything that goes wrong and to help the person with depression realize that there are many reasons for things to go wrong, not just one's presence in the world. The technique has also been called "de-responsibilitizing" because it assists in relieving the client of the burden of total responsibility for everything in his or her life.

This technique requires that the client keep a record that consists of four columns with the following head-

---

CLINICAL APPLICATION
Cognitive Therapy

The following is Peggy's "homework" and is an example of reattribution technique.

Situation	Emotions	Automatic Thoughts	Other Interpretations
Kids were late for school.	Upset/shame. I made a mistake.	I should have helped them more in morning. I did something wrong.	They dawdled (wasted time) on the way. The clocks are off.
I forgot name of person I was introducing to friend.	Embarrassed. Humiliated.	I'm losing my mind. I can't do anything right. I'm socially inept.	Everybody forgets sometimes. I'd only met her once, over a month ago.
Burned cookies.	Shamed. Sad.	I'm a failure. I can't even do simple things.	Buzzer didn't go off. Kids didn't call me.

ings: Situation; Emotions; Automatic Thoughts; Other Interpretations.

The client records situations that trigger negative feelings and records these feelings and the automatic thoughts associated with them. The client is then challenged to come up with other possible explanations regarding the situation and, by so doing, begins to evaluate and modify the automatic thoughts.

Behavioral Techniques

Beck emphasizes that behavioral techniques are used to supplement the cognitive work. One of the main reasons for using a behavioral technique is to demonstrate to the client that the negative assumptions and conclusions are incorrect and thus pave the way for improvement in performance in those aspects of life that are important to the client.

After the therapist has assisted the client with identification of appropriate data to be studied, he or she designs an experiment to help the client become more specific in his or her observations and thinking and to recognize gradations. For example, the therapist may ask the client to keep an activity schedule to test the hypothesis that inactivity increases negative thinking. If so, then perhaps activity would decrease such thoughts. The client's task is to make a schedule of daily activities and record their effect on cognition, as well as any changes in the level of depressed thinking that accompanies the activity. The point is to get the client to observe (not evaluate) how much is accomplished by the client throughout the day.

Such an "experiment" implies many things, such as the following: the client can organize activities; there are subtleties to reactions that the client may be missing; and the despair may be influenced by activities. None of this is "told" to the client, but rather left for the client to discover through the homework and the skillful questioning of the therapist.

Mastery and Pleasure Technique

The next step may be the mastery and pleasure technique. Mastery refers to the sense of accomplishment one feels after a task completion, and pleasure refers to the pleasant feeling associated with it. In this technique the client rates a certain activity in terms of his or her mastery over it and pleasure in doing the task. This technique begins to counteract the client's unidimensional thinking by having him or her notice even small variations in successes and pleasures (Beck et al, 1979).

Cognitive Rehearsal

In cognitive rehearsal the client is asked to imagine all of the steps required to complete a task. This is useful in breaking down the repetitive thought patterns that so often prevent a depressed client from accomplishing things.

When the client has demonstrated the ability to observe his or her actions and thoughts, the therapist moves to the higher level of cognitive techniques, to assist the client in discovering his or her own thinking and in testing the validity of his or her automatic thoughts. It is here that the therapist and client act as true collaborators as the client learns to observe and record his or her thoughts, images, and self-talk, and the therapist continues to help the client to observe and identify the dysfunctional thinking. After the client has identified an automatic thought, the therapist poses questions that help the client ascertain the connection between the thought and certain behaviors the client has identified, especially those in recent experiences. Homework is assigned to further assist the client in this task.

The therapy continues until the client is able to identify his or her automatic thoughts, recognize their effects on feelings and behaviors, and develop more balanced cognitions and self-statements more reflective of reality.

STRATEGIC THERAPY

Communication theorists propose that the actual structure of language creates reality for individuals. They suggest that the choice, use, and organization of words influence one's perceptions of one's experiences. In fact, many theorists propose that defining an experience with words limits and confines the experience (Box 3-3). Consequently, communication theorists have extensively investigated how language can influence a person's perceptions and reactions and, in a therapeutic sense, how the use of words can promote health.

Strategic therapy, a form of communication therapy, is considered an effective and time-efficient approach to treatment. There are variations of strategic therapy (i.e., solution-focused therapy, brief therapy), but all types trace their beginnings to the pioneering work of Gregory Bateson, Don Jackson, Paul Watzlawick, John Weakland, and Richard Fisch at the Mental Research Institute (MRI) in Palo Alto, California, in the 1950s and 1960s. This group took a decidedly different approach in its attempt to decrease the time of treatment for individuals and families. They studied the process of change itself. The "Palo Alto Group" examined problem formulation and maintenance in human systems and how best to promote change in that system (Greene, 1991).

Box 3-3   Strategic Therapy Exercise

Become aware of the position your body is in now: the various points of pressure, the feel of the clothing on your skin, the position of the muscles. To name it "sitting," "standing," or "lying" certainly identifies it but limits the nuances. This is also the nature of more complex social interactions.

THEORETIC OVERVIEW

Strategic therapy represents a departure from medical model–based approaches. In the medical model the healer diagnoses a disorder or dysfunction and then treats it. Strategic therapy is based on the approach of one of its founders, anthropologist Gregory Bateson. While working with clients with psychosis at a Veterans Administration (VA) hospital, Bateson would ask, "In what human context does this 'crazy' behavior fit?" The anthropologic position is that behavior makes sense in the context in which it occurs. This is one of the underlying assumptions of strategic therapy. The corollary to this is that behavior is continually being shaped and reinforced by the individual's support system (i.e., the family), and vice versa. This is called the **interactive context of behavior** (Fisch, Weakland, and Segal, 1986). Over time, behavior patterns arise between people, and some patterns may be viewed as problematic. A strategic therapist always examines the problem behavior in the context of the surrounding behaviors.

The MRI group theorizes that the reason behaviors are viewed as problematic has to do with people's perception of reality. Most people assume that there is one reality that is based on objective truths and that their own thinking reflects this. If this assumption is valid, then it would follow that anyone with a different view of reality than their own must be either "mad" or "bad" (Watzlawick, 1977). The MRI Group proposes that there is no *one* reality. Each person creates his or her own reality through communication with others (Watzlawick, 1977). For example, a child's behavior may be called "stubborn" by one individual and "determined" by another. Each definition creates a different "reality" for the child and other. If the child's behavior is seen as "stubborn," it may also be viewed as problematic and requiring treatment. If it is seen as "determined," it may become a source of pride and esteem. As Shakespeare said, "Nothing is good or bad, but thinking makes it so." The concept of reality as a function of one's communication is essential. Following this, change is approached within the framework of communication and the complainant's* view of reality. To promote change, the strategic therapist must learn the individual's view of the reality of the problem.

The MRI group has done a considerable amount of research on change, and it has defined two types: first-order change and second-order change. *First-order change* is defined as a change within the system that remains unchanged. *Second-order change* is that which changes the system itself. Second-order change is discontinuous and therefore appears illogical from within the system (Watzlawick, 1974). One of MRI's classic examples will help to illustrate first- and second-order changes. *Example of first-order change:* A dreamer is caught in a nightmare.

Within her dream, she does many things to end the nightmare: she runs, hides, and tries to change its course. This is first-order change, since the dreamer is attempting to change the course of the dream from within the dream. *Example of second-order change:* The only way the dreamer can change the dream is to awaken and be in a different state altogether. This is second-order change because it changes the system itself from without (Watzlawick, 1974).

Strategic therapy creates second-order change in human systems, and these changes seem illogical from within the system. Strategic therapists propose that insight is not a necessary prerequisite for change. Rather, people must learn how to act in a different way if they are to see things in a different way. This is congruent with thinking that reality is created through communication and behaviors are a form of communication.

BASIC CONCEPTS

To work within this orientation, it is necessary to understand two concepts: *attempted solutions* and *position*.

Attempted Solutions

Basic to this approach is the view of problem development and maintenance. The MRI model defines a problem as a client's concern about some behavior (action, thought, or feeling) in the self, or another behavior that is described as deviant or distressing in some way. Furthermore, *all of the client's efforts to stop or change this behavior have failed*, and the client is seeking the therapist's help to change the situation (Fisch, Weakland, and Segal, 1986). There are two important points here: (1) the client's repeated and best attempts at change have failed; and (2) the request for assistance is for a specific problem, not a personality makeover. The strategic therapy approach focuses on change in relation to the identified problem.

In the MRI model, problems are the result of mishandled or wrong attempts at changing an area of difficulty. In other words, it is the attempted solutions that create the problem. An attempted solution is simply the client's best attempt to change a troublesome situation, but the attempt repeatedly fails and further aggravates the situation. Most attempted solutions are first-order changes and are simply repetitions of a theme. For example, a couple presents with complaints of family distress based on their perception of their teenage son's defiant stance toward them, as demonstrated by his consistent disregard of curfew. They scolded and disciplined him to get him to comply with rules, only to see him increase his defiance as a result of their attempts. Their attempted solutions were variations on the theme "You Will Obey Us," and only served to maintain the problem and possibly aggravate it.

There are three ways to mishandle a difficulty: (1) an action is necessary but none is taken (as in the case of denial); (2) an action is taken when it should not be (as in the case of a nonproblem being defined as a problem); and (3)

Complainant refers to the person who presents with a complaint and is requesting assistance.

an action is taken at the wrong level (i.e., a first-order change is attempted when a second-order change is necessary) (Watzlawick, 1974).

Attempted solutions are *problem-maintaining behaviors* in that the attempts to solve the problem actually aggravate it despite the reasonableness of the approach. The MRI group believes that people continue problem-maintaining behavior inadvertently and often with the best of intentions. They do not view the presence of a problem as an indicator of a pathologic condition (Fisch, Weakland, and Segal, 1986). Because it is the attempted solution that is noted to worsen (or at least maintain) the problem, strategic therapists aim their interventions at the attempted solutions rather than the problem itself (Watzlawick, 1974).

Position

To know how to intervene, it is important that the therapist understand the client's position on the problem—the values, beliefs, and priorities of the client (Fisch, Weakland, and Segal, 1986). In brief, the client's position is his or her view of the "reality" of the situation and is demonstrated by the client's language, perception of the problem, and motivations. It is essential that strategic therapists understand the client's position in order to present the intervention in a way that the client will accept and use (Greene, 1991). One of the most basic positions to note is whether the client is "benevolently concerned" about the behavior or is feeling victimized. Benevolent concern implies that the problem behavior is not willfully done (i.e., it is caused by a sickness, illness, or weakness). Victimization implies a willful enactment of the behavior and is viewed as "bad" by the client. In the example of the teenage boy, the parents' position was that their son was "bad" (i.e., willfully stayed out) and that he had control over his behavior. The same case would present differently if their view was that the behavior was out of their son's control as a result of some infirmity, such as being stressed over schoolwork or being unable to tell time because of a learning disability. The therapist's intervention must always be congruent with the client's position.

TECHNIQUES

The techniques of strategic therapy are designed to provide the client with a "chance occurrence" that provides a new frame of reference with which to view the problem. Watzlawick (1977) tells the following story to explain chance occurrences.

Suppose a man presents in therapy with a fear of elephants. To keep elephants away, he has begun incessant hand clapping. There are several ways the therapist can deal with this: the therapist can develop a trusting relationship with the man so that when the therapist says there is no reason to fear elephants, the man believes the therapist; the therapist can work to uncover the cause of this fear of elephants, with the assumption that under-

standing the source of the fear will stop the fear; or the therapist can introduce elephants into the therapy and demonstrate that there is no reason to fear them. Or suppose that one day, on the way to therapy, the man is involved in an accident in which both his hands are broken. Despite the fact that he cannot clap, no elephants approach, and he learns that he no longer needs to apply his solution of hand clapping. This unplanned occurrence provides a corrective emotional experience. The goal of strategic interventions is to create planned chance occurrences that lead to corrective emotional experiences. Planned chance occurrences are accomplished by either interrupting the problem-maintaining behavior or altering the client's view of the problem so it no longer causes distress (Fisch, Weakland, and Segal, 1986).

Symptom Prescription

Symptom prescription involves the therapist prescribing the very symptom from which the client is seeking relief. Symptom prescription is useful when the attempted solution has been to force something that can only occur spontaneously. This often occurs with bodily functions in which normal fluctuations are defined as problems (e.g., sexual preference, insomnia, memory blocks, gastrointestinal and urinary functions). The symptom is perceived by the client as spontaneous and out of the client's control (e.g., "I'm frigid," "I'm impotent," "I can't sleep," "I can't remember," "I wet my pants"), and yet clients work very hard to stop these behaviors. However, the attempted solution maintains the symptomatic behavior. Symptom prescription is aimed at having the client stop the attempted solutions by directing the client to perform another behavior. The strategic therapist provides a rationale and directions to fail at "attempted solutions" behaviors. The client is often instructed to bring on the symptom for diagnostic purposes or as a beginning step toward behavioral control (Fisch, Weakland, and Segal, 1986).

For example, the impotent man is instructed to maintain his impotence so that he can study his thoughts during intercourse. He is unable to maintain his impotence and enjoys intercourse. Thus the "attempted solution" ("I have to have an erection") is interrupted with the direction, "Do not, under any circumstances, have an erection," and as a result normal functioning returns.

Another variation of symptom prescription can be employed when the attempted solution revolves around mastering a feared event by avoiding it. This is often the case with fear and anxiety states (e.g., phobias, performance blocks, fear of public speaking or of beginning relationships). In these situations the client is exposed to the task but instructed not to master it (Fisch, Weakland, and Segal, 1986). For example, the client with a driving phobia is instructed to sit in the car for 30 minutes a day and consider the hazards of driving. During this time, the driver must never consider the pleasures of driving and does not actually drive at all. This again stops the client's attempted solution of avoiding the task while pushing himself or herself to master it by being presented with an alternate behavior to perform.

Reframing

Reframing is a powerful verbal tool used to create a second-order change. It involves changing the conceptual and/or emotional setting or viewpoint in which a situation is seen and placing it "in another frame that fits the facts of the situation equally well or even better, and thereby change its entire meaning" (Watzlawick, 1974). A reframe does not change anything about the client's view of the problem situation. It works by making the client's old view (or frame) absolute. To work, the reframe must always fit the client's position and be congruent with his or her understanding of the situation. However, the reframe changes the way that the situation is viewed.

For example, a 40-year-old woman is hospitalized with suicidal depression. She is despondent because she never seems to be able to please her parents, and the staff observes her parents frequently criticizing and belittling her. She continues to please them, only to be told that she will never be as good as her brothers and sisters who have moved away. In this situation the attempted solution was the client's repeated attempts to please. A reframe of the situation was initiated and proved very successful. The client was congratulated on being such a fine and caring daughter. Obviously, her parents feared an end to their parental role, and she provided them an opportunity to continue this role. By allowing them to criticize her, she reassured them that their job was not done and that their parental role could continue.

CLINICAL APPLICATION
Strategic Therapy

Peggy is having her second meeting with a strategic therapist.

Peggy:	I just can't do anything right. I'm a total failure.
Therapist:	What do you fail at?
Peggy:	Life! You name it, I fail at it. I burn cookies, oversleep, lose my job and my car keys. I don't seem to be able to do anything right. Everybody notices; they're just too nice to say anything.
Therapist:	Well, I have a suggestion, but it may be too much for you to do because you seem to be a perfectionist, and perfectionists have a hard time with this.
Peggy:	Tell me; I'll do anything.
Therapist:	This will be difficult for you to do. I want you to plan three perfect mistakes, or failures, as you call them. Now, these failures must be a secret, and you must not tell anyone what you've planned. You tell your family you're going to make these mistakes that day and ask them to figure out what they are.
Peggy:	I already make three mistakes a day.
Therapist:	Yes, but I want you to plan these mistakes, not leave them to chance.

When Peggy returns in 2 weeks, she delightedly reports that no one even noticed her planned failures.

Table 3-1   Summary of Theoretic Approaches

	Psychoanalytic	Adlerian	Transactional Analysis	Gestalt	Client-Centered	Behavioral	Rational Emotive Therapy	Cognitive	Strategic
Basic Orientation	All behavior is meaningful. Behavior is influenced by unconscious impulses and conflicts	Behavior is socially based, purposeful, and conscious	Life stance reflected in changing communication patterns. Can enhance effectiveness and decrease dysfunction by clarifying communication	Intrapsychic conflicts arise from interactions with society	Human beings move toward constructive change and integration	Behavior is learned	Individuals can choose thoughts and behaviors that promote or limit self-acceptance	Individual's affect and behavior are determined by his or her organization of world through thoughts and assumptions	Reality is created through communication with others
Concepts	Id, ego, superego. Unconscious and preconscious	Phenomenologic approach. Final goal. Gemeinschaftsgefühl	Ego states: parent, adult, child. Games. Script analysis	Organism; top dog and underdog. Figure-background formation	Interpersonal relationships are basis for health and neurosis	Conditioning. Separation of client from problem	ABCs of interaction	Cognitive triad. Schemas. Faulty information processing	Attempted solutions. Position

Goal

Uncover unconscious conflict and empower the ego to deal with it	Become a more fully functioning person	Interact from role-appropriate ego state	Mutual acknowledgment and integration of organisms top dog and underdog through completion of unfinished situation	Bring aspects of self into awareness and acceptance	Modify observable behavior	Provide skills to scientifically challenge irrational premises and change behavior	Develop balanced cognitions and self-statements	To decrease pain that a person is experiencing as a result of his or her view of a situation

Techniques

Dream analysis Free association	Socratic questioning Encouragement	Structural analysis Transactional analysis Game analysis Script analysis	Chair work Dream work	Unconditional and positive regard Therapeutic relationships Alter ego	Systematic desensitization Relaxation training	Cognitive approach Behavioral: Role-playing Progressive tasks Questioning	Cognitive: Questioning Reattribution Behavioral: Activity schedule Cognitive rehearsal	Reframing Symptom prescription

Summary of Key Concepts

1. Theories of human behavior are developed with the goal of producing frameworks that enhance understanding of the complexities of human behavior and somehow define or interpret them and thus base effective interventions (Table 3-1).
2. The psychoanalytic approach to treatment is based on the belief that all behavior is meaningful and is influenced by unconscious impulses and conflicts represented by the id, ego, superego, unconscious, and preconscious.
3. Adlerian therapy views humans as socially based, capable of developing unique lifestyles rather than being shaped by their childhood experiences.
4. Transactional analysis is based on the belief that the individual's life stance is reflected in communication and that dysfunction can be decreased by clarifying the communication in the specified ego state.
5. Gestalt therapy is based on the belief that intrapsychic conflicts arise from interactions with society and that only integration of all the organisms can offer completion.
6. The client-centered approach to mental health is based on the belief that human beings move toward constructive change and integration and that interpersonal relationships are the basis for health and neurosis.
7. The behavioral approach maintains that behavior is learned; therefore conditioning and separation of the client from the problem through systematic desensitization and relaxation training can modify undesirable behavior.
8. Rational emotive therapy is based on the belief that individuals can choose thoughts and behaviors and thus select to sometimes promote or limit self-acceptance. Through cognitive tasks, a therapist can provide the skills to scientifically challenge irrational premises and change behavior.
9. Cognitive (Beck's) therapy is based on the belief that an individual's behavior is influenced by the way he or she structures the world, through thoughts and assumptions. Through cognitive and behavioral activities, one can develop balanced thoughts and self-statements.
10. Strategic therapy assumes that reality for each person is created through communication with others, affecting his or her view of every situation.
11. Each theory outlines various techniques for promoting desirable behavior.

REFERENCES

Beck AT: *Depression: clinical, experimental and theoretical aspects*, New York, 1967, Harper & Row.

Beck AT: *Depression: causes and treatment*, Philadelphia, 1971, University of Pennsylvania Press.

Beck AT: *The diagnosis and management of depression*, Philadelphia, 1973, University of Pennsylvania Press.

Beck AT et al: *Cognitive therapy of depression*, New York, 1979, Guilford Press.

Berne E: *Games people play*, New York, 1964, Ballantine.

Berne E: *What do you say after you say "Hello"?* New York, 1972, Grove Press.

Corey G: *Theory and practice of counseling and psychotherapy*, ed 4, Pacific Grove, Calif, 1991, Brooks/Cole Publishing.

Ellis A: *Humanistic psychotherapy*, New York, 1973, McGraw-Hill.

Ellis A: *Handbook of rational-emotive therapy*, New York, 1977, Springer Publishing.

Ellis A: *The practice of rational-emotive therapy*, New York, 1987, Springer Publishing.

Fisch R, Weakland J, Segal: *The tactics of change*, San Francisco, 1986, Jossey-Bass.

Freud A: *Introduction to psychoanalysis for teachers*, London, 1931, George Allen.

Freud A: *The writings of Anna Freud*, New York, 1967, International Universities Press.

Freud A: *Psychoanalysis for teachers and parents: introductory lectures*, New York, 1979, WW Norton.

Freud S: *The ego and the id*, New York, 1960, Norton Library.

Goulding M, Goulding R: *Changing lives through redecision therapy*, New York, 1979, Grove Press.

Greene RL: Brief strategic treatment: the tactical promotion of change, *Newsletter, Academy of San Diego Psychologists*, pp 1-4, May 1991.

Kovel J: *A complete guide to therapy from psychoanalysis to behavior modification*, New York, 1976, Pantheon Books.

Rogers CP: *Client centered therapy*, Boston, 1951, Houghton Mifflin.

Rogers CP: *On becoming a person*, Boston, 1961, Houghton Mifflin.

Rogers CR: *Person to person, the problem of being human*, Walnut Creek, Calif, 1967, Real People Press.

Rogers P, Reich R, Nicholi AM Jr, editors: Psychosomatic medicine and consultation-liaison psychiatry. In *The new Harvard guide to psychiatry*, Cambridge, Mass, 1988, Belknap Press of Harvard University Press.

Skinner BF: *Science and human behavior,* New York, 1953, MacMillan.

Stein H, Edwards M: Classical Adlerian theory and practice. In Marcus P, Rosenberg A, editors: *Philosophies of life and their impact on practice,* New York, 1998, NYU Press.

Stevens O, editor: *Gestalt is—addresses, essays, lectures,* Moab, Utah, 1975, Real People Press.

Watzlawick P, Weakland J, Fisch R: *Change,* New York, 1974, WW Norton.

Watzlawick P: *How real is real?* New York, 1977, Vintage Books.

INTERNET SOURCES

Internet Mental Health, *http://www.mentalhealth.com/copy/html*

Mental Health Info Source, *http://www.mhsource.com/edu/index.html*

PsychoPro Online, *http://www.onlinepsych.com*

CHAPTER 4

Psychobiology

Kathleen M. Walker and James M. Turnbull

OBJECTIVES

- Identify the basic anatomic structures of the central nervous system.

- Describe the physiologic functions of the central nervous system.

- Describe normal functioning of neurons.

- Discuss the role of common neurotransmitters in the functioning of the central nervous system.

- Describe the electrochemical mechanism of the central nervous system.

- Identify common client care concerns for patients having neuroimaging testing.

- Identify the common behavioral symptoms demonstrated by clients with brain-based abnormalities who are diagnosed with mental disorders.

- Formulate potential areas for further nursing research related to neurobiology.

Action potential A wave of electrical depolarization that travels down a neuron to transfer information; when the impulse reaches the end of the neuron, it stimulates the production and release of chemical compounds called neurotransmitters.

Amygdala The part of the limbic system that modulates common emotional states such as feelings of anger and aggression, love, and comfort in social settings.

Association cortex The part of the cerebral frontal lobe that performs many of the activities that make us human, such as reasoning, planning, working memory, insight, inhibition, and judgment; the area of the brain most responsible for personality.

Axon The part of the neuron that transmits signals from the neuron's cell body to connect with other neurons and cells.

Basal ganglia An area of the central nervous system made up of cell bodies and that is responsible for motor functions and association.

Central nervous system A division of the human nervous system containing the brain and spinal cord.

Cerebral cortex The thin layer of gray matter that makes up the surface of the two cerebral hemispheres; the area where information related to sensation, speech, thinking, voluntary motor function, and perception is merged.

Cerebrum The largest structure in the central nervous system; can be subdivided into right and left hemispheres and contains four main lobes.

Corpus callosum A large bundle of white matter that connects the right and left sides of the cerebral cortex.

Dendrites The part of the neuron designed to collect incoming signals from other neurons and send the signal to the neuron's cell body.

Extrapyramidal motor system A collection of nerve fibers responsible for much of the involuntary motor functioning of the central nervous system; can be adversely impacted by drugs used to treat mental illness.

Fissures Grooves on the surface of the brain that extend deep into the brain.

Frontal lobe The largest of the four lobes of the cerebrum; responsible for motor function, higher thought, memory, and judgment.

Gray matter Brain tissue composed of nerve cell bodies and dendrites.

Gyri Raised convolutions visible on the cerebral cortex surface.

Hippocampus The area located in the inside fold of the temporal lobe below the thalamus; the site of the intersection between the storage of memories and their reproduction of emotional coloring.

Hypothalamus The part of the limbic system that rests deep within the brain and helps regulate basic human functions such as sleep-rest patterns, body temperature, and physical drives of hunger and sex.

Limbic system A group of structures found deep in the brain; responsible for modulation of instincts, drives, needs, and emotions.

Motor cortex The part of the frontal lobe responsible for controlling voluntary motor activity of specific muscles.

Neuron A nerve cell, the elemental functioning unit in the brain; composed of a cell body, an axon, and connecting dendrite branches.

Neurotransmitter A chemical substance released by presynaptic cells when stimulated that functions to activate postsynaptic cells and thus cause them to act as messengers in the central nervous system. Common neurotransmitters are acetylcholine, dopamine, norepinephrine, serotonin, and γ-aminobutyric acid (GABA).

Occipital lobe A division of the cerebrum that is responsible for visual functioning.

Parietal lobe A division of the cerebrum that functions as a processing center.

Peripheral nervous system A division of the nervous system that includes all nerves not in the brain or spinal cord and includes the cranial nerves.

Premotor area The part of the frontal lobe responsible for coordinated voluntary movement of multiple muscles.

Sulci Shallow grooves in the surface of the cerebrum running between gyri.

Temporal lobe One of the four lobes of the cerebrum responsible for hearing and receiving auditory information.

Thalamus Part of the limbic system and primarily a regulatory structure that relays all sensory information, except smell, from the peripheral nervous system to the cortex of the central nervous system.

White matter Brain tissue composed of the myelinated axons of neurons.

The 1990s have been referred to as the "decade of the brain." Certainly, at no time in the past has so much been known about the most complex organ in the human body. New technologies have increased researchers' ability to examine the brain and understand the complex manner in which the brain works. Accelerated learning about the brain has led to better understanding of the biologic basis of mental disorders. The explosion of new knowledge about the brain has greatly influenced the care of the mentally disordered and the role of the psychiatric mental health nurse. Today's psychiatric mental health nurse is faced with significantly different patient care issues from those of nurses even 10 years ago. Mental disorders are beginning to be understood as "brain-based" illnesses, lay publications are devoting volumes to helping the public understand the chemistry of the brain, and medical and nursing treatments are increasingly specific to targeted brain areas in attempts to correct brain-based anomalies. Psychiatric mental health nurses need to be aware of the anatomy and physiology of the brain and increasingly must be aware of psychobiologic approaches to treating the mentally disordered.

UNDERSTANDING NEUROBIOLOGIC FUNCTIONS

Although approaches to understanding the psychobiologic model of mental disorders date back to the time of the classical Greeks, modern understanding of this biology has been shaped by current neuroscience (Carpenter and Buchanan, 1994). Psychobiologic models of nursing care incorporate information from many fields, including neuroanatomy, neurophysiology, neuropharmacology, neuroimaging (such as computed tomography [CT], positron emission tomography [PET], magnetic resonance imaging [MRI], and single photon emission computed tomography [SPECT] scans), neurochemistry, and neuropsychology. New, emerging fields are becoming more critical in understanding mental disorders and include neuroendocrinology (the study of the impact of normally occurring substances on brain functioning), psychoimmunology (the study of the impact of psychosocial events on a person's biologic functioning), and genetics, the study of the role of genes in the development of mental disorders) (Collins, 1997).

The biologic model has been increasingly used by nurses as a means of understanding and treating clients with serious mental disorders. The symptoms associated with mental disorders are often manifested behaviorally. Clients with mental disorders frequently do not behave in ways society considers normal. They may express their disorders through behavior such as hearing voices, considering suicide, or wearing a winter coat on a hot summer day. Understanding the structural or neurochemical defect experienced by clients with mental disorders allows

psychiatric mental health nurses to assess these clients' behaviors and plan interventions to improve health. The best psychiatric mental health nursing care begins with understanding normal brain functioning and how it has been altered by illness. Whether a client has bipolar disorder, schizophrenia, panic disorder, major depression, or dementia, the basis for all aspects of nursing care in clients with these brain-based illnesses starts with understanding the normal brain and how it operates.

NEUROANATOMY AND NEUROPHYSIOLOGY OF THE HUMAN NERVOUS SYSTEM

Human thoughts, feelings, and actions begin in the nervous system. Although it weighs only 3 to 5 pounds, the brain contains over 100 billion neurons, making it the most complex and vital of human organs (Haines, 1997). The nervous system of human beings is composed of two separate but interconnected divisions. The first division, the **central nervous system** (CNS), is composed of the spinal cord and the brain and is commonly thought of as any nervous system tissue that is protected by the bones of either the skull or the vertebrae. The second division, the **peripheral nervous system** (PNS), contains peripheral nerves and includes the cranial nerves starting from just outside of the brain stem.

Although the peripheral nervous system is of critical importance to human functioning, understanding of mental disorders most often involves in-depth understanding of the structure and function of the CNS. For that reason, the rest of this chapter focuses on understanding the CNS and how that knowledge can be used to provide nursing care to the mentally disordered.

NEUROANATOMY

Understanding the normal structures of the brain and their functions in directing human behavior is one of the best ways to comprehend the complexity of the brain. Brain tissue is categorized as either white or gray matter. **White matter** is the myelinated axons of neurons, and **gray matter** is composed of nerve cell bodies and dendrites. The gray matter is the working area of the brain, and because the gray matter contains the cell bodies, it also contains the synapses between the cell bodies.

CEREBRUM

The **cerebrum,** the largest part of the brain, is divided into two halves called cerebral hemispheres. The cerebral hemispheres compose the bulk of the CNS and include the cerebral cortex, limbic system, and basal ganglia. These structures are described in more detail within this chapter. Figure 4-1 shows these divisions of the CNS.

The cerebral hemispheres account for over 70% of the neurons in the CNS and are responsible for functions such

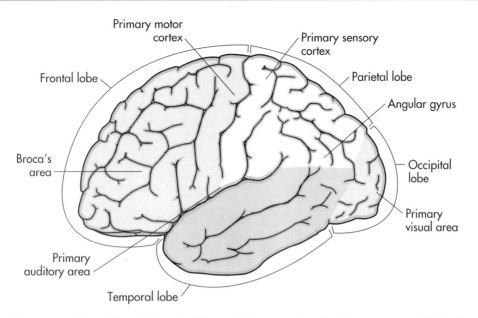

Figure 4-1   Map of the cortex. (From Hamdy R et al: *Alzheimer's disease: a handbook for caregivers,* ed 3, St. Louis, 1998, Mosby.)

as hearing and vision. In most people one hemisphere is dominant and is responsible for language expression. The left hemisphere, dominant in almost 95% of people, controls functions mainly on the right side of the body. The right hemisphere, dominant in only about 5% of people, controls functions on the left side of the body. Most right-handed people, as well as about half of left-handed people, have a dominant left hemisphere. In rare cases people may have mixed dominance, with one side dominant for language expression and the other for motor functions such as handwriting.

Although differences between the hemispheres have been of interest to researchers, effective coordinated human activity requires a complex interrelationship and communication between the two hemispheres. The hemispheres are connected by a large bundle of white matter referred to as the **corpus callosum.** Sensorimotor information constantly flows between the two hemispheres via nerve pathways that are contained in the corpus collosum. Since information from one hemisphere is continuously transmitted to the other hemisphere via this connection, the corpus callosum must be intact for full, smooth, and coordinated bilateral behavior.

The **cerebral cortex** is the thin layer of gray matter that makes up the surface of the two hemispheres. The cerebral cortex is responsible for much of the behavior that makes us human. Areas of the brain that are responsible for sensations, speech, thinking, voluntary motor function, and perceptions merge in this area of the CNS. Cortical brain tissue, regardless of where it is located, performs one of four functions: primary sensory function, primary motor function, secondary sensory function, or association function.

The outermost surface of the brain cortex contains corrugated wrinkles with many grooves and indentations. Shallow grooves are called **sulci,** and the deeper groves extending deep into the brain are called **fissures.** The raised areas are called **gyri.** These fissures, sulci, and gyri give the brain its characteristic look and provide identifiable landmarks indicating specific areas of the brain. The wrinkles and grooves also dramatically increase the overall surface area of the cerebral cortex. Because the brain has wrinkles and grooves, the cerebral cortex contains almost 70% of the total neurons in the CNS, with over 70 miles of axons and dendrites; the surface area, if spread out, equals almost 2.5 square feet.

The cerebrum can be further divided into four distinct regions referred to as lobes. These are the frontal lobe, the temporal lobe, the occipital lobe, and the parietal lobe. Although these lobes work in an interrelated manner, each of the lobes has a distinct function. Many of the symptoms exhibited by clients with mental illness can be understood as a disturbance in the normal functioning of one or more of these lobes. The normal functions of each lobe, along with typical symptoms of disturbances in each cerebral region of the brain, are shown in Table 4-1.

The **frontal lobe** is the largest lobe, and human beings as a species have the best-developed frontal lobes of all mammals. Much of what makes human behavior unique can be explained by the functioning of the frontal lobe. The frontal lobe contains several important structures that give it its important function. The motor strip, or **motor cortex,** lies in front of a large sulci and is also called the precentral gyrus. The motor cortex of the frontal lobe is responsible for controlling voluntary motor activity of specific muscles. Nerves from the frontal lobe can be directly traced to the peripheral nerves that innervate the muscles of the body; they form a pyramid-shaped bulge

Table 4-1		Normal Functions and Symptoms of Dysfunction of the Cerebrum	
Lobe	Location	Normal Function	Symptoms of Alterations in Brain Functioning
Frontal	Anterior, or front area, of brain	Programming and execution of motor functions Higher thought processes, such as planning, ability to abstract, trial-and-error learning, and decision making Intellectual insight, judgment Expression of emotion	Changes in affect, such as flattening Alteration in language production Alteration in motor functioning Impulsive behavior Impaired decision making Concrete thinking
Parietal	Lies beneath skull, posterior to central sulcus	Sensory perception, taking in information from environment, organizing it, and communicating this information to rest of brain Association areas that allow for such things as accurately following directions on a map, reading a clock, building a birdhouse, or dressing oneself	Altered sensory perceptions, such as decreased consciousness of pain sensation Difficulty with time concepts, such as inability to keep appointment times Alteration in personal hygiene Alteration in ability to calculate numbers Inability to adequately perform common motor actions of writing Mixing up right and left Poor attention span
Temporal	Lies beneath skull on both sides; commonly called the temple	Primarily responsible for hearing and receiving information via ears	Auditory hallucinations Increased sexual focus Decreased motivation Alterations in memory Altered emotional responses
Occipital	Most posterior of brain lobes—back of head	Primarily responsible for seeing and receiving information via eyes	Visual hallucinations

called the corticospinal nerve tract. This system of nerves, because of its unique shape, is also referred to as the pyramidal tract. The pyramidal tract passes through the intersection of the medulla and spinal cord. It is at this point that the nerve tract crosses over, or decussates. This helps to explain why the right motor cortex actually controls voluntary motor activity on the left side of the body and the left motor cortex controls motor activity on the right side of the body.

The frontal lobe also contains two other important structures, the **premotor area,** which is responsible for coordinated movement of multiple muscles, and the **association cortex.** The association cortex performs many of the activities that make us human and is the area of the brain most responsible for personality. Damage to this area of the frontal lobe causes changes in personality. Reasoning, planning, working memory, insight, inhibition, and judgment, commonly labeled executive functions, are all functions of the association cortex. These executive functions help suppress and

modulate more primitive impulses and actions. The outcome of difficulty in performing these executive function activities often manifests as symptoms of mental disorder (Crow, 1997).

The **temporal lobe** is most involved with language, memory, and emotion. Wernicke's area is a specialized area of the temporal lobe responsible for speech capacity. Written speech, verbal speech, and the visual recognition that is critical to communication are all functions of the temporal lobe. Aphasia occurs when there is damage to the temporal lobe. Other structures of the temporal lobe are involved with memory, especially those connected to visual and auditory cues.

The **occipital lobe** is most responsible for visual functioning. Color recognition, the ability to recognize and name objects, and the ability to track moving objects are a function of the occipital lobe. The occipital lobe is sensitive to hypoxia, and trauma to this region of the brain can result in blindness even if the optic nerves remain intact. Lesions of the occipital lobe can cause visual hallucinations and other abnormalities of visual functioning, such as alexia (the inability to read).

The **parietal lobe** of the brain functions as a processing center. Sensory information such as visual, tactile, and auditory information is interpreted in the sensory strip area of the parietal lobe.

Basal Ganglia

The **basal ganglia** are made up of cell bodies closely involved with motor functions and association. The basal ganglia interpret movements, such as walking, while it is happening and modulate and correct muscle functioning to allow movements to occur. The basal ganglia lie beneath the frontal cortex and have many connections to both the cortex above and the midbrain structures below. The basal ganglia are involved in the learning and programming of behavior. Activities that are well learned and rehearsed over the course of one's life often become automatic. Complex motor skills involved in walking, eating, or driving become so ingrained that one does not have to think consciously to perform them. Much of these complex activities are functions of the basal ganglia. This helps to explain why some of these complex behaviors are retained in people with dementia long after the severe loss of memory or language has occurred as a result of damaged frontal lobes. Alterations in this area also help explain odd associations or loose and illogical associations often seen as a symptom of severe mental disorders such as schizophrenia (Crow, 1997).

The **extrapyramidal motor system,** a collection of nerve fibers responsible for much of the involuntary motor functioning of the CNS, is a nerve pathway starting in and connecting the basal ganglia with the thalamus and the cerebral cortex. Muscle tone, common reflexes, and automatic motor functioning of walking (posture) are controlled by this nerve track. The extrapyramidal tract works by maintaining balance between excitatory and inhibitory neurons. Diseases such as Huntington's and Parkinson's cause dysfunction of this motor track and produce symptoms of abnormal muscle movements.

Alteration in functioning of the basal ganglia is also seen as a consequence of medications used to treat mental disorders. Hypertonicity, for example, is seen as a common side effect of the older neuroleptic antipsychotic medications such as chlorpromazine (Thorazine) and haloperidol (Haldol).

Limbic System

Instincts, drives, needs, and emotions are considered part of the functions of the deeper structures of the brain called the **limbic system** or limbic lobe. It is often called a "system" because its functions are thought to be a result of the interrelated, closely coordinated actions of its various structures. Table 4-2 and Figure 4-2 identify the structural components of the limbic system.

Part of the limbic system, the **amygdala,** is instrumen-

Table 4-2	Structures of the Limbic System
Structure	**Function**
Amygdala	Modulate emotional states Regulate affective responses to events
Thalamus	Relay all sensory information, except smell Filter incoming information regarding emotions, mood, and memory to prevent cortex from becoming overloaded
Hypothalamus	Regulate basic human functions such as sleep-rest patterns, body temperature, and physical drives of hunger and sex
Hippocampus	Control learning and recall of an event with its associated memory

tal in emotional functioning and in regulating affective responses to events. The amygdala modulates common emotional states such as feelings of anger and aggression, love, and comfort in social settings. The amygdala has direct connection to areas of the brain involved with smell. The limbic system's function of emotional regulation is integrally linked with the olfactory pathways that connect to the amygdala. Primitive drives such as sexual arousal and aggression are also functions of the amygdala. This area of the limbic system has been of increasing interest to researchers trying to identify the biologic etiology of bipolar disorder. Some researchers have hypothesized that rapid misfiring of neurons in the amygdala are instrumental in the development of the typical symptoms of bipolar disorder.

The **thalamus** is another part of the limbic system and is primarily a regulatory structure that acts as the gateway to the cerebral cortex. The thalamus functions to relay all sensory information, except smell, from the PNS to the cortex of the CNS. This critical structure helps to filter incoming information to prevent the cortex from becoming overloaded. Most incoming information regarding emotions, mood, and memory passes through and is regulated by the thalamus.

The **hypothalamus** is another part of the limbic system that rests deep within the brain and helps regulate some of the most basic human functions, such as sleep-rest patterns, body temperature, and physical drives of hunger and sex. Dysfunction of this structure is common in many mental disorders. Appetite and sleep problems seen in the depressed client, the seasonal mood changes of seasonal affective disorder, and temperature regulation problems often manifested in clients with schizophrenia (e.g., wear-

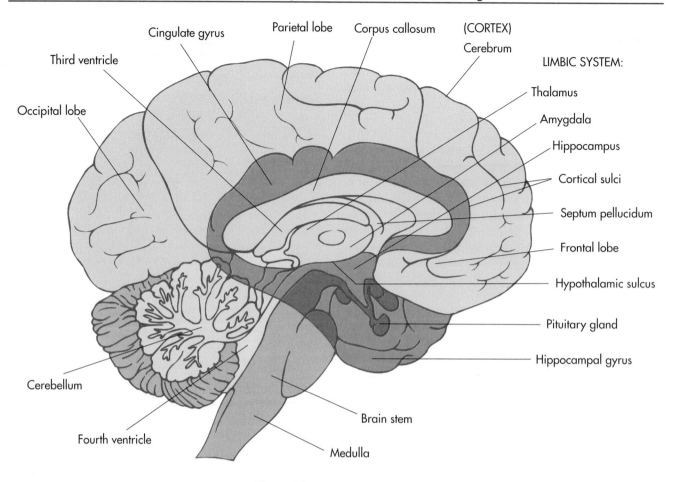

Figure 4-2   The limbic system.

ing winter coats in the summer) can be understood in part as hypothalamic dysregulation.

The **hippocampus** is located in the inside fold of each temporal lobe below the thalamus. It has direct connections with the hypothalamus and the amygdala. The hypothalamus is the site of the intersection between the storage of memories and their reproduction with emotional coloring. The hippocampus allows us to recall an event with its associated memory, allowing a memory to make us cry or cause us to laugh. It plays a major role in the encoding, consolidation, and retrieval of memories. Alzheimer's disease causes damage to the hippocampus, resulting in defects and difficulties with short-term memory and learning ability.

NEUROPHYSIOLOGY

The brain is made up of approximately 140 billion nerve cells. Twenty billion of these cells are directly involved in information processing. Each of these cells has up to 15,000 direct physical connections to other brain cells. This massive network of brain cell connections is what allows the many different areas of the brain to communicate with one another. Nerve stimuli are constantly being sent

and received within these cells, and those stimuli or messages turn on and off the various structures of the brain. This constant brain nerve cell activity accounts for the intricate perceptions and behaviors that make us human. The vast number of synaptic interconnections also help us to understand why the brain is far more complex and sophisticated than any man-made computer that has been constructed at this time.

Each nerve cell (**neuron**) has a cell body, a stem (axon), and connecting dendrite branches. The **dendrites** collect incoming signals from other neurons and send the signal to the neuron's cell body. The **axon** transmits signals from the neuron's cell body to connect with other neurons and cells. Figure 4-3 shows the complex nature of neuron connections.

Nerve Cell Electrical Functioning

Neurons within the brain are interconnected and operate both via electrical impulses and chemical activity. When a neuron is stimulated, by chemical or physical stimuli, it sends an **action potential** wave of electrical depolarization down the neuron. These electrical impulses move along the nerve cell, and when an impulse reaches the end of the

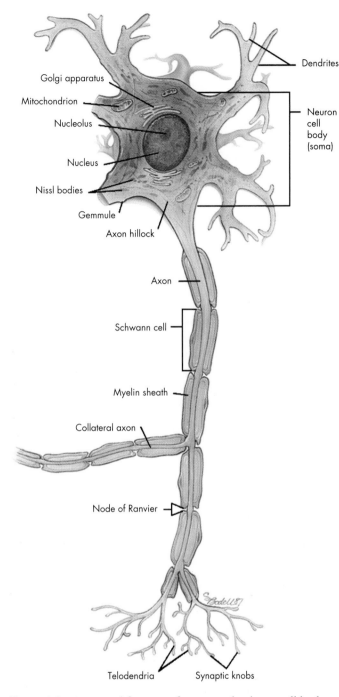

Figure 4-3   Structural features of neurons: dendrites, cell body, and axons. (From Lewis SM et al: *Medical-surgical nursing: assessment and management of clinical problems*, ed 4, St. Louis, 1996, Mosby.)

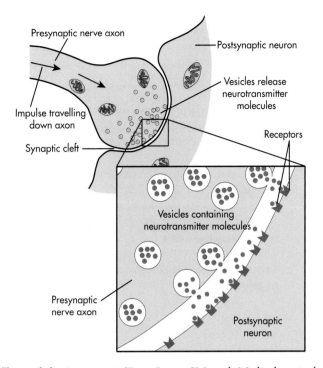

Figure 4-4   A synapse. (From Lewis SM et al: *Medical-surgical nursing: assessment and management of clinical problems*, ed 4, St. Louis, 1996, Mosby.)

and reaches the dendrite of an adjacent neuron, that cell is stimulated. This newly stimulated neuron will then transmit an impulse via depolarization waves down the axon to the synaptic space, or cleft. The stimuli, now in the form of a chemical messenger, goes across the synapse and in this way will stimulate neighboring cells. This process is repeated billions of times a day and allows for the complex working of the structures of the CNS.

Many of the medications used to treat mental disorders operate at the cellular level by impacting the ability of neurons to initiate impulses through cell membrane depolarization. The neuron's cell membrane action potential, or ability to depolarize, can be increased or decreased by medication. When a medication decreases the membrane potential of neurons, it is said to have an *excitatory* action that makes the neuron more easily stimulated. Conversely, medications that increase the membrane potential, making it harder to stimulate the neuron, are *inhibitory* in nature.

Neurotransmitters: Nerve Cell Chemical Functioning

Many new advances in the understanding and treatment of mental disorders are related to increased understanding of neurotransmitters. As the depolarization of neurons reaches the synapse, the stimuli transfer from an intracellular electrical signal to an extracellular chemical signal. Therefore medications that are used to treat mental disor-

neuron, it stimulates the production and release of chemical compounds called **neurotransmitters.** These neurotransmitters move across the synaptic gap, or cleft, between neurons and cause the adjacent neuron to be stimulated to produce an action potential. This space, less than 20 nm in size, separates one neuron from another. This process is shown in Figure 4-4.

When a neurotransmitter moves across the synapse

ders operate in and around the synaptic cleft and have action at the neurotransmitter level. The discovery of new drugs has been concerned mainly with the study of neurotransmitters that make up the chemical messenger system of the brain.

Once a neurotransmitter has done its job by transferring a stimulus to an adjacent neuron, the chemical messenger is removed from the synaptic area by one of three naturally occurring processes:

1. The neurotransmitter leaves the area through natural diffusion of a substance from an area of high concentration to one of low concentration.
2. The neurotransmitter can be broken down by enzymatic degradation.
3. The neurotransmitter can undergo reuptake and be transported back into storage in the presynaptic neuron.

Many medications used to treat mental disorders involve these three mechanisms. The selective serotonin reuptake inhibitor (SSRI) class of antidepressants works by influencing the reuptake mechanism, whereas monoamine oxidase inhibitors (MAOIs) affect the degree of enzyme degradation that occurs in the synaptic cleft.

Neurotransmitters carry two different types of messages. Some neurotransmitters carry excitatory messages, whereas others carry inhibitory messages. Nerve cells stimulated by an excitatory neurotransmitter will be "turned on," or stimulated to start some action. Nerve cells stimulated by an inhibitory neurotransmitter will be "turned off," causing slowing or stopping of actions. (Antianxiety medications are an example of inhibitory transmitters.) Many antianxiety medications act on the γ-aminobutyric acid (GABA) system. GABA is an inhibitory neurotransmitter, which has a calming action when taken by clients experiencing anxiety.

The intricate interaction of nerve cells in different areas of the brain is the basis for all complex activities of the CNS. Different neurotransmitters are found in different regions and areas of the brain, allowing for highly differentiated functions of brain tissue. Interruptions in the normal functioning of the brain can be caused by dysfunction in either the structure or the chemistry of the brain. Problems with either structure or chemistry interrupt the nor-

---

Box 4-1   Criteria for a Substance to Be Labeled as a Neurotransmitter

1. The chemical must be synthesized in the neuron.
2. The chemical must be present in the presynaptic terminal and released in amounts sufficient to exert a particular effect on a receptor neuron.
3. When applied exogenously (as a drug) in a reasonable concentration, the drug mimics exactly the action of the endogenously released neurotransmitter.
4. A specific mechanism exists for removing it from its site of action, the synaptic cleft.

---

mal flow of impulses and stimuli and result in symptoms of mental disorders that manifest as unusual behaviors.

Over 100 substances have been identified as actual or potential chemical messengers in the CNS. Not all of these can be considered neurotransmitters. Sir Henry Dale formulated a fundamental rule about synaptic transmission: any given neuron produces the same transmitter substance at all of its synapses. This rule has led to the identification of four criteria that must be met before a chemical substance can be considered a neurotransmitter. Box 4-1 outlines these criteria.

Neurotransmitters can be classified into one of three groups: the biogenic amines, the amino acids, and the peptides. Five common neurotransmitters are important to the understanding of mental disorders. Table 4-3 describes these common neurotransmitters.

Acetylcholine was the first substance discovered to be a neurotransmitter. It can be found almost everywhere in the brain, but particularly high concentrations occur in the basal ganglia and motor cortex of the brain. Acetylcholine is the neurotransmitter primarily involved in Alzheimer's disease. Decreased levels of the neurotransmitter are thought to produce many of the behavioral manifestations of the disease. This helps to explain why drugs such as donepezil (Aricept) are useful in the treatment of Alzheimer's disease. Aricept and other similar drugs inhibit cholinesterase (the enzyme that degrades or breaks down acetylcholine), thus increasing the amount of available acetylcholine to improve symptoms of Alzheimer's disease (Selkoe, 1992).

Table 4-3	**Neurotransmitters**			
Neurotransmitter	**Type**	**Action**	**Synthesis Substrate**	**Synthesis Location**
Acetylcholine	Monoamine	Excitatory	Acetyl Coenzyme + choline	Nucleus basalis in cortex
Dopamine	Monoamine	Excitatory	Tyrosine	Substantia nigra
Norepinephrine	Monoamine	Excitatory	Tyrosine	Locus ceruleus
Serotonin	Monoamine	Excitatory	Tryptophan	Raphe nuclei in brain stem
γ-Aminobutyric acid (GABA)	Amino acid	Inhibitory	Glutamate	No localized cell bodies

Acetylcholine receptors can be divided into two types: muscarinic and nicotinic. Many drugs will interact with acetylcholine and its receptor sites, such as the older neuroleptic antipsychotics, to produce anticholinergic side effects. These occur when muscarinic acetylcholine receptors are blocked, and the side effects that are experienced by the client include dry mouth, blurred vision, constipation, and urinary retention. These side effects can be troubling to clients and are a common reason for noncompliance with treatment. In severe cases muscarinic receptor blockade can produce confusion and delirium in clients, especially in the elderly. Good client teaching and nursing care designed to manage the side effects are a significant aspect of psychiatric mental health nursing.

The neurotransmitter dopamine is well localized in the CNS. Dopaminergic pathways include the substantia nigra, the midbrain, and the hypothalamus. Dopamine-containing cells in the midbrain project to the limbic cortex, which is thought to be the part of the brain that is disturbed in schizophrenia. Dopamine levels are thought to be excessively elevated in some patients suffering from schizophrenia, and most of the drugs used to treat schizophrenia act in part by decreasing dopamine levels or transmission.

Norepinephrine or noradrenaline is concentrated in a small area of the brain known as the locus ceruleus. It has some modulating effect, and there are many studies now that indicate that patients suffering from mood disorders, particularly major depression, may suffer from a deficit of norepinephrine. Norepinephrine is found in heavy concentrations in sympathetic nerves, which helps to explain its role in the "fight or flight" response.

Serotonin has a pattern of action very similar to norepinephrine. Serotonin production begins in the brain stem and is primarily concentrated in the raphe nuclei, but it is also widely dispersed throughout the cerebral cortex. Serotonin is involved with many functions that we all take for granted. Maintaining a normal body temperature, having a normal sleep-rest pattern, eating well, and having normal moods are all dependent in large measure on adequate levels of serotonin. Clinically significant problems occur when clients have too little serotonin, and many behavioral symptoms common to such disorders as depression occur when available serotonin levels are low.

The illness of depression is helpful in demonstrating the role that neurotransmitters play in the development of mental illness. It is widely believed that there are two subtypes of major depression: one caused by abnormal norepinephrine balance and the other by abnormal serotonin balance. These are discussed in greater length in Chapter 13. The two major classes of antidepressants—tricyclic and SSRI agents—differ primarily in their effect on either norepinephrine or serotonin levels. This explains why certain drugs that specifically target serotonin, such as fluoxetine or paroxetine, do not work for some clients but work well for others.

DIAGNOSTIC AND EVALUATION PROCEDURES
NEUROIMAGING

Within the last 20 years the development of imaging techniques has dramatically altered our understanding of brain functioning. Brain anatomy can now be mapped in exquisite detail, providing valuable information. The techniques that permit observation of the brain can be divided into two groups:

1. Techniques that measure structure (anatomic imaging)
2. Techniques that measure function (functional imaging)

Anatomic imaging techniques include computed tomography (CT) and magnetic resonance imaging (MRI). Functional imaging techniques include single photon emission computed tomography (SPECT) and position emission tomography (PET), which measure metabolic and neurotransmitter functions (Margolin, 1993).

ANATOMIC IMAGING
Computed Tomography

The first of these new neuroimaging techniques was discovered by scientists at Electronic Music Industry (EMI), a branch of Capitol Records, who were funded in part by money from the sale of records of the Beatles. A CT scan of the brain provides a three-dimensional view of brain structures that can differentiate fine densities, unlike a normal x-ray film. Abnormalities in CT scans are not specific to any type of mental disorder and do not serve as a specific test for disorders. They do, however, provide suggestive evidence of brain-based problems. Nonspecific abnormalities in CT scans have been found in patients with schizophrenia, bipolar disorder, other mood disorders, alcoholism, multiinfarct dementia, and Alzheimer's disease. The CT scan is widely used because it is very available and costs relatively little. Its disadvantages include lack of sensitivity, underestimation of brain atrophy, and inability to image in the sagittal and coronal views.

Magnetic Resonance Imaging

MRI is unaffected by bone and, unlike CT, can view brain structures close to the skull and can separate white matter from gray matter tissue. MRI is now readily available in most hospitals. It cannot, however, be performed with all clients because of several contraindications to its use that have been identified. Box 4-2 indicates the client groups who must avoid MRIs.

Clients with claustrophobia are often unable to complete the study because of the design of the machinery for the MRI. The MRI machine is an enclosed tubelike structure in which clients are required to lie still. Because of the

| | Table 4-4 | Nursing Considerations With Neuroimaging Procedures | | |

Test	General Considerations	Common Nursing Care	Common Contraindications
Anatomic Imaging			
Computed tomography (CT)	Three-dimensional view of structures of brain Differentiate fine-density structures, unlike normal x-ray film Examination time: 15-30 min Clear fluids meal before test	Explain purpose of test and all procedures. Reassure client that test is safe and that radiation exposure is not a concern. Assess client's anxiety level and monitor for symptoms of claustrophobia. Reassure client that monotonous noise is commonly heard. Instruct client on need to lie very still to ensure good imaging. If contrast iodine is used, monitor for gastrointestinal upset, flushing, and perceptions of excess warmth.	Allergy to iodine (not all CT requires iodine) Inability to lie completely still Claustrophobia
Magnetic resonance imaging (MRI)	Separates view of white matter from gray matter tissue Examination time: 15-60 min	Explain purpose of test and all procedures. Reassure client that test uses magnets, not radiation. Radiation exposure is not a concern. Assess client's anxiety level and monitor for symptoms of claustrophobia. Instruct client on need to lie very still to ensure good imaging. Instruct client that a clear plastic helmet with antenna will be put over head. Reassure client that monotonous noise is commonly heard.	Inability to lie completely still Claustrophobia Pacemakers Metallic implants, plates, screws, or pacemakers Life-support equipment needed for client Infusion pumps Generally not used when client is pregnant

| Box 4-2 | Patient Group Contraindications for MRI |

Individuals with pacemakers
Individuals with metallic objects such as screws, prostheses, and orthopedic devices
Patients on life-support systems

confining environment of the machine, focused client teaching is necessary before testing, and close monitoring of anxiety levels occurs during testing. MRIs have demonstrated neuroanatomic changes present in clients with schizophrenia. Changes include increased size of ventricles, temporal lobe reductions, hippocampal reductions, and cortical atrophy.

FUNCTIONAL IMAGING

The basis of PET and SPECT scanning is resultant information about blood flow to the brain. Both PET scans and

Table 4-4	Nursing Considerations With Neuroimaging Procedures—cont'd		
Test	**General Considerations**	**Common Nursing Care**	**Common Contraindications**
Functional Imaging			
Positron emission tomography (PET)	Two-dimensional image Measures physiologic and chemical functioning such as glucose uptake by cells in brain, as well as information on anatomic structures Examination time: 45-60 min	Explain purpose of test and all procedures. Reassure client that test uses magnets. Radiation exposure is not a concern. Assess client's anxiety level and monitor for symptoms of claustrophobia. Explain that there will be time interval of about 45 min between injection of isotope and scanning procedure. Explain that client may be blindfolded and have earplugs to decrease environmental stimulus during testing. Instruct client on need to lie very still to ensure good imaging. Client should not fall asleep during procedure—test results will be affected.	Inability to lie completely still Claustrophobia Severe anxiety level Recent use of sedating/tranquilizing medication because these medications alter cellular glucose use patterns Breast-feeding Requires expensive cyclotron machine
Single photon emission computed tomography (SPECT)	Long half-life isotopes used No on-site cyclotron required		Breast-feeding Inability to lie completely still Claustrophobia

SPECT scans use radiopharmaceuticals that readily cross the intact blood-brain barrier. PET scanning remains at the forefront in neuroimaging procedures because of the resultant information it provides. PET scans are, however, extremely expensive because they require use of a cyclotron machine.

Positron Emission Tomography
PET relies on "coincidence scanning." Images of the brain are produced when a positron-emitting radionuclei interacts with an electron. Both particles cease to exist and are converted into two photons that travel in opposite directions. Positron-emitting radionuclei can only be produced by a cyclotron. The machine and procedure requires a support team of physicists, chemists, and computer experts.

Single Photon Emission Computed Tomography
SPECT is more widely available and less expensive than PET. SPECT scans have detected abnormalities in the frontal cortex, occipital and temporal lobes, and parahippocampal gyrus in patients with panic disorders.

Table 4-4 identifies the common nursing considerations for clients having a neuroimaging test.

PUTTING IT ALL TOGETHER
UNDERSTANDING NEUROANATOMY, NEUROCHEMISTRY, BEHAVIOR, AND MENTAL DISORDERS
Each structure and each chemical produced and used by the brain has a specific function. Disease may cause alteration in structures or functions of the brain. As illness affects different areas of the brain, certain abnormalities in normal brain activity will be produced, and these will frequently manifest in clients as alterations in behavior. Table 4-5 shows, in an abbreviated way, the link between neurotransmitter dysfunction and the expression of symptoms of mental disorders.

Table 4-5		Relationship of Neurotransmitter Dysfunction to Mental Disorders
Neurotransmitter	**Dysfunction**	**Mental Disorder**
Dopamine	Increase	Schizophrenia
Serotonin	Decrease	Depression
Norepinephrine	Decrease	Depression
γ-Aminobutyric acid (GABA)	Decrease	Anxiety disorders
Acetylcholine	Decrease	Alzheimer's disease

Psychiatric mental health nursing provides nursing care to clients with brain-based illnesses. All steps of the nursing process need to occur within the context of the nurse's understanding of the client's biochemical problem. By putting together the findings of the nursing assessment discussed in Chapter 7 and the nurse's understanding of normal psychobiology, effective nursing care can assist clients in achieving wellness.

Psychiatric mental health nurses are increasingly required to apply principles of psychobiology to their care of clients with mental disorders. The American Nurses Association (1994) has emphasized the importance of nurses having a strong background in neurobiology as part of the standards of practice for psychiatric mental health nursing. Much of the stigma that has been attached to mental illness has come from a lack of understanding regarding the biologic basis of these disorders. Client teaching is an important function of the role of the psychiatric mental health nurse as new information is discovered regarding the structures and functioning of the CNS. The Client & Family Teaching Guidelines box displays the highlights of effective client teaching regarding the biologic basis of mental disorders.

New research findings continue to alter the care of the mentally disordered. The Understanding & Applying Research box highlights the critical thinking needed by psychiatric mental health nurses as they encounter these alterations in care based on new research findings.

The explosion of information regarding the structure and functioning of the brain will continue. Because of this, the role and function of the psychiatric mental health nurse is expected to continue to evolve. Knowledge of the psychobiologic basis of mental disorders is now essential in effective psychiatric mental health nursing practice. All aspects of nursing care, from assessment to evaluation, need to incorporate biologic principles for comprehensive and quality nursing care to occur.

Client & Family TEACHING GUIDELINES

Determine a mutually acceptable time and location for the teaching session.

Identify the client's readiness for learning.

Identify the client's motivation for learning.

Identify what the client already knows about the topic and the accuracy of that knowledge.

Mutually identify with the client what content learning is requested.

Mutually define a measurable outcome that will be used to determine that learning has occurred.

Define the evaluation method used to determine the efficacy of teaching.

Use multiple teaching-learning approaches such as visual and auditory.

Monitor the client's anxiety level during the teaching session, since increased anxiety will decrease information processing.

Identify alternative resources available to the client to increase learning potential.

Identify the process for the client to access support persons if the client is having difficulty with learned content.

Understanding & Applying Research

ISSUES OF BIOLOGY AND PSYCHIATRIC MENTAL HEALTH NURSING

It has been reported that the brains of individuals who commit suicide are different from the brains of individuals who have died of natural causes (Gross-Isseroff et al, 1998). Postmortem examination of the receptor/transport binding sites of the brain tissue of suicide victims and of individuals who have died of natural causes shows that the brains of suicide victims have unique, specific neurochemical characteristics that make "suicide brains" different from brains of individuals who have died of natural causes. Such studies are being used to formulate a hypothesis of the molecular markers that could help define and identify individuals at risk for suicidal behavior. Tests to measure such identified markers are expected in the near future. Once these markers are identified and prove to be reliable in their ability to predict suicidal behavior, the test is expected to become a routine aspect of mental health evaluation.

Psychobiology

Tremendous advances have been made in the field of cognitive (brain) neurobiologic research related to mental disorders. Discoveries about the mechanisms and role of the neurotransmitters, their functions, and their pathways have revolutionized the treatment of a variety of psychiatric illnesses from schizophrenia to eating disorders. These discoveries have brought about a whole new market of antipsychotic, antidepressant, and related drugs for the treatment of mental disorders and other behavioral problems.

Because of the rapid advances in neurobiology and/or diseases of the brain, newer psychiatric nursing paradigms are emerging. These paradigms stress the integration of this neurobiologic perspective into community-based treatment and clinical practice approaches. The integration of neurobiologic concepts, along with psychosocial and spiritual dimensions of care, will truly move our practice toward holistic models of working more intimately with our clients in the community.

In addition to medication education related to brain malfunction, social skills training must have a greater impact. Supportive nursing interventions for meeting these deficits must be very basic (e.g., how to introduce oneself, how to stay focused and make small talk, when to join in a conversation and when to stay quiet and just listen—all important survival skills for living and fitting into the community). No amount of psychopharmaceutical medication will reverse social skills deficits. Cognitive approaches such as reframing and better interpersonal communication for changing maladaptive core beliefs will be the norm.

Also, in working with our clients using these newer paradigms, we must be able to deal with disease/symptom management and, more important, the ever-present economic realities of managed care and capitation. Mental health experts are already pointing out that behavioral care systems are becoming multidisciplinary, integrated systems for the delivery of care. This will require that all disciplines involved in the care of the mentally disordered be more resourceful in allocating and coordinating services to client groups. No longer will one discipline have a monopoly on providing all services to this group.

The significant opening of the scientific frontier of "diseases of the brain" means that we will have to deal with our client's behavioral limitations, their cognitive deficits, and their emotional responses in new and more meaningful ways.

Summary of Key Concepts

1. The last decade of the twentieth century was designated by Congress as the "Decade of the Brain."
2. More has been learned about brain function in the last 15 years than was learned in all preceding time.
3. The brain is the most complex organ in the human body and one of the most important because of its many functions.
4. Mental disorders are beginning to be understood as brain-based illnesses that have anatomic and/or physiologic components. It is therefore imperative that nurses understand the anatomy and physiology of the brain and other systems that interact with the nervous system and become familiar with psychobiologic approaches to treat mental disorders.
5. This chapter begins to explain human brain structure and function and names some of the disorders that may occur when these systems are disrupted.
6. Modern neuroimaging techniques have greatly expanded the capacity to understand mental illnesses and are presented in this text.

REFERENCES

Amen DG: Brain SPECT imaging in psychiatry, *Prim Psychiatry* 5:83, 1998.

American Nurses Association: *Psychopharmacology guidelines for psychiatric mental health nurses: psychiatric mental health nursing psychopharmacology project*, Washington, DC, 1994, The Association.

Andreasen NC: Brain imaging in psychiatry, *Science,* 239:1381, 1988.

Andreasen NC, Black DW: *Introductory textbook of psychiatry*, Washington, DC, 1995, American Psychiatric Press.

Arango, V et al: Localized alterations in pre- and post-synaptic serotonin binding sites in the ventrolateral prefrontal cortex of suicide victims, *Brain Res* 688:121, 1995.

Bear MF, Connors, BW, Paradiso MA: *Neuroscience: exploring the brain*, Baltimore, 1996, Williams & Wilkens.

Carpenter WT, Buchanan RW: Medical progress: schizophrenia, *N Engl J Med* 330:681, 1994.

Collins RC: *Neurology*, Philadelphia, 1997, WB Saunders.

Cooper JR, Bloom FE, Roth RH: *The biochemical basis of neuropharmacology*, ed 7, New York, 1995, Oxford University Press.

Crow TJ: Schizophrenia as failure of hemisphere dominance for language, *TINS* 20:339, 1997.

Davidson RJ: Anterior cerebral asymmetry and the nature of emotions, *Brain Cogn* 20:125, 1992.

Davis M: The role of the amygdala in fear and anxiety, *Annu Rev Neurosci* 15:353, 1992.

Gross-Isseroff R et al: The suicide brain: a review of postmortem receptor transporter binding studies, *Neurosci Biobehav Rev* 22(5):653, 1998.

Haines DE: *Fundamental neuroscience*, New York, 1997, Churchill Livingstone.

Kaplan HI, Sadock BJ: *Comprehensive textbook of psychiatry*, ed 6, Baltimore, 1995, Williams & Wilkens.

Keltner NL: Pathoanatomy of schizophrenia, *Perspect Psychiatr Care* 32(2):32, 1996.

Keltner NL et al: *Psychobiological foundations of psychiatric care*, St. Louis, 1998, Mosby.

Margolin R. In Sadovoy J, Lazarus L, Jarvik L, editors: *Neuroimaging*, Washington, DC, 1993, American Psychiatric Press.

Roberts GW, Leigh PN, Weinberger DR: *Neuropsychiatric disorders*, London, 1993, Mosby-Wolfe.

Selkoe D: Aging brain, aging mind, *Sci Am* 267:135, 1992.

Thibodeau G, Patton K: *Anatomy and physiology*, ed 4, St. Louis, 1998, Mosby.

Yates M et al: $5HT_2$ receptor changes in major depression, *Biol Psychiatry* 27:489, 1990.

Yudofsky SC, Hales RE: *The American psychiatric press textbook of neuropsychiatry*, Washington DC, 1992, American Psychiatric Press.

Notes

Legal-Ethical Issues

Joyce K. Laben

HISTORICAL REVIEW

According to Sales and Shuman (1994), law and mental health have been intertwined for many years. Even in ancient Rome the law was concerned about the legal status of the mentally disabled. Should the individual have a guardian? Could the individual enter into a contract? According to Roman law, the person with a mental disability could not form a marriage contract and if made a ward could not have any legal capacity (Brakel, Parry, and Weiner, 1985).

During the Middle Ages people with mental illnesses were considered to be possessed by demons. The king could hold custody of property of these people. The profits were applied to the maintenance of the individuals and their households. When a person was thought to be incompetent because of mental illness, a jury of 12 men would decide whether to commit the individual to the care of a friend, who would receive an allowance for maintenance (Brakel, Parry, and Weiner, 1985).

In the American colonies of the seventeenth century, the lack of facilities meant that families were expected to care for people with mental illnesses. If a person had no family or friends, the individual might wander from town to town—in some instances in the company of transient groups. There was no distinguishing between a vagrant and a person with a mental illness; therefore, all were treated as itinerant poor persons. As early as 1676, a law was passed in the state of Massachusetts to manage people who were considered to have mental illnesses and be dangerous. The individual could be detained, but generally no procedures for commitment of a person with a mental illness were instigated at this time (Brakel, Parry, and Weiner, 1985).

It was not until 1752 that Pennsylvania Hospital in Philadelphia opened to treat people with mental illnesses (Laben and MacLean,

KEY TERMS

Autonomy Self-determination, self-governance.

Beneficence Doing good, preventing harm.

Clear and convincing evidence A burden of proof that requires more than that used in a civil proceeding and less than that used in a criminal proceeding. Civil proceedings call for merely a preponderance of evidence, whereas criminal proceedings require proof beyond a reasonable doubt.

Commitment Court order certifying that an individual is to be confined to a mental health facility for treatment.

Competency to stand trial The ability of the individual to understand the charges and their consequences, to comprehend the nature and object of the legal proceedings, and to advise an attorney and assist in the defense.

Distributive justice Allotment of benefits and burdens according to fairness on what the individual is owed.

Duty to warn Legal obligation of a mental health professional to warn an intended victim of potential harm from a mental health client.

Expert witness Someone with education and experience on a specialized subject who is qualified as an expert and is allowed to testify, thereby assisting the jury in understanding technical information.

Least restrictive alternative Providing the least restrictive treatment in the least restrictive setting for a mental health client.

Legal duty Something that an individual is required to do by law.

Mandatory outpatient treatment An individual is legally required to undergo mental health treatment in an outpatient setting. The individual usually has been noncompliant and allegedly has a propensity for dangerous acts.

Privileged communication Communication between a professional and a client is confidential and protected from forced disclosure in court unless authorized by the client. The privilege is delegated by statutes in various states.

1989). In Williamsburg, Virginia, in 1773, a facility was opened by the state especially for treatment of people with mental illnesses. The next state institution erected was in Lexington, Kentucky, in 1824 (Brakel, Parry, and Weiner, 1985).

In 1841 Dorothea Dix began her crusade for placing individuals with mental illnesses in specially built hospitals rather than placing them in almshouses and jails. During the following years, Dix traveled throughout the United States, pressing for moral and humanistic treatment of people with mental illnesses (Laben and MacLean, 1989).

During the late nineteenth and early twentieth centuries, laws were passed by various states enacting civil commitment procedures for people with mental illnesses. From 1900 to 1955, the population in mental institutions grew from 150,000 to 819,000 inpatients in state and county mental hospitals (LaFond, 1994). Passage of the Community Mental Health Centers Act of 1963 authorized monies to build community treatment centers. Shortly thereafter, civil rights lawyers began to challenge the treatment of people with mental illnesses. During the Vietnam War era, a distrust of government emerged. Judicial activism began with concern about the treatment of people with mental illnesses and maintenance of their rights. More consideration was given to individual rights; especially questioned was the long-standing practice of hospitalizing individuals for many years, in some instances without much treatment (LaFond, 1994).

Commitment to mental hospitals was no longer seen as a medical decision but rather as a decision to be entrusted to a neutral decision maker, such as a judge. Many laws were changed at this time to encompass not only mental illness but also dangerousness. In addition to this criteria, individuals with mental illnesses who were unable to care for themselves were labeled "gravely disabled" and were committed.

Large numbers of individuals were released into the community, raising concerns that there were not appropriate facilities and services to adequately care for them within the community. Because of the increasing number of people with mental illnesses in the community and the appointment of more conservative judges, who were reluctant to become involved in the administration of hospitals, recommendations for expanding the mental health commitment laws emerged. A tendency developed in some jurisdictions, such as the state of Washington, where more individuals were committed under the gravely disabled criteria rather than the dangerousness criteria.

There is growing concern about mentally ill individuals in jails and prisons. Studies seem to indicate that up to 15% of inmates in jails and prisons have severe mental illnesses. In an extensive review of the literature Lamb and Weinberger (1998) attribute this problem to deinstitutionalization, lack of needed community support, and inability to access community treatment, including reluctance of facilities to provide care, lack of understanding by police officers and the general population, and the creation of rigid civil commitment standards.

A major issue that has many ethical and legal ramifications is the impact on mental health care by managed behavioral health care organizations. In an effort to control spiraling health care costs, employers and several states have turned to behavioral health organizations to manage mental health care. Although some preliminary studies have been completed, the total impact of this change has not been fully documented (Dee, van Servellen, and Brecht, 1998). The legal and ethical implications of managed care organizations applying pressure to discharge a client from an inpatient facility prematurely are mounting (Simon, 1998).

COMMITMENT
LEAST RESTRICTIVE ALTERNATIVE

When an individual enters mental health treatment, determining the best location for the individual's treatment is crucial. The concept of **least restrictive alternative** means providing mental health treatment in the least restrictive environment, using the least restrictive treatment. About 30 years ago an elderly woman who was hospitalized at St. Elizabeth's in Washington, D.C., filed a writ of habeas corpus so that she could be released into the community. At that time, there were few alternatives to hospitals for treatment. The court ruled that there should be alternatives to inpatient facilities, including halfway houses, nursing homes, and day treatment programs (*Lake v. Cameron*, 1966).

Developing a treatment plan involves consideration of all alternatives, including such options as inpatient treatment, day treatment, and respite, foster, and home health care. An individual residing in a community that has developed many care options is the least likely to be hospitalized. Currently, health care costs are closely monitored. The most cost-effective, as well as the most appropriate, intervention to assist the client should be selected.

VOLUNTARY ADMISSIONS

Legally, **commitment** refers to a court order certifying that an individual is to be confined to a mental health facility for treatment. Generally, there are three types of commitments in each of the states: an emergency commitment, a voluntary commitment, and an involuntary indefinite commitment. The details may vary from state to state as do the mechanisms for admission. Nurses are most familiar with the voluntary admission: individuals come to the hospital and agree to be treated.

INFORMED CONSENT

On admission, clients should be informed about the treatments involving material risks (i.e., risks that a reasonable person would consider significant). For example, the side effect tardive dyskinesia can occur with neurologic drugs and, in some instances, is irreversible and would be considered a material risk. In addition, the client should know alternatives to the treatment and possible side effects of these alternatives. If the individual agrees to a treatment, the consent can be revoked at any time (Laben and MacLean, 1989).

The emphasis should be placed on including the individual in the decision-making process. The problem with admissions into a mental health facility is that in some instances the individual's ability to make an informed decision is questionable. Generally, unless the person has been declared incompetent to manage personal matters, the individual is considered able to give consent.

However, in emergency situations, where clients require treatment as result of behavior that is dangerous to themselves or others, treatment can be provided without the clients' consent. State laws vary, both in emergency and judicial commitment statutes, regarding the limits of such treatment. Under any other conditions, if a person cannot give informed consent, a guardian must be appointed. It is difficult to maintain that a person who is acutely psychotic has the ability to make an informed decision. It is, however, incumbent on mental health professionals to continually inform clients about treatment and to provide a list of client rights at the time of admission or soon after.

One incident that generated national interest concerned individuals with schizophrenia who were selected to be in a research study. A controversy ensued when some of the clients were withdrawn from antipsychotic medication and suffered severe exacerbations as a result. One individual committed suicide. The purpose of the study was to observe the client's behavior when withdrawn from medication. The question has arisen as to whether the clients were sufficiently informed about the severity of the symptoms that might occur if withdrawn from medication. Some ethicists have stated that it was not ethical to withdraw the medication when, most assuredly, psychotic symptoms were sure to reoccur (Hilts, 1994).

INVOLUNTARY ADMISSIONS

When some individuals become mentally ill, they refuse to seek treatment for a variety of reasons. A person could be suffering from paranoid delusions that someone is going to inflict harm, and therefore help is rejected because of the psychiatric symptomatology. In some instances the individual may be at risk for violent behavior because of suicidal ideation or commanding hallucinatory voices that instruct the client to harm others. This situation poses a likelihood of serious harm to the individual, as well as to other members of the community. Under these circumstances an emergency commitment might be appropriate.

EMERGENCY COMMITMENT

Emergency commitment is different from a judicial or indefinite commitment in that it is for a shorter period of time and generally has more restrictive criteria for admission. Usually, a state will require that the individual be seen initially by a mental health official, such as a physician, psychologist, social worker, or advanced practice nurse. Some states require a licensed physician. The examining professional cannot be on the staff of the admitting facility. Once the individual is brought to the inpatient unit, examination by a second mental health professional, usually a physician, must take place. This procedure protects the rights of the individuals. Usually, within a short period (5 days or less, excluding weekends and holidays) a probable cause hearing must take place to continue the person's hospitalization. For emergency admissions the standard criterion for an involuntary commitment is like-

lihood of harm to self or to others. In some jurisdictions, the term *gravely disabled* has come into use (Appelbaum, 1994; Laben and MacLean, 1989).

In Alabama an individual with paranoid schizophrenia contended that his commitment into a psychiatric facility was not proper because he had not perpetrated any recent dangerous acts. The mental health professional (a psychologist) testified that the client had threatened to harm others on previous occasions, was not compliant with medication, and had threatened a woman who had terminated her relationship with him. The court upheld the commitment because of the clear and convincing evidence that he needed continued inpatient treatment (*Mink v. Alabama Department of Mental Health and Mental Retardation*, 1993).

The standard of proof that must be offered to uphold a commitment proceeding is **clear and convincing evidence.** A U.S. Supreme Court decision ruled that the civil standard of preponderance of evidence, as used in civil lawsuits, was insufficient to use in a commitment hearing that deprived a person of liberty. The criminal standard of "beyond a reasonable doubt" was not used because the purpose of a commitment was not to punish but to treat the individual (*Addington v. Texas*, 1979). Therefore the middle standard of clear and convincing evidence was deemed sufficient.

CIVIL OR JUDICIAL COMMITMENT

An indefinite judicial or civil commitment is for a longer period of time than an emergency commitment. The legal basis for detention of an individual for treatment lies in the *parens patriae* power of the state to protect and care for individuals with disabilities and the police power of the state to protect the community from persons who pose a threat. A judicial commitment allows for involuntary hospitalization not only of persons dangerous to themselves or others but also of people with other kinds of behavioral problems—such as inability to provide self-care because of mental illness (Laben and MacLean, 1989).

For a judicial commitment the individual must be given time to prepare a defense to state why hospitalization is not necessary. The client has the right to have his or her attorney cross-examine the mental health professionals regarding the necessity for inpatient treatment. The client may also appeal a decision of a lower court (see Understanding & Applying Research box).

PREVENTIVE OR MANDATORY OUTPATIENT TREATMENT

In recent years, because of the concept of least restrictive alternative, long-term hospitalization, especially in state hospitals, has decreased. A dilemma has arisen about what to do with individuals who, on discharge from an inpatient treatment facility, discontinue medication, deteriorate,

---

Understanding & Applying Research

Researchers describe commitment proceedings at a large state hospital in Virginia over a 3-month period in 1988. More than half of the 190 individuals were at the initial commitment hearing, and 184 were at recommitment hearings. As the individuals' time in the hospital increased, attorneys were less likely to consult with the client/respondent to review the information in the charts or to cross-examine the clinical examiner. Judges were less likely to inform the respondents of their right to legal counsel or the right to appeal or to contemplate a voluntary admission.

Based on this information, nurses must take steps to ensure that clients are not confined to mental health facilities for long periods without meaningful treatment and frequent assessments of their ability to be discharged to a less restrictive environment.

Parry DH, Turkheimer E: Length of hospitalization and outcome of commitment and recommitment hearings, *Hosp Community Psychiatry* 43:65, 1992.

---

and exhibit dangerous behavior. Legislation for preventive commitment or involuntary outpatient treatment has subsequently been enacted. According to Torrey and Kaplan (1995), 35 states have such laws. In Tennessee an individual must be judicially committed and **mandatory outpatient treatment** ordered before discharge. If the individual does not remain in compliance with the treatment agreement, the treating professional files an affidavit with the court, and the client is ordered to appear in court before a judge and to state why compliance has not been maintained. The individual can be returned to the hospital for noncompliance with the treatment plan (Tenn Ann Code §33-6-201). Other states do not have a hearing for noncompliance as a criteria for rehospitalization (*Rhode Island Department of Mental Health, Retardation, and Hospitals v. RB*, 1988). The standard for rehospitalization does not have to be dangerousness or likelihood of serious harm, although this is usually a potential result of noncompliance. It is the treating professionals' responsibility to closely follow the individuals mandated to receive treatment. If these clients become compliant and no longer need the surveillance demanded by mandatory outpatient treatment, in some instances the treating professionals can remove them from this requirement by writing a letter to the court.

CONFIDENTIALITY

Confidentiality of information is a concept that nurses learn early in their education. Information given to them by clients is considered private and should not be disseminated, either verbally or in writing, without the permission of the client or guardian. Confidentiality of client information is clearly defined in the American Nurses Association Code of Ethics.

A recent court decision was related to a confidentiality issue. A doctor revealed a client's HIV status to the attorney of the client's employer. The individual, a flight attendant, was HIV positive and sought treatment from a physician for an ear and sinus infection. The flight attendant explicitly stated that the HIV status was not to be included on insurance forms because it might endanger his employment. The doctor agreed to this specification. One month later, the client filed a claim with a state workers' compensation board. A subpoena from another state was sent to the physician along with authorization from the client for two earlier workers' compensation claims, but not for this claim. The doctor sent the record with the HIV status to the attorney. A New York appeals court ruled that by revealing the client information to the requesting parties, the doctor had not acted in good faith. The subpoena was voluntary and from another state. This case illustrates that even with a subpoena, a health care professional should not release information without consulting with an attorney from the facility where employed (*Doe v. Roe*, 1993).

Questions have been raised also about the confidentiality limits of group therapy. Currently there are no known laws requiring clients to respect the confidentiality of other group members. However, it is important to stress to group members the importance of not revealing information outside of the therapy session. The participants should consider themselves co-therapists who help to ensure the comfort and safety of other group members. In group therapy perhaps each member should sign a contract relative to confidentiality (Appelbaum and Greer, 1993).

Confidentiality must be considered with changing technology. Computer-generated records will become more and more prevalent. They are time efficient for the provider, and generation of data is useful for utilization review, diagnosing, treatment planning, and communicating through various networks. It is paramount that information be secure; a system of passwords should be included to gain entry into the system. Those who have accessed the network should be monitored (Mordai and Rabinowitz, 1993).

PRIVILEGED COMMUNICATION

Privileged communication is different from confidentiality. It is enacted by statute to designated professionals, such as the clergy, attorneys, psychologists, or physicians. Privilege extends to information elicited in the therapeutic relationship. In many states nurses are not included. The provisions of these statutes allow certain information given to the professionals by clients to remain secret during any litigation. The privilege belongs to the client and can be asserted or waived only by the client. These statutes exclude reporting child and elder abuse (in some in-

---

Legal Case Report: Clinical Case Implications
Sexually Violent Predator: Commitment Standard
Kansas v. Hendricks (1997)

In a controversial 5-to-4 decision the U.S. Supreme Court upheld a statute enacted by the state of Kansas. Leroy Hendricks had been convicted of sexual offenses against children. He had a 40-year history of sexual involvement with children, for which he had been convicted on several occasions. Before his release, the state of Kansas petitioned to have Hendricks civilly committed under the state's Sexually Violent Predator Act. When he was stressed or pressured, he was unable to control his impulses. A jury in a lower state court found him to be a sexually violent predator, and the court civilly committed him. The court defined his pedophilia as a mental abnormality, but on appeal to the Kansas State Supreme Court, the commitment was invalidated on the basis of an assessment that a mental abnormality did not meet the commitment standard, which was predicated on mental illness.

On appeal to the U.S. Supreme Court, the justices commented that "states, have over the years, developed numerous specialized terms to define mental health concepts. Often these definitions do not fit precisely with the definitions employed by the medical community." The court maintained that the person must have an inability to control behavior and can be held until he or she is no longer dangerous to others. Hendricks had admitted at the jury trial that he could not control his behavior. "This admitted lack of volitional control, coupled with a prediction of future dangerousness, adequately distinguishes Hendricks from other dangerous persons who are perhaps more properly dealt with exclusively through criminal proceedings. Hendricks' diagnosis as a pedophile, which qualifies as a 'mental abnormality' under the Act, thus plainly suffices for due process purposes."

Because no effective treatment was being offered at this point, treatment was "nonexistent." The court asserted, "We have never held that the constitution prevents a state from civilly detaining those for whom no treatment is available, but nevertheless pose a danger to others." Treatment is not required for those who are dangerously mentally ill. There are built-in safeguards to ensure against an indefinite duration. The commitment is reviewed annually, and if the person can demonstrate in the future that there is no longer dangerous behavior, release can be granted.

The dissenting opinion focused on several issues; the Act was meant to segregate violent sexual offenders and be a meaningful attempt to provide treatment. This had not been accomplished. "As of the time of Hendricks' commitment, the state had not funded treatment, it had not entered into treatment contracts, and it had little, if any, qualified staff." Offenders were not committed until sentences were near completion, there were no less restrictive alternatives, and any treatment available was not offered until the sentence had been completed.

Since this ruling, some states have moved toward enacting laws that would place sexual offenders who have completed their sentences, in mental health facilities. This action places a responsibility on mental health professionals to develop programs of intervention that will lead to diminution of symptoms of these sexual offenders.

---

stances), domestic violence, some communicable diseases, and information that could prevent the commission of a felony, such as murder.

RELEASE OF INFORMATION

States have specific statutes related to release of mental health records. Nurses practicing in this clinical area should be aware of the state and federal statutes and guidelines relative to release of information. When clients are admitted to mental health facilities and have been treated on prior occasions, a request is usually extended to the client to authorize release of prior records. The kind of records requested, and for what period of time, should be clearly spelled out on the authorization form. Contents of records should not be released over the telephone unless the health care professional has a release signed by the client and is familiar with the other professional to whom the information is being given. Courts have generally considered that information contained in health records belongs to the client and that the actual record is the prop-

---

Legal Case Report: Clinical Case Implications
Privileged Communication
Jaffee v. Redmond (1996)

In a U.S. Supreme Court decision the justices ruled that a social worker, according to Illinois law and the Federal Rule of Evidence 501, did have privileged communication and that her client could invoke privilege in keeping communications between them confidential. The client, Mary Lu Redmond, a police officer, had in the process of her duties shot and killed Ricky Allen. In a wrongful death lawsuit filed by Allen's estate after his death, the social worker and Redmond declined to answer questions concerning what transpired in the therapeutic sessions. The judge directed the jury that it could deduce that notes concerning the sessions must be negative in relation to the defendant. The jury sent back a verdict of $545,000 against the defendant, Redmond, on state and federal claims. Even though the therapist was not an advanced practice nurse, if a state has a nurse therapist–client privilege, it seems likely that federal courts, on the basis of this decision, would recognize the privilege. Nurses should be cognizant of the privileged communication in the state where practicing.

erty of the treating professional or health care facility (Laben and MacLean, 1989). Most individuals no longer have problems obtaining records; however, obtaining the information can be expensive.

DUTY TO WARN AND PROTECT

Twenty years ago a case came to the forefront that changed the manner in which mental health professionals dealt with warning their clients' potential victims. The landmark decision, *Tarasoff v. Regents of the University of California* (1976), concerned a young man from India, Prosenjit Poddar, who was attending the University of California. He had formed a relationship with Tatiana Tarasoff and had misinterpreted a New Year's Eve kiss as a serious romantic gesture. After several months had passed, she conveyed to him that she wished to date other men and that she did not view their relationship as serious. He subsequently became depressed and sought mental health counseling. He communicated to his therapist that he might harm Tarasoff, who at that time was in South America. One day he ran out of the therapist's office and was detained by the campus police and released. After Tarasoff's return, he went to her home and fatally wounded her with a knife. The family of the victim brought suit against the University of California, and after the case reached the Supreme Court of California, the justices ruled that "protective privilege ends where the public peril begins." This ruling, **duty to warn**, established the responsibility of a treating mental health professional to notify an intended, identifiable victim.

Since this time many states and federal jurisdictions have promulgated decisions and passed statutes that delineate the duty to warn potential identifiable victims. In Vermont the court imposed the duty to warn when an individual posed a threat of potential harm to property. Mr. Peck was seen by an outpatient counselor to whom he communicated that he was angry with his father and wanted to set fire to his father's barn. The next day a family session was held with the father present. Five days later Peck again stated that he wanted to set fire to his father's barn. He promised the therapist that he would not burn down the barn; however, despite this agreement, he did later ignite the structure. The court ruled that the therapist had a duty to inform the parents of the threat to their property (*Peck v. the Counseling Service of Addison County, Inc.*, 1985).

Nurses should be aware of any case law related to this matter within their jurisdiction. In addition, several states have passed statutes in relation to this issue defining the responsibility of mental health professionals and the duty to warn potential victims (Cal Civ Code §43.92, Tenn Ann Code §33-10-103). Nurses, especially advanced practice nurses, should also know when to refer a patient for commitment in order to protect family and community members (see Legal Case Report on *Estates of Morgan v. Fairfield Family Counseling Center* on p. 96).

RIGHTS OF CLIENTS

According to Wexler and Winick (1992), mental health law based on the constitutional premise of protecting client rights is a little more than 20 years old. Before that time, there was little litigation or attention paid to the rights of individuals in mental health facilities.

Although the number of lawsuits that emerged in the 1970s and 1980s has decreased, certain rights not afforded to people with mental illnesses in institutions before that time are now taken for granted. Currently, when individuals enter a mental hospital, it is a rarity (not a probability) that the individuals have had their civil rights removed. Therefore these individuals have retained the right to vote, to manage financial matters, and to assert the constitutional right to seek the advice of an attorney. Other rights usually include the rights to receive mail, to wear one's own clothes, and to receive visitors (although, in forensic units, a limitation on the days and hours could be delineated).

The state of Pennsylvania requires that voluntary clients receive a summary of their rights on admission to an inpatient facility and a more inclusive manual of the rights within 72 hours. A study that was conducted in an urban university-affiliated hospital with 50 subjects concluded that only a minority of the subjects understood their rights after having them read by a nurse, followed up by a written copy. The implications are that, as part of the treatment plan, discussion and reinforcement of client rights should be an ongoing process (Wolpe, Schwartz, and Sanford, 1991). The state of Washington provides for a list of rights to be posted in the facility (Wash Ann Code §71.05.370). (See Nursing Care in the Community box for a discussion of legal issues and community psychiatric nursing.)

ACCESS TO CLIENT RECORDS AND CONFIDENTIALITY

The majority of states provide for client access to records. Generally, there is a procedure to be followed. Release forms should be signed if information is provided to a third party (Lyon, Levine, and Susman, 1982). When a relative or significant other desires information about the client, a release form should be signed by the client before any information is released. Especially with people with serious and persistent mental illnesses who have family members involved with their care, it is important to collaborate with the family on treatment to maintain the individual in the community without frequent exacerbations. With the shorter length of stay in a hospital and, in some areas, the lack of wide-based community alternatives, coordination of care with significant others is important. "The issue of confidentiality must be carefully considered but not used as an artificial barrier to collaboration. Formal and informal strategies can resolve the conflict between the patient's confidentiality and the family's compelling need for information fundamental to

Legal and Ethical Issues

The expansion of nursing mental health care into the community presents unique legal and ethical concerns. The community psychiatric mental health nurse's role is greatly limited by laws that were originally intended to promote and protect the rights of the individual client. Often, the right of the individual to receive treatment seems to conflict with the right of the individual to refuse treatment. The right to refuse treatment usually takes precedence unless the client is deemed by law to be a danger to self or others or to be in some way gravely disabled. The nurse often makes decisions balancing the expressed desire of the client against what would be in the client's best interest mentally, emotionally, and physically.

These decisions may challenge the trust implicit in the nurse-client therapeutic relationship. A broader impact may be felt in the community, since other individuals might respond defensively regarding the involuntary hospitalization of a friend. A nurse's commitment to advocacy may be called into question, jeopardizing her position in the mental health community. Alternative solutions should be thoroughly explored to ensure that the principle of least restrictive environment for the individual is upheld while maintaining the integrity of the environment for the surrounding community.

Nurses may also experience an internal conflict between the expectations of meeting legal requirements, containing costs, and satisfying personal ethical values. Psychiatric mental health nurses practicing in the community have expanded independence, which demands increased responsibility. Their documentation must be rigorous, thorough, and accurate, leaving no opportunity for challenge, especially in the current managed care environment.

Treatment plans are required to be clear and concise, including rationales and anticipated outcomes. The standards of care and outcomes should be measurable in concrete ways and treated as if they were part of a research study. The nurse's ethical ideals will be mollified by painstaking attention to the details of patient care in accordance with the requirements of the law. An adequate support system should be in place for addressing these issues, including a consultant to explore legal ramifications of specific interventions and a working collegial network in which to discuss and explore treatment options.

---

successful caregiving" (Reinhard, 1994). This stance does not negate the signing for release of information by the client for relatives to receive information but instead stresses the importance of the family in caregiving.

SECLUSION AND RESTRAINTS

Seclusion and restraint were major issues in two well-known cases: the right to treatment suit in Alabama (*Wyatt v. Stickney*, 1972) and the evaluation of seclusion practices at a state hospital in Massachusetts (*Rogers v. Okin*, 1980). In the latter case, seclusion had been insti-

gated when there was no immediate threat of violence or threatening behavior. *Wyatt v. Stickney* (1972) outlines guidelines for instituting seclusion and restraint. The original 20-year-old guidelines were updated by a federal judge. These standards include the instruction that clients should only be restrained to prevent "physical injury to themselves or others." Only a psychiatrist or other licensed physician can order nonemergency seclusion or restraint, and the physician must be present and evaluate the client before writing the order (News and Notes, 1992). The new guidelines set 8 hours instead of 24 as the maximum time limit for the original order. The client must be observed every 15 minutes instead of every hour as previously outlined. An order for seclusion and restraint can be issued by a nurse for 1 hour, but the nurse must be physically present and document observations in the client's chart. A qualified physician must be notified after the emergency and see the client within 4 hours; however, 1 hour is preferred. Although these guidelines are only binding in Alabama, when originally disseminated, they were used as guidelines in other states and mental health organizations (News and Notes, 1992).

Although research is limited in guiding the nurse about the implementation of seclusion, Outlaw and Lowery (1992) recommend that seclusion be used only when necessary and not for events such as refusing to take medications, participating in activities, or making loud noises. Research shows that secluding a client is viewed by the staff as upsetting. Some clients also see seclusion as a very negative experience, whereas others view it as a reward.

Norris and Kennedy (1992) recommend that explanations about what is happening be given to the isolated individual and that special attention be given to assessing the individual's physical needs. Every attempt should be made to minimize a struggle, and the person should be placed in seclusion or restraints in the least restrictive manner. Afterward, talking with the client can help decrease the psychologic impact.

Nurses should be familiar with the seclusion and restraint rules and regulations of the agency where practicing. Clear documentation delineating the reasons for seclusion and restraint and the less restrictive alternatives initially attempted should be outlined. Recording of the client's behavior, including the nurse's verbal interventions to decrease the behavior that prompted the intervention, is important. If a staff member or other client is injured during an incident related to seclusion or restraint, a debriefing of the incident should take place to assess what happened and to plan for more appropriate interventions in the future.

RIGHT TO TREATMENT

More than 20 years ago a movement began in Alabama that was directed at the right to treatment for people with mental illnesses. With financial constraints within the mental health system, employees at Bryce Hospital were

Understanding & Applying Research

A phenomenologic study was conducted with 10 adult participants—5 men and 5 women—relating to their experiences of being restrained. Interviews were transcribed in their entirety. All of the participants had been controlled with leather restraints on a psychiatric unit. Generally, the attitude of psychiatric nurses had been that assisting clients with external limits helped them to feel safe and protected. Usually the restraint resulted from failure to conform to unit rules, or from a feeling on the part of the staff that the behavior of these clients was escalating and out of control. The results of the study indicated that the participants felt coerced, vulnerable, helpless, and dehumanized. Johnson comments that "We need to use restraints as a last resort."

This study aptly supports the need to use least restrictive interventions before physical restraint whenever possible.

Johnson ME: Being restrained: a study of power and powerlessness, *Issues Ment Health Nurs* 19(3):191, 1998.

laid off because of a budget shortfall. As a result of this situation, a class action suit on behalf of the employees and clients was filed, alleging that with fewer employees the clients could not receive the proper treatment. Eventually, the Fifth Circuit Court of Appeals upheld a right to treatment, and the state of Alabama was placed in receivership to be monitored by the federal system. The case was settled by consent decree in 1986. Although the right to treatment concept applies to this particular federal circuit, the guidelines for treatment promulgated by Judge Johnson of the Federal District Court have been followed in many jurisdictions. Some of the standards specified include the right to privacy and dignity, the right to the least restrictive treatment, and individual treatment plans that include a statement of problems and intermediate and long-range treatment goals (with a timetable for attainment with rationale for the specified treatment) (Laben and MacLean, 1989; *Wyatt v. Stickney*, 1972).

In a U.S. Supreme Court decision it was ruled that an individual cannot be kept in a mental hospital without treatment if he or she is nondangerous and capable of surviving in the community. Mr. Donaldson had been hospitalized in Florida for over 14 years and desired to be released. Because of his religion, he declined to take medication or other treatment. He was denied the privilege of going out on the grounds. He had a friend who was willing to assist him on discharge from the hospital. The ruling was very limited, but it did set forth the premise that the state cannot detain individuals who are nondangerous without providing some mode of treatment (*O'Connor v. Donaldson*, 1975).

In the later decision *Youngberg v. Romeo* (1982), the U.S. Supreme Court ruled that a young man with profound retardation was entitled to "minimally adequate training" to provide him with safe conditions. The court stated that a qualified professional's judgment about this matter is considered "presumptively valid." There was great concern at the time that the right-to-treatment movement was over, but that has not proved to be true: courts have upheld the concept of providing adequate treatment (*Woe v. Cuomo*, 1986, and Appelbaum, 1987). Stefan (1993), however, reports that "conditions and treatment in many state institutions are still so appalling that plaintiffs still can establish a departure from professional judgment in a well-litigated case."

RIGHT TO REFUSE TREATMENT

In the late 1970s and early 1980s, two well-known cases were litigated in the states of Massachusetts and New Jersey, based on the right to refuse psychotropic medication. In the New Jersey case, Mr. Rennie was diagnosed with a psychotic disorder (schizophrenia) at one point and manic depression at another time. There was no unanimous conclusion about the appropriate medication to be administered to him. He was given fluphenazine (Prolixin) and chlorpromazine (Thorazine) at different times. He suffered from such side effects as akathisia and wormlike movements of the tongue. He refused to take his medication. Rennie filed suit in court to prevent the involuntary administration of medications. After the suit was heard on four different occasions, it was decided that voluntary and involuntary clients had the right to refuse medication. During emergency situations, if potential danger is involved, clients can be forcibly medicated. In the case of an involuntary client, as long as due process guidelines are followed as established and the administration complies with accepted professional judgment, medication can be given (*Rennie v. Klein*, 1979, 1981). The administrative procedure includes the physician communicating with the clients about their mental health condition and outlining the plan of care with the client when possible. If the client refuses, the medical director of the facility reviews the treatment recommendations and is authorized to call in an outside psychiatrist for consultation (Weiner and Wettstein, 1993).

Rogers v. Okin was originally filed in 1975 as a class action suit to enjoin a state hospital from certain seclusion practices and forcibly medicating clients. In this case, the courts reached a different conclusion. Instead of deferring to administrative procedures that rely on professional judgment, the right to refuse treatment is upheld if the client is involuntary and competent. If the person is ruled incompetent, the judge will use the substituted judgment standard to determine administration of medication. The judge will look at whether the client, if competent, would have chosen medication administration. In this decision the court ruled that only a judicial authority, and not the decision of the physician or the guardian, was paramount (Weiner and Wettstein, 1993).

Later the Massachusetts Supreme Court ruled that once a client becomes competent, the substituted judg-

Legal Case Report: Clinical Case Implications
Involuntary Commitment
In the Interest of R.A.J (1996)

In a recent case a son petitioned for involuntary commitment of his 62-year-old father, R.A.J. The court found probable cause at a preliminary hearing to commit R.A.J. for no more than 14 days to the state hospital. At the hospital he was diagnosed with bipolar disorder and alcohol abuse. At a later hearing it was not concluded that he had a chemical dependency, but a judgment was issued that he was mentally ill, had impairment, and could be hospitalized for up to an additional 90 days. Because he was refusing to take medication, the court ordered that this intervention was the least restrictive and that he could be involuntarily medicated with haloperidol (Haldol) and carbamazepine (Tegretol), or with risperidone (Risperdal) and carbamazepine, for 90 days. R.A.J. then appealed the decision related to the forced medication order. R.A.J. contended that he had agreed to take the risperidone but not the other medication. The hospital argued that if one medication was refused, the client had "effectively refused necessary treatment." The court noted that it must find by clear and convincing evidence that the treatment was necessary, that the client refused it, that medication was the least restrictive alternative, and that the benefits outweighed the risks. The following items also had to be taken into consideration:

- The danger that the client represented to himself or others
- The client's current condition
- The client's past treatment history
- The results of previous medication trials
- The efficacy of current or past treatment modalities concerning the client
- The client's prognosis
- The effect of the client's mental condition on his capacity to consent

The court ruled that refusal to take one medication instead of the two prescribed amounted to refusal of treatment for the "purposes of the forced medication statute." The medication haloperidol could be given in injectable form if R.A.J. refused the oral risperidone. The benefits outweighed the risks and was the least restrictive form of treatment.

ment should be terminated. The court also ruled that substituted judgment treatment orders should be reviewed periodically to be in compliance with the current treatment plan. All substituted judgment orders should in the future include a termination (*Guardianship of Weedon*, 1992).

Nurses practicing in mental health facilities should be aware of the state and case laws and policies and procedures for that jurisdiction relative to administration of medication to refusing clients. Frequent checks for side effects and listening carefully to clients' complaints about side effects are imperative for adjustment and changing of medication. The reason for the refusal of medication should be carefully analyzed: is it because of the denial of the illness or symptomatology of the psychosis, or is it because of side effects or anger with the treatment staff? Education of the client and a reassuring therapeutic relationship can assist in diminishing a client's refusal (Laben and MacLean, 1989).

ELECTROCONVULSIVE THERAPY AND PSYCHOSURGERY

The administration of electroconvulsive therapy (ECT) continues to be controversial; however, in certain instances, it can be a viable treatment. One major issue that arises is providing informed consent for the procedure. The procedure, including the risks and benefits, should be carefully explained to the client. A major side effect continues to be loss of memory, which may not later be recovered.

There has been some concern about ECT being given to the elderly. Texas is the only state to keep statistics on the numbers of people undergoing ECT. It has been pointed out that 65-year-olds get 360% more shock therapy than 64-year-olds in Texas. This may be due to the payment by Medicare (Cauchon, 1995). It is essential to follow established pre-ECT guidelines to make sure that it is safe to send the patient for ECT no matter what the age. There are some medical conditions where it is contradicted, such as recent myocardial infarction with continued unstable cardiac function (Fitzsimons, 1995) and a history of increased intracranial pressure related to brain tumor or other space-occupying lesions.

Another issue is, who can give consent? The American Psychiatric Association (1978) advises that if an incompetent client cannot give informed consent, a relative of the client should be sufficient. Parry (1985) however, states that if there is a question of competency, legal consultation or court guidance should take place.

In the state of Washington a client has the right to refuse such treatment unless there is clear and convincing evidence that it is needed. The state must have compelling evidence that ECT is necessary and would be effective, and that other forms of treatment have not been beneficial or are not available (Washington; Antipsychotic Medication; ECT, 1993). Some states, such as Tennessee, have regulations related to administration of ECT to minors (Tenn Ann Code §33-3-105). Other states limit the number of treatments that can be given to an individual within a certain time frame (Weiner and Wettstein, 1993).

RESEARCH

Guidelines have been established by the federal government that apply to research on human subjects. The major objective is to provide informed consent to the person who has agreed to participate in research projects. Some of the guidelines include a clear statement of the following: the purpose of the research, the risks and possible discomforts to the subject, the possible benefits to the individual or to others, alternative treatment procedures, confidentiality of records, sources for further information, and availability of compensation if injury occurs. Perhaps the most important fact to convey is that the research is voluntary (45 CFR §46.116).

Alzheimer's disease and other dementias will increase in numbers as the population ages. Because there are no animal models of this degenerative process, human experimentation is necessary (Dukoff and Sunderland, 1997). The National Institutes of Health has discovered that clients in the early stages of dementia can select health care proxies despite some "minimal memory problems and word-finding difficulties"; in the early stages they continue to "possess the capacity to make independent decisions." As a safeguard to this process, all clients are assessed by a bioethicist. In this manner, as the disease progresses and informed consent can no longer be given by the participant in the research, the client will have a health care proxy to speak for him or her.

Nurses should be aware of these guidelines, especially when completing research projects to fulfill educational requirements. Many health care facilities are encouraging staff nurses to participate in research, and awareness of these guidelines is imperative.

THE AMERICANS WITH DISABILITIES ACT

The Americans With Disabilities Act (42 USC §12101) is a substantial breakthrough in discrimination against people with mental illnesses; however, there are specific exclusions. The definition includes mental impediments that limit the ability of the individual in one or more major activities. Enforcement of the statute depends on the person's limitations. It has been ruled that if a person's mental condition is stabilized, there is no disability (*Mackie v. Runyon*, 1992). Such people are protected, however, if the fact that they once had a mental disability (such as depression) is used against them in the employment situation. Some exclusions include persons who use controlled substances for unlawful purposes and individuals who take prescribed drugs without the supervision of a health care professional (Parry, 1985). In addition, people who pose a direct threat to others are excluded. However, it is important to recognize that this must be based on actual behavior of the individual and not on the mental disability itself.

A person cannot be asked about a prior history of mental health treatment as part of an application process for employment. The individual can be evaluated as to the ability to perform the job functions. Questions about prior use of health care insurance coverage are also not permissible (Weiner and Wettstein, 1993).

ADVOCACY

The term *advocacy* refers to speaking in favor of or arguing for a cause (American Heritage Dictionary, 1993).

As a result of the mental health movement begun in the 1970s, states developed advocacy programs for clients. Internal grievance procedures allowing clients to express views on their treatment have been initiated in many states. Under the Protection and Advocacy for Mentally Ill Individuals Act of 1986, all states were required to designate an agency that is responsible for maintaining the rights of people with mental illnesses. The names vary from state to state. For example, in Tennessee, Effective Advocacy for Citizens With Handicaps, Inc. (EACH) is the organization responsible for implementation of this act. There has been some controversy over this movement; some mental health professionals say that advocacy sets up adversarial relationships. Advocates should have some understanding of the nature of mental illness and how the mental health system works (Laben and MacLean, 1989).

With the increasing prevalence of managed care, advocacy may become more and more a part of the nurse's responsibility, especially in the case of nurse psychotherapists who are seeking appropriate care for their clients from third-party payers. Simon (1998) writes that psychiatrists must advocate with managed care organizations for the care they consider necessary. This strategy includes nurses calling for authorization from managed care companies. Nurses should be informed about the client's right to appeal denial of services that a mental health provider believes is a "medical necessity." Appeals should be pursued with zeal, particularly in a case where the client is living in the community and the mental health provider thinks there is a potential for violence. Documentation that the client has been informed of these rights is also advisable. In addition to the responsibility to pursue appeals, the nurse may be responsible for providing adequate data on which a utilization reviewer can base an informed decision.

At the least, nurses should have some understanding of each client's rights and should report to administration when those rights are observed to be violated. Nursing has a long history of advocating for the client, and this should be continued, taking into account changing laws and guidelines relative to mental health treatment.

FORENSIC EVALUATIONS

Individuals who have mental health problems and who are charged with or convicted of crimes fall within the category of forensic mental health services. In the 1960s and 1970s exposés of treatment of these individuals were prevalent in the professional journals and newspapers. In many instances persons were sent to institutions for evaluation and remained for many years in these facilities without resolution of criminal charges. Procedural due process for many was nonexistent. Many forensic units were isolated and provided inadequate treatment. These conditions began to change in 1972 with the landmark decision *Jackson v. Indiana*. Jackson was mentally challenged and hearing and speech impaired. He was found incompetent to stand trial. Because of his disabilities, he probably would never become competent to stand trial. At that time Indiana required hospitalization in a mental hospital until return to competency. Jackson was not going to become competent, so hospitalization would literally sentence him to a form of detention for life. His criminal charge was robbery for a total of $9.

The U.S. Supreme Court ruled that an individual could be hospitalized only for a reasonable length of time (not defined) and that the 3½ years that Jackson had been detained was too long. If the state wanted to hospitalize him longer, he had to be civilly committed, meeting commitment standards. Otherwise, he had to be released. Because of this ruling in the state of Tennessee, the population of the forensic unit went from 185 to 50 within 2 years (Laben and Spencer, 1976).

COMPETENCY TO STAND TRIAL

Competency to stand trial is a very narrow concept. The criteria include the following: Does the individual charged with the crime understand the criminal charges? Is there an understanding of the legal process and the consequences of the charges? Can the individual advise an attorney and defend the charges? Essentially, it is the person's awareness of the legal process that must be evaluated by the mental health professional.

If the judge, prosecuting attorney, or defense attorney believes that competency is an issue, a request by the attorney results in a court order asking for the evaluation of the person's competency to stand trial. Many states recognize not only the psychiatrist as the competent evaluator on this issue but also psychologists, social workers, and advanced practice psychiatric nurses who have been educated and trained in this evaluation process. Many evaluations are now performed on an outpatient basis, resulting in return to the courts and a more timely resolution of the charges (Laben and MacLean, 1989).

CRIMINAL RESPONSIBILITY (INSANITY DEFENSE)

Competency to stand trial relates to the present mental condition of the defendants and their current ability to make a defense in court. The insanity defense relates to the state of mind at the time of the offense. This concept stems from the legal doctrine of *mens rea*. For a person to be found guilty, the individual must be able to form intent. If, because of mental illness, intent cannot be formed and the person is possibly responding to hallucinatory voices, there is no guilt involved (Shah, 1986).

The first well-known case came from England where the M'Naghten Rule was promulgated. The set of circumstances involved Daniel M'Naghten, who shot and mistakenly murdered the secretary to the prime minister instead of his intended victim, Sir Robert Peel. M'Naghten was found not guilty by reason of insanity, and this caused great consternation in that country. Subsequently, a panel of 15 judges met and defined what has become known as the M'Naghten Rule. An accused will not be held responsible if at the time of the commission of the act, he was "laboring under such a defect of reason, from disease of the mind, as to not know the nature and quality of the act he was doing, or if he did know it, that he did not know he was doing what was wrong" (Shah, 1986).

Much criticism of this doctrine emerged in the 1960s and 1970s, and some states subsequently adopted a modern interpretation of the insanity defense, which states that a person is not responsible for criminal conduct if at the time of such conduct, as a result of mental disease or defect, the person lacks substantial capacity either to appreciate the criminality (wrongfulness) of the conduct or to conform his or her conduct to the requirements of the law (*Graham v. State of Tennessee*, 1977). This definition is derived from the Model Penal Code.

Once a person is found not guilty by reason of insanity, he or she is usually hospitalized and sent to a psychiatric unit for evaluation of commitability. Many states have stricter release standards for individuals found not guilty by reason of insanity because, although they have been found not guilty, they have committed a criminal act (Laben and MacLean, 1989).

GUILTY BUT MENTALLY ILL

Recently several states have adopted a new plea of guilty but mentally ill (GBMI). The individual is found guilty, but because of the plea that mental illness caused commission of the crime, is sent to prison and treated for the mental illness. It was thought that fewer people would adopt an insanity defense with the GBMI plea. This has

Understanding & Applying Research

A survey was completed of Massachusetts district court judges related to forensic evaluations. Fifty-eight of 160 responded. The question presented to the judges was, when civil commitment was available and the charge was a minor offense, why were individuals committed for a 20-day forensic evaluation for competency to stand trial? An overwhelming majority (93.1%) admitted concerns about the treatment of individuals in a civil commitment to a mental health facility. Some of the reasons for this strategy included that the defendant did not meet commitment standards and that on some occasions psychiatric hospitals deny admission to offenders who meet commitment criteria unless the court orders the admission. A forensic commitment does not allow for early discharge; the defendant must remain for 20 days and must appear in court before discharge. "This study confirms suspicions that judges order pretrial evaluations to fill perceived gaps in the civil system."

Applebaum KL, Fisher WH: Judges' assumptions about the appropriateness of civil and forensic commitment, *Psychiatr Serv* 48(5):710, 1997.

not always proved to be the case; in Michigan the numbers of those pleading this form of the insanity defense increased, although in Georgia the numbers have decreased (Callahan et al, 1992).

NURSING RESPONSIBILITIES IN THE CRIMINAL JUSTICE SYSTEM

In at least one state, advanced practice nurses can testify to the issue of competency to stand trial. This should not be undertaken lightly, and special education should be sought out before testifying on this issue. In most states, psychologists with doctoral degrees and psychiatrists testify concerning the insanity defense.

MALPRACTICE

Because of the irreversible side effects of some medications given to individuals with mental health problems and the trend of short-term hospitalizations, nurses working in psychiatric settings must be aware of situations that might later lead to a malpractice lawsuit. Negligence, the

primary basis for malpractice lawsuits, is a civil dispute between two or more citizens or a health care facility. A person alleges that a professional omitted or committed an act that a reasonably prudent professional would not do. The action of the professional causes injury resulting in measurable damages.

ELEMENTS OF A MALPRACTICE SUIT BASED ON NEGLIGENCE

To bring a suit, the plaintiff must establish that a nurse had a **legal duty** to that person to provide a certain standard of care. The care is measured by the reasonably prudent nurse standard: What would another nurse working in a mental health facility have done in the same situation? Usually **expert witnesses** are brought in to testify to the standard of care. Some jurisdictions look to a reasonably prudent nurse standard; however, with the development of standards by the American Nurses Association in relationship to psychiatric nursing practice, these guidelines could be adopted in a lawsuit (Statement on Psychiatric Mental Health Nursing Practice, 1994). The next element

---

Legal Case Report: Clinical Case Implications
Nurse's Responsibility
Hatley v. Kassen (1992)

Pennie Johnson had been mentally ill for 10 years. She had been an outpatient in a forensic unit, because long-term inpatient treatment was considered nontherapeutic. Because of her long-term history, a difficult client file had been established to assist treating physicians. In February of 1988 she was picked up by a state trooper on a tollway road, at which time she threatened suicide. She was taken to a county hospital. In the nursing assessment Johnson stated that she was feeling increasingly depressed and had ingested medication that exceeded the prescribed dosage. She continued to take this medication in front of the hospital staff, at which time it was removed from her.

She was examined by Dr. Kalra, who decided to discharge her because he thought her condition had not changed. Johnson asked both the nurse who assessed her and the nursing supervisor, Ms. Kassen, RN, to return her medication. She announced that if the medication was not returned, she would throw herself in front of a car. Kassen told Johnson that if she would return home in a taxicab paid for by the hospital, Kassen would return the medication. Johnson declined the offer. A security officer was instructed to escort her out of the hospital. There was disputed testimony as to whether the physician knew of her threats. Thirty minutes after leaving the hospital, Johnson stepped in front of a truck and was killed.

An action for damages was brought by Johnson's parents. In the lower court decision, a summary judgment (granted when no genuine issue of material fact is presented) was awarded to the physician and the hospital, and a directed verdict in favor of Kassen (a decision that is directed to the jury by the judge because the opposing party has not sufficiently presented its case) (Weiner and Wettstein, 1993). The Court of Appeals of Texas reversed the decision and remanded the case back to the lower

court for further litigation, stating that the doctor and the nurse were not entitled to official immunity because of employment at a government hospital.

The court, in its decision, did note the testimony of three expert witnesses regarding Kassen's nursing care. Two nurse experts testified that Kassen's actions were substandard once she knew that Johnson had communicated suicidal intentions with a specific plan. A psychiatric expert in the field of suicidology testified that Kassen should have sought the advice of the physician or supervisor before releasing Johnson after the suicidal threats.

One judge wrote a dissenting opinion. This justice believed that Johnson had threatened for 10 years to commit suicide and had never done so; therefore it was not foreseeable that Johnson would follow through with her threat, and therefore it was not negligence on Kassen's part. "I would hold that threats of suicide cannot enslave the intended victim to either submission or damages—especially threats that have been 'empty' for years."

This case was remanded for retrial, so the final results are unknown. However, elements of the case can be analyzed. The nurses and doctor had a duty to a client who was brought to the emergency department. Several experts testified that once a client has a suicide plan, some form of hospitalization should be instituted, or—at the least—a supervisor notified or another discussion held with the physician. Based on this testimony, it might be concluded that the nurse fell below the standard of care. Because the nurse permitted the client to leave the hospital, she could be targeted as a causal agent in the resulting death. Damages could be awarded for the incident (Weiner and Wettstein, 1993).

that is explored is whether or not the injury was foreseeable based on the nurse's behavior and the set of circumstances that followed. The court explores whether the nurse was the causal link in the injury that ensued. For example, did the nurse give the wrong medication or did the nurse not know about drug interactions with certain medications that led to the injury? The last element that must be determined is whether or not there is a proven injury because of the nurse's behavior.

DOCUMENTATION

The information that must be kept in a mental health record is often regulated by the state or the mental health facility where the nurse is practicing. Many mental health professionals view charting as a burden. However, it is not just a record of the care of the client; it is also a legal document that might be very valuable in any litigation that might take place.

Adequate documentation is the best means of defense against a lawsuit and the best way to validate that the nurse provided a safe standard of care. It is important to be specific and to document symptoms by writing in quotes what the client expresses to you, such as, "I am hearing voices that say I am a bad person." Recording the actual words of the client is more definitive than simply noting, "The client is hallucinating," especially if the words are destructive to the client or others. Charting should be done in a timely manner. Recording at the time something happens is considered more adequate than block charting, which is usually more brief and not as definitive (Nurse's Handbook of Law and Ethics, 1992). A client's record is a sequential document; thus space should not be "saved" for late entries. Late entries should be labeled as such and initialed.

In a mental health record it is especially important to document when the person has achieved the goals outlined in the treatment plan. If the individual has an exacerbation of the illness, the treatment plan should reflect the change. Informed consent concerning the giving of psychiatric medications is an important aspect of the chart, especially medications such as some neuroleptics, which can cause irreversible side effects.

Records are an excellent source for communicating with other mental health professionals on the staff of a facility, as well as other agencies where the client is being treated. It is also validation for reimbursement that care was given for particular symptoms. Since managed care is becoming prevalent, a clear outline of all of the client's symptoms should be carefully recorded to document a necessity for continued hospitalization. For example, if routine hospitalization is for 5 days, but the client continues to verbalize suicidal thoughts daily, recording of this information is critical for extended permission to continue the hospitalization.

Improper abbreviations not authorized by the agency should not be used. Records from other facilities or other treating professionals should be obtained to provide an accurate long-term picture of how the client was treated on prior occasions.

Any client teaching, aftercare plans, or referral to other agencies for care should be written. Accurate recording of blood pressure is essential, especially in relation to the taking of medications. Any nursing assessments that are required by the organization should be completed. Words should be spelled correctly and sentences should be grammatically correct. Errors in documentation should be noted by placing a single line through the words without obliterating them and then initialing each instance.

SEXUAL MISCONDUCT

In studies that have been conducted with social workers, psychiatrists, and psychologists, it is estimated that up to 14% of these professionals have had a sexual relationship with a client (Weiner and Wettstein, 1993). There has been no known study of nurses; however, cases for removal of a nursing license for such activity are recorded (*Heinecke v. Department of Commerce*, 1991). All mental health professions consider such behavior unethical, and in many states this behavior is considered criminal, especially if it is within a few months of the therapeutic relationship. Some states have mandatory reporting laws for a second therapist who becomes knowledgeable about such behavior (Strasburger, Jorgenson, and Randles, 1991).

Many of the cases are settled out of court (*Hall v. Schulte*, 1992). When information about the relationship is presented to a jury, members tend to be sympathetic to the client, except when a client appears to have encouraged the relationship. Because the client comes to a therapist with a problem, the issue of the transference phenomenon becomes pronounced, resulting in true lack of consent to become involved with the therapist (Weiner and Wettstein, 1993).

SUICIDE AND HOMICIDE

Malpractice suits and wrongful death actions for homicidal clients' injury to a third party and death from suicide have become prevalent. Some states have ruled that individuals working in government agencies have sovereign immunity and can be protected from liability in malpractice situations (*Poss v. Department of Human Resources*, 1992; *Smith v. King*, 1993). It should be noted, however, that when an individual threatens suicide and communicates this information to a mental health provider, the appropriate steps, including involuntary commitment, must be taken to escape liability. If there is a question, legal consultation should be sought. However, "clinicians are not liable for errors of clinical judgment; they are liable only for departures from the relevant standard of care, given the clinical situation" (Weiner and Wettstein, 1993).

Because of the previously described decision re *Tarasoff v. Regents of the University of California*, it is important to communicate with the mental health treatment team

Legal Case Report: Clinical Case Implications
Responsibilities of Treating Therapists
Estates of Morgan v. Fairfield Family Counseling Center (1997)

Matt Morgan was playing a card game with his parents and sister when he left the room, returned with a gun, and shot and killed his parents. His sister was injured but survived. Matt had problems in his senior year in high school and after graduation had difficulty retaining employment. He was "verbally abusive" to his parents, and they had become afraid of him. In January of 1990 he was removed from his home by police as he was attempting to fight with his father.

After a period of wandering, Matt eventually presented to the emergency department at a hospital in Philadelphia. He was diagnosed with schizophreniform disorder and was transferred to a mental health facility. He had delusions that the government was affecting his body and the air waves, so that he was unable to watch television or listen to tapes or radio, and he had delusions of persecution, ideas of reference, and thought broadcasting. He was given thiothixene (Navane) and was admitted to a respite unit.

During the 12-week stay at the respite unit, Matt continued to receive thiothixene and intensive therapy. He had paranoia concerning his family, but this decreased, and he was able to admit that the medication assisted him in managing his symptoms. He acknowledged that his conflicts with his family, especially his relationship with his father, could be attributed to his mental illness. The treating physician thought it would be in Matt's best interest to return to his home and be followed at the Fairfield Family Counseling Center (FFCC). His parents came to get him at the end of June 1990, and he was first seen in the FFCC on July 16, 1990.

He was initially seen by a psychotherapist and was then referred to Dr. Brown, a contract psychiatrist for medication evaluation, on July 19, 1990. Dr. Brown reported that Matt had been in a mental health unit "of some sort" in Philadelphia and that he was out of medication. He wrote, "He comes to the mental health clinic for his medication, continued care and help in completing a Social Security Disability form." Dr. Brown concluded that Matt had some form of atypical psychosis and did not appear to have a thought disorder or schizophrenia. Dr. Brown also noted that he thought Matt might be malingering in an attempt to obtain disability. Dr. Brown wrote that it was "wise to defer diagnosis, continue the medication, obtain Matt's records from Philadelphia and schedule another appointment for a month later." When Matt returned for his appointment, the records from the mental health unit in Philadelphia were available, but the court reported that it was clear from Dr. Brown's testimony that he never read them or attempted to contact the treating physician.

Dr. Brown reduced the dosage of thiothixene and wrote again about the possibility of malingering. Dr. Brown saw Matt on October 11, 1990, for the last time; he prescribed a tapering and discontinuation of the thiothixene. He stated that Matt would continue in psychotherapy. Matt was referred to a vocational counselor to assist him in finding employment. Between October and January 1991, Matt remained in psychotherapy and vocational counseling. His mother reported, however, that Matt's condition was deteriorating, as evidenced by his pacing, quiet demeanor, withdrawal, and irritability. She asked that he be placed back on medication and shared that Matt had given a deposit toward the purchase of a gun. The vocational counselor thought that the mother was overprotective. When Matt failed to keep his appointment with the psychotherapist in January of 1991, it was decided that the only person who should see him was the vocational counselor. Matt continued to decompensate, his parents became afraid of him, and he once again developed symptoms of paranoia. During the month of May 1991, Matt's mother continued to report Matt's deterioration. An appointment was scheduled with Dr. Brown, but Matt did not keep it. Matt's employer also reported that he was "too weak to push a lawnmower, was on the verge of passing out, and did not seem to be totally in touch with reality." On June 14, 1991, Matt's mother wrote a letter to FFCC seeking assistance with her son. She explained her concerns about his potential violence. An assessment was conducted by the vocational counselor and a licensed social worker. FFCC had an unwritten policy that no involuntary commitment would be initiated without family involvement, but when the family attempted such course of action, the probate court informed them that it would need the vocational counselor's approval.

On July 20, 1991, Matt's parents sent a letter to a psychologist employed at FFCC who reviewed the record, talked with the vocational counselor and social worker, and determined that Matt could not be given medication against his will and could not be hospitalized. Another social worker commented on July 25, 1991, that Matt was losing weight and deteriorating. That evening Matt shot his family.

In an action for negligence brought by the parents' estate, expert witnesses for the plaintiffs, the Morgan estates, testified that Dr. Brown's treatment of Matt was negligent for failure to read the prior treatment reports, for failure to diagnose, for discontinuing needed medication, and for failure to closely monitor Matt after discontinuation of the medication. The fact that a vocational therapist was making commitment decisions was of particular concern. One expert testified that it was foreseeable that without medication, a potential for violent behavior was created. "The only reason Matt killed his parents is because he was taken off medication and didn't receive good care."

The expert witnesses testified that at the point that Matt refused medication, because of his deteriorating condition, the action should have included "strong family involvement, making Matt's participation in vocational therapy contingent upon continued treatment, and telling Matt that he faced involuntary hospitalization unless he resumed taking his medication."

The court in its ruling stated that "a relationship between the psychotherapist and the patient in the outpatient setting constitutes a special relationship justifying the imposition of a duty upon the psychotherapist to protect against the patient's violent propensities. The outpatient setting embodies sufficient elements of control to warrant the imposition of such a duty, and such a duty would serve the public's interest in protection from the violently inclined mental patient in a manner that is consistent with Ohio law."

The trial court had dismissed this action, and the Court of Appeals affirmed in part and reversed in part. The Supreme Court held that the psychotherapist had a duty to protect against the client's potentially violent behavior. The case was returned to the trial court to settle the issues of whether the defendants were negligent and whether a summary judgment in the defendant's favor was warranted.

What can be learned from this case is that any treating therapist must be aware of the duty to hospitalize and protect families and the public when appropriate. Consultation by nurse clinicians with mental health professionals who have legal authority to commit is essential.

when a client threatens to harm someone. Many states require that a potential victim and/or police be notified of this occurrence. Some states have limited the warning to include only identifiable victims (*Leonard v. Iowa*, 1992; Rudegair and Appelbaum, 1992). Failure to comply with the required notification could lead to liability.

ETHICAL ISSUES

Ethical issues are closely tied to legal implications for nursing care. *Ethics* is that body of knowledge that explores the moral problems that are raised about specific issues. In nursing practice one should look at the rules, principles, and ethical guidelines that have been developed by the nursing profession to guide conduct (Davis and Aroskar, 1991). Laws reflect the moral fiber of a society and are developed (hopefully) with an ethical basis; therefore ethical principles should be taken into consideration when evaluating a dilemma. Many problems are raised in the area of mental health law when statutes conflict with a nurse's personal beliefs.

AUTONOMY

The term **autonomy** refers to having respect for an individual's decision or self-determination about health care issues. This point is especially important with problems such as the right to die and, in mental health, treatment in the least restrictive alternative. When involuntary commitment is necessary, it is very difficult for mental health providers to have to follow the law rather than what the client currently desires. On one hand the caregiver may want to allow the client to make decisions, but, if the individual is threatening suicide with an active plan, proceeding against the wishes of the person may be necessary for safety and compliance with the law. This kind of decision in ethical terms is called a *paternalistic decision*, or *parentalism* (Purtilo, 1993). This can cause a great deal of inner turmoil for the health care professional who is just beginning to participate in this kind of decision making.

In addition, it is sometimes very difficult for families when the member who is mentally ill and refusing treatment has to be involuntarily hospitalized. Educating the family about the illness, being supportive, and allowing all of the family to ventilate their frustration, anxieties, and (perhaps) anger can be helpful in this time of crisis for the family.

Olsen (1998) has raised an interesting question about autonomy and privacy in relation to video monitoring of psychiatric clients who are placed in seclusion. One loses autonomy when secluded or restrained, and compounding this situation with video monitoring can be very threatening to a client. To justify the use of such strategies, Olsen recommends that there should be a record that a monitor is being used and the therapeutic reason for such use. The client should be informed of the monitoring, perhaps by placing a sign in the seclusion room. Olsen contends that only staff with clinical responsibility for care of the client should have access to the monitor, that only clinically competent staff should be monitoring clients, and that personal visualization and contact with the client should be carried out by the nurse. "Ethical treatment means balancing the good of a safer environment with the potential of harm from a loss of privacy."

BENEFICENCE

Individuals who work in the health care field have a special duty and responsibility to act in a manner that is going to benefit and not harm clients. The term **beneficence** refers to bringing about good (Purtilo, 1993). The goal in mental health treatment is to assist individuals in returning to a mentally healthy way of life.

The moral imperative of *primum no nocere* ("first do no harm") should be paramount in clinical interventions with persons with mental illnesses. Situations in which this issue might arise include giving neuroleptic medications when it is known that certain side effects may be irreversible. Another instance is the consideration of giving ECT to a client who has failed to respond to antidepressive medication and continues to be suicidal. It is known that memory loss can be a side effect. Do the beneficial aspects of the treatment outweigh the possible side effects? This dilemma can cause anxiety for the client, the family, and the mental health professional in the decision-making process.

Certainly, when a mental health professional considers a sexual relationship with a client, preventing harm should be the major consideration. According to the literature, the professional who becomes involved with a client uses denial and rationalization that the client desires the relationship, that the therapeutic relationship has been discontinued, or that it took place outside of the therapeutic time (Russell, 1993). Russell writes that it is important for students to become aware of their own sexual feelings and possible attraction to a client, and that this be an important part of the mental health curriculum, especially for students who later hope to specialize in this area.

DISTRIBUTIVE JUSTICE

According to Purtilo (1993), **distributive justice** refers to the "comparative treatment of individuals in the allotment of benefits and burdens."

"The principle of justice holds that a person should be treated according to what is fair, given what is due or owed" (Chally and Loriz, 1998). During times of health care cost constraints, who is going to get treatment and for how much are frequently asked questions. In managed care, provisions for mental health care are not always treated equally with provisions for physical health; the mental health needs of clients can be compromised. The nurses working in a mental health setting may find that it is necessary to become an advocate for the client with the primary care provider to access mental health care. When there is a yearly cap on the amount of money that a managed care organization is allowing for each individual in a health care plan, resistance to treating a person with a serious and persistent mental illness can arise, especially when this person needs a variety of services over a long period of time.

A major question is the treatment site for individuals with medical and mental health problems. It is not uncommon for a mental health unit to not want to admit a person with serious physical health problems, and a medical unit might not want to admit someone with severe mental health problems who also has a physical problem. These issues are going to become more prevalent as the nation moves more toward managed care to control health costs. How is the health care dollar going to be divided, and where will the individuals with mental illnesses fit into the picture when it comes to the division of resources (Lazarus, 1994)?

In an editorial in the *American Journal of Psychiatry*, it was reported that "under managed care, the actual dollar amounts spent on all mental illness treatment have gone down." There is growing concern that because people with the diagnosis of major depression have high rates of health care utilization, they will be "dumped" by the managed care organizations or not provided with adequate care, resulting in longer incapacity.

Mental health parity bills have been introduced and passed in some states. In addition, some states have passed their own statutes giving clients a bill of rights in relation to reimbursement for mental health care. Maryland has a law that requires coverage for mental health and substance abuse care (Goldstein, 1998).

Summary of Key Concepts

1. Balancing the rights of the mentally ill versus the community has been and continues to be a struggle.
2. Alternatives to inpatient mental health treatment should consider the least restrictive environment utilizing the least restrictive treatment.
3. There are three types of commitments for a client with a mental illness: an emergency commitment, a voluntary commitment, and an involuntary indefinite commitment.
4. Clients should be informed about treatment, including risks and alternatives, on admission.
5. A civil or judicial commitment of a client is legally based in *parens patriae*, the power of the state to protect and care for disabled individuals, and the police power of the state to protect the community from persons who pose a threat.
6. Half of the states in the United States have enacted preventive or mandatory outpatient treatment, in which clients can be returned to the hospital if they discontinue treatment medication, deteriorate, and/or exhibit dangerous behavior after discharge.
7. Clients with mental illnesses retain their civil rights on entering a mental hospital or other inpatient treatment center. Clients should receive a summary of their rights on admission.
8. Clients should be restrained only to prevent physical injury to themselves or others, and only a psychiatrist or licensed physician can order nonemergency seclusion or restraint.
9. Clients who are ruled competent and are voluntarily or involuntarily committed have a right to refuse treatment and medication.
10. The U.S. Supreme Court ruled that individuals charged with or convicted of a crime could only be hospitalized for a reasonable length of time. To be committed longer requires a person to be civilly committed or released.
11. Competency to stand trial is based on a person's current awareness of the legal process as evaluated by a mental health professional.
12. The insanity defense stems from the concept that for a person to be found guilty, the person must be able to form intent and relate to his or her state of mind at the time of the offense.
13. A new plea, guilty but mentally ill (GBMI), has recently been adopted by several states. Because of the plea that states mental illness caused the commission of the crime, the person is sent to prison and treated for mental illness.
14. Nurses working in psychiatric settings must be aware of situations that may lead to potential malpractice lawsuits.

REFERENCES

Addington v. Texas, 441 US 418 (1979).

American heritage dictionary, 1993.

American Nurses Association: *Code for nurses,* Kansas City, Mo, 1982, The Association.

American Psychiatric Association: *Electroconvulsive therapy: task force report 14,* Washington, DC, 1978, The Association.

Americans With Disabilities Act (42 USC §12101).

Appelbaum P: Resurrecting the right to treatment, *Hosp Community Psychiatry* 38(7):703, 1987.

Appelbaum PS: *Almost a revolution: mental health law and the limits of change,* New York, 1994, Oxford University Press.

Appelbaum PS, Greer A: Confidentiality in group therapy, *Hosp Community Psychiatry* 44(4):311, 1993.

Black's law dictionary, St. Paul, Minn, 1990, West Publishing.

Brakel SJ, Parry J, Weiner BA: *The mentally disabled and the law,* ed 3, Chicago, 1985, American Bar Foundation.

Cal Civ Code §43.92.

Callahan LA et al: Measuring the effects of the guilty but mentally ill (GBMI) verdict, *Law Hum Behav* 16(4):441, 1992.

Cauchon D: Patients often aren't informed of full danger, *USA Today,* p 1A, December 6, 1995.

Chally PS, Loriz L: Ethics in the trenches: decision making in practice, *Am J Nurs* 98(6):17, 1998.

45 CFR §46.116.

Davis AJ, Aroskar MA: *Ethical dilemmas and nursing practice,* ed 3, Norwalk, Conn, 1991, Appleton & Lange.

Dee V, van Servellen G, Brecht ML: Managed behavioral health care patients and their nursing care problems, level of functioning and impairment on discharge, *J Am Psychiatr Nurses Assoc* 4(2):57, 1998.

Doe v. Roe, 599 NYS2d 350 (NY App Div 1993).

Dukoff R, Sunderland T: Durable power of attorney and informed consent with Alzheimer's disease patients: a clinical study, *Am J Psychiatry* 154(8):1070, 1997.

Estates of Morgan v. Fairfield Family Counseling Center, 673 NE2d 1311 (Ohio 1997).

Fitzsimons L: Electroconvulsive therapy: what nurses need to know, *J Psychosoc Nurs* 33(12):14, 1995.

Geller J: Rx: a tincture of coercion in outpatient treatment? *Hosp Community Psychiatry* 42(10):1068, 1991.

Goldstein A: Ahead of the fed: How some states are already regulating managed care, *Time,* p 30, July 13, 1998.

Graham v. State of Tennessee, 541 SW2d 531 (Tenn 1977).

Guardianship of Weedon, 565 NE2d 432 (MA 1992).

Hall v. Schulte, 836 P2d 989 (Ariz Or of App 1992).

Hatley v. Kassen, 859 SW2d 367 (Tex App Dallas 1992).

Heinecke v. Department of Commerce, 810 P2d 459 (Utah App 1991).

Hilts PJ: Agency faults a U.C.L.A. study for suffering of mental patients, *New York Times,* p A1, March 10, 1994.

In the Interest of RAJ, 554 NW2d 809 (ND 1996).

Jackson v. Indiana, 406 US 715 (1972).

Jaffee v. Redmond, 116 S Ct 1923 (1996).

Kansas v. Hendricks, 117 S Ct 2072 (US Sup Ct 1997).

Laben JK, MacLean CP: *Legal issues and guidelines for nurses who care for the mentally ill,* Owings Mills, Md, 1989, National Health Publishing.

Laben JK, Spencer LD: Decentralization of forensic services, *Community Ment Health J* 12(4):405, 1976.

LaFond JQ: Law and the delivery of involuntary mental health services, *Am J Orthopsychiatry* 64(2):409, 1994.

Lake v. Cameron, 364 F2d 657 (DC Cir 1966 *en banc*).

Lamb HR, Weinberger LE: Persons with severe mental illness in jails and prisons: a review, *Psychiatr Serv* 49(4):483, 1998.

Lazarus A: Disputes over payment for hospitalization under mental health "carve-out" programs, *Hosp Community Psychiatry* 45(2):115, 1994.

Leonard v. Iowa, 491 NW2d 508 (Iowa Sup Ct 1992).

Lyon M, Levine ML, Susman J: Patient's bill of rights: a survey of state statutes, *Ment Phys Disabil Law Rep* 6(3):178, 1982.

Mackie v. Runyon, 804 F Supp 1508 (1992).

Mink v. Alabama Department of Mental Health and Mental Retardation, 620 So2d 22 (1993).

Mordai MD, Rabinowitz IJ: Why and how to establish computerized system for psychiatric case records, *Hosp Community Psychiatry* 44(11):1091, 1993.

News and notes, *Hosp Community Psychiatry* 43(8):851, 1992.

Norris MK, Kennedy CW: How patients perceive the seclusion process, *J Psychosoc Nurs Ment Health Serv* 30(3):7, 1992.

Nurse's handbook of law and ethics, Springhouse, Penn, 1992, Springhouse.

O'Connor v. Donaldson, 422 U5 563 (1975).

Olsen DP: Ethical consideration of video monitoring psychiatric patients in seclusion and restraint, *Arch Psychiatr Nurs* 12(2):90, 1998.

Outlaw FJ, Lowery BJ: Seclusion: the nursing challenge, *J Psychosoc Nurs Ment Health Serv* 30(4):13, 1992.

Parry J: Mental disabilities under the APA: a difficult path to follow, *Ment Phys Disabil Law Rep* 17(1):100, 1985.

Peck v. the Counseling Service of Addison County, Inc., 449A2d 422 (Vt 1985).

Poss v. Department of Human Resources, 426 SE2d 635 (Go Or App 1992).

Purtilo R: *Ethical dimensions in the health professions,* ed 2, Philadelphia, 1993, WB Saunders.

Reinhard SC: Perspectives of the family's caregiving experience in mental illness, *Image: J Nurs Sch* 26(1):70, 1994.

Rennie v. Klein 416 F Supp 1294 (1979); 653 F2d 836 (3rd Cir 1981); 454 US 1978 (1982).

Rhode Island Department of Mental Health, Retardation, and Hospitals v. RB, 541 A2d (RI 1988).

Rogers v. Okin 478 F Supp 1342 (D Mass 1979).

Rogers v. Okin 634 F2d 650 (1980).

Rudegair TS, Applebaum PS: On the duty to protect: an evolutionary perspective, *Bull Am Acad Psychiatry Law* 20(4):419, 1992.

Russell J: *Out of bounds sexual exploitation in counseling and therapy,* London, 1993, Sage Publications.

Sales BD, Shuman DW: Mental health law and mental health care: introduction, *Am J Orthopsychiatry* 64(2):172, 1994.

Shah S: *Criminal responsibility in forensic psychiatry and psychology*, Philadelphia, 1986, FA Davis.

Simon RI: Psychiatrists' duties in discharging sicker and potentially violent inpatients in the managed care era, *Psychiatr Serv* 49(1):62, 1998.

Smith v. King, 615 So2s 69 (Ala Sup Ct 1993).

Statement on psychiatric mental health nursing practice and standards of psychiatric mental health clinical nursing practice, Washington, DC, 1994, American Nurses Publishing.

Stefan S: What constitutes departure from professional judgment? *Ment Phys Disabil Law Rep* 17(2):207, 1993.

Strasburger L, Jorgenson L, Randles R: Criminalization of psychotherapist-patient sex, *Am J Psychiatry* 148:859, 1991.

Tarasoff v. Regents of the University of California, 529 P2d 553 (Cal 1974) and 551 P2d 334 (Cal 1976).

Tenn Ann Code §33-6-201, 33-10-103, 33-3-105.

Tooke SR, Brown JS: Perceptions of seclusion: comparing patient and staff reactions, *J Psychosoc Nurs Ment Health Serv* 30(8):23, 1992.

Torrey EF, Kaplan RS: A national survey of the use of outpatient commitment, *Psychiatr Serv* 46(8):778, 1995.

Treatment for major depression in managed care and fee-for-service systems, *Am J Psychiatry* 155:859, 1998.

Wash Ann Code §71.05.370.

Washington; antipsychotic medication; ECT: legislative and regulatory developments, *Ment Phys Disabil Law Rep* 17(2):206, 1993.

Weiner BA, Wettstein RM: *Legal issues in mental health care*, New York, 1993, Plenum Press.

Wexler DB, Winick BJ: Therapeutic jurisprudence and criminal justice mental health issues, *Ment Phys Disabil Law Rep* 16(2):225, 1992.

Woe v. Cuomo 638 F Supp 1506 (ED NY 1986).

Wolpe PR, Schwartz SL, Sanford B: Psychiatric inpatients' knowledge of their rights, *Hosp Community Psychiatry* 42(11):1168, 1991.

Wyatt v. Stickney 344 F Supp 373 (1972).

Youngberg v. Romeo 461 US 308 (1982).

CHAPTER 6

Cultural Issues

Merry A. Armstrong

OBJECTIVES

- Discuss the need for a nurse's self-evaluation when providing care to patients from other sociocultural backgrounds.

- Analyze socialization issues—acculturation, assimilation, ethnocentrism, and xenophobia—as they interrelate with heritage and mental health.

- Compare and contrast cultural issues that define mental health perspectives.

- Differentiate general examples of both health and illness and mental health beliefs and practices of various ethnic and cultural groups.

- Identify selected social issues that interface with mental health beliefs and practices.

- Perform a cultural assessment using the Heritage Assessment Tool.

- Formulate potential nursing diagnoses related to a client's cultural or ethnic orientation.

- Discuss ways in which planning and implementation of nursing interventions can be adapted to a client's cultural or ethnic orientation.

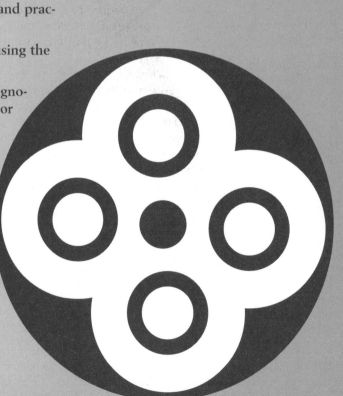

All health care takes place within a social structure. Represented within the social structure of the United States, and most other countries, are multiplicities of cultures, traditions, and ethnicities. Becoming familiar with concepts of psychiatric mental health nursing within a cultural and social context is a professional responsibility (American Nurses Association, 1993, 1994) and supports an enriched professional nursing practice that evolves and deepens through appreciation and understanding of one's own culture and the culture of others.

Orientation to cultural issues in psychiatric mental health nursing will provide the reader with cultural awareness and tools for accomplishing a cultural assessment. This chapter presents ideas about culture and describes several predominant types of cultural organizations as a beginning point of inquiry in this area. The professional nurse will strive to become acquainted with cultural and ethnic criteria that identify clients in his or her geographic area and the predominant thinking and perception of mental health and illness in that area. Likewise, the nurse should be able to think critically about his or her own ideas, values, and assumptions regarding mental health and illness. This sensitivity to his or her own world views can help the nurse to avoid **ethnocentrism,** a universal human characteristic of judging others by one's own standards of believing, acting, thinking, and valuing. Without inclusion of the cultural perspective of self and others, it is impossible to provide adequate psychiatric nursing care. Actualizing social and cultural theory is evidenced in a caring clinical practice and can be defined as cultural competence, which is discussed at a later point in the chapter.

THE NEED FOR CULTURAL UNDERSTANDING

It may be a cliché to say that America is a land of immigrants; however, except for native peoples, this is true. One in every 13 residents in the United States is foreign born (Figure 6-1) (Information please, 1995). Some geographic areas in the country are more diverse than others, but wherever nursing care occurs, cultural differences among and between persons exist. This is not to say that the majority of cultural variations occur with clients who are foreign born, because cultural variations among people in the United States also occur as a result of regional differences and the influences of individual heritage. In particular dimensions of culture, differences between people sharing the same culture may be greater than differences across the culture in general (Hofstede, 1991). For example, Kevin and Nadia live in the same city, belong to the same political party, and share the same American culture, but each possesses characteristics that make each of them unique individuals. It is clearly an erroneous belief that one can generalize about individuals according to culture or ethnicity.

Regional differences and the increase of a diverse and aging population support the notion that cultural realities in the United States are complex and will likely become even more varied. In 1996 foreign residents totaled 24.5 million people, or 9.3% of the population. Since 1970 the percentage of foreign-born African-Americans doubled to 8.7 and Asians and Pacific Islanders tripled to 28.6; Hispanics make up 43% of immigrants (Minehan, 1997). In the year 2006 the United States workforce is expected to be 73% white, 11% African-American, 10% Hispanic, and 5% Asian. A dramatic increase in workers age 45 to 64 is expected, with that age group representing 22% of the U.S. population by the year 2000 and 26% by 2010 (Greco, 1998). Figure 6-1 depicts population comparisons for the years 1980 and 1990.

The process of **acculturation** occurs when a member of a cultural group adapts to the new dominant culture in order to survive. This involuntary process evolves, but the person usually can be identified, through language or some other characteristic, as a member of a nondominant culture. The model of second-culture acquisition is what an individual experiences when he or she lives within or between cultures (LaFromboise, Coleman, and Gerton, 1993).

KEY TERMS

Acculturation The process of adapting to another culture.

Assimilation To become absorbed into another culture and adopt its characteristics.

Cultural competence Standard of practice that ensures that clients of all cultures receive information that they can understand.

Culture The collective process of acquiring shared beliefs, dominant patterns of behavior, values, and attitudes learned through socialization.

Ethnicity A specific cultural group's sense of identification associated with its common social and cultural heritage.

Ethnocentrism
The tendency of members of one cultural group to view the members of other cultural groups in terms of the standards of behavior, attitudes, and values of their own group; belief in the superiority of one's own group.

Heritage consistency The observance of the beliefs and practices of one's traditional cultural belief system.

Socialization The process of being raised within a culture and acquiring the characteristics of the given group.

Xenophobia
A morbid fear of strangers and those who are not of one's own ethnic group.

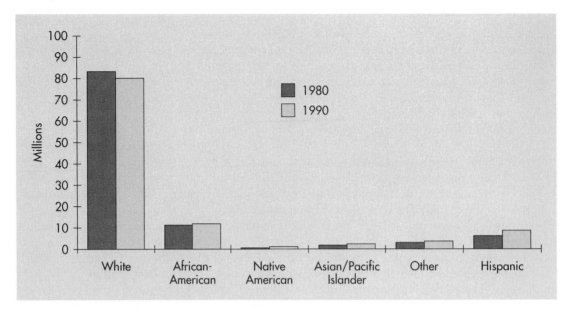

Figure 6-1   United States population comparison: 1980 and 1990, including Hispanic origin population. (Data from U.S. Bureau of the Census: *Current population reports: 1980 general social and economic characteristics, part 1, United States summary, PC 80-1-C1, United States*, Washington, DC, 1983, U.S. Government Printing Office; and U.S. Bureau of the Census: *Current population reports, 1990 census of population and housing: summary populations and housing characteristics, United States*, Washington, DC, 1991, U.S. Government Printing Office.)

Assimilation is the process of developing a new cultural identity. Assimilation means becoming, in all ways, like the members of the dominant culture. The process comprises several stages, such as cultural or behavioral assimilation, marital assimilation, identification assimilation, and civic assimilation. The underlying assumption is that the person loses his or her original cultural identity to acquire the new one. However, this is not always possible, and the process of assimilation may cause stress and anxiety (LaFromboise, Coleman, and Gerton, 1993). Stress and anxiety may bring this individual into the mental health system for care. How are nurses prepared to serve this diverse population? One effective way to begin the study of culture is to become familiar with one's own culture. Understanding the differences between culture and ethnicity is a beginning point for exploration.

ETHNICITY VERSUS CULTURE

The term **ethnicity** refers to people from common geographic origins who share language and religion, among other characteristics. Ethnic identification may be considered an internal and personal identification or distinctiveness (Mensah, 1993). The terms *ethnicity* and *culture* are sometimes used interchangeably, but it is important to understand the differences. **Culture** is a broad term that is related to but is not the same as, or as specific as, ethnicity. For example, one may be culturally American and also share an ethnic relatedness, through traditions, language, and customs, to others who have, for example, Hispanic

ancestry. Knowing that someone is from Louisiana does not indicate their ethnicity, which may be Cajun, Indian, Middle Eastern, Native American, Germanic, Scandinavian, Hmong, or that of any other group.

Culture is acquired, transmitted from generation to generation, and shared. It is the whole collective process of acquiring shared beliefs, dominant patterns of behavior, values, and attitudes learned through **socialization.** Culture determines appropriate dress, language, values, norms for behavior, economics, politics, law and social control, technology, and health care (Germain, 1992). Although people from individual cultures share many aspects of that culture, every person has a unique response to and relation to that culture. A culture does not indicate a "king-sized personality" (Hofstede, 1994) but rather refers to a social group that encompasses many different and interdependent people. Culture is influenced by the environment of the area in which people live and has been likened to a biotype in biology, or the population that belongs to a particular ecosystem (Hofstede, 1994).

An entire society, or subgroups within that society including lifestyles and habits, can be described in terms of culture. For example, the culture of a high school may contain subsets of persons involved and identified with sports, computers, drama, music, or academics. Members of those subsets may have their own special ways of talking about areas of interest, probably select friends among those interested in similar activities, and value certain activities above others. Considering society in greater depth, Geuss (1981) further considers aspects of culture to be ar-

Box 6-1	Common Prejudices or Biases
Racism	The belief that members of one race are superior to those of other races.
Sexism	The belief that members of one sex are superior to the other sex.
Heterosexism	The belief that everyone is or should be heterosexual and that heterosexuality is best, normal, and superior.
Ageism	The belief that members of one age-group are superior to those of other ages.
Ethnocentrism	The belief that one's own cultural, ethnic, or professional group is superior to that of others. One judges others by his or her own "yardstick" and is unable or unwilling to see what the other group is really about.
Xenophobia	The morbid fear of strangers and those who are not of one's own ethnic group.

From American Nurses Association: *Multicultural issues in the nursing workforce*, Washington, DC, 1993, The Association.

eas of beliefs, concepts, attitudes and psychologic dispositions, desires, works of art, and religions and religious rituals. Included in this view of culture are values, principles, and standards that guide a person's actions in the world. For example, one's culture provides rules for touching; styles of communication, including appropriate eye contact; and relationships with others. The values set forth in a culture connect us to (and/or set us apart from) our families, communities, and social groups. In addition to positive values, negative values are manifested in "isms" or phobias: racism, sexism, ageism, classism, **xenophobia**, homophobia, anti-Semitism, and others. "Isms" are often reflected as stereotypes that we have about different others that can manifest as prejudicial thinking and behavior (Box 6-1).

CULTURE AND MENTAL HEALTH

Persons of a particular culture deem what behavior is normal and what behavior is aberrant, what beliefs are tolerable and acceptable, and what beliefs are not acceptable. These collective beliefs change over time and are influenced by many factors. Cultural assumptions become the basis for decisions and actions, are part of one's fundamental psychologic realities, are deeply ingrained, are difficult to identify, and are difficult to change (Fielo and Degazon, 1997). Definitions of mental health and illness, as well as entire concepts of mental health and illness, may be different in different societal structures. To illustrate this point, note that Appendix I of *The Diagnostic and Statistical Manual*, fourth edition (American Psychiatric Association, 1994), provides information about syndromes that are predominantly found in particular cultures (culture-

bound syndromes) that may be of interest to nursing students. This appendix also notes that certain psychiatric syndromes are found in the Chinese Classification of Mental Disorders, illustrating that different cultures regard normal and abnormal behaviors in different ways. Because of differences in pharmacokinetics and pharmacodynamics, culture may be a variable when considering drug therapy (Keltner and Folks, 1992).

INFLUENCE OF CULTURE ON MENTAL HEALTH AND MENTAL ILLNESS

It is important to think about what each mental health team member contributes to the care of the client and how that person's particular worldview influences mental health care. Examining definitions of mental health and illness can be done from the perspective of the individual, the perspective of the family or immediate social group, and the perspective of the trained professional. Kleinman (1980), a medical sociologist, proposes that perceptions of normal and abnormal behavior are influenced and shaped by culture. Kleinman defines three aspects of illness that are useful to consider when discussing cultural aspects of health care. These three ways of considering the occurrence of illness help us to understand different perspectives of the illness experience and the interrelationships of culture, illness, and the provision of health care. This is a particularly useful framework for considering the event of mental illness because many social systems are involved in the care of the mentally ill.

Illness

Illness is defined as the way in which a sick person and members of the family or social network perceive, live with, and respond to symptoms and disability. Using this framework, the illness experience is always culturally shaped. To apply critical thinking to this situation, examine the ways that your family deals with an ill family member. Were you, as a child with the flu, permitted to camp out on the sofa and watch television, or were you confined to your bed? Did your mother or another family member prepare soothing foods and give you medications or a unique "cure" to alleviate symptoms? (As an example, an Appalachian treatment for colds is to administer teaspoonfuls of a mixture of lemon juice, Kentucky bourbon, and honey—an incentive to feel better quickly!) What happened if both of your parents worked? What if multiple siblings were ill at the same time? What happens now when you or your spouse becomes ill? What happens when an extended family member becomes ill? Who becomes the caretaker? What are acceptable behaviors of the ill person in your household? What special tasks do others perform in the presence of illness? What happens to relatives or members of your immediate family who may have a mental problem? How does your family talk about this person? Does your family include or exclude this person? Are illnesses associated with accidents such as a broken arm approached differently than chronic diseases such as diabetes or mental illness?

Sickness

Sickness, according to Kleinman (1988), is the understanding of a disease in relation to economic, political, and institutional forces. Examples of sickness are the higher incidence of lead poisoning in children living in poverty and higher incidences of clinical depression in the poor and in people who abuse drugs and alcohol. How does our society interpret and respond to increased incidences of sickness in certain populations? Research monies are allotted differently to study the causes and treatment of certain diseases such as breast cancer, testicular cancer, and HIV infection. What are insurance companies' policies regarding reimbursement for certain medications? How do forces in our society influence or change these policies? What provisions do health insurance companies make for treatment of mental illness? For promotion of mental health?

Disease

According to Kleinman (1988), disease is seeing the disorder through the framework of one's professional training. For example, after examining a client and completing a psychiatric examination, a psychiatrist might arrive at a diagnosis of major depressive disorder. The nurse who treats the same client later in the hospital might arrive at a nursing diagnosis of sleep pattern disturbance. We all "see" the client and interpret symptoms from the viewpoint of our professional training. The client experiences the symptoms, the physician names the symptoms or syndrome according to the taxonomy of psychiatric disease, and the nurse names the client's response to the illness according to nursing taxonomy. All three team members (client, physician, and nurse) consider the client's problems in a slightly different way—according to the experience of the problem, according to professional preparation, and according to society's determination of what is normal and abnormal. Like mental health and illness, behaviors and perceptions that are normal exist on a continuum. Within and among different cultures and ethnic groups, there are wide variations in defining and determining the limits of normality.

CULTURAL COMPETENCE

Cultural competence refers to a set of practice standards developed and instituted by county health and county mental health departments in states across the country. These standards are required by specific managed care and other health care payers. The purpose of cultural competence is to ensure that patients of all cultures are given every opportunity to receive information about treatment in ways that they understand, considering their education, acculturation, and language.

How do nurses approach thinking about culture and mental illness, illness, sickness and disease? Why is a working knowledge of cultural influences in mental health important? The experience of illness from the individual and family point of view can be ascertained in various ways. Health care practices, including health-seeking behaviors, responsibility for health care, folklore practices, barriers to health care, and cultural responses to health and illness, including mental illness, are summarized in Box 6-2.

Another helpful tool is Spector's Heritage Assessment Tool (Box 6-3), which may be used when assessing persons who identify with a traditional culture within the modern American culture. As the nurse begins to develop skills in this form of assessment, it is suggested that the initial assessment of an individual be a personal one, followed by assessments of the individual's parents, family members, and friends. Since most clients (especially those in

---

Box 6-2   **Health Care Practices**

Health-Seeking Beliefs and Behaviors

Identify predominant beliefs that influence health care practices.

Describe the influences of health promotion and prevention practices.

Responsibility for Health Care

Describe the focus of acute care practice (curative or fatalistic).

Explore who assumes responsibility for health care in this culture.

Describe the role of health insurance in this culture.

Explore behaviors associated with the use of over-the-counter medications.

Folklore Practices

Explore combinations of magicoreligious beliefs, folklore, and traditional beliefs that influence health care behaviors.

Barriers to Health Care

Identify barriers to health care such as language, economics, and geography for this group.

Cultural Responses to Health and Illness

Explore cultural beliefs and responses to pain that influence interventions. Does pain have a special meaning?

Describe beliefs and views about mental illness in this culture.

Differentiate between the perceptions of mentally and physically handicapped in this culture.

Describe cultural beliefs and practices related to chronicity and rehabilitation.

Identify cultural perceptions of the sick role in this group.

Modified from Purnell L, Paulanka B: *Transcultural health care: a culturally competent approach*, Philadelphia, 1998, FA Davis.

Box 6-3   Heritage Assessment Tool

1. Where was your mother born?
2. Where was your father born?
3. Where were your grandparents born?
   a. Your mother's mother?
   b. Your mother's father?
   c. Your father's mother?
   d. Your father's father?
4. How many brothers and sisters do you have?
5. What setting did you grow up in?
   a. Urban
   b. Rural
   c. Suburban
6. What country did your parents grow up in?
   a. Father
   b. Mother
7. How old were you when you came to the United States?
8. How old were your parents when they came to the United States?
   a. Mother
   b. Father
9. When you were growing up, who lived with you? (ask this way)
   a. Nuclear family
   b. Extended family
   c. Single-parent family
   d. Other
10. Have you maintained contact with:
    a. Aunts, uncles, cousins?   (1) Yes   (2) No
    b. Brothers and sisters?   (1) Yes   (2) No
    c. Parents?   (1) Yes   (2) No
    d. Your own children?   (1) Yes   (2) No
11. Did most of your aunts, uncles, and cousins live near to your home when you were growing up?
    a. Yes
    b. No
12. Approximately how often did you visit your family members who lived outside of your home when you were young?
    a. Daily
    b. Weekly
    c. Monthly
    d. Once a year or less
    e. Never
13. Was your original family name changed?
    a. Yes
    b. No
14. Do you have a religious preference?
    a. Yes (if yes, please specify)
    b. No (1 point for yes, but 0 for no)
15. Is your spouse the same religion as you?
    a. Yes
    b. No
16. Is your spouse the same ethnic background as you?
    a. Yes
    b. No
17. What kind of school did you go to?
    a. Public (0)
    b. Private
    c. Parochial

18. As an adult, do you live in a neighborhood where the neighbors are the same religion and/or ethnic background as yourself?
    a. Religion   (1) Yes   (2) No
    b. Ethnicity (1) Yes   (2) No
19. Do you belong to a religious institution?
    a. Yes
    b. No
20. Would you describe yourself as an active member?
    a. Yes
    b. No
21. How often do you attend your religious institution?
    a. More than once a week
    b. Weekly
    c. Monthly (0)
    d. Special holidays only (0)
    e. Never
22. Do you practice your religion in your home?
    a. Yes (please specify, 1 point for each example)
    b. Praying
    c. Bible reading
    d. Diet
    e. Celebrating religious holidays
    f. No
23. Do you prepare foods of your ethnic background?
    a. Yes
    b. No
24. Do you participate in ethnic activities?
    a. Yes (if yes, please specify, 1 point for each)
    b. Singing
    c. Holiday celebrations
    d. Dancing
    e. Festivals
    f. Costumes
    g. Other
    h. No
25. Are your friends from the same religious background as you?
    a. Yes
    b. No
26. Are your friends from the same ethnic background as you?
    a. Yes
    b. No
27. What is your native language (the language your parents may have spoken other than English)?
28. Do you speak this language?
    a. Prefer
    b. Occasionally (0)
    c. Rarely (0)
29. Do you read this language?
    a. Yes
    b. No

The greater the number of yes answers, the more likely the client is to strongly identify with a traditional heritage. (The one no answer that indicates heritage identity is "Was your name changed?") This assessment may be scored 1 point for each yes from question 10, except where noted (0), and 2 points for no if the person's family name was not Americanized. Again, a high score, usually greater than 15 points, is indicative of identification with a traditional background.

From Spector RE: *Cultural diversity in health and illness,* ed 4, Norwalk, Conn, 1996, Appleton & Lange.

mental health settings) often do not react well to pencil-and-paper questionnaires, it is helpful to memorize the scope and nature of these questions and then piece together the information needed to determine a client's level of **heritage consistency.**

CONSIDERING SELF IN CULTURAL COMPETENCE

It is impossible to appreciate the importance of becoming culturally competent without some awareness of our own framework through which we understand and view life. We all are challenged to understand our own culture, which is perhaps the most difficult aspect of becoming culturally competent caregivers (Leininger, 1991; Lester, 1998; Tripp-Reimer, 1995). Pertinent questions that nurses may ask themselves about their own cultural perspective are found in Box 6-4.

Camphina-Bacote (1994) suggests that nurses think of themselves as being continually in the process of becoming culturally competent, rather than as being culturally competent. This suggestion implies that we are lifelong learners about culture and constantly work to understand individuals, and ourselves, as part of a culture and within that culture. Purnell and Paulanka (1998) define a person who is culturally competent as one who:

1. Develops an awareness of his or her own existence, sensations, thoughts, and other environment without letting it have an undue influence on those from other backgrounds
2. Demonstrates knowledge and understanding of the client's culture
3. Accepts and respects cultural differences
4. Adapts care to be congruent with the client's culture

This model presumes that one progresses from unconscious incompetence (not being aware at all of lacking information about other cultures) to conscious incompetence (being aware that one lacks information about other cultures), to conscious competence (actively learning about other cultures and verifying this information), and finally to unconscious competence, when one automatically provides culturally competent care. These authors believe that most caregivers achieve conscious competence but must always be on the alert for ethnocentrism and the effect of deeply held values on attitudes and behaviors toward others. Being culturally competent is an expectation of professionals working in the United States and is a requirement of accrediting bodies that examine the quality of care in health care institutions. Having a culturally competent practice means that one is able to render care in a cultural environment different from one's own and that one can relate, communicate, and sensitively provide care in a manner appropriate for clients and their families.

> **Box 6-4   Cultural Self-Assessment for Nurses**
>
> Who am I with respect to my cultural identity?
> What is my personal heritage, and how deeply do I adhere to it?
> What is my nursing heritage, and how deeply do I adhere to it?
> What biases and assumptions do I have, and how do these affect my ability to interact with clients?
> What do I know about mental health and illness from my formative years?
> What have I learned about mental health and illness in nursing?

Developing cultural competence can be a rewarding experience that many nurses share with others. The use of literature (Bartol and Richardson, 1998) and sharing of information with other nurses through paradigm cases and unique experiences can forward one's clinical practice (Lester, 1998). Information can be gained through reading, through in-service education, by developing a model for cultural assessment, and through sensitivity to the uniqueness of others while engaging in practice (Box 6-5).

In the current multilingual and ethnically diverse environment, the nurse and other health care providers are important advocates in helping clients and families understand and comply with treatment. This is particularly critical in the area of mental health, given the complex terminology and myriad behaviors and symptoms that require accurate interpretation by a culturally aware staff. Interpreters must be able to attach accurate meaning and purpose to a client's language so that nursing implications for effective treatment are clearly understood. Cultural diversity helps nurses and professionals in other health care disciplines recognize that people are more alike than different and that everyone deserves the best possible physical and psychologic treatment regardless of language, culture, and ethnicity.

COMMUNICATION

One of the primary functions of a psychiatric mental health nurse is to communicate with clients, families, and teammates. As health professionals, we communicate through words, through gestures, and through our dress and deportment. For example, at one hospital, recent Southeast Asian immigrants were distressed by the white uniforms of the nurses. Although it took some time to figure out that this was a problem, one nurse asked them why they looked away from her white uniform. Through a trained health care interpreter, they stated that white symbolized death and was often used in funerals. Their associations with the color white and a place where very ill persons were being cared for was a confusing combina-

| Box 6-5 | Summary of Cultural Competence Standards in Clinical Practice |

- Availability of professional interpreters who are capable of effectively communicating with the population they serve
- A multicultural, multilingual staff who effectively represent the community they serve
- Psychologic testing that is culturally sound and appropriate for the ethnically diverse population
- Cultural components as part of the patient admission interview, treatment plan, education plan, interventions, and discharge plan
- Use of resources, including family and community, in helping patients meet cultural needs
- Physician recognition that cultural factors play a role in treatment compliance
- Involvement in culturally competent community research and training
- Provider involvement in ongoing cultural competence self-assessment
- Agency/facility involvement in ongoing cultural competence self-assessment.

Each cultural competence standard is accompanied by a series of objectives and outcomes for that standard. Methods of outcome measurement include the following:

- Submission of written protocols such as documentation in the medical record of how the language needs of the client were met
- Quarterly and annual reports, including an annual program review of the bilingual proficiency of staff and other agency support positions
- Periodic site reviews by designated county reviewers
- Client satisfaction survey reports in culturally sensitive areas
- Documentation in the medical record of client orientation, education, treatment goals, legal issues, program expectations of the client and provider, and confidentiality that meet cultural needs
- Availability of a clinic/hospital brochure describing treatment services in the preferred language of the client
- Minimum of 4 hours required for staff training per year, with submission of a report listing staff names and hours of cultural competence training (Staff training log must be kept on site.)
- Procedure/protocol for psychologists to access consultation when needed for assessment of ethnically diverse clients. (This is to be documented in the client's medical record.)

tion. Shortly afterward, personnel in the neonatal intensive care unit began to wear colors.

Written, spoken, and nonverbal forms of language are equally important aspects in communicating with clients. More information is transmitted nonverbally than verbally. Nonverbal communication provides the process and context through which messages are communicated and is used very extensively for much of the world's population. Although generalizing about individuals solely on the basis of their culture is impossible, understanding low- and high-context cultures will help the nurse understand barriers to dynamic communication and expression.

LOW- AND HIGH-CONTEXT CULTURES

A concept helpful in examining behavioral and communication aspects of culture considers societies whose foundations are low context (or individualistic) or high context (collectivistic). This sociologic framework suggests that one universal characteristic of culture is the way that individuals relate to one another. Hofstede (1991) suggests that an individualistic, or low-context, society is one in which people are expected to care for themselves and their immediate family. Low-context societies emphasize thinking and values that are centered on the individual: autonomy, individual initiative, the right to privacy, emotional independence, and universalism (arriving at rules of conduct that are applied to everyone). Although there are wide variations among persons in any culture, these qualities are generally characteristic of persons who function in a democratic environment in which most members of the

society have a legal voice and are expected to advocate for themselves. These cultures emphasize individual thinking and an analytic style of approaching a situation without considering the context or social situation in which the individual is acting. In general, this kind of thinking is typically American and is found in other Western cultures. Successful communication in this type of culture includes being assertive (including making direct eye contact), advocating for oneself, thinking through problems independently, and arguing for a point of view. It is typical for Americans to use this type of interactional style as a standard; however, many of the world's peoples do not function with these understandings.

In contrast, a high-context society is one in which people are included in strong, cohesive groups throughout their lifetime. These persons stress a "we" consciousness, collective identity, group solidarity, sharing, group decision making, collective duties and obligations, emotional dependence, and particularism (arriving at rules of conduct that are applied to persons depending on their particular role in society) (Hofstede, 1980; Kim, 1994). These cultures are referred to as high context because the emphasis is on the individual as part of a societal structure and within relationships whose rules may be inferred by those who are part of that culture.

Those from a high-context culture orientation tend to use communication that is more global and based on standards external to the person, such as social position. Successful communication in this culture may depend on the physical context and the cultural information internalized in the communicators. More of the message is developed from nonverbal symbolization and cultural roles in the society.

This kind of cultural environment supports the development of persons who base their decisions on group input, may not want to argue in public, may use indirect language to communicate, and may also be hesitant to make direct eye contact. Asian, some South American, Hispanic, African-American, and some Native American cultures may share high-context culture characteristics. Roles of women and men in some cultures may dictate appropriate interaction with professional persons or those outside the family. (However, it must be remembered that wide individual variations exist within any culture, and knowing that a client is from a particular culture is just a starting point.)

Several examples of high-context culture responses may provide perspective. A client from a high-context culture stated that he could not offer an opinion about treatment because he did not know what to say. This stance was not due to lack of information or intellectual ability but was based on his lack of training in making arguments and inability to refute or question another's opinion. His culture had taught him that important statements were based on authority, which as a client he did not possess. Thus he believed that his own observations and feelings were not appropriate to verbalize. Another client thought that she could not speak in public because she might be wrong and would embarass her family by this action. It is important to ascertain clients' levels of comfort in speaking for themselves. Some questions suggested by Swanson (1993) are:

When is it appropriate to express yourself publicly?
What subjects are appropriate to express publicly?
When is it appropriate to disagree?
When do you think it is appropriate to express disagreement?
To whom is it appropriate to express disagreement?

These two styles of communication and relationship to society are important to include in one's assessment of culture because clients may come from a high-context culture and find themselves as clients in a low-context culture. For the nurse to appreciate the experience of illness as defined by Kleinman (1988), investigation of the client's comfort level in a high- or low-context culture must occur, because the American system of health care requires individuals to speak for themselves, articulate a dissenting opinion, and function apart from their families. Those from cultures who function with different assumptions can present real nursing challenges (Lester, 1998). The nurse's role as a client advocate may be of the utmost importance in this situation, since clients with chronic mental illness often have low self-esteem, have difficulty

processing information, and may thus have a great deal of difficulty speaking for themselves. If the caregivers are from a low-context culture (analytic and objective) and the client is from a high-context culture (identification with a group and symbolic meanings), these problems may be intensified.

OBTAINING TRANSLATION SERVICES

Because nurses are often in the position of using translation services, it is important to have guidelines for directing this process. Especially in mental health, it is important to acquire accurate translation, using a trained translator if possible. Using a family member or ancillary hospital staff is often convenient but not recommended, because the client may wish to avoid embarrassing the translator or reveal information that would be culturally inappropriate. Accuracy of translation may be affected by many factors, and care must be taken to avoid bias on the part of the translator. It is a good idea to use standard communication techniques when asking questions through an interpreter, beginning with general information and asking sensitive questions after communication has been established. Communication patterns in low-context cultures may be characterized by fewer words and more nonverbal communication. Therefore the translator may seem not to be asking the questions posed by the interviewer. It is important to consider the communication context and preference of the client and translator. Persons of Hindu culture tend to speak quietly, and those of Arabic cultures may speak loudly; both may be misinterpreted if the interviewer is not sensitive to these differences (Purnell and Paulanka, 1998). If the client is hospitalized, it may be impossible to provide 8 hours of translation for groups or activities. The care team needs to incorporate a plan of adequate translator involvement for adequate ongoing assessment of the client's status. Box 6-6 provides suggestions for communicating with and obtaining translation for clients who speak other languages.

In addition to language, dietary needs should be addressed if the client is hospitalized and not accustomed to American foods. Reading materials, especially client education materials, need to be provided in the client's language. Leisure activities such as listening to music should also be tailored to suit the client's preferences. Some hospitals with large populations have specific units for clients with specific cultural needs (Foster, 1990).

PASTORAL CARE

Akin to obtaining translation services is the provision of spiritual support or pastoral counseling to psychiatric clients. It is helpful for clients when the nurse obtains a representative of traditional faith to offer them support. In general, one of the pastoral services offered by institutions or within communities is to contact the appropriate representatives. Having these services available is often of great comfort to the mentally ill. Certified Pastoral Coun-

Box 6-6   **Communicating With Patients Who Speak a Foreign Language**

Use interpreters rather than translators. Translators just restate the words from one language to another. An interpreter decodes the words and provides the meaning behind the message.

Use dialect-specific interpreters whenever possible.

Use interpreters trained in the health care field.

Give the interpreter time alone with the client.

Provide time for translation and interpretation.

Be aware that interpreters may affect the reporting of symptoms, insert their own ideas, or omit information.

Avoid the use of relatives who may distort information or not be objective.

Avoid using children as interpreters, especially with sensitive topics.

Use same-age and same-gender interpreters whenever possible.

Maintain eye contact with both the client and the interpreter to elicit feedback and read nonverbal cues.

Remember that clients can usually understand more than they can express; thus they need time to think in their own language. They are alert to the health care provider's body language, and they may forget some or all of their English in times of stress.

Speak slowly without exaggerated mouthing, allow time for translation, use the active rather than the passive tense, wait for feedback, and restate the message. Do not rush; do not speak loudly. Use a reference book with common phrases, such as *Roget's International Thesaurus* or *Taber's Cyclopedic Medical Dictionary.*

Use as many words as possible in the client's language, and use nonverbal communication when you and the client are unable to understand each other's language.

If an interpreter is unavailable, the use of a translator may be acceptable. The difficulty with translation is omission of parts of the message, distortion of the message, transmission of information not given by the speaker, and messages not being fully understood.

NOTE: Social class differences between the interpreter and the client may result in the interpreter's not reporting information that he or she perceives as superstitious or unimportant.

selors are skilled in communicating with mentally ill patients (see Chapter 34).

CROSS-CULTURAL PERSPECTIVES OF MENTAL HEALTH

Beliefs, values, and behaviors of persons of various cultures and ethnic groups can be generalized only with the cautionary statement that *vast* differences occur among individuals. The nurse will provide sensitive, culturally com-

petent care by first completing a thorough assessment that identifies these individual differences. Table 6-1 provides the beginning point for approaching persons from different cultural groups, but making the assumption that every person in a particular group shares these characteristics is cultural stereotyping (Foster, 1990) and is to be avoided. The degree to which people are influenced by other people and cultures may influence their beliefs about mental illness. Although persons with mental illness are still negatively viewed in much of the world (Purnell and Paulanka, 1998), advances in neuroscience that promote the biochemical model of mental illness are helping to alleviate this social response.

The following discussion presents an overview of mental health beliefs and practices from different selected cultures. This information is not intended to stereotype any group but merely to describe the known traditional means by which an individual member or family of a given group may cope with a mental health problem.

The nurse's understanding of a client's cultural norms serves as a framework for understanding the client's world. The nurse cannot begin to understand a client with only previously held views of that client's cultural group. Sincere dialogue and genuine interest in the client and his or her culture are necessary elements for beginning the process.

AFRICAN-AMERICANS

Members of the African-American communities in the United States have their origins in Africa and a cultural heritage that is a mixture of the Caribbean cultures, Native American cultures, and northern European cultures (Baker, 1994). In 1990 there were 29,986,000 African-Americans in the United States, or 11.7% of the total population. The following is a brief demographic sketch of this population (Go, 1994):

Median age is 27.9 years
71.9% of the men and 77.9% of the women have a high school education
50.2% are married couples
70.1% of the men and 57.8% of the women are employed
Median earning for a family is $20,210
30.7% of this group are below the poverty level

The family often has a matriarchal structure, and there are many single-parent households headed by women. There are strong, large, extended family networks. There is a continuation of tradition and a strong religious affiliation within the community. Many African-Americans tend to use traditional medicines and healers when they are knowledgeable in this area and have access to this resource.

Traditional African-Americans may choose to be treated by a traditional voodoo priest, "old lady" ("granny"

Table 6-1 Cross-Cultural Examples of Selected Communication Phenomena That Affect Nursing Care

Nations of Origin	Language	Space	Time Orientation	Mental Illness*
Asian Origin China Hawaii Philippines Korea Japan Southeast Asia Laos Cambodia Vietnam	National language preference Dialects, written characters Use of silence Nonverbal and contextual cuing	Noncontact people	Present	Metabolic imbalance and organic problem Evaluate (many other beliefs)
African Origin West Coast (as slaves) Many African countries West Indian islands Dominican Republic Haiti Jamaica	National languages Dialect Pidgin Creole Spanish French	Close personal space	Present over future	Spiritual distress Evaluate for religious beliefs Evaluate (many other beliefs)
European Origin Germany England Italy Ireland Other European countries	National languages Many learn English immediately	Noncontact people Aloof Distant Southern countries: closer contact and touch	Future over present	Evaluate (many beliefs)
Native American 170 Native American tribes Aleuts Eskimos	Tribal languages Many learn English immediately	Space is very important and has no boundaries	Future over present	Placing of a curse (Navajo) Evaluate (many other beliefs)
Hispanic Origin Spain Cuba Mexico Central and South America	Spanish or Portuguese primary languages	Tactile relationships Touch Handshakes Embracing Values physical presence	Present	Spells or bad spirits Evaluate (many other beliefs)
Arab Origin Yemen Lebanon-occupied Palestine Oman Saudi Arabia Morocco Tunisia Algeria Sudan Libya Egypt Syria Jordan Iraq Kuwait Bahrain Qatar United Arab Emirates	Arabic Colloquial Arabic and dialects in many areas	Variable; many customs, formal manners	Assess for religion	Consequence of physical or emotional trauma Attributed to supernatural beings Evaluate (many other beliefs)

Data from Spector RE: *Cultural diversity in health and illness*, ed 4, Norwalk, Conn, 1996, Appleton & Lange; Giger JN, Davidhizar RE: *Transcultural nursing*, ed 3, St. Louis, 1999, Mosby; and Purnell L, Paulanka B: *Transcultural health care*, Philadelphia, 1998, FA Davis.
*See DSM-IV for culture-bound syndromes.

Understanding & Applying Research

This single case study explored the conflict that occurred when a male African-American client displayed behavior that seemed incongruent to staff. Using several nursing models explaining cross-cultural influences, staff were able to determine that the client's behaviors were congruent with his cultural beliefs, thereby averting a conflict with the client. Comparing and contrasting African-American and Anglo-American values and beliefs through an explanatory model interview helped clarify confusing aspects of caring for this client. (An explanatory model interview seeks to discover any cultural values or beliefs that might explain behavior.) In this case the client referred to several historical events and beliefs that explained his behavior. A plan of care was instituted to address the client's anxiety during particular activities and to engage in client education activities, including stress management techniques. A potentially difficult client care situation was resolved using cultural assessment and subsequent treatment modifications.

Simond M: Case analysis: cross-cultural conflict in the psychiatric setting, *J Multicult Nurs Health* 2(3):38, 1996.

or "Mrs. Markus"), or other traditional healer, and herbs are frequently used to treat mental symptoms. Several diagnostic techniques include the use of Biblical phrases and material from folk medicine books, observation, and entering the spirit of the client. The therapeutic measures include various rituals such as the reading of bones, wearing of special garments, or some rituals from voodoo (Spurlock, 1988).

ASIAN-AMERICANS

Members of the Asian–Pacific Island communities in the United States have their origins in China, Hawaii, the Philippines, Korea, Japan, and Southeast Asia (Cambodia, Laos, and Vietnam). In 1990 there were 7,273,662 Asian-Americans in the United States, or 3% of the total population. The following is a brief demographic sketch of this population (Go, 1994):

Median age is 30.4 years
82% of the members have a high school education
80% are married couples
72% of the men and 56% of the women are employed
Median earning for a family is $42,250
11% of this group are below the poverty level

The family has a hierarchical structure, and loyalty among members is valued. There is a devotion to tradition; many religions, including Taoism, Buddhism, Islam, and Christianity, are practiced. Many people tend to use traditional medicines and healers such as the "Chinese doctor" or other traditional healers; herbs are frequently used to treat mental symptoms.

Little knowledge or skill in mental health therapy is seen in the Asian communities. There are two points that must be noted: the importance placed on the family in caring for the mentally ill and the fact that people may tend to describe mental illness in somatic terms. There is a tremendous amount of stigma attached to mental illness. Asian clients tend to come to the attention of mental health workers late in the course of their illness, and they come with a feeling of hopelessness (Lin, 1982).

One example of cross-cultural therapy is the Japanese practice of Morita therapy. This 70-year-old treatment originated from a treatment for shinkeishitsu, a form of compulsive neurosis with aspects of neurasthenia. The client is separated from the family for 1 to 2 weeks and taught that one's feelings are the same as the Japanese sky and instantly changeable. One cannot be responsible for how one feels, only for what one does. At the end of therapy, the client focuses outside of the self and less on inner feelings, symptoms, concerns, or obsessive thoughts (Yamamoto, 1982).

HISPANICS

Members of the Hispanic community have their origins in Spain, Cuba, Central and South America, Mexico, Puerto Rico, and other Spanish-speaking countries. In 1990 there were 22,354,059 Hispanics in the United States, or 9% of the total population. Hispanics are now the most rapidly growing ethnic group in the American population. The following is a brief demographic sketch of this population (Go, 1994):

Median age is 26.2 years
51% of the members have a high school education
56.7% are married couples
78% of the men and 51% of the women are employed
Median earning for a family is $23,400
25% of this group are below the poverty level

The family often has a nuclear structure, with strong, large, extended family networks and compadrazzo (godparents). There is a continuation of tradition and a strong church affiliation within the community. Many Hispanics are Catholic. Many tend to use traditional medicines and healers and are knowledgeable about these resources.

People may be treated by a traditional healer such as a curandero, santero, or señora, and herbs are frequently used to treat mental symptoms. Diagnostic techniques include the use of divination (foretelling the future), observation, and exorcism.

NATIVE AMERICANS

The ancestors of Native Americans living in the United States today immigrated to this land long before the Europeans and other immigrants. Today there are approximately 170 Native American nations, or tribes, located mostly in the western states. Many Native Americans have remained on reservations, whereas others live in urban and rural areas off the reservations on the East Coast. In 1990 there were 1.9 million Native Americans in the United States, or 0.7% of the total population. They now compose the smallest ethnic group in the American population. The following is a brief demographic sketch of this population (Go, 1994):

> Median age is 23.5 years
> 56% of the members have a high school education
> Median earning for a family is $20,025
> 23.7% of this group are below the poverty level

The family often has a nuclear structure, with strong, large, extended family networks. Children are taught to respect traditions and community organizations that provide social and cultural services. Many Native Americans tend to use traditional medicines and healers and are knowledgeable about these resources. People may frequently be treated by a traditional medicine man, and

herbs are frequently used to treat mental symptoms. Diagnostic techniques include the following:

> Divination (foretelling events or revealing secrets)
> Conjuring (summoning information)
> Stargazing ("reading" the stars to find answers to questions)

The basis of Native American philosophy is that all of nature, including the holistic person—body, mind, and spirit—is related. If one aspect of this relationship is not in balance, then health cannot exist.

HEALTH CARE OUTCOMES OF MINORITY POPULATIONS

High degrees of poverty and stress result in an increased incidence of physical and mental illness (American Nurses Association, 1997). The cultural expression and personal experience of illness (Kleinman, 1980) may be misinterpreted by the health care practitioner who diagnoses disease using a Western medical model. It is possible that some diagnosticians are limited in their application of cross-cultural differences (Davis, 1995) as evidenced by the disproportionate number of diagnoses of schizophrenia given to African-Americans and Hispanics (Davis, 1995; Mandersheid and Sonnenachein, 1996). Kleinman's findings about illness relate to poverty and mental illness, because persons in poverty are apt to experience more stress and are diagnosed with more severe disorders than those not in poverty situations.

Frequently persons from minority groups are handicapped when seeking employment. Since employment is tied to most health care plans, many persons from minority cultures either lack access to health care or have access only to very limited health care that often excludes mental health care. In addition, among adults considered poor according to defined federal guidelines for poverty, there was a 1.92 greater probability for the development of new (Axis I) psychiatric disorders than among the nonpoor population (Bruce, Takeuchi, and Leaf, 1991). Different cultural and ethnic presentations of symptoms contribute to this disparity, and persons who are less acculturated are not adept at gaining entry into a caregiving system (Ruiz, Venegas-Samuels, and Alarcon, 1995). Therapeutic and treatment issues are also affected if the client is treated by someone not culturally competent (Fielo, 1997). It is estimated that one third to two thirds of clients discharged from psychiatric hospitals return to their families (Cook, 1988; Goldman, 1982; Lefley, 1987). How are these clients managed if their family members are not able to negotiate the often-complicated mental health system or do not agree with the diagnosis? The cycle of poverty depicted in Figure 6-2 perpetuates a closed social and economic system that includes an increased incidence of mental illness, physical illness, and substance abuse.

Understanding & Applying Research

This case study illustrates the conflicts that arose when a 90-year-old Orthodox Jewish South African woman was referred to a nursing center in the United States. Placement in a nursing home was not acceptable to the client because she could not choose who would care for her. The client had been raised in Praetoria, South Africa, while apartheid was prevalent. She was accustomed to thinking of Africans as being in service positions and largely uneducated. Although caregivers visited her home, the client ignored those who were Hispanic or Afro-Carribean, or otherwise made them feel uncomfortable. These conflicts were addressed by the nursing director. The Jamaican nurse felt rejected but at the same time honored the client's right to choose who would care for her. The nurse appreciated opportunities in the United States and was learning to cope with expressions of discrimination. Her verbalizations that this situation was not troublesome was doubted by some other team members. Team conferences were held that included the client and her son. The conferences centered on open discussions on thinking processes and were not intended to influence the client to accept care from someone she found problematic. A compromise was reached when a British-born nursing student offered to help with this client's care. This was acceptable to all, and the plan of care continued until the client had further health problems.

This case study presents a difficult situation and a plan to address that difficulty. The author encourages clear commitment to fostering a climate that recognizes cultural needs and to establishing clear policies to encourage problem solving and decision making.

Fielo S: When cultures collide: decision making in a multicultural environment: an elder-care case study illustrates the concept of culturally competent nursing care and its implications for nurse-client relationships, *Nurs Health Perspect* 18(5):238, 1997.

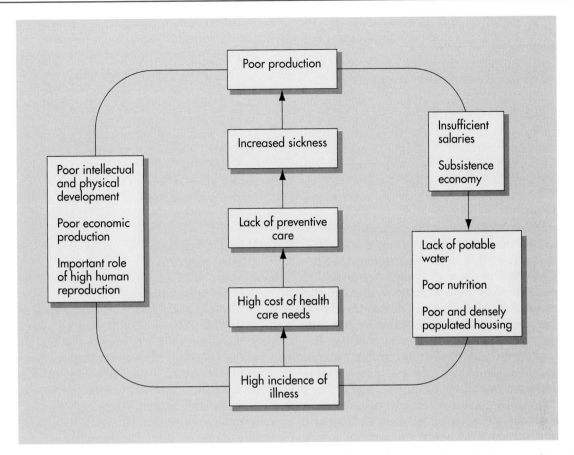

Figure 6-2   The cycle of poverty. (From Spector RE: *Cultural diversity in health and illness*, ed 4, Norwalk, Conn, Appleton & Lange.)

CULTURAL FACTORS AND THE NURSING PROCESS

Understanding the significance of culture and its impact on clients' mental and physical health is of foundational importance for nurses in all settings of health care delivery. This understanding and awareness are integral to the nursing process; they affect assessment, diagnosis, outcome identification, planning, intervention, and evaluation of clients.

The principal nursing tool in mental health is the therapeutic use of self. It is in the relationship between the nurse and client that the sensitive and usually embedded cultural issues manifest themselves and impact client care.

As the nurse applies the nursing process in the mental health setting, understanding the meanings of the health care problem from both the client's and the nurses's cultural perspective is important. Each step of the nursing process is impacted by an understanding of the complex cultural issues that affect clients and their interpretation of life events.

ASSESSMENT

The assessment process is foundational to all other steps of the nursing process. It is during assessment that the nurse formulates a perspective of the client's needs and issues.

CASE STUDY

Maria, a 20-year-old Hispanic woman, is seen in the psychiatric unit to rule out schizophrenia. She was admitted after she was found screaming in her front yard and acting irrationally. She sat in her room and was well-groomed and quiet. She isolated herself from other clients and appeared suspicious of staff. She had poor eye contact and spoke softly when questioned by the nurse. She remarked that her mother, who has been deceased 3 years, appears to her and speaks to her. The nature of these "appearances" is comforting; no commands are given.

Critical Thinking—Assessment

1. What culture-specific issues may be influencing Maria?
2. How might the assessment process be improved with an understanding of Maria's cultural heritage?
3. It is known that Hispanic people often report hearing the voice of deceased relatives in times of stress. How could the nurse differentiate between this cultural phenomenon and a psychotic thought process?
4. What communication barriers may be operating between Maria and the nurse?

Far from being objective, this process is colored by the nurse's personal biases, assumptions, cultural meanings, and nursing experience.

Numerous researchers have described cultural factors that influence assessment. Race in particular can alter the assessment of symptoms and level of functioning. Lawson et al (1994) describe how racial differences between client and clinician can lead to a failure to appreciate cultural differences in the presentation of symptoms and thus lead to misdiagnosis. In addition, clients from minority groups may delay seeking treatment because of mistrust of the system, which can lead to the application of more serious diagnostic labels.

The nurse must be as informed and as sensitive as possible. This enables the client to be truly "heard" and allows for accurate diagnosis. It helps prevent stereotyping and labeling, major problems in mental health care today.

The nurse needs to be aware of his or her own personal and professional cultural heritage, as well as the client's cultural heritage and what mental health means in its context. The use of the Heritage Assessment Tool (see Box 6-3) in assessing the client is an entry point for gathering culture-specific data. In addition, the following questions may be asked to gather cultural data:

1. *Cultural background.* What is the client's ethnic, religious, spiritual, and racial heritage? If unfamiliar with the client's culture, the nurse should seek information about the specific cultural group by interviewing the client's family and members of the group.

2. *Values orientation.* What are the attitudes of the given client, family, or community, based on their cultural heritage, in regard to this mental health problem?

3. *Cultural sanction and restrictions.* What are the "rules" in this client's cultural background with respect to this mental health problem? Does the client identify with a high-context or low-context culture?

4. *Communication.* What primary language does this client speak? If necessary, the nurse should obtain an interpreter.

5. *Health/illness beliefs and practices.* What cultural factors do the client and family associate with the identified problem? What types of traditional healers are available to the family?

6. *Nutrition.* What are the specific dietary restrictions to consider, if any?

7. *Economic considerations.* What economic resources are available to the family?

8. *Educational background.* What is the level of education of both the client and family? Are they able to read, understand, and follow instructions in English or in their native language? Where have they attended schools and for how long? Have they attended schools in the United States? What role does informal education play in their lives?

9. *Spiritual or religious affiliation.* What role does spirituality or religion play in the life of the client and family? Is a spiritual advisor or a member of the clergy readily available? What are the religious views of this client and family? Do they have special prayers?

NURSING DIAGNOSIS

The nursing diagnoses are much the same for clients from diverse cultural backgrounds, with a few exceptions. The nurse should be as specific as possible in conducting an assessment to determine that a problem is individualized to the client. Actual culture-related nursing diagnoses include those related to communication barriers, sociocultural dissonance, language barriers, and differences in health and illness beliefs and practices.

CASE STUDY

Mr. Looie is a 40-year-old Native American who has been diagnosed and treated for paranoid schizophrenia for about 20 years. During an acute phase of his illness, he is hospitalized. While hospitalized, he wishes to have his fan of eagle feathers in order to control his auditory hallucinations. He waves the fan in front of himself and talks to himself in his native language when he is distressed. This activity frightens some of the other clients. Some of the staff think that the fan should be taken away because it disturbs other clients, but other staff think Mr. Looie has a right to keep the fan if it helps him cope with his symptoms.

Critical Thinking—Intervention

1. How can the nurse balance the needs of Mr. Looie and the needs of the other clients?
2. Should the nurse support Mr. Looie in the use of this device?
3. What should the nurse's intervention be, if any, when Mr. Looie is seen using his fan?
4. What is the meaning of the fan to Mr. Looie?
5. What other cultural supports might be available to Mr. Looie during his hospitalization?

CLINICAL ALERT

Mrs. Williams is a 50-year-old woman whose husband died about 14 months ago of a myocardial infarction. She has come to the family practice clinic because she has begun to have chest pain and wonders if she might also have cardiac problems. While obtaining a history, the practitioner notices that Mrs. Williams is still dressed in black and adds the diagnosis of delayed bereavement to the history. The practitioner failed to assess Mrs. Williams in terms of her cultural expression of grief. Mrs. Williams is Hispanic, and it is customary for people of many Hispanic cultures to wear black for a year or longer. It would be socially unacceptable for Mrs. Williams to do otherwise.

The process of assigning a nursing diagnosis is an important one. These diagnostic categories often enable other staff to "frame" a client's health concerns. They must be as accurate as possible and reflect the unique cultural perspective of the client. In other words, they must be culturally congruent.

Often, a nursing diagnosis is chosen on the basis of an inaccurate assessment. The nurse, viewing client behavior through an ethnocentric lens, interprets the client's behavior as dysfunctional. Box 6-6 describes common nursing diagnoses that are often misapplied to clients as a result of culture-related misunderstandings.

OUTCOME IDENTIFICATION

Client outcomes in the mental health setting are determined on the basis of the assessment and diagnostic process. An understanding of cultural issues is crucial to ensure that the determination of outcomes of nursing care uses client input and is congruent with the clients' needs and wishes. Often clients fail to achieve the desired outcomes because such outcomes are inconsistent with their cultural worldview. Many clients will defer to the nurse, whom they see as the "expert." In reality, however, the clients do not plan to follow through with the client educational and discharge planning because it does not make sense to them and is not relevant to their problems from their perspective. This may lead to further misdiagnosis, especially the diagnosis of noncompliance. This happens most often when a client wants to use a traditional healing method or other culture-specific approach and sees the allopathic-oriented nursing intervention as conflicting with the traditional ways of achieving health.

PLANNING

When establishing goals of care and planning nursing interventions, the nurse considers each client's variables. The family is generally included in the client's treatment plan and, as often as possible, the client's community as well. A client's beliefs will more likely be included in a client's mental health care plan when the nurse is aware of the meaning of the client's behavior and verbalizations in the context of his or her culture and tradition.

IMPLEMENTATION

The implementation of nursing care plans that are holistic and culturally sensitive, congruent, and competent evolves over time and includes the following goals:

1. Maintain the client's cultural mental health practices as much as possible. For example, if the client is using ethnomedications, determine what type and how they react with conventional medications.
2. Maintain effective verbal and nonverbal communication between the client and caregivers and obtain an interpreter if necessary.
3. Promote the client's understanding of the allopathic system and the rationale behind the care that is being delivered.

The nurse must be aware that trust issues are important in mental health nursing care. Clients who are members of cultural communities may have a deep-seated mistrust of the system in general and the nurse in particular, especially if the nurse comes from a different cultural background. Researchers have noted that race, for example, is a powerful issue in treatment. In particular, it can affect how medication is administered, the level and frequency of interventions, and the outcome of intervention.

In a study of the psychiatric treatment of older African-American clients, Baker (1994) noted that the use of social support mechanisms in the intervention process was crucial in effectively caring for these elderly clients. This study is typical of many that suggest that mental health intervention must be done within the framework of culture if it is to be effective (Friedman, Paradis, and

---

Box 6-6   **Commonly Misapplied Nursing Diagnoses**

Common NANDA nursing diagnoses frequently misapplied because of a lack of understanding of cultural issues:

Coping, Defensive, and Noncompliance
Clients from minority cultures that have experienced discrimination, bias, and stereotyping may be resistant to appropriate nursing interventions, especially in the area of teaching and discharge planning. Suspicion and mistrust may cause the nurse to misunderstand a client's behaviors and mislabel them.

Role Performance, Altered, and Parenting, Altered
Use of these diagnoses requires an understanding of the client's culture-specific roles and parenting activities. They may be different from those of the nurse and the majority culture.

Social Interaction, Impaired, and Communication, Impaired Verbal
Misunderstanding occurs when the nurse fails to take into account culture-specific interaction patterns. Silence, infrequent eye contact, shame, fear, and language barriers all affect clients' ability to interact. The gender of the nurse and the gender of the client may also influence communication because many cultures have specific gender-role behavioral codes.

Thought Processes, Altered
Thought patterns and processes that may appear to be distorted can be related to culture-specific expressions of anxiety and fear. Careful assessment will enable the nurse to accurately diagnose anxiety or fear in many clients, rather than assume that underlying thought processes are altered.

Hatch, 1994; Hickling and Griffith, 1994; Morris and Si-love, 1992; Nelson et al, 1992). Use of family members and other members of the client's cultural group in the assessment, planning, and intervention process can facilitate nursing care and ensure more effective client outcomes.

EVALUATION

The nurse evaluates mental health care from a multicultural nursing perspective by determining if the client outcomes have been achieved.

It is important to evaluate whether or not the client has been able to maintain his or her cultural beliefs regarding mental health and illness. The client's needs and beliefs should be respected with open lines of communication. The discharge plan should be realistic and culturally congruent. If the client does not feel invested in the treatment choices, he or she is less likely to be effective after discharge. Thus evaluation of nursing interventions is based on the attainment of client outcomes that have been determined to be culturally sensitive and realistic.

Summary of Key Concepts

1. Psychiatric mental health nurses must assess and evaluate clients and implement care plans with a holistic and culturally sensitive perspective toward care.
2. Multicultural nursing in mental health involves an understanding of many issues, including demographic change, heritage consistency, socialization, acculturation, and assimilation.
3. To effectively assist someone from another culture, nurses need to have an awareness of their own cultural heritage.
4. Heritage consistency is the concept that describes the degree to which a person identifies with his or her cultural background.
5. The Heritage Assessment Tool can assist nurses in assessing a client's heritage consistency.
6. Health can be viewed as three-dimensional, encompassing the body, mind, and spirit.
7. The communication aspects of language, space, and time orientation have various practices among different cultures.

REFERENCES

American Nurses Association: *Multicultural issues in the nursing workforce,* Washington, DC, 1993, The Association.

American Nurses Association: Addressing cultural diversity in the profession, *Am Nurse* 30(1):25, 1994.

American Nurses Association: Improving minority health outcomes through culturally specific care, *Nurs Trends Issues* 2(3):1, 1997.

American Psychiatric Association: *Diagnostic and statistical manual of mental disorders,* ed 4, Washington, DC, 1994, The Association.

Baker F: Psychiatric treatment of older African-Americans, *Hosp Community Psychiatry* 45(32), 1994.

Bartol G, Richardson L: Using literature to create cultural competence, *Image: J Nurs Sch* 30(1):75, 1998.

Bruce M, Takeuchi E, Leaf P: Poverty and psychiatric status: longitudinal evidence from the New Haven Epidemiologic Catchment Area Study, *Arch Gen Psychiatry* 48:470, 1991.

Camphina-Bacote J: Cultural competence in psychiatric mental health nursing: a conceptual model, *Nurs Clin North Am* 29(1), 1994.

Cook J: Who "mothers" the chronically mentally ill? *Fam Relations* 37:42, 1988.

Davis K: *Mental health training and black colleges: identifying the need.* Keynote speaker at the September African-American Behavioral Health Conference in Atlanta, 1995.

Fielo S, Degazon C: When cultures collide: decision making in a multicultural environment, *Nurs Health Care Perspect* 18(5):238, 1997.

Foster S: The pragmatics of culture: the rhetoric of difference in psychiatric nursing, *Arch Psychiatr Nurs* 4(5):292, 1990.

Friedman S, Paradis C, Hatch M: Characteristics of African-American and white patients with panic disorder and agoraphobia, *Hosp Community Psychiatry* 45, 1994.

Germain C: Cultural care: a bridge between sickness, illness, and disease, *Holistic Nurs Pract* 6(3):1-9, 1992.

Geuss R: *The idea of a critical theory,* New York, 1981, Cambridge University Press.

Go H: Changing populations and health. In Edelman CL, Mandle CL, editors: *Health promotion throughout the lifespan,* ed 3, St. Louis, 1994, Mosby.

Goldman H: Mental illness and family burden: a public health perspective, *Hosp Community Psychiatry* 33:557, 1982.

Greco J: America's changing workforce, *J Bus Strategy* 19(2):43, 1998.

Hickling F, Griffith E: Clinical perspectives on the Rastafari movement, *Hosp Community Psychiatry* 45, 1994.

Hofstede G: *Culture's consequences: international differences in work-related values,* Thousand Oaks, Calif, 1980, Sage Publications.

Hofstede G: *Cultures and organizations: software of the mind,* New York, 1991, McGraw-Hill.

Hofstede G: In Kim U et al, editors: *Individualism and collectivism: theory, method, and applications,* Thousand Oaks, Calif, 1994, Sage Publications.

Information please: almanac 1995, Boston, 1995, Houghton Mifflin.

Keltner N, Folks D: Psychopharmacology update, *Perspect Psychiatr Care* 28(1):33, 1992.

Kim U: Individualism and collectivism: conceptual clarification and elaboration. In Kim U et al, editors: *Individualism and collectivism: theory, method and applications,* Thousand Oaks, Calif, 1994, Sage Publications.

Kleinman A: *Patients and healers in the context of culture,* Berkeley, Calif, 1980, University of California Press.

Kleinman A: *The illness narratives: suffering, healing, and the human condition,* New York, 1988, Basic Books.

LaFromboise T, Coleman H, Gerton J: Psychological impact of biculturalism: evidence and theory, *Psychol Bull* 14:395, 1993.

Lawson W et al: Race as a factor in inpatient and outpatient admissions and diagnoses, *Hosp Community Psychiatry* 45(72), 1994.

Lefley H: The family's response to mental illness in a relative. In Hatfield A, editor: *Families of the mentally ill,* New York, 1987, Guilford Press.

Leininger M: *Culture, care, diversity, and universality: a theory of nursing,* New York, 1991, National League of Nursing.

Lester N: Cultural competence: a nursing dialogue, *Am J Nurs* 98(8):26, 1998.

Lin K: Cultural aspects of mental health for Asian Americans. In Gaw A, editor: *Cross-cultural psychiatry,* Boston, 1982, John Wright.

Mandersheid R, Sonnenachein M: Percentage of clinically trained mental health personnel. In *Mental health, United States,* Washington, DC, 1996, U.S. Department of Health and Human Services.

Mensah L: Transcultural, cross-cultural, and multicultural health perspectives in focus. In Masi R, Mensah L, McLeod K, editors: *Health and cultures: exploring the relationships,* vol 1, New York, 1993, Mosaic Press.

Minehan M: Increasing immigration will diversify issues, *Human Resources Magazine* 42(11):160, 1997.

Morris P, Silove D: Cultural influences in psychotherapy with refugee survivors of torture and trauma, *Hosp Community Psychiatry* 43(3), 1992.

Nelson S et al: An overview of mental health services for American Indians and Alaska natives in the 1990s, *Hosp Community Psychiatry* 43(3), 1992.

Purnell L, Paulanka B: *Transcultural health care: a culturally competent approach,* Philadelphia, 1998, FA Davis.

Ruiz P, Venegas-Samuels K, Alarcon R: The economics of pain: mental health care costs among minorities, *Psychiatr Clin North Am* 18(3):659, 1995.

Spector RE: *Cultural diversity in health and illness,* ed 4, Norwalk, Conn, 1996, Appleton & Lange.

Spurlock J: Black Americans. In Comas-Diaz L, Griffith E, editors: *Cross-cultural mental health,* New York, 1988, John Wiley & Sons.

Swanson D: *Considering the communication traits of expressiveness, advocacy, and argumentativeness in the multicultural student population at the University of Guam,* 1993, Unpublished manuscript.

Tripp-Remier T: *Cultural assessment: a multidimensional approach,* Monterey, Calif, 1995, Wadsworth.

Yamamoto J: Japanese Americans. In Gaw A, editor: *Cross-cultural psychiatry,* Boston, 1982, John Wright.

PART TWO

Dynamics of Nursing Practice

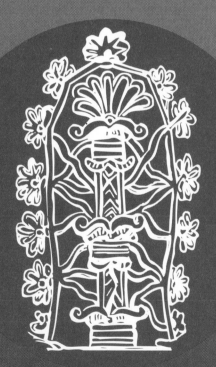

Tree of Life
Ancient Babylonia

This symbol represents a tree of life and knowledge and appears throughout the world in various forms. It signifies the perpetual nature of life, knowledge, and learning. The chapters in Part Two discuss key concepts in the application of psychiatric nursing principles to life situations as perpetuated through the nursing process and principles of communication.

CHAPTER 7

The Nursing Process

Katherine M. Fortinash

OBJECTIVES

- Discuss the roles of intuition, expertise, and critical thinking and their application to the nursing process in mental health.

- Describe the cyclic nature of the American Nurses Association six-step nursing process.

- Compare and contrast nursing and medical assessment frameworks, with particular focus on the NANDA taxonomy.

- Differentiate actual, risk, and wellness diagnoses with emphasis on the most current NANDA labels, etiologies, risk factors, and defining characteristics.

- Identify outcomes that accurately measure clients' achievable behaviors based on their nursing diagnoses.

- Describe nursing-sensitive outcomes and the Nursing Outcomes Classification (NOC) and their influence on the nursing process.

- Formulate nursing interventions that are prescriptive and directive, for both actual and risk diagnoses.

- Define the Nursing Interventions Classification (NIC) and its relationship to the nursing process.

- Construct rationale statements for each proposed nursing intervention.

- Develop evaluations for outcomes that effectively measure client progress within an appropriate time frame.

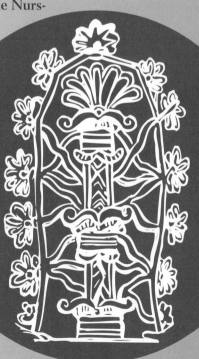

The nursing process is a time-tested, organized method that consists of a series of planned steps and actions designed to help nurses treat and evaluate human responses to actual or potential health problems. Originally a five-step process, the nursing process has been revised to a six-step process in recent years, according to the American Nurses Association (ANA) Standards of Practice (ANA, 1991). See comparison below:

Five-Step Process
Standard I—Assessment
Standard II—Nursing Diagnosis
Standard III—Planning
Standard IV—Implementation
Standard V—Evaluation

Six-Step Process
Standard I—Assessment
Standard II—Nursing Diagnosis
Standard III—Outcome Identification
Standard IV—Planning
Standard V—Implementation
Standard VI—Evaluation

To maintain the most current practice standards, the six-step process is used throughout this text, although the authors recognize the merits of the five-step process and realize that it is still in use. In the six-step process, outcome identification is featured as a separate step, since some believe it may be useful to list outcomes directly after nursing diagnoses and before the planning phase. They contend that the planning phase incorporates measures that assist clients in achieving outcomes. Outcome achievement can be accomplished more readily if outcomes have already been selected. In the five-step process the planning phase exists in part to plan outcomes, so that outcomes are actually part of the planning phase and therefore not singled out as a separate step.

In recent times outcomes, whether client centered or organizational, have emerged as a major focus

for accrediting bodies and managed care companies. The current trend toward cost-effective quality outcomes and methods of achievement is a major component of health care delivery systems.

The **Nursing Outcomes Classification (NOC)** was developed by the Iowa Outcomes Project in part to assist nursing in identifying those outcomes that are essentially influenced by the actions of nurses. For nurses to work effectively with managed care organizations to improve quality and reduce costs, they must be able to measure and document the patient outcomes that are most sensitive to nursing care (Johnson and Maas, 1997).

Regardless of the method used, the nursing process remains a forceful, systematic, problem-solving method that encompasses all of the significant components necessary to care for clients, with attention given to families, significant others, and the community. Many nursing theorists concur that the nursing process is even more than an organized, systematic approach

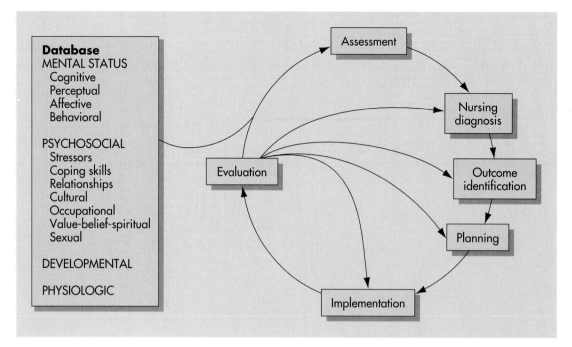

Figure 7-1   Cyclic nature of the nursing process. (From Fortinash KM, Holoday-Worret PA: *Psychiatric nursing care plans,* ed 3, St. Louis, 1999, Mosby.)

to clinical problems. Unlike most episodic or linear problem-solving methods, in which a problem is identified, diagnosed, treated, and resolved (thus the problem ends with a resolution), the nursing process is an ongoing, multidimensional, cyclic approach in which data are continually collected, critically analyzed, and incorporated into the treatment plan according to the client's fluctuating responses to health and illness. Figure 7-1 shows the cyclic nature of the nursing process.

The steps in the nursing process are not necessarily taken in strict sequence (beginning with assessment and ending with evaluation). They may be taken concurrently, since nurses may be evaluating their assessment or even their plan of action at any given time.

Since the client's health status is dynamic rather than static, so, too, is the nursing process. This challenges the seasoned nurse to make sound, clinical judgments and decisions, and guides the novice toward practicing and mastering clear, analytic thinking and keen organizational skills. The steps of the nursing process create a circular pattern of continuous interpretation of data and management of client care.

Kritek (1978) states that the phases of the nursing process are interactive as well as continual. Thus the phases influence each other and the client at the same time. There are points throughout the process in which the phases converge. The nurse can attend the client at any point throughout this interactive, fluid process.

NOC, which developed the first comprehensive, standardized language describing patient outcomes that are responsive to nursing interventions, defines nursing-sensitive outcomes as neutral concepts that can be measured on a continuum. Neutral concepts, such as mobility and hydration (physical states), or coping and grieving (psychologic states), differ from discrete goals that are either met or unmet (Johnson and Maas, 1997).

For psychiatric mental health nurses, whether students, new graduates, or seasoned clinicians, the use of the nursing process presents significant challenges that can be mastered. In the world of mental health, the nursing process focuses primarily on the client's behavior and its meaning beyond the spoken word, including psychosocial stressors. A client's psychic strength, vulnerability, coping skills, and ego defense mechanisms are among the major components that are the psychiatric nurse's primary focus for the nursing process.

The psychiatric mental health component of holistic client assessment includes the Mental Status Examination and psychosocial criteria (Box 7-1), which consist of an organized collection of data that reflects an individual's functioning at the time of the interview. It is a basis for subsequent medical and nursing diagnoses and management of care by all disciplines that interface with psychiatric mental health nursing.

Components of the Mental Status Examination, such as mood, affect, thoughts, and perceptions, are the psychiatric mental health nurse's major focus in treating mental or emotional disorders. However, psychiatric mental

Box 7-1   **Components of Assessment: Mental Status and Psychosocial Criteria**

Mental Status Examination

Appearance
Dress, grooming, hygiene, cosmetics, apparent age, posture, facial expression

Behavior/activity
Hypoactivity or hyperactivity, rigid, relaxed, restless or agitated motor movements, gait and coordination, facial grimacing, gestures, mannerisms, passive, combative, bizarre

Attitude
Interactions with the interviewer: cooperative, resistive, friendly, hostile, ingratiating

Speech
Quantity: Poverty of speech, poverty of content, voluminous
Quality: Articulate, congruent, monotonous, talkative, repetitious, spontaneous, circumlocutory, confabulations, tangential, pressured, stereotypic
Rate: Slowed, rapid

Mood and affect
Mood (intensity, depth, duration): Sad, fearful, depressed, angry, anxious, ambivalent, happy, ecstatic, grandiose
Affect (intensity, depth, duration): Appropriate, apathetic, constricted, blunted, flat, labile, euphoric, bizarre

Perceptions
Hallucinations, illusions, depersonalization, derealization, distortions

Thoughts
Form and content: Logical versus illogical, loose associations, flight of ideas, autistic, blocking, broadcasting, neologisms, word salad, obsessions, ruminations, delusions, abstract versus concrete

Sensorium/cognition
Levels of consciousness, orientation, attention span, recent and remote memory, concentration; ability to comprehend and process information; intelligence

Judgment
Ability to assess and evaluate situations, make rational decisions, understand consequences of behavior, and take responsibility for actions

Insight
Ability to perceive and understand the cause and nature of own and others' situations

Reliability
Interviewer's impression that individual reported information accurately and completely

Psychosocial Criteria

Stressors
Internal: Psychiatric or medical illness, perceived loss, such as loss of self-concept/self-esteem
External: Actual loss (e.g., death of a loved one, divorce, lack of support systems, job or financial loss, retirement, dysfunctional family system)

Coping skills
Adaptation to internal and external stressors; use of functional, adaptive coping mechanisms and techniques; management of activities of daily living

Relationships
Attainment and maintenance of satisfying, interpersonal relationships congruent with developmental stage; includes sexual relationship as appropriate for age and status

Cultural
Ability to adapt and conform to prescribed norms, rules, ethics, and mores of an identified group

Spiritual (value-belief)
Presence of a self-satisfying value-belief system that the individual regards as right, desirable, worthwhile, and comforting

Occupational
Engagement in useful, rewarding activity, congruent with developmental stage and societal standards (work, school, recreation)

From Fortinash KM, Holoday-Worret PA: *Psychiatric nursing care plans*, ed 3, St. Louis, 1999, Mosby.

health nurses must be equally prepared to conduct a multisystem assessment, similar to that used in a medical-surgical setting. Many clients have physical symptoms caused by medication effects, self-neglect, or self-harm. Some clients require placement in a special medical unit within the psychiatric facility. These are generally older adults with multiple physical problems or clients experiencing symptoms related to alcohol or other substance-induced disorders. Psychiatric mental health nurses should be keenly aware that clients are biopsychosocial beings and that all symptoms may affect both the mind and the body.

Although it is unlikely that clients treated in a psychiatric facility will be attached to intravenous tubing, oxygen, or a cardiac monitor, their wounds are equally painful and just as profoundly debilitating. It is the nurse's challenge to discover the source of these wounds by applying critical thinking and decision-making skills while following the familiar guidelines of the nursing process, combined with a uniqueness of self and experiential wisdom.

Even with the help of the nursing process and the current Nursing Interventions Classification (NIC) and NOC systems, there will be times when psychiatric mental health nurses are unsure of which approach to take for certain client behaviors. Unlike the medical-surgical field, there are not always specific interventions for specific client behaviors, and clients may not always respond predictably to standard approaches. As such, psychiatric mental health clients may be resistant to even the most carefully designed treatment plan, whereby a variety of treatment approaches is generally applied before a response is elicited.

The nursing process, like other decision-making methods, does not guarantee instant improvement of symptoms. Psychiatric clients seldom leave the hospital completely symptom free, given the complex nature of mental illness. However, it is hoped that clients will achieve a higher level of functioning because of nurses who are willing to try a variety of acceptable, time-tested approaches with patience, understanding, and hope. In the final analysis it is the nurse, with his or her unique spirit, who adds a critical dimension to the nursing process and brings it to life.

HISTORY AND PERSPECTIVES OF THE NURSING PROCESS

The nursing process is the long-standing method by which nurses make critical decisions for clinical care. It is influenced by such important elements as intuition, expertise, and critical thinking.

INTUITION AND THE NURSING PROCESS

Intuition, also known as intuitive reasoning, is an individual's insight into a situation without the benefit of critical analysis. A strong "hunch" and a "gut feeling" are examples of intuition. It is often proposed that a person operating on intuition needs little data to support his or her insights (Wescott, 1968). It is generally acknowledged that, in the past, nurses relied strongly on intuition for their nursing assessments and actions. With the advent of nursing as a science, intuitive reasoning fell into disfavor as a method by which to make critical decisions. Intuitiveness came to be viewed as unscientific. As technology grew and the pendulum swung toward scientific reasoning as a method of knowing and away from the intuitive approach, intuition was devalued (Munhall and Oiler, 1993).

As a result of this scientific revolution, nursing resisted using intuitive terms and instead opted for a more concrete, linear problem-solving method considered to be gender neutral and relatively safe. More recently, intuition has appeared in nursing journals as a valid component of the complex nature of clinical reasoning. Some now consider intuition as a component of critical thinking.

Benner's significant work, *From Novice to Expert: Excellence and Power in Clinical Nursing Practice* (1984), described the role of intuition in critical care nurses and concluded that many of them were not consciously aware of the higher-level reasoning processes they used to assess and deliver client care. Yet the nursing interventions based on these intuitive forces reflected superior insights and sound judgments. Smith (1988) noted that these nurses somehow had the ability to sense impending deterioration in their clients before such crises actually occurred.

Given this information, it makes sense that in the psychiatric mental health arena, where clients' fluctuating behaviors are the main focus for nursing assessment, diagnosis, and interventions, nurses inevitably incorporate judgments based on intuitive reasoning to make clinical decisions. It seems obvious, then, that intuition has a role in influencing the phases of the nursing process and has strongly resurfaced as a major force in clinical reasoning. Although the mental mechanisms by which intuition works remain in part mysterious and elusive, the results as measured by client outcomes have nonetheless been impressive. Intuitive reasoning most decidedly has a place in the future of clinical nursing research and practice.

Example of a nurse's use of intuition: A nurse retreats from an intense interview with a client and focuses on less volatile topics. When asked about her strategy, she stated that she experienced a "gut" feeling that prompted her to change the topic. When questioned later about his feelings during the interview, the client stated that he experienced a buildup of anger, although he was not fully aware of it at the time.

EXPERTISE AND THE NURSING PROCESS

Expertise is another component necessary for sound clinical judgments. Only through clinical experience can nurses develop expertise in selected specialty areas of practice (Benner, 1984). Expertise, like intuition, influences the phases of the nursing process. Although it is said that intuition cannot be taught, it can nonetheless be learned through clinical practice. The exact process by which this occurs, however, remains elusive and complex. Both expertise and intuition are worthwhile goals that nurses should continue to develop and pursue throughout their professional lives. Expertise can incorporate intuitiveness in clinical practice.

CRITICAL THINKING IN THE NURSING PROCESS

Critical thinking is most important in the nursing process and contains many of the components of keen judgment, intuition, and expertise. Critical thinking skills enhance and become a part of the nurse's continually expanding knowledge base and help the nurse decide which data are meaningful and which take priority.

When using the nursing process, the nurse incorporates experience and knowledge from nursing and other courses to apply theories and principles in practice. Knowledge of basic human needs, anatomy and physiology, disease processes, growth and development, sociologic patterns and trends, and various cultures, religions, and philosophies are all crucial components of the critical thinking framework. The following critical thinking skills are used in all phases of the nursing process (Wilkinson, 1992):

Observing (observations should be planned and ongoing versus casual and singular)
Distinguishing relevant from irrelevant data
Validating data through observations and communication
Organizing data into meaningful parts
Categorizing data for efficient retrieval and communication

Critical thinking embodies much more than the skills of logical analysis. It involves questioning the assumptions underlying one's customary, habitual ways of thinking and behaving, and subsequently being willing to think and act differently as a result of this critical thinking.

ASSESSMENT

Assessment, the initial phase of the nursing process, is perhaps the most critical component because it is the phase in which nurses collect enormous amounts of data about clients' holistic health status. *Holistic assessment provides nurses with relevant data from which to accurately formulate and prioritize nursing diagnoses, the crux of treatment planning, according to clients' needs or immediate conditions.* Throughout the assessment phase, nurses collect data through learned, time-proven, interactive and interviewing skills and observations of verbal and nonverbal behaviors, based on a broad biopsychosociocultural background and knowledge of functional and dysfunctional behaviors (Fortinash and Holoday-Worret, 1999).

In psychiatric mental health nursing, assessment takes place in a number of settings (e.g., inpatient, outpatient, or community and home environments). This gives the nurse many opportunities to observe the client and modify assessment data in accordance with the client's continued adjustment to the milieu and progress made throughout hospitalization. Ideally, the client is the primary source of information during the assessment phase. Occasionally, however, the client may be unable to offer a complete or accurate health history, given the acuity of his or her illness. In such cases, a reliable source may be interviewed on the client's behalf, with the understanding that such infor-

mation will be evaluated in terms of that person's relationship with the client (Fortinash, 1990).

Assessment of the individual includes the following criteria: physical, psychiatric, psychosocial, mental status, developmental, cultural, spiritual, and sexual. The method of assessment includes the client's subjective report of symptoms and problems and the nurse's objective findings (Fortinash, 1990; Fortinash and Holoday-Worret, 1999). Box 7-1 details mental status and psychosocial criteria that should be covered during assessment.

A major focus of a client's mental status is identification of his or her strengths and capabilities for interaction with and within the environment. This includes the ability to initiate interactions, sustain meaningful communication and relationships, and attain satisfaction congruent with his or her developmental and sociocultural lifestyle. Knowledge and appreciation of the psychodynamics and psychopathology of human behavior are essential for effective assessment of the individual's adjustment or maladjustment to internal and external life stressors (Fortinash and Holoday-Worret, 1999).

THE NURSE-CLIENT INTERVIEW

The interview is the most critical process involved in gathering information related to the overall health status of clients with psychiatric disorders. It is a more meaningful, flexible method of collecting important data than are questionnaires or computers, and it allows the examiner to use all of the senses to explore specific topics and key themes or concerns expressed by the client through verbal and nonverbal responses. Box 7-2 lists samples of some general questions that can be asked during the nurse-client interview.

In assessing a client's mental status, the primary instrument, or "tool," of evaluation is the nurse interviewer. The success of the interview depends in large part on the development of trust, rapport, and respect between the nurse and the client and between the nurse and the family. Keen therapeutic communication skills such as active listening and reflective questioning are used throughout the interview in an effort to determine the client's immediate needs and actively engage him or her in treatment (Fortinash, 1990; Fortinash and Holoday-Worret, 1999). See Chapter 8 for more information on development of good communication skills.

ASSESSMENT FRAMEWORKS

Assessment frameworks are not new or unique to nursing. As a result of nursing's orientation and commitment to holistic assessment, nurses collect large amounts of data about a client's biopsychosociocultural health status. Assessment frameworks are organizational systems by which to store data for easier access to information. Such frameworks can also serve as guides for assessment, since their compartments consist of categories that correspond to those qualities accepted by nurses as constituting the na-

Box 7-2   The Nurse-Client Interview: Sample General Questions

Presenting Problem
Tell me the reason you are here (in treatment).

Present Illness
When did you first notice the problem?
What changes have you noticed in yourself?
What do you think is causing the problem?
Have you had any troubling feelings or thoughts?

Family History
How would you describe your relationship with your
    parents?
Did either of your parents have emotional or mental prob-
    lems?
Were either of your parents treated by a psychiatrist or
    therapist?
Did their treatment include medication or ECT?
Were they helped by their treatment?

Childhood/Premorbid History
How did you get along with your family and friends?
How would you describe yourself as a child?

Medical History
Do you have any serious medical problems?
How have they affected your current problem?

Psychosocial/Psychiatric History
Have you ever been treated for an emotional or psychiatric
    problem? Have you been diagnosed with a mental
    illness?
Have you ever been a patient in a psychiatric hospital?
Have you ever been in counseling/therapy for an emotional
    or psychiatric problem?
Have you ever taken prescribed medications for an emo-
    tional problem or mental illness? Did you ever have
    ECT?
If so, did the medication or ECT help your symptoms/
    problem?
How frequently do your symptoms occur? (About every 6
    months? Once a year? Every 5 years? First episode?)
How long are you generally able to function well in
    between onset of symptoms? (Weeks? Months? Years?)
What do you feel, if anything, may have contributed to
    your symptoms? (Nothing? Stopped taking medications?
    Began using alcohol? Street drugs?)

Recent Stressors/Losses
Have you had any recent stressors or losses in your life?
What are your relationships like?
How do you get along with people at work?

Education
How did you do in school?
How did you feel about school?

Legal
Have you ever been in trouble with the law?

Marital History
How do you feel about your marriage? (If client is married)
How would you describe your relationship with your chil-
    dren? (If client has children)
What kinds of things do you do as a family?

Social History
Tell me about your friends, your social activities.
How would you describe your relationship with your
    friends?

Support Systems
Who would you turn to if you were in trouble?
Do you feel you need someone to turn to now?

Insight
Do you consider yourself different now from the way you
    were before your problem began? In what way?
Do you think you have an emotional problem or mental
    illness?
Do you think you need help for your problem?
What are your goals for yourself?

Value-Belief System (Including Spiritual)
What kinds of things give you comfort and peace of mind?
Will those things be helpful to you now?

Special Needs (Including Cultural)
How can staff help you during your treatment?
What kinds of things will be most helpful to you now?

Discharge Goals
How do you want to feel by the time you're ready for dis-
    charge?
What do you think you can do to help yourself reach that
    goal?
What things will you do differently from the way you did
    them before?
What things can you do to help prevent your symptoms
    from reoccurring and stay out of the hospital?
What are your goals for daily medication compliance?
How will you manage your leisure time?

Modified from Fortinash KM, Holoday-Worret PA: *Psychiatric nursing care plans*, ed 3, St. Louis, 1999, Mosby; and Fortinash KM: Assessment of mental states. In Malasanos L, Barkauskas V, Stoltenberg-Allen K, editors: *Health assessment*, ed 4, St. Louis, 1990, Mosby.

Table 7-1	Comparison of Medical and Nursing Assessment Frameworks	
Medical Model	**Nursing Models**	
Body Systems	**NANDA Taxonomy I–Revised**	**Functional Health Patterns (Gordon, 1994)**
Cardiovascular	Exchanging	Health perception/health management
Respiratory	Communicating	Nutritional/metabolic
Neurologic	Relating	Elimination
Endocrine	Valuing	Activity/exercise
Metabolic	Choosing	Sleep/rest
Hematopoietic	Moving	Cognitive/perceptual
Integumentary	Perceiving	Self-perception/self-concept
Gastrointestinal	Feeling	Role/relationship
Genitourinary	Knowing	Sexuality/reproductive
Reproductive		Coping/stress tolerance
Psychiatric		Value-belief

From Davie JK: The nursing process. In Thelan LA et al, editors: *Critical care nursing: diagnosis and management*, ed 3, St. Louis, 1998, Mosby.

ture of humans, health, illness, and nursing. Table 7-1 depicts three separate assessment frameworks. The traditional medical framework model is now considered insufficient for the holistic assessment required in psychiatric mental health nursing and, most likely, in other nursing specialty areas. The other two columns describe the two frameworks most commonly used in today's nursing practice, which are discussed below.

Functional Health Pattern Framework

Developed by Marjory Gordon, functional health patterns are categories of human, biologic, physiologic, psychologic, developmental, cultural, social, and spiritual assessments. Health patterns related to these categories are assessed over a time sequence as either functional or dysfunctional. Functional patterns reflect the client's strengths and adaptive coping strategies, whereas dysfunctional patterns form the basis for client problems and nursing diagnoses (Gordon, 1994). Functional health patterns are currently widely accepted framework methods in both educational and practice settings.

NANDA Taxonomy

At the seventh conference of the North American Nursing Diagnosis Association (NANDA) in 1986, a classification system for nursing diagnoses was officially formulated. It is currently called Taxonomy I—Revised (NANDA, 1999). This system is NANDA's conceptual framework. It replaces the previously used alphabetized list of diagnoses (a collection of names) as a method of categorizing.

A **taxonomy** classifies phenomena under a hierarchic structure and also helps guide new phenomena. Both the taxonomy and the diagnostic terminology guide nurses toward building a solid scientific foundation for the profession. It also provides nursing with a standardized, more efficient method of communication (NANDA, 1999).

Frameworks are necessary tools with which to process the large amount of data collected by nurses in assessing clients. Frameworks form a basis for diagnostic reasoning (discussed later) by gathering assessment information and organizing it into manageable pieces. An organized collection system ensures easier retrieval of critical client information and shows important relationships among the data. The selection of one framework over another is an individual choice (Fortinash and Holoday-Worret, 1999).

NURSING DIAGNOSIS

The formulation of nursing diagnoses involves the interpretation of data collected in the assessment phase and the application of standardized labels to clients' health problems and responses to illness and life events. Nursing diagnoses are written as statements that describe an individual's health state or an actual or potential alteration (known as a risk diagnosis) in a person's life process. The nursing diagnosis statement may reflect one's biologic, psychologic, sociocultural, developmental, spiritual, or sexual process (Table 7-2). At NANDA's ninth conference (1990), nursing diagnosis was defined as ". . . a clinical judgment about individual, family, or community responses to actual or potential health problems/life processes. Nursing diagnoses provide the basis for selection of nursing interventions to achieve outcomes for which the nurse is accountable."

The development and refinement of nursing diagnoses are still in the early stages and are continuously being revised. This challenging task is evident in the 19 newest diagnostic labels endorsed at NANDA's tenth conference in 1994. A list of the most current NANDA diagnoses (1999) is found on the inside front cover of this book.

Nursing diagnoses provide nurses with a vocabulary that is distinctive to nursing. Nursing diagnosis language

Table 7-2	Nursing Diagnosis Statements in Relationship to Life Processes	
Nursing Diagnoses	**Life Processes**
Nutrition, altered	Biologic
Self-esteem disturbance	Psychologic
Social interaction, impaired	Sociocultural
Growth and development, altered	Developmental
Spiritual distress (distress of the human spirit)	Spiritual
Sexuality patterns, altered	Sexual

enhances communication among nurses and clarity of purpose to other health care disciplines in relation to the problems nurses assess and treat. By using its own vocabulary, nursing grows as a profession and gains respectability. Carpenito (1996) states that NANDA's attempt to upgrade nursing's status as a profession by its unifying vocabulary, which enhances communication among nurses, is as much for purposes of a social policy as it is for "clarifying nursing for nurses."

DIAGNOSTIC REASONING

Once the data have been collected and recorded, the next step is interpretation of what the data actually mean in terms of the client's health-illness status. Critical thinking in diagnostic reasoning consists of the following two major cognitive processes (Wilkinson, 1992):

Analysis: Taking apart the collected data to examine and interpret each piece and identify variations from typical behaviors or responses. Analysis also includes discovering patterns or relationships in the data that may be cues that require further investigation.
Synthesis: Combining several parts of relevant data into a single piece of information. Synthesis also involves comparing behavioral patterns with learned theories or typical patterns of behavior in order to identify strengths and seek explanations for symptoms.

The term *inference* has been defined as "the process of arriving at a conclusion by reasoning from evidence." However, inherent in the use of inference is a tendency to assume that the evidence is slight or has not been fully examined. Therefore in order to avoid (as much as possible) a rush to judgment or an "inferential leap," the nurse reaches conclusions and formulates diagnoses based on logical and factual data. This can be achieved by limiting the amount of bias that can influence the diagnostic process and by remaining as objective as possible (Benner, 1984; Carnevali and Thomas, 1993; Tanner et al, 1987).

DEFINITIONS OF HEALTH PROBLEMS

Nearly all approved diagnoses are accompanied by definitions that more clearly describe or explain the health problem. This feature is useful for students who may need more specific clarification of the problem than the label alone conveys. The following examples present definitions for two sets of similar diagnoses that are often confused with one another:

Fear: "Feeling of dread related to an identifiable source which the person validates" (NANDA, 1999)
Anxiety: "A vague, uneasy feeling whose source is often nonspecific or unknown to the individual" (NANDA, 1999)
Powerlessness: "Perception that one's actions will not significantly affect an outcome; a perceived lack of control over a current situation or immediate happening" (NANDA, 1999)
Hopelessness: "A subjective state in which an individual sees limited or no alternatives or personal choices available and is unable to mobilize energy on own behalf" (NANDA, 1999)

QUALIFYING STATEMENTS

For additional clarity, some nursing diagnoses require qualifying statements based on the nature of the health problem as it is manifested in each particular client response or situation.

It is considered inadvisable to cite medical diagnoses as etiologies for nursing problems. It is more difficult for nurses to treat an etiology that is stated as a medical diagnosis, such as schizophrenia, since that type of label suggests a whole array of treatment strategies that are not uniquely nursing.

However, many symptoms and behaviors resulting from mental disorders and medical conditions are of great concern to nurses and require management and treatment by nurses. Some examples are:

Communication, impaired verbal, as a result of bipolar disorders
Nutrition, altered: less than body requirements, as a result of anorexia nervosa
Thought processes, altered, as a result of the schizophrenic process

In such situations the nurse isolates those aspects that contribute to the symptoms that can be treated by nursing interventions and cites them as etiologies. Some examples are the following:

Communication, impaired verbal, related to:
  Rapid thought processes secondary to manic state
Nutrition, altered: less than body requirements, related to:
  Inadequate intake and hypermetabolic need
  Loss of appetite secondary to constipation
Thought processes, altered, related to:
  Internal and external stressors
  Impaired ability to process internal and external stimuli

The above-cited etiologic factors that accompany the nursing diagnoses more clearly specify the focus of care for nursing interventions.

GUIDELINES FOR DEFINING CHARACTERISTICS

Defining characteristics, also known as signs and symptoms and labeled "as evidenced by" (AEB) in the nursing care plan, are the observable, measurable manifestations of clients' responses to the identified health problems (nursing diagnoses). As with diagnoses and etiologies, defining characteristics are generally in nonspecific terms and often need to be modified to reflect the particular situation or response presented by the client. For example, the diagnosis of coping, ineffective individual, has as one of its defining characteristics "ineffective problem solving" (NANDA, 1999). The nurse can clarify the defining characteristic statements by quoting the client. Examples of ineffective problem solving:

"I can't decide if I should stay with my family or move to a board-and-care home."
"I can't decide what to do first—get a job or begin day treatment."

Therefore defining characteristics, when applicable, should be present in the nurse's assessment criteria to give some validity to the health problem that is being diagnosed. Some examples of defining characteristics used to define the diagnosis of self-esteem, chronic low, are the following:

Self-negating verbalization
Expression of shame or guilt
Evaluation of self as unable to deal with events
Hesitancy to try new things or situations

RISK DIAGNOSES*

Risk factors are used in assessing potential health problems. They describe existing risk states that may contribute to the potential problem becoming actual. There are no defining characteristics in a risk diagnosis, since the actual problem has not been manifested. Also, there are no etiologies in a risk or potential problem, since etiologies reflect causality, and cause cannot exist without effect. Thus a risk diagnosis carries a two-part statement, whereas an actual nursing diagnosis consists of a three-part statement. Box 7-3 presents the two types of nursing diagnosis formats, using two examples of each type (NANDA, 1999).

---

*Current NANDA terminology; formerly known as high-risk diagnoses.

Box 7-3   Format of Nursing Diagnosis

Two-Part Statements
Risk problem (two-part statement)
Part 1   Nursing diagnosis
Violence, risk for: directed at others

Part 2   Risk factors (predictors of risk problem)
History of violence
Hyperactivity secondary to manic state
Low impulse control
Aggressive verbal remarks

Risk problem (two-part statement)
Part 1   Nursing diagnosis
Loneliness, risk for

Part 2   Risk factors (predictors of risk problem)
Social isolation
Deprivation of love/affection
Physical isolation
Long-term institutionalization

Three-Part Statements
Actual problem (three-part statement)
Part 1   Nursing diagnosis
Posttrauma syndrome

Part 2   Etiologic factor(s) (related to)
Overwhelming anxiety secondary to:

Rape or other assault
Catastrophic illness
Disasters
War

Part 3   Defining characteristics
Reexperience of traumatic event (flashbacks)
Repetitive dreams or nightmares
Intrusive thoughts about traumatic event
Excess verbalization about traumatic event

Actual problem (three-part statement)
Part 1   Nursing diagnosis
Confusion, chronic

Part 2   Etiologic factors (related to)
Disorientation secondary to Alzheimer's disease
Psychosis secondary to Korsakoff's syndrome
Trauma secondary to recent head injury
Memory loss secondary to dementia

Part 3   Defining characteristics
Altered interpretation/response to stimuli
Progressive long-standing cognitive impairment
No change in level of consciousness
Impaired socialization
Impaired short-term memory

The prediction of a risk problem in a particular client requires an estimation of probability of occurrence. Risk problems can be assigned to almost any individual in a compromised health state. For example, a client taking a tricyclic antidepressant medication may be at risk for several potential problems as a result of the actions of these drugs on many of the body systems, such as risk for injury (hypotension, dizziness, blurred vision), risk for constipation, risk for urinary retention, or risk for altered mucous membranes (dry mouth).

Examples of a risk diagnosis:

Part 1	Nursing diagnosis:	Constipation, risk for
Part 2	Risk factors:	Tricyclic antidepressant medications
		Refusal to drink water, juice, etc.
		Noncompliance to high-fiber foods

Several of the approved diagnoses address potential dysfunctional states and cite risk factors. The following are examples of such diagnoses:

Injury, risk for
Parenting, altered, risk for
Trauma, risk for
Violence, risk for

In addition to those diagnoses formally listed as risk diagnoses, any actual diagnosis from the approved list can be stated as a risk diagnosis if it meets the criteria for an "at risk" problem. For example, self-esteem disturbance can be written as "risk for self-esteem disturbance" by virtue of the presence of risk factors for (but not as yet the actual existence of) the health problem (NANDA, 1999).

GUIDELINES FOR WELLNESS DIAGNOSES

Wellness nursing diagnoses represent clinical judgments about an individual, family, or community in transition from a specific level of wellness to a higher level of wellness or functioning. Most wellness diagnoses are one-part statements (e.g., spiritual well-being, potential for enhanced; coping, family: potential for growth). Some of the latest (NANDA, 1994) wellness diagnostic statements, however, are accompanied by either defining characteristics or both defining characteristics and etiologic factors (e.g., spiritual well-being, potential for enhanced, and community coping, potential for enhanced). (See NANDA listing on inside front cover of this book.)

OUTCOME IDENTIFICATION

Outcome statements consist of highly specific, measurable indicators that are used by nurses in the evaluation phase as criteria to illustrate the following:

The actual nursing diagnosis has been resolved or reduced.
The risk diagnosis has not occurred.

Box 7-4   **Examples of Outcome Statements**

Client will:
Verbalize absence of suicidal thoughts and plans
Demonstrate absence of self-mutilation and other self-destructive behaviors
Interpret environmental stimuli accurately
Interact socially with clients and staff
Participate actively in group discussions
Seek staff when experiencing troubling thoughts and feelings
Comply with treatment and medication regimen

Outcomes derive from nursing diagnosis statements and are projections of the expected influence that the nursing interventions will have on the client in relation to the identified diagnosis. Figure 7-2 shows the nursing process depicting the actual and risk diagnosis format of the six-step process. Outcomes are often confused with client goals or nursing goals, but they are more specific, descriptive, and measurable. Outcomes also do not describe nursing interventions. Box 7-4 lists examples of outcome statements.

Outcome criteria for an actual diagnosis are generally considered the opposite of the defining characteristics. In other words, the signs and symptoms discovered in the assessment phase to help establish the nursing diagnosis are also used to identify outcomes for improvement or resolution (Figure 7-3). For example:

Nursing Diagnosis	Outcomes
Self-care deficit, bathing/hygiene; dressing/grooming	Neat, clean appearance
	Cleans and grooms self
Related to: Psychotic state	
As evidenced by: Disheveled appearance; poor hygiene/grooming	

Outcome criteria for a risk diagnosis are developed from the risk factors that replace the defining characteristics found in an actual diagnosis. Clinical symptoms are absent in a risk diagnosis, since it is a two-part statement (Figure 7-4). For example:

Nursing Diagnosis	Outcomes
Violence, risk for: self-directed	Verbalizes absence of suicidal intent
	Absent demonstration of suicidal gestures/acts

Risk Factors
History of suicide attempts
Verbalizes suicidal intent

Measurable outcomes should include client statements, behaviors, and/or psychosocial or physical condi-

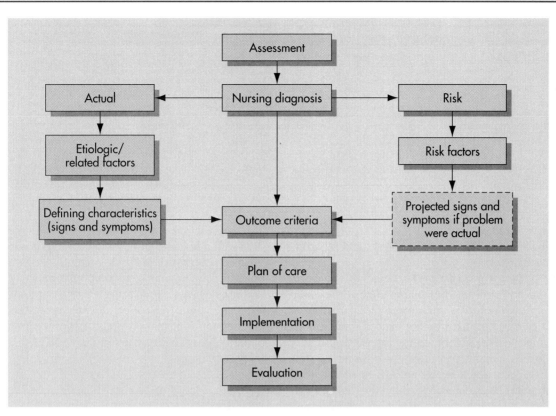

Figure 7-2 Nursing process depicting actual and risk diagnosis format of the six-step process. (Modified from Fortinash KM, Holoday-Worret PA: *Psychiatric nursing care plans*, ed 3, St. Louis, 1999, Mosby.)

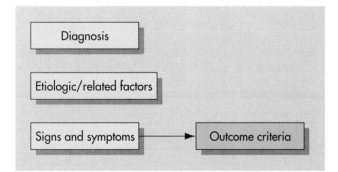

Figure 7-3 Developing outcome criteria for an actual diagnosis. (Modified from Davie JK: The nursing process. In Thelan LA et al: *Critical care nursing: diagnosis and management*, ed 3, St. Louis, 1998, Mosby.)

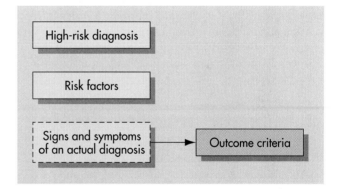

Figure 7-4 Developing outcome criteria for a risk diagnosis. (Modified from Davie JK: The nursing process. In Thelan LA et al: *Critical care nursing: diagnosis and management*, ed 3, St. Louis, 1998, Mosby.)

tions or parameters that are observable. This presents a challenge to psychiatric mental health nurses, however, since concepts such as anxiety, hopelessness, powerlessness, ineffective coping, or self-concept disturbance require the client's subjective perceptions and often resist measurability. Outcome statements such as "reduced anxiety," "more hopeful," or "copes effectively" offer minimal criteria for measuring client outcome achievements. Therefore when measuring client behaviors, the psychiat-

ric mental health nurse should do the following:

Phrase the outcomes so that they clearly describe client behavioral activity

Use the client's own words to describe feelings and thoughts whenever relevant

Incorporate some type of measurement tool or parameters by which to quantify client progress or resolution of problem/symptoms

Table 7-3	Correct and Incorrect Outcome Statements	
Nursing Diagnosis	**Incorrect Outcome**	**Correct Outcome**
Anxiety	Exhibits decreased anxiety; engages in stress reduction	Verbalizes feeling calm, relaxed, with absence of muscle tension and diaphoresis; practices deep breathing
Coping, ineffective individual	Demonstrates effective coping abilities	Makes own decisions to attend groups; seeks staff for interactions versus remaining isolated in room
Hopelessness	Expresses increased feelings of hope	Makes plans for the future (e.g., to continue therapy after discharge); states, "My kids need me to be well."

Table 7-3 provides examples of correct and incorrect outcome statements.

In some instances, nurses place a specific target date for each outcome criterion as a means of predicting the evaluation time for each outcome attainment. Designated dates ensure that certain problems do not exceed specified, acceptable time periods. The outcome criteria throughout this text do not include projected target dates or time lines, since this practice is better applied to actual situations, not hypothetic client symptoms and behaviors. Developing clear, measurable outcomes assists the nurse in managing, resolving, preventing, and improving clients' multiple health and illness states. Effective client outcomes also justify reimbursement for nurses and ensure quality client care (Olsen, Rickles, and Travlik, 1995).

As previously stated, NOC stresses the importance of developing outcomes that are sensitive to nursing intervention and influenced by nursing actions. The Iowa Outcomes Project reports that the precise impact that nursing care generates on client outcomes and satisfaction helps distinguish the role of nursing as a major contributor to quality patient care. NOC is currently working on developing precise client satisfaction outcomes with concomitant nursing care. NOC states that no outcome can represent the total range of client states, behaviors, or perceptions that make up a comprehensive assessment. Table 7-4 gives a comparison of NANDA diagnoses and NOC outcomes.

PLANNING

The planning phase consists of the total planning of the client's overall treatment in order to achieve quality outcomes in a safe, effective, timely manner. Nursing interventions with rationales are selected in the planning phase, based on the client's identified risk factors and defining characteristics. The process of planning includes the following:

Collaboration by the nurse with clients, significant others, and treatment team members

Identification of priorities of care

Critical decisions regarding the use of psychotherapeutic principles and practices

Coordination and delegation of responsibilities according to the treatment team's expertise as it relates to client needs

Planning client care builds on the prior phases of the nursing process and is vital for the ultimate selection of relevant nursing interventions by which to achieve successful client outcomes.

INTERDISCIPLINARY TREATMENT TEAM PLANNING

Interdisciplinary treatment team planning is a typical method used to plan and monitor a client's treatment. The treatment plan is generally constructed on a standard form and consists of various sections in which to document diverse information relevant to client care, such as strengths, legal status, discharge plans, medical and nursing diagnoses, therapies, and social work data.

Table 7-4	Comparison of NANDA Diagnoses and NOC Outcomes
NANDA Diagnosis	**NOC Outcome**
Impaired physical mobility	Mobility level
Hopelessness	Hope
Knowledge deficit	Knowledge: disease process
	Knowledge: medication
	Knowledge: health behaviors
	Knowledge: treatment regimen
Constipation	Bowel elimination
Diarrhea	
Bowel incontinence	Bowel continence
	Symptom control
	Well-being
	Will to live

From Johnson M, Maas ML: *Nursing outcomes classification (NOC)*, St. Louis, 1997, Mosby.

BEHAVIORAL HEALTH INTERDISCIPLINARY TREATMENT PLAN

THIS PLAN WAS FORMULATED AT THE INTERDISCIPLINARY TREATMENT MEETING:

DATE _1/1/96_   REVIEW DATES _1/4/96, 1/7/96_

RECORDER _Roseann Giordano, R.N. BSN_

ATTENDING PHYSICIAN _Dr. Jones_

Present at Meeting: MD _Dr. Jones_   RN _Mary Webster, MS, RN, CS_

Social Worker _Maggie Barker, LCSW_

Other _John Clark, Student Nurse_   Therapy Services _Beth Trottier, OTR_

PRIMARY CONTACT

Name _Jane Smith_   Relationship _temporary conservator_   Tel. # _123-4567_

REASON FOR ADMISSION: _Striking out at other clients and staff at Board and Care facility. Has refused to take meds X 3 days._

LEGAL STATUS: [√] Voluntary

[√] 72°h   Exp. Date ___
[ ] 14 d.h.   Exp. Date ___
Conservator   [√] Temp.   [ ] Perm.
Date filed _1/1/96_   Name _Jane Smith_

PATIENT STRENGTHS

[√] Verbal
[√] Intelligent
[√] Intact Physical Health
[ ] Consistent Work History
[ ] Compliant with Treatment

[√] Adequate Financial Resources
[ ] Recognizes Own Problems
[√] Supportive Friends
[ ] Resourceful
[√] History of Independent Functioning

[ ] Supportive Family
[ ] Employed

[√] Other _Cooperative and functional when taking medications regularly_

PRELIMINARY DISCHARGE PLAN

Admission Date _12/30/95_

Anticipated Length of Stay _8 days_

Anticipated Services Required:

[ ] Financial Counseling
[√] Board & Care   [ ] SNF Placement
[ ] Home Health Nurse
[ ] Crisis House
[ ] Recovery Home/Sober Living
[√] Self-Help Group

[ ] Payee   [√] Conservatorship
[√] Partial Hospitalization Referral
[ ] Psychotherapy, Marital/Family
[√] Medication Monitoring
[ ] Other

ADDRESSOGRAPH

Patient name: B. Brown

Figure 7-5   Example of an interdisciplinary treatment plan for a client with bipolar disorder. (Courtesy Tri-City Medical Center Mental Health Department, Oceanside, Calif.)

Continued

PATIENT NAME: B. Brown
PHYSICIAN:
SIGNATURE:

DIAGNOSIS   AXIS   I   Bipolar Disorder I
II   Deferred
III   None known
IV   mod-sev. (3-4)
V   30/60

DATE	PROBLEMS	PATIENT OUTCOME	GOAL DATE	INTERVENTION	DATE REVIEWED	DATE MET
12/30	Risk for Violence	Demonstrates absence of aggression	12/30	Provide safety by least restrictive means	12/31	12/31
12/30	Altered Thought Processes	Verbalizes clear realistic thoughts	1/3	Orient to reality in brief contacts	12/31	1/3
12/30	Self-Care Deficit	Demonstrates improved grooming: hygiene	1/3	Assist in grooming: hygiene as needed	1/1	1/3
12/30	Knowledge Deficit (disorder)	States understanding of diagnosis	1/5	Teach signs/symptoms of diagnosis	1/3	1/6

NURSING: SIGNATURE:
NURSING ADMISSION DATA BASE   Completed On
STANDARD NURSING PATIENT CARE PLAN (Title):
Additional Nursing Diagnosis:
1. Noncompliance, medications
2. Ineffective Individual Coping
3. Self-Esteem Disturbance
4.
5.
6.

The complete and individualized Standards of Patient Care are located in the Nursing section of the Patient Care Record.

THERAPY SERVICES   O.T. SIGNATURE: _____   T.R. SIGNATURE: _____

PROBLEMS	PATIENT OUTCOME	GOAL DATE	INTERVENTION	DATE REVIEWED	DATE MET
[√] Impaired Cognitive Skills:	OT/TR: - Demonstrates logical thought processes	1/3	[√] Task Skills Group Helps perform tasks	1/1	1/3
[√] Attention Span	Demonstrates increased attention span	1/2	[√] Living Skills Group Engages in living skills	1/2	1/5
[√] Concentration	Concentrates on unit tasks/activities	1/2	[ ] Creative Arts		
[√] Reality Testing	Tests reality appropriately	1/3	[√] Coping Skills Assists with coping skills	1/3	1/5
[√] Disorganization	Structures and organizes routine ADLs	1/4	[ ] ADL Training		
[√] Safety/Judgment	Utilizes safe judgment/behaviors	1/4	[√] Goal Setting Assists with simple goals	1/2	1/4
[ ] Orientation			[√] 1:1 Engages in 1:1 interactions	12/30	12/31
[√] Decreased Participation in Functional Activities	Increased participation in tasks/groups	1/3	[√] Leisure Education Engages in leisure ed	1/2	1/3
[√] Ineffective Coping Skills	Demonstrates effective coping skills	1/5	[√] Communication Skills Helps in group interactives	1/2	1/3
[ ] Social Withdrawal			[ ] Sensory Motor		
[√] Self-Destructive Behavior	Demonstrates absence of self-harm	12/31	[ ] Hygiene/Grooming		
[√] Low Self-Esteem	Verbalizes positive self-qualities	1/5	[√] Community Outings Accompany on outings	1/3	1/3
[ ] Other _____			[ ] Other: _____		
ACL Score: _____			1-2X wk Frequency		
			30-45 min Duration		

Figure 7-5—cont'd   For legend see p. 135.

SOCIAL WORK

SIGNATURE: _____

IDENTIFIED NEEDS/PROBLEMS	DATE REVIEWED	DATE MET
[√] Family Dysfunction		
[ ] Placement		
[ ] Placement		
[ ] Financial		
[ ] Employment		
[ ] Daily Structure		
[ ] Substance Abuse		
[√] Limited Functioning		
[ ] Spiritual		
[√] Inadequate Coping		
[√] Inadequate Support System		
[ ] Other _____		

REFERRALS/INTERVENTIONS (Family resistant to help)	DATE REVIEWED	DATE MET
[√] Family Contact (Family resistant to help)		
[ ] Family Session		
[ ] Social Service Group		
[ ] CPS/APS		
[√] Board & Care		
[ ] SNF		
√ PHP/Day Treatment (To increase support base)		
[ ] AA/NA/Alanon		
[ ] Home Health		
[ ] Clergy		
[ ] Voc. Rehabilitation		
[ ] MediCare/MediCal/SSI		
[ ] Other _____		
[√] Extended Psychosocial Assessment (See SW notes)		
Assessment/Recommendations:		
Attend all groups; interactions q shift		

PSYCHOSOCIAL DATA BASE

Appearance   *SL. disheveled; hyperactive; inappropriate dress for age*

Age *42*   Marital Status [ ]S [ ]M [√]D [ ]W

Children (N) / Y

Status of Current Family *Former spouse remarried; moved out of state; no contact*
Parents elderly - unwilling or unable to help. Ø other known family.

Religion [ ] Catholic [√] Protestant [ ] Jewish [ ] Other

Military Service N / (Y)

Place of Birth *U.S.A.*

Family of Origin *American*

Occupation *Unemployed*   Employer _____

Financial Support: Rep. Payee _____
Manages Own Funds _____
√ Receives Assistance   Type: *SSI*

Living Arrangement [ ] Home [ ] Apt. [ ] Hotel [ ] Shelter
[√] Board & Care [ ]S.N.F. [ ] None Known [ ] Other: _____

Pt. Cooperative N / Y

Lives [ ] By Self [ ] W/Family [ ] W/Friends
Case Manager/Conservator N / (Y) Name *Jane Smith*
Tel. # _____

Education: [ ] Did not complete high school   [ ] College degree
[√] High school degree   [ ] Graduate degree
[√] Some college

Primary Language *English*

Requires Interpretation Services (N) / Y

Past Psychiatric Hospitalizations N / (Y)
Dates _____ Locations _____
Contact: Name(s) *Jane Smith, Conservator*
Tel. # _____

Patient's Goal for this Admission

1. *To maintain control over aggressive impulses*
2. *To comply with medication regimen*
3. *To utilize effective coping skills & solve problems*
4. *To increase self-esteem*
5. *To return to baseline or higher level of function*

Discharge Plan: *D/C to Board and Care with partial hospitalization referral*

Tentative D/C Date: *1/7/96*

ROOM	NAME	AGE	ADMIT DATE	DOCTOR
10-A	*B. Brown*	*42*	*12/30/95*	*J. Jones*

Figure 7-5—cont'd For legend see p. 135.

BEHAVIORAL HEALTH SERVICES
PATIENT CARE PLAN

BIPOLAR DISORDER

STANDARD OF CARE ON PATIENTS

TITLE:

INITIATED Date	INITIATED RN	NURSING DIAGNOSIS	PATIENT OUTCOMES	EVALUATION Documentation	INTERVENTIONS	RESOLVED Date	RESOLVED RN	NOT RESOLVED Date	NOT RESOLVED RN
12/30	RG	1. Alteration in thought processes R/T psychosis, paranoia, or delusions.	Patient will demonstrate logical, goal-directed speech and behaviors with an absence of psychosis, paranoia, or delusions.	q shift	1. Assess patient for: a. Nature and content of thought processes. b. Risk for harm to self or others. c. Ability to participate in groups/milieu. d. Ability to perform ADLs. 2. Report to physician: a. Actual or escalating risk for harm to self or others. b. Refusal to eat/drink. c. Refusal to take medication. 3. Record assessments in the Progress Notes on Patient Care Record. 4. Implement the following interventions: a. Frequent supportive contacts with gentle reality orientation as tolerated. b. Limit-setting to control inappropriate sexual, financial, or potentially harmful interpersonal behaviors. c. Encourage participation in milieu groups consistent with patient's attention span. 5. Implement the following protocols: a. Hallucinations/Delusions Management b. Lithium Management c. Antipsychotic Medication Therapy Management 6. Validate that outcome is met when patient has demonstrated goal-directed/logical speech and behaviors x 48°.	1/3	RG		
12/30	MW	2. Risk for Violence: Self-directed or directed at others. Risk Factors: Delusions, hyperactivity, irritability	Patient will not harm self or others.	q shift	1. Implement the following protocols in increasing order of restrictiveness: a. Agitated/Assaultive Behavior Management b. Time-out c. Seclusion d. Restraint Management (only when it is least restrictive measure.) 2. Validate that outcome is met when patient demonstrates freedom from behaviors harmful to self/others x 72°.	12/31	MW		

Figure 7-6   Example of the first page of a care plan for a client with bipolar disorder. (Courtesy Tri-City Medical Center Mental Health Department, Oceanside, Calif.)

The treatment plan is implemented the first time the treatment team meets to discuss the client (ideally, no later than 3 days following the client's admission). The team is generally represented by nursing, social work, occupational and recreational therapy, and the client's physician. The client may also be present during a portion of the meeting unless contraindicated. Each team member is given an opportunity to discuss the client from the perspective of his or her own discipline and expertise. The treatment plan may be updated after the initial treatment team meeting as each discipline has more opportunity to spend time with the client and elaborate on its specific criteria.

The interdisciplinary treatment plan for a client with bipolar disorder in Figure 7-5 was developed in conjunction with the sample standard care plan in Figure 7-6. The information on each form should be reflected on the other. For example, the nursing diagnoses identified during the treatment team meeting should be the same diagnoses initiated on the client's standard care plan. Thus client assessment and treatment will flow from one document to the other, illustrating consistency and reliability. Treatment plans are generally updated as often as the team meets to discuss a particular client. Ideally, the second team meeting should occur not later than 3 to 4 days after the first meeting. With the current trend toward shorter lengths of stay for all acute care clients, treatment team planning needs to occur in a timely fashion in order to effectively address each client's specific needs.

STANDARDIZED CARE PLANNING

One method used to plan and measure client care is known as standardized care planning (see Figure 7-6). In this type of documentation, NANDA diagnoses, client outcomes, and interventions are formulated according to the identified DSM-IV diagnostic categories in a standardized format. This standard format style is gaining popularity with nurses for the following reasons:

The need to create new care plans for each client is reduced or eliminated.

Consistency of care is encouraged through standardized guidelines.

It requires a minimum of writing, thus freeing the nurse to spend more time interacting with clients.

Standards of care are upheld, ensuring safe, effective treatment over time.

It addresses managed care criteria for quality outcomes and length of stay.

Problems are primarily initiated, evaluated, and resolved by nursing.

Standardized care plans do not preclude individualized treatment for each client, nor do they replace relevant narrative documentation.

CLINICAL PATHWAYS

A **clinical pathway** (also known as a critical pathway, care path, or CareMap) is a standardized format used to provide and monitor client care and progress by way of the case management, interdisciplinary health care delivery system. Although nursing is a primary proponent of the clinical pathway method, other disciplines responsible for client care in the psychiatric mental health setting are actively involved in the development of each individualized clinical pathway. Such disciplines include social services, occupational therapy, therapeutic recreation, and dietary services, with strong collaborative input from psychiatrists. Consultations may be provided by psychologists, family practice physicians, or other professionals, depending on the special needs of the client.

A clinical pathway refers primarily to a written clinical process that identifies projected caregiver behaviors and interventions and expected client outcomes, based on the client's mental disorder as defined in the DSM-IV. The pathway is mapped out along a continuum that depicts chronologic milestones, generally the number of days that reflects the client's estimated length of stay for each specific diagnosis.

The pathway is a projection of the client's entire length of treatment, detailing interdisciplinary interventions or processes and client outcomes each day, from admission through discharge. A pathway may be extended to include the client's transfer to home care or another type of treatment facility. The pathway would then continue for as long as necessary. Clinical pathways may originate for clients in a home care situation and would then be developed by the interdisciplinary home care team.

Variances

Variances (also known as outliers) occur when a client's response to interventions is different from what is typically expected. A variance may therefore be considered an unexpected client response that "falls off" the pathway, requiring separate documentation and further investigation by the interdisciplinary team. Causes of pathway variances may be related to the client/family, caregivers, hospital, community, and payers (including insurance companies, health maintenance organizations, or managed care organizations).

A variance may be positive or negative and affect the client's length of stay and/or outcomes. An example of a positive variance would be a client who responds more rapidly to medication or other forms of treatment than expected and leaves the hospital before the estimated length of stay. An example of a negative variance would be a client who fails to achieve the desired nonmanic state or therapeutic lithium level in accordance with the time line designated on the clinical pathway continuum (generally by date of discharge), and whose length of stay is therefore prolonged.

Clinical Pathway: Mania
DRG #430 - LOS - 8 Days

Interval		Day of Admit	Day 2	Day 3	Day 4
	Location				
OUTCOMES	Physiologic	*Takes adequate nutrition, fluids with assistance *Complies with lithium level evaluation	*Demonstrates increased sleep/rest time *Demonstrates adequate elimination	*Takes adequate nutrition/fluid with reminders *Demonstrates adequate elimination	*Sleeping 4–6 hours *Demonstrates adequate elimination
	Psychologic	*Involved in stimulation-reducing activities with staff supervision	*Oriented to person and place	*Demonstrates reduction in: movement racing thoughts grandiosity/euphoria irritability	*Demonstrates increased attention span *Reality tests with staff *Oriented to person, place, time, and situation
	Functional Status/Role	*Tolerated orientation to the unit *Refrains from harming self/others with assistance	*Interacting with staff as told *Attends to hygiene/grooming needs with assistance *Refrains from harming self/others with assistance	*Engages in unit activities with staff supervision	*Maintains impulses with reminders *Complies with meds with reminders
	Family/Community Reintegration		*Identifies significant others to staff	*Attends community meetings with staff supervision	*Significant others involved in treatment/discharge planning
PROCESSES	Discharge Planning	*SW Assessment *Identify DC Placement *ELOS, contact family/SO *Nursing Assessment *Identify H/O chronicity *Med compliance, strengths, needs, knowledge deficit	*Team: Involved in D/C Planning Discuss with MD *UR notify managed care ( )	*SW eval completed *Treatment Team meeting #1 ( ) *Specific D/C plans, placement facility identified ( )	*Involve family/SO in DC plans *Review DC plans with patient
	Education	*Orient to unit *Inform of patient's rights *Assess patient's and family's/SO knowledge of disorder/meds	*Assist with symptom recognition and importance of compliance *Teach family/SO as needed	*Continue with symptom recognition *Continue assessing patient and family/SO learning needs	*Assist in linking symptoms with precipitating events
	Psychosocial/Spiritual	*Assess: Safety ( ) *Mental status ( ) Spirituality ( ) *Legal status: Vol ( ) 72 hour hold ( ) *Revise Writ ( ) Payor ( ) Conservator ( )	*Continue to assess: Safety issues Mental status Spiritual needs Legal status	*Continue to assess: Safety issues Mental status (e.g. racing thoughts, grandiosity, euphoria, irritability) Spiritual/Legal needs	*Continue to assess: Safety issues Mental status (e.g. racing thoughts, grandiosity, euphoria, irritability) Spiritual/Legal needs
	Consults	*Physical exam within 24 hours	*Other consults as needed	*Other consults as needed	*Other consults as needed
	Tests/Procedures	*Lithium level ( ) *Tegretol level ( ) *Drug screen ( ) *Thyroid function ( ) *CBC/SMAC ( ) *Other ( )	*Tests/Procedures as ordered	*Tests/Procedures as ordered	*Tests/Procedures as ordered
	Treatment	*Monitor: I&O *Sleep/Rest patterns *Level A ( ) *Reduce milieu stimulation *S&R yes( ) no( ) *Other	*Monitor: I&O *Sleep/Rest patterns *Level A ( ) *Reduce milieu stimulation *S&R yes( ) no( ) *Other	*Move to level B ( ) *Continue with treatment plan: Monitor: I&O Sleep/Rest Other	*Move to level B ( ) *Continue with treatment plan: Monitor: I&O Sleep/Rest Other
	Medications (IV & Others)	*Medications as ordered *See relevant protocols: Lithium *Other *Monitor side effects *Toxicity	*Medications as ordered *Continue to monitor side effects/toxicity	*Medications as ordered *Continue to monitor side effects/toxicity	*Medications as ordered *Continue to monitor side effects/toxicity
	Activity	*OT assessment *1:1 brief contacts *Reality orientation *Intervene to manage impulses: prevent harm to self/others	*Engage in stimulation-reducing activities as tolerated *Assist with hygiene, grooming, ADLs *Prevent harm to self/others during activities	*OT eval completed *Encourage hygiene, grooming, ADLs with reminders *Prevent harm to self/others during activities	*Engage in 2 groups per day *Increase group stimulation as tolerated *Prevent harm to self/others during activities
	Diet/Nutrition	*Offer adequate nutrition and fluids; normal salt intake	*Provide simple meals, finger foods, easy to carry drinks	*Encourage meals in patient community as tolerated with staff supervision	*Encourage meals in patient community as tolerated with staff supervision

Figure 7-7 Clinical pathway for a client with bipolar disorder mania. (Courtesy Sharp HealthCare Behavioral Health Services, San Diego, Calif.)

Interval	Day 5	Day 6	Day 7	Day 8
Location				
OUTCOMES				
Physiologic	*Takes adequate nutrition/fluid *Sleeps 4–6 hours *Lithium level in therapeutic range *Other drug level in therapeutic range	*Sleeps 5–8 hours *Absence of drug toxicity	*Sleeps 5–8 hours	*Sleeps 5–8 hours *Able to manage food and activity requirements independently
Psychologic	*Demonstrates more reality based thoughts *Able to focus on one topic x5–10 minutes	*Demonstrates enthymic mood *Able to focus on one topic x5–10 minutes	*Able to complete activities and unit assignments	*Able to complete activities and unit assignments independently *Able to plan and structure day
Functional Status/Role	*Demonstrates less intrusive behaviors	*Able to interact with peers *Able to make simple decisions	*Demonstrates safe appropriate activities/behaviors *Independently complies with medical regimen	*Verbalizes need for ongoing medication compliance
Family/Community Reintegration	*Identifies discharge needs	*Identifies discharge needs	*Identifies discharge needs *Able to identify supports and their appropriate use	*Able to utilize supports and lists ways to access them *States specific plans to manage symptoms, comply with medications, and aftercare
PROCESSES				
Discharge Planning	*Assist patient/family/SO to identify discharge needs *UR contact managed care as needed ( )	*Continue to problem-solve discharge needs with patient, family/SO	*Treatment team meeting #2 ( ) *Transition to Day Treatment if indicated *Assist patient, family/SO in finalizing discharge plans	*Discharge to least restrictive environment completed *UR inform managed care as needed ( )
Education	*Teach patient/family/SO about medication effects on symptom management *Instruct in medication, diet, exercise regimen	*Emphasize importance of compliance with meds after discharge *Teach about drug-to-drug effects on symptom management	*Develop aftercare plan to manage symptoms and contact supports	*Reinforce aftercare teaching plan with patient, family/SO as needed
Psychosocial/ Spiritual	*Continue to assess: Safety issues Mental status Spirituality Voluntary status	*Continue to assess: Safety issues Mental status Spirituality Voluntary status	*Continue to assess: Safety issues Mental status Spirituality Voluntary status	*Complete assessments confirm: Safety Mental status Spirituality Legal status
Consults	*Complete consults as ordered *Arrange for aftercare consults as ordered	*Complete consults as ordered *Arrange for aftercare consults as ordered	*Complete consults as ordered *Arrange for aftercare consults as ordered	*Complete consults as ordered *Arrange for aftercare consults as ordered
Tests/ Procedures	*Check lithium level for therapeutic range *Check other drug levels for therapeutic range as needed *Tests/Procedures as needed	*Check lithium level for therapeutic range *Check other drug levels within therapeutic range as needed *Tests/Procedures as needed	*Check lithium level for therapeutic range *Check other drug levels within therapeutic range as needed *Tests/Procedures as needed	*Confirm lithium level for therapeutic range *Confirm other drug levels within therapeutic range as needed *Tests/Procedures as ordered aftercare
Treatment	*Move to level C ( ) *Continue with treatment plan I&O Sleep/Rest Other	*Move to level C ( ) *Continue with treatment plan I&O Sleep/Rest Other	*Transfer to open unit ( ) *Aftercare treatment instructions reviewed with patient, family/SO as needed	*D/C with aftercare treatment instructions
Medications (IV & Others)	*Medications as ordered *Contact managed care if any change in medication regimen	*Medications as ordered *Contact managed care if any change in medication regimen	*Medications as ordered *Review of medications with patient, family/SO as needed	*D/C with medications and instructions as ordered
Activity	*Encourage: Independent hygiene and grooming Independent ADLs Increased participation in groups	*Engage in all unit activities and groups *Encourage independent decision-making	*Reinforce active participation in all unit activities and groups; independent decision-making	*Confirm: Ability to complete activity assignments independently Ability to make decisions independently
Diet/Nutrition	*Teach family/SO importance of adequate foods/fluids/salt intake	*Teach family/SO importance of adequate foods/fluids/salt intake	*Reinforce adequate nutrition fluids and normal salt intake	*Confirm patient/SO/family knowledge of adequate foods/fluids/salt intake

Figure 7-7—cont'd For legend see opposite page.

Clinical pathways help ensure timely lengths of stay, prevention of complications, cost-effectiveness, and continued quality assurance. Also, overall coordinated management of each client's care and progress by the nurse case manager and the interdisciplinary team is ensured.

Figure 7-7 is an example of a clinical pathway describing a client with bipolar disorder mania, with a length of stay of 8 days. The upper columns list client outcomes. The larger lower columns consist of categories of care known as processes. Evaluation of client progress is measured daily along the pathway time lines. Clinical pathways continue to be developed, improved, and instituted in a variety of health care settings and are expected to reflect the changing trends and complexities of current health care delivery systems.

IMPLEMENTATION

In the implementation phase the nurse actually sets in motion the interventions prescribed in the planning phase. Some general nursing considerations directed toward clients and families during this phase include the following:

> Promote health and safety.
> Monitor medication regimen/effects.
> Provide adequate nutrition/hydration.
> Facilitate a nurturing, therapeutic environment.
> Build self-esteem, trust, and dignity.
> Engage in therapeutic groups/activities.
> Develop strengths/coping methods.
> Enhance communication/social skills.
> Use family/community support systems.
> Educate according to identified learning needs.
> Prevent relapse through effective discharge planning.

NURSING INTERVENTIONS

Nursing interventions (also known as nursing orders or nursing prescriptions) are critical action components of the implementation phase and are the most powerful pieces of the nursing process. They make up the management and treatment approach to an identified health problem. Interventions are selected to achieve client outcomes and to prevent or reduce problems. Some flaws noted in nursing interventions, both in the literature and in clinical practice, are that they are often weak, vague, and nonspecific.

The **Nursing Interventions Classification (NIC)** is the first comprehensive standardized classification of treatments and interventions performed by nurses. These interventions can be physiologic, such as airway suctioning and decubitus ulcer care, or psychosocial, such as anxiety reduction and assisting with coping strategies. They can prevent falls or self-harm and promote health, education, good nutrition, and stress reduction. The purpose of NIC is to identify and refine nursing actions from groups of

data found throughout the literature and construct a taxonomy in which interventions are organized with clear rules and principles for the interventions selected (McCloskey and Bulechek, 1996).

For nursing interventions to be prescriptive, they must prescribe a course of action and not simply support the existing regimen. The interventions listed throughout this text reflect both actual and typical nursing responses and behaviors derived from educational preparation and a wide range of clinical experience.

In the psychiatric mental health setting, treatment frequently incorporates verbal communication skills, a major source of psychosocial interventions. Such treatments are intended to effect a change in the client's present condition, not merely to maintain the problem in its present state. Nursing interventions should explicitly describe a course of therapeutic activity that helps mobilize the client toward a more functional state. The following are some descriptive examples:

> Gradually engage the client in interactions with other clients, beginning with individual contacts and progressing to informal gatherings and eventually to structured group activities.
> Teach the client and family/significant other that therapeutic effects of antidepressant medications may take up to 2 weeks and that uncomfortable effects may begin immediately.
> Praise the client for attempts to seek out staff and other clients for interactions and activities, and to respond to others' attempts to engage the client in interactions and activities.

Nondescriptive examples include:

> Assist the client to interact with others.
> Teach client and family about medications.
> Praise the client for socializing.

Note the clarity and substance demonstrated in the descriptive examples, as opposed to the weaker, more vague statements in the nondescriptive examples.

Nursing interventions that simply repeat physician's orders are not substantive enough to treat or manage the health problem effectively. The following are nonsubstantive examples:

> Monitor the client's progress.
> Check lithium levels.
> Notify social services.
> Obtain the client's consent form.
> Report changes in mood and affect.

Effective nursing interventions should have the capability of moving the client to a more functional health state by virtue of their clarity, substance, and direction. In

Table 7-5 Comparison of NIC With Major Coded Classifications

	ICD-10	DSM-IV	HCPCS	NANDA ICD Code	NIC
Stands for	*International Statistical Classification of Diseases and Related Health Problems*, tenth edition	*Diagnostic and Statistical Manual of Mental Disorders*, fourth edition	*HCFA Common Procedure Coding System*	*North American Nursing Diagnosis Association Translation of Taxonomy I, revised*	*Nursing Interventions Classification*
Published by	World Health Organization	American Psychiatric Association	Practice Management Information Corporation	North American Nursing Diagnosis Association	Mosby
Codes for	Diseases and morbid entities	Psychiatric diagnoses	Supplies, materials, injections, and certain services and procedures in Medicare	Nursing diagnoses	Nursing interventions
Structured	Has three volumes 1. Tabular list: the classification itself; diseases are listed by system; also has pregnancy, conditions originating in perinatal period, congenital malformations, symptoms not elsewhere classified, injury, external causes of morbidity and mortality, and factors influencing health status 2. Instruction manual 3. Alphabetic index	Consists of five axes: I. Clinical disorders and other conditions that may be a focus of clinical attention II. Personality disorders and mental retardation III. General medical conditions IV. Psychosocial and environmental problems V. Global assessment of functioning	Builds on the CPT (Level I) This is Level II—2400 national standardized codes divided into 18 sections, including: transportation services, chiropractic services, medical and surgical supplies, dental procedures, rehabilitative services, drugs administered other than orally, medical services, pathology and laboratory, vision services, hearing services Level III are local codes assigned and maintained by local medical carriers	NANDA's nine patterns arranged alphabetically are the classification structure NANDA's fourth, fifth, and sixth levels are collapsed to two levels of diagnostic utility	Over 400 interventions are located within 27 classes and six domains: physiologic: basic; physiologic: complex; behavioral; safety; family; health system Each intervention is composed of a label, a definition, and a set of activities a nurse does to carry out the intervention

Modified from McCloskey JC, Bulechek GM: *Nursing interventions classification (NIC)*, ed 2, St. Louis, 1996, Mosby.

the psychiatric mental health setting, nurses constantly assess, diagnose, and treat clients' health states. Therefore the challenge for nurses is to formulate strong, effective nursing interventions that address and modify the client's health problem and are based on researched, independent nursing therapies.

The interventions in NIC are effective in the treatment of physical and psychiatric illnesses (e.g., hypertension or cognitive disorders). They are equally effective in preventing various types of trauma, such as falls or self-harm. NIC interventions are also used in health promotion and education. The purpose of NIC is to identify and refine nursing actions from groups of data found throughout the literature and construct a taxonomy such as NANDA and NOC, in which interventions are systematically organized, with clear rules and principles for the interventions selected. Table 7-5 provides a comparison of NIC with some other major coded classifications (NOC is absent, since it was published in 1997).

INTERVENTIONS' IMPACT ON ETIOLOGIES

Interventions have the greatest impact when they are focused toward etiologies (related factors) that accompany the nursing diagnosis or, if the problem is a risk nursing diagnosis, when they are aimed at the risk factors. (Figure 7-8 illustrates the former, Figure 7-9 the latter.) This suggests that nursing can modify or affect the etiologies of a problem. It makes sense, considering that etiologies are in some respects causal factors that greatly affect or provoke the health problem (nursing diagnosis). By the same token, risk diagnoses are less likely to become actual if interventions are aimed primarily at their accompanying risk factors. To achieve the most favorable client outcomes, etiologic factors associated with the problems (nursing diagnoses) should be examined meticulously and interventions carefully selected to modify each of them.

INTERVENTIONS AND MEDICAL ACTIONS

Interventions can include medically focused actions, such as the administration of medications. However, *the major focus of nursing interventions should emphasize nursing actions, judgments, treatments, and directives.* Examples of nontherapeutic, medically focused interventions include:

Administer antipsychotic medications as prescribed.
Observe for extrapyramidal effects.
Initiate benztropine (Cogentin) as ordered.

Note in the above examples the obvious absence of any prescribed nursing actions that would influence the client's health state.

RATIONALE STATEMENTS

A rationale statement is the reason for the nursing intervention. Rationales are not usually listed as part of a written care plan in clinical practice; however, they are generally part of the overall discussion of interventions in treatment team meetings. Rationales reflect nurses' accountability for their actions. Clear, descriptive rationale statements (in italics following the interventions) are provided in the disorders chapters in this text to enhance the reader's overall understanding of the selected interventions. For example:

Actively listen, observe, and respond to the client's verbal and nonverbal expressions *to let the client know he or she is worthwhile and respected.*
Initiate brief, frequent contacts with the client throughout the day *to let the client know he or she is an important part of the community.*
Praise the client for attempts to interact with others and for participating in group activities *to increase self-esteem and reinforce repetition of healthy, functional behaviors.*

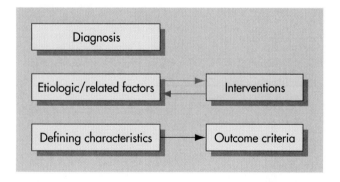

Figure 7-8 Developing interventions for an actual diagnosis. The red arrow indicates interventions for an actual diagnosis, and the blue arrow indicates the impact of the interventions on etiologies. (Modified from Davie JK: The nursing process. In Thelan LA et al: *Critical care nursing: diagnosis and management,* ed 3, St. Louis, 1998, Mosby.)

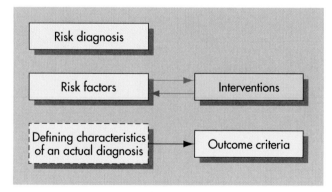

Figure 7-9 Developing interventions for a risk diagnosis. The red arrow indicates interventions for a risk diagnosis, and the blue arrow indicates the impact of the interventions on risk factors. (Modified from Davie JK: The nursing process. In Thelan LA et al: *Critical care nursing: diagnosis and management,* ed 3, St. Louis, 1998, Mosby.)

EVALUATION

Evaluation of achieved expected client outcomes must occur at various intervals as designated in the outcome criteria, with the capability and health state of each client as a primary consideration. There are two steps in the evaluation phase:

1. *The nurse compares the client's current mental health state or condition with that described in the outcome criteria.* Is the client's anxiety reduced to a tolerable level? (For example, can the client sit calmly for 10 minutes, attend a simple recreational activity for 10 minutes, and engage in one-to-one interaction with staff for 5 minutes without distractions? Is there a significant reduction in pacing, fidgeting, or scanning? Were these outcomes attained within the times originally projected?) The degree to which client outcomes are achieved or not achieved is also an evaluation of the effectiveness of nursing.
2. *The nurse considers all of the possible reasons why nursing outcomes were not achieved, if this is the case.* For example, perhaps it is too soon to evaluate, and the plan of action needs further implementation. (For example, the client needed another 2 days of one-to-one interactions before attending client group activities.) Or perhaps the interventions were too forceful and frequent or too weak and infrequent. It may be that the outcomes were unattainable, impractical, or just not feasible for this client, or perhaps they were not within the client's scope and capabilities on a developmental or sociocultural level. What about the validity of the nursing diagnosis? Was it developed with a questionable or faulty database? Are more data required? What were the conditions during the assessment phase? Was it too hurried? Were conclusions drawn too quickly?

Were there any language, cultural, or other communication barriers?

Specific recommendations are then made based on conclusions drawn from the above questions. They include either continuing implementation of the plan of action or review of the previous phases of the nursing process (assessment, nursing diagnosis, outcome identification, planning, or implementation). Evaluation of the client's progress and the nursing activities involved in the process are critical because they require that nursing be accountable for the standards of care defined by its own discipline. Informal evaluation of the client's progress, much like that of the nursing process, takes place continuously.

Figures 7-10 and 7-11 show how evaluation is determined according to the identified outcomes and is also the measurement tool used to appraise outcome attainment for both actual and risk diagnoses, respectively.

THE NURSING PROCESS IN COMMUNITY AND HOME SETTINGS

In the past, the nursing process and its multistep format have been most associated with the care of hospitalized clients. Current trends in health care delivery systems have shifted from inpatient facilities to community and home-based settings and provide yet another important avenue for use of the nursing process. Home health care is a primary alternative to hospitalization, and the nursing process continues to be a major factor in the effective management of home client care.

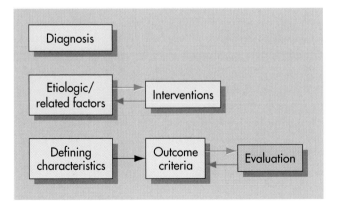

Figure 7-10 Evaluation process in an actual diagnosis. The arrows show how evaluation is determined according to identified outcomes. (Modified from Davie JK: The nursing process. In Thelan LA et al: *Critical care nursing: diagnosis and management,* ed 3, St. Louis, 1998, Mosby.)

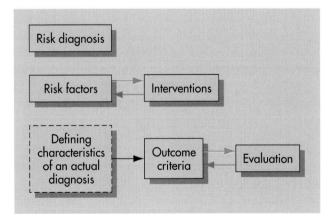

Figure 7-11 Evaluation process in a risk diagnosis. The arrows show how evaluation is determined according to identified outcomes. (Modified from Davie JK: The nursing process. In Thelan LA et al: *Critical care nursing: diagnosis and management,* ed 3, St. Louis, 1998, Mosby.)

PSYCHIATRIC HOME HEALTH CARE CASE MANAGEMENT SYSTEM

The changes in today's health care delivery system have resulted in several trends in health care reform designed to bring about cost-effective quality care. Although the case management concept has existed for years in acute care settings and public health arenas, only recently has the private home health model subscribed to total case management, and only more recently has psychiatric home care been incorporated under the case management umbrella.

Psychiatric home care case management is a method by which a client is identified as a candidate for home care and treated on a health care continuum in the familiar surroundings of the home. The interdisciplinary home care team, facilitated by a registered nurse, coordinates all available resources to meet its goals for treatment and to achieve the client's expected outcomes in a quality and cost-effective manner. At one end of the continuum is the highest degree of independent wellness within the client's capacity, and at the other end of the continuum is death, with varying levels of wellness-illness in between.

Critical to successful use of case management is the accurate placement of the client at the entry point on the continuum, and a clear understanding of the team's best estimate for the date of termination of home care services (Provancha and Hurst, 1994).

Summary of Key Concepts

1. The nursing process is a decision-making method used by nurses for clinical care. As defined by the ANA, it has six steps: assessment, diagnosis, outcome identification, planning, implementation, and evaluation.
2. The nursing process is an ongoing, multidimensional, cyclic approach in which data are continually collected, analyzed, and incorporated into a treatment plan.
3. Intuition, expertise, and critical thinking are important elements in the nursing process.
4. The two most common nursing assessment frameworks are the NANDA taxonomy and Gordon's Functional Health Patterns.
5. NIC and NOC are two current nursing classification systems that complement NANDA and also represent taxonomies for effective interventions and outcomes.
6. Nursing diagnoses provide nurses with a vocabulary that is distinctive to its own discipline and encourage nursing's theory and science-building efforts.

NANDA diagnoses are the most common and accepted diagnoses used in nursing.
7. Nursing diagnoses can have two formats: two-part statements that describe potential or risk problems and three-part statements that describe an actual problem.
8. Outcome statements are highly specific, measurable indicators derived from nursing diagnoses and used to evaluate client progress.
9. The planning phase consists of the total planning of the client's treatment regimen. Nursing interventions are selected in the planning phase.
10. A clinical pathway is an interdisciplinary standardized format used to provide and monitor client care and progress.
11. The implementation phase involves the actual setting into motion of the interventions that have been prescribed in the planning phase.
12. Evaluation of the achieved expected client outcomes as designated by the outcome criteria should occur at various levels.

REFERENCES

American Health Consultants: Monthly update on hospital-based care planning and critical pathways, *Hosp Case Manage* 1(10):173, 1993.

American Nurses Association: *Nursing, a social policy statement*, Kansas City, Mo, 1990, The Association.

American Nurses Association: *Standards of clinical nursing practice*, Kansas City, Mo, 1991, The Association.

American Psychiatric Association: *Diagnostic and statistical manual of mental disorders*, ed 4, Washington, DC, 1994, The Association.

Benner P: *From novice to expert: excellence and power in clinical nursing practice*, Menlo Park, Calif, 1984, Addison-Wesley.

Boomsa J, Dingemans CAJ, Dassen TWN: The nursing process in crisis-oriented home care, *J Psychiatr Ment Health Nurs* 4:295, 1997.

Bulechek GM, McCloskey JC: Nursing interventions, *Nurs Clin North Am* 27:289, 1992a.

Bulechek GM, McCloskey JC, editors: *Nursing interventions: essential nursing treatments*, ed 2, Philadelphia, 1992b, WB Saunders.

Carnevali DL, Thomas MD: *Diagnostic reasoning and treatment decision-making in nursing*, Philadelphia, 1993, JB Lippincott.

Carpenito LJ: *Nursing diagnosis: application to clinical practice*, ed 6, Philadelphia, 1996, JB Lippincott.

Carrol-Johnson R: *Classification of nursing diagnosis: proceedings of the eighth conference*, Philadelphia, 1993, JB Lippincott.

Davie JK: The nursing process. In Thelan LA et al, editors: *Critical care nursing: diagnosis and management*, ed 3, St Louis, 1998, Mosby.

Fortinash KM: Assessment of mental status. In Malasanos L, Barkauskas V, and Stoltenberg-Allen K, editors: *Health assessment*, ed 4, St Louis, 1990, Mosby.

Fortinash KM, Holoday-Worret PA: *Psychiatric nursing care plans*, ed 3, St Louis, 1999, Mosby.

Gordon M: *Nursing diagnosis: process and application*, ed 3, St. Louis, 1994, Mosby.

Johnson M, Maas ML: *Nursing outcomes classification (NOC)*, St. Louis, 1997, Mosby.

Kaplan H: *The comprehensive textbook of psychiatry*, ed 6, Baltimore, 1995, Williams & Wilkins.

Kaplan H, Sadock B: *Synopsis of psychiatry–behavioral science–clinical psychiatry*, ed 8, Baltimore, 1998, Williams & Wilkins.

Kritek PB: Generation and classification of nursing diagnoses: toward a theory of nursing, *Image J Nurs Sch* 10:73, 1978.

McCloskey JC, Bulechek GM: *Nursing interventions classification*, ed 2, St. Louis, 1996, Mosby.

McCloskey JC et al: Standardizing the language for nursing treatments: an overview of the issues, *Nurs Outlook* 42:56, 1994.

Medina L: Clinical pathways: sharp home health, *Home Care*, October 1995.

Munhall PL, Oiler CJ: *Nursing research*, ed 2, New York, 1993, National League for Nursing.

North American Nursing Diagnosis Association: *Taxonomy I–revised–1990, with official diagnostic categories*, St. Louis, 1990, NANDA.

North American Nursing Diagnosis Association: *NANDA, nursing diagnoses: definitions and classification, 1995-1996*, Philadelphia, 1994, The Association.

North American Nursing Diagnosis Association: *Taxonomy I–revised–1999, with official diagnostic categories*, St. Louis, 1999, NANDA.

Olsen DP, Rickles H, Travlik K: A treatment team model of managed mental health care, *Psychiatr Serv* 46(3):252, 1995.

Provancha LE, Hurst S: Home health case management: an old approach to a new system, *NSI Home Health Newsletter* 1994.

Smith SK: An analysis of the phenomenon of deterioration in the critically ill, *Image J Nurs Sch* 20:12, 1988.

Southwick K et al: Strategies for health care excellence: care paths for psychiatric patients, *COR Health Care Resources*, 8(2):1, 1995.

Tanner C et al: Diagnostic reasoning strategies of nurses and nursing students, *Nurs Res* 36:358, 1987.

Wescott MR: *Antecedents and consequences of intuitive thinking: final report to U.S. Department of Health, Education and Welfare*, Poughkeepsie, NY, 1968, Vassar College.

Wilkinson J: *Nursing process in action: a critical thinking approach*, Redwood City, Calif, 1992, Addison-Wesley.

CHAPTER 8

Principles of Communication

Susan Fertig McDonald

OBJECTIVES

- Describe the components of communication.

- Discuss factors that influence communication.

- Compare and contrast social, intimate, collegial, and therapeutic communication.

- Describe the characteristics of effective helpers.

- Discuss the core qualities of the nurse and the various roles the nurse plays in interacting therapeutically with clients.

- Explain the principles of therapeutic communication.

- Compare and contrast the communication techniques that enhance and hinder therapeutic communication.

- Examine therapeutic communication in the context of the nursing process.

- Discuss three special communication challenges and their implications for the future.

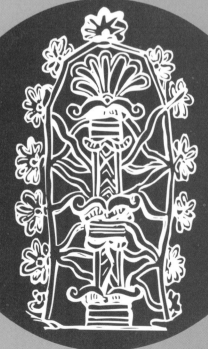

Communication is a dynamic, two-way, circular process in which all types of information are shared between two or more people and their environment. Since we learn how to communicate at an early age, it might be thought of as quite simple. However, communication is a complex process requiring much practice in order to do it effectively.

Communication is the most powerful tool a psychiatric nurse can have. It is the basic component of the therapeutic nurse-client relationship and the medium through which the nursing process occurs. Communication is critical to the successful outcome of nursing interventions, for without effective communication, a therapeutic nurse-client relationship would not be possible. Therefore the nurse must understand and master the general principles of communication, as well as the specific principles of therapeutic communication.

COMPONENTS OF COMMUNICATION

Communication consists of several components: the stimulus (reason for communication), the sender, the message, the medium, the receiver, and feedback. Usually there is a stimulus, a need or reason for the communication to occur. The individual who initiates the transmission of information is the **sender.** Each transmission is both verbal and nonverbal. The information being sent and received, such as feelings or ideas, is the **message.** The method by which the message is sent is the **medium,** which can be written (seen), verbal (heard), scent (smelled), or tactile (felt). For example, a note or letter is *sent;* a shout, scream, or whisper is *heard;* the scent of perfume or body odor is *smelled;* a hug or pat on the back is *felt.*

The **receiver** both receives and interprets the message that has been

Boundary violations Going beyond the established therapeutic relationship standards.

Communication A reciprocal process of sending and receiving messages between two or more people and their environment; the vehicle for establishing a therapeutic relationship.

Congruence Consistency or agreement between verbal and nonverbal behavior.

Confidentiality The right of the psychiatric client to keep information from people outside the health care team.

Countertransference The nurse's unconscious and inappropriate responses to a client who is associated with a significant person in the nurse's life.

Empathy Projecting sensitivity and understanding of another's feelings and communicating the understanding in a way the client comprehends.

Feedback The measure by which the effectiveness of the message is gauged.

Genuineness A quality of an effective nurse that encompasses openness, honesty, and sincerity.

Interpersonal communication Communication between two or more persons containing both verbal and nonverbal messages.

Intrapersonal communication Communication occurring within oneself that can be functional or dysfunctional.

Medium Method by which a message is sent, which can be written, verbal, or tactile.

Message The information (feelings or ideas) being sent and received.

Nonverbal communication Nonverbal behaviors displayed by individuals during the process of an interaction.

Positive regard Acceptance of and respect for a client.

Receiver The individual who both receives and interprets the message.

Resistance The inability, whether conscious or unconscious, to accept change; denial of new problems.

Sender The individual who initiates the transmission of information.

Therapeutic communication Communication that takes place between the nurse and client; the content has meaning and focuses on the client's concerns.

Transference An unconscious response whereby a client associates the nurse with someone significant in his or her life and acts on those feelings.

Verbal communication Spoken or written words that make up the symbols of language.

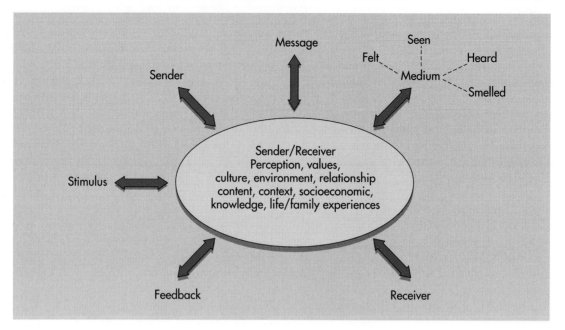

Figure 8-1   Model of the communication process

sent. Ideally, the receiver interprets the message exactly as the sender meant to give it, thus producing effective communication. The **feedback** that the receiver gives back to the sender is the measure by which the effectiveness of the message is gauged. Feedback is a continual process because it is a response to the message and provides a new stimulus to the sender, whereupon the original sender then becomes the receiver. Therefore in any interaction the sender and receiver continually reverse roles. Figure 8-1 shows a model of the communication process.

FACTORS THAT INFLUENCE COMMUNICATION

Communication is a learned process influenced by several factors, including the environment, the relationship between the sender and the receiver, the content of the message, and the context in which the message takes place. Other factors include one's own attitude, ethnic background, socioeconomic status, family dynamics, other life experience, knowledge level, ability to relate to others, and value perceptions.

Environmental factors that control the effectiveness of communication include time, place, noise, privacy, comfort, and temperature. Timing of interaction can be very important. The phrase "counting to ten" describes a waiting or "cooling off" period necessary for some individuals to ensure that they can rationally discuss a "hot" topic or understand a critical concept. Consider the nurse who chooses to wait for an appropriate period of time to begin teaching a client about medications, since the client has just experienced an emotional outburst in the medication-

teaching group and is unable to concentrate in that environment. A carefully chosen time can mean the difference between successful and unsuccessful client learning.

The place of the interaction can be instrumental in conveying the sincerity or importance of communication. Consider the man who wishes to propose marriage to a woman and chooses a mutually predetermined, romantic place in which to do it. A carefully chosen location could mean the difference between a "yes," "maybe," or "no" answer. If the location is noisy and other people are present, messages in the conversation may not be heard, resulting in ineffective communication. Therefore the type, quality, and perceived importance of the specific message conveyed depend in part on the general comfort of the environment.

The *relationship* between two people in a conversation greatly influences the communication. For example, a casual friend can give the same message to an individual as an intimate friend, but the receiver may react quite differently to each person according to the nature of each relationship.

The *context*, as well as the content, of the message also influences the receiver's response. The context, or circumstances in which the message is given, must be appropriate to the type of interaction. Individuals need to feel safe in their environment in order to disclose highly personal information.

Interaction is also affected by *attitude*, which determines how one person generally responds to another person and includes one's biases, past experiences, and levels of openness and acceptance. Also, people from one socioeconomic class, ethnic background, or family background often have difficulty communicating with individuals from a different background or class, possibly because of language or knowledge barriers. For example, both eye contact and personal space may vary greatly from one culture to another.

Communication is greatly influenced by one's upbringing and those aspects of communication that were encouraged, modeled, and discouraged by significant others. Boys in traditional households are often taught that "boys don't cry" and may grow up unable to easily express sad emotions. A teenager who is continually told to "shut up" for "talking too much" may develop a quiet or nonassertive style of communication as an adult.

Knowledge differences can create a deficiency in understanding during communication. If the sender has a greater knowledge of the subject matter than the receiver, it is the responsibility of the sender to ensure that the receiver understands the message. This is always one of the challenges in teaching students or clients important concepts. Some people have an ability to relate with ease to a variety of people and can explain complex information in simple, concrete terms. Some have a great deal of difficulty with this task and are easily intimidated by others. People can learn to communicate more easily and clearly and feel secure about it, with knowledge about communication techniques, with practice and with feedback about their efforts.

Perception is an individual's subjective experience that influences how the message is interpreted. Because misperceptions create problems in communication, the sender must be certain that the receiver has a clear understanding of the message. Thus effective communication depends on understanding what is being communicated, interpreting the message as it was meant to be given, and providing feedback that supports the correct interpretation.

MODES OF COMMUNICATION
WRITTEN COMMUNICATION

Written communication is primarily for the purpose of sharing information. The reader reads for knowledge, pleasure, and understanding. The reader who is able to understand the written word as it appears and comprehend its meaning is prepared to absorb the meaning. It is important that the nurse be able to clearly convey ideas on paper through documentation in the medical record, on statistical reports, and through the use of computers (e.g., computerized reports). The ability to write legibly, spell correctly, use proper grammar, and organize ideas clearly are critical skills for the nurse and cannot be replaced by technology.

VERBAL COMMUNICATION

Verbal communication commonly refers to the spoken words that encompass the symbols of language. Precise verbal communication is important because spoken words often mean different things to different people. Many words or phrases have slang meanings or have developed

new meanings. Words or phrases may also have different meanings for different groups. Figures of speech, jokes, clichés, colloquialisms, and other terms or special phrases have a variety of meanings. For example, "It is a blue Monday" could mean it is a sad day to a person who has the ability to think on an abstract level, but to a client with schizophrenia who interprets concretely and literally, it could mean that the sky is blue. "Don't rain on my parade" means "don't spoil my fun" to one person but to the client with psychosis, who may have loose associations, it prompts the question regarding whether a parade is actually occurring or the question, "Why would I rain on a parade?"

In interactions with individuals from different cultures, slang phrases and idioms such as "double dipping," "making good bread," "rad," "cool," and "let's party" would not be understood and therefore would be misinterpreted. It is easy to assume that other people understand intended meanings. Thus it is necessary to periodically check their interpretation, including examining the cues obtained from their nonverbal responses.

It is increasingly important for nurses to develop a greater sensitivity to the cultural aspects of communication. It is clearly a challenge to learn how to communicate effectively with psychiatric clients who not only have difficulty communicating in a clear, logical, or reasonable manner because of their mental disorder but are also from another culture. (Chapter 6 further discusses issues of communication with those from cultural groups different from one's own.)

NONVERBAL COMMUNICATION

Nonverbal communication is believed by many communication theorists to be the most important part of any message. It includes elements such as tone of voice, hand and body movements, facial expressions, auditory noises that do not involve actual words, and other movements and expressions. Nonverbal cues involve all five senses. They add to the meaning of verbal messages by performing several functions such as expression of feelings, the contradiction or validation of verbal messages, and the preservation of both the ego and the relationship. As a general rule, nonverbal behavior is more revealing and truthful than verbal communication. Therefore it is important for the nurse to observe and consider the client's entire message, both verbal and nonverbal, before arriving at a conclusion.

Ninety percent of a communication is thought to be nonverbal. To have effective communication, nonverbal cues should have **congruence,** or be consistent, with the verbal message.

An example of congruent communication follows:

Verbal: "I have been waiting a long time and was worried about you."
Nonverbal: Concerned facial expression, warm, friendly, outstretched hand

An example of incongruent communication follows:

Verbal: "I have been waiting a long time and was worried about you."
Nonverbal: Frowning, cold, sarcastic voice, no physical contact

Nonverbal cues are grouped into four categories: body cues (kinesics), space (proxemics), touch, and appearance (Northouse and Northouse, 1992).

Body Cues

Body cues comprise facial expressions, reflexes, body posture, hand gestures, eye movement, mannerisms, touch, and other body motions. Body posture and facial expressions, including eye movements, are two of the most important cues to determine how a person is responding to the message. When a client who is frowning, with clenched teeth and fists, narrowed eyes, and a red face, says "I really enjoy my mother visiting me," there is a contradiction between verbal and nonverbal cues that needs to be addressed. A slumped or stooped posture can mean a client is depressed or, at the very least, feeling sad or dejected. A closed posture with arms folded may indicate a client is withdrawing or possibly feeling some anger or angst. An erect posture with shoulders back can mean that the client feels more confident or may be attempting to portray confidence. The gait of an individual as it relates to posture can also indicate one's self-concept. The person who bounces along in a self-assured manner may be perceived as more "upbeat" than the individual who walks at a slow-moving pace.

Nurses should carefully observe hand gestures, since they may also signal anger, restlessness, frustration, giving up, relaxation, or apathy. The nurse needs to be aware of impending anger so that early interventions can be implemented to prevent a situation from becoming quickly out of control. The old adage "when in doubt, observe what people do, not only what they say" is especially important when dealing with psychiatric clients, because what they say and what they do may often be incongruent.

Paralinguistics (paralanguage) behavior includes any audible sound that is not a spoken word. It includes voice tone, inflection, word spacing, rate, emphasis or intensity, groaning, coughing, laughing, crying, grunting, moaning, and other audible sounds. Along with the silent cues, these audible nonverbal cues are very important in assessing clients.

Space

The use of space is another nonverbal cue. Each person has a "comfort zone," or space boundary, that invisibly surrounds him or her when interacting with others. The boundary becomes larger or smaller depending on the nature of the relationship. *Intimate space* is the closest distance between two individuals. *Personal space* is for close relationships within touching distance. *Consultive space* is farther apart than personal space, requiring louder speech. *Public space* is used for public gatherings such as speeches and is usually seen in a large hall or auditorium.

Space as a concept of boundaries and safety is important to understand because the nurse and the client need to respect the distance each one needs. For successful communication to occur, both parties need to feel comfortable. Some clients have problems with their boundaries and may "invade" other clients' own "safe zone." Clients who perceive this as threatening may react aggressively to such boundary violations. At such times the nurse may need to help the client understand the appropriate distance by actually stating the boundary for the client in inches or feet, as needed. When the client violates the nurse's own comfortable space, the nurse may need to set a limit for the client after the initial intrusion.

Touch

Touch is a nonverbal message that involves both action and personal space. Touch typically conveys a message to connect with another person. In nursing, touch has been used to convey messages of concern and empathy. The nurse must be careful when deciding whether to touch a psychiatric client. Not all clients want to be touched. They may perceive it as a threat and respond with aggression, or interpret it as an intimate move and respond by withdrawal or inappropriate sexual response. Touch as communication is discussed in more detail later in the chapter.

Appearance

Appearance communicates a particular image, as well as a clue to one's mental status. Appearance refers to the way an individual uses clothing, makeup, hairstyle, jewelry, and other items such as hats, purses, or glasses, as well as grooming and hygiene. These nonverbal cues often disclose how the person wishes to be viewed by others. For example, a nurse who comes to work wearing a revealing blouse, tight slacks, and high-heeled shoes exhibits a look more suitable for a social engagement than one representing professional nursing.

Another example is an individual who comes in for a supervisory job interview wearing shorts, a wrinkled knit shirt, and sandals; his hair is uncombed and his beard untrimmed. On first glance, the employer wonders if the job candidate is serious about being hired, since his appearance is sloppy and projects an unfavorable image. A third example is an elderly woman who is admitted to the hospital wearing dirty, wrinkled clothing. She was found by the home health nurse in a filthy apartment and has not bathed in several weeks. On further assessment, it is revealed that her husband died 2 months ago, and she was subsequently diagnosed as depressed. Therefore her appearance is a result of her obvious unresolved grief response, which has incapacitated her.

Nurses must try to interpret a client's nonverbal behavior when evaluating the verbal content. They then need to incorporate this evaluation into the assessment and plan of care.

Finally, nurses need to be aware of their own nonverbal cues. For effective communication to occur, these nonverbal messages should communicate genuine interest and respect.

TYPES OF COMMUNICATION
INTRAPERSONAL COMMUNICATION

In **intrapersonal communication,** self-talk occurs, during which individuals give themselves all types of positive and negative messages. Self-talk can be helpful if the messages one gives oneself are helpful or positive. Intrapersonal communication can be functional or dysfunctional.

For example, a 45-year-old client spends a session with the nurse developing a realistic set of goals for her hospital stay. The client subsequently tells herself she is pleased that she has finally accomplished a useful task and is clear about what she needs to do before she leaves the hospital. In this situation, she gives herself positive messages that assist her in her recovery.

An example of dysfunctional self-talk occurs if this same individual persists in giving herself negative, self-defeating messages (e.g., "I can never do anything right," or "I'll never get well"). This type of self-talk can impede recovery.

In another example, a client with a diagnosis of schizophrenia continually hears many internal voices that tell him he is cursed and evil, and that he must kill himself as the only way out. These internal voices, displayed through auditory hallucinations, are considered dysfunctional self-talk.

INTERPERSONAL COMMUNICATION

Interpersonal communication occurs between two or more individuals and contains both verbal and nonverbal messages. It is a complex process consisting of a variety of factors affecting its outcome. The nurse communicates on an interpersonal level with a variety of individuals and groups throughout the day. Emphasis is placed on *therapeutic* and *collegial* communication when the nurse is at work. *Social communication,* primarily used away from work, is discussed only briefly. The characteristics of social and therapeutic communication are listed in Table 8-1.

Social Communication

Social communication occurs in everyday situations, usually away from the work setting. This type of interaction may include discussions regarding family business, social activities, family issues, vacations, school, and church. Much of this interaction is superficial and light, and it may not have a goal. The purpose of much social communication is to maintain a relationship and for enjoyment, and it is primarily done for the mutual benefit of all involved.

Varying levels of intimacy exist in social communication. Communication between parent and child carries a level of intimacy different from communication between parent and teacher. Self-disclosure occurs at varying levels, but superficiality is more the norm, since there are no real expectations of help. When help is the expected outcome

Table 8-1	Characteristics of Social and Therapeutic Communication	
	Social	**Therapeutic**
Who	Friends, family, acquaintances	Helper and client
Setting	Home, away from work, any type of setting	Clinical setting; private, quiet, confidential, safe environment
Purpose	Maintain relationships; mutual sharing of information, thoughts, beliefs, ideas, feelings	Promote growth and change in clients
Content	Social talk, focus on children, vacations, family, leisure, church, doing a favor, giving advice	Therapeutic talk; client expresses thoughts, beliefs, feelings, anxieties, fears, problems; client identifies needs
Characteristics	Superficial, light, not necessarily goal directed; spontaneous, enjoyable; two-way, focusing on both sender and receiver, giving suggestions, advice; personal or intimate relationship occurs	Learned skill; purposeful, client-focused; client sets goals; planned, difficult, intense; disclosure of personal information by client; meaningful and personal (but not intimate) relationship occurs
Skills	Uses a variety of resources during socialization	Uses specialized professional skills, primarily therapeutic interpersonal communication

of social communication, it is typically given in the form of suggestions and advice by friends and family. This differs dramatically from the help given to the client in therapeutic communication.

Collegial Communication

The purpose of collegial communication is professional collaboration. Collegial communication occurs among colleagues in the professional work setting.

The nurse may also be involved in professional nursing groups within the work setting and in the community. This type of collegial communication is called intradisciplinary.

When psychiatric nurses interact with members of the unit's treatment team, it is referred to as interdisciplinary collegial communication. The interdisciplinary team has regularly scheduled treatment team meetings designed to develop, review, and revise the client's treatment plan. It is vital that all members involved in the client's treatment attend and actively participate in the meeting. Members are assigned roles critical to the success of the treatment team process. The nurse can be the designated leader who facilitates the meeting and is expected to clearly communicate with all members of the team. The nurse can also be assigned the role of recorder, the person responsible for documenting the pertinent information discussed in the client's treatment plan. This role requires skillful written communication techniques. Within a nursing professional group, the intent is to share knowledge, collaborate on a project, or in other ways enhance or improve the profession.

Effective collaboration has the advantage of breaking through power issues and competition that arise when teams of professionals are brought together. In the collaborative process no member is more important than another member or the group as a whole. Each member's contribution is important to the success of the project, purpose, or goal.

The nurse therefore communicates in the collegial arena with supervisors, co-workers, physicians, outside consultants, and other members of the treatment team. These relationships exist within the profession of nursing and outside it. Simultaneously, the psychiatric nurse communicates on a therapeutic level with clients and their family members or significant others.

Therapeutic Communication

Therapeutic communication occurs between the nurse (helper) and the client (recipient). It is the psychiatric mental health nurse's single most important tool. The art of interacting therapeutically is a learned skill involving both nonverbal and verbal communication; its purpose is to promote client growth. It is the medium through which health promotion interventions occur.

Therapeutic communication is client focused, whereas social communication consists of sharing information equally between two or more individuals. Even though the nurse may engage in some social interaction with the client, such as greeting the client at the beginning of the shift, the progress toward a greater level of health occurs through the therapeutic interaction between the nurse and client.

This therapeutic interaction involves the disclosure of personal information by the client. It may include hurtful memories and situations that stir up painful emotions. Sharing such feelings can be extremely beneficial for the client because it allows him or her to identify and discuss experiences and accompanying feelings in a safe, therapeutic setting. The nurse provides a confidential and quiet setting in which the interaction takes place, encourages the client to openly discuss thoughts and feelings, and practices active listening, acceptance, and empathy.

Therapeutic communication can be intimidating not only for the client but also for the nurse. Intense negative feelings are not easy to discuss. Many clients have not previously discussed them for fear of undesired responses such as a lack of understanding on the part of the listener, retaliation, feelings of being unworthy, and inadequacy in explaining them. The intensity of the client's feelings or verbal responses may frighten or catch the new nurse off guard—especially when a client openly discusses such issues as wanting to die because life is not worth living. The nurse may also feel uneasy when a client discusses an emotion or feeling similar to the nurse's personal experience. The nurse's own anxiety level may rise if she or he has not dealt with personal problems effectively.

In summary, therapeutic communication has three essential purposes:

1. To allow the client to express thoughts, feelings, behaviors, and life experiences in a meaningful way in order to promote healthy growth
2. To understand the significance of the client's problem(s) and the role the client and the significant people in his or her life play in perpetuating those problems
3. To assist in the identification and resolution processes of the client's problem areas

The nurse's therapeutic use of communication is the mechanism by which clients can achieve successful outcomes to the problems currently preventing them from achieving optimum health.

PERSONAL ELEMENTS IMPORTANT FOR THERAPEUTIC COMMUNICATION

The nurse's use of self as the primary tool in psychiatric nursing is similar to the singer's use of voice as an instrument to create music. All of the elements essential to helping another individual are within the nurse. This is both exciting and challenging.

The therapeutic use of self begins with *knowing oneself.* Nurses will not be able to help others unless they are first able to help themselves. Knowing the self is a complex and lifelong learning process. It is essential to have self-knowledge before use of the therapeutic self.

At the core of self-knowledge is the nurse's ability to correctly identify negative or unresolved issues of the self. Nurses need to know what values and beliefs they hold. It is also important for them to know and understand their own family background, including dynamic, cultural, and social issues; values; and biases and prejudices.

Nurses also need to be aware of unresolved family life issues and make every effort to resolve them as soon as they are recognized. For example, consider a female nurse who has a long-held belief regarding men and alcohol dependency. She believes they can stop drinking if they really want to. Her belief developed because her maternal grandfather had died from alcohol-related liver disease. The nurse may be unaware that she holds this belief until the first alcohol-dependent male client is assigned to her. It is only when the nurse understands and resolves her issues that she can truly succeed in the necessary separation of her own issues from those of the client.

Since therapeutic communication occurs for the purpose of helping others, it is vital that nurses *understand what motivates them to help others.* Nurse's emotional needs must be recognized so that they do not interfere with the ability to relate therapeutically to clients. Since clients do not take care of nurse's emotional needs, nurses must meet their own emotional needs outside of work. A well-balanced, multifaceted lifestyle satisfies one's emotional needs. When the nurse's needs are met, he or she can better assist the client through therapeutic communication.

Nurses who are *in control of their own lives and emotions* can engage the client in effective communication while maintaining therapeutic control of the conversation, especially when a client is attempting to be intimidating, manipulative, or threatening.

Also, nurses who are comfortable with themselves will be able to put the client's needs first by listening attentively and recognizing emotions in the client that may hinder a therapeutic exchange. For example, high anxiety can produce "tunnel vision" in a client, which can impair communication.

Finally, the nurse needs to be able to *conduct a periodic self evaluation of his or her responses to the client.* Questions to ask oneself may include (Shives, 1994):

Am I open or closed minded regarding this issue?
Am I accepting? Or am I rejecting?
Am I being supportive? Or am I being nonsupportive?
Am I being objective? Or am I allowing my biases to interfere with the interaction?
Am I remaining calm and in control of my own feelings? Or am I allowing my anxiety, sympathy, or anger to surface?

What are my true feelings? Do my nonverbal cues match my verbal communication?

ROLES OF THE NURSE IN THERAPEUTIC COMMUNICATION

Nurses assume many roles during therapeutic communication with clients, such as the professional role and the model role. In the professional role the nurse acts as teacher, socializer, technician, advocate, parent, counselor, and therapist. As a role model the nurse is looked up to by staff, students, and the community. The nurse models therapeutic communication for clients, staff, and students. In the community, as well as in the health care setting, the nurse serves as a professional role model against which nursing, as a profession, is judged.

Clients learn about their illnesses and treatment modalities from the nurse as a teacher. As a teacher, the nurse uses excellent communication to train staff and educate clients. The nurse as a socializer brings clients together for activities to prevent social isolation during hospital treatment. In the technician role the nurse changes the intravenous line, administers medications, or takes vital signs. As an advocate the nurse informs the client of his or her rights and responsibilities and supports the client in decision making. The advocate nurse also serves as a liaison between the client and other members of the mental health team, ensuring that the client's rights, either legal or human, are not violated (Fontaine and Fletcher, 1995). The nurse in the parent role does not mean that the nurse becomes the parent, but rather performs traditional nurturing tasks such as feeding, bathing, or comforting. As a counselor the nurse can assist the client with personal problems, such as a disagreement between the client and a family member. With advanced education the nurse can take on the role of a therapist, conducting individual, group, or family therapy sessions in the hospital, clinic, or community setting.

In any relationship with a client, the nurse may take on part or all of these roles. The number of roles the nurse assumes will vary according to the type and length of the individual nurse-client relationship, as well as the setting of the interactions.

TRAITS OF THERAPEUTIC COMMUNICATION

The following are traits of effective therapeutic communication: genuineness, positive regard, empathy, trustworthiness, clarity, responsibility, and assertiveness. These characteristics allow the nurse to influence growth and change in others because they incorporate verbal and nonverbal behaviors, as well as attitudes, beliefs, and feelings behind the communication. Thus they are necessary for therapeutic communication to take place.

GENUINENESS

Genuineness is demonstrated by congruence between the nurse's verbal and nonverbal behavior. Consistent verbal and nonverbal behavior implies that the nurse is open, honest, and sincere. Genuineness is necessary for clients to develop trust in the nurse. Trust is built when the nurse does not appear mechanical but rather responds with sincerity. Genuine interaction does not mean that the nurse must disclose personal information or relate to the client in a social manner. Rather, the nurse remains focused on the client and responds therapeutically. Nurses cannot expect a client to be open and honest if they do not display these characteristics themselves.

POSITIVE REGARD

Positive regard refers to respect and acceptance. Nurses can show that they view their clients as worthy, for example, by addressing clients by names they prefer. Nurses accept clients for who they are and do not expect them to change except in a therapeutic way.

Positive regard is communicated in a variety of ways. It can be conveyed by sitting and listening to a client, by expressing appropriate emotion about events affecting a client, by validating the client's feelings, or by effectively responding to a client's inappropriate behavior. For example, a client who has just been through the admission process is found on his bed openly masturbating. After assessing the situation and understanding that this activity is not harmful to others, the nurse explains to the client that this behavior should be private. The nurse closes the door to allow the client to continue, but out of the view of others.

Part of positive regard is being nonjudgmental. The nurse should avoid harsh judgment of clients' behavior and feelings because both are real and cannot be argued with, discounted, or criticized. Clients must not be made to feel wrong. Labeling behaviors based on one's own value system is not useful. Instead, the nurse should help clients explore their behavior by discussing the thoughts and feelings that determine the behavior. When clients realize that they are not being judged, they may feel free to express their most intimate thoughts and feelings. A nonjudgmental attitude in the nurse relaxes clients by removing fears of being misunderstood or rejected. This open relationship can occur only when nurses identify their own thoughts and feelings regarding clients' behavior.

EMPATHY

Empathy, or empathic understanding, is the nurse's ability to see things from the client's viewpoint and to communicate this understanding to the client. There are two types of empathy. The first type—*natural, trait,* or *basic empathy*—implies that empathy is an inherent human trait apparent in varying degrees in everyone. Some research suggests that trait empathy is a naturally inherited potential that matures during growth. This viewpoint suggests that we all have an instinctual sensitivity that unfolds in a person, as is the case with other characteristics of human development (Alligood, 1992).

The second type, *trained* or *clinical empathy,* is said to build on the nurse's own natural level of empathy. Trained empathy is a tool or skill used consciously to achieve a therapeutic intervention (Pike, 1990). Some researchers suggest that nursing students should be tested for their level of basic or natural empathy before being taught the clinical empathy techniques to determine potential problematic levels that are either too low or too high (Alligood, 1992; Williams, 1990). Testing would give a baseline indicator before any empathy training to determine the effectiveness of the instruction. High levels of natural empathy may indicate that the nurse has a tendency to overidentify and thus become too involved with clients' problems. Low levels may indicate that the nurse may not be able to demonstrate enough genuine concern for clients.

Empathy should not be confused with sympathy. Sympathy is overinvolvement and sharing one's own feelings after hearing about another person's similar experience. It is not objective, and its primary purpose is to decrease one's own personal distress.

An empathic response involves an appreciation and awareness of the client's feelings and keeps the focus on the client. For example, a client reveals to the nurse that her father died in an automobile accident 1 month before her arrival at the hospital. The nurse responds sympathetically by saying that her own mother died in a small plane crash and that it had made the nurse feel sad for a year afterward. Here the focus is on the nurse, and the client may not know how to respond. An empathic response by the nurse would be: "I can understand how difficult that would be for you. Tell me how it made you feel and how you have been coping with the loss." Now the focus is on the client, and the client is better able to reply.

The development of empathy poses a challenge for the psychiatric mental health nurse in the hospital setting, who typically has a brief time frame with clients and must primarily use crisis intervention principles. Lower levels of empathy from the nurse are healthier for clients in the beginning stage of the relationship. However, it has been shown through research that empathy, especially if it is expressed early in a relationship, is clearly related to positive outcomes.

Empathy consists of two stages. If a client shares important and uncomfortable emotions, nurses should first be receptive to and understand the client's communication by putting themselves in the client's place. This does not mean that nurses need to have had the same problem or feeling. Then, after stepping back into the professional role, nurses must be able to communicate understanding, which demonstrates objectivity and sensitivity to the client. This understanding mirrors the client's identity and is the process by which the client makes changes to achieve positive outcomes. The following skills help nurses develop greater empathic responses:

Attending to the client physically, by sitting in front of the client, at a slight angle, leaning slightly forward with hands and arms in an open stance

Attending to the client emotionally by clearing one's mind of other personal or work-related business and focusing one's full attention on the client

Listening and providing a response to each of the client's verbal and nonverbal communications

Focusing on the client's strengths

Conveying caring, warmth, interest, and concern through nonverbal behaviors

Picking out the most important point of what the client is trying to say

Demonstrating congruence between one's own nonverbal and verbal communication

Checking whether or not one's empathic responses are effective by looking for verbal and nonverbal clues

Closely aligned with empathy is *active listening*, because it incorporates both nonverbal and verbal behaviors necessary for therapeutic communication. Nonverbally, the nurse leans slightly forward, facing the client; uses comfortable, intermittent eye contact; nods; and uses verbal phrases such as "uh huh" or "I hear you." Active listening results in articulation of the client's feelings, specifically providing the client with the knowledge that the nurse accepts how the client is feeling and attempts to understand this (Smith, 1990). A nurse who listens actively also displays interest. A client who is trying to work through problems needs to know that the nurse is there to help and wants to help.

TRUSTWORTHINESS

Trustworthiness is another essential characteristic of an effective nurse. Being trustworthy means being responsible and dependable. Trustworthy nurses adhere to commitments, keep promises, and are consistent in their approach and response to clients. Clients need to learn they can rely on the nurse so that trust can be built. Trustworthy nurses respect the client's privacy, rights, and the need for confidentiality. Clients need to be convinced that the information they share will not go beyond the health care team.

CLARITY

Nurses must communicate clearly. Often, psychiatric clients have difficulty processing information. If the nurse is specific and detailed, there will be less room for miscommunication. Clear communication involves selecting concise words when speaking, and asking questions to clarify meaning. Although using medical jargon is part of the nurse's way of life, the nurse should remember that clients might not speak the same language. Everyday terms such as "taking your vitals," "NPO after midnight," or "take these meds," could be misunderstood, especially by psychiatric clients who may not be thinking clearly as a result of their disorders. Problems may arise if instructions or information is relayed in a highly technical manner, because the client may be too embarrassed to ask for clarification.

A study conducted at the University of Alberta Hospital revealed that clients frequently do not understand or often misunderstand professional jargon (Cochrane et al, 1992). For 2 weeks, several nurses listened to themselves and other nurses in conversation with clients. Each time a word or phrase considered to be medical jargon was used, it was recorded. Thirty-four of the most common medical words or phrases were selected for the study. One hundred one adult clients, both newly admitted and those on their fourth day of hospitalization, were surveyed. The results of the study showed that most of the words were defined correctly by more than half of the respondents. For example, 98% of the respondents knew what "OR" (operating room) meant. But words that had one meaning in everyday terminology and another in the nursing profession were often misinterpreted. The newly admitted clients did not do better or worse than clients hospitalized for 4 days or those who had been hospitalized before this admission.

Thus nurses need to make a conscious effort to speak at a level the client will understand. Avoidance of abstract, lengthy explanations is also necessary.

RESPONSIBILITY

Responsible communication involves being accountable for the outcome of one's professional interactions. When nurses communicate, they need to be responsible for their part in the interaction and ensure that all messages are received and interpreted correctly. Nurses who communicate responsibly enhance growth in others. Responsibility language involves the use of "I" statements when being assertive, as described in the following section.

ASSERTIVENESS

Assertive communication is the ability to express thoughts and feelings comfortably and confidently in a positive, honest, and open manner that demonstrates respect for self while respecting others (Balzer-Riley, 1996). The nurse who communicates assertively makes a conscious choice about how to communicate with others. Communicating assertively is a style choice and can be implemented in any situation at any time. An assertive nurse should control negative feelings, which is important in communication not only with clients but also with supervisors, employees, physicians, and colleagues. Box 8-1 lists behaviors of assertive communication.

Some basic assertiveness techniques can be practiced by the nurse. First, the nurse must learn to use responsibility language using "I" instead of "you" (e.g., "I am responsible for the medication error," or "I feel hurt when you say that to me"). Blaming one's behavior on another takes away the personal power of the nurse to make changes. For example, the client who states, "My mother made me angry," or "God made me punch him," indicates that he has

---

Box 8-1   Behaviors of Assertive Communication

Assertive

Stands up for rights and respects those of others. Uses expressive, directive, self-enhancing speech. Chooses appropriate words and actions.

Aggressive

Stands up for rights but abuses those of others. Speaks in demeaning or attacking manner. Fails to monitor or control words or actions.

Acquiescent

Does not stand up for own rights and accepts the domination and bullying of others. Performs unwanted tasks and feels victimized.

Examples of Assertive Behaviors

1. "I" messages (e.g., "I need," "I feel," "I will")
2. "Eye" contact (e.g., looking directly into the eyes of the person while making or refusing a request)
3. Congruent verbal and facial expressions (e.g., making certain that the facial expression matches the intent of the spoken message. A serious message accompanied by laughter could negate the credibility of the message.)

Example of Assertive Plan for Change

1. Target the behavior that one desires to change (e.g., how to say no and mean it).
2. List approximately 10 situations in which it is difficult to say no, and order them from least to most difficult.

3. Practice saying no, using the least-threatening method first and working up to more challenging situations (e.g., imagery, tape recorder, feedback, role-playing), and practice in actual situations.
4. Say no as the first word in the practice response, since it is a clear message without excuses or apologies.
5. Follow with a clear, concise, declarative statement (e.g., "I will not rearrange my schedule; I need my day off").
6. Use eye contact appropriate to the intent of the verbal message.

   Assertiveness training is most often done in small-group sessions and has been described in detail in a variety of textbooks.

Modified from Fortinash KM, Holoday-Worret PA: *Psychiatric nursing care plans*, ed 3, St. Louis, 1999, Mosby.

---

no power or control over his behavior and takes no responsibility for his actions. Being assertive means learning how to say "no," expressing opinions and feelings, stating beliefs, and initiating conversation. Nonverbal assertive language includes giving others good eye contact when speaking to them.

Assertive messages are those in which the verbal message and nonverbal message match (congruence). For example, when relating to someone that you just witnessed a horrific automobile accident on the way to work, your voice tone and facial expression indicate shock and sadness. Sometimes clients will try to cover up their true sadness by laughing or smiling while relating a very painful experience that they do not know how to deal with appropriately.

RESPONDING TECHNIQUES THAT ENHANCE THERAPEUTIC COMMUNICATION

Techniques of responding therapeutically are methods used to encourage clients to interact in a manner that promotes their growth and moves them toward their treatment goals. These strategies create an atmosphere that promotes communication for problem solving. Table 8-2 gives examples of many of these techniques.

Silence is an important listening skill for psychiatric nurses to develop. It is not the absence of communication, but rather a useful and purposeful communication tool to give the client time to feel comfortable and respond when ready to do so. Silence must be used to serve a particular function and not to frighten or discomfort the already-anxious client. A successful interview is largely dependent on the nurse's ability to remain silent long enough to allow the client to share relevant information. Silence gives the client an opportunity to consider what is being said, weigh alternatives, and formulate an answer.

Support and reassurance are provided in a genuine and honest manner. Clients need to be in an atmosphere where they can safely disclose information that may be of a sensitive nature. Nurses can offer both verbal and nonverbal support so that the client feels free to share thoughts and feelings, which is necessary for progress toward mental health to occur.

Sharing observations made by the nurse is important in order to increase the client's self-understanding. It also demonstrates to the client that the nurse is actively listening.

Acknowledging feelings is a form of client support. It is important to let the client know that his or her feelings are valid and important. There are no right or wrong answers when it comes to feelings. They cannot be taken away, or argued with, or discounted.

Table 8-2	**Therapeutic Responding Techniques as Related to Steps of the Nursing Process and Phases of the Therapeutic Relationship**		
Therapeutic Relationship Phase	**Nursing Process Step**	**Technique**	**Examples**
Orientation	Assessment and nursing diagnosis	*Introducing* self when the client is admitted.	"Hi, my name is Susan. I will be your nurse today."
		Offering self. The nurse demonstrates an honest, open posture, making self available to demonstrate concern and interest.	"I have some information to gather. Let's sit here so we can begin your admission."
		Active listening is practiced by using both verbal and nonverbal skills that show the nurse is giving full attention to the client.	The nurse faces the client and takes an open position, maintains eye contact, and uses verbal and nonverbal messages to demonstrate that the client has the nurse's full attention. "Go on. I hear what you are saying."
		Questioning. The nurse skillfully asks open-ended questions during the initial admission. Interviewing skills are necessary to avoid asking too many personal questions in one session. Questions are geared to achieve relevance and depth. Closed questions are used to gather factual information.	"How many children do you have?" "Has this ever happened before?" "How come you stopped taking your medications?" "What is that all about?" "Tell me how you feel now."
		Waiting in silence is used frequently so that the client has time to verbalize thoughts and feelings. It is planned and used to draw out the client. Silence should be comfortable for both client and nurse.	Sit quietly, maintain comfortable eye contact, demonstrate interest using nonverbal nods and expressive facial movements.
		Empathizing. The nurse demonstrates warmth and acknowledges the client's feelings.	"I know how hurt you must have felt. It sounds like that made you sad."
		Reality orienting/providing information. The nurse explains to the client the type of unit, gives a brief tour, and provides the client with unit information and admission paperwork.	"John, here is a copy of the unit rules. Let's go over a few important items." "You are on the locked unit now." "Today is Friday. You were admitted yesterday afternoon."
		Restating. The nurse repeats what the client says to show understanding and to review what was said.	"You say you are saddened by your friend's death." "You became depressed soon after the accident?"
		Clarifying. The nurse asks specific questions to help clear up a specific point the client makes.	"Did it help when you tried any of the techniques you mentioned?" "Which technique helped the most?" "So your mother remarried soon after you were born?"
		Offering reality. The nurse presents a realistic view to the client in a reasonable manner.	"I know you think people are out to get you. I do not think that. You are safe here, and we are here to help you. This medication will help decrease those thoughts."

Continued

Table 8-2

Table 8-2 Therapeutic Responding Techniques as Related to Steps of the Nursing Process and Phases of the Therapeutic Relationship—cont'd

Therapeutic Relationship Phase	Nursing Process Step	Technique	Examples
Orientation	Assessment and nursing diagnosis	*Stating observations.* The nurse offers a view of what is seen or heard to increase verbalization.	"I see you are quite anxious." "I noticed you had trouble sleeping last night."
		Fostering description of perceptions. The nurse requests clients to describe their situation.	"Help me to understand how this is affecting you right now." "What is the voice telling you?"
		Placing event in time and order: The nurse asks questions to determine the relationships of events, and the nurse helps put events in perspective.	"Was the birth of your first child before or after your mother came to live with you?" "Did your alcohol abuse begin immediately after your divorce?"
		Voicing doubt. The nurse discusses any uncertainty of the client's perceptions.	"I find it hard to believe that you felt no joy on hearing that she survived." "Are you sure you were in bed for 1 full year after that?"
		Identifying themes. The nurse voices issues that arise again and again in the course of conversation.	"It sounds like that is very important to you. You've mentioned it a few times." "When this happens over and over, how do you feel?"
		Encouraging comparisons. The nurse asks for similarities and differences among feelings, thoughts, behaviors, and various life situations.	"Is this feeling the same as or different from what you felt the last time it happened?"
		Summarizing. The nurse verbalizes a compilation of what has been expressed on a particular subject or event.	"Let me see if I understand your anxiety about . . ." "From what you describe, your family seems . . ."
		Focusing zeroes in on a subject until the important points come into clear view for both the client and the nurse.	"When you talk about loss, tell me more about the losses you've experienced." "You touched on his drinking. Tell me more about that."
Working	Outcome identification, planning, and implementation	*Evaluating.* The nurse encourages the client to express the importance of an event.	"What does this type of behavior mean to you?" "After thinking about it all, how does it affect you?"
		Encouraging plan formulation helps the client develop steps to make changes and solve problems.	"What are the steps you'll need to take to achieve that?"
		Assisting in goal setting encourages client to set goals during hospitalization and after hospitalization.	"I will help you set some achievable goals during your hospital stay. What are your ideas?"
		Providing information offers data that will help the client in setting goals and developing a plan of action.	"This list and description of crisis houses may help you decide on which one will be best for you after discharge."

Therapeutic Relationship Phase	Nursing Process Step	Technique	Examples
			"I have a problem-solving guide that helps people go through the necessary steps to follow in solving big problems."
		Fostering decision making encourages the client to work on arriving at healthy, growth-producing decisions.	"Looking over these pros and cons, which alternative would be best for you?"
			"What would be your best choice, given this situation?"
		Role playing. The nurse plays the part of a person the client needs to say something to, in order to help the client practice what he or she wants to say.	"Let's go over what you want to say to her."
			"I'll play your father, and you play yourself."
			"Sometimes it helps to say it in the mirror a few times before the real encounter."
		Providing feedback. The nurse provides the client with supportive comments in reaction to behaviors or statements made.	"Tell me what you want to say; I'll listen and give you my honest reaction."
			"When you walked away, I felt . . ."
			"You may anger some people with a response like that."
		Confronting. The nurse supports the client but directly challenges inaction on the part of the client.	"I know this is hard to do, but I believe it will help you to make a decision."
			"I understand your concerns; however, you have to take some action now."
		Setting limits. The nurse provides the client with external boundaries to an expressed thought, feeling, or behavior.	"You became very angry again. In order to stay in the day room, you'll need to act calmer. You can walk in the hallway if you need to get up."
Termination	Evaluation	*Evaluating actions* encourages clients to look at their behavior and the outcomes it produces.	"When you tried to do that, how well did it work?"
			"When you told her to leave, how did she react?"
			"Was that useful for you?"
		Reinforcing healthy behaviors offers positive responses to the client who is trying out new growth-producing behaviors and making helpful decisions.	"It sounds like you have made a healthy choice."
			"Standing up for yourself is new."
			"You've successfully tried it, so now keep practicing it."
		Encouraging posthospital transition helps the client see that new thoughts and actions can be accomplished after discharge.	"I know you will continue to practice being assertive."
			"What situations will you run into that will make this new action necessary?"
			"How can that stress reduction plan assist you at home?"
			"Which techniques will be useful to you after you return home?"

Broad, open-ended statements allow the client to assume some control over topics to be discussed. However, the nurse should not allow the client to discuss only non-relevant topics or engage in a conversation with a superficial or social content. The nurse should frequently ask the client questions that will not produce one-word answers. Open-ended questions result in fuller, more revealing answers, which typically stimulate further questions by the nurse.

Information giving is an ongoing process for the nurse. Information is provided to enhance the client's knowledge about a variety of topics on his or her illness and treatment. Information may decrease fears and anxiety and increase the client's fund of resources and support for his or her problem. Examples may include information regarding the client's disorder, medication, aftercare support groups, structured living options, or treatment alternatives. Information should be given according to the client's level of understanding and willingness to receive it.

Interpretation of what is being shared by clients is useful to help them see the real meaning behind their message. The nurse must be careful when using this technique. A client may disagree with the nurse's interpretation, which may set up a roadblock. Helping clients *focus* to pursue a particular topic allows them to spend their time discussing subjects of most importance. *Identification of themes* is necessary to help clients see what they repeatedly bring up in the conversation. *Placing events in order and time* is also important to help clients develop a greater perspective on events in their lives.

Clients often need to be encouraged to *describe their perceptions* regarding their thoughts and feelings. For example, some psychiatric clients hear imaginary voices telling them to hurt themselves or others. The nurse asks such clients to tell the staff when this occurs so that the nurse can intervene and prevent clients' attempts to harm themselves or others. Treatment strategies can then be introduced to reduce this perception and therefore minimize the client's dysfunctional behavior.

To develop a sense of clients' past and current behavior, the nurse may ask clients to *compare* their present anxiety to that of their last hospitalization. Or the nurse may ask clients if they have ever experienced before what they are telling the nurse now.

Restating what clients say lets them know that the nurse heard and understands them. It is an active listening technique.

Reflecting is a technique used to turn a question around to obtain a response from the client. Forcing clients to answer a question best answered by clients themselves helps them accept their own ideas and feelings regarding an important event or behavior.

Clarifying is a method used to ask the client to elaborate or restate something just said. It serves to increase the nurse's understanding and to allow the client to rethink and restate the thought or feeling.

Confrontation in an accepting manner is necessary for the client to be more aware of incongruent thoughts, feelings, and behaviors. This helps to bring the issue into focus and should be used only after a good rapport has been established (Fortinash and Holoday-Worret, 1999).

When a client is struggling to explore and solve a problem but can only see one or two solutions, the nurse may *offer alternatives*. Suggesting to the client other possible solutions to the problem is not the same as giving advice. It uses introductions such as "What have you thought about . . ." "Other clients have solved it using this solution," and "Other alternatives might be . . ." The nurse avoids phrases such as "You should," and "I think you need to solve it the way I did" (giving advice).

Voicing doubt is a technique to use when the client is having difficulty relating in a way that sounds believable. Voicing some doubt may help the client to be more realistic about perceptions and conclusions of events. Voicing doubt is used cautiously, since it could set up a barrier between the client and nurse.

On a regular basis the nurse will need to *summarize* the information the client provides. Summarizing the main points of what a client has been discussing helps focus on the most important issues related to the client's life situation. After the summary is provided, the client can agree or disagree with any point, and then together the nurse and client will agree on a final summary.

Role-playing provides a place for the client to act out a particular event, problem, or situation in a safe environment. The nurse can play the other part or role. He or she can also provide feedback to the client on a variety of components within the dialogue, such as voice tone, use of assertive language, identification of feelings, emotion expressed, and nonverbal behavior exhibited (Fortinash and Holoday-Worret, 1999).

SPECIAL COMMUNICATION TECHNIQUES
SELF-DISCLOSURE

Self-disclosure is opening up oneself to another and can be an effective therapeutic skill if it is fully understood and used carefully. Experienced nurses reveal their thoughts, feelings, and life events to demonstrate to the client that they understand what the client is going through.

Disclosing one's own personal beliefs, views, and life experiences occurs in social relationships on a continual basis. In intimate relationships, what is revealed is very personal. Because a professional nurse-client therapeutic relationship exists for the purpose of helping the client, whatever the nurse discloses needs to be carefully thought out before being revealed. Since self-disclosure by the nurse is *always* for the client's benefit and *never* for the nurse's, it is important to explore the what, where, why, and when of self-disclosing to see what purpose it serves (Balzer-Riley, 1996).

Criteria have been developed to help the nurse discern appropriate use of self-disclosure. The purpose of the self-disclosure should be one or more of the following (Stricker and Fisher, 1990):

> *To model and educate.* Will clients learn more about themselves and be able to deal better with the problems in their lives?
> *To build the therapeutic partnership.* Will disclosure foster a greater nurse-client alliance by obtaining a greater amount of cooperation?
> *To validate reality.* Will clients be supported in their natural feelings in response to an event?
> *To foster clients' autonomy.* Will the disclosure help clients to express previously held feelings on their own?

The use of self-disclosure requires that the nurse and client have a therapeutic relationship. The rationale for using self-disclosure comes from the belief that in doing so, the client will in turn self-disclose. Both the amount and the relevance of the nurse's own self-disclosure need to be monitored. If the self-disclosure is too lengthy, it may decrease the time the client has for disclosure and may result in a breakdown in the interaction.

If the disclosure is irrelevant to the client's problem, the client may become distracted and feel alienated from the nurse. Table 8-3 compares an example of therapeutic versus nontherapeutic self-disclosure.

Both research and literature have indicated that self-disclosure can be an important tool for client growth. The nurse must realize that not all self-disclosure is revealing personal information. It can simply be sharing a feeling. Genuine, open communication that creates a therapeutic alliance can be achieved without the use of self-disclosure. Self-disclosure can enhance that alliance only when the nurse feels comfortable with its use and when it will benefit the client.

TOUCH

Touch is a nonverbal method of communication that may convey many messages. Handshaking, holding hands, hugging, and kissing all demonstrate positive feelings for another human being. Nonessential touch is purposeful physical contact with the client other than the touch necessary for a procedure. Nonprocedural touches range from a light touch on the arm or a handshake to holding the hand or a full embrace. For touch to convey warmth, the nurse must be comfortable with it.

Touch carries a different meaning for each person. Several variables influence the intended message of the touch, including the length of the touch, the part of the body touched, the way in which the client is touched, and the frequency of the touch.

The nurse should use caution when touching clients in a psychiatric setting. Reactions to touch are influenced by the age and gender of the client, the client's interpretation of the gesture, the client's cultural background, and the appropriateness of the touch.

The nurse needs to take potential reactions into consideration when deciding which clients to touch and what type of touch to use, if any. For example, a depressed client may respond positively to touch as a gesture of concern. An elderly, frail client or a client who is dying may also be comforted by the nurse's touch. However, a paranoid, hostile client may misinterpret touch to mean confrontation and may strike out at the nurse. An abused client may pull away and feel frightened by a hand on the shoulder.

Procedural touch may include positioning the arm of a client when taking a blood pressure or drawing blood for laboratory work (Figure 8-2, *A*), turning a client to change a dressing or diaper, lifting or assisting a client from the bed to a wheelchair, or performing a seclusion or restraint procedure on a highly agitated and hostile client. *Nonproc-*

Table 8-3 **Self-Disclosure**	
Therapeutic	**Nontherapeutic**
Client: "I'm real upset that I have to leave the hospital today." *Nurse:* "I have enjoyed working with you. I realize endings can be sad. It is important for you to use the tools you have learned when you go home." *Discussion:* The nurse is using self-disclosure in the termination phase of the relationship. She is validating the client's feelings and is also validating the alliance with the purpose of encouraging the client to transfer what has been learned in treatment to life after discharge.	*Client:* "That jerk of a husband had to leave me with three children to support, and it is hard." *Nurse:* "I know how you feel because my husband was just like that, leaving me 5 years ago with two small children when he ran off with another woman. He gives me no support and doesn't see his children. I get angry a lot, too." *Discussion:* The nurse is using self-disclosure in the admission interview or beginning phase of the relationship, when no rapport has been established. In addition, it reveals too much personal information and is too lengthy. It seems to serve the nurse's purpose, rather than the client's, to share the incident.

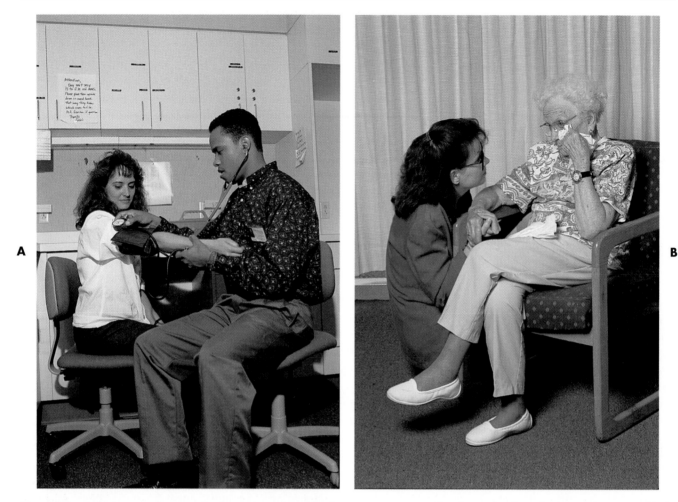

Figure 8-2 **A,** Positioning the arm of a client when taking blood pressure is an example of procedural touch. **B,** Comforting an elderly client as she grieves over her husband's death is an example of nonprocedural touch. (Copyright Cathy Lander-Goldberg, Lander Photographics.)

edural touch may include holding an elderly client's hand as she is conveying sadness over her husband's death (Figure 8-2, *B*), hugging an adolescent client as he leaves the hospital, shaking the hand of new clients as they are introduced by another nurse during their transfer to your unit, or giving a back rub to a long-term, bedridden client.

The use of touch is an individual preference by the nurse because not all practitioners feel comfortable doing it. Much depends on the nurse's comfort level, the ability to correctly interpret the situation, and the appropriate use of touch. Using touch can be highly beneficial to the client's progress by enhancing the nurse-client relationship and promoting health (see Understanding & Applying Research box).

HUMOR

Humor can be a useful tool in psychiatric nursing. Humor is defined as the quality that makes something seem funny, amusing, or ludicrous. It is the ability to perceive, appreciate, and express what is funny, amusing, or absurd. Use of humor has been controversial in psychiatric settings and is seen by some as unprofessional and inappropriate. Healthy humor elicits laughter between people; it encourages laughing *with* others and not *at* them. It includes others, is appropriate to the situation, respects others, and preserves their dignity. Harmful humor excludes others. It singles out people from a group and ridicules them.

A good sense of humor is considered to be a mature coping mechanism and can help the nurse adequately handle difficult situations. It also assists in gaining a different perspective on the problem by lightening a serious mood for a few moments.

Physiologically, humor has been known to improve the circulatory system, stimulate the respiratory system, and increase blood oxygen levels and heart rate. These changes result in a rise in the epinephrine levels, which makes one feel more alert and offers a sense of well-being. Laughing and having positive social interactions during mealtimes has been reported to aid digestion. The psychologic benefits of laughter decrease fears and anxiety, lessen negative

The purpose of this study was to identify and describe the ways and reasons registered nurses use nonprocedural touch in the inpatient psychiatric setting. Natural setting observation and nurse interviews were used to examine the nurses' reasons for touch.

Twenty-six incidents of nonprocedural touch initiated by 13 registered nurses with 17 psychiatric clients were recorded over 27.5 hours of observation. Observations were made on one adolescent unit and two adult psychiatric units in a large university teaching hospital.

Of the 30 nurses who agreed to participate in the study, 24 were observed. Of those 24 nurses, 13 touched clients. Several elements went into the decision to touch. Both the client and the nurse were taken into account. Client characteristics such as age, gender, needs, and the nurse's knowledge of the client were involved in the decision to touch. Also, the nurses' feelings, beliefs, intuition, style, and role expectations were acknowledged.

Ninety-two percent of the touches recorded were used in a purposeful, therapeutic manner. The nurses' intentions for using touch were to establish contact with the client, enhance communication, convey warmth and caring, show interest and recognition, and offer reassurance and comfort.

Nonprocedural touch can be very effective in conveying therapeutic messages, and nurses should use touch whenever therapeutically appropriate.

Tommasini NR: The use of touch with the hospitalized psychiatric patient, *Arch Psych Nurs* 4(4):213, 1990.

emotions, and decrease stress and tension (Ferguson and Campinha-Bacote, 1989).

The nurse should assess the degree to which a client has a sense of humor. In depressed clients the outward expression of laughter and pleasure is usually missing. Clients with paranoid features are unable to laugh. In fact, they may view others' laughter as a personal attack. This is important to remember. For example, nurses in the nursing station may choose not to laugh and joke behind a glass partition where paranoid clients can see them and interpret the behavior as a personal affront. On the other hand, manic clients may laugh at everything, whether or not it is actually humorous. This exaggerated sense of well-being demonstrates a lack of judgment on the part of the client, and it can turn into biting sarcasm that can hurt others.

Clinicians who have studied humor as an important indicator of a person's health believe that asking clients simple questions such as what their favorite joke is, how often they laugh, and how their patterns of laughter have changed offers the nurse new insights into their illness (Ferguson and Campinha-Bacote, 1989).

The psychiatric mental health nurse can use humor as a therapeutic tool in a variety of ways. For example, it can be used to teach the client the difference between hurtful and healthy humor, to encourage healthy humor on the unit by role modeling, and to introduce humor in formal and informal groups and individually. The use of humor can increase the flexibility of interactions and create a more relaxed environment. It can enhance the client's insight and facilitate the type of interaction that is difficult for the client, in a safe, low-keyed setting.

OBSTACLES TO THERAPEUTIC COMMUNICATION

Certain obstacles can occur in the client-nurse relationship that affect the nature of the communication. Some obstacles are due to the client's disorder or lack of knowledge, and some have to do with the nurse's own inability to be effective because of inexperience, lack of knowledge, or personal problems. For the relationship to grow in a healthy manner, these obstacles must be overcome.

Four key therapeutic obstacles are introduced here for discussion: resistance, transference, countertransference, and boundary violations.

RESISTANCE

Resistance occurs in clients who consciously or unconsciously maintain a lack of awareness of problems they are having to avoid anxiety. It can take the form of a natural and short-lived reservation about accepting a problem, or a long-term, firmly stated denial that there are problems. This resistance to change is a part of human nature but must be addressed and dealt with by both the client and the nurse for positive growth to occur. Nurses can help clients overcome resistance by pointing out their progress and strengths.

For example, a nurse can assure a client who resists impending discharge because of fear of failure, abandonment, or loneliness that such fears are not uncommon at the time of termination or discharge. The nurse can then remind the client of progress made (e.g., "You've been a big part of the success of the activities, and you even facilitated a few groups; these are accomplishments you didn't believe possible when you first arrived at this facility"). Such observations build the client's confidence and offer hope that will counteract resistance.

TRANSFERENCE

Transference is the unconscious response whereby clients associate the nurse with someone significant in their lives. Feelings and attitudes about the other person are transferred to the nurse. For example, a male client sees a female nurse as a mother figure because she has a mannerism that reminds him of his own mother. The client may have negative feelings about his mother and, without provocation, becomes angry or bothered by the nurse's interaction with him because of the resemblance. Often, the client's intense response does not match the situation or the content of the interaction. The interaction will come to a standstill if the nurse does not address and examine the client's reasons for transference.

The nurse can deal with both resistance and transference by being prepared to hear a client's irrational and highly charged responses to the nurse. The nurse must truly listen to the client and then use the therapeutic techniques of clarifying and reflecting to begin problem solving. The goal is for the client to gain awareness and recognition of what lies behind the resistance.

COUNTERTRANSFERENCE

Countertransference is initiated by the nurse's emotional response to a specific client. The response is irrational, inappropriate, highly charged, and generated by certain qualities of the client. It is simply the nurse's own transference. Nurses have a natural response to each client and will like or dislike some more than others. Countertransference occurs when the feelings are intense—either positive or negative—and are not based on reality. Because it will impede the nurse's ability to be therapeutically effective, the nurse must always observe for signs of its occurrence.

From time to time, countertransference issues are bound to surface. Even though it is natural, it can be destructive if ignored by the nurse or treated as insignificant. The nurse most often encounters countertransference when the client is displaying disruptive, aggressive, irritating, or resistive behaviors. If the nurse remains angry with the client as a result of these behaviors, the degree of objectivity needed to promote healthy change is lost. Nurses may also find themselves attracted positively to clients in excessive ways and should recognize and take steps to avoid countertransference.

To deal with countertransference, the nurse should conduct an honest self-appraisal throughout the course of the therapeutic relationship while gaining a good understanding of the client's background and issues. If the self-appraisal reveals any problems, the nurse should explore why these feelings are occurring. This work needs to be done as soon as the problem is recognized. The nurse may not be able to handle these feelings alone and may need some clinical supervision time to deal with them.

BOUNDARY VIOLATIONS

Boundary violations occur when the nurse goes beyond the established therapeutic relationship standards and enters into a social or personal relationship with the client. A client can also attempt to violate the boundaries of the nurse-client relationship. A client may ask the nurse, "How old are you?" or "Are you married?" or may try to touch the nurse inappropriately. Violations can also occur if the nurse treats the client at odd hours or in an unusual set-

ting, if the nurse accepts compensation or gifts for treatment, if the nurse's language or clothing are inappropriate, or if the nurse's self-disclosure or physical contact lack therapeutic value. For example, the nurse calls the client from her home after he leaves the hospital, just to "talk" or because she is "concerned" about him.

RESPONDING TECHNIQUES THAT HINDER THERAPEUTIC COMMUNICATION

Therapeutic skills that have enhanced the communication process are presented earlier in the chapter. There are also many responses that are counterproductive to healthy outcomes and are therefore considered nontherapeutic.

There are several reasons why nurses fail to interact effectively. The inexperienced nurse's insecurity is one factor. A certain amount of experience and maturity greatly helps the nurse deal effectively with the difficult and complex behaviors psychiatric clients often display.

Other explanations for nontherapeutic communication are that the nurse has allowed necessary skills to stagnate or diminish. Or the nurse may have developed personal problems that have not been dealt with sufficiently and are thus interfering with his or her ability to focus on the client and the client's needs (Table 8-4).

It is important that nurses build on the knowledge they possess by continually practicing and perfecting skills and attending skills-building classes and therapeutic communication in-service workshops to refresh and enhance skills they already possess. It is also important that they know when to obtain outside help for their own life problems so that those problems do not interfere with work.

There are other potential instances for a nurse's ineffective responses. A nurse may display anger toward the client for not behaving in a socially acceptable manner or for not doing what is asked. Or the nurse may take personally what the client says. A client may be angry, delusional, and display out-of-control behavior, and may say something to the nurse that hurts the nurse's feelings. For example, a client may say to the overweight nurse placing him in seclusion, "Get out of here, you big fat . . ." The nurse, upset by the client's statement, may respond angrily or defensively if the nurse is not able to detach from the statement and realize that the client is angry at his own behavior, and is projecting it to the nurse in the form of a personal statement.

COMMUNICATION AND THE NURSING PROCESS

There are many opportunities to communicate therapeutically throughout the nursing process. Each step of the nursing process—assessment, nursing diagnosis, outcome identification, implementation, planning, and evalua-

Table 8-4	Ineffective Responses That Hinder Therapeutic Communication		
Response	Discussion	Nontherapeutic Response	Therapeutic Response
Offering false reassurance	The nurse, in an effort to be supportive and to make the client's pain disappear, offers reassuring clichés. This response is not based on fact. It brushes aside the client's feelings and closes off communication. Often, it is due to the nurse's inability to listen to the client's negative emotions. No one can predict the outcome of a situation.	"Don't worry, everything will be OK." "Things will be better soon; you'll see."	"I know you have a lot going on right now. Let's make a list and begin to discuss them one at a time. Working toward solutions will help you to get through this."
Not listening	The nurse is preoccupied with other work that needs to be done, is distracted by noise in the area, or is thinking about personal problems.	"I'm sorry, what did you say?" "Could you start again? I was listening to the other nurse."	"That is interesting. Please elaborate." "I really hear what you are saying . . . it must be difficult."
Offering approval	It is most important how the client feels about what he or she said or did. The client ultimately must approve of his or her own actions.	"That's good." "I agree—I think you should have told him."	"What do you think about what you said to him?" "How do you feel about it?"
Minimizing the problem	The nurse may use this when it is difficult to hear the enormity of a particular problem. This is used in an effort to try to make the client feel better. It cuts off communication.	"That's nothing compared to that other client's problem." "Everyone feels that way at times, it's not a big deal."	"That is a very difficult problem for you." "That sounds pretty important for you to deal with."
Offering advice	This response undermines clients' ability to solve their own problems. It serves to render them dependent and helpless. If the solution provided by the nurse does not work, the client may blame the outcome on the nurse. Clients do not take responsibility for developing outcomes. The nurse maintains control and at the same time devalues the client.	"I think you should . . ." "In my opinion, it would be wise to . . ." "Why don't you do . . ." "The best solution is . . ."	"What do *you* think you should do?" "There can be several alternatives—let's talk about some. However, the final decision must be yours. I will listen to your problem and help you see it clearly. We can develop a pros and cons list that may assist you in solving the problem."
Giving literal responses	The nurse feeds into the client's delusions or hallucinations and denies the client the opportunity to see reality. This does not provide a healthy response toward growth.	*Client:* "That TV is talking to me." *Nurse:* "What is it saying to you?" *Client:* "There is nuclear power coming through the air ducts." *Nurse:* "I'll turn off the air conditioner for a while."	*Nurse:* "The TV is on for everyone." *Nurse:* "There is cool air blowing from the vents. It is the air conditioning system."
Changing the subject	The nurse changes the topic at a crucial time because the discussion is too uncomfortable. It negates what the client seems interested in discussing. Communication will remain superficial.	*Client:* "My mother always puts me down." *Nurse:* "That's interesting, but let's talk about . . ."	*Nurse:* "Tell me about that."

Continued

Table 8-4	Ineffective Responses That Hinder Therapeutic Communication—cont'd		
Response	**Discussion**	**Nontherapeutic Response**	**Therapeutic Response**
Belittling	The nurse puts down the client's expressed feelings to avoid having to deal with painful feelings.	*Client:* "I don't want to live anymore now that my child is gone." *Nurse:* "Anyone would be sad, but that's no reason to want to die."	*Nurse:* "The death must be very difficult for you. Tell me more about how you are feeling."
Disagreeing	The nurse criticizes the client who is seeking support.	"I definitely do not agree with your view." "I really don't believe that."	"Let's talk about the way you see that." "It seems hard to believe. Please explain further."
Judging	The nurse's responses are filled with his or her own values and judgments. This demonstrates a lack of acceptance of the client's differences. It will provide a barrier to further disclosures.	"You are not married. Do you think having this baby will solve your problems?" "This is certainly not the Christian thing to do." "You are thinking about divorce when you have three children?"	"What will having this baby provide for you?" "What do you think about what you are attempting to do?" "Let's discuss this option," or "Let's discuss other options."
Excessive probing	This serves to control the nature of the client's responses. The nurse asks many questions of clients before they are ready to provide the information. This is self-protective to the nurse by avoiding the anxiety of uncomfortable silences. The client feels overwhelmed and may withdraw. The use of the "why" question places the client in a defensive position and may block further communication.	"Why do you do this?" "What do you think was the real cause?" "Why do you feel this way?" "Why do you think that way?"	"Tell me how this is upsetting to you." "Tell me what you believe to be the cause." "Tell me how you feel when that happens." "Explain your thinking on this if you can."
Challenging	This stems from the nurse's belief that if clients are challenged regarding their unrealistic beliefs, they will be coerced into seeing reality. The client may feel threatened when challenged, holding onto the beliefs even more strongly.	"You are not the Queen of England." "If your leg is missing, then why can you walk up and down this hall?"	"You sound like you want to be important." "It seems to you like you are missing a leg. Tell me more about that."
Superficial comments	The nurse gives simple or meaningless responses to clients. It suggests a lack of understanding regarding the client as an individual. The interactions remain superficial, maintaining distance between the nurse and client. Nothing of significance gets communicated.	"Great day, huh!" "You should be feeling good; you are being discharged today." "Keep the faith; your doctor should be coming anytime now."	"What kind of day are you having?" "How are you feeling about leaving the hospital today?" "You look worried. Your doctor called and said he would be here within the hour."

Table 8-4	Ineffective Responses That Hinder Therapeutic Communication—cont'd		
Response	**Discussion**	**Nontherapeutic Response**	**Therapeutic Response**
Defending	The nurse may believe that he or she must defend herself or himself, the staff, or the hospital. The nurse may not take the time to listen to the client's concerns. Efforts need to be made to explore the client's thoughts and feelings.	"Your doctor is a good doctor. He would never say that." "We have a very experienced staff here. They would not ever do that."	"What has you so upset about your doctor?" "Tell me what happened on the evening shift."
Self-focusing	The nurse focuses attention away from the client by thinking about sharing his or her own thoughts, feelings, or problems. The focus is taken away from the client, who is seeking help. The nurse is more interested in what to say next instead of actively listening to the client.	"That may have happened to you last year, but it happened to me twice this month, which hurt me a great deal and . . ." "Excuse me but could you say that again? I have a response to make, but I want to be sure of what you said."	"Tell me about your incident and how it might relate to your sadness now." "If I heard you accurately, you said . . ."
Criticism of others	The nurse puts down others.	*Client:* "The staff members on the day shift let me smoke two cigarettes." *Nurse:* "The day shift is always breaking the rules. On this shift we follow the one-cigarette policy." *Client:* "My daughter is hateful to me." *Nurse:* "She must be just awful to live with."	*Nurse:* "The policy is one cigarette, which we will follow." *Nurse:* "It sounds like you are having a rough time right now with your daughter."
Premature interpretation	The nurse does not wait until the client fully expresses thoughts and feelings related to a particular problem. This rushes the client and disregards his or her input. The nurse may miss what the client wants to explain.	"I think this is what you really mean." "You may think that way consciously, but your unconscious believes . . ."	"What do you think this means?" "So you think . . ."

tion—corresponds with the three phases of the therapeutic relationship—orientation, working, and termination. Therapeutic responding techniques unique to each step and phase are used throughout.

The nurse's first communication task is to greet the client on admission. The nurse communicates the nature of his or her role. This orientation phase begins with the initial contact, continues with the admission interview and assessment, and ends with the formulation of a nursing diagnosis. This phase can last one or more sessions because much of highly personal data must be collected, and it occurs when the client is in the most need of help and may be displaying highly dysfunctional behavior.

In the working phase of the relationship when the care plan with outcome criteria is being developed and implemented with the client and treatment team, many therapeutic responding techniques can be used. The therapeutic communication skills the nurse uses during this phase are designed to help clients deal with the issues that brought them into the hospital.

During the termination phase both evaluation and discharge planning are predominant. The nurse uses communication techniques associated with assisting the client toward discharge and aftercare. Throughout the nurse-client relationship, the nurse must avoid responding in ways that hinder therapeutic communication (see Table 8-4).

The phases of the therapeutic relationship are discussed in greater detail in Chapter 22.

CHALLENGES IN COMMUNICATION
LEGAL ISSUES

Confidentiality and informed consent are legal issues that impact nurse-client communication. They are discussed briefly here as they relate to this relationship. They are discussed in detail in Chapter 5.

Confidentiality

All client information the nurse obtains is protected by the client's right to privacy, or **confidentiality.** Information can be shared with the health care team so that the most effective plan of care can be developed. However, the nurse must fiercely protect the client's right to privacy and the right to keep that information from individuals outside the health care team.

All communication is therefore considered confidential or privileged. In the initial interview the nurse has the responsibility to inform the client of the confidential nature of the disclosure. The client also has the right to know with whom the nurse will share the disclosed information. The nurse needs to explain that the information may be shared with team members such as the social worker, the physician, and other nursing staff, but not the client's family members or friends. If information is to be shared with them, it is usually done by the physician with express permission from the client.

Often clients with mental illness have difficulty trusting others. To encourage clients to confide in the nurse, the nurse must gain the client's trust through honest, open, and congruent communication and by doing what he or she says will be done. However, the client may wish to confide something that the nurse needs to share. It is the nurse's responsibility to tell the client that secrets cannot be kept. Therefore it is most important for the nurse to inform the client that shared information essential to the client's own or others' safety or treatment plan will be discussed with various members of the health care team.

For example, a client shares with a nursing student that he wishes to gain access to a sharp object to cut himself when everyone has gone to bed because he is feeling even more depressed than on the previous day. The student explains that this type of disclosure must be shared with the charge nurse. The client then begs the student not to tell the physician. The student replies that the charge nurse must communicate to the client's physician all disclosures that reveal behavior harmful to the client.

Legal Status and Rights

There is much opportunity for the nurse to communicate with clients regarding their legal status. For example, a client is brought into the hospital by the police, who have placed the client on a legal "hold." A client may not understand this term, which can seem confusing. It is often the nurse who communicates to the client the exact nature of his or her legal status, explaining the implications and rights associated with the status. Clients' specific legal rights are discussed in Chapter 5.

Informed Consent

Informed consent simply means that a legal document must outline any procedure to be conducted or specific types of medication to be given to the client. The client must be informed fully by his or her physician in an understandable manner so that he or she can decide whether to have the procedure or take the specific medication considered helpful to treatment. The nurse must verify with the physician that the client has a basic understanding of the informed consent regarding treatment, medication, alternative therapies, and/or the client's prognosis with or without treatment. The nurse can then obtain the client's signature and sign as witness to the signature.

Effective nurse-client communication is extremely helpful in processing legal paperwork, especially with clients who have difficulty trusting. The nurse must be honest, open, congruent, and clear in all messages given to the client regarding all communication of a legal nature, thus preparing a client to be well informed and to consent to treatment.

LENGTH OF STAY

Another communication challenge comes with brief hospital stays. For the chemically dependent client, for example, the length of stay could be as short as 3 days. For the client with schizophrenia, it could be a 3- to 7-day stay. Communication must then be geared toward a crisis intervention style of relating, where the initial phase of the relationship takes on a new meaning. The data gathering must be accomplished within hours. Thus the nurse needs to establish rapport quickly. If the client's behavior is not conducive to working quickly, then rest and medication can be provided to calm the client so that the preliminary interview and data gathering can occur.

PHYSICAL IMPAIRMENTS

Other issues affecting communication are special client care needs. Consider, for example, the client with hearing impairment. If the client reads lips or the nurse "signs," then communication is possible. The nurse should sit in a manner that facilitates the communication. The nurse may wish to inform the other clients what is being done and why. This is especially helpful in a group setting.

COMMUNICATING WITH CHILDREN AND ADOLESCENTS

Communicating with children and adolescents presents unique challenges. Often the nurse is in a position of caring for infants, children, and adolescents through the age of 18. In caring for patients in these age-groups, the nurse will need to adapt his or her communication level to the developmental age of the child or adolescent to match the young client's ability to comprehend. Therefore it is important for the nurse to understand the developmental age of the child with whom he or she is trying to communicate so that not only the language, but also the examples and educational materials, can be adapted to basic concepts that the young client can easily grasp.

Because the child's capacity to grasp language does not begin until the second year of life, until then, the nurse needs to rely on nonverbal skills, using kind and gentle facial expressions and a nurturing and caring attitude, with soothing voice tones. Having the parents participate in the child's care can be helpful and may reduce their anxiety. Between the ages of 2 and 6 years, the child is in the beginning stage of language development and the nurse can begin to communicate verbally with the child, using simple explanations and instructions and keeping the interactions in the here and now. The nurse may use pictures or storybooks to provide information and clarify meanings.

During the juvenile stage, between the ages of 6 and 10, the nurse usually experiences less difficulty communicating with the child. During this stage the child is accustomed to adults other than the parents, such as teachers and coaches, giving instruction and assistance. By this time the child has developed a more mature mode of communication and has a need for close relationships, both of which are helpful when interacting with the child. Concrete examples, as well as simple videotapes and books suitable for the child's age, can be used with success.

During preadolescence, from the ages of 10 to 12 or 13, when the onset of puberty begins, the preadolescent remains receptive to adults and their influence. The nurse may begin to use some of the preadolescent's own language to communicate more effectively. Keeping explanations relevant, brief, and at a level commensurate with the preteen's understanding may help the process.

The adolescent stage begins with puberty, ordinarily ages 12 or 13 through ages 18 or 19. During the early adolescent years the child is trying to form a self-identity and feel comfortable with himself or herself. The adolescent may be very self-conscious and easily embarrassed. The nurse needs to respect the adolescent's privacy. The nurse also needs to relate more directly with the adolescent and less through the parents, since the adolescent is trying to separate emotionally from the parents and become independent, a significant characteristic of adolescence. The early-age adolescent begins to develop abstract thinking and can now not only grasp past and present events but also think about and discuss future events. The nurse can use these skills in his or her interactions with the early-age adolescent. As the adolescent reaches 14 or 15, the nurse may find that doing an activity with the adolescent while communicating allows the adolescent to feel more comfortable with the adult. The fact that the nurse is not the adolescent's parent is an advantage and will assist in the communication process. Regardless of the age of the child, the nurse needs to present a verbal and nonverbal environment in which the child feels comfortable. The degree of success that the nurse will have in communicating with a child or adolescent greatly depends on the nurse's understanding of the developmental age of the child.

With clients who are visually challenged, the nurse must physically assist the clients to and from activities, groups, and their rooms. These actions communicate caring and concern, as does sitting near the client when speaking. When approaching the visually impaired client, the nurse must proceed slowly and speak in soft tones to avoid startling the client. Communicating is challenging, but it can be effective with the help of the client and the nurse's own sensitivity.

LANGUAGE AND CULTURAL DIFFERENCES

Since the United States is one of the most diverse societies in the world and part of a rapidly changing and growing multicultural world, it is imperative that nurses become culturally competent to best deal with the diverse cultures and multicultural patients. Cultural competence is defined as the ability of a system, agency, or individual to respond to the unique needs of populations whose cultures are different from that of the dominant or mainstream society (Lester, 1998a). Demographers state that there were 12 million new arrivals to the United States in the past 10 years, the largest since the period between 1905 and 1914, when 10 million immigrants came to the United States (Leininger, 1997).

Communication is one of six areas of cultural uniqueness that needs to be assessed in the initial nursing assessment, because communication and culture are intertwined. Oral and written language, gestures, facial expressions, and body language are the means by which culture is conveyed and preserved.

Cultural patterns of communication are set early in life and affect the way in which a person communicates ideas and feelings. It also affects decision making and communication methods (Lester, 1998a). Even though a cultural group shares the same communication pattern, the nurse should not assume that all members of the cultural group use the same method of expression. Cultural competence does not suggest that the nurse needs to know everything about every culture. Rather, it is thought of as the ability to develop working relationships with those who are different from the nurse. This encompasses self-awareness, cultural knowledge about illness and healing practices, intercultural communication skills, and behavioral flexibility (Lester, 1998b).

The nurse needs to be aware of the potential language barriers to effective intercultural communication. As in any attempt to establish a good nurse-client relationship, the nurse should try to understand the client's point of view and frame of reference. Respecting and allowing a free exchange of the client's and family's ideas, thoughts, and feelings can facilitate effective intercultural communication.

For clients who are not native English speakers, verbal and nonverbal barriers to effective communication can inhibit the following:

An accurate understanding of their diagnosis, progress, and prognosis

The assurance of knowing what is going on and what procedures will be done

The assurance of the expertise of the nurse and other health care providers

The ability to explain their symptoms to the nurse, to assist in their diagnosis and treatment

Therefore nurses need to make a special effort to provide these essentials to clients, such as locating an interpreter who can not only speak the client's language but also translate at the level required.

Most hospitals have lists of local interpreters who offer their services and who can communicate technical terminology to the client. For nontechnical, uncomplicated translation, the nurse can usually locate a hospital staff member who communicates in the client's own language. (Chapter 6 discusses this in greater detail.)

DIFFICULT CLIENTS

Nurses may find it difficult to communicate with clients who are aggressive, unpopular, or distressed.

Clients who exhibit *aggressive* behaviors are hostile, verbally or physically abusive, rejecting, and manipulative. These are unpleasant behaviors that are difficult to be around. This attacking style of behavior demonstrates a general lack of consideration and respect for others, and the natural response is to protect the self and reject the client. Even though the nurse's self-esteem and personal safety are under attack, they must meet the aggression assertively by setting firm limits that do not embarrass themselves or the client. Most facilities offer assault response training and education to help staff members manage these behaviors.

Unpopular clients have a variety of characteristics. Nurses naturally have likes and dislikes regarding client behaviors. The behavior that one nurse enjoys working with may be another nurse's displeasure. Some general characteristics of unpopular clients are shown in Box 8-2.

When dealing with unpopular clients, nurses often feel frustrated, angry, or fearful. These clients may be ignored, labeled as troublemakers or problems, medicated more often, admonished, and generally given less care than other clients.

Box 8-2   **General Characteristics of Unpopular Clients**

Clients who:
Claim they are more ill than nurses believe
Express their dislike of the hospital
Take up much of the nurse's time and attention
Misuse hospitalization
Are uncooperative and argumentative
Have severe, complicated problems and a poor prognosis
Have problems brought on by themselves (e.g., alcohol-related disease)
Have low morals or social stigmas
Produce feelings of incompetence in the nurse

Distressed clients express their emotional pain both verbally and nonverbally, and sometimes continuously. Becoming too involved with a client's distress can overwhelm the nurse and interfere with effective communication. Often the nurse feels inadequate dealing with severe emotional distress. It is important for the nurse to remain clearheaded and to responsibly communicate understanding and concern without becoming judgmental.

Not only must the nurse deal effectively with clients who are distressed, aggressive, and unpopular, but there are also times when the nurse has to deal with health care professionals exhibiting this same behavior. Health care can be emotionally and physically demanding, which produces stress and conflict in the health care environment. There are times when colleagues become irritated, angry, and argumentative, and occasionally even verbally abusive.

The nurse can use similar effective communication techniques when dealing with conflict in professional relationships. Conflict in health care settings has to do with responsibility conflicts, role differences and uncertainty, power issues and beliefs, and value differences. Effective communication skills are necessary to deal with a variety of conflicting professional relationships. Win-win solutions are necessary for a growth-producing outcome. Thus both parties must employ creative problem-solving techniques. Communication efforts are geared toward understanding the other person and the issues involved, employing compromise and collaboration, and avoiding competition. In these situations, nurses should communicate both assertively and responsibly, owning their part of the conflict (Northouse and Northouse, 1992).

The nurse should have the skills necessary to communicate therapeutically with clients and their families, as well as the responsibility to communicate effectively with other health professionals and throughout the health care setting using some of these same learned skills.

Summary of Key Concepts

1. The components of communication are the stimulus (reason), the sender, the message, the medium, the receiver, and feedback.
2. Communication can be influenced by environmental factors, the relationship between the sender and the receiver, the context of the communication, and the individuals' attitudes, knowledge, and perception.
3. Nonverbal communication cues involve all five senses. Ninety percent of communication is thought to be nonverbal. Verbal and nonverbal communication must be congruent for the communication to be effective.
4. Interpersonal communication—communication between two or more people—can be collegial, social, or therapeutic.
5. The three purposes of therapeutic communication are to allow the client self-expression to promote healthy growth, to understand the significance of the client's problems, and to assist in the identification and resolution of the problems.
6. Empathy is an important quality of therapeutic communication and is necessary to the success of the nurse-client relationship.
7. Some responding techniques that enhance therapeutic communication are silence, support and reassurance, giving information, restating, reflecting, clarifying, and role-playing.
8. Self-disclosure by the nurse can be an effective technique if used for the right reasons.
9. Resistance, transference, countertransference, and boundary violations can be obstacles to therapeutic communication.
10. Certain therapeutic responding techniques correspond to specific steps of the nursing process and phases of the nurse-client relationship.
11. Effective communication can be challenged by issues relating to a client's length of stay in treatment, a client's physical impairments, or language and cultural differences.

REFERENCES

Alligood MR: Empathy: the importance of recognizing two types, *J Psychosoc Nurs* 30:3, 1992.

Armstrong MA, Kelly AE: Enhancing staff nurses' interpersonal skills: theory to practice, *Clin Nurse Spec* 7:6, 1993.

Balzer-Riley J: *Communications in nursing*, ed 3, St. Louis, 1996, Mosby.

Cochrane DA et al: Patient education: do they really understand us? *Am J Nurs*, July 1992.

Ferguson MS, Campinha-Bacote J: Humor in nursing, *J Psychosoc Nurs* 26(4):29, 1989.

Fontaine KL, Fletcher JS: *Essentials of mental health nursing*, ed 2, Reading, Mass, 1995, Addison-Wesley.

Fortinash KM, Holoday-Worret PA: *Psychiatric nursing care plans*, ed 3, St. Louis, 1999, Mosby.

Kemper BJ: Therapeutic listening: developing the concept, *J Psychosoc Nurs* 30:7, 1992.

Kirkham S: Nurses' descriptions of caring for culturally diverse clients, *Clin Nurs Res* (7):125, 1998.

Leininger M: Overview of the theory of culture care with the ethnonursing research method, *J Transcult Nurs* 8(2):32, 1997.

Lester N: Cultural competence: a nursing dialogue, part I, *Am J Nurs* 98(8):26, 1998a.

Lester N: Cultural competence: a nursing dialogue, part II, *Am J Nurs* 98(9):36, 1998b.

Morse J et al: Exploring empathy: a conceptual fit for nursing practice? *Image: J Nurs Sch* 24:4, 1992.

Northouse PG, Northouse LL: *Health communication: strategies for health professionals*, ed 2, East Norwalk, Conn, 1992, Appleton & Lange.

Pike AW: On the nature and place of empathy in clinical nursing practice, *J Prof Nurs* 6(4):235, 1990.

Rowland-Morin PA, Carroll JG: Verbal communication skills and the patient satisfaction survey, *Evaluation Health Prof* 13:2, 1990.

Shives LR: *Basic concepts of psychiatric mental health nursing*, ed 3, Philadelphia, 1994, JB Lippincott.

Smith J: Privileged communication: psychiatric mental health nurses and the law, *Perspect Psychiatr Care* 26:4, 1990.

Stern SB: Privileged communication: an ethical and legal right of psychiatric clients, *Perspect Psychiatr Care* 26:4, 1990.

Stewart M: Nurses need to strengthen cultural competence for next century to ensure quality patient care, *Am Nurse*, January/February 1998.

Stricker G, Fisher M: *Self-disclosure in the therapeutic relationship*, New York, 1990, Plenum Press.

Tommasini NR: The use of touch with the hospitalized psychiatric patient, *Arch Psych Nurs* 4(4):213, 1990.

Trossman S: Diversity: a continuing challenge, *Am Nurse*, January/February 1998.

Williams C: Biopsychosocial elements of empathy: a multidimensional model, *Issues Ment Health Nurs* 11:155, 1990.

Developmental Aspects Across the Life Span

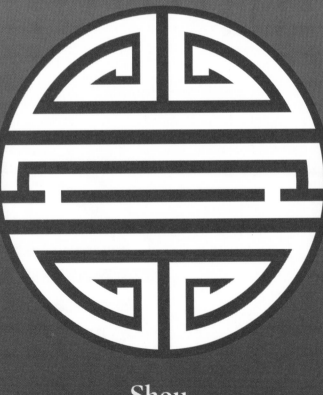

Shou
China

The Chinese Shou symbol is one of the oldest and most frequently used symbols for longevity. Included in the representation is quality of life, from birth to death. The chapters in Part Three discuss developmental issues related to children and adolescents, adults, and the elderly.

CHAPTER 9

Children and Adolescents

Diane Podsedly Oran

OBJECTIVES

- Examine the process of developmental change and the factors that influence development.

- Discuss important historical perspectives that have influenced modern ideas about development.

- Compare and contrast developmental theories and use them in trying to understand developmental progression.

- Describe the difference between normal, abnormal, resilient, and vulnerable developmental pathways.

- Discuss the effects of both genetics/nature and environment/nurture on developmental change.

Adaptation The adjustment of an individual to changing life conditions.

Autonomy versus shame and doubt Erikson's term for the second developmental crisis. Parental encouragement toward self-sufficiency in basic tasks of toileting, dressing, and feeding foster autonomy. Thwarted efforts by undercontrolling or overcontrolling parents result in the polar opposite, or shame and doubt. Shame is rage turned against the self. Doubt is an internal feeling of badness.

Behavioral reorganization A view of development emphasizing that new developmental capabilities are fitted together with previous capabilities in an orderly, patterned, and predictable fashion that builds in a cumulative manner from earlier capabilities toward greater complexity.

Concrete operations period Piaget's term for the third stage of cognitive development, in which the child begins to think and reason in logical ways about the present and past.

Conventional level of morality Kohlberg's second stage of morality, in which moral decisions consider the perspective of the victim and are first based on a desire for approval from others to avoid guilt and are later based on defined rights, assigned duty, rules of the community, and respect for authority.

Developmental contexts The necessary circumstances that must exist for development to occur. Some circumstances are related to nature (genes, inheritance), and others are related to nurture (environment).

Formal operations period Piaget's term for the fourth stage of cognitive development, in which the child learns to think in abstract and hypothetical ways about future events and learns to develop strategies for solving complex problems.

Identity versus role confusion Erikson's term for the fifth developmental crisis. Self-assurance of the previous stage leads to the adolescent's gaining a self-identity and the ability to determine where the adolescent fits in society. Failure to develop a self-identity leads to role confusion, poor self-confidence, and alienation.

Industry versus inferiority Erikson's term for the fourth developmental crisis. From the initiative achieved in the previous stage, the child develops an ability to master learning and develop peer relationships, which leads to self-assurance or industry. Failure to master academic and social pursuits leads to inferiority and hinders attempts to try new things.

Initiative versus guilt Erikson's term for the third developmental crisis. Self-sufficiency allows the child to undertake and plan tasks and join with others in cooperative effort resulting in increased initiative. If the child's desire to show initiative causes excessive conflict in the family, guilt results.

Postconventional level of morality Kohlberg's third stage of morality, in which moral decisions reflect underlying ethical principles that consider societal needs and are first based on a sense of community respect and disrespect and are later based on principles of justice, the reciprocity and quality of human rights, and respect for the dignity of human beings as individuals.

Preconventional level of morality Kohlberg's first stage of morality, in which moral decisions are self-centered and the child's behavior is first based on avoidance of punishment and is later based on a desire to gain rewards or benefits.

Preoperational period Piaget's term for the second stage of cognitive development, in which the child remains egocentric, is oriented in the present, and only guesses about cause and effect.

Self-system Sullivan's term for the system that infants develop to cope with anxiety associated with the interpersonal process of need satisfaction and security. The individual develops self-appraisal as a result of significant others' responses to actions by the individual. Actions that cause anxiety result in "bad me" self-appraisals. Actions that cause no anxiety result in "good me" self-appraisals. Actions of disapproval cause severe anxiety, emotional withdrawal, and "not me" self-appraisals.

Sensorimotor period Piaget's term for the first stage of cognitive development, in which children use their senses and motor skills to manipulate the environment and develop the ability to differentiate self from objects.

Social learning The process by which children acquire the behaviors they need to survive and function in society. The behaviors result from repeated interactions in their environments.

Trust versus mistrust Erikson's term for the first developmental crisis that the child tries to resolve. Consistent, predictable, and continuous care results in developing a sense of trust in oneself, others, and the world. Inconsistent, unpredictable, or discontinuous care results in the polar opposite, or mistrust of oneself, others, and the world.

This chapter discusses development from birth through adolescence, focusing on both traditional theories of child development and emerging new theories from current research. Human development involves complex variables and processes. The purpose of this chapter is to help readers understand some of these variables and processes, and integrate knowledge of development into their overall understanding of psychiatric mental health nursing.

THEORETIC AND HISTORICAL PERSPECTIVES OF DEVELOPMENT

A developmental perspective includes several views of the ways in which children grow and change over time. At any one time children are expected to achieve certain tasks called milestones. In addition to milestones, developmental theorists have identified stages or life periods during which changes in emotional, cognitive, and social development emerge. Understanding how children develop involves more than knowing what a child should be achieving at a particular time. Developmental changes occur in an orderly fashion, building in a cumulative manner from the capacities that the child accrued earlier, in a direction of greater complexity. The rate and manner in which the individual develops and changes is coherent and remains relatively consistent. The 1-year-old child who walked and began pointing at an early age will probably be running in a coordinated manner and talking with more sophisticated sentences earlier than another child who may have been generally slower. Through a process called **behavioral reorganization,** the toddling of a 1-year-old paves the way for the running of the same child at age 3. The 1-year-old's pointing builds up to the 3-year-old's more complex communication of using sentences. The threads of continuity over time are as much a part of development as is change (Stroufe, Cooper, and DeHart, 1992).

Development has been observed to occur with remarkable consistency and orderliness through generations of observations. Developmental change depends on three factors: (1) a preexisting developmental plan built into the organism, (2) the individual's prior developmental history, and (3) supportive environmental conditions (Stroufe, Cooper, and DeHart, 1992). Each individual has a set of genes that are expressed in a time frame that has been set in motion since birth. The exact moment specific genes are expressed in observable developmental changes (phenotype) depends on current environmental support (e.g., nutrients, opportunity, challenges, encouragement, circumstances). Scar (1992) described examples of gene-environment interactions: "Feeding a well-nourished but short-statured genotype will not give them the stature of a basketball player. Feeding a below-average intellect more information will not make them brilliant. Exposing a shy child to socially demanding events will not make them feel less shy. The child with below-average intellect and

the shy child may gain some specific skills and helpful knowledge of how to behave in specific situations, but their enduring intellectual and personality characteristics will not be fundamentally changed."

The mechanism by which genetics and environment interact to produce developmental change is still not fully understood; however, important clues can be traced back to the evolutionary theory of Charles Darwin.

Darwin's work focused on evolution of various animal species. Two views of human development regarding heredity and environment can be traced to the philosophies of John Locke and Jean-Jacques Rousseau. Locke saw the human infant as a *tabula rasa*, a blank slate to be written on by life's experiences. Rousseau saw children as individuals from birth and believed that human development unfolds naturally. Rousseau believed that maturation takes a natural course without much need for shaping from parents or caretakers. Locke's work can be traced to contemporary social learning theory, which stresses the importance of rewards and punishments in shaping development. Rousseau's work can be traced to modern maturational theories, which focus on stage-specific development (Stroufe, Cooper, and DeHart, 1992).

There has been and continues to be a debate regarding how much of development is related to nature versus nurture and biology versus culture (Baumrind, 1993; Jackson, 1993; Scar, 1993). This debate is discussed under Developmental Contexts.

THEORIES OF DEVELOPMENT

There are several theories that try to explain how and why children develop. Several theories of development are presented here.

PSYCHOSEXUAL THEORY

The psychosexual theory of development was formed by Sigmund Freud (1856-1939). Freud's ideas of development resulted from his work with adult clients who suffered from hysterias and unexplained paralyses. In trying to understand the cause of his adult clients' illnesses, he encouraged clients to talk about and explore childhood experiences, using various techniques such as asking them to talk freely about childhood memories and hypnosis. Freud suspected that the root of their problems could be traced to early childhood traumas. He believed that early trauma causes intense feelings but, because the child is immature, these feelings cannot be expressed.

In describing how the personality develops, Freud believed that the infant begins life in a selfish, internal, uncivilized state with basic instincts that are aimed at self-preservation and self-gratification. Through interactions with parents the infant learns that selfish behaviors are not always tolerated, which causes conflict.

Within the first few years of life, according to Freud,

Table 9-1	Psychosexual Theory—Freud		

Development results from sexual aim or biologic need for tension reduction. The goal of development is maximizing need gratification while minimizing punishment and guilt, using defenses to control anxiety.

Stage	Age (Yr)	Basic Concepts	Developmental Issues
Oral	0-1	Id	Internalized, selfish, unable to delay gratification of needs. Primary activities: receiving and taking; major conflict: feeding
Anal	2-3	Ego	Develops ability to delay gratification of impulses and self-control; responds to external limits. Primary activity: giving and withholding; major conflict: bowel training.
Phallic	3-5	Superego	Learns values and rules from parents; development of guilt and self-esteem. Primary activity: heterosexual interactions; major conflicts: Oedipus/Electra in boys and girls, respectively.
Latency	6-12	Sexuality repressed	Mastery of learning: focus is on relationship with same-sex peers.
Genital	13	Mature sexuality	Combines learning of pregenital stages; develops ability to love and work.

the ego evolves and is the individual's sense of reality. The ego serves as mediator between the id (primitive drives) and the superego (conscience and values). Freud's psychoanalytic theory is described in Chapter 3.

According to Freud's early theory, all behavior is motivated by a desire to satisfy biologic needs and release tension. The amount of frustration or gratification the child wishes to release is expressed through different body zones during the course of development. Freud described development in terms of psychosexual stages (Maddi, 1972). A summary of Freud's theory is found in Table 9-1.

Freud (1923) believed that conflict shapes a person's life. Human beings are caught in opposition of the two great forces: one force being the selfish, evil individual and the other force being the good society. Life, according to Freud, is at best a compromise. In attempting to maximize instinctual gratification while minimizing punishment and guilt, the individual employs defenses. Whenever an instinct (need) becomes strong enough to make a difference, an alarm reaction occurs in the form of anxiety. This anxiety reaction represents the anticipation of punishment and guilt based on remembrance of past punishment and guilt and triggers the defensive process. The defensive process balances the two conflicting forces, thereby leading to tolerance of life.

When the inevitable conflict encountered at each psychosexual stage is minimal in intensity, the stage is successfully passed through. However, when the parents or caretakers intensify the conflict by depriving or indulging the child unduly or inconsistently, growth is arrested, or stopped, through the occurrence of massive defensiveness aimed at avoiding anxiety through avoiding conflict. Therefore conflict in manageable doses encourages maturation, whereas conflict in massive doses arrests development and causes immaturity or fixation at that level of development. If growth is fixated at one particular stage of development, the individual will operate and adapt to the defenses at the stage in which he or she is fixated. The

stage in which one becomes fixated determines the character one carries through life.

The major defenses of the oral character are projection (attributing to others an objectionable quality that the individual possesses), denial (failing to perceive some threatening object in the external world), and introjection (becoming like another person to avoid threats posed by the other person or by one's own needs).

The major defenses of the anal character are intellectualization (making socially acceptable excuses for one's wishes or actions), reaction formation (substituting the direct opposite wishes or feelings for one's true wishes or feelings), isolation (severing the links between thoughts and feelings to enable one to consciously tolerate an unpleasant or threatening situation), and undoing or restitution (using certain thoughts and actions to cancel out or atone for previous thoughts or actions).

The major defense of the phallic character is repression (the active removal from consciousness of instinctual wishes and actions that are threatening). The genital character has sublimation as its major defense (socially unacceptable impulses are channeled into socially acceptable activities).

PSYCHOSOCIAL THEORY

Unlike Freud, who believed that the personality is completely formed in childhood, Erik Erikson (1963) believed that development continues throughout the life span. Whereas Freud attributed development to a sexual aim or biologic need for tension reduction expressed through different body zones, Erikson attributed development to social interactions and relationships. Erikson rejected Freud's belief that a child is fixated in a developmental stage as a result of not having his or her needs met. Erikson, instead, described a series of developmental tasks or lessons that all individuals must face and resolve. Failure to resolve the task at a particular stage of the life cycle results in an extension of the developmental period but allows for

Table 9-2	Psychosocial Theory—Erikson			
Development results from social aims or conflicts arising from feelings, parent-child interaction, and social relationships.				
Stage	**Age (Yr)**	**Virtue**	**Developmental Issues**	
Trust versus mistrust	0-1	Sense of hope	Care that satisfies basic oral and sensory needs (feeding, cuddling, and bowel relaxation) develops trust in self and world. Inconsistent, unpredictable, discontinuous care develops mistrust in self and world.	
Autonomy versus shame and doubt	1-3	Sense of willpower	Satisfying needs for autonomy and free choice results in child's developing impulse control and mastery of toileting, dressing, feeding, and separation from parents. Undercontrolling or overcontrolling parental behavior results in shame and doubt in abilities.	
Initiative versus guilt	3-6	Sense of purpose	Learns to plan tasks and join with others in cooperation and pretend play. Accepts responsibility and is enthusiastic about helping. If desire to show initiative causes excessive conflict in family, guilt results.	
Industry versus inferiority	7-11	Sense of competence	Focus on learning and mastery of skills. Success in peer interactions leads to self-assurance. Failure to master academic and social pursuits leads to inferiority and hinders attempts to try new things.	
Identity versus role confusion	12-18	Sense of fidelity	Concerned with how others view him or her. Begins to make occupational choices and fit in society. Development of self-identity leads to making long-term goals, self-esteem, and emotional stability. Failure to develop self-identity leads to role confusion, poor self-confidence, alienation, acting out, and no occupational choice.	

a gradual movement toward later developmental issues. Furthermore, Erikson placed more emphasis on the quality of parent-child interaction and the responsiveness and dependability of parents in fostering development, rather than merely emphasizing the quantity of gratification or lack of gratification. Erikson described development in terms of eight psychosocial crises or stages. Along with each stage, Erikson associated a specific psychosocial strength or basic virtue that emerges from the struggles that occur during each stage (Erikson, 1982). Erikson's psychosocial theory is summarized in Table 9-2.

Trust versus mistrust occurs during the first year of life. Through satisfying basic oral and sensory needs, the infant's ability to demonstrate social trust is noted in the ease in feeding, depth of sleep, and relaxation of the bowels (Erikson, 1963). Infants who receive outer predictable, consistent, and continuous care develop a sense of trust and feelings of inner goodness, or beginnings of self-worth. Infants who receive inconsistent, unpredictable, or discontinuous care may grow to mistrust themselves and the people in their world. The infant's first social achievement is the willingness to let the primary caretaker out of sight without undue anxiety or rage because of the inner conflict that develops from the outer predictability of consistent care. This is the beginning of the development of the

ego, or self. The psychosocial strength that emerges from a basic trust in the world is a sense of hope. If children do not resolve the issue of basic trust in themselves and the world, they will have a mistrustful disposition toward the challenges that must be confronted in the next stage of development.

Autonomy versus shame and doubt occurs during the first through the third year of life. The child's ability to develop muscular maturation (including anal) sets the stage for experimentation in the social area of holding on and letting go. Children learn a sense of impulse control and conforming to social rules if they are provided with parental guidance in the areas of autonomy and free choice. These opportunities for parent-supported autonomy lead to self-sufficiency in mastering tasks such as toileting, dressing, and feeding themselves, and a gradual ability to separate from their parents. Children whose efforts toward autonomy are thwarted by undercontrolling or overcontrolling parental behavior are not allowed to develop mutual regulation in the parent-child relationship. This lack of child autonomy results in feelings of shame and doubt for the child. Erikson (1963) described shame as rage turned against the self. A shamed child does not wish to be seen. Doubt is the internal feeling of badness that accompanies shame. This stage, according to Erikson, be-

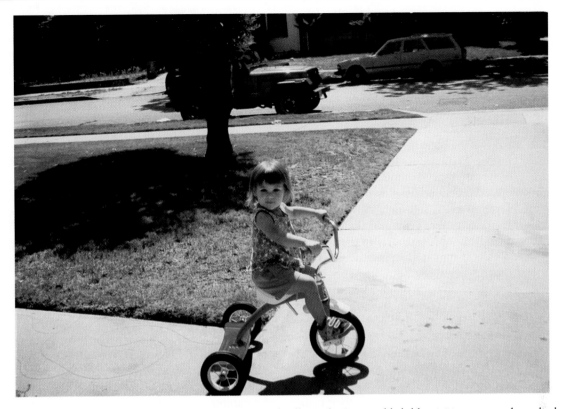

Figure 9-1   Self-sufficiency in mastering basic tasks autonomously allows the 3-year-old child to initiate new tasks and take pleasure in being active.

comes important for the child's development in the ability to develop a balance between love and hate, cooperation and willfulness, and freedom of expression or suppression. The psychosocial strength that emerges from a sense of self-control and autonomy without loss of self-esteem and without shame and doubt is a sense of willpower.

Initiative versus guilt occurs during the third to sixth year of life. At this stage children have a burst of energy. This energy allows them to add initiative to the autonomy gained in the previous stage (Figure 9-1). Initiative involves the ability to undertake and plan tasks, the ability to take pleasure in being active, and the development of a sense of purpose. Children take pleasure in attack and conquest, which leads to developing sexual identity and roles. The child's developing conscience helps to control initiative. The child learns to join with other children in a cooperative effort through pretend play and begins to identify with adults and imitate adult-desired behaviors. They recognize adult roles, functions, and responsibilities, and they begin to develop a work identification by showing interest in adult occupations. For example, children at this stage generally show excitement in the presence of a police officer, fire fighter, physician, or nurse. The child begins to accept responsibility and has an enthusiastic desire to help with household chores. Sometimes the child's desire for initiative creates conflicts with other family members, and these conflicts can create guilt. For instance, a

3-year-old child may show an intense interest in wanting to help a parent wash expensive china after a holiday meal. This desire may conflict with the parent's concern that the china may get broken. A parent who wishes to foster the child's initiative might allow the child to simultaneously wash unbreakable dishes. Excessive guilt inhibits initiative. Children resolve the crises by learning to balance initiative against parental demands (Stroufe, Cooper, and DeHart, 1992). The psychosocial strength that develops from initiative without excessive guilt is a sense of purpose.

Industry versus inferiority occurs during the seventh through the eleventh year of life. From the initiative and budding interest in work identification of the earlier stage, children are able to focus on the tasks of learning and of preparation for a career. In all cultures, at this stage children receive systematic instruction. The major task achieved is industry, or the ability to master increasingly difficult skills. Because industry involves doing things with others, it is a decisive and important stage in the development of social interaction with peers (Erikson, 1963). Children whose industry enables them to succeed in peer interactions and academic performance develop a sense of mastery and self-assurance. Children who fail to master academic and social pursuits develop a sense of inferiority and inadequacy, which hinders their attempts to try new activities. The psychosocial strength that develops from industry rather than inferiority is a sense of competence.

Identity versus role confusion occurs during the twelfth through the eighteenth year. With the mastery of social and academic skills of the previous stage and the onset of puberty, childhood ends and adolescence begins. Adolescents are primarily concerned with how they are perceived in the eyes of others compared with how they feel about themselves (Erikson, 1963). They also begin to apply the skills learned at earlier stages and connect them to occupational choices. The task of the adolescent is to develop an identity, which involves finding one's place in society, committing to a career, and developing a confident sense of self. Developing a strong self-identity results in an ability to work toward long-term goals and the development of self-esteem and emotional stability. In their search for an identity, adolescents may temporarily overidentify with cliques and crowds. They can be remarkably petty, clannish, and cruel in their exclusion of others who are different in color, manner, or dress, and they tend to develop "in crowds" and "out crowds" (Erikson, 1963). Adolescents who fail to develop a self-identity or who already have self-doubts as to where they fit in society run the risk of role confusion, and they may lack self-confidence, feel alienated, display acting-out behaviors, and feel confused regarding occupational choices and the roles they must perform as adults. The psychosocial strength that emerges from the development of identity rather than role confusion is fidelity or loyalty.

Erikson's psychosocial theory can be visualized as a bucket. At each stage, new developmental achievements are added to the bucket. If trust is added to the bucket, it is fuller than if mistrust is added, but the bucket can still be added to. If there is trust, the bucket will likely be filled fuller with autonomy, initiative, industry, and identity. If there is mistrust, the bucket will likely be filled fuller with shame and doubt, guilt, inferiority, and role confusion. This is an important concept in psychosocial theory. Although children may experience developmental stalls, they do not necessarily get fixated at any one stage; they still move on, but their developmental bucket may not be as full if each developmental challenge is not resolved. Unsuccessful resolution of each developmental challenge may present difficulties for the child in accomplishing the positive tasks of the next stage.

INTERPERSONAL THEORY

The interpersonal theory was developed by Harry Stack Sullivan (1882-1949). Sullivan was one of the first prominent American-born psychiatrists. Much of his work in understanding development came from his work with adult clients with schizophrenia and neuroses. He believed that individuals' development results from their interpersonal relationships with others. Whereas Freud viewed development in terms of an intrapersonal process of maximizing instinctual gratification while minimizing punishment and guilt, Sullivan believed that an individual's development results from interpersonal relationships in which satisfaction of needs is maximized while insecurity is minimized (Maddi, 1972). According to Sullivan, satisfaction includes biologic needs such as food, water, air, sex, and excretion. Satisfaction also includes psychologic needs such as desire for power and physical closeness. In trying to meet individual or selfish needs, there is an unavoidable interpersonal conflict from others in the form of disapproval. A fear of disapproval threatens the individual's sense of security, creating anxiety. The individual develops mechanisms to cope with anxiety. Thus an individual's development is motivated by a need for social conformity and a desire to satisfy biologic and psychologic needs with minimal disapproval from others and minimal loss of security. Rather than describing development in terms of stages, Sullivan described development in six eras. Sullivan's eras are summarized in Table 9-3.

The *infancy era* occurs during the first 2 years of life and ends with maturation of language capacity. Infants are essentially dependent on others for meeting biologic survival needs. Infants are in a *prototaxic mode* (unable to differentiate themselves from the outside world). The parents' moods are communicated to the child by an empathic process in which the child feels anxiety when the parents are annoyed by the infant's neediness or crying, and feels good when the parents show approval in the form of tenderness. Gradually the infant learns to differentiate self from others and determines that comfort and discomfort are connected to the caregiver. Sullivan termed this differentiation the *parataxic mode*. The infant develops a **self-system** to cope with anxiety surrounding need gratification. When the "good mother" meets the infant's needs and shows a positive mood and approval, the child develops a sense that Sullivan called "the good me." When needs are not met and the caregiver shows a negative mood and mild disapproval, the child develops a sense that Sullivan called "the bad me" with accompanying anxiety. The infant is trained through repeated interactions (trial and error) to avoid negative parental mood and the accompanying anxiety it carries for the infant. For example, during toilet training, at first the infant has no control over the bowels. Gradually, as children show signs of an ability to toilet (physical maturation and motor skills of being able to pull their pants up and down), parents introduce toileting and praise the child for desired toileting. When inevitable accidents occur, most parents show a mild level of frustration with having to change soiled clothes. This parental mood is transformed into anxiety for the child. In an attempt to avoid anxiety and relieve the tension of excretion, the child learns that "potty makes Mommy happy and me too." This mild form of anxiety helps to train the child. On the other hand, if the child experiences extreme disapproval and parental frustration and unrealistic or excessively punitive responses, the child may develop a sense that Sullivan termed the "not me." This causes severe anxiety and emotional withdrawal.

Table 9-3	**Interpersonal Theory—Sullivan**		

Development results from interpersonal relationships with others in maximizing satisfaction of needs while minimizing insecurity.

Era	Age (Yr)	Basic Concepts	Developmental Issues
Infancy	0-2	Trial-and-error learning from parental interactions of tenderness or annoyance molds development; ends with language development	Infant learns to differentiate self from others and that comfort and discomfort are connected to caregiver: parataxic mode. Develops self-system: "good me" from positive parental mood, "bad me" from negative parental mood with mild anxiety, and "not me" from extreme parental disapproval with severe anxiety and emotional withdrawal.
Childhood	2-6	Language development allows child to be educated, not trained	Language takes on symbolic function of communication. Self-system continues to develop with sublimation (expression of impulses in socially acceptable ways) or develops malevolent transformation (a feeling of living among enemies).
Juvenile	6-10	Relations with peers allow children to see themselves objectively	Increased peer interactions help to give child feedback from others and widen sphere of interactions to include society. Develops conscience. Self-system develops internalized reputation and cultural stereotypes. Able to distinguish fantasy and reality and develop syntaxic communication (a mature method of communicating): their own behavior is connected to others' opinions of them.
Preadolescent	10-13	Develops same-sex chums	Transition from egocentrism to love. Development of chumships helps to validate personal worth through collaboration and mutual satisfaction of needs. Able to work with peers toward a common goal and develop sense of oneness. All for one and one for all.
Adolescent	13-17	Lust: interest in sexual activity	Sexual attractions allow adolescent to test the waters of intimacy. If attractions are severely discouraged or thwarted by adults, the adolescent will feel insecure and lonely.
Late adolescent	17-19	Personality integration	Able to become genuinely intimate with others by integrating needs of society without excessive insecurity or anxiety. Inability to achieve personality integration results in regression and egocentrism for life.

Without either good or bad emotions, the infant is confused and does not know what to do.

If potty training begins too early or the child receives excessively punitive responses to soiling, the child's anxiety will interfere with training, and the child will not be able to associate the parent's mood with release of excretion or any other form of relief.

The *childhood era* begins in the second year with the onset of language development and ends around the sixth year or when the child develops a need for peers. With language development, the child can be educated rather than merely trained through trial and error. Language takes on a symbolic function of communication. The self-system ("good me," "bad me," "not me") continues to develop under the influence of the caregivers. If relations with caregivers are in the range of tenderness and mild disapproval ("good me" and "bad me") without continuous extreme disapproval ("not me"), the child develops the unconscious defense mechanism of sublimation (expression of impulses in socially acceptable ways). One especially important negative development, which Sullivan termed *malevolent transformation* (a feeling of living among enemies), can occur during the childhood era. With the continued development in the self-system via parental influence, the child develops feelings of fear of disapproval, anger, and resentment. If these feelings become too strong, the child is unable to respond positively to the affectionate advances of others (Maddi, 1972). Sullivan (1953) described these children as mischievous, who may progress to become bullies who take out their anger and resentment on younger family members, pets, or other children. Parent-communicated malevolence educates the child to become malevolent (malicious, spiteful, ill willed).

The *juvenile era* begins around age 6 years with the emergence of a need for peers and lasts through most of the elementary school years; it ends around the tenth year when there is a need for close relationships. During this era the child is surrounded by peers and adults other than their parents, such as teachers and neighbors. With this widening social sphere of experience, juveniles are able to look at themselves more objectively, develop a conscience, and begin to function in society. Along with increased peer interaction comes the development of rivalry, competition, and compromise. School-age children develop "in groups" and "out groups" and engage in various forms of ostracism among their group members. At this stage security is not based solely on parental approval, but it also involves a reputation in a broader social sense (Maddi, 1972). In the juvenile era cultural stereotypes with relation to the self-system develop. The youngster begins to see the self in terms of being a Protestant, a Jew, a tough guy, or a nice guy (Maddi, 1972; Sullivan, 1953). The juvenile also learns to distinguish more clearly between fantasy and reality and develops the mature mode of communicating and experiencing, termed *syntaxis*. This mode is characterized by a full appreciation of the logical interrelatedness of various symbols and the recognition and acceptance of their consensual meaning. The child realizes that similar behaviors result in similar opinions about their behavior, from parents and other adults, as well as from peers.

Sullivan described what he called supervisory patterns that emerge from the self-system and the developing personality during the juvenile era. Sullivan termed the first supervisory pattern *the hearer*. The hearer judges the approval of what one says to others. The hearer develops an internal sense of the extent to which others want to listen to what the juvenile has to say. The second supervisory pattern is *the spectator*. The spectator pays attention to what is shown to others and done with others. It warns the self-system when interactions are not right or if there is a need to cover up for breaches in relating. The third supervisory pattern is *the reader*. This pattern pays attention to others' responses to what one writes. Sullivan believed that he was a poor writer and thus wrote almost nothing. Most of Sullivan's work came through others' interpretations of what he lectured or taught. Sullivan (1953) believed that these supervisory patterns, developed in the juvenile era, remain (with some refinements) with each individual from that time on.

The *preadolescent era* begins around age 10 and ends with the onset of puberty and beginning interest in the opposite sex around the age of 12 or 13. The preadolescent makes the transition from egocentrism to love (Maddi, 1972). The basis for the transition comes from the need to develop relationships with same-sex friends. These friendships help validate personal worth through collaboration.

The collaborative relationship is based on a process of learning to adjust to the needs of others, as well as one's own needs and reaching mutual satisfaction of needs. The preadolescent is able to work with peers toward a common goal and develop a sense of oneness (e.g., the success of "our" team or dislike of "our" teacher) (Sullivan, 1953). The peer relationships of this era are marked by equality, mutuality, and reciprocity. From these peer experiences, the preadolescent is able to transcend the stereotypes of the juvenile era (Maddi, 1972).

The early *adolescent era* begins with puberty, genital interest, and sexual attractions. Sullivan termed this attraction *lust*. Sullivan believed that lust was often on a collision course with other needs for personal security, freedom from anxiety, and intimacy. Lust, according to Sullivan, is extremely powerful and creates anxiety in connection with the adolescent's newfound motivation toward sexual activity. If attractions are not met or are severely prevented by parents, there may be a loss of self-esteem and personal worth, thereby threatening one's personal security and needs for intimacy. For example, the early adolescent has lustful attractions; however, parents may severely ridicule and prohibit interactions because of their fears of sexually transmitted diseases or pregnancy. Without opportunities to "test the waters" of intimacy, the adolescent is left feeling lonely. Sullivan also described the collision between lust and needs for personal security, freedom from anxiety, and intimacy when the early adolescent is labeled a "good" or "bad" girl in regard to sexual experimentation. For example, the young girl may be viewed as "good" by adults if she does not experiment sexually. On the other hand, she may be viewed unfavorably or "bad" by peers who have had sexual experiences, and therefore be made to feel that she does not meet their expectations, as a result of her sexual inexperience.

The *late adolescent era* begins when the adolescent is able to integrate the needs of society without being overwhelmed with anxiety. The adolescent who does not experience extreme opposition during the previous eras is able to become genuinely intimate with others. The adolescent who is presented with problems in personality integration that are extremely difficult to solve may regress to the juvenile era, thereby losing the values of the preadolescent era. This results in a personality that is essentially egocentric for life (Maddi, 1972). An individual with an egocentric perspective would have difficulty meeting the need for social conformity, which Sullivan believed was at the core of developing satisfactory interpersonal relationships. Sullivan believed that human development primarily results from the learning that individuals gain from their interpersonal relationships within the context of their environments.

COGNITIVE THEORY

Jean Piaget (1896-1980) was a Swiss psychologist whose work centered primarily on how humans develop intelligence in terms of structure and function. Unlike Freud, who studied adult clients, Piaget directly observed how infants and children develop intelligence, which he believed then allows them to have increasingly effective and more organized interactions with the environment. Piaget believed that all individuals are born with a tendency to organize and adapt to the environment, and he described the basic organizational units of learning as schemas. A *schema* is a mental image or action pattern. Schemas may be simple, such as an innate reflex, or complicated, such as a task requiring several steps. Piaget believed that environmental adaptation occurs in observable periods through the complementary processes of assimilation and accommodation. Assimilation occurs when new experiences are incorporated into preexisting experiences. Accommodation occurs when a new experience requires some new way of thinking or a modification of preexisting experiences. For instance, when a child who has been fed solely baby formula is introduced to apple juice, the child may assimilate the introduction of apple juice (a new experience) into the preexisting experience of formula. However, when the child is introduced to solid food, the child must accommodate to the new experience because a

spoon and a different texture are introduced. Piaget defined cognitive development in four general periods, with each period building cumulatively from the one before. Piaget believed that a complete mastery of period-specific achievements was not necessary for development to progress to the next period. He was more interested in the process of development of cognitive skills than in time frames. Piaget's cognitive theory is summarized in Table 9-4.

The **sensorimotor period** occurs from birth to 2 years. Initially the infant is unable to differentiate self from others or objects and shows only innate, preprogrammed reflexes such as grasping and sucking. Intelligence emerges when the baby begins to recognize objects and grasp for them and begins to suck on a nipple or pacifier for need gratification rather than from a reflex action (Figure 9-2). The discovery of how actions can lead to outcomes develops through trial and error. Piaget termed this discovery *instrumentality*. By the end of the sensorimotor period, the infant is able to differentiate self from objects, a process known as *decentering*, and develops *object permanence*, which means that the child realizes that an object is in a given area even when it is thrust out of the child's visual

Table 9-4	**Cognitive Development—Piaget**		

Development results from a tendency to organize and adapt to the environment. Intelligence development allows children to have increasingly effective and more organized interactions with the environment.

Stage	Age (Yr)	Basic Concepts	Developmental Issues
Sensorimotor	0-2	In-the-moment thinking: ability to differentiate self from objects	Child moves from reflexive action to instrumentability: actions lead to outcomes through trial and error. Develops decentering: ability to differentiate self from objects. Develops object permanence: ability to hold mental representations when objects or people are out of sight.
Preoperational	2-7	Here-and-now thinking: uses symbols and words to represent objects, actions, people, and places not present	Engages in pretend (symbolic) play. Remains egocentric: unable to take another's point of view. Cannot distinguish reality from fantasy. Acquires language. Only intuitively guesses about cause and effect. Time is oriented in present only. Can only focus on one emotion at a time. Beginning development of self-system. Noncontested respect for authority.
Concrete operational	7-11	Past and present thinking	Able to conserve: understands that physical properties such as volume and length remain the same when there are changes in shape, group, or position. Able to reverse operations. Able to decenter: relates two classifications at one time. Able to think about past and present events but not future. Begins to appreciate perspective of others.
Formal operational	11-16	Future thinking	Able to think in abstract and hypothetical terms. Able to ponder what might be rather than just what is. Can think of future events and develop strategies for solving complex problems.

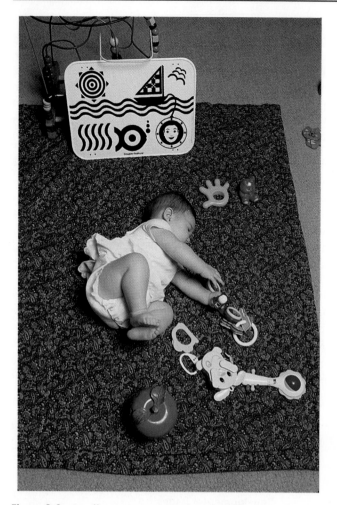

Figure 9-2 Intelligence emerges when the baby starts to recognize objects and reach for them. (Copyright Cathy Lander-Goldberg, Lander Photographics)

to understand symbolic representation enables the child to remember emotions longer in the absence of provocative conditions. There is a beginning ability to experience feelings of inferiority and superiority toward the self (self-esteem). A noncontested respect for authority begins to emerge.

The **concrete operations period** occurs during ages 7 to 11. The child is able to understand the concept of conservation and can recognize that manipulation of objects is reversible. The child is able to decenter (focus on and coordinate) two or more concepts, such as height and width or longer and shorter, at one time. The child can recognize that a dimension such as narrowness compensates for the dimension of height. The child is able to imagine a series of events and think about past and present events but cannot envision future events or what might be. He or she is unable to think logically or abstractly. The child begins to appreciate the perspective of others and develops moral sentiments such as feelings of justice, honesty, and camaraderie. He or she develops an ability to integrate and experience more than one emotion at the same time.

The **formal operations period** emerges at around age 11 and fully develops by age 16, although some adults never completely develop formal operations (Sternberg, 1990). During this period the child learns to think in abstract and hypothetical terms rather than merely concretely. The child develops an ability to understand ideas about what might be rather than simply what is (Stroufe, Cooper, and DeHart, 1992). The child learns to think of future events and can develop systematic strategies for solving abstract and complex problems. Teenagers learn to take on the role of devil's advocate and are able to construct logical arguments and see errors in others' logic.

ADAPTATION THEORY

John Bowlby (1908-1990) was an English psychiatrist who was influenced by Freud and Meyer. Bowlby gave credit to Freud for his ideas that an individual's internal world influences the way people learn to think, feel, and behave in terms of how they perceive, construe, and structure events and situations they encounter (Bowlby, 1988a, 1988b). In addition to Freud's theory of internal drives influencing development, Bowlby gave credit to Adolf Meyer for Meyer's emphasis on the role of events and situations people experience and how environment can influence development.

Bowlby believed that the crux of human development lies in the strength of the infant's attachment to the caretaker and in the strength of the caretaker's bond with the infant (Figure 9-3). Bowlby was also influenced by Darwin's evolutionary theory and believed that the infant and caretaker are preprogrammed. The infant gives out signals of distress, and the caretaker responds in relation to the intensity of the infant's signal. Sometimes the signal is of low intensity, and the caretaker's response of coming closer to the infant will generally satisfy the infant. At other times

field. Thus if a toy is hidden or dropped from a high chair, the 2-year-old child will look for the object. Where the infant operated under the assumption of "out of sight, out of mind," the 2-year-old child begins to hold mental representations when objects or people are out of sight.

The second period is the **preoperational period,** which occurs from ages 2 through 7. During this period the child is able to use mental symbols and words to represent objects and actions, and people and places not present. The child can now engage in pretend (symbolic) play. The child remains egocentric and is unable to take another's point of view, and he or she has difficulties distinguishing reality from fantasy. There is an acquisition of language. Intelligence is intuitive, and the child only guesses about cause and effect. The child is unable to relate two classifications at one time (centrality). Time is oriented in the present only. Emotional states fluctuate, and the child can focus on only one emotion at a time (e.g., either love or hate). One minute the child loves his or her parents, and the next minute the child hates them. The child's ability

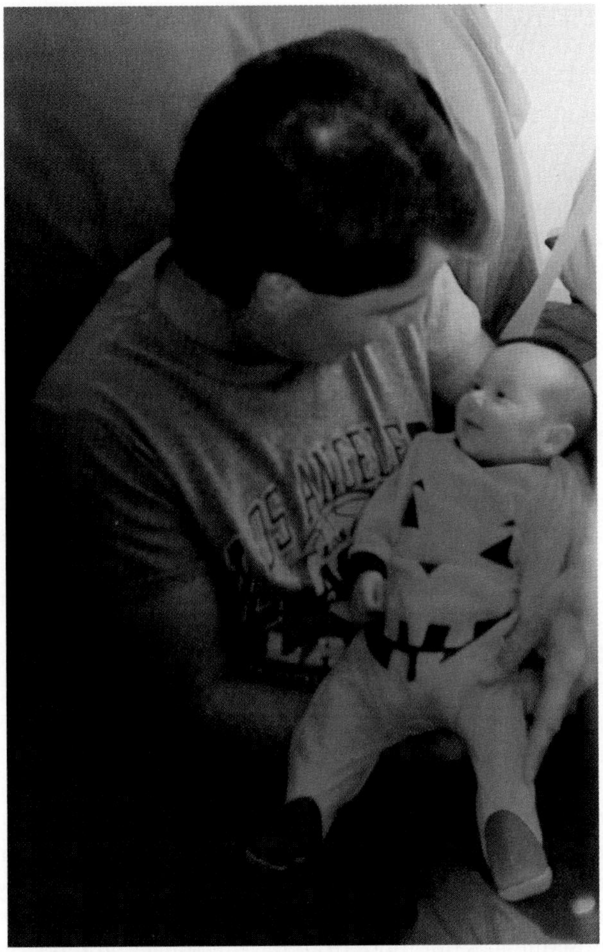

Figure 9-3 The crux of human development lies in the strength of the infant's attachment to the caretaker and in the strength of the caretaker's bond to the infant.

the signal is of high intensity, and nothing but a prolonged cuddle will do. The biologic function of this signal response pattern was postulated to be protection, especially protection from predators (Bowlby, 1988a, 1988b). Through hours of repeated interactions of signals and responses, the infant develops a generalized expectation about caretaker responses and the infant's own role in producing these reactions. Bowlby called these expectations internal working models of self and parent and believed that, once formed, they guide future social interactions (Stroufe, Cooper, and DeHart, 1992). When parenting behavior is consistent and responsive, the infant develops a sense that he or she has a secure base, or attachment. When parenting is inconsistent, nonresponsive, or overresponsive, an insecure attachment results. Bowlby believed that secure or insecure attachments are profoundly influenced by the way parents treat the child. Bowlby's (1988a, 1988b) central concept of parenting was that both parents need to provide a secure base from which a child or an adolescent can travel into the outside world, and to which he or she can return, knowing that he or she

will be welcomed when returning home, nourished physically and emotionally, comforted if distressed, and reassured if frightened. The parenting role is one of being available, ready to respond when asked to encourage and perhaps assist, but intervening actively only when clearly necessary. Without a secure attachment and feeling of security, the individual develops anxiety about exploring the world, or feels that he or she will be rebuffed or rejected.

Bowlby described securely attached children as cheerful, cooperative, popular, resilient, and resourceful, and insecurely attached children as hostile, antisocial, impulsive, passive, helpless, or attention seeking.

Although Bowlby considered the security of the child's base as central to normal development, he recognized that developmental pathways can be influenced by changing life conditions. For instance, an insecurely attached child who has an internal working model of helplessness and defeatism may be positively influenced by a caring teacher whose encouragement, support, and nurturing help promote a healthy developmental pathway. Conversely, a child with a secure base who loses a parent through death may select a vulnerable pathway. Bowlby termed this process of life **adaptation.**

A recent example of the adaptation theory can be seen in the life of Olympic figure skating gold medal winner Oksana Baiul. Oksana's father abandoned her when she was young, and she was raised as an only child by her mother, who helped form a secure base for Oksana. When Oksana was 16, her mother died of ovarian cancer. Oksana was left vulnerable without a secure base. Her developmental pathway had the potential to deviate from normal. However, her life situation changed, and her base became secure again when her figure skating coach assumed the role of "mother." Oksana's resiliency (obtained from her early secure base with her natural mother) allowed her to face extreme adversity (losing her mother) and become an Olympic champion. After winning her gold medal, she said that through all the stress of competition and loss, her mother was always with her. Oksana, according to Bowlby's theory, was able to adapt (although she experienced some troubling episodes after her victory) because she had an inner working model that promoted resiliency even during periods of vulnerability. Bowlby (1988a, 1988b) believed that a person's degree of vulnerability to stressors is strongly influenced by his or her development and the current state of his or her intimate relationships.

SOCIAL LEARNING THEORY

From birth, parents try to help infants learn what they will need to survive and function in society. An important aspect of human development, called *socialization*, occurs when parents help to mold their children's behaviors to make them effective members of society. The process by which children acquire these behaviors is called **social learning** (Fischer and Lazerson, 1984). Social learning theorists believe that behaviors are gradually learned and modified as a result of repeated interactions with the environment. Children are socialized not because of an inner developmental mechanism but from environmental responses. According to social learning theory, behaviors that are rewarded will be repeated and behaviors that have been punished will be avoided. This includes desirable and undesirable behaviors. A 4-year-old child who wants a toy from another child can ask for it politely or grab it rudely from the child and get the same result—possession of the desired toy. However, there may be undesirable consequences for rudely grabbing a toy, such as severe emotional reactions in the form of crying from other children and unwanted reprimands from adults. Social learning theorists would argue that the child would gradually opt for the more rewarding behavior of asking for the toy to avoid the undesirable consequences of crying and reprimands.

Classical Conditioning

Social learning theory was influenced by the work of American psychologist John B. Watson (1878-1958). Watson believed that psychologists cannot measure introspective processes such as thoughts and feelings and should limit themselves to the study of observable behavior. Using an experimental technique developed in the early 1900s by Russian physiologist Ivan Pavlov, Watson tried to establish that new human behaviors can be learned through a process called *classical conditioning*. In his original experiment, Pavlov produced a salivation reflex in dogs by giving them food and ringing a bell at the same time. Eventually the bell alone made the dogs salivate. Pavlov conditioned the dogs to salivate in response to a stimulus (bell) that normally would not produce a salivation response. Watson replicated the classical conditioning experiment with an 11-month-old child named Albert. Watson conditioned Albert to fear a white rat (conditioned stimulus) by pairing the rat with a sudden loud noise (unconditioned stimulus). Eventually Albert became fearful whenever he saw a white rat (conditioned response). Watson demonstrated that the behavioral change in Albert (fear in response to a white rat) was due to learning and not to some extraneous factor or innate internal mechanism.

Operant Conditioning

B.F. Skinner (1904-1990), another American psychologist, further influenced social learning theory by demonstrating that learning is due less to classical conditioning and more to what Skinner called *operant conditioning*. Skinner believed that behavior is influenced most strongly in response to its consequences. Skinner defined operant behavior as voluntary action. Classical conditioning demonstrated that an antecedent event can influence a developmental outcome. Operant conditioning expanded this idea with an emphasis on consequences of behaviors in learning.

There are three basic outcome controls in operant conditioning: reinforcement, punishment, and extinction. *Reinforcement*, a pleasant or favorable response, increases the future frequency of behaviors. *Punishment*, an unpleasant or unfavorable response, decreases the future frequency of behaviors. *Extinction* eliminates a behavior by decreasing reinforcement to a point where its frequency gradually stops. Skinner believed that behaviors can be modified or shaped by varying the schedule of reinforcement. Continuous reinforcement refers to rewarding the behavior each time it occurs. Intermittent or partial reinforcement refers to occasional reinforcement that is given once the behavior is learned. For example, a 5-year-old child can learn to comply with adult requests when adults reinforce the compliance with positive responses such as praise or hugs each time the child demonstrates correct behavior. Conversely, when the child does not comply, the child can be punished by being scolded, being sent to his or her room, or being made to sit quietly in a corner. Both reinforcing the desired behavior and punishing the undesired behavior result in increased compliance by the child. Eventually, compliance will only need to be rewarded occasionally for it to continue, and noncompliance will be extinguished.

Modern Cognitive Conditioning

Albert Bandura (1986) expanded classical and operant conditioning approaches by stating that learning and development proceed not merely from reinforcement or consequences but more from the influence that modeling plays in learning. Rather than viewing development as a series of trial-and-error events that are either strengthened or weakened by reinforcement or consequences, Bandura believed that much of social learning is fostered by observing the actions of others and the consequences of their actions. Therefore people can learn by one-trial learning through observation without ever having been reinforced. Like Piaget, Bandura believed that observational learning depends on one's developmental level. Very young children are limited mostly to spontaneous imitation, whereas delayed modeling of complex behaviors requires the development of the ability to use symbols (Figure 9-4). Unlike Piaget, he believed that new learning is not restricted by preexisting mental schemes but rather is more a function of attentional, retention, motor, and motivational processes. People, according to Bandura, cannot learn much by observation unless they attend to, and accurately perceive, the relevant aspects of modeled activities. People cannot be influenced by observation if they do not remember or retain modeled behavior in a symbolic form that can be retrieved. They cannot model behaviors if they do not have the motor capabilities to carry out the behavior. People are also more motivated to exhibit modeled behavior if it results in valued outcomes than if it yields unrewarding or punishing effects. More recently, Bandura (1989) has focused on the cognitive factors of self-efficacy

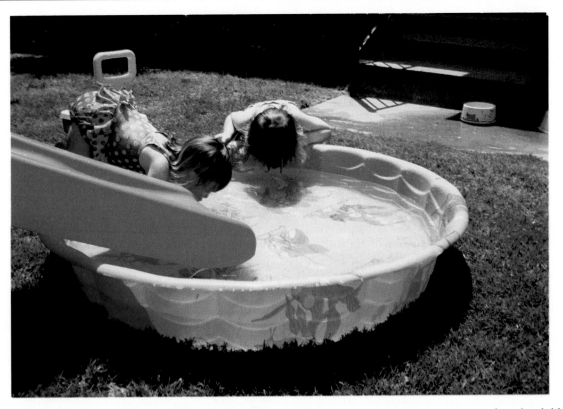

Figure 9-4 Learning for the very young child is initially limited primarily to spontaneous imitation. Later, when the child develops increased symbolic ability, delayed modeling of complex behaviors emerges.

or reinforcement. According to his later work, if one thinks of oneself as capable and effective, one is more likely to overcome failures and master and exercise control over potential threats and challenges. An example of Bandura's approach can be seen in a preschool child whose baby sibling is crying in the playpen. Without being told, the preschooler runs to the refrigerator, gets a bottle of formula, and gives it to the baby. The mother is surprised when she returns from another room to see the baby with the bottle. The preschooler smiles and says that "the baby was crying and now is not." The mother says, "How nice of you to help the baby." In this example the preschooler attends to the parental modeling, retains and retrieves the information, has the motor ability to get the bottle, and is rewarded by the mother's praise and the baby's comfort.

MORAL DEVELOPMENT

The main theorists who have studied the development of moral judgment or reasoning are Jean Piaget, Lawrence Kohlberg, Carol Gilligan, and Robert Coles. The development of moral judgment or reasoning is the process of thinking and making judgments about the right and wrong courses of action in a given situation (Stroufe, Cooper, and DeHart, 1992).

Piaget's model begins with an *amoral stage* and lasts

until age 7. With the emergence of concrete operations, the child moves to the stage of *moral realism*. At this stage behavior is seen in concrete terms as either totally right or totally wrong. When asked whether an action is right or wrong, children at this stage base their answers on the consequences of the action and ignore the intentions behind the action. When asked if it is right or wrong to take something that does not belong to them, children may say it is wrong because they will get in trouble. Children in the moral realism stage also believe in imminent justice. If they break a moral precept, they think that God or some moral authority will provide retribution. The next stage is called *autonomous morality* and is usually attained during late middle childhood or early adolescence. During this stage, children are able to consider consequences and intentions when making moral judgments. They begin to consider rules as a result of social agreement rather than as absolute right or wrong. Rather than viewing theft as wrong merely because they will get in trouble, children in this stage know that they may make another person feel bad or that others might view them as untrustworthy.

According to Piaget, moral development occurs as a result of both cognitive development and increased social experience. For instance, as children move into concrete operations, they are able to appreciate the perspectives of others, which allows them to make moral judgments based on social agreement. The child who has developed formal operations has an ability to think in hypothetical and future terms, which allows him or her to look critically at different moral viewpoints regarding the same situation (Stroufe, Cooper, and DeHart, 1992).

Lawrence Kohlberg also identified stages of moral development. He empirically studied how morality develops at different ages by presenting hypothetical moral dilemmas to children at various ages. Kohlberg (1983) identified three levels of moral development: preconventional, conventional, and postconventional. Kohlberg's stages are summarized in Table 9-5.

At the **preconventional level of morality** the first stage is the punishment-obedience orientation stage. Moral decisions are based on avoiding punishment by authority. The second stage is hedonistic and instrumental orientation. Moral decisions are motivated by a desire for rewards or benefits rather than to avoid punishment. There is also a belief in helping others in order to get help in return: "You scratch my back and I'll scratch yours."

At the **conventional level of morality** the third stage is good boy/nice girl orientation. Actions at this stage are motivated by a sense of wanting approval from others. Disapproval is avoided not because of a fear of punishment but because of guilt that is experienced by not doing the right thing. When asked why stealing is wrong, a child

at this stage might say, "Because people would think you were bad and did not come from a good family." The fourth stage is the law-and-order orientation. In this stage the moral judgments are defined by rights, assigned duty, and rules of the community. At this stage, when asked about stealing, the child would likely say, "You'd be mad, too, if you worked for something and someone just came along and stole it." At both stages of the conventional level, the child is able to see the perspective of the victim; however, the good girl/boy expresses disapproval of the thief as a bad or unloved individual, whereas the child at the law-and-order stage expresses a sense that the victim's rights as a community member have been violated.

At the **postconventional level of morality** individuals move beyond conventional reasoning and begin to focus on more abstract principles underlying right and wrong rather than moral rules. The child at the postconventional level is able to accept the possibility of conflict between norms. The fifth stage is *social contract orientation*. Moral judgments are motivated by a sense of community respect and disrespect. Even if a person does not believe in a rule or sees the rule as arbitrary, he or she will follow the rule to maintain community harmony. The sixth stage is the *hierarchy of principles orientation*. The hallmark of this stage is that moral principles are abstract and ethical. Moral judgments are based on principles of justice, the reciprocity

Table 9-5	**Moral Development—Kohlberg**		
Moral development is influenced by the child's motivation or need, the child's opportunity to learn social roles, and the forms of justice the child encounters in the social institutions where he or she lives.			
Level	**Age (Yr)**	**Stage**	**Development Issues**
I. Preconventional (self-centered orientation)	4-10	1. Punishment-obedience orientation	Moral decisions are based on avoidance of punishment.
		2. Hedonistic and instrumental orientation	Moral decisions are motivated by desire for rewards rather than avoiding punishment, and belief that by helping others they will get help in return.
II. Conventional (able to see victim's perspective)	10-13 but can go into adolescence	3. Good boy/girl orientation	Moral decisions are based on desire for approval from others and on avoiding guilt experienced by not doing the right thing.
		4. Law-and-order orientation	Moral decisions are defined by rights, assigned duty, rules of the community, and respect for authority.
III. Postconventional (underlying ethical principles are considered that take into account societal needs)		5. Social contract orientation	Moral decisions are based on a sense of community respect and disrespect. Rules should be followed to maintain community harmony.
		6. Hierarchy of principles orientation	Moral judgments are based on principles of justice, the reciprocity and quality of human rights, and respect for the dignity of human beings as individual persons: Golden rule—do to others as you would have them do to you.

and quality of human rights, and respect for the dignity of human beings as individual persons. Examples of principles at this stage are the Golden Rule (do to others as you would have them do to you), the utilitarian principle (the greatest good for the greatest number), and Kant's categoric imperative (a moral principle is an ideal rule of choice between legitimate alternatives, rather than a concrete prescription of action) (Kohlberg, 1983). According to Kohlberg, moral development is influenced by three important factors: (1) the child's motivation or need, (2) the child's opportunity to learn social roles, and (3) the forms of justice that the child encounters in the social institutions where he or she lives.

Carol Gilligan also studied moral development; however, she focused on the perspective of women and moral development. Kohlberg believed that women reach stages five and six (postconventional) less often than men. Gilligan (1982) suggested that this observation may reflect social roles ascribed to women that are less than full realization of moral development. Women, according to Gilligan, are more likely to respond to moral dilemmas based on concepts such as caring, personal relationships, and interpersonal obligations—concepts that are scored according to Kohlberg at stage three. Men, in contrast, are more likely to respond to abstract concepts such as justice and equity—concepts that are scored at stage five or six. Further research has shown no consistent sex differences in relation to Kohlberg's dilemmas, and when there are differences, women actually tend to score higher than men (Stroufe, Cooper, and DeHart, 1992).

Robert Coles (1986) also studied the moral lives of children. He observed numerous children in stressful life situations. He believed that the moral lives of children may not follow a prescribed developmental sequence but may result more from unique life experiences. He observed that even very young children can express advanced moral development in unique and stressful situations. Coles believed that unique experiences that foster moral and ethical development depend heavily on the models to which the child is exposed.

DEVELOPMENTAL CONTEXTS

Spring in California begins in March. The tulips and daffodils are in full bloom by Easter. To a native Californian who has moved to Maine, spring is a long-overdue event. The winter thaw in Maine starts nearly 2 months later than in California, and spring erupts in its magnificent beauty in May. It is hard to imagine the beauty that lies beneath the frozen cover, but it is there, waiting for the right circumstances to make the springtime greenery burst. There must be just the right conditions for spring to emerge. The sun melts the snow away and supplies the energy for budding and blossoming, and the soil must supply nutrients. **Developmental contexts** are like spring. A child must be given the right circumstances to grow and blos-

som in the process of development. Some of these circumstances are related to nature (genes, inheritance), and some are related to nurture (environment). The significance of both nature and nurture is a topic of continuous discussion.

The nature versus nurture debate is alive and well. In her presidential address to the Society for Research in Child Development (SRCD), Sandra Scar (1992) proposed that developmental research during the past 25 years supports the idea that normal genes and normal environments promote species-typical development and that, given a wide range of opportunities, individuals make their own environments on the basis of their own inherited characteristics. Scar (1992) cited the example that smiling, cheerful infants who evoke positive social interactions from parents and other adults seem likely to form positive impressions of the social world and its attractions. Conversely, infants who are fussy and irritable and who experience negative or neutral interactions with their caregivers and others are less likely to interpret social interactions as a positive source of reinforcement. Therefore Scar supported the idea that individuals' inherited temperament (genotype) influences their social world and ultimately the environment in which they will grow. The central theme here is that individuals create their own environments based on the inherited characteristics they are dealt from birth.

Baumrind (1993) provided a lively response to Scar's address. According to Baumrind, Scar's assertion that individuals create their own environment undermines parents' belief in their own effectiveness as nurturers. She believes that caretakers construct the external environment to which the young child must then accommodate. Baumrind cited Piaget's work to counter Scar's assertions. Piaget contended that the child assimilates and accommodates to environmental input. For Piaget, children's construction of their world is based on experiences that the caregiver provides. Baumrind's contention is that "parent's denial of responsibility for child outcomes is associated with negative child outcomes." She believes that an environmentalistic perspective helps to empower parents to reinforce their sense of responsibility to their children. In addition, Baumrind (1993) cites Patterson's (Patterson and Capaldi, 1991) demonstrations that parents can be taught how to respond in more constructive ways to difficult children or those with special needs. According to Baumrind (1993), negative, hostile, and coercive responses by parents to their difficult children, although natural, are neither inevitable nor helpful.

ECOLOGIC SYSTEMS MODEL

The ecologic systems model describes developmental contexts in a way that identifies factors that help shape development and their relationships to each other. The ecologic systems model contains four contexts in concentric rings, with each ring influencing those inside. As can be

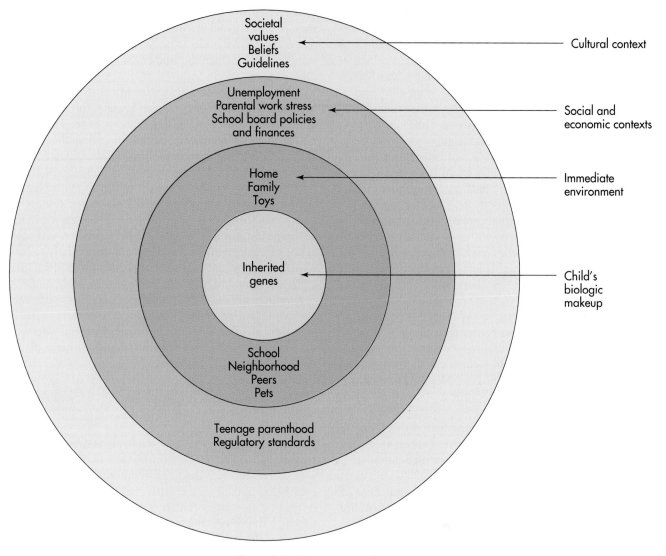

Figure 9-5 Developmental contexts.

seen in Figure 9-5, the child is placed in the center of the ring and brings to development the *biologic context* that he or she inherited. Surrounding the child's biologic context is the child's *immediate environment*, which contains all of the settings, people, and objects that touch the child in a direct way. For example, the immediate environment contains the child's home. The home may be a single house, an apartment, a battered women's shelter, or a housing project. The immediate environment also includes the family. In the family there are parents, siblings, and perhaps other relatives. The family may be a single-parent family, a blended family, or a traditional family. Other examples of immediate environments are the child's toys, school (teachers, classroom, library), neighborhood (peers, playgrounds), and pets. Each of these different immediate environments provide different opportunities and challenges that influence development.

The people, settings, and objects of the immediate environment are found within a larger *social and economic context*. The home may be indirectly influenced by the parents' employment situation in terms of economic resources for the family or demands placed on the parent at work. A parent who is stressed at work may bring the stress from the social and economic context to the immediate home environment. The parent who is stressed from work may be tired and emotionally unavailable or irritable and impatient. A single teenage mother may have less economic resources to share than a two-income intact family. The child's school is influenced by the finances and policies of the local school board. If the child's school district has limited resources, the child may not get exposure to a wide variety of educational tools with which to enhance development. The neighborhood is part of the larger city, county, or state context. There may be high levels of unemployment in a city or state that have an influence on social situations such as poverty and crime. The toys in the home may have been subject to regulatory standards for safety. The child's dog may be regulated by animal control standards and must have a rabies vaccination.

At the outer rung of the ring in Figure 9-5 is the *cultural context*. It contains all of the beliefs, values, and guidelines that people in society share. For instance, most adults in the United States share the belief that mothers are important in shaping a child's development; however, current research (Coley, 1998) (see Understanding & Applying Research box) underlines the belief that fathers should take an active role, too.

Our culture is in a state of constant change. The contexts of development provide the foundation and support for development to occur. A change in cultural expectations can have an impact on development. According to Rutter (1998), "one of the most striking features of the past half-century has been the extent to which the prevalence of many psychosocial disorders in young people living in the industrialized world has increased over time. This increase is perhaps most obvious in the case of crime and drug problems, but it is also evident in cases of suicide, attempted suicide, and depression." Rutter (1998) suggests that current cultural research variables related to this increase in the prevalence of disorders may include a change in the age people begin engaging in sexual activity, in teenage pregnancy, in mental dysfunctions, and in scholastic achievement.

• • •

This chapter has outlined many variables and processes important for understanding development. Developmental knowledge is crucial in the practice of psychiatric mental health nursing, since it shows us where we have been, where we are currently, and where we need to go in promoting mental health.

Understanding & Applying Research

Most studies of the influence of parental relationships on children's cognitive, social, and behavioral functioning have historically focused almost exclusively on the impact of mothers. In this research, the impact of children's experiences of warmth and control provided by fathers and other male father figures and their effects on children's cognitive, social, and behavioral functioning were explored. The research sample included 111 third- and fourth-grade children residing with unmarried mothers. The children were allowed to nominate adults who were important to them and then answered numerous questions concerning specific warm emotional and social interactions. The majority of nonpaternal men named by the children were not extended relatives but rather partners or boyfriends of the children's mothers. Academic achievement, social behaviors, and emotional development were measured using established instruments. After controlling for demographic variables and the influence of maternal parenting, the results showed that children who reported more positive and warm social interactions with their non-residential fathers received higher achievement scores in standardized school tests, and that children with nonpaternal men who played significant disciplinary and regulatory roles showed better behaviors. Teachers rated children who had more positive and warm interactions with significant males as having fewer behavior problems in school, and their peers rated them as being more helpful than their counterparts with little adult male contact. These results were even more significant for girls, which ran counter to previous research that found links between fathers and other male relatives and children's functioning for boys, but not for girls.

This research supports the importance of social policies that help to increase single-parented children's exposure to, and close relationships with, fathers and father figures, since these relationships can be an integral part of their system of social resources.

Coley R: Children's socialization experiences and functioning in single-mother households: the importance of fathers and other men, *Child Dev* 69:219, 1998.

Summary of Key Concepts

1. Psychosexual, psychosocial, interpersonal, cognitive, adaptation, social learning, and information processing are all theories that try to explain how and why children develop.

2. Freud's psychosexual theory holds that the root of adult problems can be traced back to childhood trauma.

3. The stages in Freud's psychosexual theory include the oral, anal, phallic, latency, and genital stages.

4. Erikson's psychosocial theory states that all individuals must face and resolve a series of developmental tasks or issues during the life span, including trust versus mistrust, autonomy versus shame and doubt, initiative versus guilt, industry versus inferiority, and identity versus role confusion.

5. Sullivan believes that development results from interpersonal relationships in the infancy, childhood, juvenile, preadolescent, adolescent, and late adolescent eras.

6. Piaget's cognitive theory includes four periods that build on each other during the life span: sensorimotor, preoperational, concrete operational, and formal operational.

7. Bowlby's adaptation theory states that the crux of human development lies in the strength of an infant's attachment to the caretaker, and the strength of the caretaker's bond with the infant.

8. The social learning theory states that behaviors are gradually learned and modified as a result of repeated interactions with the environment.

9. The moral development theory by Kohlberg includes three levels: preconventional (self-centered), conventional (victim awareness), and postconventional (society awareness).

REFERENCES

Bandura A: *Social foundations of thought and action: a social cognitive theory*, Englewood Cliffs, NJ, 1986, Prentice-Hall.

Bandura A: Human agency in social cognitive theory, *Am Psychol* 44:1175, 1989.

Baumrind D: The average expectable environment is not good enough: a response to Scar, *Child Dev* 64:1299, 1993.

Bowlby J: Developmental psychiatry comes of age. *Am J Psychiatry* 145:1, 1988a.

Bowlby J: *A secure base*, New York, 1988b, Basic Books.

Coles R: *The moral life of children*, Boston, 1986, Atlantic Monthly Press.

Coley R: Children's socialization experiences and functioning in single-mother households: the importance of fathers and other men, *Child Dev* 69:219, 1998.

Erikson E: *Childhood and society*, New York, 1963, WW Norton.

Erikson E: *The life cycle completed*, New York, 1982, WW Norton.

Fischer K, Lazerson A: *Human development from conception through adolescence*, New York, 1984, WH Freeman.

Freud S: *The ego and the id*, New York, 1923, WW Norton.

Gilligan C: *In a different voice*, Cambridge, Mass, 1982, Harvard University Press.

Jackson J: Human behavioral genetics, Scar's theory, and her views on interventions: a critical review and commentary on their implications for African-American children, *Child Dev* 64:1318, 1993.

Kohlberg L: The development of children's orientations toward a moral order. In Damon W, editor: *Social and personality development essays on the growth of the child*, New York, 1983, WW Norton.

Maddi S: *Personality theories: a comparative analysis*, Homewood, Ill, 1972, Dorsey Press.

Patterson G, Capaldi D: Antisocial parents: unskilled and vulnerable. In Cowan PE, Hetherington M, editors: *Family transitions*, Hillsdale, NJ, 1991, Lawrence Erlbaum.

Rutter M: Some research considerations on intergenerational continuities and discontinuities: comment on the special section, *Dev Psychol* 34:6:1269, 1998.

Scar S: Developmental theories for the 1990s: development and individual differences, *Child Dev* 63:1, 1992.

Scar S: Biological and cultural diversity: the legacy of Darwin for development, *Child Dev* 64:1333, 1993.

Sternberg R: *Metaphors of the mind: conceptions of the nature of intelligence*, New York, 1990, Cambridge University Press.

Stroufe A, Cooper R, DeHart G: *Child development: its nature and course*, New York, 1992, McGraw-Hill.

Sullivan H: *The interpersonal theory of psychiatry*, New York, 1953, WW Norton.

Notes

CHAPTER 10

The Adult

Margaret T. Barker

OBJECTIVES

- Discuss early and contemporary theories of adult development.

- Recognize and apply Erikson's psychosocial stages in client assessment and care.

- Identify the major life span transitions.

- Discuss life span transitions and their biologic, psychologic, and social aspects.

- Compare and contrast mature and immature developmental defense mechanisms for success in transitional crises.

- Debate how Gail Sheehy's description of the three stages of adulthood provides new challenges for traditional theorists and researchers of adult development.

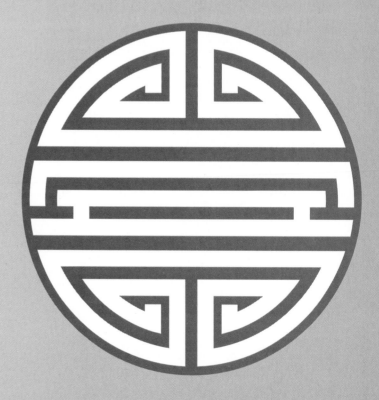

ADULT DEVELOPMENT OVERVIEW

Because many mental health crises result from life span issues or transitions and are affected by the individual's developmental maturity, it is essential for the psychiatric mental health nurse to have a clear understanding of both child and adult developmental stages. Furthermore, many mental health disorders characteristically develop or are detected at certain stages of life. For example, schizophrenia generally begins in the late teenage years and early adulthood and rarely occurs after age 50. Although depressive disorders may occur at any time, they generally begin between the ages of 20 and 50, with 40 as the mean age of onset for depression.

Throughout the ages, humans have yearned to grasp an understanding of life, its meaning, and their place in the universe. Questions such as "Where are we going? And what is our purpose?" have perplexed humanity since the beginning of time. Confucius (511-479 BC) saw his own life as representative of man's journey. For example, at age 15 came learning; at age 30 Confucius established stability (planting one's feet on the ground); at age 40 he no longer suffered from his perplexities; at age 50 he knew the bidding of heaven; and at 60 he could "follow the dictates of his own heart, for what [he] desired no longer overstepped the boundaries of right." The relevant central themes of ancient writings can be summarized as follows (Colarusso and Nemiroff, 1981):

- A comprehensive, chronologic life cycle is described.
- Adulthood is not static; the adult is in a constant state of dynamic change and flux, always "becoming" or "finding the way."
- Development in adulthood is contiguous with that in childhood and old age.

Defense A means or method of protecting oneself; an unconscious mental activity or mental structure (e.g., defense mechanism) that protects the ego from anxiety.

Defense mechanism A structure of the psyche that protects the ego against anxiety, unpleasant feelings, or impulses. Defense mechanisms are unconscious and deny, falsify, or distort reality.

Generativity In Erikson's personality theory, the positive outcome of one of the stages of adult personality development; the ability to do creative work or to contribute to the raising of one's children; the opposite of stagnation.

Marker events Human life events such as leaving the primary family, first job, first marriage, first child, empty nest, retirement, widowhood, and death, described by Sheehy as predictable life stages.

Metaneed The need for belonging and love that emerges as physiologic and safety needs are met.

Psychosocial stages Erikson's eight stages in a person's social development. Each stage is marked by a particular type of crisis resulting from the ego's attempt to meet the demands of social reality.

Rites of passage Rituals such as puberty, marriage, birth, and death that facilitate maturational development; associated with life transition. These rites commonly consist of three stages: separation, transition, and incorporation.

Self-actualization A concept developed by Maslow as an ongoing actualization of potentials, capacities, and talents as fulfillment of a mission and as a greater knowledge and acceptance of one's own intrinsic nature.

There is a continual need to define the adult self, especially with regard to the integrity of the inner person versus his or her external environment.
Adults must come to terms with their limited life span and individual mortality. A preoccupation with time is an expression of these concerns.
The development and maintenance of the adult body and its relationship to the mind is a universal preoccupation.
Narcissism (love of self) versus responsibility to the society in which one lives, and the individuals in that society for whom one bears responsibility as an adult, is a central issue in all civilized cultures.

Studies in adult development continue to lag behind, in contrast to the research in infancy, childhood, and adolescence. Stevens-Long (1992) believed that this lag is attributable to economic, social, and psychologic issues. With the introduction of compulsory education, it became imperative to study child development to provide optimum teaching methods and environments. Biologists and psychologists stressed the relevance of child development research as an important source of information regarding the evolution of the species.

The average life span has increased from 45 years at the turn of the century to well beyond 70 years in the 1990s. Longitudinal child studies and gerontologic studies are now meeting in the middle (Neugarten, 1979), providing a much-needed focus on the adult years.

ADULT DEVELOPMENTAL THEORISTS

PIONEER ADULT DEVELOPMENTALISTS

Before this century there was little written on a scientific level regarding adult changes and development. It took the writings of four men—Arnold Van Gennep, Sigmund Freud, Carl Gustav Jung, and Erik H. Erikson—to stimulate this discourse. Three of these—Freud, Jung, and Erikson—became the main theorists on adult development, and their work became the cornerstone of later work. The fourth, Van Gennep, in his landmark text *The Rites of Passage* (1960), described the importance and meaning of the rituals surrounding life span transitions (e.g., pregnancy, childbirth, menarche, betrothal, marriage, and death).

Freud's developmental ideas formed the basis for psychoanalysis and much subsequent theoretic work. Before Freud, issues of adult development were viewed essentially as the "unwinding meaning of hidden springs" within an organism. Freud was both a biologist and a neurologist.

As such, he emphasized the interaction of biologic and psychologic variables and described development as the interaction between focus within the biologic organism and the individual's world, which is the psychologic experience.

Whereas Freud focused on the developmental sequences in childhood, Jung, a disciple of Freud's, was the first psychoanalyst to study the second half of life. Jung viewed adult development as continuous throughout the life cycle. Jung wrote that adults in their twenties and thirties continue to work on separation and personality individuation from their primary families, at the same time that they are trying to establish a family. Jung was one of the first to write a psychologic description of midlife transition, with its often growing awareness of the masculine and feminine aspects of personality.

To support Jung's view, many women in contemporary society have awakened to social responsibility and assertiveness, whereas men in their forties and fifties have become more aware of their nurturing sides. The reversal of

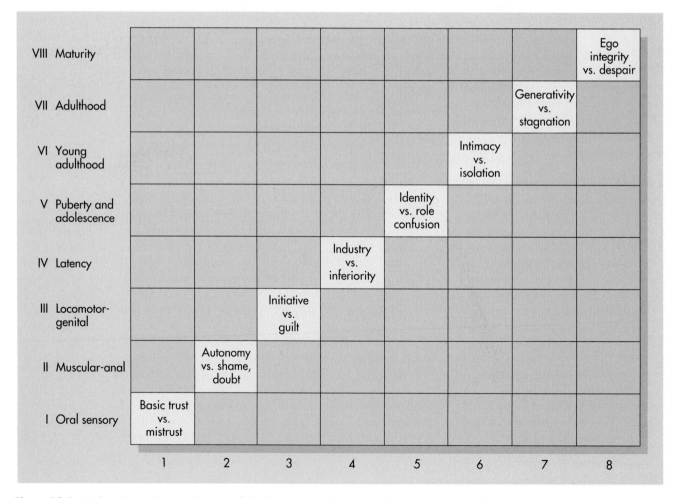

Figure 10-1 Erikson's psychosocial stages of development and corresponding developmental issues for the individual. (Modified from Erikson EH: *Childhood and society*, ed 2, New York, 1974, WW Norton.)

the individual's ego identity may be accompanied by self-examination and ego dissonance "when the husband discovers his tender feelings, and the wife, her sharpness of mind."

PSYCHOSOCIAL STAGES

Erikson was the first to define a developmental outlook for the life span. His eight stages of development were a significant theoretic advance, since it was the first time developmental concepts were validated for the entire life span (Figure 10-1). Before this time, development was thought to be complete after adolescence. Contemporary developmentalists base their hypothesis on Erikson's concepts, and Erikson continues to have enormous influence in many fields, including nursing, psychology, psychiatry, psychoanalysis, the social sciences, and the humanities.

Erikson and later contemporary developmentalists believed that development is lifelong and that adulthood is a time of dynamic growth and change. Each of Erikson's **psychosocial stages** is organized around a critical developmental issue for the individual self and its relationship to the social world. The issue is described as a polarity (i.e., two opposites on a continuum), creating intrapsychic tension that results in a unique, growing experience for the individual. Each human being must pass eight great tests. Chapter 9 deals in depth with the first five psychosocial stages. At this point it is relevant to touch on the earlier stages to reinforce that the resolution of each stage is interlinked and dependent on the prior stages.

At the first stage (Freud's oral stage) the crisis is one of basic trust or mistrust, the source of "both primal hope and doom throughout life" (Erikson, 1963). This critical stage is a stepping-stone for successful resolution of subsequent stages. The mature, postadolescent personality is a combination of successful or unsuccessful outcomes of the preceding crises. At worst, a person at the negative extreme would be completely mistrustful, full of shame and doubt, riddled with guilt and feelings of failure, confused about his or her roles, and isolated from humanity. At the other (positive) extreme, the individual would be completely trusting, autonomous, able to initiate, competent, and intimate with humanity. It is obvious that most people's personalities reflect experiences of both successes and failures. In his sixth, seventh, and eighth stages, Erikson discussed the key crises of young adulthood, adulthood, and old age. Erikson brought psychology and psychiatry beyond a constricted view of the life span to a more comprehensive, lifelong view of development.

Adult Development Within the Psychosocial Stages

Adult developmental stages incorporate the sixth and seventh stages of life. During the sixth (or young adult) stage, individuals struggle with issues of intimacy versus self-absorption. As in each of the other stages, how one resolved the preceding crises plays an important role in the individual's approach to, and resolution of, the current task. Successful resolution of the earlier developmental tasks is particularly important for the achievement of intimacy versus self-absorption. To achieve true intimacy, the individual must experience another person's needs and concerns as being equally important as his or her own. To have genuine concern for another, one needs a cohesive sense of personal self and minimal fear or anxiety about losing oneself in giving to another, whether in the emotional, intellectual, or sexual domain.

Intimacy requires a comfortable sense of fusing one's identity with that of another. To achieve that in any relationship, whether the relationship is sexual, between parent and child, with friends, or in marriage, one must be able to tolerate the threat of some ego loss. If one cannot allow oneself to experience another individual on this level, one faces the possibility of isolation and self-absorption (Colarusso and Nemiroff, 1981).

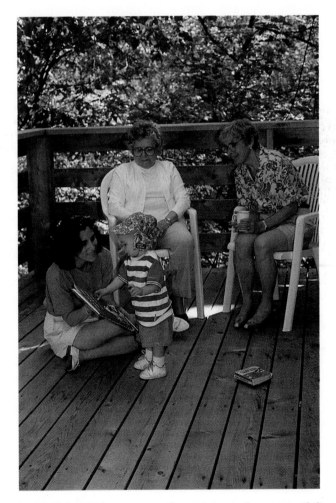

Figure 10-2 Each generation faces unique roles, responsibilities, and conflicts. Generativity is the concern for establishing and guiding the next generation, something that adults face at midlife. (Copyright Cathy Lander-Goldberg, Lander Photographics.)

During the seventh stage, or the midlife period, the conflict between **generativity** and stagnation emerges (Figure 10-2). For Erikson, successful generativity is simply the concern for establishing and guiding the next generation. This is the midlife, the generation between developing adolescents and aging parents. As early adulthood ends and middle adulthood begins, there is a new and necessary awareness of the generational sequence. As children become more independent, aging parents become more dependent; therefore the adult at midlife is faced with new generational roles, responsibilities, and conflicts. Erikson addresses this as the seventh stage of ego development, the stage of generativity versus stagnation. Generativity includes the ability to evaluate and appreciate one's past life, embrace the future, assume new responsibilities and new relationships, and acknowledge and use one's creativity, in contrast to stagnation in a life of unfulfilling sameness and emotional isolation. When such enrichment and emotional self-knowledge is absent, the individual can regress to an obsessive need for pseudointimacy, stagnation, boredom, and interpersonal impoverishment.

The eighth and final psychosocial stage, ego integrity versus despair, is described in Chapter 11. Briefly, those individuals who have taken care of people and effectively adapted themselves to life's triumphs and disappointments will not be threatened with the despair of an empty, fruitless old age. Such individuals truly personify the healthy, cumulative outcome of the previous seven stages.

The possessor of integrity is ready to defend the dignity of his or her own lifestyle against all physical and economic threats. Without successful accomplishments of the earlier developmental tasks, the individual lacks this accumulated ego integration and, as such, may be preoccupied with fear of death and/or a sense of bitterness owing to an unfulfilled life. With the inevitability of death, feelings of despair and worthlessness ensue, rather than satisfaction with a life well lived. Time is generally too short to try alternatives, and the individual is stagnated in despair.

CONTEMPORARY THEORISTS

In adult life, developmental issues of childhood continue as central themes, but the adult's developmental focus is the ability to interact with transitional aspects of the life span and the environment. A central theme in childhood is the development of trust, autonomy, and individuation. Integral to adult development in middle and later life is the recognition and acceptance of the finiteness of time and the inevitability of death.

In *The Seasons of a Man's Life*, Daniel Levinson (a psychosocial theorist), and associates (1986) looked at life from the aspect of stages that move from early adulthood into middle and late adulthood. The stages are broadly based on Erikson's stages of ego development, but Levinson's group focused less on changes occurring within the person and more on the interface between the self and the

interpersonal world. This requires an assessing of one's self within the world, the functioning of the individual self, and one's relationship to one's world (Newton and Levinson, 1979).

Levinson's psychosocial theory of adult development proposes a universal life cycle consisting of specific eras in a set sequence from birth to old age. The basic unit of the life cycle is the era, which lasts about 20 years (e.g., preadulthood, 0 to 20 years; early adulthood, 20 to 40 years; middle adulthood, 40 to 60 years; late adulthood, 60 to 80 years to death) (Figure 10-3).

In systematic alternating sequences, stable periods of 6 to 7 years are followed by transitional intervals of 4 to 5 years, each with its specific tasks to be met and mastered. Clinicians find the concept of stable periods followed by transitional periods useful because, for many individuals, internal conflict during the transitional times is an impetus for seeking treatment.

The Harvard Grant Longitudinal Study has followed the life course of 268 undergraduate students from 1939 to the present. The current director of the Grant study, George Vaillant, has used these data to study adaptation in adulthood, particularly in terms of ego **defense mechanisms.** The interviews and collected data have supported Erikson's concept of the life cycle. The study has examined the qualities that distinguished effective adaptation and how problems were resolved rather than the absence of problems.

Vaillant's study focused on the intrapsychic styles of adaptation first described by Freud. These ego mechanisms of defense are a major means of managing instinct and affect. They are unconsciously activated, discrete from one another, dynamic, and reversible, and they can be adaptive as well as pathologic. Building on Freud's work and using data collected from the Harvard study, Vaillant devised a theoretic hierarchy, grouping 18 defenses according to their relative maturity and pathology (Box 10-1).

Central to Vaillant's work is the thesis that if individuals are to master conflict gracefully and are to be successful and efficient in their choices, ego defense mechanisms must change and mature throughout the life cycle. What distinguishes effective adaptations are how problems are dealt with, not the absence of problems.

In looking at the change in specific **defenses** over time, Vaillant's group traced the decline of the defense mechanisms of fantasy and acting out with the emergence of maturity and an accompanying increase in suppression. Dissociation, repression, sublimation, and altruism increase in midlife, whereas projection, hypochondriasis, and masochism are most common in adolescence. Vaillant points out that the decade from 25 to 35 years is a guilty period, in which defenses of reaction formation and repression are used with greater frequency.

Vaillant compared men who were considered generative (i.e., more psychosocially mature in Eriksonian terms) with a group of "perpetual boys" (i.e., men who retained

Developmental Periods

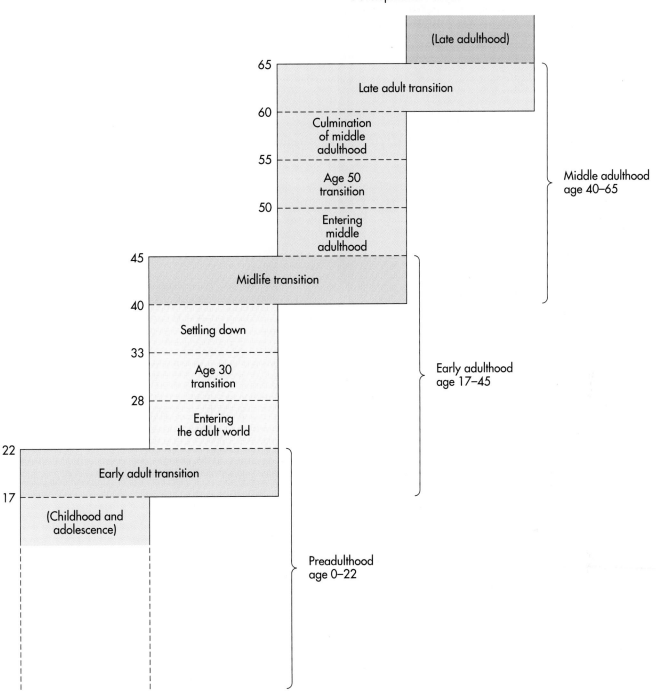

Figure 10-3 Levinson's psychosocial theory of adult development. (From Levinson DJ et al: *The seasons of a man's life*, New York, 1986, Ballantine Books.)

immature qualities). Over time, the perpetual boys failed to show any significant shift in their adaptive patterns, unlike the pattern seen in the generative men (Vaillant, 1977).

Vaillant described the association between adult maturity and external adjustment. He contrasted the subjects with the best and worst outcomes in negotiating Erikson's psychosocial stages of development. Vaillant was able to

document that difficulties for those with worse outcomes began in childhood, with events perceived as traumatic and interfering with the establishment of basic trust, autonomy, and initiative.

Those men who had difficulty with the earlier psychosocial stages appeared to be less well integrated in adolescence, and subsequently their identities were less secure as adults. They were also less likely to have internalized their

---

Box 10-1   **Vaillant's Hierarchy of Adaptive Mechanisms**

Level I: Psychotic Mechanisms (Common in Psychosis, Dreams, Childhood)
Denial (of external reality)
Distortion
Delusional projection

Level II: Immature Mechanisms (Common in Severe Depression, Personality Disorders, and Adolescence)
Fantasy (schizoid withdrawal, denial through fantasy)
Projection
Hypochondriasis
Passive-aggressive behavior (masochism, turning against the self)
Acting out (compulsive delinquency, perversion)

Level III: Neurotic Mechanisms (Common in Everyone)
Intellectualization (isolation, obsessive behavior, undoing, rationalization)
Repression
Reaction formation
Displacement (conversion, phobias, wit)
Dissociation (neurotic denial)

Level IV: Mature Mechanisms (Common in "Healthy" Adults)
Sublimination
Altruism
Suppression
Anticipation
Humor

From Vaillant GE: *Adaptation to life*, Boston, 1977, Little, Brown.

---

and behavior. It is understood that later experiences and environmental conditions can either reinforce or reverse early influences as they interact with the personality (Blanck and Blanck, 1979; Millon, 1987).

The inflexible, maladaptive life patterns that are the hallmark of personality disorders can be viewed as originally developing as defensive survival patterns. However dysfunctional the personality style, it seems safe to observe that at one time such behavior was the individual's safeguard against intolerable anxiety, self-hate, helplessness, and insecurity created by the early developmental environment. These behaviors and personality styles were a means of fending off unacceptable sexual or hostile impulses. At the time in one's life that these defensive styles were developed to protect against inner and outer threats, they may have been the most adaptive alternative mechanisms available to the young person unconsciously initiating them.

Defensive life patterns can prevent the development and emergence of healthy defense mechanisms. For example, the individual with a dependent personality disorder or dependent traits may never have successfully developed defenses against separation anxiety, which is necessary for autonomy, individuation, and the ability to deal effectively with reality (Bowlby, 1988; Millon, 1987).

Defensive personality traits may be converted into assets. Many nurses have strong caregiving qualities, which may have been defensive adaptations in early life. Perhaps as a young child, the nurse defended himself or herself against feelings of insecurity by eventually becoming a protective caregiver for dependent, vulnerable, mentally or physically frail adults.

A more comprehensive review of the literature regarding personality disorders can be found in Chapter 15.

fathers as role models and still seemed dependent on their mothers. Finally, both at age 30 and at 50, these individuals were still having trouble with intimacy. Their marriages and friendships were more likely to be problematic, and they seemed to be considerably less generative in the sense of being willing to assume responsibility for other adults.

PERSONALITY DISORDERS: AN ADULT DEVELOPMENT PERSPECTIVE

Many mental health professionals have little interest in exploring the relationship between personality, behavior, and early childhood influences. The roles of heredity and environmental factors continue to be subject to disagreement. However, despite the different viewpoints, psychoanalytic and psychosocial experts concur that the child's earliest years critically affect subsequent development

LIFE SPAN TRANSITIONS
TRANSITIONS

Normative adult life transitions consist of leaving one's original family, forming new relationships, starting a family, having and raising children, children leaving home, reforming as a couple, becoming adult caregivers for the older generation, and retiring. Throughout these normal life stressors, an individual's ability to use learned coping strategies and unconscious ego defense mechanisms to resolve crises or transitions depends on earlier accomplishments of developmental tasks. Any of the above can become extraordinary life stressors if they occur out of sequence to life's expected developmental pattern. Individuals who seek help often have a combination of poor mastery of developmental tasks and a life stressor that is unexpected (e.g., an out-of-sequence life event such as the premature death of a parent or child), which results in ego dissonance and crisis. All individuals need added support at these times, and individuals with fragile ego develop-

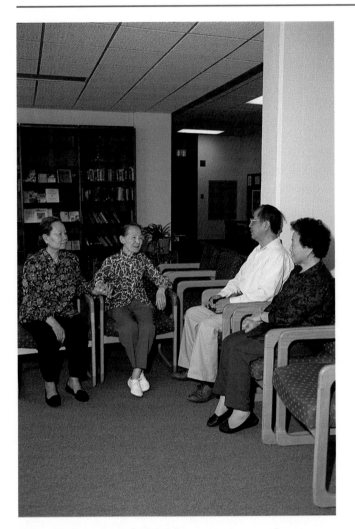

Figure 10-4 A normal adult life transition is providing support and care for one's parents as they age. (Copyright Cathy Lander-Goldberg, Lander Photographics.)

ment tend to need more intensive support, perhaps even hospitalization, during these crises (Figure 10-4).

MIDLIFE TRANSITIONS

The term *midlife crisis* is a misnomer; many changes that occur at midlife are not crises. Transitions generate a range of feelings and events in individuals, from a private, low-key introspection to a more obvious transition, but few experience dramatic midlife change and possibly a crisis. Levinson et al (1986) prefer the term *midlife transitions* because it includes aspects of crisis, process, and change. According to Levinson et al, approximately 80% of individuals experience the period of midlife—the years crossing the third and fourth decades—as a time marked by tumultuous struggles within the individual and the external world.

During the years between the late thirties or early forties and continuing at an individual-specific rate throughout the life span, the beginnings of expected midlife biologic changes occur. These include alterations in strength and endurance, skin and muscle tone, hearing, and vision.

Reaction time may also be affected, as well as graying or loss of hair and sexual function. These changes affect individuals differently, often depending on how one has achieved the earlier developmental tasks and one's level of knowledge and self-acceptance. Integral to acceptance and mastery of these changes is the individual's ability to incorporate the concept of death and perception of time in such a way as to accept it as a part of life. Neugarten (1979) described a shift in thinking from asking oneself "How long have I lived?" to asking, "How long do I have left?"

RITES OF PASSAGE: MEANING AND PURPOSE

Although much of our socialization takes place gradually, during certain transitional periods the shaping of adult development within the context of the social structure is accelerated, often creating a feeling of anxiety and crisis. Some of these transitions may be closely associated with biologic developments such as menstruation and menopause, and others are influenced by sociocultural factors such as school graduation, marriage, or retirement.

Transitions are frequently occasions for ceremonies that focus on the importance of the person's change in status and affirm his or her new place in society. Rituals, or ceremonies, are stepping-stones toward resolving conflict and facilitating maturational development and change through life transitions such as puberty, marriage, birth, and death. Rituals can contribute to a person's identity and help make change manageable. The rituals associated with these life transitions are known as **rites of passage.** These rites commonly comprise three stages: separation, transition, and incorporation (Van Gennep, 1960).

The marriage ceremony in many Western cultures provides a clear example of the stages of a rite of passage. In the first stage the bride is separated physically from the groom until the ceremony, and during this stage she prepares herself for her change in status; she is separated symbolically by the veil over her face, which shields her against the external world. The transitional stage is the ceremony, or ritual, in which the bride and groom are suspended between the old existence and the new. During the ceremony spiritual leaders often offer guidance for the new life that is to follow. Vows and rings are exchanged to bind the couple together as a unit. Finally, the newly married couple is reintroduced to the wedding party and guests as husband and wife, which indicates their new unified status. The honeymoon follows, where the couple has a chance to adapt to their new status and new roles before they return to the routine of everyday life.

Rites of passage are cross-cultural. Van Gennep (1960) describes these rites as necessary to facilitate the transition from group to group and from one social situation to the next. They are considered critical to an individual's and a society's existence. In all cultures men's and women's lives are made up of a succession of stages with similar ends and beginnings: birth, puberty, marriage, parenthood, advancement to a higher social class, occupational specialization, and death. For each of these events there are ceremonies whose essential purpose is to enable the individual to pass from one defined position to another equally defined position.

Many contemporary social scientists and clinicians believe that with each life transitional crisis, these unique social rituals help an individual achieve his or her potential and obtain group support in the transition. With the decline in sacred rituals and ceremonies, individuals and social groups are forced to accomplish their life tasks during transitional periods, essentially alone, often failing or not completing the needed maturational development. As a result, their individual potential and development may be compromised, and the family and society may also be adversely affected (Colarusso and Nemiroff, 1981).

GENDER DIFFERENCE IN ADULT DEVELOPMENT

There are important basic similarities between adult male and female development, but there are also significant differences. These differences have only recently been recognized, because all early studies on adult development were carried out with male subjects. Only recently have studies included women or examined gender differences.

PSYCHOLOGIC DIFFERENCES

There are significant differences in how men and women respond to four natural transitions (i.e., leaving one's primary family, starting a family, children leaving home, and retiring) (Lowenthal, Turner, and Cheroboga, 1975). These differences become more apparent with age, indicating that the development is parallel throughout adolescence and early childhood but diverges through the late twenties. At age 30, when most people reassess their life structure, women seem to struggle between two major life choices: whether to marry and start a family or work on a career first. Those who attempt to do both at the same time may deal with consequences such as guilt, anxiety, and fatigue. Those who postpone either the family or the career may fear that time is running out and that one of their life choices will be sacrificed. Women facing such a choice have been quoted as saying, "My biologic clock is ticking." Such beliefs may influence a critical decision in a woman's life.

HORMONAL DIFFERENCES

Hormonal differences and their relationship to mood have been studied extensively. Postpartum psychosis and postpartum depression have been related to the precipitous postpartum reduction in gonadotropins (Vandenbergh, 1980). Bardwick (1976) hypothesized that premenstrual depression is related to low levels of estrogen, which has been shown to induce high levels of monoamine oxidase (MAO). Estrogen appears to be the most potent of the gonadal hormones affecting MAO levels. High levels of MAO at the synapse are associated with low levels of catecholamines, a state associated with certain types of depression. An increase in estrogen, which elevates mood, may act to decrease the quantity of MAO or to increase the levels of catecholamines. It is important for the psychiatric mental health nurse to be aware of this, especially with clients who have had an oophorectomy or a total hysterectomy, or who are in their late thirties through early fifties. Certainly, with a first-time depression during this age range, the possibility of a hormonal imbalance should be ruled out. Studies have shown that the rate of depression is twice as high for women as for men in the United States and in Western societies. Depression resembles grief because feelings of loss and sadness dominate the emotions. Depression has components involving self-esteem, cognition, sleep, appetite, energy level, and behavior (American Psychiatric Association, 1994; Bardwick, 1976).

As mood and the endocrine system are interrelated, so is the gender response to the tricyclic antidepressants. Women not only become depressed more often than men but also demonstrate slower responses to tricyclic antidepressants. The emergence of newer, more effective antidepressants such as selective serotonin reuptake inhibitors (SSRIs) has been helpful in these instances. (See Chapter 13 for more comprehensive information in this area.)

The developmental stages for women appear to be characterized not by successive stages of separation and individuation as are men's, but by differing forms of connection within relationships. Women are most affected by losses involving close relationships, whereas men tend to become depressed with the loss of an ideal, an achievement-related goal, or a performance issue. Developmental arrest occurs in women generally as a result of failure to remain connected while developing a distinct sense of self rather than as a result of failure to separate (Gilligan, 1977, 1990). Many middle-age women experience the loss of their youth by becoming painfully preoccupied with the physical signs of aging. Society's overvaluation of the youthful female body results in fears of being "unsexed" by the aging process and losing love as a consequence. Men generally are not confronted as brutally with this issue, because male sexuality is depicted by society as continuing well beyond midlife.

SOCIAL DIFFERENCES

Women appear to be more pressured and restricted than men by what Neugarten (1979) terms a socially *defined sense of time*, or a sense of the temporal appropriateness of major events. Such socially defined standards are based on the male life cycle, which places career as the dominant component. Women who have raised a family are viewed as being out of synchrony with current standards. Often, where there is a shift between one's career goals and the desire to start a family, this change in goals can result in a serious midlife reappraisal of career, marriage, goals, life, and an individual's essential values.

Depression occurring at this stage, as in any other transitional phase, requires a mourning period to enable the individual to move and grow beyond the confusion of the developmental crisis.

HIERARCHY OF NEEDS

The construct of human need satisfaction has played an important role in nursing theory, education, and practice. A chapter on adult development would be incomplete without a review of Maslow's theory of the hierarchy of needs (Maslow, 1968, 1970). The existence of unmet needs and the desire to achieve optimum self-potential are fundamental sources of human motivation. Essential needs constitute an inexact hierarchy of relative predominance, beginning with the most urgent physiologic necessities and culminating in the search for self-actualization.

Physiologic needs include the somatically based drives of hunger, thirst, sexual desire, and the need for activity, exercise, sleep, rest, and sensory pleasure. With the gratification of these most basic needs, other higher needs emerge, such as more socially oriented goals and the predominance of the need for safety and security, including stability, protection, and freedom from fear, anxiety, and chaos. People with unmet safety needs experience their world as hostile or threatening. Individuals with met safety needs perceive their world as trustworthy and are more self-directed, autonomous, and interested in others.

As the physiologic needs are met, the need for belonging and love emerges; these **metaneeds** include the yearnings for affection, intimacy, and establishing relationships with others in order to find a place in one's peer group. The person with unmet love and intimacy needs is likely to experience feelings of desolation, alienation, and rejection.

The fourth level of Maslow's hierarchy describes the need for self-esteem, as well as respect and esteem from others. Self-esteem needs include a desire for adequacy, self-respect, competence, independence, and freedom. The need to acquire esteem or respect from others includes the desire for recognition, dignity, and appreciation.

When any of the four levels of human needs ([1] physiologic, [2] safety or security, [3] social or affiliation, and [4] esteem) are frustrated, a deficiency in one's motivation predominates. Individuals with deficient motivation experience feelings of threat, anxiety, and tension, and they tend to use immature defense mechanisms, such as projection, in an effort to gratify the prevailing need. In contrast, individuals whose physiologic and safety needs have been met are characterized by a predominance of challenge (Maslow, 1970).

The final need to emerge, when all prior needs are relatively satisfied, is the desire for **self-actualization.** This is defined as an ongoing actualization of potentials, capacities, and talents; as fulfillment of a mission (or call, fate,

Understanding & Applying Research

The focus of this study was on the patterns of individual behaviors that influence relationships and interactions. Behavioral patterns studied were dependence, independence, and interdependence. The purpose of the study was to:
1. Determine the defining characteristics for interdependence and dysfunctional independence.
2. Determine the prevalence of the behavior patterns according to gender and race.
3. Generate questions for hypothesis testing.
4. Add to the nursing taxonomy.

Over 100 certified psychiatric mental health clinical nurse specialists who encounter these behaviors in their clients participated in three rounds of a Delphi study. The Delphi technique was used because it has been found to be useful for generating, analyzing, and synthesizing expert opinions about controversial or intangible content. From a collection of judgments, this technique achieves a uniform opinion through repetition and controlled feedback.

The results suggest that there is agreement on the behavior patterns and characteristics of dependence, independence, and interdependence. It confirmed a set of defining characteristics for interdependence and dysfunctional independence. Nurses can use these defining characteristics as criteria against which to measure client behaviors and to establish client goals.

Anderson-Whiting S: A Delphi study to determine defining characteristics of interdependence and dysfunctional independence as potential nursing diagnoses, *Ment Health Nurs* 115:37, 1994.

destiny, or vocation); and as a greater knowledge and acceptance of the individual's intrinsic nature. Therefore this need is not environmentally dependent. Rather, it is a process of growth and development from within that is considered rewarding and exciting. Although this higher-level need develops only as lower needs are satisfied, the need for self-actualization can become relatively independent of those fundamental desires, since the sense of satisfaction develops through the self-actualization process and becomes well established (Maslow, 1970).

Most individuals are partially satisfied and partially unsatisfied in their basic needs at any given time. An individual can be helped to meet the basic and metaneeds through support, reassurance, acceptance, education, and protection. These actions are the therapeutic essence of nursing practice and the core of many nursing theories (see Understanding & Applying Research box).

CHANGING TIMES

According to *Current Population Reports* (U.S. Bureau of the Census), we must rethink and redesign our life course as a result of the lengthening life expectancy and changing standards for expected life events. An example is that it is becoming almost commonplace for women in their fifties and sixties to proudly announce that they have given

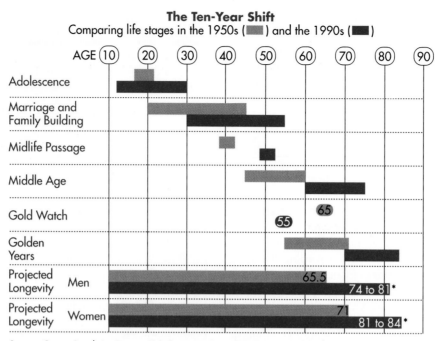

Source: Current Population Reports, U.S. Commerce Dept. Ages are approximated.

*The higher figure is the average projected life expectancy for those who have reached age 65.

Figure 10-5 The ten-year shift. (From U.S. Bureau of the Census: Life expectancy at birth and at age 65, by race and sex: 1950 to 2080. In *Current Population Reports*, Washington, DC, U.S. Department of Commerce, Economics and Statistics Administration.)

birth. Medical ethicist and lawyer George Annas of Boston University states that the fact that a woman can be fertile indefinitely "makes the life course incoherent."

Gail Sheehy in *New Passages* (1995) urges us to look at how we divide the human life into ages and stages. What she and many researchers are finding is that **marker events** of life, such as leaving the primary family, first job, first marriage, first child, empty nest, retirement, widowhood, and death, have occurred at predictable points in life until now, when there appears to be a 10-year shift in events when comparing population reports from 1950 to the 1990s (Figure 10-5). Sheehy describes the three periods of adulthood as:

Provisional adulthood (18-30)
First adulthood (30-45)
Second adulthood (45-85++)

This does not compute with our old time tables and can lead to a sense of disorientation and anxiety, and it is cer-

tainly not what our parents and grandparents led us to expect from life.

OPTIMUM GROWTH

Erikson (1974a, 1974b) put it well when he wrote about optimum opportunity for growth and a person's ability to continue to grow and mature, individually and within an institution. He wrote that from the stages of life come faith, willpower, purposefulness, competence, fidelity, love, care, and wisdom—all criteria of vital individual strengths that also flow into institutions. Without these strengths, institutions wilt; however, without the spirit of institutions and training, no strengths can emerge for the coming generations. Psychosocial strength depends on a total process that regulates the individual's life cycles, the sequence of generations, and the structure of society simultaneously.

Summary of Key Concepts

1. Freud believed that development is the result of biologic and psychologic interactions.
2. Jung viewed adult development as continuous throughout the life cycle.
3. Erikson's eight psychosocial stages of development are as follows:
   Trust versus mistrust (infancy)
   Automony versus shame and doubt (toddlerhood)
   Initiative versus guilt (preschool)
   Industry versus inferiority (school age)
   Identity versus role confusion (puberty to adolescence)
   Intimacy versus isolation (young adulthood)
   Generativity versus stagnation (middle adulthood)
   Ego integrity versus despair (older adulthood)
4. Successful resolution of earlier crises determines the likelihood of resolution of current crises.
5. Generativity, the task of the seventh psychosocial stage, includes the ability to evaluate and appreciate one's past life, embrace the future, assume new responsibilities and relationships, and acknowledge and utilize one's creativity.
6. Modern theorists view adult development as an ongoing dynamic process.
7. Adult development is concerned with the continued evolution of that structure previously developed in childhood.
8. Vaillant's theory holds that if individuals are to master conflict gracefully, and to be successful and efficient in their life choices, ego defense mechanisms must change and mature throughout the life cycle.
9. Defensive personality traits may prevent the development of healthy defense mechanisms and/or be converted into assets.
10. In *New Passages* (1995), Gail Sheehy describes the three periods of adulthood as provisional adulthood (18 to 30 years of age), first adulthood (30 to 45 years of age), and second adulthood (45 to 85+ years of age).

REFERENCES

American Psychiatric Association: *Diagnostic and statistical manual of mental disorders*, ed 4, Washington, DC, 1994, The Association.

Anderson-Whiting S: A Delphi study to determine defining characteristics of interdependence and dysfunctional independence as potential nursing diagnoses, *Ment Health Nurs* 115:37, 1994.

Bardwick J: Psychological correlates of the menstrual cycle and oral contraceptive medication. In Sachar E, editor: *Hormones, behavior, and psychopathology*, New York, 1976, Raven Press.

Blanck G, Blanck R: *Ego psychology*, ed 11, New York, 1979, Columbia University Press.

Bowlby J: *A secure base: clinical applications of attachment theory*, London, 1988, Routledge.

Colarusso CA, Nemiroff RA: *Adult development*, New York, 1981, Plenum Press.

Erikson EH: *Eight stages of man in childhood and society*, New York, 1963, WW Norton.

Erikson EH: *Childhood and society*, ed 2, New York, 1974a, WW Norton.

Erikson EH: *Dimensions of a new identity: Jefferson lectures*, New York, 1974b, WW Norton.

Gilligan C: In a different voice: women's conceptions of self and of morality, *Harvard Educ Rev* 47:481, 1977.

Gilligan C: Joining the resistances: psychology, politics, girls and women, *Mich Q Rev* 29:501, 1990.

Kolata G: Reproductive revolution is jolting old views, *New York Times*, January 11, 1994.

Levinson DJ et al: *The seasons of a man's life*, New York, 1986, Ballantine Books.

Lowenthal MF, Turner M, Cheroboga D: *Four stages of life: a comparative study of men and women facing transitions*, San Francisco, 1975, Jossey-Bass.

Maslow AH: *Toward a psychology of being*, New York, 1968, D. Van Nostrand.

Maslow AH: *Motivation and personality*, New York, 1970, Harper & Row.

Millon T: *Millon clinical multi axial inventory manual*, ed 3, Minneapolis, 1987, National Computer Systems.

Neugarten BL: Time, age, and the life cycle, *Am J Psychiatry* 136:887, 1979.

Newton PM, Levinson DJ: Crisis in adult development. In Lazare A, editor: *Outpatient psychiatry: diagnosis and treatment*, Baltimore, 1979, Williams & Wilkins.

Sheehy G: *New passages: mapping your life across time*, New York, 1995, Ballantine Books.

Stevens-Long J: *Adult life: developmental processes*, ed 4, Palo Alto, Calif, 1992, Mayfield.

U.S. Bureau of the Census: Life expectancy at birth and at age 65, by race and sex: 1950 to 2080. In *Current Population Reports*, Washington, DC, U.S. Department of Commerce, Economics and Statistics Administration.

Vaillant GE: *Adaptation to life*, Boston, 1977, Little, Brown.

Van Gennep A: *The rites of passage*, Chicago, 1960, University of Chicago Press.

Vandenbergh RL: Postpartum depression, *Clin Obstet Gynocol* 23:1105, 1980.

CHAPTER 11

The Elderly

Linda Hollinger-Smith

OBJECTIVES

- Describe characteristics of the biologic, social, and psychologic theories of aging from a developmental perspective.

- Distinguish between normal and abnormal physical and psychosocial processes of aging.

- Discuss the process of functional assessment as related to the elderly client.

- Explore the meaning of health and wellness for the elderly.

- Examine how negative attitudes toward the elderly have influenced others' behaviors.

- Compare the developmental tasks of aging with tasks of younger cohorts.

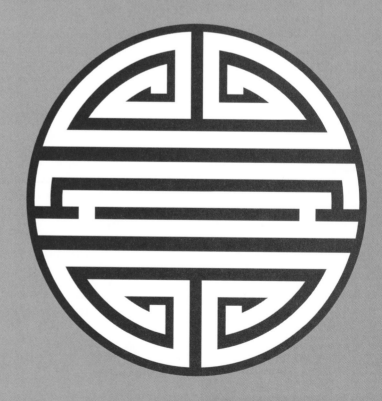

Advances in health care sciences have ensured that a larger proportion of people will be living longer with a better quality of life. More than ever as we enter the twenty-first century, aging is viewed as an evolutionary process. Aging is a complex process involving biologic, psychologic, social, and environmental factors. How a person adapts to aging is very individualized, and no single theory adequately explains the effects of aging from a developmental perspective. New theories of aging are attempting to integrate biologic and behavioral changes in order to view aging as a series of life events.

The process of aging is described as a series of physiologic and psychosocial changes. It is important that psychiatric nurses understand normal and abnormal aging changes and their impact on such factors as daily living activities, mental processes, social supports, sexuality, and role development. For the elderly, their physical and mental health represents the summation of health care beliefs and practices across the years. The psychiatric mental health nurse needs to consider the older person's perceptions of health and wellness as key information in the assessment and management of care.

Changing attitudes and images of aging have important implications for the psychiatric mental health nurse. Carl Jung stated that we would not grow to be 70 or 80 years old if this longevity had no meaning for the species. Two decades ago that concept was poetically stated as follows: "The afternoon of human life must also have a significance of its own and cannot be merely a pitiful appendage to life's morning" (Campbell, 1979). This is even more significant as we enter the new millennium. Scientists are beginning to heed those words, focusing on successful aging processes as reality rather than an ideal.

Activities of daily living (ADL) Categories of personal care (e.g., bathing, grooming, toileting).

Activity theory Theory that supports the idea that maintaining an active lifestyle and social roles offsets the negative effects of aging.

Ageism Systematic stereotyping and discrimination against the elderly.

Cohort A group having one or more factors in common.

Continuity theory Theory that promotes the premise that people become "more like themselves" as they age, maintaining continuity of habits, beliefs, and values.

Dependency ratio The number of individuals under age 18 and over age 64 who are dependent on persons ages 18 to 64 years.

Disengagement theory Process of mutual withdrawal between the aging individual and society.

Dystonic Pertaining to unstable states or to some disorder.

Geriatrics The provision of health care services to the elderly.

Gerontology The study of the aging process involving multiple disciplines and settings.

Instrumental activities of daily living (IADL) Activities required of an individual to function in the community (e.g., shopping, preparing meals, getting around).

Intraphysic Pertaining to the mind or mental processes.

Life expectancy The estimated length of human life from a given point in time.

Life span The maximum length of human life from birth to death.

Locus of control An aspect of personality that deals with the degree of control one perceives to have over one's own destiny. *Internal locus of control* refers to the ability to actively control one's destiny. *External locus of control* refers to the inability to control one's destiny.

Metamemory One's self-perceptions of memory changes.

Psyche The mind as the center of thought processes, emotions, and behavior.

Selective attention The ability to discriminate and focus on relevant information.

Syntonic Pertaining to a state of stability.

Vigilance The ability to sustain attention.

OVERVIEW OF THE ELDERLY POPULATION

Since over 70% of all health care resources are used by those age 65 years and older, an imperative for all health care professionals is an understanding of basic gerontology (U.S. Bureau of the Census, 1996). **Gerontology** is defined as the study of the aging process across multiple disciplines and settings. Gerontologists, who receive specialized training and education in the field of aging, may be found in many disciplines, including nursing, medicine, psychiatry, social services, pharmacology, biology, and the humanities. The term **geriatrics** broadly refers to the health care and human services that are provided to the elderly (Eliopoulos, 1993).

DEMOGRAPHICS

Over the past 100 years, the average growth rate of the population age 65 and older has greatly surpassed the overall population rate according to the U.S. Census Bureau (1992). From 1900 to 1994 the elderly population increased elevenfold, from 3 million to 33 million. In comparison, the total population over that same period tripled. By 2050, projections show a marked increased in the elderly population to more than 80 million persons. With the aging of the baby boomers, 1 in 5 individuals will be over the age of 65 in the year 2030. Elderly minority groups, including African-Americans, Asians and Pacific Islanders, Native Americans, and Hispanics, will see substantial population growth into the middle of the twenty-first century.

The most rapidly growing group of the elderly population are those age 85 and older, termed the *oldest old*. Currently 1.3% of the U.S. population is in this age cohort. By 2050 this group will grow to 19 million, or almost one quarter of the entire elderly population (U.S. Bureau of the Census, 1996). Table 11-1 presents highlights of findings from the recent report "65+ in the United States," showing several important characteristics of the elderly population today and in the future.

HEALTH STATUS

Overall, the elderly report that their health is good to excellent (Rowe and Kahn, 1998). Socioeconomic status and availability of social support have direct effects on reports of health. Minority groups and those with low incomes consistently report poorer health, even when age is controlled. Because both males and females are living longer, a greater proportion of couples are surviving into old age. The elderly of today are more educated, with a greater portion having completed some college. Over 22% of persons age 65 years and older completed at least 1 year of college, compared with 12.5% in 1970. The elderly also maintain better health care practices than some of their younger-age cohorts. The most recent data from the U.S. Department of Health and Human Services (1993) reported that elderly persons had better dietary habits and smoked and consumed alcohol to a lesser extent than those less than 65 years of age. Only in the area of physical exercise did the elderly report less activity than younger age-groups.

Although a majority of the elderly across all settings suffer from at least one chronic condition, illness in itself does not appear to influence individual perception of health status, if functional abilities are not impaired. Functional ability is categorized as activities of daily living (ADL) and instrumental activities of daily living (IADL). Physical and psychosocial functions are included in a functional assessment. Assessing functional abilities of the elderly is discussed later in this chapter.

Table 11-1	Profile of the Elderly U.S. Population: 1990 and 2050 Comparisons	
	Elderly Population in 1994 (%)	Elderly Population in 2050 (%)
Ethnic group proportions		
Caucasian	87	67
African-American	7	10
Native American	<1	<1
Asian, Pacific Islander	3	7
Hispanic	3	16

Other Facts

Sex ratios will continue to decline (number of males per 100 females) as age increases:
   Ratio of 82 for males 65-69 years of age
   Ratio of 44 for males 85-89 years of age
   Ratio of 26 for males 95-99 years of age
Eight states will double their elderly population by 2020: Nevada, Arizona, Georgia, Washington, Alaska, Utah, Colorado, and
   California
Increasing numbers of elderly women live in poverty compared with elderly men:
   Currently 16% of elderly women are at or below poverty level, compared with 9% of men
   2 million of the 2.3 million elderly poor living alone are women
   Poverty rates are higher for elderly minorities

Modified from U.S. Bureau of the Census: Sixty-five plus in the United States. In *Current Population Reports*, P23-190, No. 178RV, special studies, Washington, DC, 1996, U.S. Department of Commerce, Economics and Statistics Administration.

LIFE EXPECTANCY VERSUS LIFE SPAN

Life expectancy and life span are terms that require differentiation. **Life expectancy** is defined as the expected number of years of life. Several factors affect life expectancy, including gender, race, and environmental conditions.

The average life expectancy in the United States is 75 years (Centers for Disease Control, 1990). Women outlive men by about 6.9 years, and this difference is not expected to change dramatically over the next 30 years. Both male and female African-Americans have a shorter life expectancy than whites.

Researchers disagree about the possibility of significant increases in life expectancy. Some researchers predict that life expectancy will increase an additional 10 years by the year 2040 as a result of medical advancements and decreased mortality. The primary focus of all health care providers must be to provide comprehensive and affordable medical care to this growing population.

Life span refers to the maximum length of survival, which is genetically fixed for each species. Most scientists consider 100 to 115 years as the maximum verified human life span. Increases in life expectancy are a result of increases in survival rates of infants and children to a much greater extent than increases in survival rates for those over age 50.

The **dependency ratio** is another measure used to describe the demographic characteristics of a population. Dependency ratio is defined as the number of individuals under age 18 and over age 64 who are dependent on persons ages 18 to 64 years. The ratio is an estimate of the main workforce required to provide health, education, social, and recreational resources to the young and old.

Any factors that cause shifts in the population, such as an increased or decreased birthrate, will alter the dependency ratio. A major decrease in the dependency ratio will occur in the early part of the twenty-first century as a result of the Social Security Amendment of 1983, which adjusts the retirement ages to 66 years of age by the year 2000 and to 67 years of age by the year 2027.

A LIFE SPAN PERSPECTIVE OF AGING

Gerontologists in a variety of scientific fields have attempted to explain the developmental processes of aging from biologic and behavioral perspectives. A variety of theories on aging exist because scientists do not agree on a single definition of aging. Chronologic, biologic, psychologic, and social definitions of aging have been extensively described in the literature but are inadequate in describing the process of aging. Therefore scientists and philosophers have developed theories to explain the meaning, causes, and factors related to the aging process.

BIOLOGIC THEORIES OF AGING

Biologic theories of aging are classified into various categories based on causative factors. Most biologic theories view the process of aging as either a normal, gradual wearing down of all systems or an abnormal series of cellular damage or mutations eventually leading to the body's inability to make repairs (Schneider and Rowe, 1990).

One method of classifying biologic theories of aging relates to categorizing predisposing factors as intrinsic or extrinsic to the organism. Intrinsic, or genetic, theories focus on the process of aging as internal to the organism. It is estimated that up to 30% of one's life expectancy is genetically determined, with lifestyle and environmental influences having more profound effects on aging than what was earlier believed (Finch and Tanzi, 1997). Certain genetic diseases, including several types of cancers and high cholesterol syndromes that lead to heart disease, have a negative impact on life expectancy (Rowe and Kahn, 1998).

Extrinsic, or nongenetic, theories propose that aging occurs as a result of environmental factors acting on the organism, such as radiation, ozone, drugs, and toxic substances, which have been theorized to damage cellular structures, leading to aging and death.

Researchers have not agreed on any single biologic theory to explain the aging process. A combination of genetic and environmental factors may best explain why individuals age differently. Four of the biologic theories of aging most examined by researchers follow.

Genetic Theory

The genetic theory of aging represents a group of intrinsic aging theories, all of which focus on an internal genetic code that drives the aging process. The premise of the theory is that genes are categorized as juvenescent or senescent. *Juvenescent* genes promote and maintain growth and vigor through the adult years, whereas *senescent* genes become active in middle adult and later years and initiate a process of decline and deterioration. Empiric evidence to support the theory of this "aging" gene is lacking.

Another popular genetic theory is known as the *biologic clock theory* (Schneider and Rowe, 1990) and suggests that an organism's development and subsequent decline are regulated by some programmed internal genetic clock. This internal clock runs down over a predetermined length of time. Supporters of this theory point to certain normal physiologic changes in humans that appear to be correlated with time, such as hair graying and menopause.

Although the biologic clock theory gives dramatic evidence for boundaries of the human life span, there are limitations to this theory. One limitation is the inability to generalize in vitro studies to in vivo studies. Second, the theory does not explain what factor triggers the end of cellular replication and the beginning of cellular degeneration. Finally, the theory does not explain extreme cases of longevity.

A final genetic theory, *error theory*, has been suggested to explain the development of harmful genes that interfere with biologic processes such as protein synthesis (Hayflick, 1985). Damage to biologic synthesis results in the development of damaged cells that interfere with normal biologic functions. The proliferation of cancerous cells is an example of a process in which normal cells become aberrant through some error process.

Immunologic Theory

Most biologists agree that changes in the immunologic system after puberty influence the process of aging. Antibody production declines, and autoimmune responses change in response to the decline. The result is that the body's ability to differentiate normal and abnormal or foreign substances fails. This response is sometimes seen in cases of tissue rejection in organ transplantation.

Immune function significantly declines with aging. By age 85 an individual's immune system functions at 5% to 10% of the system's level at puberty. Rheumatoid arthritis and mature-onset diabetes are two diseases commonly experienced in older age that are caused by alterations to the immune system. Although it is not exactly known how or why the immune system exhibits a functional decline with aging, the appearance of autoantibodies in the serum of elderly persons is common. Autoantibodies are antibodies particular to an individual's own normal serum or tissue. It is hypothesized that their appearance signals declines in immune system function (Mille, 1996).

Cross-Linkage Theory

Collagen tissue, an important component of connective tissue that maintains the structure of cells, tissues, and organs, undergoes changes with aging. Collagen provides the elasticity necessary in many types of tissue, such as cardiac and muscle. With age, the combination of chemical changes and external stimuli cause the formation of molecular bonds in collagen, or cross-links, which tend to stabilize the collagen fibers, resulting in rigid, fragile tissue. Scientists do not understand the mechanism that triggers the formation of cross-links, but it is believed that the most active period of cross-link development is between 30 and 50 years of age.

Cross-links also form in elastin in connective tissue. Elastin is similar to collagen in that it maintains tissue flexibility and permeability. The effects of cross-linking in elastin fibers are most pronounced in the changes in facial skin with aging. Skin becomes brittle, dry, saggy, and appears translucent. The formation of cross-links is probably not the sole cause of aging, but structural and functional changes associated with aging are impacted by collagen alterations at the cellular level.

Free Radical Theory

Biologists theorize that some environmental stimuli, such as radiation, ozone, and certain chemicals, interfere with cellular activity, resulting in the production of free radicals, which are compounds produced in cells as a result of environmental stimuli. They may interact with various cellular structures, causing damage to normal cellular function. Free radicals are also formed during the normal process of cellular oxygenation when the cell removes waste products. Although the cell is capable of neutralizing and removing such by-products, it is theorized that over time the cell loses its capacity to eliminate waste and repair itself. Researchers are continuing to study the potential effectiveness of antioxidants, such as vitamins A, C, and E, in protecting cellular structures (Packer and Glazer, 1990).

SOCIOLOGIC THEORIES OF AGING

Sociologists have observed that an individual's role, relationships, and social experiences change as he or she ages. Sociologic theories of aging attempt to explain the social aspects of the aging process. Three of the earliest theories were developed in the 1960s. These three theories, *disengagement*, *continuity*, and *activity*, all take a different approach to the social aspects of aging. Common to the three theories is the focus on action and adaptation by the individual (i.e., the aging person needs to change or adjust to new situations). Relocation to a nursing home is often traumatic for the elderly person who cannot adjust to the highly structured institutional routines. Social theories that focus more on the interaction between the aging individual and the environment have evolved.

Disengagement Theory

The **disengagement theory** was the first sociologic aging theory developed by social gerontologists. In 1961 Cumming and Henry published the results of their exploratory study of 275 healthy, financially stable persons, ages 50 to 95, who lived in Kansas City. They theorized that a process of mutual withdrawal naturally occurs between the aging individual and society that is inevitable and universal in its occurrence. The retirement process is an example of this disengagement. Society clearly identifies the age of 65 years as the time for retirement. Identifying a retirement marker, or target, is also a mechanism for society to open the opportunity for a young person to enter the workforce. According to Cumming and Henry (1961), if the older person is prepared for retirement, he or she will have an easier time "disengaging" from society. The elderly person's social ties continue to shrink, perpetuating the individual's further withdrawal into self.

The disengagement theory has been the most controversial of the social aging theories. Most of the criticism focuses on its presumed universality and on the fact that it does not allow for biologic or personality differences between individuals. In addition, it presumes that the individual will see disengagement as an obligation to society. How ready and accepting elderly persons are to change roles determines their ability to adjust and, subsequently, their life satisfaction.

Havighurst, Neugarten, and Tobin (1968) reexamined the original data used to formulate the disengagement theory and arrived at different conclusions in support of disengagement. For example, they found that individual personality traits and past experiences influence how an individual in society adapts to aging. A person who is withdrawn early in life will probably continue to withdraw and adapt if his or her social ties also support withdrawal behaviors. Society today is less insistent that elderly persons completely disengage. For example, some industries are hiring retired persons on a part-time or per diem basis or using them as expert consultants. It is more of a combination of one's personal preferences and the needs of society that dictates the degree and pattern of disengagement rather than personal preference or societal needs alone.

Continuity Theory

The **continuity theory** was developed out of Havighurst, Neugarten, and Tobin's reformulation of the disengagement theory (1968). The basic premise behind the continuity theory is that people adapt best when they are allowed to be who they are and that, with aging, people become "more like themselves"; that is, as an individual ages, he or she attempts to maintain continuity and consistency of habits, beliefs, norms, values, and other aspects of the personality. If a person is having difficulties adjusting to changes such as retirement or relocation, the continuity theory holds that it is not the process of aging that interferes with adaptation, but rather personality factors or the individual's social environment that influences adaptation. The continuity theory allows for individual differences in the aging process and theorizes that each individual's personality contains a self-maintaining component, meaning that the individual's longstanding behavior patterns enhance coping and adjustments to new situations across the life span (Atchley, 1989).

Activity Theory

The supporters of the **activity theory** believe that maintaining an active lifestyle and social roles offsets the negative effects of aging (Figure 11-1). By retaining a high level of participation in his or her socioenvironment, activity theorists postulated that the elderly individual would report a higher level of overall life satisfaction and a more positive self-concept. Four propositions were initially identified in the conceptualization of the activity theory (Lemon, Bengston, and Peterson, 1972):

1. The greater the loss in social roles (both formal and informal), the less the activity participation.

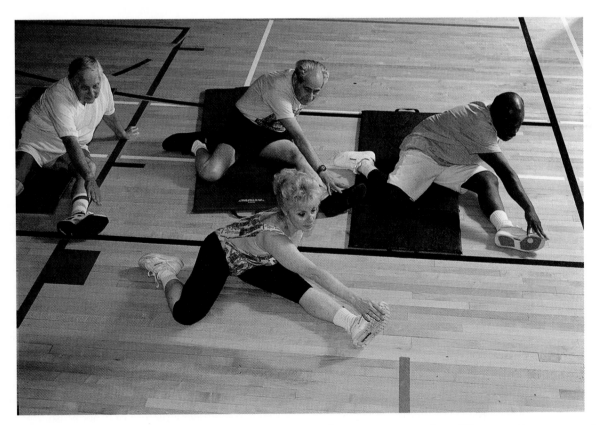

Figure 11-1   Supervised physical exercise is good for the elderly, as it is for any age-group, and would be viewed by an activity theorist as possibly offsetting the negative effects of aging. (Copyright Cathy Lander-Goldberg, Lander Photographics.)

2. The more activity maintained, the greater the social role support for the older person.

3. Maintaining stability of social roles supports a person's positive self-concept.

4. The more positive a person's self-concept, the greater the degree of life satisfaction experienced.

Wider acceptance of the activity theory is hindered by the lack of empiric evidence to support these postulates. The importance, type, and availability of a particular activity as perceived by the elderly person is an important consideration affecting self-concept and life satisfaction. The activity theory may only apply to elderly persons who enjoy and have the opportunity to participate in meaningful activities and social interactions.

PSYCHOLOGIC THEORIES OF AGING

Studying human behavior and attempting to explain why persons act the way they do have been the focus of developmental psychologists since Freud, the founder of psychoanalysis. Because in many cases the elderly do not exhibit the same patterns of behavior as their younger counterparts, theorists developed psychologic theories and models of aging. Whereas sociologic theories of aging focus more on the interaction between the aging individual and his or her socioenvironment within an age **cohort** (group with one or more factors in common) or a culture, developmental psychologists examine human development from an **intrapsychic** or mental viewpoint. Few of the human development theories address characteristics of developmental change in the elderly. Most of the developmental theories focus on a single area of one's **psyche**, or the center of thought processes, emotions, and behavior. For example, Freud's theory and practice focused on sexual aspects across the human life span. A focus on cycles or stages during which key developmental tasks or events are carried out is apparent in most of the developmental theories.

Life Stage Theories

Several life stage theories have been advanced over the past several years. These theories divide the life span into a series of sequential transitions. Individuals who are adjusted and happy are able to achieve age-appropriate developmental tasks at each stage.

Jung's life stage theory (1971) was based on psychoanalytic theory that states that as one goes through life, one develops inner exploratory abilities that add meaning to life. He also postulated that personality differences between males and females become less distinct as people age. The final life stage deals with maintaining a balance between wisdom and senility in old age. The elderly person who is successful in life does not attempt to compete with youth but rather is able to deal with age changes.

Erikson, a social psychoanalyst, is the most well known of the life stage theorists and identified eight stages of psychologic development. Each stage of development involves maintaining a balance between the **syntonic** (state of stability) and **dystonic** (state of disorder) (Erikson, Erikson, and Kiunick, 1986) in order to adjust and move forward to the next level. In describing the final stage of life, Erickson stated that "the process of bringing into balance feelings of integrity and despair involves a review of and a coming to terms with the life one has lived thus far" (Erikson, Erikson, and Kiunick, 1986).

More recently, a psychologic model encompassing life span development, called *selective optimization with compensation*, has been developed (Baltes, Smith, and Staudinger, 1992). This theoretic framework focuses on managing age-related gains and losses for successful aging. Individuals who age successfully are those who select and modify activities that enrich their lives despite energy declines.

Human Motivation and Development Theory

Maslow's motivation and development theory (1962) is widely viewed as a valuable framework to understand human needs and values from a holistic point of reference. Maslow's theoretic construct is described as a hierarchy of needs and is diagrammed in the form of a pyramid. Five levels of needs are identified, the most basic representing the base of the pyramid. From the most basic (1) to the highest (5) level, these needs include the following:

1. Biologic and physiologic
2. Safety and security
3. Affiliation or sense of belonging
4. Self-esteem
5. Self-actualization

Ebersole and Hess (1999) have conceptualized Maslow's hierarchy of needs and applied his theory to identification of special needs of the elderly at each level. Table 11-2 identifies some of these specific needs of the older adult and potential strategies to meet those needs.

Adaptation Theory

The adaptation theory as described by Vaillant (1977) is more of a conceptual model that categorizes the changes brought about by aging. Vaillant identified a series of shifts and trade-offs that occur during the aging process. What is critical to successful adaptation is the ability of the individual to let go of parts of the past while pursuing quality-of-life components. For example, the elderly person often experiences sensory losses, especially in the areas of vision and hearing, and adapts to such losses by facilitating the quality of the remaining sensory perceptions. For instance, the use of large-print books, direct lighting, or hearing aids would enhance the older person's remaining sight and hearing. Encouraging the use of other sensory perceptual systems such as touch or taste would be another way for the older individual to gather pertinent information from the environment.

Table 11-2	Special Needs of the Elderly According to Maslow's Hierarchy of Needs	
Needs of the Elderly	**Maslow's Hierarchy of Needs**	**Strategies to Meet Needs**
Finding meaning in life and death Transcendence over aging processes Creativity and mastery	Self-actualization	Identify value and contributions of individual Encourage continuity of participation in decision-making processes Reminisce about past in relation to present and future
Responsible roles Social supports Locus of control Cognitive awareness	Self-esteem	Maintain aspects of roles important to individual Facilitate socialization Promote physical appearance Facilitate decision making
Relationships Intimacy Affiliations	Belonging	Identify impact of loss on individual Support needs for intimacy and sexuality Facilitate changes in lifestyle
Sensory awareness Environmental safety Legal and economic issues	Safety and security	Obtain necessary equipment or supplies for home independence Assist with obtaining legal or financial help Educate elderly person and family regarding home safety
Biologic needs Comfort needs	Biologic integrity	Provide for physical comfort Provide for nutritional needs

From Ebersole P, Hess P: *Toward healthy aging: human needs and nursing responses,* ed 5, St. Louis, 1999, Mosby.

NEW THEORIES OF AGING

In the realm of theory, theories of aging are considered to be in their infancy. This is especially true with psychologic theories, most of which were developed after World War II. New theories of aging include behavioral genetics, gerotranscendence, and gerodynamics theories.

Behavioral genetics theory examines the relevant impact of genetic and environmental factors on biologic and behavioral differences among individuals across the life span (Pedersen, 1996). *Gerotranscendence theory* looks at aging from three levels: cosmic, the self, and social relations. The theory implies that aging brings on changes such as (1) changes in time perception, (2) acceptance of the mysteries of life and death, (3) altruistic behavior, and (4) increased need for solitude and reflection (Tornstam, 1994). *Gerodynamics theory* is based on several physics theories, including general systems theory and chaos theory. Gerodynamics postulates that individuals pass through a series of transformations, or life events, and are thereby changed in some way (Schroots, 1995). Individuals respond differently and are either weakened or strengthened by the events. Those who age successfully have the ability to cope with traumatic events and maintain healthy lifestyles. As yet, these theories need additional empiric testing to support these concepts.

PROCESS OF AGING

The process of aging incorporates physiologic and psychosocial changes within the individual. As described in sev-

eral of the biologic and psychosocial theories of aging, external or environmental factors affect aging in many ways. The physiologic changes that come with aging are universal. Because the changes that characterize normal physiologic aging mirror pathologic changes, normal and abnormal aging processes are often confused. Although aging is ultimately irreversible, disease and disability can be significantly delayed even into very old age (Rowe and Kahn, 1998).

Psychosocial changes during aging in the areas of cognition, personality, social interactions, sexuality, and roles are even less distinct. Personality and socioenvironmental factors play a huge role in determining psychosocial aging changes. Particular aspects of such processes as cognition and memory may decline with aging, whereas other aspects may remain the same or even be enhanced with advanced age.

PHYSIOLOGIC AGING

The physiologic aging changes considered part of normal aging affect all body systems, but not necessarily at the same rates. It is important to have an understanding of the common physiologic aging changes, since some of these changes may indicate the development of pathologic conditions. Many of these changes begin as early as the fourth and fifth decades of life. There are also individual differences in the rates of aging of some biologic systems due to factors such as heredity, environment, lifestyle, and nutrition (Steinberg, 1983).

Musculoskeletal System

Aging changes occur in bone and muscle mass, tendon and joint flexibility, and cartilage structure (Meier, 1988). It appears that bone continues to grow up to the eighth decade in some bony structures, but the reabsorption of the interior of flat and long bones occurs at a greater rate than bone growth. Also, bone minerals and proteins are lost from the bone matrix. Osteoporosis, or loss of bone mass, and loss of minerals, especially calcium, increase the possibility of fractures and subsequent immobility. Women are affected by osteoporosis twice as often as men.

Changes in joints begin about the third decade and continue throughout the remainder of the life span. With severe loss of cartilage and fluids, bones may begin to rub together, resulting in painful, slow movements. Changes in the vertebral column combined with osteoporosis cause a loss of sitting height with aging.

Cardiovascular System

Changes in the cardiovascular system as a result of aging are complex. Some of the changes that have been attributed to disease may be part of normal aging; thus it is difficult for researchers to separate normal versus abnormal cardiovascular changes to a great extent (Lakatta, 1988).

With normal aging, the size of the heart may decrease slightly as a result of loss of muscle cells. In the heart, muscle cells are replaced with fat cells and connective tissue that causes rigidity in the heart muscle. This results in a slower heart rate and decreased cardiac output. A decrease in oxygen consumption by the heart reflects decreased effectiveness of the heart. Changes in the structure of the heart muscle fibers may result in changes in heart rhythm. Atrial dysrhythmias, including atrial fibrillation and atrial flutter, are common.

Blood pressure may increase to compensate for changes in atrial circulation. The structure of arteries changes with aging. Collagen fibers, lipids, and minerals increase in the walls of arteries and in veins. These arterial changes also affect the baroreceptors that are important in moderating blood pressure during postural changes. This is reflected in the elderly person's complaint of dizziness when standing quickly.

Respiratory System

The respiratory system exhibits changes in its structure and function with aging (Kumpe et al, 1985). The diameter of the chest wall increases with age as a result of loss of lung resiliency and muscle strength, giving the appearance of a "barrel" chest. Lung compliance increases with aging, but the work of breathing increases because the chest wall compliance decreases. The ability to remove secretions through ciliary movement and coughing decreases with aging. The lungs of older adults stay partially inflated at rest as a result of an increase in residual volume. It is believed that changes in lung tissue with aging decrease pulmonary diffusion capacity, which results in

decreased oxygen saturation. Under normal circumstances the older person puts less stress on the lungs; thus a slight decrease in oxygen use balances out the decrease in oxygen availability.

Gastrointestinal System

Changes in the gastrointestinal system with aging are not well understood. Most of the gastrointestinal changes are primarily due to disease rather than to aging alone.

Decreased motility of the esophagus may lead to spasm and reflux. Delayed emptying of stomach contents may occur as a result of decreased motility and acid secretion. Decreased absorption of vitamins, nutrients, and water also results from diminished muscle tone and changes in vascular perfusion (Bowman and Rosenberg, 1983).

The size of the liver decreases with age and results in decreased blood flow, protein synthesis, and metabolism of some drugs. The potential for serious toxic effects of drugs that are metabolized in the liver should be closely monitored through blood levels.

The formation of stones in the gallbladder increases with aging. It is believed that the absorption of cholesterol is less efficient as one ages, resulting in stone production. Changes in the pancreas with aging primarily affect enzyme production, but not to a degree that significantly affects normal digestive processes in the absence of disease.

Integumentary System

Changes in the skin, hair, and nails are most pronounced with advancing age. A loss of subcutaneous fat, thinning of the dermis and epidermis, and loss of elastin flexibility are responsible for the wrinkling and saggy appearance of the skin. Fragility of the dermal vasculature causes "senile purpura," a condition that appears as bruises under the skin.

Sometimes the loss of skin turgor in the elderly is mistaken for dehydration. Decreased skin turgor results from a combination of less body water and subcutaneous fat and a loss of flexibility of the skin's elastin. Dryness of the skin also increases with aging as a result of a decrease in the number and size of sweat glands and reduced hormonal levels.

Changes in hair production and appearance occur with aging. Decreased melanin production results in the appearance of gray hair. Genetics influence the onset of gray hair. Hair also grows more slowly with aging and be-

⚠ CLINICAL ALERT

Because many drugs are excreted through the kidneys, it is important to test creatinine clearance, which is an indicator of the proportion of muscle mass. Reduced creatinine clearance indicates a decrease in muscle mass, so dosages of medications that are absorbed by the kidneys may need to be reduced for older clients.

comes coarse and thick in such areas as the nose, ears, and eyebrows, whereas general body hair thins.

The growth of nail tissue also decreases with aging. Years of use or injury may cause changes in the appearance of nails. Yellowing, the formation of ridges, or thickening of the nails may be observed in older individuals.

Immune System

The ability of the body to form antibodies to some antigens such as pneumococcal and influenza vaccines is greatly reduced in the elderly. Delays in hypersensitive reactions also come with aging. Across the life span, the elderly individual's immune system was required to fight off exposure to many pathogens, with the additive effect resulting in more frequent and severe infections in the elderly.

The thymus, a small organ above the heart, is important to the development of the immune system. The thymus produces hormones that assist with the maturation of T lymphocytes, which are one type of lymph cell that may ward off cancer cells. The actual number of T lymphocytes does not decline with aging, but their ability to proliferate in the presence of particular viruses decreases significantly. Therefore the elderly person has a more difficult time developing defense mechanisms to infections such as pneumonia, bronchitis, and bloodstream infections.

Renal System

The renal system is critical in the removal of a variety of waste products and drugs and in the regulation of fluid volume in extracellular space. With normal aging, the functioning of the renal system decreases significantly, although the remaining kidney functions are usually adequate. Changes to the kidney as a result of aging include loss of glomeruli, loss of total kidney tissue mass, and a decreased glomerular filtration rate. Glomeruli are small structures in the kidney made up of clusters of blood capillaries. The rate and degree of changes to the kidneys are highly variable; therefore researchers believe that aging is not the chief cause of the structural and functional changes. Because cardiac output decreases as a result of aging, the elimination of waste products is affected.

Nervous System

Unlike cells of other body systems, the cells of the nervous system do not reproduce. There is a loss of nerve cells with normal aging, but the degree of loss differs, depending on the structure of the nervous system. The aging pigment, lipofuscin, is deposited in nerve cells, and neurofibrillary plaques and tangles form in the aging brain. These plaques and tangles may indicate Alzheimer's disease but are found in normal aging brains in the absence of dementia (see Chapter 17).

The amount of neurotransmitters also decreases with normal aging. Changes in cognitive functioning such as memory storage may be affected by a decrease in acetyl-

> **⚠ CLINICAL ALERT**
>
> The use of sedatives over an extended period of time should be discouraged, because the older person's normal pattern of sleep usually recurs after only a few nights of sedative use. Frequent periods of sleeplessness should be monitored, since the possibility of an underlying physiologic or psychologic problem may be a precipitating factor.

choline and epinephrine. Because of the redundancy of nerve cells, it is impossible to generalize that all elderly persons have diminished memory or cognitive abilities. Decreases in another neurotransmitter, serotonin, is also part of normal aging. Serotonin is important in the regulation of activities such as sleeping, drinking, and breathing. Serotonin also affects temperature regulation, heart rate, and affect. Reductions in the amount of serotonin result in the elderly person's inability to respond to physical and psychologic stressors in an appropriate manner (see Chapters 12 and 22).

The sleep cycle is influenced as a result of the normal aging process. The elderly usually complain of frequent periods of restlessness or insomnia. They may go to the bathroom often during the night and, as a result, they may nap during the day to make up for the loss of night sleep. Periods of rapid eye movement (REM) sleep are also decreased with aging.

Reproductive System

In females menopause, or the permanent cessation of menses, occurs at around age 51 years. Ovarian estrogen ceases to be produced, but adrenal estrogens continue to be manufactured. Menopausal women commonly complain of hot flashes, or intermittent sensations of warmth and palpations in the upper body. Hot flashes lessen in frequency with aging. There is a narrowing of the vagina and a decrease in vaginal secretions. The uterus, ovaries, and cervix also decrease in size as a result of vascular and muscular changes.

In males the production of androgen hormones decreases with aging. The consequences of reductions in androgen to aging are not yet known. Androgens may affect the libido and nocturnal erections, but they do not appear to influence erections due to the presence of erotic stimuli. The changes in testosterone levels with aging are not agreed on at this time. Although not well studied, the production of sperm, or spermatogenesis, seems to be sustained well into old age in the absence of disease. Physically, the testes and penis may decrease in size, whereas the scrotal sac becomes pendulous.

Many health care providers erroneously believe that the physiologic changes to the reproductive system due to aging mean that the elderly person's sexuality is also impaired. This has become a self-fulfilling prophecy for some elderly individuals who think that sexual pleasures are taboo in the later years. Many elderly persons do enjoy various forms and degrees of intimacy, and caregivers need to encourage such feelings (see Chapter 20).

Endocrine System

Changes in the endocrine organs and the hormones they secrete vary with aging. The endocrine organs are highly interrelated; thus a change in one system usually impacts the others. Researchers believe that focusing on preventing some endocrine changes may hold the greatest promise for reducing the occurrence of disabilities and disorders of the aged.

The endocrine system is made up of the following organs:

> Adrenal glands
> Thyroid gland
> Parathyroid glands
> Pancreas
> Pituitary gland

The adrenal glands appear to decrease in size with aging. The major hormones secreted by the adrenal glands (i.e., cortisol, aldosterone, and the adrenal androgens) decrease in amounts, but the functional implications of these reductions are not well understood.

The thyroid gland atrophies with aging and undergoes some structural changes such as the development of fibrotic tissue and nodules. Thyroid hormonal production decreases with aging, but the impact appears to be minimal, since there is less need for these hormones into old age. The parathyroid hormone may decrease or increase with aging. It appears that the parathyroid hormone increases in the presence of osteoporosis, since it is a factor stimulating bone demineralization.

The secretion of the hormone insulin by the pancreas appears to decrease with aging, resulting in a decreased ability of the elderly to metabolize glucose. Insulin is necessary to the metabolism of blood glucose and for maintenance of normal blood glucose levels in the body. Recent studies have demonstrated that the amount of total insulin produced by the body remains the same across the life span; thus the problem for the elderly may be that release of the available insulin is delayed in some still-unknown manner.

The pituitary gland, which secretes several hormones, undergoes structural changes with aging in its cellular and vascular components. With aging there is a decline in growth hormone and an increase in levels of follicle-stimulating and luteinizing hormones. Alterations in mechanisms that regulate the secretion of thyroid-stimulating hormones, adrenocorticotropic hormones, and antidiuretic hormones are believed to occur with aging, but further research is needed before determining the significance of these changes for the elderly.

Sensory System

The senses of vision and hearing decline with aging. Everyone experiences some visual changes as a part of the normal aging process. The lens of the eye continues to grow throughout aging, but the appearance of the lens changes. The lens becomes rigid and transparent and loses the ability to accommodate or adjust to changing distances—a condition commonly known as presbyopia. The pupil decreases in size and becomes less responsive to light. The ability to discriminate color in the blue, green, and violet hues becomes less distinct (Carter, 1982). Decreases in the lacrimal secretions result in feelings of dryness in the eyes. Arcus senilus, a condition that appears as a white circle around the iris, is due to lipid deposits and is considered a definite normal result of aging.

Hearing loss is gradual with aging and occurs in about one third of individuals age 75 years and older (Olsho, Harkins, and Harmon, 1985). Diminished ability in hearing acuity related to perception of tones is known as presbycusis. Increases in earwax in the ear canal and external noise also contribute to presbycusis.

It is believed that taste sensation is not markedly changed as a result of normal aging and that changes in taste sensation may be due to individual perceptions. The sense of smell appears to have minor decreases with aging, although environmental exposures to smoke or chemicals influence changes in the sense of smell over the life span.

Changes in the sense of touch during aging are complex and highly individualized. There are few changes to tactile nerve endings, but dermal changes may decrease touch sensation acuity in the elderly. Although some elderly persons experience a decreased pain threshold, others experience an increased pain threshold, and it appears that past experiences with pain are an influential factor in pain perception.

The sense of proprioception, or kinesthetics, refers to the individual's sense of balance and orientation in space. As a result of skeletal and inner ear structural changes with aging, the person's sense of orientation, and especially of balance, may be severely compromised. The older person also has difficulty regaining a sense of balance.

FUNCTIONAL ASSESSMENT

In view of all of the physiologic changes the elderly experience throughout the life span, most individuals are able to cope with the minor aches and pains attributed to normal aging. It is when the elderly person's ability to function and carry out activities of daily living independently is hindered that coping mechanisms may fail. Most situations that bring the elderly person to the primary care practitioner involve an inability to carry out specific functional tasks. Therefore it is important to assess the elderly person's functional status and its effect on the person's daily life (Table 11-3).

Functional assessment usually consists of evaluating two areas. The first area, **activities of daily living (ADL),**

Table 11-3   Functional Assessment of Common Physiologic Aging Changes

System	Normal Aging Changes	Areas for Functional Assessment
Musculoskeletal	↓Muscle strength ↓Body mass ↑Fat deposit ↓Bone mass ↓Joint mobility ↓Sitting height	Activity/exercise tolerance Joint pain on movement Gait, balance, and posture Susceptibility to falls Ability to perform ADL and IADL
Cardiovascular	↓Cardiac output ↓Basal metabolic rate ↓Cardiac performance ↓Arterial circulation ↑Peripheral resistance ↑Systolic blood pressure	Adaptation to stress Activity/exercise tolerance Orthostatic hypotension
Respiratory	↓Elasticity of chest walls ↑Anteroposterior diameter of chest ↓Intercostal muscle strength ↑Rigidity of lung tissue ↑Residual capacity ↓Cough reflex	Cough reflex Ability to blow out candle with open mouth Use of accessory muscles
Gastrointestinal	↓Saliva production ↓Motility ↓Gastric acid production ↓Absorption of nutrients ↓Drug metabolism	Condition of teeth/denture fit Dental hygiene Swallow reflex Frequency/size of meals Pattern of elimination Drug blood levels (metabolized by liver) History of constipation
Integument	↑Wrinkling of skin ↑Dryness of skin ↓Skin turgor ↑Thinning, graying body hair ↓Nail growth ↑Nails thicken, yellow	Assess for skin breakdown, especially over bony prominences Assess hydration status Susceptibility to infection
Immune	↓Size of thymus gland ↓Antibodies ↑Healing time	Assess for secondary infections History of allergies
Renal	↓Mass of kidney ↓Nephrons ↓Glomerular filtration rate ↓Nitrogen waste removal	Criterion for renal function is creatinine clearance Maintain adequate hydration Assess for incontinence
Nervous	↓Nerve cells ↓Neurotransmitters ↓Blood flow to central nervous system ↑Lipofuscin ↑Plaques and tangles ↓REM sleep	Response to pain is highly individualized Diminished deep tendon reflexes Complaint of restlessness/frequently go to bathroom May have memory changes
Reproductive	↓Estrogen production ↓Size of clitoris, cervix, uterus, and ovaries ↓Free testosterone ↓Penis and testes size	Support need for intimacy/sexuality Hormonal replacement
Endocrine	↓Production of adrenal gland hormones ↓Insulin release ↓Thyroid structure ↓↑Mixed changes to pituitary hormones	Response to stressors may be diminished
Sensory	↓Vision (loss of depth perception, accommodation, and visual acuity; increased glare) ↓Hearing (loss of sound conduction) ↓Odor recognition ↓↑Changes in pain threshold ↓Sense of balance	Need for increased illumination Need for corrective appliances Avoidance of night driving Assess tolerance to pain Assess thresholds for hot/cold Safety precautions

Table 11-4	ADL and IADL Functional Assessment Categories
ADL Categories	**IADL Categories**
Bathing	Shopping
Dressing	Meal preparation
Hair care	Transportation
Mouth care	Use of telephone
Nutrition/assist with feeding	Medication usage
Ambulation/mobility	Housekeeping
Mental status	Laundry
Elimination	Financial management

includes categories of personal care such as bathing, grooming, toileting, and transferring. The second area, **instrumental activities of daily living (IADL)**, addresses activities important for the individual to function in the community. IADL include shopping, preparing meals, and getting around. Table 11-4 highlights the major categories of ADL and IADL assessment.

Activities of Daily Living

ADL focus on the physical skills necessary to function from day to day. A recent study by the U.S. Department of Health and Human Services (1993) reported that 12.9% of the total population age 65 years or older reported having at least one ADL problem. Elderly African-Americans and Hispanics tended to have more difficulties with ADLs (U.S. Bureau of the Census, 1996). The elderly reported having the greatest amount of difficulty bathing, walking, and transferring between the bed and chair.

Several ADL assessment instruments are available. A good ADL instrument should be able to discriminate between physical and cognitive sources of the limitations. ADL scales typically categorize activity limitations in one of two ways. One type of ADL scale classifies limitations as present or absent. This scale fails to differentiate degrees of ADL limitations. The value of an ADL assessment tool is in its ability to identify areas for interventions. The *Katz Index of ADL* (Katz et al, 1963) is a valid, objective tool that measures six areas of function: (1) bathing, (2) dressing, (3) toileting, (4) transferring, (5) continence, and (6) feeding. The degree of limitation in each category is measurable. For example, in assessing transfer ability, the caregiver selects from one of the following three choices:

1. Moves in and out of bed or chair without assistance (may be using an object for support such as a cane or walker)
2. Moves in or out of bed or chair with assistance
3. Does not get out of bed

The Katz Index of ADL was developed and tested with elderly subjects across a variety of settings and is considered a reliable measure of function in the aged.

Instrumental Activities of Daily Living

The ability of the individual to function in the community is an important aspect of the functional assessment. Approximately 17.5% of the elderly report difficulty with at least one IADL (U.S. Department of Health and Human Services, 1993). Transportation, or getting around in the community, was most often identified as a problem area, followed by difficulty with shopping and light household chores.

There is a subjective, as well as objective, component of IADL. Assessing the ability of the older person to perform daily skills needed to function in the community is important. In addition, the meaning of the activity to the individual needs to be assessed. For example, taking care of shopping needs may not be as important to an individual as housekeeping or meal preparation. An older individual who fears going out into the community because of safety issues may essentially become isolated. Another elderly person may have difficulty with chewing and swallowing, so that meal preparation seems like a difficult task.

Both aspects of the functional assessment, ADL and IADL, are relevant indicators for identifying outcomes of illness, both physical and mental. Often, changes in ADL and IADL may be the forerunner of a new illness. Individuals respond differently to physical aging changes, so the ability to function independently is more predictive of outcomes of aging than physical aging changes alone.

PSYCHOSOCIAL AGING

Psychosocial aging changes typically focus on an individual's responses to particular events across the life span. Past coping mechanisms may not be effective in adjusting to stressful events in later life. The reason adaptation may be more difficult for the elderly is that the life events of old age differ from those of younger ages. Miller (1990) distinguished the life events of the elderly as follows:

They are viewed as losses, rather than gains.
They are most likely to occur close together with less time to adjust to each event.
They are more intense and demand greater energy in the coping process.
They are longer lasting and often become chronic problems.
They are inevitable and evoke a feeling of powerlessness.

Preparing for some life events may facilitate adjustment in old age. For instance, some employers offer preretirement counseling for older employees in preparation for retirement. Psychosocial aging changes are reflected in several areas, including cognition and memory, personality, social support, sexuality, and role status. From a developmental perspective, the meaningfulness of life events is important in determining patterns of psychosocial aging in these particular areas. There is a great deal of research needed before any conclusion may be drawn regarding normal versus abnormal psychosocial aging. The following section explores the current state of knowledge on psychosocial aging from a developmental perspective.

Cognition and Memory

There is probably no other area of aging research that has been studied to such an extent as cognition, especially in the areas of intelligence and memory. Evidence on the development of cognitive functions into old age is coming to light with studies that have followed elderly subjects over time. It is now apparent that cognitive functioning shows as much variability in aging as do physiologic indicators (Christensen et al, 1994).

Several factors may contribute to the variability in cognitive functioning observed in the elderly. These factors include health status, genetic profile, socioeconomic status, education, and lifestyle behaviors (Herzog and Wallace, 1997). In turn, cognitive losses often result in functional impairment and physical disabilities, causing a spiraling decline for the aged person.

Cognitive behaviors are divided into several interrelated processes, including intelligence, memory, attention, reaction time, and problem solving. These divisions are arbitrary and are based on the ways researchers typically study cognitive behaviors.

Studies of intelligence during the 1940s reported that the elderly experience declines in all aspects of intelligence, including knowledge acquisition, calculating, vocabulary, and abstract thought. The problem with these early studies was that the cross-sectional method was used to collect the data, with younger-age cohorts being compared with elderly cohorts in these studies. The younger-age cohorts consistently had higher intelligence scores on the various tests, prompting researchers to conclude that intelligence declines with aging (Woodruff, 1983). Later longitudinal studies, which followed the same older subjects over a period of time, found that intelligence showed little or no decline in healthy aging persons. Declines that occurred were in the oldest age cohorts (Schaie and Willis, 1991).

Horn and Cattell (1967) theorized that age-related differences in intelligence may be due to distinctions between two types of intelligence that seem to develop from birth. *Crystallized intelligence* develops from knowledge gained through the accumulation of experience and education. Crystallized intelligence may decline slightly, remain the same, or even increase with aging, depending on one's life experiences. On the other hand, *fluid intelligence* is affected by neurophysiologic processes across the life span. Declines in the nervous system with aging that affect one's attention span or reaction time reflect a loss of fluid intelligence. Instruments that measure intelligence using performance standards show declines in intelligence with aging (Birren and Schaie, 1985); and even these conclusions have been questioned by some gerontologists. The

increased reaction time by the elderly in intelligence performance tests may be because they are more cautious and take additional time to make correct choices.

Much aging research is devoted to the study of memory processes during aging. It is unfortunate that society equates aging with memory loss. Elderly persons are often portrayed on television or in movies as forgetful. A common joke is, "There are three telltale signs you are getting old. The first is loss of memory, and the other two . . . I forget." There is much that is still unknown about the process of memory perception, storage, and retrieval.

Most of the early theories of memory focused on the three components of memory (i.e., perception or encoding, storage, and retrieval). Memory was categorized as short or long term, or as primary, secondary, or tertiary. These categorizations were based on the length of storage time and the process of retrieval.

Other memory theories focused on the encoding processes, which yield different types of information in various ways. For instance, information that is processed in a more complex manner, such as algebraic equations, is stored in a deeper area of memory and will last longer. Information that is easily recognized requires less attention, thus tasks such as starting a car are performed almost automatically. It is believed that automatic processing of information does not change with aging (Botwinick, 1984). Offering cues to the elderly may help them recall information stored in deeper areas of memory.

Contextual theory of memory was developed from the information-processing model. This expands the information-processing model by including individual factors that may impact memory, such as learning behaviors, past experiences, personality, degree of motivation, physical health, and socioeconomic status (Perlmutter et al, 1987).

Certain types of memory decline as a part of normal aging. *Explicit memory*, the ability to recall a specific name or place, tends to decline in aging (Rowe and Kahn, 1998). *Working memory*, the type of memory needed to perform daily activities, does not show an aging decline. Because the elderly may take longer to process information (also normal to aging) and have some specific recall problems, they often fear that this is a harbinger of Alzheimer's disease. It is important to dispel this myth and to encourage the elderly to seek ways to improve cognitive functioning through training and practice.

Self-perception of memory changes and self-efficacy also influence memory performance (Ryan, 1992; Ryan and See, 1993). The concept of **metamemory** refers to one's self-perceptions of memory changes and their effect on memory processes (Hertzog, Dixon, and Hultsch, 1990). For example, an elderly person may falsely believe that memory loss is part of aging and perceive that forgetfulness indicates the start of memory decline. In reality, forgetting information may be due to a lack of attention to detail in a particular situation. Further study is needed to determine whether an individual can mentally control or influence the development of memory across the life span.

Attention span refers to the ability to concentrate throughout the performance of some task. With aging, the ability to maintain the attention span through completion of complex tasks diminishes. This is due to the fact that complex tasks require dividing one's attention among several tasks at the same time. Some of these normal aging changes with the attention span are misinterpreted as dementia. Two other segments of attention also show some decrements in aging. **Vigilance,** or the ability to sustain attention over longer periods of time, and **selective attention,** or the ability to discriminate and focus on relevant information, are less acute in the elderly.

Increased reaction time/decreased speed of performance on intelligence tests is one of the most agreed on changes in normal aging, but its mechanism is not well understood. Unfamiliarity with performance tests or increased cautiousness due to a fear of failure resulting in test anxiety may affect reaction time in the elderly.

Problem-solving ability is considered a higher cognitive function. The complexity of the problem, past experiences, the amount of information that is irrelevant to a situation, and the individual's level of education are factors that influence problem solving. There is little known about changes in higher cognitive functioning during aging. Most elderly persons are able to live and function effectively in the community.

Personality

Personality traits develop over the life span and are influenced by internal and external environmental factors. Personality is molded by an individual's ability to cope with stress and adapt to change. It is reflected in how individuals perceive themselves in what is referred to as *self-concept.* In general, most personality traits remain stable during the aging process. Personality influences how an individual interacts and reacts within the socioenvironment (see Chapter 14).

Personality theorists have attempted to identify specific traits that predict successful aging. Individuals described as introverted are more self-centered and internalize behaviors and responses. Extroverted personalities focus more on the outside world and are described as outgoing. Certain personality traits may assist individuals in adapting to aging better than others. Successful aging is determined more by the individual's ability to adapt to change than by a particular category of personality traits.

Some traits may intensify with aging, such as that of cautiousness, which may be an effective safety mechanism for the elderly. For example, the elderly person may tend to drive a car with more caution, drive only in daylight hours, or avoid high speeds. In unfamiliar situations or when several choices are available, the elderly tend to act more cautiously. They also tend to prefer familiar tasks, places, or situations.

Locus of control is another aspect of personality that remains stable over time (Reid, Haas, and Hawkings, 1977). Individuals with an *internal locus of control* perceive that they actively control their own destiny. On the other hand, individuals with an *external locus of control* believe they have no control over their destiny and think that their behaviors have no effect on any outcomes. Another phenomenon, that of *secondary locus of control*, describes individuals with an external locus of control who learn to adapt to their beliefs. This has also been termed *learned helplessness*. These individuals learn dependency and prefer others to decide for them.

Social Support and Interactions

In an extensive review of the literature, Broadhead et al (1983) presented Kahn and Antonucci's comprehensive definition of social support as interpersonal transactions that include one or more of the following behaviors: (1) expression of positive affect between individuals, (2) affirmation or endorsement of another person's behaviors, and (3) providing direct aid or assistance to another. Different individuals within one's social network may provide different types of support.

Hyde (1988) suggested that the quality, rather than the quantity, of social relationships is significantly related to life satisfaction among older adults. The quality of social support is a key area for interventions in the training of health care providers. Social support has been conceptualized as a communication process, in which facilitation of communication skills improves the quality of support (Albrecht and Adelman, 1984).

Social networks are generally viewed as the web of social ties that surround a person and include several characteristics important in the study of health and well-being of the elderly, including:

Size of the social network
Frequency of social contacts
Density of the interactions
Intimacy or closeness among members
Durability of ties
Geographic dispersion of members
Reciprocity of assistance

Social networks and social supports are different concepts. Considering the network as the web or structure, social support refers to the emotional or tangible assistance obtained from the social resource network. Not all social ties are supportive, and not all social supports come from the closest social network, such as a son or daughter living near elderly parents. Oxman and Berkman (1990) proposed a three-component model of social relationships that incorporates the quantitative and qualitative nature of social relationships. Because social relationships have been associated with subsequent physical and mental illness in the elderly, an assessment tool that addresses the

Table 11-5	Social Relationship Components and Characteristics	
Component	**Characteristics**	**Sample Questions**
Social network Structure and composition	Marital status/confidant	Are you married? Is there any one special person that you feel very close and intimate with?
	Number, kinship	How many children do you have?
	Proximity	How many live within an hour's drive?
	Frequency and type of contact	How many do you have phone or letter contact with at least once per month?
Type and amount of social support function	Emotional	How frequently did someone try and make you feel better about your illness in the past month?
	Tangible aid	How frequently did someone help you get your medications in the past month?
	Guidance	How frequently did someone suggest that you call the doctor in the past month?
Perceived adequacy of social support	General	In the past year could you have used more help with daily tasks than you received?
	Specific	How helpful was it for your children to try and make you feel better about your illness?

From Oxman T, Berkman L: Assessment of social relationships in elderly patients, *Int J Psychiatry Med* 20:65, 1990.

multidimensional aspects of social relationships is important. An example of some of the questions according to the dimensions being assessed is presented in Table 11-5 (Oxman and Berkman, 1990).

Sexuality and Intimacy

Physical aging changes related to the reproductive system occur in men and women. Psychologic aspects of sexuality and intimacy in the elderly are influenced by several factors, including past experiences, attitudes toward intimacy, societal views about sexuality in the elderly, and functional status.

Many elderly feel a newfound freedom in their sexual behaviors because they no longer need to focus on concerns regarding pregnancy. Hindering such feelings may be the unavailability of an acceptable partner, stereotypes that the elderly are asexual, or fears of inability to initiate and maintain sexual performance. Elderly women probably experience the greatest effects because many become widowed or there may exist long-standing values about sexual taboos.

It has only been in recent years that elderly persons, and especially those over 80 years, have been subjects of studies of sexuality. Bretschneider and McCoy (1988) reviewed the available studies of psychosocial aspects of sexuality and aging. The following summarizes some of their findings:

1. The frequency of sexual activity decreases with aging, but the interest and ability in sexual function does not necessarily decline with aging. Older individuals who are in normal health and functioning have the ability to maintain sexual activity.

2. Declines in sexual activity are mostly related to lack of a partner, especially for women.
3. Psychosocial factors that may impede sexual activity by the elderly include stereotypic beliefs, attitudes, and personality factors.
4. Sexual behaviors and beliefs generally remain stable across the life span.
5. Men remain more sexually active than women across the life span.

Role Transitions

Accompanying the aging changes are changes in roles for the older person. Some of these role changes are more obvious than others, and individuals adapt to role changes in different ways. The degree of importance attributed to a particular role by the individual influences how well the older person is able to cope with a role transition. From a developmental perspective, roles contain various tasks one must carry out in life. Each role carries with it different life tasks. Some tasks may be new to the person if the role is a completely new one, and other tasks may be similar to ones carried out early in life, as in role reversals.

Retirement implies a major role transition for many individuals. Since individuals live longer and retire earlier, the retirement period may last for 30 to 40 years. Only recently have researchers begun to explore gender differences in adaptation to retirement. Adaptation to retirement appears to be affected more by the life events surrounding retirement than by the retirement process itself (Szinovacz and Washo, 1992). Particular life events may even precipitate retirement. For instance, a middle-age woman may take an early retirement because she needs to care for her elderly mother at home who has Alzheimer's disease. This individual's adjustment to retirement may be negatively affected because of a conflict between the woman's role in the workforce and her caregiver role.

A major role transition occurs after loss of one's spouse, when adaptation requires the survivor to assume tasks previously performed by the partner. Couples who have shared responsibilities across the life span have less difficulty with the role changes. Personality traits seem to influence adjustment to widowhood. For example, the husband who lost his wife may not have learned how to cook or clean, but if the husband can adapt to change, he will rapidly adjust and learn these tasks. The widower may also find himself the center of attention by family members who want to assist him, as well as by widows looking for male companionship.

The role of the grandparent is another transition. The grandparent who adjusts successfully can provide grand-children with a viewpoint that may differ from the parents but be equally positive. Many grandparents take on the role of full- or part-time surrogate parents.

In the presence of physical or mental deterioration, the roles of the parent and child may be reversed. Most often the oldest female child, on reaching middle age, may need to provide care for the incapacitated elderly parent. This is an especially difficult transition for the female middle-age child who has just completed raising her own children and who was planning her own retirement in a few years. If the caregiver is a middle-age man, it is often an awkward situation, because his wife is called on to adapt to a role for which she may have no emotional connection in caring for the elderly parent-in-law. Supporting the caregiver is as important as supporting the care receiver under these circumstances. Table 11-6 summarizes some normal aging changes discussed in this section and areas for functional assessment.

Table 11-6	**Functional Assessment of Common Psychosocial Aging Changes**	
Area	**Normal Aging Changes**	**Areas for Functional Assessment**
Cognition and memory	Normal crystallized intelligence ↓Fluid intelligence (slight, gradual) ↑Reaction time ↓Divided attention ↓Vigilance ↓Selected attention ↑Information-processing time ↑Cautiousness	Degree of external stimulation Environmental distraction Assess barriers to learning (e.g., sensory impairments, relevancy/level of information, learning environment) Assess factors influencing memory process (e.g., education level, learning style, past experiences, physical/mental health, motivation)
Personality	Stability of most personality traits ↑Cautiousness ↑Rigidity (slight)	Adaptive coping mechanisms Decision-making processes Adjustment to change (e.g., retirement, relocation, loss)
Social support and interactions	Perceived social support impacted by several factors (personality, health status, past experiences, coping style) Changes in social network (size, intimacy, geographic dispersion, reciprocity of assistance) Changes in source of social support with aging	Attitude/perception of social support Past experience with social support Social network ties Types of social support needed Sources of social support
Sexuality and intimacy	Sexual behaviors/interests maintained across life span in absence of physical/mental disorders ↓Sexual activity in males ↓Intensity of sexual responses Lack of partner is greatest factor affecting sexual activity	Attitudes toward expressions of sexuality and intimacy Means to maintain sexual behaviors/interests Availability of privacy in environment Risk factors impeding sexual behaviors
Role transitions	Retirement Widowhood Grandparenting	Importance of past roles/tasks Responses to retirement Relation of life events to retirement Effects of retirement on spouses Impact of loss of spouse Ability to take on new tasks in ADL/IADL Social supports/network Relationships with children/grandchildren Parenting role

Mini-Mental State Examination

Maximum Score	Score	
		Orientation
5	( )	What is the (year)(season)(date)(day)(month)?
5	( )	Where are we (state)(country)(town or city)(place)(floor)?
		Registration
3	( )	Name three random objects, taking one second to say each one. Then ask the patient to name all three objects (apple, table, penny) after you have said them.
		Give 1 point for each correct answer. Count the number of trials and record the number. (number of trials _____).
		Attention and Calculation
5	( )	Begin with 100, and count backward by 7 (stop after 5 answers): 93, 86, 79, 72, 65. Score one point for each correct answer.
		If the patient will not perform this task, ask the patient to spell "world" backwards (dlrow). Record the patient's spelling. Score 1 point for each correctly placed letter.
		Recall
3	( )	Ask the patient to repeat the names of the objects learned in the Registration section. Give one point for each object correctly named.
		Language – Naming
2	( )	Show a pencil and a watch, and ask the patient to name them.
		Repetition
1	( )	Ask the patient to repeat, "No ifs, ands, or buts."
		Three-stage Command
3	( )	Have the patient follow a three-stage command: "Take this paper in your right hand, fold the paper in half, and put the paper on the table."
		Reading
1	( )	Ask the patient to read and obey the following command: **CLOSE YOUR EYES.**
		Writing
1	( )	Have the patient write a sentence of his or her choice. The sentence should contain a subject and an object and should make sense. Ignore spelling errors when scoring.
		Construction/Copying
1	( )	Enlarge the design given below to 1.5 cm per side and have the patient copy it. Give one point if all sides and angles are preserved and if the intersecting sides form a quadrangle.
30	_____	**Total**

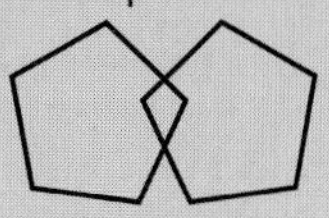

Scoring: 0–12 (severe), 13–22 (moderate), 23–24 (mild), 25–30 (none). These ranges vary depending on a person's age, education, and language background.

Reprinted with permission from *J Psychiatric Research*, Vol. 12, p. 189–198, Folstein MF, Folstein SE, and McHugh PR, Mini-mental state examination: A practical method of grading the cognitive state of patients for the clinician, 1975, Elsevier Science Ltd., Pergamon Imprint, Oxford, England.

Figure 11-2 Mini-mental state (MMS) examination. (From Folstein M, Folstein S, McHugh P: "Mini-mental state": a practical method of grading the cognitive state of patients for the clinician, *J Psychiatr Res* 12:189, 1975.)

MENTAL ASSESSMENT

Assessment of mental status and cognitive functioning is an area where gerontologists are attempting to develop adequate standardized tests specifically for the elderly. Designing reliable instruments for the elderly continues to be a challenge because of the interrelationships among several factors, including health status, physical/mental aging changes, socioenvironmental variables, and life events. Thus the context of what is considered normal development for an elderly individual should be the focus of any mental status assessment.

Several mental status assessment instruments have been designed to evaluate mental and cognitive functions. Most instruments examine mental status in view of the in-

Instructions:

Ask questions 1–10 in this list, and record all answers. Ask question 4A only if patient does not have a telephone. Record total number of errors based on ten questions.

1.   What is the date today? (month, day, year)

2.   What day of the week is it?

3.   What is the name of this place?

4.   What is your telephone number?

4a.   What is your street address? (Ask only if patient does not have a telephone.)

5.   What is your street address?

6.   When were you born? (month, day, year)

7.   Who is the president of the United States now? (last name)

8.   Who was president just before him? (last name)

9.   What was your mother's maiden name?

10.   Subtract 3 from 20 and keep subtracting 3 from each new number, all the way down.

Scoring

For Caucasian subjects with at least some high school education, but not more than high school education, the following criteria have been established:

0–2 errors	Intact intellectual functioning
3–4 errors	Mild intellectual impairment
5–7 errors	Moderate intellectual impairment
8–10 errors	Severe intellectual impairment

Allow one more error if subject has only grade school education.

Allow one more error for African = American subjects, using identical education criteria.

Allow one less error if subject has education beyond high school.

Figure 11-3   Short portable mental status questionnaire (SPMSQ). (From Pfeiffer E: A short portable mental status questionnaire for the assessment of organic brain deficit in elderly patients, *J Am Geriatr Soc* 23:433, 1975.)

dividual's ability to function in daily living activities. However, the mental status assessment is not sufficient to provide a diagnosis of a disorder. Other sources of information, such as the health history, physical examination, diagnostic/laboratory tests, and psychosocial factors, are required for diagnosing (see Chapters 7 and 17.)

The mental status assessment of the elderly includes the following areas: appearance, mood, communication, thought processes, perceptual motor abilities, attention, memory, consciousness, and orientation. Appearance, behaviors, and responses of the elderly client should be areas for attention by the health care provider performing the assessment. For instance, the older person may state that he or she has no suicidal ideations, but appearance may indicate self-neglect and behaviors may include withdrawing from social networks and accumulating drugs. Such discrepancies are important to identify.

Several screening instruments are available for the health care provider to provide a quick assessment of mental status. Each instrument addresses different areas of the mental status examination. Often these brief instruments provide an initial baseline of cognitive functioning, to be used for further in-depth assessment and screening for diagnosis and subsequent interventions.

The Mini-Mental State (MMS) examination continues to be one of the most commonly used instruments to screen for cognitive disorders in the elderly (Folstein, Folstein, and McHugh, 1975) (Figure 11-2). Several dimensions of cognitive function are assessed, including orientation, memory, attention, and speech. Out of a total score of 30, normal persons score 25 and above, whereas individuals diagnosed with dementia score lower than 20 points.

Another commonly used instrument is the Short Portable Mental Status Questionnaire (SPMSQ) (Pfeiffer, 1975). Although it is not adequate to provide a diagnosis of dementia, this tool provides a rapid assessment of mental status. Areas of cognitive function assessed by the SPMSQ include orientation, immediate and remote memory, thought processes, and attention span. The scoring also allows for differences in education and race (Figure 11-3).

REFOCUSING ON HEALTHY AGING

Perceptions of health and wellness develop across the life span and affect attitudes and behaviors related to health care practices. For the elderly, their physical and mental health represent the summation of health care beliefs and practices across the years. The majority of elderly persons consider their health to be good to excellent (74.3% of those ages 65 to 74 and 66.8% of those ages 75 and older) (U.S. Bureau of the Census, 1996). Perceived health has been shown to affect disease and disability among the el-

derly. Rogers (1995) found that in elderly persons suffering from multiple chronic conditions and disability, those who perceived their overall health as very good to excellent lived longer than persons who considered themselves to be in poor health.

The MacArthur Foundation Study (Rowe and Kahn, 1998) has brought together 10 years of scientific knowledge and expertise related to aging. They identify three components necessary for successful aging:

1. Avoidance of disease and risk factors
2. Maintaining high cognitive and physical abilities
3. Engagement with life through productive relationships and behaviors

Early identification of risk factors and disease prevention/health promotion behaviors can have a significant impact on the development and progress of several chronic diseases. For example, exercise is very beneficial to the elderly in prevention of heart disease, hypertension, and diabetes. A regular, moderate program of aerobic and strength training for the elderly is both safe and effective in improving function.

Challenging the mind as well as the body is important to maintain mental capabilities. Not all cognitive processes decline in aging, and most of these changes occur very late in life. Older persons who maintain a high level of self-efficacy, a measure of one's self-esteem, appear to manage well both mentally and physically.

Maintaining social relationships and continuing some sort of meaningful activities contribute positively to aging. Social networks often shrink for the elderly who outlive their peers and relatives. Elderly persons find support in reciprocal relationships with friends or family members. Grandparents find joy in having their grandchildren visit for extended periods, offering a respite to the parents. In terms of productive activities, many older retirees remark that they are much more busy after retirement, with new projects and volunteer work. With the aging of the baby boomers over the next 30 years, the focus on successful aging may be more of a reality than an ideal.

IMAGES OF AGING

The images of aging and attitudes of society toward the elderly have been changing over the past several years. Unfortunately, society has always focused on the negative aspects of aging. The term **ageism** has been used to describe the stereotypic views of the elderly (Butler, 1987). The myth of the "burden of the elderly" has been gradually dispelled with the growing body of scientific evidence disproving that "to be old is to be sick" (Rowe and Kahn, 1998).

In 1995 the American Association of Retired Persons (AARP) published a study entitled *Images of Aging in America* (Speas and Obenshain, 1995). The purpose of

Table 11-7	AARP Report on Knowledge, Perceptions, and Attitudes Toward Aging
Area	**Key Findings From Respondents**
Knowledge of aging	Most answered correctly 50% of the items from the Facts on Aging Quiz. Misconceptions related to the financial status of the elderly, perceptions that most elderly persons are lonely or bored, that 10% of all elderly persons are institutionalized, and that the overall health of the elderly will decline in the future. Respondents with more incorrect answers held more negative views of the elderly; those with more correct answers held more positive views of the elderly. A low level of knowledge was related to a low socioeconomic status and high anxiety about aging.
Stereotypes of the aged	Poor health, disabilities, isolation, and financial problems were most often identified as problems for the elderly. Younger respondents thought the elderly did not receive the respect they deserved; older respondents thought they received the right amount of respect. Younger respondents overestimated the number of serious problems experienced by the elderly. Personal experience with the elderly had the greatest impact on perceived images of aging. Younger respondents described old age in chronologic years; older respondents saw old age in terms of health, attitudes, and level of activity. Respondents with less education and high anxiety about aging held more negative stereotypes about the elderly.
Perceptions of the aging process	Physical dependency was the number one cause for anxiety related to aging for younger respondents. Minorities and low-income persons tended to be more anxious about aging. At least one half of respondents had some anxiety about health, independence, and finances in their future.

Modified from Speas K, Obenshain B: *Images of aging in America: final report*, American Association of Retired Persons, Chapel Hill, NC, 1995, FGI Integrated Marketing.

this report was to examine knowledge, perceptions, and attitudes about aging. Key results of this study are listed in Table 11-7. One's personal experience with the elderly was the strongest predictor of perceptions and attitudes toward aging. Most Americans had misconceptions about the elderly, reflecting a lack of knowledge about aging. On a positive note, there was a lack of stereotypes and myths of aging subscribed to by the respondents. These findings have important implications for health care professionals who work with the elderly.

CULTURAL IMPACT

Cultural beliefs also influence one's attitudes toward the elderly. Culture influences the responses of the elderly to health, illness, and treatment. Some cultures subscribe to health care practices or home remedies that may be in direct opposition to modern health care practices. The health care professional needs to examine his or her own feelings toward differing cultural beliefs and health care practices of elderly clients. The incorporation of some home remedies into the elderly client's care plan may increase compliance, given that these remedies are not in conflict with treatment.

Various cultures hold different views regarding aging. Since ancient times, the contributions of the elderly to a society affect the status of the aged within a particular cultural group. For example, Far Eastern cultures value the wisdom of their elders and thus hold the aged in high esteem. In contrast, some primitive cultures may have considered the elderly a burden, unable to hunt and provide for the tribe. Such cultures have been known to banish the elderly from the tribe.

In the current Western culture there is greater support for views of successful aging. The focus on age has presented the public with issues that future elderly persons will experience, relating to functional, economic, and political aspects of aging. The situation of today's elderly may be the most optimistic in terms of availability of social and economic resources, but future generations of elderly persons may face difficult resource issues (Conrad, 1992). The costs may outweigh the contributions by future elderly persons in society, and cultural values toward the elderly may change.

Summary of Key Concepts

1. The elderly population is growing in number and proportion of the entire U.S. population, especially those in minority groups; thus health care providers need to have an understanding of biologic, social, and psychologic aging processes.

2. The process of aging is a period of decreases in function, but the elderly have great reserves to adapt to loss and change.

3. The major theories that attempt to explain developmental processes of aging can be divided into biologic, sociologic, and psychologic theories of aging.

4. Many physiologic and psychosocial changes occur as a result of aging.

5. Most elderly perceive their overall health as good to excellent.

REFERENCES

Albrecht T, Adelman M: Social support and life stress: new directions for communication research, *Hum Communication Res* 11:3, 1984.

Atchley R: A continuity theory of normal aging, *Gerontologist* 29:183, 1989.

Baltes P, Smith J, Staudinger U: Life-span developmental psychology, *Ann Rev Psychol* 23:65, 1992.

Bennett N, Garson L: Extraordinary longevity in the Soviet Union: fact or artifact? *Gerontologist* 26:358, 1986.

Birren J, Schaie K: *Handbook of the psychology of aging*, ed 2, New York, 1985, Van Nostrand Reinhold.

Botwinick J: *Aging and behavior*, ed 3, New York, 1984, Springer.

Bowman B, Rosenberg I: Digestive function and aging, *Hum Nutr Clin Nutr* 27C:75, 1983.

Bretschneider J, McCoy N: Sexual interest and behavior in healthy 80 to 102 year olds. *Arch Sex Behav* 17:109, 1988.

Broadhead W et al: The epidemiologic evidence for a relationship between social support and health, *Am J Epidemiol* 117:521, 1983.

Brower H: Social organization and nurses' attitudes toward older persons, *J Gerontol Nurs* 7:293, 1981.

Brower H: Do nurses stereotype the aged? *J Gerontol Nurs* 11:17, 1985.

Buschmann M, Burns E, Jones F: Student nurses' attitudes towards the elderly, *J Nurs Educ* 20:7, 1981.

Butler R: Ageism. In Maddox G, editor: *The encyclopedia of aging*, New York, 1987, Springer.

Campbell J: *The portable Jung*, New York, 1979, Penguin Books.

Campbell M: Study of the attitudes of nursing personnel toward the geriatric patient, *Nurs Res* 20:127, 1971.

Carter J: The effects of aging upon selected visual functions: color vision, glare sensitivity, field of vision, and accommodation. In Sekuler R, Kline D, Dismukes K, editors: *Aging and human visual function*, New York, 1982, Oxford University Press.

Centers for Disease Control: *Life expectancy in 33 developing countries*, Atlanta, April 7, 1990, The Centers.

Christiansen H et al: Age differences and interindividual variation in cognition in community-dwelling elderly, *Psychol Aging* 9:381, 1994.

Conrad C: Old age in the modern and postmodern western world. In Cole T, Van Tassel D, Kastenbaum R, editors: *Handbook of the humanities and aging*, New York, 1992, Springer.

Cumming E, Henry W: *Growing old: the process of disengagement*, New York, 1961, Basic Books.

Ebersole P, Hess P: *Toward healthy aging: human needs and nursing responses*, ed 5, St. Louis, 1999, Mosby.

Eliopoulos C: *Gerontological nursing*, ed 3, Philadelphia, 1993, JB Lippincott.

Enloe C: Managing daily living with diminishing resources and losses. In Carnevali D, Patrick M, editors: *Nursing management for the elderly*, ed 3, Philadelphia, 1993, JB Lippincott.

Erikson E, Erikson J, Kiunick H: *Vital involvement in old age: the experience of old age in our time*, New York, 1986, WW Norton.

Fielding P: An exploratory investigation of self concept in the institutionalized elderly, and a comparison with nurses' conceptions and attitudes, *Int J Nurs Stud* 16:345, 1979.

Finch C, Tanzi R: Genetics of aging, *Science* 278:407, 1997.

Folstein M, Folstein S, McHugh P: "Mini-mental state": a practical method of grading the cognitive state of patients for the clinician, *J Psychiatr Res* 12:189, 1975.

Havighurst R, Neugarten B, Tobin S: Disengagement and patterns of aging. In Neugarten B, editor: *Middle age and aging*, Chicago, 1968, University of Chicago Press.

Hayflick L: Theories of biological aging. In Andres R, Bierman E, Hazzard W, editors: *Principles of geriatric medicine*, New York, 1985, McGraw-Hill.

Herzog A, Wallace R: Measures of cognitive functioning in the AHEAD study, *J Gerontol* 52B:37, 1997.

Hertzog C, Dixon R, Hultsch D: Relationships between metamemory, memory predictions, and memory task performance in adults, *Psychol Aging* 5:215, 1990.

Hollinger L, Buschmann M: Factors influencing the perception of touch by elderly nursing home residents and their health caregivers, *Int J Nurs Stud* 30:445, 1993.

Horn J, Cattell R: Age differences in fluid and crystallized intelligence, *Acta Psychol* 26:107, 1967.

Hyde R: Facilitative communication skills training: social support for elderly people, *Gerontologist* 28:418, 1988.

Jung C: The stages of life. In Campbell J, editor: *The portable Jung*, New York, 1971, Viking Press.

Katz S et al: Studies of illness in the aged: the Index of ADL, a standardized measure of biological and psychological function, *JAMA* 185:914, 1963.

Kumpe P et al: The aging respiratory system, *Clin Geriatr Med* 1:143, 1985.

Lakatta E: Cardiovascular system aging. In Kent B, Butler R, editors: *Human aging research: concepts and techniques*, New York, 1988, Raven Press.

Lee H: Why I won't retire, *Reader's Digest* 122:61, 1983.

Lemon B, Bengston V, Peterson J: An exploration of the activity theory of aging: activity types and life satisfaction among inmovers to a retirement community, *J Gerontol* 27:511, 1972.

Levin J, Levin W: *Ageism: prejudice and discrimination against the elderly*, Belmont, Calif, 1980, Wadsworth.

Maslow A: *Toward a psychology of being*, New York, 1962, Van Nostrand.

Meier D: Skeletal aging. In Kent B, Butler R, editors: *Human aging research: concepts and techniques*, New York, 1988, Raven Press.

Mille R: The aging immune system: primer and prospectus, *Science* 273:70, 1996.

Miller C: *Nursing care of older adults: theory and practice*, Glenview, Ill, 1990, Scott, Foresman.

Olsho L, Harkins S, Harmon B: Aging and the auditory system. In Birren J, Schaie K, editors: *Handbook of the psychology of aging*, ed 2, New York, 1985, Van Nostrand Reinhold.

Oxman T, Berkman L: Assessment of social relationships in elderly patients, *Int J Psychiatry Med* 20:65, 1990.

Packer L, Glazer A: *Oxygen radicals in biological systems*, part B, *Oxygen radicals and antioxidants*, San Diego, 1990, Academic Press.

Pederson N: Gerontological behavior genetics. In Birren JE, Schaie K, editors: *Handbook of the psychology of aging*, ed 3, San Diego, 1996, Academic Press.

Perlmutter M et al: Aging and memory, *Annu Rev Gerontol Geriatr* 7:57, 1987.

Pfeiffer E: A short portable mental status questionnaire for the assessment of organic brain deficit in elderly patients, *J Am Geriatr Soc* 23:433, 1975.

Reid D, Haas G, Hawkings D: Locus of desired control and positive self-concept of the elderly, *J Gerontol* 32:441, 1977.

Rogers R: Sociodemographic characteristics of long-lived and healthy individuals, *Popul Dev Rev* 21:33, 1995.

Rosenkoetter M: Role change after retirement, *J Gerontol Nurs* 11:21, 1985.

Rowe J, Kahn R: *Successful aging: the MacArthur Foundation Study*, New York, 1998, Pantheon Books.

Ryan E: Beliefs about memory changes across the adult life span, *J Gerontol* 47:41, 1992.

Ryan E, See S: Age-based beliefs about memory changes for self and others across adulthood, *J Gerontol* 48:199, 1993.

Schaie K, Willis S: *Adult development and aging*, Boston, 1991, Little, Brown.

Schneider E, Rowe J: *Handbook of the biology of aging*, ed 3, San Diego, 1990, Academic Press.

Schroots J: Gerodynamics: toward a branching theory of aging, *Can J Aging* 14:74, 1995.

Smith L: Retirement options: pack up or stay put, *Grandparents*, p 62, Spring 1987.

Speas K, Obenshain B: *Images of aging in America: final report*, American Association of Retired Persons, Chapel Hill, NC, 1995, FGI Integrated Marketing.

Steinberg F: The aging of organs and organ systems. In Steinberg F, editor: *Care of the geriatric patient*, ed 6, St. Louis, 1983, Mosby.

Szinovacz M, Washo C: Gender differences in exposure to life events and adaptation to retirement, *J Gerontol* 47:191, 1992.

Taylor K, Harned T: Attitudes toward old people: a study of nurses who care for the elderly, *J Gerontol Nurs* 4:43, 1978.

Tornstam H: Gero-transcendence: a theoretical and empirical exploration. In Thomas L, Eisenhandler S, editors: *Aging and the religious dimension*, Westport, Conn, 1994, Auburn House.

U.S. Bureau of the Census: How we're changing: demographic state of the nation, 1990. In *Current Population Reports*, P23, No. 170. Washington, DC, 1991, U.S. Department of Commerce, Economics and Statistics Administration.

U.S. Bureau of the Census: *Census of population: general population characteristics (1990)*, Washington, DC, 1992, U.S. Department of Commerce, Economics and Statistics Administration.

U.S. Bureau of the Census: Sixty-five plus in the United States. In *Current Population Reports*, P23-190, No. 178RV, special studies, Washington, DC, 1996, U.S. Department of Commerce, Economics and Statistics Administration.

U.S. Department of Health and Human Services, Public Health Service: *Healthy people 2000*, DHHS Publ No. (PHS) 91-50213, 1990.

U.S. Department of Health and Human Services: *Health data on older Americans*, Hyattsville, Md., Public Health Service, Centers for Disease Control and Prevention, National Center for Health Statistics, No. PHS93-1411, 1993.

Vaillant G: *Adaptation to life*, Boston, 1977, Little, Brown.

Woodruff D: A review of aging and cognitive processes, *Res Aging* 5:139, 1983.

Psychiatric Disorders

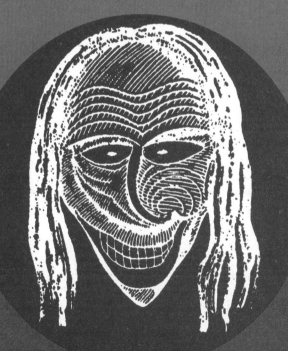

**False Face Mask
Iroquois**

The highly organized Iroquois Indians carved masks into trees that were alive and growing and then cut them away from the tree. The masks were used in ceremonies to heal individuals' mental, emotional, or physical disorders or to protect the entire tribe from illness. The chapters in Part Four discuss the major mental disorders and treatment according to an interdisciplinary process.

CHAPTER 12

Anxiety and Related Disorders

Monica Molloy

OBJECTIVES

- Employ two of the etiologic paradigms to explain the four stages of anxiety.

- Use the defining characteristics of anxiety in the NANDA classification to differentiate between circumscribed and pervasive anxiety disorders.

- Design a teaching plan for family members of clients with agoraphobia.

- Appraise the coping mechanisms of trauma victims to evaluate risk for post-traumatic stress disorder.

- Apply a cost-benefit approach to weigh the advantages of inpatient and outpatient treatment of dissociative identity disorder (formerly multiple personality disorder).

- Evaluate the advantages of the humanistic nursing model in providing care to clients experiencing varying levels of anxiety.

- Discuss the usefulness of clinical rating scales in evaluating collaborative treatment outcomes of inpatients with anxiety disorders and obsessive compulsive disorder.

- Relate the biologic paradigm to target symptoms and therapeutic agents for psychopharmacologic intervention in anxiety and related disorders.

ANXIETY AND RELATED DISORDERS

Anxiety is an integral part of the universal human experience. For most people, most of the time, it is a vague, subjective, nonspecific feeling of uneasiness with no identifiable object, resulting from an external threat to one's integrity. The function of anxiety is to warn the individual of impending threat, conflict, or danger. Anxiety is also a state of tension, dread, or impending doom, arising from external influences that threaten to be overwhelming. When an individual receives a signal of approaching danger, he or she is motivated to action: flee the threatening situation or control dangerous impulses. The person may even freeze to the spot, immobilized.

Defense mechanisms (see Box 1-2) are the primary methods the ego uses in an attempt to control or manage anxiety. Defenses protect the individual from threats to the biologic, psychologic, and social aspects of the self. The consequence of ignoring anxiety signals is the threat of being destroyed, or of no longer existing. Anxiety responses exist on a continuum (Table 12-1), and individuals are more or less successful at using various methods to control their own anxiety experiences. Those who are less successful, or who rely primarily on less adaptive defense mechanisms, such as dissociation in the case of dissociative identity disorder or projection in the case of paranoid schizophrenia, develop the defining characteristics of the anxiety disorders.

KEY TERMS

Agoraphobia Fear of open spaces or public spaces, related to feelings of loss of control, which may be associated with panic.

Anxiety A vague, nonspecific feeling of uneasiness, tension, apprehension, and sometimes dread or pending doom. Anxiety occurs as a result of a threat to one's biologic, psychologic, or social integrity, arising from external sources. It is a universal experience and part of the human condition.

Anxiolytic Anxiety-reducing effects, such as those resulting from antianxiety medications.

Compulsion An unremitting, repetitive impulse to perform a behavior, such as hand washing, checking, cleaning, or putting things in order; or mental acts, such as praying, counting, or repeating words silently. The goal of the behavior is to prevent or reduce anxiety or distress, not to provide pleasure or gratification. Compulsive acts often occur to reduce the distress that accompanies an obsession or to prevent some dreaded event or situation.

Defense mechanisms
Also known as ego defenses. Automatic and semiautomatic mental processes to protect the ego (person) against anxiety resulting from feelings and impulses that threaten psychologic harm, conflict, or exposure, for example, denial and repression.

Denial Avoidance of reality that threatens an individual's self-concept. Denial is demonstrated by ignoring or deemphasizing the importance of an event, observation, or feeling. At times, denial helps one survive life stressors.

Depersonalization Feelings of unreality or alienation. Individuals experiencing depersonalization have difficulty distinguishing themselves from others. Depersonalization may occur in extreme anxiety.

Dissociation The separation of an overwhelming event from one's conscious awareness; a prominent defense mechanism in dissociative identity disorder (formerly known as multiple personality disorder).

Humanistic nursing A view of nursing as an interactive process, developed by nursing theorists Patterson and Zderad, that occurs between two persons: one needing help and the other willing to give help.

Obsessions
Persistent ideas, thoughts, impulses, or images about death, sexual matters, religion, or any themes that lead to the person's efforts to resist them. They result in marked anxiety or distress.

Panic A circumscribed period of extreme anxiety. During panic one's perceptions are distorted and the ability to integrate and separate environmental stimuli is impaired.

Panic attacks Discrete periods of panic that are characterized by several cognitive and physiologic symptoms.

Phobias A group of disorders primarily characterized by avoidance of a specific situation or object, or by escape if the situation or object is unexpectedly encountered.

Repression Involuntary exclusion of a painful, threatening experience. It begins in infancy and continues throughout life. It underlies all other defense mechanisms but also operates as its own defense mechanism.

Stress Defined by Selye (1956) as "the nonspecific response of the body to any demand made on it, regardless of whether the demand is pleasant or unpleasant."

Table 12-1	Responses to Anxiety		
Anxiety Level	**Physiologic**	**Cognitive/Perceptual**	**Emotional/Behavioral**
Mild	Vital signs normal. Minimal muscle tension. Pupils normal, constricted.	Perceptual field is broad. Awareness of multiple environmental and internal stimuli. Thoughts may be random, but controlled.	Feelings of relative comfort and safety. Relaxed, calm appearance and voice. Performance is automatic; habitual behaviors occur here.
Moderate	Vital signs normal or slightly elevated. Tension experienced; may be uncomfortable or pleasurable (labeled as "tense" or "excited").	Alert; perception narrowed, focused. Optimum state for problem solving and learning. Attentive.	Feelings of readiness and challenge; energized. Engage in competitive activity and learn new skills. Voice, facial expression interested or concerned.
Severe	"Fight or flight" response. Autonomic nervous system excessively stimulated (vital signs increased, diaphoresis increased, urinary urgency and frequency, diarrhea, dry mouth, appetite decreased, pupils dilated). Muscles rigid, tense. Senses affected; hearing decreased, pain sensation decreased.	Perceptual field greatly narrowed. Problem solving difficult. Selective attention (focus on one detail). Selective inattention (block out threatening stimuli). Distortion of time (things seem faster or slower than actual). Dissociative tendencies; vigilambulism (automatic behavior).	Feels threatened, startles with new stimuli; feels on "overload." Activity may increase or decrease (may pace, run away, wring hands, moan, shake, stutter, become very disorganized or withdrawn, freeze in position/be unable to move). May appear and feel depressed. Demonstrates denial; may complain of aches or pains; may be agitated or irritable. Need for space increased. Eyes may dart around room, or gaze may be fixed. May close eyes to shut out environment.
Panic	Above symptoms escalate until sympathetic nervous system release occurs. Person may become pale; blood pressure decreases; hypotension. Muscle coordination poor. Pain, hearing sensations minimal.	Perception totally scattered or closed. Unable to take in stimuli. Problem solving and logical thinking highly improbable. Perception of unreality about self, environment, or event. Dissociation may occur.	Feels helpless with total loss of control. May be angry, terrified; may become combative or totally withdrawn, cry, or run. Completely disorganized. Behavior is usually extremely active or inactive.

From Fortinash K, Holoday-Worret P: *Psychiatric nursing care plans*, ed 3, St. Louis, 1999, Mosby.

HISTORICAL AND THEORETIC PERSPECTIVES

In *Interpersonal Relations in Nursing*, Hildegard Peplau (1952), a pioneer of psychiatric mental health nursing, identifies four stages of anxiety on a continuum in order to illustrate the view of anxiety and tension developed by Harry Stack Sullivan (1882-1949), an early, prominent, American-born psychiatrist and expert in developmental theory. These stages of anxiety—mild, moderate, severe, and panic—are described and expanded on in Figure 12-1. Optimally functioning people generally function in the mild range of anxiety. This stage of anxiety facilitates learning, creativity, and personal growth, an important point for nursing students and other learners to acknowl-

edge as they strive to excel in their work. Occasional movement to the moderate stage may also be an adaptive mechanism to cope with stressful situations, whether they are pleasant or unpleasant. A nursing student who is giving an important oral presentation or who is involved in a challenging situation with a client may be experiencing moderate anxiety. When the stressor is managed, the adapted person moves back along the continuum to mild anxiety. Moderate and severe anxiety can be acute or chronic. In severe anxiety, energy is focused primarily on reducing the pain and discomfort of anxiety, rather than on coping with the environment. Consequently, the individual's level of function is impaired, and the person may need help to reverse the situation. In panic anxiety the in-

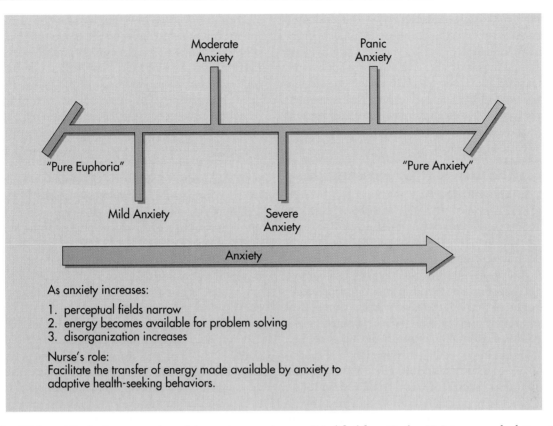

Figure 12-1   Hildegard Peplau's construction of the anxiety continuum. (Modified from Peplau H: *Interpersonal relations in nursing: a conceptual frame of reference for psychodynamic nursing,* New York, 1991, Springer.)

dividual is disorganized, with increased motor activity, a distorted visual-perceptual field, loss of rational thought, and decreased ability to relate to others. Responses to the stages of anxiety are more fully explained in Table 12-1.

In *The Meaning of Anxiety,* Rollo May (1979) distinguishes between fear and anxiety by differentiating anxiety from all other affects. According to May, fear is a threat to the periphery of an individual existence, but anxiety is a threat to the foundation and center of existence. The experience of anxiety confirms the existence of a measure of freedom (Hall and Lindzey, 1978).

In addition to describing anxiety by degree, anxiety can also be differentiated by type. Signal anxiety is the type of anxiety experienced when a precipitant is identified. It is important to note that although signal anxiety is learned, it results from situations that have been successfully repressed, or coped with, by using another defense mechanism. Consequently, the precipitant is successfully excluded from one's consciousness. Signal anxiety is the predominant etiologic factor in phobic disorders.

Trait anxiety is a function of personality structure. As a part of the developmental processes or events, some individuals have more traumatic experiences or have less success in coping with these events, resulting in unresolved conflict or confusion. These individuals are described as

having an anxiety diathesis, or predisposition to anxiety when stressed. Situations that recreate or represent the original conflict or experience evoke a more severe anxiety response in persons with a higher level of trait anxiety. For example, a woman whose mother was chronically ill for much of her childhood may worry excessively about her own children being injured or catching colds. As a result, she limits their activity and is anxious and overprotective.

State anxiety develops in situations identified as conflictual or stressful and in which the individual experiences limited control. This is often perceived as anxiety that has occurred before. The "butterflies" experienced by a student before an important examination is an example of mild state anxiety. The increased heart rate that a person who has been bitten by a dog in the past may experience when confronted by a Great Dane is a more moderate form of state anxiety. A woman with a strong family history of cancer who delays making an appointment with her primary health care provider after noticing a lump in her breast demonstrates severe and maladaptive state anxiety. Free-floating anxiety is characterized by a pervasive sense of dread or doom that cannot be attached to any idea or event. This type of anxiety may result in a panic state if stressors exceed the person's ability to cope.

State and trait anxiety are important concepts for

nurses because they can be differentiated and estimated by a rating scale known as the State/Trait Anxiety Inventory. Persons with high levels of trait anxiety are likely to experience higher levels of state anxiety when confronted with significant stressors. Nurses who are able to estimate their clients' levels of trait anxiety during the assessment process are better able to promptly institute interventions directed at helping clients cope with high state anxiety responses to identified stressors.

ANXIETY IN THE CONTEXT OF PSYCHIATRIC MENTAL HEALTH NURSING

The term *anxiety* is employed in such a variety of contexts that it is important to be precise in its use. One definition of anxiety is "the inability to choose among potentials" (May, 1979). Inherent in all nurse-client relationships is the nurse's role in facilitating meaning and becoming within the relationship. Another important nursing goal is to facilitate choices through the relationship. Although all relationships are not nursing, the basis for all nursing is a relationship. The phenomenon of a relationship as applied to nursing does not imply equal participation or responsibility on the part of the nurse and the client but rather the nurse's intention to establish a connection. Caring for an unconscious, anesthetized client or for an individual experiencing psychosis or dementia establishes a connection; therefore it is a relationship. For psychiatric mental health nurses, the primary goal of the nurse-client relationship is to become available to the individual. Through establishing a relationship, both the client and the nurse have the opportunity to develop their potentials as human beings, with the understanding that the focus of therapy is the client. Recognizing and managing anxiety and making appropriate choices are critical for both the client and the nurse in the relationship.

INFLUENCE OF HILDEGARD PEPLAU

In the 1950s Peplau described the nurse in a relationship as a person who is "to" the client rather than "with" the client. She presented the phases of the nurse-client relationship in a social learning model that today appears maternalistic but was nonetheless consistent with the meaning of developmental theory and mental health nursing practice at the time. In fact, Peplau is considered by both seasoned and novice colleagues as the "matriarch" of psychiatric mental health nursing.

According to Peplau, it is critical that nurses recognize the choices or potentials that exist in the emerging relationship between the client and the nurse. In *Interpersonal Relations in Nursing*, Peplau (1952) addresses the term *unexplained discomfort*, which includes the needs, frustrations, and conflicts that arise within the relationship. She considers them experiences that influence behavior by providing energy to the relationship. According to Peplau, anxiety needs to be examined as it occurs in nurses and clients and in the communication of the interpersonal relationship.

Peplau also presents a method for the nurse to examine the relationship between the nurse and the client. This method is known as process recording. Process recording helps nurses develop self-awareness about the way they relate to clients and underscores the value of the nurse-client relationship. This method is currently widely used in educating nurses, despite the technologic advances of videotape. In process recording, the nurse simply "records" or writes the interaction that occurred between nurse and client as the nurse remembers it. It is best to record the words directly following the interaction so that the recalled information is as valid as possible. The nurse then "processes" the interaction with a professor or clinical supervisor so as to analyze the responses of the nurse and client, the intent of the client's statements, and the overall effectiveness of the nurse in interacting with the client. It is important to note that recording always takes place after the interaction and not with the client present. However, as part of developing a relationship with the client, the nurse recorder and the client need to agree that the client is part of a valuable learning experience and that confidentiality outside of the learning experience will be protected. It is important to observe the protocols of the individual facilities. The defining purpose of process recording is to provide a practical vehicle for nurses to reflect on the content of the interaction in a safe, effective manner. As nurses review their responses to clients or "the nursed," Peplau's position is that nurses will develop a growing awareness of their responses, which is a critical factor in helping clients to achieve their goals and to function optimally. Peplau's anxiety continuum is a theory that is widely used in the treatment of anxiety disorders.

HUMANISTIC NURSING THEORY

Humanistic nursing theory can also be applied in treating anxiety and anxiety disorders. Patterson and Zderad (1976) developed a theory of **humanistic nursing** based on existential theory and the phenomenologic method. The cornerstone of their theory is an interactive process that occurs between two persons: one needing help and one willing to give help. Nurses and clients interact; the client "calls," and the nurse "responds." Humanistic nursing differs from Peplau's interpersonal nursing in that in humanistic theory the nurse is clearly identified as a participant in the process. The nurse strives to be fully present in the process and is described in relationship "with" the client, rather than "to" the client, as defined in Peplau's theory. In humanistic theory the nurse's availability to the client is critical to the process of nursing.

ANXIETY IN PSYCHIATRIC PRACTICE

Descriptions of anxiety as a phenomenon of concern in mental health are relatively recent. Psychiatry as a medical specialty had its origins in France in the late eighteenth century. Before that time, care for the insane (lunatics) fell to the law or to the church. Foucault (1988) has asserted that "madness" replaced death as a major theme in human experience. During the Age of Reason and into the nineteenth century, early psychiatric practitioners concerned themselves with the psychoses, those mental disorders believed to pose the greatest risk to society. However, in the second half of the nineteenth century, as the roots of psychoanalytic theory developed, anxiety (or "neuroses") emerged as a source of a variety of emotional and behavioral disturbances.

PHILOSOPHIC ROOTS OF ANXIETY

The philosophers most commonly associated with the concept of anxiety are the existentialists. However, Kierkegaard, a Danish philosopher (1813-1855), antedated the existentialists, and his work influenced them profoundly in some instances. His concept of anxiety is a seminal work on the subject from a theologic perspective. Kierkegaard was supportive of the phenomenologic method from the standpoint of "te unum noris omnes," meaning "if you know one, you know all, and hold fast to the one that actually is all." Kierkegaard went on to write from his own experience: "The one that actually is all, is the self" (Kierkegaard, 1980). His philosophic discussion of anxiety begins by considering innocence and, through a dialectic, develops the idea that anxiety is the qualitative leap (i.e., the "nothingness") between innocence and guilt. Kierkegaard viewed anxiety as the questioning of one's existence; the potential **denial** of self.

Martin Heidegger, a German phenomenologist and existentialist (1889-1976), stated that existential being (self-relatedness) is the only door to *being* itself. To Heidegger, being in the world projects itself entirely on possibilities. He viewed anxiety as "not being at home, therefore it is a state of discomfort; but nonetheless, anxiety is a condition of being" (Heidegger, 1962).

ETIOLOGY
BIOLOGIC MODEL

Roots of the biologic model for anxiety disorders date back to the nineteenth-century writings of Charles Darwin. Darwin postulated that emotional expression and anatomic structures both changed in the course of evolution to enable the species to adapt to its environment. Darwin further identified certain emotions as being universally demonstrated through expression, using motor and postural changes. In the early part of the twentieth century, investigators linked the endocrine system with emotions, first through establishing the relationship of the adrenal medulla in the production of epinephrine, resulting in the "fight or flight" response.

Selye built on this work after World War II, using observations of stress and anxiety demonstrated by soldiers who served in combat. A new conceptualization of stress replaced the former "psychic trauma." Selye expanded on the notion that the endocrine system and the central nervous system (CNS), particularly the hypothalamus and pituitary gland, have a reciprocal relationship. At the same time, important investigations were conducted regarding the neuropharmacology of the autonomic nervous system (ANS) in regulating cardiovascular, gastrointestinal, and motor responses. The ANS, particularly the sympathetic nervous system, was shown to be responsive to environmental stimuli, including emotional states. These biologic investigations found a continuity between normal states of fear and anxiety and the clinical disorders (Klerman, 1990). Today, psychopharmacologic interventions target the serotonin, noradrenergic, and γ-aminobutyric acid (GABA) systems primarily (see Chapter 4).

PSYCHODYNAMIC MODEL

In psychoanalytic terms, anxiety is conceptualized as a warning to the ego that it is in peril from either an internal or an external threat. Anxiety is involved in the development of personality and personality functioning and in the development and treatment of neuroses and psychoses. Freud's work is the basis for anxiety neurosis existing as a separate classification.

Three types of anxiety are identified in psychoanalytic theory: reality anxiety, moral anxiety, and neurotic anxiety. Reality anxiety is a painful emotional experience resulting from the perception of danger in the external world. Fear is the response to external danger; consequently, anxiety parallels fear. Moral anxiety is the ego's experience of guilt or shame. Neurotic anxiety is the perception of a threat according to one's instincts (Hall, 1954). According to Freud's theory of "signal anxiety," anxiety is a signal of impending emergence of threatening, unconscious mental content. Neurotic symptoms develop in an attempt to defend against anxiety—including hysterical symptoms, obsessions, compulsions, and phobias.

INTERPERSONAL MODEL

Both the interpersonal and the social psychiatry models view anxiety as a response to the individual's external environment, rather than the relatively simple psychoanalytic view of a response to instinctual drives. Interpersonal theorists, particularly Sullivan, regarded symptom formation as a result of expectations, insecurities, frustrations, and conflicts between individuals and primary groups. Primary groups include families, work colleagues, and social associates.

Like psychoanalytic theorists, interpersonal theorists place a great deal of emphasis on early development and experiences in relation to future mental health. According to Sullivan, the individual's first experience of anxiety is the infant's perception of the anxiety of the mothering person. The self system develops in the context of approval or disapproval from significant others. Disapproval results in a threat to the self system, a fear of rejection; in other words, anxiety.

Interpersonal theorists define anxiety broadly. According to Sullivan, anxiety is the first great educative experience in living. Also according to Sullivan, one of the great tasks of psychology is to discover the basic vulnerabilities to anxiety in interpersonal relations, rather than to try to deal with the symptoms of anxiety.

SOCIAL PSYCHIATRY: ENVIRONMENTAL MODEL

Social theorists emphasize the role of social conditions in deviant behavior and assert that symptoms, including anxiety and its manifestations, result from the dynamic relationship between individuals and their environment. Social psychiatry evolved after World War II and began to be defined by the large number of community and epidemiologic surveys designed to develop a model for understanding the role of vulnerability, predisposition, and stressors in symptom formation. Social psychiatry views factors such as socioeconomic status, racial inequalities, and migration as stressors equivalent to combat in the military. Individuals respond to the environment on a continuum, either adaptively or with symptom formation—mental illness or physical illness. The mediating factor in this response is the individual's ability to manage anxiety. Social psychiatric influences, particularly with respect to sampling methodology and the use of standardized questionnaires and scales, have contributed significantly to the current research base for the anxiety disorders.

BEHAVIORAL MODEL

Behavioral models in psychiatry and psychology were proposed by clinicians who were stimulated by the shortcomings of the psychoanalytic model and methods. They identified experimental psychology as a resource for ideas from which to develop new treatments. In behavioral models, based on learning theory, the etiology of anxiety symptoms is a generalization from an earlier traumatic experience to a benign setting or object. An example is an awkward child, ridiculed by parents while bowling, who associates embarrassment and shame with sports events in indoor facilities and develops panic attacks during basketball games. The same kinds of cognitive operations that link embarrassment with sporting events link cognitions of the expectation of embarrassment with the idea of a sporting event, and the individual begins to experience panic attacks while reading the sports page. Consequently, in this model, anxiety occurs when an individual encounters a signal that "predicts" a painful or feared event.

Early behavioral therapists directed their efforts at the anxiety disorders. In 1958 Wolpe, a South African physician working with soldiers experiencing symptoms of what is now classified as posttraumatic stress disorder (PTSD), reported success using systematic desensitization applied to simple phobias (Wolpe, 1973). Systematic desensitization is a method derived from learning theory in which the deeply relaxed client is exposed to a graded hierarchy of phobic stimuli. This method has been refined further into a method termed *in vivo desensitization*, whereby the individual is exposed to progressively more anxiety-provoking situations, often accompanied by a

therapist. These live exposure treatments can take a variety of forms, including graded practice, participant modeling, and prolonged or brief duration. In 1981 behaviorists demonstrated that 60% to 79% of patients with agoraphobia experienced clinically significant improvement by using the methods of systematic desensitization.

EPIDEMIOLOGY
SEX RATIO

The Environmental Catchment Area (ECA) study has emphasized the extensiveness of the anxiety disorders in terms of short-term and lifetime prevalence. According to Ross et al (1988), the 6-month prevalence of anxiety disorders in the general population ranges from 6% to 8%, with a phobic anxiety rate of about 1.5%. The lifetime prevalence of anxiety disorders is estimated to exceed 15%. The rates of panic disorder are higher in women, in persons ages 24 to 44, and in separated and divorced persons.

Almost all clients presenting with agoraphobia in clinical samples have a current diagnosis or history of panic disorder. In contrast, epidemiologic samples identify more clients with agoraphobia without a history of panic disor-

Table 12-2	Clinical Manifestations of Anxiety: Symptoms and Responses
Manifestation	**Symptom/Response**
PHYSIOLOGIC	
Cardiovascular system	Palpitations, racing heart, increased blood pressure, fainting, decreased pulse, decreased blood pressure
Respiratory system	Rapid, shallow breathing, pressure in chest, shortness of breath, gasping, lump in throat
Gastrointestinal system	Loss of appetite or increased appetite, abdominal discomfort or feeling of fullness, nausea, heartburn, diarrhea
Neuromuscular system	Hyperreflexia, insomnia, tremors, pacing, clumsiness, restlessness, flushing, sweating, muscle tension
Genitourinary system	Decreased libido, frequency or urgency of urination
COGNITIVE	Decreased attention, inability to concentrate, forgetfulness, impaired judgment, thought blocking, fear of injury or death
BEHAVIORAL	Rapid speech, muscle tension, fine hand tremors, restlessness, pacing, hyperventilation
AFFECTIVE	Irritability, impatience, nervousness, fear, uneasiness

der. Agoraphobia is diagnosed more often in women than in men.

Simple phobia is common in the general population, with reported lifetime prevalence rates of 10% to 12% (American Psychiatric Association [APA], 1994). Overall, the prevalence of simple phobia is higher for women than for men. However, with fear of heights and blood injection injury, the percentage of males is higher, from 30% to 45%, as compared with 10% to 25% in other categories.

In contrast to other anxiety disorders, in clinical samples, equal numbers of men and women seek treatment for social phobia. However, in community-based samples, social phobia is more common among women. Lifetime prevalence rates vary from 3% to 13% (APA, 1994). In outpatient treatment settings, rates of social phobia range from 10% to 20% of persons seeking treatment for anxiety disorders. Similarly, obsessive-compulsive disorder (OCD) is equally common in men and women; the lifetime prevalence is estimated at 2.5% (APA, 1994).

Estimates for the prevalence of PTSD range from 3% to 58% of at-risk individuals, with this wide variability being due to both sampling methods and the population assessed. Community-based samples for prevalence range from 1% to 14% (APA, 1994).

The prevalence of dissociative disorders is difficult to estimate. The diagnosis is usually made after an individual seeks treatment. There is still substantial controversy surrounding dissociative disorders. The lack of epidemiologic data reflects both case-finding difficulty and clinician bias. The disorder is more commonly diagnosed in women.

AGE OF ONSET

In general, anxiety disorders develop during adolescence and early adulthood. The typical age of onset for panic disorder varies from late adolescence to the mid-thirties. Rare cases have an onset in childhood, and a small number develop symptoms after age 45. Acute and posttraumatic stress disorders can develop at any age.

The age of onset for specific phobias, situational type, is bimodally distributed. There is a peak of onset in childhood and another peak in early adulthood. Other types of phobias usually have an onset in childhood.

CULTURAL VARIANCE

Most of the research supporting the development of the DSM-IV classification was done in the United States; consequently, symptoms defining disorders are representative of that culture. However, care should be taken to establish cultural norms when evaluating clients for anxiety and related disorders. For example, some cultures restrict women's participation in public activities; thus agoraphobia is less commonly diagnosed. Fears of magic or spirits are present in many cultures and should only be considered pathologic when the fear is excessive in the context of that culture. Many cultures prescribe rituals to mark important events in peoples' lives. The observation of these rituals is not considered indicative of OCD unless it exceeds norms for that culture, is exhibited at times or places inappropriate for that culture, or interferes with social functioning.

It seems that with the exception of OCD and social phobia, anxiety and related disorders exhibit a higher prevalence among women than among men. This observation may represent a cultural variation. Overall, women are more likely than men to present for treatment or come in contact with health care providers.

COMORBIDITY

Anxiety disorders do not exist in a clinical vacuum. In one study of a general medical practice, Katon et al (1986) determined that 13% of patients presenting for treatment met criteria for panic disorder. In the same sample, another 25% had past histories of panic disorder or less severe anxiety syndromes.

An early estimate of the comorbidity between anxiety and depression was offered in 1959 by Rosh, who estimated that half of the patients suffering from the "phobic-anxiety depersonalization syndrome" experienced variable degrees of depression (Stein and Unde, 1990). ECA risk ratios were not quite as high. Clients with major depression were found to have an 18.8% increased risk of panic and a 15.3% increased risk of agoraphobia. There is substantial comorbidity between substance abuse disorders and anxiety disorders.

OCD exists with other anxiety disorders, as well as substance abuse, major depression, and eating disorders. In Tourette's disorder, 30% to 50% of clients also have OCD; however, the rate of Tourette's disorder among OCD clients is lower, with estimates ranging from 5% to 7%.

Acute and posttraumatic stress disorders are associated with increased risk for major depression, other anxiety disorders, somatization disorder, and substance abuse disorders. Because of the nature of the disorder and its presentation after a significant event, it is difficult to determine whether the comorbid condition developed before the stress disorder or as a consequence of it. The epidemiology of anxiety disorders is summarized in Box 12-1.

CLINICAL DESCRIPTIONS
ANXIETY DISORDERS

The anxiety disorders as they are described in this chapter are categorized by whether they have circumscribed or limited symptom complexes or whether their symptoms are pervasive (Table 12-2).

Panic

In the nineteenth century, clinical syndromes similar to those we now label panic disorder and agoraphobia began to appear in the literature. In 1871 an American physician, Dr. Jacob Da Costa, described panic attacks occurring in soldiers who served in the Civil War. Around the same time, Westphal, a German physician, presented clinical data on four patients with classic agoraphobic syndromes. Freud first named panic attacks as occurring when "the connection between anxiety and threatened danger is entirely lost from view . . . spontaneous attacks . . . represented by intensely developed symptoms . . . tremor, vertigo, palpitations of the heart" (Freud, 1963). Freud also noted the comorbidity of the anxiety disorders and depression.

World Wars I and II contributed to the development of the knowledge base of the anxiety disorders, as did the work of the noted cardiologist Dr. Paul Dudley White. White and colleagues collected data on a number of patients referred to them at Massachusetts General Hospital who did not have organic heart disease, and they named the clinical syndrome *neurocirculatory asthenia*. In the same institution, neuropsychiatrists identified a similar symptom complex and named it *anxiety neurosis*. Both the cardiologists and the neuropsychiatrists were describing what we call panic disorder today.

Panic anxiety refers to anxiety symptoms that occur during panic attacks. Panic anxiety is differentiated from generalized anxiety by the sudden onset of distressing physical symptoms, combined with thoughts of dread, impending doom, death, and fear of being trapped. However, despite the gains made in describing the condition, the analytic conceptualization of anxiety neurosis remained intact until 1980.

Panic attack.   It is important to note that in and of themselves, panic attacks are not listed in the DSM-IV classification as psychiatric illnesses. Rather, **panic attacks** are symptoms, potentially meeting some of the defining characteristics of many of the disorders described in this chapter. Panic attacks are sudden, spontaneous episodes accompanied by symptoms such as a racing heart or palpitations, dizziness, dyspnea, and a feeling that death is imminent.

With the publication of DSM-III in 1980, the APA launched its effort to standardize the diagnostic criteria for each psychiatric disorder. One of the sweeping changes made in DSM-III was the introduction of panic disorder and generalized anxiety disorder as distinct clinical syndromes replacing anxiety neurosis. To meet the criteria for a panic attack four of the symptoms describing a panic attack must be present. Episodes of panic anxiety with fewer than four symptoms are considered limited-symptom attacks.

Panic attacks occur in a variety of anxiety disorders, including panic disorder, social phobia, simple phobia, and PTSD. Panic attacks can occur in specific, cued situations (as with simple phobias) or be unexpected (uncued) (APA, 1994). The DSM-IV Criteria box on p. 241 lists the symptoms of a panic attack.

Panic disorder.   There have been some changes in the criteria for panic disorder in DSM-IV. In both DSM-III-R and DSM-IV the trend has been to become more inclusive, particularly with respect to the frequency of panic attacks. To meet the DSM-III-R criteria for panic disorder, a person must have had four or more panic attacks during a 1-month period or one attack followed by a month of worry. The focus of that worry must be on having another attack.

In DSM-IV, published in 1994, an individual may be diagnosed with panic disorder if the following two criteria are met: (1) recent and unexpected panic attacks are present, and (2) at least one of the attacks has been followed for 1 or more months by (a) persistent concern about having additional attacks, (b) worry about the implications of the attack or its consequences (e.g., losing control, having a heart attack, "going crazy"), or (c) a significant change in behavior related to the attacks.

In panic disorder without agoraphobia, the individual is free from agoraphobic symptoms, the panic attacks are not related to direct effects of a substance (illicit drugs,

Panic Attack

A discrete period of intense fear or discomfort in which four or more of the following symptoms developed abruptly and reached a peak within 10 minutes:

1. Palpitations, pounding heart, accelerated heart rate
2. Sweating
3. Trembling or shaking
4. Sensations of shortness of breath or smothering
5. Feeling of choking
6. Chest pain or discomfort
7. Nausea or abdominal distress
8. Feeling dizzy, unsteady, lightheaded, or faint
9. Derealization or depersonalization
10. Fear of losing control or going crazy
11. Fear of dying
12. Parasthesias
13. Chills or hot flashes

From American Psychiatric Association: *Diagnostic and statistical manual of mental disorders*, ed 4, Washington, DC, 1994, The Association.

medication), and they are not due to a physiologic condition (e.g., hyperthyroidism). In addition, the anxiety is not better accounted for by another mental disorder, such as OCD (fear of contamination) or PTSD (e.g., in response to stimuli associated with a severe stressor).

Classified with phobias in DSM-III, agoraphobia is treated as a special complication of panic disorder in DSM-III-R and DSM-IV. Some controversy still exists surrounding the relationship of panic disorder and agoraphobia. To be diagnosed with panic disorder with agoraphobia, the individual must meet the criteria for panic disorder, as well as experience debilitating agoraphobic symptoms.

Panic disorder is primarily seen in ambulatory settings. Nurses are among the first health care providers that clients with new-onset panic disorder come in contact with, either in a clinic or physician's office or, more typically, a hospital emergency department. The sudden onset of physical symptoms and the pervasive feelings of impending doom are frightening, and the client often responds by seeking reassurance from a caregiver. However, it is not uncommon for clients with panic disorder to have been ill for 8 to 10 years before presenting for treatment and to have experienced one or two attacks per week. In addition, clients have learned to avoid those situations that trigger attacks. The attack may begin with a feeling of general unease that is quickly followed (in a few seconds to minutes) by the onset of the physical symptoms.

Phobias

The prominent features of phobic disorders, or **phobias,** are that the patient experiences panic attacks in response to particular situations or learns to avoid the situations that evoke panic attacks.

Agoraphobia. To meet the first DSM-IV criterion for panic disorder with agoraphobia, the person must experience recurrent, unexpected panic attacks, with at least one attack followed by one of the following for a month: (a) persistent concern about having additional attacks, (b) worry about the implications or its consequences, or (c) a significant change in behavior related to the attacks. The second criterion is that the individual experiences **agoraphobia** (i.e., anxiety about being in places or situations from which escape may be difficult [or embarrassing] or in which help might not be readily available in the event of an unexpected or situationally predisposed panic attack). Agoraphobic fears typically involve characteristic clusters of situations that include being outside the home alone, being in a crowd or standing in line, being on a bridge, and traveling in a bus, train, or car. The third criterion is that agoraphobic situations are avoided or endured with distress or anxiety about having a panic attack, or the individual requires the presence of a companion. The fourth criterion stipulates that panic attacks are not due to the direct effects of a substance or a general medical condition. Finally, the anxiety or phobic avoidance is not better accounted for by another mental disorder, as described in the panic disorder section (APA, 1994).

Agoraphobia can exist apart from panic disorder according to DSM-IV criteria. The individual with agoraphobia without a history of panic disorder meets the criteria for agoraphobia as just described but has no history of panic attacks. The description of agoraphobia is expanded to include "in the event of suddenly developing paniclike symptoms that the individual fears could be incapacitating or extremely embarrassing, for example, fear of going outside because of fear of having a sudden episode of dizziness or a sudden attack of diarrhea." If the individual has a comorbid medical condition, the fear described is clearly in excess of the fear usually associated with that disorder.

Specific phobias. The DSM-IV criteria define a specific phobia as a marked and persistent fear that is excessive or unreasonable, cued by the presence or anticipation of a specific object or situation, such as animals, insects, heights, flying, or seeing blood. Exposure to the phobic stimulus invariably provokes an anxiety response, which may take the form of a cued panic attack (i.e., the individual experiences symptoms listed in the DSM-IV Criteria box above. Children with a specific phobia may express their anxiety by crying, throwing tantrums, freezing, or clinging. Persons with a simple phobia (except children) recognize that their fear is excessive or unreasonable. Phobic situations are avoided, or endured with distress. The avoidance, anticipatory anxiety, or distress interferes significantly with the person's routine, occupational or social functioning; or there is marked distress about having the phobia. Finally, as with panic disorder and agoraphobia, the condition cannot be better accounted for by another Axis I mental disorder. (APA, 1994).

Social phobia.   Social phobia, or social anxiety disorder, is characterized by a marked and persistent fear of one or more social or performance situations in which the person is exposed to unfamiliar people or to possible scrutiny by others. The individual fears that he or she will act in a way (or show anxiety symptoms) that will be humiliating or embarrassing. To make this diagnosis in a child, the child must demonstrate the capacity for social relationships with familiar people, and the anxiety must occur in interactions with peers. In addition, the exposure to the feared social situation almost invariably provokes anxiety, which

CASE STUDY

Neil is a 19-year-old freshman at a local college. He is brought to the emergency department from a fraternity party one Saturday night with acute alcohol intoxication. He is referred to the college health service.

During his initial evaluation, the nurse asks Neil about his patterns of drinking. He reports that he began drinking at age 14 when one of his friends suggested having a beer or two before attending a school dance. He reported that ever since he started school, he was unable to participate in the easy banter, the "social chit-chat" common among fellow students. However, he did not have the same experience with family members. He was afraid that he wouldn't have anything to contribute to the conversation. He began to worry about his appearance, and his tendency to trip over his own feet.

When Neil reached high school, he found that this uneasiness was beginning to isolate him from others in his age-group. At home his parents usually began dinner parties with a glass of wine or a cocktail, so when his friend suggested a beer before the dance, Neil eagerly accepted. To his surprise, he found that once he arrived at the dance, he was relaxed and able to interact. He was even able to ask two girls to dance!

He continued to drink before arriving at parties, dances, football games, and just about any other social activity. He was worried that he was an alcoholic. The clinical specialist at the health service talked with Neil at length about social phobia and prescribed imipramine. Neil also began attending a group focused on behavioral strategies to cope with anxiety.

Critical Thinking—Nursing Diagnosis
1. What cues does Neil offer that will lead to the most appropriate nursing diagnoses for him?
2. List two beliefs Neil may have formed that led to his experience at the fraternity party.
3. Using information in this chapter and information in Chapter 16, what would be the prognosis for Neil?
4. Identify an alternative pharmacologic choice for Neil (see Chapter 23).
5. How would you describe the advantages of group therapy to Neil?

may take the form of a situationally bound panic attack. Children may express their fear by crying or exhibiting tantrumlike behavior. Adults acknowledge that their fear is excessive or unreasonable. Individuals with social phobia avoid social or performance situations or endure them with intense anxiety or distress (APA, 1994) (see Case Study box at left).

Posttraumatic Stress Disorder

Posttraumatic stress disorder (PSTD) was first defined as a diagnostic category in DSM-III. Before that time, the pattern of responses following traumatic events were most commonly found in soldiers and the syndrome was called "shell shock" or "combat fatigue." Psychiatric diagnosis currently relies on a simple description of predictable symptoms to define a disorder.

PTSD is a model diagnostic category for psychiatric disorders from a theoretic perspective: the causal factors are identifiable. Recently investigators have begun to adapt the PTSD model to traumatic events in human experience beyond combat, including the experiences of adult and child survivors of sexual abuse, physical abuse, disasters, and the grieving process. Controversy still exists in refining the level of intensity required of an event or an experience to meet the definition of "trauma" and in separating PTSD symptoms from other comorbid disorders, including substance abuse, depression, and anxiety. Since the comorbidity is high, the distinction of PTSD as a separate disorder remains to be firmly established.

To be diagnosed with PTSD, the individual must have experienced a traumatic event before the onset of symptoms. The individual must have either experienced the event, witnessed the event, or been confronted with an event that involved actual or threatened death or serious injury, or a threat to the physical integrity of self or others. The individual's response must have involved intense fear, helplessness, or horror. Children may express their response with agitated or disorganized behavior.

The second group of defining criteria for PTSD involves various mechanisms of reexperiencing the event. One of the following must be present: recurrent and intrusive disturbing recollections of the event, including thoughts, images, or perceptions; recurrent dreams of the event; acting or feeling as though the event were recurring; the experience of psychologic distress when internal or external cues resemble the event; and/or physiologic reactivity on exposure to internal or external cues that resemble the event.

Furthermore, the individual avoids stimuli associated with the trauma and experiences a numbing of general responsiveness (that was not present before the trauma). This numbing and avoidance are marked by at least three of the following: efforts to avoid thoughts, feelings, or conversations about the trauma; efforts to avoid persons or places that evoke memories of the trauma; an inability to remember an important aspect of the trauma **(repression)**;

diminished interest or participation in significant activities; a feeling of estrangement or detachment from others; restricted range of affect; and/or a sense of a foreshortened future (no expectation of a career or normal life span).

The fourth criterion is concerned with symptoms of increased arousal that were not present before the trauma. Two of the following must be present: sleep disturbances, irritability or angry outbursts, difficulty concentrating, hypervigilance, and exaggerated startle response. The symptoms must persist for more than 1 month and cause significant impairment in social or occupational or other significant areas of functioning.

PTSD can be further defined as acute if symptoms have occurred for 1 to 3 months or as chronic if the symptoms have persisted for at least 3 months or more. When the onset of symptoms is more than 6 months after the traumatic event, the further definition of delayed onset is specified (APA, 1994).

Acute Stress Disorder

Acute stress disorder is differentiated from PTSD in three ways: the individual experiences at least three symptoms indicating dissociation, the time frame of development and duration of symptoms is shorter, and the dissociative symptoms may prevent the individual from adaptively coping with the trauma. Three of the following indications of **dissociation** must be present: subjective sense of numbing or detachment, reduced awareness of surroundings (being in a daze), derealization, **depersonalization,** and dissociative amnesia. In terms of time, the symptoms may last from 2 days to a month. The onset of the dissociative experience may occur during the trauma experience or develop immediately afterward. The defining characteristic of causing significant distress or impairment in social and occupational functioning is that the individual is prevented from pursuing some necessary task, such as obtaining necessary medical or legal assistance or mobilizing personal resources.

Generalized Anxiety Disorder

Generalized anxiety disorder (GAD) is characterized by excessive anxiety and worry (apprehensive expectation) that occurs more days than not, for at least 6 months. This anxiety involves concerns about a number of events and activities. The individual finds it difficult to control the worry. Three of the following six symptoms must be present to some degree for a period of at least 6 months. These symptoms include restlessness, or feeling on edge; being easily fatigued; difficulties with concentration; irritability; muscle tension; and sleep disturbance. The focus of the anxiety and worry is not confined to features of another Axis I disorder (worry about having a panic attack, as in panic disorder, or fear of contamination, as in OCD) and is not a part of PTSD. The anxiety or worry interferes with normal social or occupational functioning and is not due to the direct effects of a substance or a general medi-

cal condition, and it does not occur exclusively in the presence of another Axis I disorder (mood disorder, psychotic disorder, or pervasive developmental disorder).

Obsessive-Compulsive Disorder

Obsessive-compulsive disorder (OCD) is characterized by the presence of either obsessions or compulsions. DSM-IV defines **obsessions** as recurrent and persistent thoughts, impulses, or images that are experienced at some time during the disturbance as intrusive and inappropriate and cause marked anxiety or distress. The thoughts, impulses, and images are not simply excessive worry about real problems. The individual attempts to suppress or ignore these thoughts and impulses or to neutralize them with some other thought or action. Finally, the individual recognizes that the obsessional thoughts are a product of his or her own mind (not imposed from without, as in thought insertion).

Compulsions are repetitive behaviors that the person feels driven to perform in response to an obsession. Examples are repeated hand washing in response to thoughts of contamination and checking over and over again to ensure that appliances are unplugged before leaving the house (see Case Study box below). The behaviors or mental acts are an attempt to prevent or reduce the distress invoked by the obsession or to prevent some dreaded threatening situation (such as a fire in the example of checking

---

CASE STUDY

Mark is a 31-year-old accountant who has been disabled from his job with a national firm for 8 months. He reports that he has been hospitalized for treatment of depression, which he has experienced since college. Despite his depression, he graduated with honors, obtained certification as a public accountant, and finished graduate school.

Mark first was treated for OCD 2 years later when he began experiencing trouble with his supervisor. A number of the firm's clients had complained that Mark was unable to either give them completed tax forms or file for the necessary extensions in a timely manner.

Mark received some relief from his counting and checking behaviors with treatment with clomipramine but presently spends his time preoccupied with thoughts about killing himself. He is unable to decide on a method of suicide that will not endanger his family's entitlement to his accidental death insurance policies. Mark has been admitted to an inpatient facility to begin a course of electroconvulsive therapy (ECT).

Critical Thinking—Planning

1. Develop an inpatient treatment plan for Mark with safety as a priority.
2. What are three collaborative treatment approaches that are important in Mark's long-term therapy?
3. Which methods can be used to measure outcomes achieved as a result of Mark's treatment?

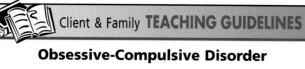

Client & Family TEACHING GUIDELINES

Obsessive-Compulsive Disorder

Teach the client's family:
1. Obsessive-compulsive disorder is a chronic anxiety disorder that responds to different treatment strategies.
2. Thoughts, impulses, and images are involuntary and may worsen with stress.

Teach the client:
1. Behavioral and cognitive strategies to manage anxiety and reduce the symptoms of the disorder.
2. Medication management is an effective treatment modality and usually involves treatment with a drug in the antidepressant category.
3. Different classes of drugs have different side effect profiles; recognizing and reporting side effects is an important part of managing the client's drug therapy.
4. Achieving symptom control through pharmacotherapy may take months.

CASE STUDY

Rita is a 28-year-old advertising account executive. She is referred to a mental health practice group by the fourth plastic surgeon with whom she has consulted regarding dermabrasion surgery to remove three 2-cm flat scars from her right upper arm. Although she lives in a coastal Florida city, Rita wears only long-sleeved jackets, blouses, and dresses. The garments are always loosely fitted. Rita is certain that people notice her "lumpy" arm and make comments about it; therefore she goes to extreme lengths to prevent this embarrassment and will bear the consequences of an extremely hot climate.

Critical Thinking—Outcome Identification
1. Develop an outcome that reflects Rita's awareness of her preoccupation with her area of concern.
2. List three outcome strategies that Rita can perform that would help reduce her exaggerated perceptions.
3. State two verbal outcome statements that would illustrate Rita's progress in managing her problem.
4. What are two behavioral outcomes that would indicate Rita's ability to better cope with her disorder?

appliances). However, these behaviors or mental processes are either not connected in a realistic way with what they are designed to prevent or are clearly excessive.

Except in children, individuals have recognized that the obsessions or compulsions are excessive or unreasonable at some point in the disorder. The obsessions or compulsions cause marked distress, are time consuming, or significantly interfere with the person's normal routine or occupational functioning. If another Axis I disorder is present, the content of obsessions or compulsions is not restricted to it (e.g., food rituals in anorexia, hair pulling in trichotillomania). Finally, the disorder is not due to the direct effects of a substance or a general medical condition (see Client & Family Teaching Guidelines box).

SOMATOFORM DISORDERS
The common focus of somatoform disorders is physical symptoms in the absence of clinically significant organic disease.

Body Dysmorphic Disorder
Body dysmorphic disorder is characterized by a preoccupation with an imagined defect in appearance. If the individual has a slight physical anomaly, the person's concern is markedly excessive. This preoccupation causes clinically significant distress or impairment in social or occupational functioning. Finally, the preoccupation is not better accounted for by another mental disorder (see Case Study box above).

Pain Disorder
The predominant focus of the clinical presentation in pain disorder is pain in one or more anatomic sites. The pain is of sufficient severity to warrant clinical attention and causes clinically significant impairment in one or more areas of functioning. Psychologic factors are judged to have an important role in the onset, severity, exacerbation, or maintenance of the pain. Finally, the pain is not better accounted for by a mood, anxiety, or psychotic disorder and does not meet the criteria for dyspareunia. The disorder can further be defined as a pain disorder associated with psychologic factors if an associated medical condition does not play a major role in the onset, severity, and maintenance of symptoms. If a general medical condition plays a major role in the maintenance of the syndrome, the disorder is termed pain disorder associated with both psychologic factors and a general medical condition. Both disorders can be specified as acute (if the duration is less than 6 months) or chronic.

Somatization Disorder
The characteristic pattern of clients presenting with somatization disorder is one of frequently seeking and obtaining medical treatment for multiple, clinically significant somatic complaints. To meet DSM-IV criteria, the complaints must begin before age 30, and the complaints cannot be adequately explained by any general medical disorder or the direct effects of a substance. For example, patients with multiple sclerosis, systemic lupus erythematosus, or other chronic debilitating diseases that have an onset in early adulthood frequently present with multisystem complaints but are not also diagnosed as having somatization disorder because a general medical condition better explains their symptom complex.

The distribution of symptoms in somatization disorder requires that symptoms have a distinct pattern that can be

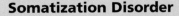

DSM-IV CRITERIA

Somatization Disorder

A. A history of many physical complaints beginning before age 30 years that occur over a period of several years and result in treatment being sought or significant impairment in social, occupational, or other important areas of functioning.

B. Each of the following criteria must have been met, with individual symptoms occurring at any time during the course of the disturbance:
1. *Four pain symptoms:* a history of pain related to at least four different sites or functions (e.g., head, abdomen, back, joints, extremities, chest, rectum, during menstruation, during sexual intercourse, or during urination)
2. *Two gastrointestinal symptoms:* a history of at least two gastrointestinal symptoms other than pain (e.g., nausea, bloating, vomiting other than during pregnancy, diarrhea, or intolerance of several different foods)
3. *One sexual symptom:* a history of at least one sexual or reproductive symptom other than pain (e.g., sexual indifference, erectile or ejaculatory dysfunction, irregular menses, excessive menstrual bleeding, vomiting throughout pregnancy)

4. *One pseudoneurological symptom:* A history of at least one symptom or deficit suggesting a neurologic condition not limited to pain (conversion symptoms such as impaired coordination or balance, paralysis or localized weakness, difficulty swallowing or lump in throat, aphonia, urinary retention, hallucinations, loss of touch or pain sensation, double vision, blindness, deafness, seizures; dissociative symptoms such as amnesia; or loss of consciousness other than fainting)

C. Either (1) or (2):
1. After appropriate investigation, each of the symptoms in Criterion B cannot be fully explained by a known general medical condition or the direct effects of a substance (e.g., a drug of abuse, a medication).
2. When there is a related general medical condition, the physical complaints or resulting social or occupational impairment are in excess of what would be expected from the history, physical examination, or laboratory findings.

D. The symptoms are not intentionally produced or feigned (as in factitious disorder or malingering).

From American Psychiatric Association: *Diagnostic and statistical manual of mental disorders,* ed 4, Washington, DC, 1994, The Association.

differentiated from general medical conditions if the following three criteria are met: (1) there is involvement of multiple organ systems (gastrointestinal, sexual/reproductive, and/or neurologic); (2) the symptoms exhibit an early onset and chronic course, without development of physical signs or structural abnormalities (e.g., degenerative changes in bones and joints associated with complaints of pain); and (3) clinical laboratory abnormalities commonly associated with general medical conditions are absent. The specific diagnostic criteria are detailed in the DSM-IV Criteria box above. Nurses in general hospital or clinic practices are more likely to encounter clients with somatization disorder than those working in inpatient psychiatric units.

Conversion Disorder

Clients who present with conversion symptoms exhibit one or more symptoms or deficits that affect voluntary motor or sensory function that appear to be related to a neurologic or general medical condition. As in somatization disorder, however, the symptom or deficit cannot be fully accounted for by a general medical condition, the direct effects of a substance, or as a culturally sanctioned behavior or experience. The symptom is not intentionally produced or feigned and is not limited to pain or sexual dysfunction; nor does it occur exclusively in the context of somatization disorder. As in other somatization disorders, the symptom causes clinically significant distress or impairment in social or occupational or other important areas of functioning (see Case Study box on p. 246).

The critical defining characteristics of conversion disorder are as follows: (1) psychologic factors are identified as being related to the onset or exacerbation of the symptom; (2) specific, identifiable conflicts or stressors precede the development of the conversion symptoms; and (3) the person demonstrates an obvious lack of concern about the seriousness of the symptoms, which is incongruent with the problem. This lack of concern is known as "la belle indifference," or "beautiful indifference."

Hypochondriasis

"Don't be such a hypochondriac!" is a common theme in American culture and perhaps other cultures as well. Parents say it to children who complain of stomachaches before school on the day of an important test. Sometimes even nursing students say it to each other as they worry about potential signs and symptoms while learning and acquiring knowledge related to medical, surgical, or psychiatric mental health nursing. However, such instances probably do not reflect true hypochondriasis as defined in the DSM-IV.

Six major criteria are associated with this diagnosis. First, the individual is preoccupied with fears of having—or the idea of having—a serious medical disorder based on the individual's misinterpretation of bodily symptoms. Second, this misinterpretation of symptoms

CASE STUDY

Carlos is a 34-year-old client on a neurologic unit in a Department of Veteran's Administration medical center. He has been treated on the psychiatric service in this facility for a number of years and was diagnosed with schizophrenia, based primarily on his prominent and constant visual and auditory hallucinations regarding his drill sergeant. In the past he has been treated with haloperidol.

Carlos was born in Puerto Rico and joined the Marines in San Juan when he turned 18. He was unable to complete basic training because he experienced a psychotic episode during which he assaulted his drill sergeant. Carlos was admitted to the neurology department when, one morning, he told his family he was unable to walk. Carlos had no recent falls or other injuries. No abnormalities were found on his physical examination or his computed tomography (CT) scan. During a mental status examination he reported that he no longer heard any voices. His assessment was also remarkable for his lack of concern about his paralysis, a seemingly serious problem. The psychiatric mental health nurse specialist was consulted and learned from Carlos's family that about a month before his admission, his appeal for a service-related disability was turned down. His family was depending on that financial supplement to help them obtain better housing, a goal they had voiced on many occasions.

Critical Thinking—Assessment

1. Describe two symptoms that indicate Carlos may be experiencing a conversion disorder.
2. How may the recent behavior of Carlos's family play a role in his current symptomatology?
3. Which symptom experienced by Carlos might be labeled "la belle indifference?"
4. Explain how Carlos's assaultive behavior during his psychotic episode may have influenced his perceived paralysis.

persists despite appropriate medical evaluation and reassurance. Third, the individual's preoccupation with symptoms is not as intense or distorted as in delusional disorder, nor is it as restricted as in body dysmorphic disorder. The fourth criterion is, as in the other somatoform disorders, that the preoccupation causes clinically significant distress or impairment in social, occupational, or other major areas of functioning. To meet the fifth criterion, the duration of the disturbance must be at least 6 months. Finally, as in other Axis I diagnoses, the condition is not better accounted for by another anxiety disorder, somataform disorder, or major depressive episode.

DISSOCIATIVE DISORDERS
Dissociative Amnesia

In persons with dissociative amnesia the defining symptom is one or more episodes of inability to recall important personal information, usually of a traumatic or stressful nature, that is too extensive to be explained by ordinary forgetting. In addition, the disturbance does not occur exclusively during the course of dissociative identity disorder and is not due to the effects of a substance (blackouts during ETOH intoxication) or as a result of a general medical condition (amnesia following head trauma).

Dissociative Fugue

Dissociative fugue is characterized by sudden, unexpected travel away from home or one's customary place of work, with an inability to recall one's past (or where one has been). The individual demonstrates confusion about personal identity or assumes a new identity, which may be partial ("filling in the blanks"). As in dissociative amnesia, the disturbance does not occur in the context of a dissociative identity disorder and is not due to the effects of a substance or to a general medical condition.

Dissociative Identity Disorder

No other disorder in current psychiatric nosology (classification) has aroused as much controversy as dissociative identity disorder (DID).

DSM-IV criteria for DID are straightforward. The first criterion is that the individual must demonstrate two or more distinct identities or personality states, each with its own relatively enduring pattern of perceiving, relating to, and thinking about the environment and self. Second, at least two of these personality states recurrently take control of the person's behavior. The individual is unable to recall important personal information that is too extensive to be accounted for by ordinary forgetting. Finally, these phenomena are not due to the effects of a substance (e.g., blackouts or chaotic behavior during alcohol intoxication) or a general medical condition (complex partial seizures). In children the symptoms are not attributable to imaginary playmates or other fantasy play.

PROGNOSIS

The prognosis for anxiety and associated disorders is related to factors specific to the disorder, the client, and the clinician. Clients treated for panic disorder with or without agoraphobia are typically described as chronic. Follow-up studies indicate that 6 to 10 years after treatment, 30% of clients are well, 40% to 50% are improved but still symptomatic, and the remaining 20% to 30% are the same or slightly worse (APA, 1994).

Specific phobias that persist into adulthood generally do not remit. The course of social phobia is often continuous with onset or reemergence after stressful or humiliating experiences. The prognosis for obsessive-compulsive disorder is similar to the other anxiety disorders, with waxing and waning symptoms related to stressors. However, 15% of clients demonstrate a chronically deteriorating course with progressive compromise of social and occupational functioning.

For acute and posttraumatic stress disorders, the prognosis is closely related to individuals' exposure to the stressful event, as well as their premorbid functioning and support systems. Persons with acute stress disorder by definition either recover in 4 weeks or are diagnosed with PTSD. Approximately half of those diagnosed with PTSD recover in 3 months; half continue to experience symptoms persisting for longer than a year after the trauma.

The somatoform disorders, with the exception of conversion disorder, are chronic and fluctuating and rarely remit fully. Conversion disorders usually remit within 2 weeks; however, there is recurrence in 20% to 25% of cases. A single recurrence of symptoms is predictive of future episodes. Factors that have been identified with a good prognosis are identifiable stressors at the time that symptoms develop, early treatment, and above-average intelligence.

The dissociative disorders have varying prognoses, ranging from a rapid, complete recovery (fugue) to both episodic and continuous chronic courses (dissociative identity disorder). Dissociative identity disorder frequently reemerges during periods of stress or relapse of substance abuse (APA, 1994).

DISCHARGE CRITERIA
Client will:

Identify situations and events that trigger anxiety and select ways to prevent or manage them.
Identify anxiety symptoms and levels of anxiety.
Discuss the connection between anxiety-provoking situations or events and anxiety symptoms.
Discuss relief behaviors openly.
Identify adaptive, positive techniques and strategies that relieve anxiety.
Demonstrate behaviors that represent reduced anxiety symptoms.
Use learned anxiety-reducing strategies.
Demonstrate ability to problem solve, concentrate, and make decisions.
Verbalize feeling relaxed.
Sleep through the night.
Use appropriate supports from the nursing and medical community, family, and friends.
Acknowledge the inevitability of occurrence of anxiety.
Discuss ability to tolerate manageable levels of anxiety.
Seek help from appropriate sources when anxiety is not manageable.
Continue postdischarge anxiety management, including medication and therapy.

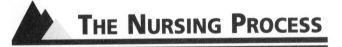

THE NURSING PROCESS

ASSESSMENT
New treatment modalities have markedly improved the quality of life and level of participation in activities for people with anxiety disorders. Nurses no longer expect to encounter clients with psychiatric disorders only in traditional psychiatric settings. It is important for all nurses to identify dysfunctional manifestations of anxiety so that treatment can be implemented promptly.

Panic disorders are primarily seen in ambulatory settings. Nurses are among the first health care providers to come in contact with clients who are experiencing their first symptoms of panic disorder, either in a clinic or physician's office or, more typically, in a hospital emergency department. The sudden onset of physical symptoms and the pervasive feelings of impending doom are frightening, and the client often responds by seeking reassurance from a caregiver. It is these physical symptoms that bring clients to the emergency department.

The client with agoraphobia may come to the attention of a nurse when preparing a client for diagnostic testing that includes a computed tomography (CT) scan or magnetic resonance imaging (MRI). The client who becomes visibly anxious at the prospect of entering a confined space when the nurse describes the procedure and the equipment may be agoraphobic.

Most often clients with anxiety symptoms do not present with anxiety as their reason for seeking treatment. Anxiety by definition is a vague, nonspecific feeling of discomfort. Nurses who use an assessment tool that addresses each identified human response pattern will obtain cues from the client experiencing anxiety that indicate further assessment is needed. The guidelines for a comprehensive nursing assessment, listed in Box 12-2, are adaptable for any practice setting. When thought of as a list of questions, an "admission interview" becomes a task for nurses and consequently an ordeal for clients. As the nurse becomes more experienced, assessment is integrated into the continuing nursing process, and inquiring about human response patterns evolves into a less threatening interaction between client and nurse.

Box 12-2   Nursing Assessment Guidelines According to Human Response Patterns

Exchanging: A Pattern Involving Mutual Giving and Receiving

Assess eating and elimination patterns. *Clients with anxiety disorders and somatization disorders have frequent appetite disturbances and such gastrointestinal complaints as gas, constipation, and diarrhea. Urinary frequency is another associated symptom.*

Communicating: A Pattern Involving Sending Messages

Observe for tics, stuttering, or other unusual speech patterns. Note whether the client maintains eye contact throughout the interview, and whether there are any instances of blushing. *There is comorbidity between Tourette's syndrome and obsessive-compulsive disorder; blushing and difficulty communicating with those the client perceives as having authority are common in social phobia.*

Relating: A Pattern Involving Established Bonds

In taking a social history, be particularly attentive to the client's affect in describing roles and role-related problems, including occupational function, financial issues, and role in the home. Ask about the client's role satisfaction and what contributes to it. Note whether the client presented alone for the appointment with the provider. If the client was accompanied, what is the client's relationship to the accompanying individual? *Clients with multiple roles are at risk for role strain, and role strain is often characterized by anxiety symptoms. Alternatively, if the individual describes an isolated existence, probe gently for contributing factors to this isolation. Clients with severe obsessive-compulsive disorder are isolated in part because their degree of involvement with rituals is a competing demand on their time available for social and occupational functioning. Clients with dissociative identity disorder also have poor role functioning, or one of the personality states may be unable to articulate its role functioning. Chronic worry about children or parents as a defining characteristic of anxiety disorders also may be expressed in exploring this pattern.*

Valuing: A Pattern Involving the Assigning of Relative Worth

Inquire about cultural background and values. *Be particularly attentive when assessing a client with a cultural experience different from your own. In addition to various culture-bound syndromes that are related to anxiety, somatization, and dissociative disorders, clients may exhibit behaviors and cognitive patterns that are adaptive and syntonic in one culture, yet labeled pathologic in another.*

Choosing: A Pattern Involving the Selection of Alternatives

Assess client's usual methods of coping with stressors. What aspects of the client's life are stressful? If the individual is part of a family unit, how does the family cope with change? Does the individual use alcohol to cope with stressful situations or public appearances? *Social phobia is often diagnosed only after a maladaptive substance use disorder is identified.* What is the client's usual method of decision making? Does the individual usually follow recommendations? What strategies does the person use to enhance success? *Clients with obsessive-compulsive disorder most often experience a disturbance in this pattern. Obsessional thinking and ritualistic behaviors are developed to cope with perceived threats (that range from intrusive thoughts to adaptive motor responses that become overgeneralized). If the nurse suspects symptoms of obsessive-compulsive disorder, the client should be asked quite frankly if she or he has any particular ways that tasks should be performed and if interruptions during the performance of these are stressful. Clients with other anxiety disorders, particularly generalized anxiety disorder, often express difficulties in coping and making choices, fearing they will make the wrong decision.*

Moving: A Pattern Involving Activity

In inquiring about an individual's history of physical disability, remember to ask about any episodes of motor dysfunction that may indicate conversion symptoms. If the client indicates past traumatic injury, ask about the circumstances. *Although posttraumatic stress disorder develops after combat situations, sexual abuse, and disasters, it also can follow less dramatic events, such as automobile accidents, and may be related to grief or bereavement as well. Questions about traveling, sports activities, and hobbies may yield content suggesting agoraphobic symptoms.*

Perceiving: A Pattern Involving the Reception of Information; and Knowing: A Pattern Involving the Meaning Associated With Information

These two patterns together compose the traditional mental status examination, formerly a touchstone for psychiatric mental health nurses. Orientation and memory questions are key to identifying anxiety, somatization, and dissociative disorders. *Look for signs of hesitation in answering questions about an individual's history that may indicate periods of dissociation. Listen carefully as the client describes past medical treatment for clusters of illnesses that suggest somatization disorder. When asking about self-perception and self-concept, be alert for responses that indicate a negative body image. Clients with body dysmorphic disorder may seek reassurance about a perceived defect if offered the opportunity and the subject is opened in a nonthreatening manner.*

Feeling: A Pattern Involving the Subjective Awareness of Information

Ask directly about experience of pain and fears. Anxiety symptoms are more easily identified if the nurse prompts the client for actual phenomena (e.g., "Are your muscles tight from time to time, is your mouth dry, do you perspire a lot—particularly when you're expecting something unpleasant?" "Have you had more difficulty concentrating lately?" "Have you ever had these feelings come out of nowhere?") *Endorsement of several of the defining characteristics of panic attack warrants a more thorough evaluation for panic disorder and agoraphobia. Explore the client's experiences of guilt and shame for signs of social phobia.*

NURSING DIAGNOSIS

To determine which nursing diagnoses will most effectively guide treatment for clients with anxiety and related disorders, the nurse relies on information obtained in the assessment process. The nurse identifies defining characteristics for the target diagnoses from the client, and the nurse and client jointly identify etiologic factors.

Etiologic factors influence selection of intervention. It is impossible to anticipate each potential diagnosis for all of the disorders discussed in this chapter. Typical diagnoses for clients with anxiety and related disorders are listed here.

NURSING DIAGNOSES FOR ANXIETY AND RELATED DISORDERS

Activity intolerance
Adjustment, impaired
Anxiety
Body image disturbance
Coping, ineffective individual
Decisional conflict
Family processes, altered
Fatigue
Fear
Hopelessness
Knowledge deficit
Mobility, impaired physical
Noncompliance
Nutrition, altered: less than body requirements
Nutrition, altered: more than body requirements
Pain, chronic
Posttrauma syndrome
Powerlessness
Rape-trauma syndrome: compound reaction
Rape-trauma syndrome: silent reaction
Relocation stress syndrome
Role performance, altered
Self-care deficit
Self-esteem, situational low
Self-mutilation, risk for
Sensory/perceptual alterations
Sexual dysfunction
Skin integrity, impaired, risk for
Sleep pattern disturbance
Social interaction, impaired
Social isolation
Spiritual distress (distress of the human spirit)
Thought processes, altered
Violence, risk for: directed at others
Violence, risk for: self-directed

OUTCOME IDENTIFICATION

Outcome criteria will differ according to the characteristics that define each client's nursing diagnoses and collaborative (DSM-IV) diagnoses (see Collaborative Diag-

COLLABORATIVE DIAGNOSES

DSM-IV Diagnoses*	NANDA Diagnoses†
Dissociative identity disorder	Personal identity disturbance
	Role performance, altered
Generalized anxiety disorder	Anxiety
	Coping, ineffective individual
Obsessive-compulsive disorder	Social interaction, impaired
	Social isolation
	Violence, risk for: self-directed
Posttraumatic stress disorder	Posttrauma syndrome
	Rape-trauma syndrome
Somatization disorder	Constipation, perceived

*From American Psychiatric Association: *Diagnostic and statistical manual of mental disorders*, ed 4, Washington, DC, 1994, The Association.
†Reprinted with permission from North American Nursing Diagnosis Association: *NANDA nursing diagnoses: definitions and classifications, 1999-2000*, Philadelphia, 1999, The Association.

noses box). Determining outcomes before implementation of the plan will guide both nursing interventions and evaluation. Nursing diagnoses are associated with outcomes (goals) to serve as a guide in outcome development. In practice, outcomes are generally determined by the patient's presentation of clinical manifestations.

OUTCOME IDENTIFICATION FOR GENERALIZED ANXIETY DISORDER

Client will:

1. Demonstrate significant decrease in physiologic, cognitive, behavioral, and emotional symptoms of anxiety.
2. Demonstrate effective coping skills.
3. Exhibit enhanced ability to make decisions and problem solve.
4. Demonstrate ability to function adaptively in mild anxiety states.

OUTCOME IDENTIFICATION FOR OBSESSIVE-COMPULSIVE DISORDER

Client will:

1. Participate actively in learned strategies to manage anxiety and decrease obsessive-compulsive behaviors.
2. Describe increasing sense of control over intrusive thoughts and ritualistic behaviors.
3. Demonstrate ability to cope effectively when ruminations or rituals are interrupted.
4. Spend less time involved in anxiety-binding activities and instead use time gained to complete tasks of daily living and participate in social/recreational activities.

5. Successfully manage times of increased stress by integrating knowledge that thoughts, impulses, and images are involuntary, thus reducing sense of responsibility and consequent anxiety.

OUTCOME IDENTIFICATION FOR POSTTRAUMATIC STRESS DISORDER

Client will:

1. Demonstrate concern for personal safety by beginning to verbalize worries.
2. Participate actively in support group.
3. Identify and involve significant support system.
4. Assume decision-making role for own health care needs.
5. Acquire and practice strategies for coping with anxiety symptoms such as breathing techniques; progressive relaxation exercises; thought, image and memory substitution; and assertive behaviors.

OUTCOME IDENTIFICATION FOR SOMATIZATION DISORDER

Client will:

1. Increase level of exercise to walking 1 mile four times a week.
2. Accurately describe the potential consequences of laxative dependence.
3. Meet with a dietitian to evaluate eating habits.
4. Keep an intake log to document fluid and fiber intake.

OUTCOME IDENTIFICATION FOR DISSOCIATIVE IDENTITY DISORDER

Client will:

1. Respond to name when addressed by a member of the treatment team.
2. Refer to self in the first-person pronoun form: "I think."
3. Identify periods of increasing anxiety.
4. Inform others of dissatisfaction in a nonthreatening manner.
5. Use assertive-response behaviors to meet needs.

PLANNING

Treatment planning for the client with anxiety and related disorders in the current health care environment is complex and varied. Clients with severe obsessive-compulsive disorder were formerly hospitalized for structured behavioral programs. Treatment for dissociative identity disorder also occurred in special units with a protracted hospitalization.

Today, both clinicians and administrators in inpatient facilities are struggling to balance effective treatment with the high costs associated with these specialty units. Increasingly, inpatient hospitalization is available only for short periods of time for clients at imminent risk to themselves or others. Rather than their traditional roles of providing direct care to clients in inpatient facilities, nurses are increasingly involved as case managers. As case managers nurses provide information on treatment alternatives to clients and families.

IMPLEMENTATION

The role of a nurse in the implementation of a care plan for clients with anxiety and related disorders depends on the setting in which the client is treated. The following interventions are useful for clients with anxiety symptoms, regardless of diagnosis or treatment setting. Specific issues community nurses may face are found in the Nursing Care in the Community box.

NURSING INTERVENTIONS

1. Assess own level of anxiety and make a conscious effort to remain calm. *Anxiety is readily transferable from one person to another.*
2. Recognize the client's use of relief behaviors (pacing, wringing of hands) as indicators of anxiety *to intervene early in managing anxiety and prevent escalation of symptoms.*
3. Inform the client of the importance of limiting caffeine, nicotine, and other central nervous system stimulants *to prevent/minimize physical symptoms of anxiety, such as rapid heart rate and jitteriness.*
4. Teach the client to distinguish between anxiety that can be connected to identifiable objects or sources (illness, prognosis, hospitalization, known stressors) and anxiety for which there is no immediate identifiable object or source. *Knowledge of anxiety and its related components increases the client's control over the disorder.*
5. Instruct the client in the following anxiety-reducing strategies:
   Progressive relaxation technique
   Slow deep-breathing exercises
   Focusing on a single object in the room
   Listening to soothing music or relaxation tapes
   Visual imagery
   Strategies help reduce anxiety in a variety of ways and distract the client from focusing on the anxiety.
6. Help the client build on previously successful coping methods to manage anxiety symptoms. *Coping methods that were successful in the past are generally effective in subsequent situations.*
7. Help the client identify support persons who can help him or her perform personal tasks and activities that present circumstances (such as hospitalization) make difficult. *A strong support system can help circumvent anxiety-provoking situations/activities.*
8. Help the client gain control of overwhelming feelings and impulses through brief, directive verbal interac-

Anxiety and Related Disorders

Anxiety disorders are seldom found in a pure form. Clients who seek help or who are found at home in a highly anxious state are usually reacting to a situational crisis that may be physical or psychologic. They may benefit from a brief intervention such as reassurance or reorientation to the environment.

Often, older adults may become extremely anxious about somatic complaints, ranging from worries about constipation to sensations of having a heart attack. Community mental health nurses may have responded to a client's repeated complaints, but these complaints should be investigated medically before psychiatric intervention is attempted. After a medical condition has been ruled out, these types of anxious persons will usually respond to cognitive interventions and/or medication. They may benefit from increased unsolicited attention and involvement of a community-based support system, such as the family, visiting nurse, and/or social worker.

The older client with progressive dementia also presents with increased anxiety or paranoia as a result of the confusional state of the disease itself. In some cases antipsychotic or antianxiety medications are prescribed and the older client must be monitored closely for hypotension and the increased risk of accidental falls.

A client with a chronic mental disorder, such as paranoid schizophrenia, may often seek reassurance from the nurse. Kindness and simple self-care suggestions for stress reduction will usually be enough to return the client's attention to normal functioning, but an adjustment in medication may also be indicated.

Occasionally the nurse will encounter a person who cannot identify a current stressor but is experiencing severe anxiety, verging on panic. Daily functions are seriously impaired, and a family member or friend must intervene to call for help or deliver the client to a care site. Such individuals may respond to **anxiolytic** medications but are not generally capable of processing cognitive therapy. They will usually continue to experience overwhelming apprehension despite reassurance and reality testing.

It is essential to recognize that the client's sensations are beyond rationality and to maintain a calm presence until the appropriate medications act to decrease pathologic activity in the brain and allow resumption of functional response patterns. The client should not be expected to supply information; situation permitting, it should be obtained from a significant other. As the client becomes calmer, the nurse may establish a therapeutic relationship, and gaps in the history may be filled and validated by the client.

If the intensity of the anxiety is not mitigated by a standard dose of medication within a reasonable time, the nurse working in the community must consider hospitalizing the client. Hospitalization will relieve the client of the pressures of family and daily maintenance behaviors until rational abilities are restored. The hospital offers a safe environment with reduced **stress** and therapeutic suggestions for more positive coping activities.

---

tions. *Individual interactions executed at appropriate intervals can help reduce/manage client's anxious feelings/impulses.*

9. Help the client structure the environment so it is less noisy. *A less stimulating environment can create a calming, stress-free atmosphere that reduces anxiety.*

10. Assess the presence and degree of depression and suicidal ideation in all clients with anxiety and related disorders *to prevent self-harm and intervene in depression early.*

11. Employ anxiolytic medication as least restrictive measure to reduce anxiety. *Appropriate medicine may be an effective adjunct to other psychosocial therapeutic interventions, when necessary, to manage stress.*

ADDITIONAL TREATMENT MODALITIES
Biologic Interventions

Pharmacologic interventions alone or in combination with cognitive behavioral interventions are among the most successful treatments for anxiety and related disorders. Since the early 1960s, benzodiazepines have been widely used in the treatment of anxiety disorders. They are relatively safe and effective for short-term use in controlling debilitating symptoms of anxiety. Longer-term treatment raises issues of tolerance abuse and dependence.

Tricyclic antidepressants (TCAs), monoamine oxidase inhibitors (MAOIs), and benzodiazepines have been effective in the treatment of panic disorder and OCD. More recently, however, after successful double-bind clinical trials, selective serotonin reuptake inhibitors (SSRIs) are widely used to treat anxiety disorders and are particularly effective in treating OCD and panic disorders.

Although other TCAs have been used to treat OCD, newer drugs such as clomipramine (Anafranil) and fluvoxamine (Luvox) have demonstrated significant efficacy in treating OCD. Dosage of antidepressant drugs required for control of symptoms of OCD may be higher than those traditionally used for depression.

Pharmacologic treatment for PTSD and dissociative identity disorder is largely symptomatic. Varying combinations of antidepressants, antipsychotics, and, to a lesser extent, benzodiazepines are used. Medications are generally avoided in somatoform disorders unless anxiety or depression is present. (For more specific information about dosages and side effect profiles, see Chapter 23.)

Electroconvulsive Therapy

The primary indication for electroconvulsive therapy (ECT) is depression. However, ECT may be used for anxiety disorders when other treatments are too high a risk or have failed. For example, in clients with OCD who have only a partial response to clomipramine and who are suicidal, ECT is a reasonable treatment alternative. The mechanism of ECT is unknown, but it is thought to be related to improving transmission of dopamine, norepinephrine, and serotonin and release of hypothalamic and pituitary hormones (Keltner and Folks, 1997).

Psychotherapy

Psychotherapeutic intervention can take place in group or in individual settings. One advantage of group therapy is the opportunity for the client to learn from the successes and failures of others with similar symptoms. Behavioral and cognitive behavioral therapies have proved to be widely effective in treating a variety of anxiety disorders.

Behavioral therapy. Behavioral treatments, including systematic desensitization, are among the most effective treatments for panic disorder with agoraphobia. First, the phobic stimulus is defined. Clients are assisted in defining a hierarchy for the phobic stimulus. The client and therapist then expose the client to events on the hierarchy that increase the client's degree of anxiety. As the client and therapist move through the hierarchy, the client experiences progressive mastery of increasing levels of anxiety until the phobic stimulus is encountered (see Chapter 3).

Cognitive behavioral therapy. Cognitive behavioral therapy is widely used in the treatment of anxiety disorders. The success of this approach centers on the client's understanding that symptoms are a learned response to thoughts or feelings about behaviors that occur in daily life. The client and therapist identify the target symptoms and then examine circumstances associated with the symptoms. Together they devise strategies to change either the cognitions or the behaviors. Cognitive behavioral therapy is short term and demands active participation on the part of both client and therapist (see Chapter 3).

• • •

Additional treatment modalities and collaborative interventions may include consultation with occupational therapists, vocational rehabilitation counselors, and psychologists, depending on the particular treatment needs of a patient. A summary of additional treatment modalities appears in the Additional Treatment Modalities box and is explored in depth in Chapter 3.

EVALUATION

One of the most difficult aspects of applying the nursing process to psychiatric mental health nursing, in particular, nursing care of clients with anxiety and related disorders, is generating measurable outcomes. Outcome criteria for clients with the more concrete nursing diagnoses, such as hyperthermia, decreased cardiac output, or even altered thought processes as evidenced by auditory hallucinations, seem clear and straightforward when compared with the more vague concept of anxiety. Fortunately, there are a number of valid, time-tested tools available that will yield such reliable information for anxiety-related disorders. Although not developed by and for nurses specifically, clinical rating scales offer a method to track changes in symptoms over time with a numeric value. These changes can be correlated with discrete interventions (such as instituting a behavioral program or a change in medication). Two rating scales commonly used with clients exhibiting anxiety disorders are the Yale-Brown Obsessive-Compulsive Scale and the Hamilton Anxiety Scale.

Ideally, nurses evaluate client progress toward the identified outcomes at every interaction with the client. If satisfactory progress is not made, the nurse either modifies the expected outcomes or the interventions. The nurse examines all factors that relate to the outcomes, including the role of the nurse in setting the expectations, the clarity of communicating about the goals with the client, and other intervening events that may have occurred since the outcomes were set.

ADDITIONAL TREATMENT MODALITIES
For Clients With Anxiety and Related Disorders

Biologic
Pharmacologic
   Benzodiazepines
   Tricyclic antidepressants
   Monoamine oxidase inhibitors
   Selective serotonin reuptake inhibitors
Electroconvulsive Therapy
Psychotherapy
   Behavioral therapy
   Cognitive therapy

▲ NURSING CARE PLAN

Sarah, a 47-year-old woman, presented to the employee health department of a teaching hospital after walking there from her office, complaining of chest pain and shortness of breath. The staff instituted the standard cardiac workup for clients with new-onset chest pain. Sarah's medical history included psoriasis. Her vital signs were remarkable for a pulse of 116; her electrocardiogram and laboratory work were within normal limits.

Sarah mentioned to the staff that her son had died 3 months ago. She was referred to a research team conducting a study on panic disorder and was seen by a clinical specialist in psychiatric mental health nursing. Sarah participated in the research protocol after giving informed consent. During the course of the interview, she revealed that her deceased son, an only child, had been an alcoholic whose death was a suicide. She was presently considering separating from her husband of 27 years who was involved in a long-term extramarital affair. Her screening was positive for limited-symptom panic attacks that were increasing in frequency. She agreed to an extended evaluation after her initial interview.

During her evaluation, Sarah and the nurse explored her symptoms of anxiety and depression, the exacerbation of her psoriasis, and her chronic headaches, which had be-come worse since her son's death. On moving back from the West Coast, Sarah had obtained her first job in 24 years. In addition to concern about financial matters and her son's alcoholism, she now worried frequently about her performance at work. She revealed that her husband's extramarital affair had been ongoing for several years and related his behavior to their sexual difficulties. The nurse recommended a medication trial. Sarah refused medication because of her fears of addiction and loss of control.

DSM-IV Diagnoses

Axis I	Generalized anxiety disorder (with limited-symptom panic attacks)
	Bereavement
	Partner relational problem
Axis II	Dependent/avoidant traits
Axis III	Psoriasis
	Headaches
Axis IV	Psychosocial stressors = moderate to severe (6 to 7)
Axis V	GAF = 60 (current)
	GAF = 75 (past year)

Nursing Diagnosis: Anxiety related to change in role functioning, recent loss of son (dysfunctional grieving), threat to socioeconomic status, and stressors exceeding ability to cope, as evidenced by uncertainty, intermittent sympathetic nervous system stimulation, restlessness, and exacerbation of medical condition (psoriasis).

Client Outcomes	Nursing Interventions	Evaluation
• Sarah will identify common situations that provoke anxiety.	• Assign "homework" to client (e.g., keeping a panic attack and headache diary). *Documenting anxiety responses helps client link symptoms with precipitating events.* • During weekly sessions, review with Sarah her log of panic symptoms. *Discussing the linking of events/situations with anxiety symptoms teaches Sarah which stressor events provoke anxiety so she can learn to manage/avoid them.*	• Sarah identifies returning home after work as a critical time for symptoms to develop. She reports that she visits her mother or does errands daily.
• Sarah will describe early warning symptoms of anxiety. • Sarah will report willingness to tolerate mild to moderate levels of anxiety. • Sarah will demonstrate adaptive coping mechanisms.	• Assist Sarah in associating her panic attack symptoms with thoughts about separation from her husband *to illustrate to Sarah specific situations in her life that result in panic anxiety.* • In weekly sessions explore with Sarah the advantages and disadvantages of separation and divorce *to help Sarah problem solve viable options that may offer some control over her anxiety.* • During weekly sessions discuss options that will allow Sarah maximum control over her choices. *Increased choices over life situations tend to minimize anxiety responses to some degree.*	• Sarah reports that she does not experience headaches when her husband is traveling. • Sarah reveals unwillingness to live alone. • Sarah informs her husband she wants a trial separation. He moves into their son's former room.

Continued

NURSING CARE PLAN —cont'd

Nursing Diagnosis: Dysfunctional grieving related to son's death, as evidenced by anxiety on returning home; alteration in sleeping patterns; expression of guilt, sadness, and crying; and difficulty with concentration.

Client Outcomes
- Sarah will return to her home directly after work, without going immediately to bed.

- Sarah will be able to talk with family and significant others about her son's death.

- Sarah will be able to use her son's former bedroom as a functional part of the house.

Nursing Interventions
- Explore with Sarah her usual patterns of behavior before her son's death. Identify possible modifications of those behaviors *to help Sarah focus on alternative activities/behaviors that would minimize dysfunctional grieving patterns and increase coping skills.*
- Promote recognition that others also experience the loss of Sarah's son *to help Sarah understand that others share her grief, which can be comforting at such times.*

- Initiate discussion of ways Sarah and her husband can plan for disposal of some of their son's possessions without feeling disloyal to his memory *to expedite the functional grieving process via discussion of feelings.*

Evaluation
- Sarah describes cooking dinner for her son. She identifies other constructive activities she could perform to modify that routine.
- Sarah is able to visit with her mother and talk about her son without experiencing panic symptoms.
- As part of their trial separation agreement, Sarah's husband moves into their son's room.

Nursing Diagnosis: Decisional conflict related to unclear personal values and beliefs, as evidenced by delayed decision making and physical signs of distress.

Client Outcomes
- Sarah will make an informed decision about her relationship with her husband.

- Sarah will identify potential outcomes of separation and divorce and prioritize them according to social, financial, and interpersonal values.

Nursing Interventions
- During weekly sessions explore with Sarah her expectations of marriage, how her relationship with her husband has changed over the course of their marriage, and what part she played in the changes *to help Sarah clarify values and expectations and her role in marriage, which can assist her in making critical life choices.*

- Review with Sarah some of the important relationships in her life. Support her considerations in the values clarification process. *It is critical that the nurse be aware of his or her own values and choices and maintain clear distinctions between his or her worldview and the client's.*

Evaluation
- Sarah describes increasing involvement with her son as his substance abuse worsened and consequent discord in an already-strained marriage. She reports frequent conflict with her husband over his own drinking.
- Sarah describes her parental relationships as conflict ridden, with her father frequently abusing alcohol. She is critical of her mother's domination of her father. She acknowledges long-standing differences with her husband over sexual issues and feelings of disgust toward her husband when he smells of beer.

NURSING CARE PLAN —cont'd

Nursing Diagnosis: Chronic low self-esteem related to unresolved developmental issues as evidenced by self-negating verbalizations, evaluation of self as unable to deal with decisions, and passive dependence on marital partner.

Client Outcomes	Nursing Interventions	Evaluation
• Sarah will exhibit a more positive self-evaluation.	• Suggest use of a diary *to record interactions with her husband that result in anxiety symptoms.* • During weekly sessions, role-play other responses that seem more satisfactory to Sarah *to help Sarah distinguish anxiety-producing interactions and modify responses through role-playing and other teaching strategies.*	• Sarah reports fewer episodes of headaches and limited-symptom panic attacks. • Sarah frequently describes reinitiating discussions with her husband that she previously identified as being unsatisfactory to her.
• Sarah will demonstrate assertive behaviors and a positive interpersonal relationship.	• Provide feedback to Sarah about behaviors observed *to give her information about her responses/behaviors so she can begin to modify/manage them.* • Help Sarah identify and label angry feelings *so she can begin to process feelings correctly and not misinterpret feelings or their meaning.*	• Sarah initiates subject of marital therapy with the nurse. • Sarah requests that her husband join her in weekly sessions to deal with issues involving the husband's use of alcohol, his extramarital affair, and their sexual difficulties.

Nursing Diagnosis: Sexual dysfunction related to values conflict, as evidenced by alteration in relationship with husband and inability to achieve desired satisfaction.

Client Outcomes	Nursing Interventions	Evaluation
• Sarah will demonstrate ability to attain an ongoing intimate relationship with her husband.	• Provide an open, neutral atmosphere where Sarah and her husband can discuss their differences regarding the level of interest in intimate relations and achievement of satisfaction *to open up sound discussion in a nonthreatening environment.*	• Sarah and her husband report increased mutually satisfying sexual encounters.

Summary of Key Concepts

1. Anxiety and related disorders encompass a wide variety of illnesses that share the common symptoms of anxiety.
2. Etiologic models for anxiety include biologic, psychosocial, psychodynamic, and social theories.
3. Anxiety disorders have high comorbidity with depression and substance abuse.
4. Anxiety disorders are more commonly diagnosed and treated among women, although obsessive-compulsive disorder is equally common with both sexes.
5. Treatment of anxiety and related disorders is multidisciplinary and usually involves more than one treatment modality.
6. Inpatient treatment of anxiety disorders is increasingly rare and is generally confined to managing acute exacerbations.
7. The nursing role in the treatment of clients with anxiety symptoms varies. Common to all treatment settings is the nurse's role in client and family education about the disorders and their treatment.
8. Nursing care plans for clients with symptoms of anxiety reflect the understanding that managing anxiety effectively is part of daily living.
9. Nurses actively participate in behavioral interventions structured to decrease phobic responses.
10. Rating scales are an effective means for nurses to measure success of strategies implemented to reduce anxiety.

REFERENCES

American Psychiatric Association: *Diagnostic and statistical manual of mental disorders*, ed 4, Washington, DC, 1994, The Association.

Bailey K, Glod CA: Post-traumatic stress disorder; a role for psychopharmacology, *J Psychosoc Nurs Ment Health Serv* 29(9):42, 1991.

Fortinash K, Holoday-Worret P: *Psychiatric nursing care plans*, ed 3, St. Louis, 1999, Mosby.

Foucault M: *Madness and civilization*, New York, 1988, Vantage.

Freud S: Introductory lectures on psychoanalysis. In *The standard edition of the complete psychological works*, London, 1963, Hogarth Press (originally published in 1917).

Freud S: *The standard edition of the complete psychological works*, London, 1963, Hogarth Press.

Gellengarg A et al: *The practitioner's guide to psychoactive drugs*, ed 3, New York, 1991, Plenum.

Hall CS: *A primer of Freudian psychology*, Cleveland, 1954, World.

Hall C, Lindzey G: *Theories of personality*, New York, 1978, Wiley.

Heidegger M: *Being and time*, New York, 1962, Harper & Row.

Katon W et al: Panic disorder epidemiology in primary care, *J Fam Pract* 23(3):233, 1986.

Keltner NL, Folks DG: *Psychotropic drugs*, ed 2, St. Louis, 1997, Mosby.

Kierkegaard S: *The concept of anxiety*, Princeton, 1980, Princeton University Press.

Kim M et al: *Pocket guide to nursing diagnosis*, ed 6, St. Louis, 1995, Mosby.

Klerman G: Modern concepts of anxiety and panic. In Ballenger J, editor: *Clinical aspects of panic disorder*, New York, 1990, Wiley-Less.

Kluft, RP: Enhancing the hospital treatment of dissociative disorder patients by developing nursing expertise in the application of hypnotic techniques without formal trance induction, *Am J Clin Hypnosis* 34(3):158, 1992.

May R: *The meaning of anxiety*, New York, 1979, Pocket Books.

Meleis A: *Theoretical nursing, development and progress*, Philadelphia, 1985, JB Lippincott.

Neziroglu FA, Yaryura-Tobias JA: A review of cognitive-behavioral and pharmacological treatment of body dysmorphic disorder, *Behav Modif* 21:324, 1997.

North American Nursing Diagnosis Association: Classification of nursing diagnosis. In *Proceedings of the ninth conference*, Philadelphia, 1991, JB Lippincott.

North American Nursing Diagnosis Association: *NANDA nursing diagnoses: definitions and classifications, 1999-2000*, Philadelphia, 1999, The Association.

Patterson JG, Zderad LT: *Humanistic nursing*, New York, 1976, Wiley.

Peplau H: *Interpersonal relations in nursing*, New York, 1952, Putnam.

Peplau H: *Interpersonal relations in nursing: a conceptual frame of reference for psychodynamic nursing*, New York, 1991, Springer.

Ross CA et al: Management of anxiety and panic attacks in immediate care facilities, *Gen Hosp Psychiatry* 10(2):120, 1988.

Roy-Byrne PP: Generalized anxiety and mixed anxiety-depression: association with disability and health care utilization, *J Clin Psychol* 57(7):86, 1996.

Selye H: *The stress of life*, New York, 1956, McGraw-Hill.

Stein M, Unde T: Panic disorder and major depression: lifetime relationship and biological markers. In Ballenger J, editor: *Clinical aspects of panic disorder*, New York, 1990, Wiley-Less.

Swenson RP, Kuch K: Clinical features of panic and related disorders. In Ballenger J, editor: *Clinical aspects of panic disorder*, New York, 1990, Wiley-Less.

Wolpe J: *The practice of behavior therapy*, ed 2, New York, 1973, Pergamon Press.

CHAPTER 13

Mood Disorders: Depression and Mania

Bonnie Hagerty

OBJECTIVES

- Describe biologic and psychosocial theories about the etiology of mood disorders.

- Compare and contrast the DSM-IV groupings of depressive disorders and bipolar disorders.

- Discuss the epidemiology and life course of depressive and bipolar disorders.

- Apply the nursing process (i.e., assessment, diagnosis, outcome identification, planning, implementation, and evaluation) for clients with mood disorders.

- Describe collaborative interventions and interventions used by nurses and other mental health professionals for clients with mood disorders.

- Examine personal feelings, thoughts, and reactions to clients with mood disorders that may affect the therapeutic relationship and management of client care.

Mood disorders are a group of common psychiatric disorders characterized by dysregulation of emotion. Persons exhibiting mood disorders demonstrate a range of emotions, from intense elation or irritability to severe depression. Mood disorders are also characterized by a constellation of symptoms, including impaired cognition, physiologic disturbances such as sleep and appetite problems, and lowered self-esteem. Mood disorders have a serious impact that results in personal and family suffering, interpersonal and occupational impairment, and expensive social costs. In recent years mood disorders, including their recurrent and cyclic nature and the disabling outcomes associated with repeated episodes, have come to be understood better. Mood disorders are now viewed as major public health problems, in terms of both economic costs and personal suffering. Depression alone has been identified as the fourth-ranked illness in the world, causing "burden," morbidity, and mortality throughout multiple countries (Murray and Lopez, 1996).

Although most people experience mood fluctuations of depression and elation, normal variations tend not to be prolonged or incapacitating. Mood fluctuation is often a normal response to life experiences and events that influence the human capacity for feeling. Grief and sadness in response to loss of a loved one and excitement at the thought of a long-awaited vacation are normal, adaptive responses. Most people experience sadness and depression with losses (e.g., of loved ones, jobs, status, possessions). This sadness may persist for days, weeks, or longer as the individual grieves the loss (see Chapter 29). Mood states become maladaptive, however, when they persist, are pervasive, incorporate additional symptoms such as impaired sleep and cognition, and interfere with usual functioning. At that point the mood dysregulation, accompa-

Affect The external manifestation of an emotional feeling or tone.

Anhedonia Loss of pleasure and interest in activities previously enjoyed, or in life itself.

Atypical depression Depression with features that include hypersomnia, weight gain, mood reactivity, and sensitivity in interpersonal relationships.

Bipolar disorder A mood disorder characterized by episodes of mania and depression.

Dysphoria Depressed, sad mood.

Dysthymia Chronic, low-level depression lasting more than 2 years that may lead to more severe depression if untreated.

Euthymia Mood that is normal and level.

Flight of ideas Rapid shifting from one idea to another without completion of the preceding idea, commonly manifested in mania.

Hypomania Mood of elation with higher than usual activity and social interaction; not as expansive as full mania.

Kindling Creation of electrophysiologic sensitivity in the brain from stress, altering neural functioning.

Learned helplessness The perception that events are uncontrollable, leading to apathy, helplessness, powerlessness, and depression.

Mania Elevated, expansive, or irritable mood accompanied by hyperactivity, grandiosity, and loss of reality.

Melancholic depression Severe depression characterized by anhedonia, feeling worse in the morning, weight loss, and psychomotor retardation.

Mood A feeling state reported by the client that can vary with external and internal changes.

Neurotransmission The process by which electrochemical signals are sent throughout the brain.

Nihilism The belief that existence is senseless and useless.

Psychomotor agitation Agitated motor activity.

Psychomotor retardation The slowing of physiologic processes, resulting in slow movement, speech, and reaction time.

Seasonal affective disorder (SAD) A type of mood disorder that occurs at a regular time each year.

Schemata The cognitive set of the self and world through which situations are perceived, coded, and interpreted.

Unipolar depression Disorder characterized by episodes of depression with no mania.

nied by a pattern of signs and symptoms, affects cognitive, behavioral, spiritual, social, and physiologic functioning.

HISTORICAL AND THEORETIC PERSPECTIVES

Disturbances in mood have been recognized for many years. It is thought that the term *melancholia* was first coined by Hippocrates when he described changing temperament. In 1896 Kraepelin distinguished between dementia praecox (now known as schizophrenia) and manic depression. He described dementia praecox as a chronic illness with progressive deterioration in the client's functioning. Kraepelin (1913, 1921) saw manic depression as cyclic abnormalities of mood, marked by a family history of similar disorders and caused by innate physical factors. This differentiation served as a primary underpinning for modern approaches to understanding and diagnosing mood disorders.

Since Kraepelin, attempts have been made to describe nuances of both depression and mania. Freud (1957) differentiated between maladaptive depression and grief in his famous paper "Mourning and Melancholia," detailing the psychodynamic genesis of depression. Leonhard (1974), a German psychiatrist, proposed the separation of manic-depressive illness into two types: bipolar (history of depression and mania) and monopolar (history of depression only). This differentiation is the basis for the current clinical depiction of **bipolar disorder** and unipolar disorders.

Throughout much of the twentieth century, various forms of bipolar and unipolar disorders have been described. **Unipolar depression,** for example, has been considered to be one of two types: reactive (exogenous) depression or endogenous depression. Reactive depression was believed to be caused by external stressors and was considered less severe than endogenous depression, which was believed to be due to physiologic dysregulation. Mental health professionals currently recognize various forms of bipolar disorders and unipolar depression. Researchers and clinicians continue to document a broad spectrum of mood disorders with varied features and clinical characteristics.

In recent years mood disorders have commanded more public attention as a result of their pervasiveness. New treatments, including use of drugs such as fluoxetine (Prozac), have created social controversy. Famous persons, including Patty Duke, William Styron, and Dick Cavett, have publicly acknowledged their struggles with mood disorders, and it is now recognized that many other prominent persons, including Abraham Lincoln, Winston Churchill, Vincent Van Gogh, Ernest Hemingway, Sylvia Plath, and Herman Melville, have experienced a mood disorder.

ETIOLOGY

Various theories have been presented to explain the development of mood disorders, but their exact cause remains unknown. Many researchers and clinicians support the premise that mood disorders have multicausal origins, in which biologic, psychologic, social, and cognitive factors converge to promote the development of depression and mania. Others contend that specific types of mood disorders may be related more to certain, specific etiologic factors. Research findings suggest that depression, for example, includes several distinct syndromes that can be differentiated clinically and over time (Kendler et al, 1996). Each theoretic perspective helps to explain some aspect of mood disorders, but none fully accounts for their development. In general, these etiologic factors can be grouped primarily as neurobiologic or psychosocial. These factors are summarized in Box 13-1.

NEUROBIOLOGIC FACTORS

Over the past decade, research on the etiology of mood disorders has focused on the biologic mechanisms that may be related to their development. Although this research has been able to identify physiologic correlates of depression and mania, direct cause-and-effect relationships have not been established. For example, a strong relationship between low mood and low systolic blood pressure was found in a study conducted in Great Britain, but no direct causal relationship was identified (Pilgrim et al, 1992). The more common biologic theories include those related to altered neurotransmission, neuroendocrine dysregulation, and genetic transmission.

Box 13-1   Etiologic Factors Related to Mood Disorders

Neurobiologic Factors
Altered neurotransmission
Neuroendocrine dysregulation
Genetic transmission

Pyschosocial Factors
Psychoanalytic theory
  Depression is a result of loss.
  Mania is a defense against depression.
Cognitive theory
  Depression is a result of negative processing of
    thoughts.
Learned helplessness
  Depression is a result of a perceived lack of control
    over events.
Life events and stress theory
  Significant life events cause stress, which results in
    depression or mania.
Personality theory
  Personality characteristics predispose an individual to
    mood disorders.

Neurotransmission

Current research on the biology of mood disorders is dominated by investigation of neurotransmitter disturbances. Interest in neurotransmission was sparked initially by investigations of the action of antidepressant drugs. In 1954 it was discovered that clients treated with reserpine for hypertension developed depression. Several years later, isoniazid was found to have an antidepressant effect on persons being treated for tuberculosis. Imipramine was introduced as an antidepressant in 1958, and research began on its mechanisms of action in the brain. The discoveries resulting from this line of research became the basis for the monoamine hypothesis of mood disorders.

Monoamine or biogenic amine neurotransmitters are crucial for sending electrical signals throughout the brain. Although there are hundreds of neurotransmitters in the brain, the biogenic amine neurotransmitters include the catecholamines of epinephrine, norepinephrine, dopamine, and acetylcholine, and the indolamine serotonin. To accomplish neurotransmission, these chemicals are released from the presynaptic neuronal terminal into the synaptic cleft. Once in the synaptic cleft, the neurotransmitter diffuses until it reaches its specific receptors on the postsynaptic membrane of the adjacent neuron, is reabsorbed through special receptors on the presynaptic membrane, or is degraded by another chemical, such as the enzyme monoamine oxidase. When the neurotransmitter locks into its receptors on the postsynaptic membrane of an adjacent neuron, it opens a gate that triggers a series of chemical actions that electrically depolarize the cell and sends an electrical impulse throughout that neuron, thus continuing the process of transmission of nerve impulses. Specialized neurons of each of the neurotransmitters project to various parts of the brain that control a wide range of functions, including appetite, sleep, and arousal.

It is believed that monoamine neurotransmitter systems, especially those of norepinephrine and serotonin, their metabolites, and their receptors are somehow altered during episodes of depression and mania. More recent research on neurotransmission has focused on the altered sensitivity of neuronal receptors and properties of neuronal membranes in mood disorders. In response to a decrease or increase in availability of neurotransmitters, it appears that, over time, there is a change in the sensitivity or density of presynaptic and postsynaptic receptors specific to a particular neurotransmitter. This results in delayed postsynaptic receptor-mediated responses.

Availability and receptor change theories propose that there is an underactivity of neurotransmission in depression and an overactivity in mania. Support for this comes from the administration of monoamine oxidase inhibitors (MAOIs) to clients with depression. MAOIs inhibit the monoamine oxidase enzyme from breaking down neurotransmitters, thus resulting in an increased supply of neurotransmitters and an accompanying decrease in clinical depression. Additional support is evident through research that demonstrates how medications such as fluoxetine, paroxetine (Paxil), and sertraline (Zoloft) (selective serotonin reuptake inhibitors [SSRIs]) selectively block serotonin reuptake in their presynaptic neuronal receptors, thus increasing the supply of serotonin in the synaptic cleft (Fuller, 1991). It can be argued that therapeutic responses to most antidepressant medications usually take several weeks, possibly because of the delayed sensitization or change in quantity of receptors.

Post (1992) has postulated that a phenomenon called **kindling** occurs, in which neurotransmission is altered initially by stress, resulting in a first episode of depression. This initial episode creates an electrophysiologic sensitivity to future stress, requiring less stress to evoke another depressive or manic episode. In essence, kindling creates new "hardwiring" of the brain or long-lasting alterations of neuronal functioning. Research with rats has demonstrated that maternal deprivation may lead to decreases in neurotrophic factors in the hippocampus, ultimately damaging brain functioning by causing early cell death (Post, 1997). It appears as though these alterations influence many cellular processes and structures, including changes in cell dendrites, and changes in cellular metabolism through second- and third-messenger systems that ultimately influence the expression of selected genes. The kindling model is consistent with the cyclic and progressive nature of mood disorders and suggests that clients be treated early for their mood episodes and remain on medication for extended periods to avoid physiologic deterioration over time.

Recent technologic advances in studying the brain provide additional support for the theory of disturbances in brain functioning during depression. The positron emission tomography (PET) scanner enables researchers to examine brain physiology of depressed persons as compared with normal controls, as well as compare brain functioning in individuals both during depression and after recovery. Figure 13-1 depicts the differences that are apparent using PET scanning of depressed, recovered, and normal control brains. Figure 13-2 indicates increased blood flow in components of the brains of persons with major depression. PET scanning has found that the prefrontal cerebral cortex and the limbic system (including the amygdala) appear to have physiologic disruptions in the brains of persons experiencing depression.

Although research continues on these biochemical theories, the complexity of the biologic structural and physiologic changes occurring with mood disorders continues to pose challenges for investigation. In addition, the research is hampered by inconsistent definitions and criteria for depression and mania, as well as the difficulties of measuring concentrations of specific neurotransmitters in selected sites in the brain and removing selected brain structures for analysis. Peripheral indicators of neurotrans-

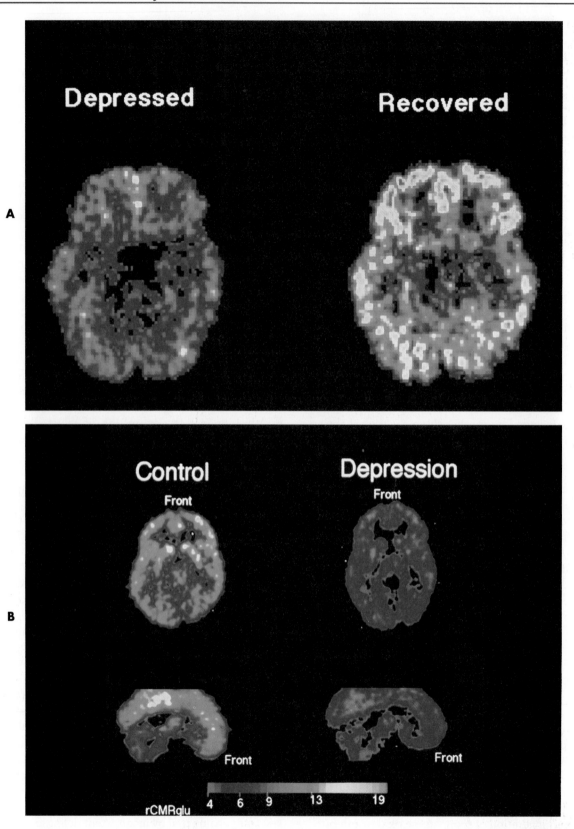

Figure 13-1   **A,** Positron emission tomography (PET) scans of the brain in the same individual during depression *(left)* and after recovery through treatment with medication *(right)*. Several brain areas, particularly the prefrontal cortex *(at top)*, show diminished activity *(darker colors)* during depression. **B,** PET scans of a normal subject *(left)* and a depressed subject *(right)* reveal reduced brain activity *(darker colors)* during depression, especially in the prefrontal cortex. A form of radioactively tagged glucose was used as a tracer to visualize levels of brain activity.   (Courtesy Mark George, MD, National Institutes of Mental Health Biological Psychiatry Branch, U.S. Department of Health and Human Services.)

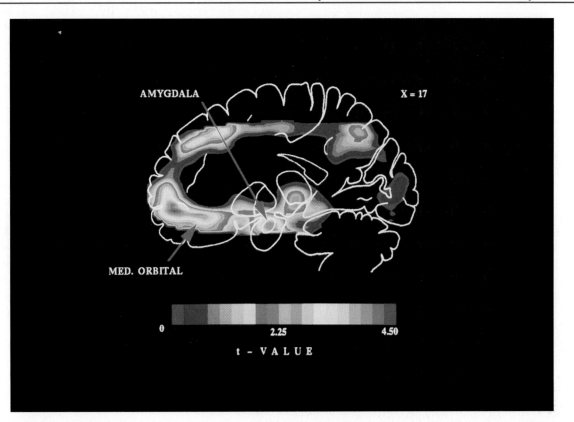

Figure 13-2   PET scan indicates increased blood flow in the amygdala and prefrontal cortex in persons with major depression of the familial pure depressive disease subtype. The scan is a composite of images of 13 individuals. (Courtesy Wayne C. Drevets, MD, Department of Psychiatry, Washington University School of Medicine, St. Louis.)

mitters and their metabolites, such as those in the blood, urine, or central spinal fluid, may not be related to their amounts or mechanisms of action in various parts of the brain. In addition, neurotransmission, as a complex activity, encompasses multiple processes such as neurotransmitter synthesis and release, receptor site function and change, interactions among the various neurotransmitters and hormones, and the action of these transmitters and hormones on genetic material via second- and third-messenger systems.

Neuroendocrine Dysregulation

Another area of research on the biologic basis of mood disorders is the role of the endocrine system. Studies indicate that dysregulation of the hypothalamic-pituitary-adrenal (HPA) axis is associated with depression. The HPA axis comprises the hypothalamus, pituitary, and adrenal glands and controls physiologic responses to stress. The hypothalamus regulates endocrine functions and the autonomic nervous system and is involved in behaviors related to fight, flight, feeding, and mating. In response to stress, the hypothalamus releases corticotropin-releasing hormone (CRH), which stimulates the anterior pituitary to secrete corticotropin. In turn, corticotropin causes the adrenal cortex to release cortisol into the blood. Through an

elaborate feedback mechanism, levels of cortisol signal the hypothalamus, via the hippocampus, to increase or decrease CRH production. The specific physiologic ways that stress signals for this process to begin are not well understood, although stress-input signals may come from the brain stem, autonomic nervous system, or cerebral cortex (Young et al, 1993).

Hyperactivity of the HPA axis is often evident in depression. Up to 50% of clients with moderate to severe depression exhibit elevated serum cortisol levels. This phenomenon led to the creation of the dexamethasone suppression test (DST), which was hoped to be a potential biologic diagnostic indicator of endogenous depression. The DST is based on the premise that when clients are given dexamethasone (synthetic cortisol) at night, a signal is sent to the hypothalamus to shut down production of CRH, leading to decreased output of corticotropin and, subsequently, cortisol by the following morning. For many clients with severe depression, measurement of this blood cortisol level the following morning revealed continued excessive amounts of cortisol production. Subsequent research regarding the DST has revealed problems with its selectivity and specificity. It is not consistent with regard to its results in persons with depression, may be affected by other variables (e.g., age, gender), and is evident in other disorders, such as alcoholism and anorexia nervosa (Zimmerman, Coryell, and Pfohl, 1986).

The functioning of the HPA axis is related to the 24-hour cycle of circadian rhythms that control physiologic processes. With mood disorders, many normal, cyclic patterns are disrupted. Blood cortisol is normally at a low level in the early morning and highest in late afternoon, although constant increases are often apparent in depression. Sleep-wake cycles are disrupted in mood disorders, and during depression clients experience decreased rapid eye movement (REM) latency and decreased shallow, slow delta wave sleep, thus fragmenting the sleep-wake cycle. Even seasonal patterns appear to have some relationship to mood disorders, with episodes of depression often occurring during periods of decreased light. Ehlers, Frank, and Kupfer (1988) proposed an interaction between behavior and environment and posited that zeitgebers (cues or stimuli from the environment) alter physiology that in turn affects mood. Research on HPA axis dysfunction continues, with special interest in the relationships between mood disorders and stress.

Genetic Transmission

Mood disorders tend to run in families, and it is commonly believed that, to some extent, genetic transmission is responsible for their manifestation. Data regarding the genetic transmission of mood disorders are derived from family, twin, and adoption studies.

In family studies, families who exhibit mood disorders are selected, and the morbid risk for developing these disorders in relatives is compared with the general population. Results of these studies consistently demonstrate that first-degree relatives of persons with bipolar disorder and unipolar depression have a greater risk for developing a mood disorder. This risk is particularly high for relatives of persons with bipolar disorder, possibly indicating a greater genetic component than that of unipolar depression (McGriffin and Katz, 1989).

Twin studies are based on the assumption that monozygotic twins share the same genes and that dizygotic twins have about 50% of their genes in common. Results of twin research provide additional evidence for the genetic transmission of mood disorders. If one monozygotic twin suffers from bipolar disorder, there is a high rate of concordance, ranging to 100% in some studies, whereby the other twin will also develop a mood disorder, usually bipolar illness. Although there are high rates of concordance for dizygotic twins, they tend to be less than those for monozygotic twins. For unipolar disorders the concordance rates continue to be higher for monozygotic twins, and both twin types have a higher concordance than the general population.

Using adoption studies, researchers can examine the contributions of both the environment and genetic transmission. In general, adoption studies also support the role of genetic factors in mood disorders. Most studies have focused specifically on bipolar disorder and have found that the biologic parents of adult adoptees diagnosed with bipolar disorder have a much higher incidence of the disorder than parents of adoptees with no mood disorder.

Although all of the above information supports the role of genetics in the development of mood disorders, particularly bipolar disorders, this research does not reveal the specific genes or genetic mechanisms involved in transmission. Early scientific reports describing the location of genetic markers on specific genes have not been replicated, although this type of research is evolving with advances in DNA and genetic analysis. The search for the specific genetic basis of mood disorders continues with special emphasis on genetic location and genetic processes, including the role of selective gene expression and neuromodulation (Barondes, 1998). Many researchers agree that genetic expressions and genetic transmission of mood disorders may hold the key to future major advances in understanding, diagnosing, and treating depression and bipolar disorders.

PSYCHOSOCIAL FACTORS

Psychosocial explanations for the development of mood disorders represent a range of theoretic positions, including psychoanalytic theory, learned helplessness, cognitive theory, life events (stress) theory, and personality theory.

Psychoanalytic Theory

The basic premise of psychoanalytic theory is that unconscious processes result in expression of symptoms, including depression and mania. Freud (1957) distinguished between depression and normal grief, citing both as a response to real or symbolic loss. According to Freud, in depression the loss generates intense, hostile feelings toward the lost object that are turned inward onto the self (anger turned inward), creating guilt and loss of self-esteem.

Thus depression is viewed together with loss and aggression. The loss of an object either physically or emotionally is compounded by the development of anger. Struggling with feelings of rejection, the child is unable to direct anger and hostility toward the lost love object for fear of more rejection and loss and because of a strong, punitive superego. The child experiences ambivalence, or both love and hate, for the lost love object. Feelings of anger and aggression are repressed, and the child interprets the loss as rejection and a reflection of his or her own lack of self-worth. As a result, patterns of low self-esteem, depression, and helplessness become established and endure as the person confronts future loss. This scenario occurs early in childhood, creating a vulnerability to real or perceived loss throughout adulthood that results in periods of depression.

Psychodynamically, mania is explained as a defense against depression. The client denies feelings of anger, low self-esteem, and worthlessness and reverses the affect such that there is a triumphant feeling of self-confidence.

Mania represents a conquered superego with little inclination to control id impulses. Yet, over time, this distorted view of reality wavers, and the client demonstrates outward hostility toward others, often focusing on the weaknesses of others that are similar to the internal weaknesses being avoided.

There are few data that support the psychodynamic theories of depression and mania, but there is some evidence that clients with depression have experienced more early childhood loss and deprivation than persons without depression (Boulby, 1969; Brown and Harris, 1978). Clinicians also note that anger is often associated with depression, although the relationship between anger and depression remains obscure. Many people who experience early childhood loss and anger never experience depression, whereas many who do not experience a visible or acknowledged loss do experience depression. The psychoanalytic theory is only one of many explanations that attempt to explain the internal dynamics of depression and mania. The relevance of this theoretic perspective may be in its references to the early childhood environment in which loss, disruption, or chaos may trigger stress that in turn triggers the physiologic mechanisms described above.

Cognitive Theory

The cognitive model of depression points to errors of logical thinking as causative factors for depression. It assumes that mood is influenced by underlying cognitive structures, some of which are not fully conscious. These cognitive structures, or schemata, may be shaped by early life experiences and are predisposed to negative processing of information. In a diatheses-stress model, when persons predisposed to depression with negative schemata encounter stress, the negative processing is activated, resulting in depressive thinking (Beck, 1967).

Beck (1967) differentiated among levels of cognition that influence depression: automatic thoughts, schemata or assumptions, and cognitive distortions. Automatic thoughts are those that can be brought into awareness, although they appear fleetingly and are usually unrecognized. They form the person's perception of a situation, and it is this perception, rather than the objective facts about the situation, that results in emotional and behavioral responses. If the perceptions are distorted, inferences and responses will be maladaptive. For example, a client expressed anger that his wife was picking vegetables from his garden and giving them to her friends. He interpreted this as an attempt to get rid of his belongings and was surprised at the suggestion that she may have been proud of his vegetables and wanted to share his accomplishment with others who appreciated good food.

Schemata are internal representations of the self and the world. They facilitate information processing because they are used to understand, code, and recall information. Beck (1967) proposed a triad of thinking (schemata) that gives rise to the development of depression:

1. Negative, self-deprecating views of self
2. Pessimistic views of the world, so that life experiences are interpreted in a negative way
3. The belief that negativity will continue into the future, promoting a negative view of future events

These mind-sets result in the misinterpretation of events and situations, so that the client's cognitive schema of self as worthless and the world and future as hopeless are supported. This faulty cognitive processing leads to assumptions and continued errors of logic that result in depressive symptoms and an ongoing negative view of life. This was evidenced by a client who began each meeting with the nurse by saying, "There is no point to this. I know things will never be better."

Cognitive distortions link schemata and automatic thoughts. Faulty information processing includes cognitive distortions, such as overgeneralization (drawing general conclusions based on isolated incidents), dichotomous thinking (perceiving events and experiences in only one of two opposite categories), and magnification (placing a distorted emphasis on a single event or error). The following example illustrates each of these types of distortion. A 42-year-old woman reported that her supervisor had not spoken directly to her at two recent company meetings. She concluded that he must be unhappy with her performance (overgeneralization). The woman stated that there were only two types of employees, good and bad, and that bad ones lost their jobs (dichotomous thinking). The woman's concern began after she forgot to give her supervisor an important message. In spite of a good work history, she was convinced that she had demonstrated what a poor employee she was (magnification).

There is considerable research support for the cognitive model of depression (Robins and Hayes, 1993). It has led to the development of specific treatment for depression using cognitive techniques. These techniques are short term and focus on changing the client's faulty negative cognition.

Learned Helplessness Theory

The learned helplessness theory is actually a variant of the cognitive theory, tracing the determinants of depression to altered cognition. The term **learned helplessness** was used first to describe the lack of motivation exhibited by dogs subjected to laboratory shocks that they were unable to control. According to the original theory as stated by Seligman (1975), stressful events that are experienced as uncontrollable result in the development of helplessness, apathy, powerlessness, and depression.

This perspective was somewhat modified by Abramson, Seligman, and Teasdale's suggestion (1978) that the primary issue is the person's expectation (cognition) that external events are uncontrollable. This causal attribution regarding current events, combined with the person's perceptions of past uncontrollable experiences, yields the expectation that the event or situation cannot be controlled. This, in turn, results in helplessness, passivity, and sadness, which lead to other symptoms of depression, such as decreased appetite and low self-esteem.

More recently, the reformulated model of learned helplessness was revised to become the hopelessness theory of depression (Abramson, Melalsy, and Alloy, 1989). This theory presents hopelessness as a sufficient cause of depression and the individual's inferred negative outcomes and negativity about self as key elements of depression. Helplessness is viewed as one component of hopelessness; perceived lack of control over events assumes a less central role. With the occurrence of an unpleasant event, persons prone to depression attribute stability (versus instability), globalization (versus specific), and importance (versus unimportance) to those events. This is exemplified by a client who perceived that his unemployment would be long lasting (stability), that his entire life had been ruined (globalization), and that his former job had been the major focus of his life (importance).

Symptoms of depression relating to apathy and lack of motivation (helplessness expectancy) and depressed, sad affect (negative outcome expectancy), as well as other symptoms of depression, are believed to flow from this condition of hopelessness. **Affect** is the external manifestation of an emotional feeling tone. Unfortunately, the specific mechanisms by which these conditions and attributions are converted into the specific symptom pattern of depression (or mania) remain elusive.

Life Events and Stress Theory

It is widely acknowledged that there appears to be some type of relationship between life events and the onset of unipolar depression. It is unclear, however, to what extent, under what conditions, and in whom external social determinants and negative life circumstances contribute to the development and course of mood disorders, particularly bipolar disorders (McPherson, Herbison, and Romans, 1993). Some episodes of depression and mania occur in the absence of any notable stressor, whereas others are clearly associated with life events. The role of life events in the onset of depression is stronger in nonendogenous depression and dysthymia. There is less evidence regarding the role of life events in the development of bipolar disorders. It appears that life events are often major precipitants of bipolar disorder only for first episodes. This supports Post's theory of electrophysiologic sensitization, or kindling, and suggests that there may be subtypes of depression and mania related more to some etiologies (e.g., biologic versus psychosocial) than to others.

In studying depression, researchers have been interested in the quantity and nature of life events and in the size and perceived supportiveness of the client's social network in relation to the initial onset and recurrence of mania and depression. Paykel (1979), for example, found that clients with depression reported three times as many life events in the 6 months before the onset of depression as persons without depression. In an enduring study, Brown and Harris (1978) reported that stressful social factors (e.g., lack of an intimate, confiding relationship with a significant other; having three or more children at home; being unemployed; and loss of one's mother before age 11) contributed significantly to vulnerability for depression. Additional evidence suggests that events involving social loss, such as the death of a loved one, have potent effects on the onset of depression. Cornelis, Ameling, and Delonghe (1989) have suggested that the emotional evaluation of an event is as important as the change it causes in daily life and that life events evoke various degrees of stress. The effect of an event is influenced by mechanisms such as social support and the person's perception of that event. Life events most likely influence the development and recurrence of depression through the psychologic and, ultimately, biologic experiences of stress.

Personality Theory

For many years psychiatric clinicians have described a depressive personality that encompasses personality traits and characteristics often seen in clients with depression. The term *depressive personality* has been used broadly to describe personality traits that (1) exist before, during, or after a depressive episode; (2) modify depression; (3) are variants of normal personality rather than reflective of a mood disorder; or (4) are indicative of enduring character and temperament (Phillips et al, 1990). Personality characteristics commonly associated with depression include negativity, pessimism, low sense of self-worth, proneness to worry and anxiety, tendency to be hypercritical toward self and others, self-denial, tendency to be serious and overly responsible, dependence on other's love and affection, demandingness, feeling of being bored and empty, hypochondriasis, quietness, incapacity for enjoyment and relaxation, and interpersonal sensitivity to rejection.

According to personality theory, these characteristics are long-standing, structural components of the person's psyche. The extent to which they predispose an individual to mood disorders, are outcomes of a depressive or manic episode, or are consistent, ongoing elements is unclear. There is some evidence that certain traits, such as interpersonal rejection sensitivity and neuroticism (worry), do increase a person's vulnerability for depression (Boyce et al, 1991). It appears, however, that these traits interact with other variables, such as age, social factors, and stressors. For example, in one prospective study, personality variables did not differentiate between subjects who did develop depression and those who did not in subjects under age 30. However, there was a differentiation for those over age 30, including drive and emotional strength, increased dependency, and increased reflection and thoughtfulness in the group that had depression (Hirshfeld et al, 1989).

Although there are advocates who support depressive personality as a DSM-IV, Axis II personality disorder, caution must be exercised not to attribute these traits to all persons with depression. The experience of depression or mania can shape behavioral characteristics or strengthen preexisting personality features.

EPIDEMIOLOGY

Mood disorders, particularly depression, are common. Recent data suggest that the lifetime prevalence of developing any affective disorder is 19.3%: 14.7% for men and 23.9% for women (Kessler et al, 1994). Since the lifetime prevalence of bipolar disorder is about equal for men and women (1.4% and 1.3%, respectively), much of this difference is due to unipolar depression. Women have a lifetime prevalence of 21.3% for major depression and 8.0% for dysthymia, whereas men have a lifetime prevalence of only 12.7% for major depression and 4.8% for dysthymia. A number of theories have been proposed to account for gender differences in the rates of depression, including hormonal or biologic differences, social roles, and cognitive processing (Nolen-Hoeksema, 1987). These gender differences for depression, however, have not been adequately explained empirically, and additional research is needed to determine why women are at higher risk for depression.

The first episode of a mood disorder seems to be occurring at younger ages. The average age for onset of bipolar illness is the mid to late twenties. Although the average age of onset for unipolar depression has been considered the middle thirties, there is some evidence that onset is occurring in younger cohorts (Lewinsohn et al, 1993). Although the most frequent age of onset for depression is the 25- to 44-year age-group, people in younger age-groups have an ever-increasing risk of developing depression. Data indicate that the onset of depression at an early age (teens or early twenties) or at age 55 or over predicts a more protracted, chronic course (Klerman and Weissman, 1992). Rates of depression do not significantly increase during menopause. The risk of developing depression and mania is increased if there is a positive family history for mood disorders (Akiskal, 1989).

Sociocultural factors may be related to the onset of depression and mania. Depression seems to occur less frequently in African-Americans than in either white or Hispanic groups in the United States. It also appears that depression may be more frequent in lower socioeconomic groups, whereas bipolar disorders are more frequent in higher socioeconomic groups. Although depression and mania occur throughout the world, the expression of symptoms is influenced by ethnicity and culture. Asians,

Box 13-2	Epidemiology of Mood Disorders

19.3% of the general population develop a mood disorder.

21.3% of women and 12.7% of men develop major depression.

Average age of onset for bipolar illness is mid to late twenties.

Average age of onset of depression is mid thirties.

Depression occurs more frequently in whites and Hispanics than in African-Americans.

Depression occurs more frequently in lower socioeconomic groups.

Bipolar disorders occur more frequently in higher socioeconomic groups.

for example, describe more somatic symptoms of depression, whereas people from Western cultures describe more mood and cognitive changes.

In an increasingly stressful society characterized by mobility, family disruptions, and economic stressors, women and younger persons are manifesting depression more than in previous generations. Unfortunately, the relationships among biologic, psychologic, developmental, and sociocultural factors and their influence on the development of mood disorders are still unclear. Epidemiology data for mood disorders are summarized in Box 13-2.

CLINICAL DESCRIPTION

Mood is defined as a feeling state reported by the client that can vary with external and internal changes. Mood disorders are defined by a pattern of episodes over time and by a pattern of symptoms in each episode. Mood disorders are classified in the DSM-IV as depressive disorders, bipolar disorders, or other mood disorders. The signs and symptoms of these disorders are described in the following sections.

DEPRESSIVE DISORDERS

Persons diagnosed with a depressive disorder have experienced only episodes of depression with no manic or hypomanic episodes. This is also referred to as unipolar depression. The DSM-IV Criteria box on p. 268 lists criteria for a major depressive episode. The clinical symptoms of depressive disorders are summarized in the Clinical Symptoms box on p. 268.

Major Depressive Episode, Single or Recurrent

An episode of major depression can be indicative of a first episode or of a recurrent episode of depression. Symptoms occur as a result of the disorder and not from the effects of

DSM-IV CRITERIA

Major Depressive Episode

A. Five (or more) of the following symptoms have been present during the same 2-week period and represent a change from previous functioning; at least one of the symptoms is either (1) depressed mood or (2) loss of interest or pleasure.
NOTE: Do not include symptoms that are clearly due to a general medical condition, or mood-incongruent delusions or hallucinations.
1. Depressed mood most of the day, nearly every day, as indicated by either subjective report (e.g., feels sad or empty) or observation made by others (e.g., appears tearful)
NOTE: In children and adolescents, can be irritable mood.
2. Markedly diminished interest or pleasure in all, or almost all, activities most of the day, nearly every day (as indicated by either subjective account or observation made by others)
3. Significant weight loss when not dieting or weight gain (e.g., a change of more than 5% of body weight in month), or decrease or increase in appetite nearly every day
NOTE: In children, consider failure to make expected weight gains.
4. Insomnia or hypersomnia nearly every day
5. Psychomotor agitation or retardation nearly every day (observable by others, not merely subjective feelings of restlessness or being slowed down)
6. Fatigue or loss of energy nearly every day
7. Feelings of worthlessness or excessive or inappropriate guilt (which may be delusional) nearly every day (not merely self-reproach or guilt about being sick)
8. Diminished ability to think or concentrate, or indecisiveness, nearly every day (either by subjective account or as observed by others)
9. Recurrent thoughts of death (not just fear of dying), recurrent suicidal ideation without a specific plan, or a suicide attempt or a specific plan for committing suicide
B. The symptoms do not meet criteria for a mixed episode.
C. The symptoms cause clinically significant distress or impairment in social, occupational, or other important areas of functioning.
D. The symptoms are not due to the direct physiologic effects of a substance (e.g., a drug of abuse, a medication) or a general medical condition (e.g., hypothyroidism).
E. The symptoms are not better accounted for by bereavement (i.e., after the loss of a loved one, the symptoms persist for longer than 2 months or are characterized by marked functional impairment, morbid preoccupation with worthlessness, suicidal ideation, psychotic symptoms, or psychomotor retardation).

From American Psychiatric Association: *Diagnostic and statistical manual of mental disorders*, ed 4, Washington, DC, 1994, The Association.

CLINICAL SYMPTOMS

Depressive Disorders

Major Depression

Emotional
Anhedonia
Depressed mood

Cognitive
Diminished ability to think, concentrate, or make decisions
Recurrent thoughts of death
Excessive focus on self-worthlessness and guilt

Behavioral
Significant weight loss or gain or change in appetite
Insomnia or hypersomnia
Psychomotor agitation or retardation
Fatigue

Social
Withdrawal from family and social interactions
Problems at work in organizing, initiating, and completing work

Dysthymic Disorder

Emotional
Depressed mood
Anhedonia
Irritability or angry mood

Cognitive
Feelings of low self-esteem and inadequacy
Feelings of guilt and brooding about the past
Difficulty with concentration, memory, and decision making
Attitudes of pessimism, despair, and hopelessness

Behavioral
Chronic fatigue

Social
Social withdrawal

a substance, medical condition, or loss of a loved one within the previous 2 months.

Emotional symptoms.   Two primary symptoms of major depression are depressed mood and **anhedonia,** or loss of interest and pleasure in activities. In order for clients to be diagnosed with major depression, one of these symptoms must be present most of the day, nearly every day, for at least 2 weeks. Clients may describe their mood as depressed, sad, empty, or numb. They may report difficulty receiving pleasure or satisfaction from their usual activities, including eating, sex, or going out with friends. Although clients may describe feelings of sadness or frequent crying, some persons with depression are unable to describe feelings and report disinterest, disconnection, or an inability to feel emotion. Anxiety, irritability, or anger may also be present. Clients may also report feelings of loneliness, helplessness, or hopelessness. The affect of a person with depression may be flat and constricted, with minimal expression, or may appear rather normal as the person attempts to camouflage his or her inner struggles.

Cognitive symptoms. Cognitive criteria for major depression include a diminished ability to think, concentrate, or make decisions; recurrent thoughts of death; and an excessive focus on self-worthlessness and guilt. Many clients describe difficulty attending to and concentrating on a task or conversation. Reading a newspaper or following the train of thought in a lecture may be overwhelming. Clients may be unable to make decisions about routine concerns, such as what clothing to put on in the morning or what to buy at the grocery store. Recurrent thoughts of death are often evident, including thoughts of suicide, death from natural causes, or existential thoughts about dying. At times, these thoughts may occupy a large portion of the client's waking hours. Negative thinking is often apparent, with feelings of worthlessness and excessive guilt. Clients ruminate about past deeds and their negative view of themselves and the world. Clients with severe depression can become delusional with fixed beliefs that cannot be changed by logic; they may focus on persecution, punishment, **nihilism,** or somatic concerns.

Behavioral symptoms. Behavioral symptoms that are criteria for major depression are significant weight loss or gain or change in appetite, insomnia or hypersomnia, **psychomotor agitation** or **psychomotor retardation,** and fatigue. Weight gain or weight loss is considered to be significant when it represents a 5% change in body weight in 1 month. Sometimes the weight change is not apparent, but the client reports a major change in appetite. Sleep disturbances are common, and clients report not being able to sleep or sleeping too much. Psychomotor agitation is evident when the client appears to be restless, paces, fidgets, or is irritable. With psychomotor retardation, the client appears to be slowed down in movement and in speech. Persons with depression may appear listless and disheveled. They may not carefully attend to their dress, appearance, or hygiene. They may exhibit a stooped posture and make little eye contact. Many clients report feelings of fatigue and loss of energy, citing an inability to accomplish tasks and an increased need for naps. They may even appear very tired. This symptom may cause many clients to visit their family physician or nurse practitioner, believing that the fatigue is indicative of a physical problem. Thus depression is often diagnosed first during a visit to the primary care provider (See the clinical pathway on p. 270).

Social symptoms. For major depression to be diagnosed, the convergence of symptoms must cause personal distress and significant impairment in social and occupational functioning. Clients may withdraw from family and social interactions. They may have problems at their job, including problems with executive functions originating in the frontal lobe of the brain, resulting in an inability to organize, begin, and complete their work. Although some are able to function at work with relatively little impairment, this often comes at great personal and family expense as their energy for social interaction is depleted. Family members begin to feel confused, angry, guilty, abandoned, and sad.

Marital distress is often a cited stressor at least 6 months before the onset of a depressive episode (Schmaling and Becker, 1991). During an episode the client's erratic behavior, mood, and cognition can alienate a loved one, who may become frustrated about how to help the partner. Unfortunately, it appears as though marital distress continues even after the acute episode subsides. Continued marital strain has been cited as a factor in episode recurrence (Schmaling and Becker, 1991).

Dysthymic Disorder

Dysthymia differs from major depression in that it is a chronic, low-level depression. To receive this diagnosis, the client must have had depressed mood and at least three of the following symptoms for most of the day, nearly every day, for at least 2 years (1 year for children and adolescents): poor appetite or overeating, insomnia or hypersomnia, low energy, low self-esteem, poor concentration or difficulty making decisions, and feelings of hopelessness. There cannot have been a manic or hypomanic episode. The client may have experienced an episode of major depression before the onset of dysthymia, provided there were at least 6 months with no signs or symptoms of depression. After 2 years of dysthymia, the client may be diagnosed with major depression superimposed on dysthymia if symptoms increase in severity. The dysthymic disorder is not due to the effects of a substance or medical condition. Psychotic features are usually not present in this disorder.

Cognitive symptoms. Cognitive symptoms of dysthymia include low self-esteem and inadequacy; guilt and brooding about the past; difficulty with concentration, memory, and decision making; and negative thinking evidenced by pessimism, despair, and hopelessness. Clients with dysthymia often have little regard for themselves and are plagued by a sense of inadequacy and a lack of self-confidence. They reflect on past actions and attribute personal guilt to their circumstances. Negativity pervades much of what they do and say; life seems hopeless, and situations are bounded by pessimism and despair. Clients often report poor memory and decreased concentration on tasks. They may have problems making decisions, but the impairment is usually not as severe as impaired decision making during major depression.

ST. JOSEPH HOSPITAL

DRG Number _____
Primary Physician _____
Physician(s) in Consult _____
Anticipated Discharge Date _____
Actual Discharge Date _____
Financial _____

MAJOR DEPRESSION CLINICAL PATHWAY©

CARE NEEDS	DAY OF ADMIT	LEVEL 1	LEVEL 2	LEVEL 3	LEVEL 4	LEVEL 5
CONSULTS/ ASSESSMENTS:	MD. CM. SW. RN. OT. Consults? Medical? Other?	Psy eval? Fam mtg? Complete all assess.	Complete family mtg. Complete psy testing if ordered.	SW/CM process family mtg w/pt. Complete psy consult if ordered.	OT reassess? Transfer summaries.	Send results of assess to out-pt Tx.
HEALTH MAINTENANCE Sleep Disturbance. ADL's. Diet. Med Dx	Chem 19. CBC. UA. Tox? T_3T_4Tsh? Pg? TCA/Li/Other? Sleep? ADL? Medical (below)? Nutri? VS ___ Ortho? ------>	Lab results? Nutri? Sleep? ADL? Review prot? Medical? VS ___ ------>	Nutri? Sleep? ADL? Review prot? Medical? VS ___ ------>	Nutri? Sleep? ADL? Review prot? Medical? VS ___ ------>	Nutri? Sleep? ADL? Review prot? Medical? Med refer to med f/u. VS ___ ------>	VS ___
PROGRAM: Target Sx ___ Meds. Teaching needs. Stressors. Compliancy. Tx	Orientation Prot. Rest 24"? Sx? Groups? Med orders? Consent form? Teaching needs? Stressors? Tx compliancy?	Shift Assess Prot. Multidis Tx plan mtg. Assess need for alt pathway. Groups per prot. Comm mtg: ___ Meds/SE? Chart to target Sx. Tx compliancy?	Shift Assess Prot. Groups per prot. ___ Tx compliancy? Med/SE? Chart to target Sx. Prov med sheets.	Shift Assess Prot. Groups per prot. Med group. D/C planning. Tx compliancy? Med/SE? Chart to target Sx. 1 unit resp.	Shift Assess Prot. Multidis Tx plan? Groups per prot. Chart to target Sx. Med/SE? Tx compl?	Daily Assess Prot. D/C Prot.
SAFETY - Harm to self, others, and destruction of property. Elopement. Potential for falls. Sexually acting out.	Suicide Prot.? Safety Prot.? SFC? Verbal contract? Mental status? E?	Suicide Prot.? Mental status? Safety Prot.? SFC? E? OW Prot.? ___	Suicide Prot.? Mental status? Safety Prot.? SFC? E? OW Prot.? ___	Suicide Prot.? Mental status? SFC? E? OW Prot.? ___	Suicide Prot.? Mental status? Safety Prot.? SFC? E? SI review opt if ret. OW Prot.? ___	Review opt if SI reoccurs. Use of support systems.
DISCHARGE PLANNING: Compliancy. F/u. Teaching. MHC Financial	CM/SW 1 data - family? placement? F/up? Release of info. LOS expectation. DSHS form? Insurance?	Housing? LOS. F/up resources? Support system? Contact fam. Assign fam. grp. Contact MHC/out-pt Tx.	Placement? MHC call liaison? Formulate f/up plan. Fam. attend sup/ed group. LOS.	Finalize f/up plan. LOS. Arrange for trans on day of D/C. Assess for therapeutic pass.	Liaison from MHC to see. Review Sx & cues to reoccurrence. Consider long-term care. Resources for meds. Coord D/C w/fam.	Check transportation & meds by 8 am for D/C by 11 am.

MAJORDEP.PIH 2/28/92

Axis I ___   Axis II ___   Axis III ___   Axis IV ___   Axis V ___

PERMANENT PART OF THE PATIENT RECORD

NOTE: This is not a Physician Order

Emotional symptoms. The predominant symptom that must be present for the diagnosis of dysthymia is depressed mood. Clients report feeling chronically "down, gloomy, sad." Many are unable to remember a time when they felt good or their usual self. Another symptom indicative of dysthymia is a generalized loss of interest or pleasure in activities, but unlike major depression, anhedonia is not a primary emotional symptom. Another symptom is irritability or angry mood. Clients may find themselves feeling impatient with family members or co-workers and demonstrating angry outbursts. Many feel bad about their irritable state but find themselves unable to control it.

Behavioral symptoms. Clients with dysthymia commonly complain of chronic fatigue. They are exhausted from usual activities and often believe that they have a physical illness or chronic fatigue syndrome. Clients may make repeated visits to their health care provider, hoping to determine the cause of their fatigue. In conjunction with the fatigue, clients display decreased activity and productivity. Everything becomes a chore, and it becomes difficult to complete tasks in the usual amount of time.

Social symptoms. Social withdrawal is common with dysthymia. Clients are tired, irritable, and depressed and no longer get satisfaction from outings or activities with family and friends. Clients' mood states and negativity may prevent people from wanting to be with them, increasing their isolation from others.

Depressive Disorders Not Otherwise Specified

There are types of depression that do not meet the criteria for the depressive disorders presented thus far. Some of these include premenstrual dysphoric disorder, minor depressive disorder, recurrent brief depressive disorder, and the postpsychotic depression of schizophrenia. **Dysphoria** refers to a depressed, sad mood. The reader is referred to the DSM-IV classification for more extensive descriptions of these diagnoses.

BIPOLAR DISORDERS

Bipolar disorders occur when the client experiences episodes of depression and episodes of **mania** or hypomania over time. Bipolar disorders are defined by the pattern of manic, hypomanic, and depressed episodes over time. The depressed and manic episodes are not due to the effects of a substance, including antidepressant medication, electroconvulsive therapy, or light therapy. Clients may be diagnosed with a bipolar I or a bipolar II disorder. The DSM-IV Criteria box above describes these bipolar patterns. Although the public continues to refer to bipolar disorders as manic depression, that term connotes a single, polarized disorder. A bipolar disorder encompasses the range of possible disturbances in mood. The clinical symptoms of bipolar disorders are summarized in the Clinical Symptoms box on p. 274.

DSM-IV CRITERIA

Bipolar I and Bipolar II Disorders

Type	Characteristics
Bipolar I Disorder	
Single manic episode	Only one manic episode
	No past major depressive episodes
Most recent episode hypomanic	Current hypomania
	At least one previous manic episode
Most recent episode manic	Current mania
	At least one previous depressive, hypomanic, or manic episode
Most recent episode mixed	Meets criteria for both manic and depressive current episode
	At least one past major depressive or hypomanic episode
Most recent episode depressed	Current depressive episode
	At least one past manic episode
Bipolar II Disorder	Must never have had full manic episode
	At least one past major depressive and past hypomanic episode

Modified from American Psychiatric Association: *Diagnostic and statistical manual of mental disorders*, ed 4, Washington, DC, 1994, The Association.

Manic Episode

Manic episodes occur when there is an abnormally and persistently elevated, expansive, or irritable mood for at least 1 week. At least three of the following symptoms must also be present: inflated self-esteem, decreased need for sleep, more than usual talkativeness, racing thoughts, distractibility, increase in goal-directed activity, and excessive involvement in pleasurable activities.

Emotional symptoms. To be diagnosed as having a manic episode, the client must exhibit an abnormally and persistently elevated, expansive, or irritable mood for at least 1 week. The client appears euphoric, with periods punctuated by irritability and anger. Some clients report minimal euphoria but describe irritability as their primary mood. Emotional lability, fluctuating between euphoria and anger, is common.

Cognitive symptoms. Inflated self-esteem and grandiosity are common symptoms of mania. Clients report that they are confident, capable, and can do things better than others. As the mania becomes more intense, clients describe themselves in glowing terms and may believe that

Barnes and Jewish Hospitals
Department of Nursing
Patient Clinical Management Path

Admission _____
D/C Date _____
Estimated LOS _____
Case Manager _____

Case Type & Number **(DRG – 430) Bipolar Affective Disorder**

	Day 1/Adm. Loc ( )	Var. n/d m u	Day 2 – 3 Loc ( )	Var. n/d m u	Day 4 – 6 Loc ( )	Var. n/d m u	Day 7 – 9 Loc ( )	Var. n/d m u
Date								
Procedure/Test	Organic Workup (MD), EEG (MD), CT (MD), MRI (MD), EKG (MD), CXR (MD), Electrolytes (MD), Lithium Level (MD), Drug Screen (MD), Thyroid Studies (MD), Routine Labs (MD), Other _____ (MD)		Lab Results (ID abnormals)		-----> Psych Testing complete		Labs _____ Tests _____ Med. Blood Levels _____	
Consults	Medical (MD) Behavior Med. (MD) Psych Testing (MD) Other _____ (MD)		ID additional consults		----->		----->	
Meds/Tx	Meds ordered per MD including PRN to control behavior. ECT (MD) – permits (Nsg) – teaching (Nsg) – team notified (Nsg)		Monitor antidepressant, lithium, tegretol, valproic acid, PRN Meds. Other anti-psychotic meds; if mania DC antidepressant ----->		-----> ----->		-----> ----->	
Activity	Voluntary/Involuntary SP/EP (MD, Nsg) Fall precautions (MS, Nsg)		Assess ADL's -----> -----> Integrate into milieu Participate in groups Individual therapy		-----> Assess precautions -----> -----> ----->		-----> -----> -----> -----> ----->	
Nutrition	Assess appetite (MD, Nsg) Assess elimination patterns (MD, Nsg)		-----> -----> Teaching diet		-----> -----> ----->		-----> -----> ----->	
Discharge Planning	Legal Guardian ID (Nsg) Assess support system (Nsg, MD, SW, AT) Initial Plan (MD/Nsg)		SW Acknowl. note Placement issues MTP signed (MD/Nsg/SW)		Family Mtg		Plans discussed with patient (MD) -----> Weekly Progress Note (MD, SW, Nsg, TR) Completes SW assess Referrals Resources MTP developed	
INTERVENTIONS: Assessment Functional Assessment	H+P & Psych orders (MD) Nsg Assessment and ADB SW notified – pt/family Proper envir. assessed Mini Mental (Nsg) Assess LOF (Nsg, SW, AT) Assess methods to control behavior (Nsg) Remove ext. stimuli (Nsg)		Ongoing assess & treatment (MD, Nsg, SW, TR) BM initial Assess. Assess for dystonia If ADL assess needed OT referral		-----> Assess: – thought patterns – orientation – cog. skills – task completion		-----> Assess task completion Encourage incr. LOF -----> Assess lifestyle changes ----->	
Patient Teaching	Orient pt/family to unit (Nsg) Bill of Rights Given (Nsg)		Ed. Pt/family to various therapies MED Educ. Primary Nurse (Nsg)		-----> ----->		-----> ----->	

Signature & Initials   Refer to Nurses Notes for documentation regarding variances.

_____ _____ _____
_____ _____ _____
_____ _____ _____
_____ _____ _____

	Day 10 – 12 Loc ( )	Var. n/d m u	Day 13 – 14 Loc ( )	Var. n/d m u	Day 15 Loc ( )	Var. n/d m u	Discharge Expected Outcome
Date							
Procedure/Test	Labs _____ Tests _____ Med. Blood Levels _____		Labs _____ Tests _____ Chart copied if appropriate		DC Orders Written		
Consults	- - - - - >		F/u appts made		- - - - - >		
Meds/Tx	- - - - - >

- - - - - > Begin ECT outpt. arrangements | | - - - - - >

- - - - - > - - - - - > | | Perscriptions written | | Pt will verbalize/ demonstrate imp. of medication +/or other therapies in maintaining optimal level of fcn after DC as evidenced by _____ |
| Activity | - - - - - > - - - - - > - - - - - > - - - - - > - - - - - > | | Do teaching r/t follow up therapy | | Plans finalized r/t outpt therapy | | |
| Nutrition | - - - - - > - - - - - >

- - - - - > | | DC teaching r/t nutrition | | - - - - - > | | |
| Discharge Planning | | | DC teaching w/family Weekly progress notes (MD, SW, TR, Nsg)

DC teaching on utilization of skills learned while in hosp and how to integrate to home.

Written information r/t resource given. | | MTP closed or remains ongoing

Final DC instructions given to pt/family

F/U appt finalized | | Pt will return to least restrictive/most supportive environment after DC with improved coping skills and identified resources as demonstrated by

_____ _____. |
| INTERVENTIONS: Assessment | - - - - - > - - - - - > | | - - - - - > - - - - - > | | Final assessments & DC summary written. | | |
| Functional Assessment | MMSE (Neg)

- - - - - > - - - - - > - - - - - > - - - - - > | | - - - - - > | | - - - - - > | | |
| Patient Teaching | - - - - - >

- - - - - > | | - - - - - >

- - - - - > DC teaching | | Final DC teaching to patient. Patient's responses to teaching documented | | |

*SW works M – F

Teaching (initial and date when complete)
1. Medication Education _____
2. Education on illness _____
3. Social Skills _____
4. Coping Skills _____
5. ADL's _____
6. Self-Esteem _____

7. Dealing with Anger _____
8. Communication Skills _____
9. Dealing with Sadness _____
10. Decision Making _____
11. Other _____
*Document patient response in progress notes

Addressograph:

CLINICAL SYMPTOMS

Bipolar Disorders

Manic Episode

Emotional
Abnormally and persistently elevated, expansive, or irritable mood

Cognitive
Feelings of inflated self-esteem and grandiosity
Thought-flow disturbance with racing thoughts and flight of ideas

Behavioral
Increased talkativeness
Increased goal-directed behavior or agitation
Excessive involvement in activities thought to be pleasurable

Social
Increased sociability
Intrusive, interruptive, and disruptive during conversations or activities
Fluctuations between euphoria and anger

Perceptual
Distractibility
Hallucinations

Cyclothymic Disorder

Behavioral
Periods of hypomania
Periods of depressed mood and anhedonia
Irritability or angry mood

Cognitive
Feelings of low self-esteem and inadequacy
Feelings of guilt and brooding about the past
Difficulty with concentration, memory, and decision-making
Attitudes of pessimism, despair, and hopelessness

Behavioral
Chronic fatigue

Social
Social withdrawal

---

they are capable of amazing feats and achievements. Delusions of grandeur may be evident during severe episodes of mania as clients believe that they possess extraordinary gifts and talents or that they are famous. These delusions of inflated self-worth and ability represent mood-congruent psychotic features of mania. Cognitively, clients with mania also experience thought-flow disturbance with racing thoughts and flight of ideas. **Flight of ideas** is a type of thought disorder in which somewhat connected thoughts occur quickly, resulting in little elaboration and

rapid changing of subjects. It becomes difficult to block out incoming stimuli, and the client becomes distractible, responding to irrelevant stimuli. Clients with mania often deny the seriousness of their status and lack judgment regarding personal, social, and occupational needs and activities.

Behavioral symptoms.   Increased talkativeness, increased goal-directed behavior or agitation, and excessive involvement in pleasurable activities are notable symptoms of mania. As the mania progresses, clients become more talkative and their speech is pressured (delivered with urgency). The rate of speech may increase and become rapid. Clients may exhibit extremes in appearance, wearing bright colors, unusual dress, and heavy makeup. Clients begin and engage in more activities, taking on additional tasks and initiating new projects. Productivity may appear to increase as the client delves into more tasks, but as the mania becomes more intense, actual productivity decreases as clients become more distractible, disorganized, and agitated. They begin to physically move faster—pacing, fidgeting, rarely letting their body stay still. As insight and judgment become more impaired, clients become involved in activities that they perceive as pleasurable, but that may carry a high risk for harm or negative consequences. Clients often report engaging in extramarital affairs, promiscuity, spending sprees, gambling, wild driving, and unwise business deals.

Social symptoms.   At first, mania seems to promote sociability, and clients become more outgoing and active; however, before long, insight and judgment fail, and these same clients become intrusive—interrupting others' conversations and activities, fluctuating from euphoria to anger, and disrupting social interactions. Clients with mania find it difficult to set both physical and emotional boundaries, infringing on the physical space and personal issues of others. The funny, witty client becomes angry and isolated as the mood escalates and intensifies.

Perceptual symptoms.   One symptom of mania is distractibility, in which attention is easily and frequently drawn to irrelevant external stimuli. Clients appear unable to screen out peripheral stimuli (e.g., noises, other voices, and visual attractions) that are not necessary or relevant to the task at hand. Distractibility interferes with attention, concentration, and memory. Perceptual disturbances can also occur in the form of hallucinations. Manic hallucinations can occur in any sensory mode but are usually auditory, with themes that pertain to grandiosity, power, and, occasionally, paranoia. These indicate manic psychosis.

Hypomanic Episode
Manic and hypomanic episodes share symptom criteria and are differentiated primarily by their severity and duration. Hypomanic episodes are not severe enough to

cause significant impairment in social and occupational functioning or to require hospitalization. However, it must be evident that the mood and behavioral disturbances of **hypomania** represent a definite change in the person's usual functioning for at least 4 days. During a hypomanic phase, clients may appear extremely happy and congenial, at ease with social conversation, and offer humorous input. Although the moments of elevated mood appear to be desirable, they represent dysfunctional affective states during which the client is not fully in control of moods and accompanying behavior.

Cyclothymic Disorder

Cyclothymic disorder is a chronic mood disturbance of at least 2 years' duration (1 year for children and adolescents), with many periods of hypomanic symptoms, depressed mood, and anhedonia. Clients with cyclothymic disorder have not been without the symptoms for more than 2 months over a period of 2 or more years; however, these symptoms are less severe or intense than those in major depressive or manic episodes.

ADDITIONAL TYPES OF MOOD DISORDERS

The DSM-IV also provides diagnostic criteria for mood disorders due to general medical conditions and to substance use. In these instances the depressed or elevated mood and accompanying symptoms can be attributed to some general medical condition or to the ingestion of or withdrawal from medications or other substances. Box 13-3 lists examples of the types of medical conditions and substances commonly associated with the development of mood disorders.

ADDITIONAL SYMPTOM FEATURES OF MOOD DISORDERS

The DSM-IV recognizes that there are features of mood disorders that may indicate various subtypes of unipolar and bipolar disorders. Persons experiencing an episode of major depression, whether it is part of a unipolar or bipolar pattern, may demonstrate melancholic, atypical, or seasonal features. Postpartum onset represents another type of mood disorder.

Features of **melancholic depression** include anhedonia and a lack of reactivity to any pleasurable stimulus; a distinct quality of mood in which the depression is perceived as different from the feeling felt after the death of a loved one; depression that is worse in the morning; sleep disturbance of early morning, awakening at least 2 hours before the usual time; marked psychomotor retardation or agitation; significant weight loss or loss of appetite; and excessive guilt.

Features of **atypical depression** include mood reactivity; loss of the ability to react to positive stimuli; significant weight gain or increase in appetite; hypersomnia; leaden paralysis or a heavy feeling in the arms and legs; and a long-standing pattern of being sensitive to interpersonal rejection.

A seasonal pattern occurs when there is a regular, temporal relationship between the onset and the remission of an episode of major depression (unipolar or bipolar) at a particular time of the year. This pattern must be evident for 2 consecutive years with no intervening, nonseasonal episodes. Seasonal episodes of altered mood must outnumber any nonseasonal episodes over a lifetime. This pattern is commonly called **seasonal affective disorder (SAD)**. Clients with SAD often develop depression during October or November and find it remitting in March or April. Atypical features may also be associated with SAD. A seasonal pattern can also occur with bipolar disorder, particularly bipolar II disorder, in which increased light triggers manic or hypomanic episodes.

Women may experience a postpartum mood disorder, including depression or mania, following the birth of a child. This usually occurs within 4 weeks of the birth and consists of symptoms of depression or mania described earlier.

A summary of clinical symptoms of these additional types of mood disorders is given in the Clinical Symptoms box on p. 276.

PROGNOSIS

Recently, more attention has been given to understanding the life course of persons with mood disorders. The bipolar disorders have historically been perceived as recurrent, with cycles of mania and depression interspersed with periods of **euthymia.** The pattern of cycles varies from person to person, with episodes of depression, mania, and euthymia varying widely in duration. The bipolar disorders have a high rate of recurrence and relapse. Factors that contribute to relapse include the number of and recovery from previous episodes, a family history of bipolar disorder, functional incapacity associated with episodes, past psychotic episodes, and past suicide attempts (Consensus Development Panel, 1985). Many recurrences, however, can be controlled with proper treatment and monitoring (Keller, 1988).

Box 13-3	**Medical Conditions and Substances Associated With the Development of a Mood Disorder**
Medical Conditions	**Substances**
Hypothyroidism/hyperthyroidism	Digitalis
Mononucleosis	Thiazide diuretics
Diabetes mellitus	Reserpine
Cushing's disease	Propranolol
Pernicious anemia	Anabolic steroids
Pancreatitis	Oral contraceptives
Hepatitis	Disulfiram
HIV	Sulfonamides
Multiple sclerosis	Alcohol
	Marijuana

CLINICAL SYMPTOMS

Additional Mood Disorders

Melancholic Depression

Emotional
Anhedonia
Increased depression in the morning

Cognitive
Excessive feelings of guilt

Behavioral
Waking at least 2 hours before normal and being unable to
    fall back asleep
Psychomotor retardation or agitation
Significant weight loss

Atypical Depression

Emotional
Mood reactivity
Ability to react to positive stimuli

Cognitive
Sensitivity to interpersonal rejection

Behavioral
Significant weight gain or increase in appetite
Hypersomnia
Leaden paralysis

Seasonal Affective Disorder

Emotional
Depression between October/November and March/April

Major depression, historically viewed as a single, acute occurrence, is now understood to be a serious, recurrent disorder for the majority of persons with major depression (Greden, 1993). Research indicates that 50% to 85% of clients with unipolar depression experience a subsequent episode and that recurrent episodes tend to be increasingly intense with shorter time periods between episodes (Angst, 1988). There are more episodes of recurrent depression than first-time episodes (Thase, 1992). Twenty percent of persons with depression are not fully recovered from an episode after 1 year (Sargeant et al, 1990). Adverse, long-term effects impair self-care, productivity, social functioning, occupational functioning, and physical health (Tweed, 1993).

These data depict the need for education, lifetime monitoring, and maintenance treatment for many persons with depression. The prognosis for major depressive disorder is good; it can be well controlled with medications, psychotherapy, and self-help strategies. However, clients need to be made aware of the recurrent nature of their disorder and educated about the importance of recognizing symptoms and seeking help early when depression begins. Unfortunately, many persons do not recognize the onset of their recurrences (Hagerty et al, 1997), and less than a third of the people who experience depression seek help, putting them at risk for future, more severe depression.

Dysthymia often continues for years before individuals seek assistance for their symptoms. Many people are unaware that the chronic, low-level depression that is depleting their energy is indeed a form of depression and can be treated. Unfortunately, over 50% of persons with dysthymia go on to develop major depression (Horwath et al, 1992).

With proper treatment, the prognosis for maintaining individual functioning with a mood disorder is favorable. Inevitably, failure to seek help, lack of education regarding the disorder, lack of adherence to treatment, or resistance of the symptoms to usual treatments means that some persons will become so impaired that their daily functioning will diminish for long periods.

DISCHARGE CRITERIA

Most clients with a mood disorder are not hospitalized. Those who are require attention to ensure that they meet the following criteria before discharge:

Verbalize plans for the future, including absence of imminent suicidal intent or behavior.

Verbalize plan for seeking help (a contract) if suicidal thoughts become intensified or thoughts progress to plans.

Demonstrate ability to manage basic self-care needs, such as personal hygiene, or verbalize strategies to acquire assistance.

Describe mood state and demonstrate ability to identify changes from euthymic mood.

Verbalize realistic perceptions of self and abilities that are positive and hopeful.

Verbalize realistic expectations for self and others.

Identify psychosocial or physical stressors that may have negative influences on mood and thinking.

State positive and helpful strategies to cope with threats, concerns, and stressors.

Identify signs and symptoms of the mood disorder, including prodromal (early) signs that might indicate the need to seek help.

Describe how to contact appropriate sources for validation and/or intervention when necessary.

Use learned techniques and strategies to prevent or minimize symptoms.

Verbalize knowledge about medication treatment and necessary self-care strategies.

Engage family or significant other as source of support.

Structure life to include appropriate activities that promote social support, minimize stress, and facilitate healthy living (e.g., diet, exercise).

THE NURSING PROCESS

ASSESSMENT

The prevalence and incidence of mood disorders demand that nurses be alert for symptoms of depression and mania. Most persons experiencing a mood disorder, particularly depression, never seek psychiatric care. More often, these individuals visit family practitioners, clinics, or emergency departments reporting symptoms of fatigue or lack of activity, or vague physical complaints. Many do not realize that they are experiencing a mood disorder.

Clients with mood disorders pose a challenge because their primary symptom is one of depression or emotional elation. Their affective dysregulation often evokes emotional responses in nurses, who find themselves feeling depressed, anxious, or angry while caring for the individual. The negativity of depression or the expansive euphoria, hyperactivity, and grandiosity of mania may also promote fatigue, irritability, and negativity in the nurse. Therefore when caring for clients with mood disorders, nurses must maintain awareness of their own personal reactions to the client and the ways in which these reactions can affect the nurse-client relationship and subsequent care.

Clients experiencing mood disorders are in emotional pain. They are unable to change their emotional state at will. Yet, many have heard people close to them make comments such as "Pull yourself up by your bootstraps . . . get a hold of yourself." These clients need validation that their emotional state is not their fault, that they are experiencing a psychiatric disorder. They should be approached with acceptance and respect.

It is important that nurses appear confident, straightforward, and hopeful. Reassuring comments such as "I know you'll feel better soon," are usually not helpful, because they may be false reassurance. It is appropriate to convey hope with comments such as "I've known many clients with depression, and they have felt better within several weeks of starting on their medications."

Communication with the person with depression depends on the severity of the depression. Clients with severe depression may be physically and cognitively slowed down and have problems with attention, concentration, and decision making. Simple, clear communication is most helpful in this situation. The nurse may need to be more directive if the person is having a difficult time making decisions (e.g., "It's time for lunch. I'll go with you," rather than "Would you like to go to lunch?"). As clients' conditions improve, they can cognitively process more complex information and make decisions more easily.

Communication with clients experiencing mania also can be difficult. Their hyperactivity, expansive or irritable mood, and inability to filter stimuli are barriers to effective communication. Nurses need to be simple, clear, direct, and firm. Clients need to know that the nurse cares about them and is concerned about their behavior. Acute episodes of mania are not appropriate times for the nurse to delve into the client's feelings and motives. Interactions should be brief and direct, with minimization of unnecessary stimuli. It is also important not to threaten or challenge a client in the turmoil of a manic episode, because the client might respond with rage.

Information from the client may be minimal or inaccurate because of their cognitive impairment, altered mood, or behavioral disturbances. A significant other can be an important source of information when the client is not reliable. Interviews may need to be short and more directive if the client is having behavioral or cognitive difficulty.

Assessment of the client with depression or mania includes information about his or her presenting problem and mental status, past psychiatric history, social and developmental history, family history, and physical health

---

CASE STUDY

James is a 55-year-old widower. He lives alone in an apartment and has a 32-year-old married daughter who lives 1000 miles away. Three months ago James was forced to take early retirement from his job in middle management at a computer firm. Over the past month he has exhibited depressed affect and has become so withdrawn that he no longer attends church or his weekly evening out with his friends. He reports difficulty falling asleep and staying asleep, agitation, a weight loss of 15 pounds in 1 month, difficulty concentrating and making decisions, and ruminations and guilt about his wife's death 10 years ago. He was admitted to the hospital after his neighbor brought him to the emergency department. There, James admitted plans to kill himself with a handgun he kept at home. He had one previous episode of major depression at age 45, about the time of his wife's death. He has never made an actual suicide attempt. James has been in the hospital for 13 days. He has been taking sertraline (Zoloft) 100 mg qd and trazodone hydrochloride 100 mg hs, and is being considered for discharge.

Critical Thinking—Evaluation

1. Which specific indicators would the nurse use to evaluate James's self-destructiveness in view of his impending discharge?
2. What outcome criteria are appropriate for evaluation of James's response to medication?
3. What outcomes might be evaluated by the nurse that would best demonstrate James's progress for a community mental health referral?

history. Assessment instruments can assist with the specificity of data collection. These instruments include the Beck Depression Inventory, Carroll Rating Scale for Depression, and Zung Self-Rating Depression Scale. Nurses can also ask clients to assess their own level of depression or mania by having them rate it on a 10-point scale (e.g., "If zero represents feeling fine and 10 represents the worst depression you have ever experienced, how would you rate your depression now?" This allows for daily comparisons of mood.)

PHYSIOLOGIC DISTURBANCES

Body physiology is altered during episodes of depression and mania. During moderate or severe depression, body processes frequently slow down. The client with depression may report and exhibit neurovegetative signs of depression, which include psychomotor retardation, fatigue, constipation, anorexia (loss of appetite), weight loss, decreased libido (sex drive), and sleep disturbances. These symptoms relate to changes in body processes that cause disruption and slowing of normal physiology. Clients may also describe vague physical symptoms, such as headache, backache, gastrointestinal pain, and nausea. Clients may seek assistance from their family health care provider,

thinking that they are experiencing some physical illness that is causing fatigue and loss of energy. Sleep disturbance is a common problem. Clients describe initial insomnia (the inability to fall asleep after going to bed), middle insomnia (waking up in the middle of the night and being unable to return to sleep easily), and terminal, or late, insomnia (waking up in the early hours of the morning and being unable to return to sleep). Another type of sleep disturbance seen in depression is hypersomnia, in which the client sleeps excessively but never feels rested. Clients with depression may have a decreased or increased appetite with corresponding changes in weight. Food is often described as tasteless.

The client experiencing mania also has difficulty sleeping. Not feeling the need for sleep, the client may sleep only a few hours a night or not at all and yet feel rested afterward. Hyperactive behavior and the inability to attend to tasks often preclude the client from eating properly, resulting in dehydration and inadequate nutrition. As the client becomes increasingly stimulated, metabolic activity increases, and vital signs may become elevated. Without proper intervention, clients with mania may be at physical risk for dehydration, hypertension, and cardiac arrest, which can lead to death.

NURSING ASSESSMENT QUESTIONS

Mood Disorders

How would you describe your mood? (To assess client's insight into feeling state)

Have you noticed a change in your behavior within the past month? (To determine client's awareness of behavioral changes)

Do you feel that people are noticing a change in your behavior, such as irritability or hyperactivity? (To determine client's sensitivity to others' observations of behavioral changes)

What activities have you found enjoyable over the past month? Did you enjoy them as much as you previously did? Can you imagine an event or situation that would give you pleasure? Have you been able to enjoy food and/or sex over the past month? (To determine client's current quality of life)

When did you first begin to feel depressed or elated? Did others comment that your mood seemed more depressed (or higher) than usual? Have you ever felt this way before? When? What was it like? (To establish behavioral patterns)

How has your sleep been? Are you able to fall asleep at night? Stay asleep? Do you find yourself waking up early and being unable to return to sleep? Are you sleeping more than usual in a 24-hour period? How much? (To determine sleep patterns)

How has your appetite been in the past month? How much weight have you lost or gained in the past month? (To determine nutritional/metabolic status)

How has your energy level been? Do you feel tired every day? Do you ever feel as though your limbs are heavy? (To assess fatigability)

How has your concentration been? Are you able to attend to things such as reading the newspaper? Can you concentrate on projects or activities to finish them? What has your decision making been like? (To evaluate cognitive abilities)

How have you felt about yourself lately? Have you felt guilty more than usual about things you have done? (To determine client's level of self-worth/self-esteem)

Have you felt particularly slowed down, or have others told you that you seemed to move or speak more slowly than usual? (To determine presence of sensorimotor retardation)

Have you felt particularly "speeded up" to the point where you noticed it or someone told you this? (To evaluate presence of mania/hypermania)

Have you had thoughts of death or suicide? How often? What specifically have you thought about doing to harm yourself? (To determine suicidal intent/plans)

What have you been doing lately to manage your feelings? Has it helped? (To assess for effective coping mechanisms/strategies)

How has your mood affected your job? Your family? Your social life? (To assess pervasiveness of client's present mood state)

NURSING DIAGNOSIS

The nurse uses objective and subjective data obtained during the assessment of clients with mood disorders to arrive at relevant nursing diagnoses. Data from all sources, including the client, significant others, and other professionals, are organized into a pattern of relationships that reflect the client's major areas of health care needs (see Nursing Assessment Questions box). The following nursing diagnoses are relevant to clients experiencing a mood disorder:

NURSING DIAGNOSES FOR DEPRESSION

Constipation
Fatigue
Hopelessness
Knowledge deficit (depression/mania, treatment)
Nutrition, altered
Powerlessness
Self-care deficit, bathing/hygiene
Self-care deficit, dressing/grooming
Self-care deficit, feeding
Sexual dysfunction
Sleep pattern disturbance
Social interaction, impaired
Spiritual distress (distress of the human spirit)
Violence, risk for: directed at others
Violence, risk for: self-directed

NURSING DIAGNOSES FOR MANIA

Communication, impaired verbal
Coping, defensive
Coping, ineffective individual
Family processes, altered
Noncompliance (therapeutic regimen)
Nutrition, altered: less than body requirements
Self-esteem disturbance
Sensory/perceptual alterations
Sleep pattern disturbance
Thought processes, altered
Violence, risk for: directed at others
Violence, risk for: self-directed

OUTCOME IDENTIFICATION

Outcome criteria for clients with mood disorders include short- and long-term client behaviors and responses that indicate improved functioning. These criteria are based on nursing diagnoses and are achieved through implementation of planned nursing care. Outcome criteria provide the nurse with direction for evaluating client response to treatment.

Client will:

1. Remain safe and free from harm.
2. Verbalize suicidal ideations and contract not to harm self or others.
3. Verbalize absence of suicidal or homicidal intent or plans.
4. Express desire to live and not harm others.
5. Make plans for self for the future, verbalizing feelings of hopefulness.
6. Engage in self-care activities in accordance with ability, health status, and developmental stage.
7. Develop a plan to manage inadequate sleep.
8. Establish a pattern of rest/activity that enables fulfillment of role and self-care demands.
9. Make decisions based on examination of options and problem solving.
10. Report absence of hallucinations/delusions.
11. Initiate satisfying social interactions with significant others or peers.
12. Demonstrate participation in milieu, group, and community activities.
13. Report increased communication and problem solving among family members regarding issues related to the disorder.
14. Describe alternative coping strategies for responses to stressors, strengths, and limitations.
15. Report increased feelings of self-worth and confidence.
16. Engage in activities and behaviors that promote confidence, belonging, and acceptance.
17. Describe information about the disorder, including the course of illness and personal symptom patterns, as well as resources.
18. Identify medications, including action, dosage, side effects, therapeutic effects, and self-care issues.
19. Adhere to prescribed professional and self-care treatment strategies.

CASE STUDY

Mrs. Jones is a 40-year-old mother of three. She was brought to the hospital by her husband, who was concerned that she had lost 15 pounds within the past several weeks and laid on the sofa much of the day, crying. The house had not been cleaned for weeks, and the children were making their own meals and doing the laundry. Mrs. Jones was dressed casually in wrinkled clothes. Her movements and verbalizations were slow. Mrs. Jones had told her husband that she thought they should buy a cemetary plot but could not explain why.

Critical Thinking—Outcome Identification
1. What additional information would be helpful for the nurse to know about Mrs. Jones in order to develop nursing diagnoses and goals?
2. Which nursing diagnoses would be relevant for Mrs. Jones?
3. What long- and short-term outcomes, based on the nursing diagnoses, might be established with Mrs. Jones?

PLANNING

Recent information about the epidemiology and recurrent course of depression and mania provides the basis for caring for clients with mood disorders in the hospital and in the community. Nursing care addresses the acute episodes of the disorder and the client's risk for recurrent episodes. Interventions during the acute depressive or manic episodes can be effective, but too often the client is left with little understanding of the importance of long-term management and self-care strategies. Interventions must be planned for each client based on his or her particular behaviors and concerns (see the clinical pathway on p. 270). Planning care not only involves the client but may also include the client's significant others and additional health care providers. Using nursing diagnoses derived from assessment data, interventions that facilitate achievement of desired client outcomes are planned (see Collaborative Diagnoses box).

COLLABORATIVE DIAGNOSES

DSM-IV Diagnoses*	NANDA Diagnosest
Bipolar I disorder, manic or hypomanic	Communication, impaired verbal
	Constipation
	Coping, defensive
Bipolar II disorder	Coping, ineffective individual
Cyclothymic disorder	Family processes, altered
Dysthymic disorder	Fatigue
Major depressive episode	Hopelessness
	Knowledge deficit
Mood disorder due to general medical condition	Noncompliance
	Nutrition, altered
	Powerlessness
Substance-induced mood disorder	Self-care deficit, bathing/hygiene
	Self-care deficit, dressing/grooming
	Self-care deficit, feeding
	Self-esteem disturbance
	Sensory/perceptual alterations
	Sexual dysfunction
	Sleep pattern disturbance
	Social interaction, impaired
	Spiritual distress (distress of the human spirit)
	Thought processes, altered
	Violence, risk for: directed at others
	Violence, risk for: self-directed

*From American Psychiatric Association: *Diagnostic and statistical manual of mental disorders*, ed 4, Washington, DC, 1994, The Association.

†From North American Nursing Diagnosis Association: *NANDA nursing diagnoses: definitions and classifications 1999-2000*, Philadelphia, 1999, The Association.

IMPLEMENTATION

The plan of action for clients with mood disorders varies depending on whether the client is depressed or manic. In the short term, nursing and collaborative interventions are available that are effective in reducing the acuity of the episode and promoting more optimal functioning. With the current trend of short-term hospitalizations, nurses in the hospital setting do not have the opportunity to observe the client's recovery from the episode. Projected treatment responses, however, should be documented and communicated to the client and to nurses, other mental health professionals, and significant others who will care for the client in the community. Nurses who work with clients in the community are able to see treatment responses over time (see Nursing Care in the Community box).

Mood disorders, although primarily a disturbance in emotional regulation, affect the whole person—physically, cognitively, socially, and spiritually. Short-term interventions in the hospital or community address priority issues, such as preventing self-harm, promoting physical health (e.g., adequate nutrition, bathing, grooming, sleep), monitoring effects of medications, and assisting with altered thought flow and impaired communication. Other concerns to be addressed include promoting social interaction, self-esteem, understanding of the disorder and its treatment, treatment compliance, and planning for discharge and continuation or discontinuation of services. Because episodes of depression and mania affect the entire family, involving the client's significant others provides an opportunity for them to understand the disorder and to support clients in their recovery. Clinical pathways for mood disorders, which specify collaborative interventions, can be found in Chapter 7.

Nursing interventions for clients with mood disorders span a wide range of biopsychosocial areas, with consideration of the effects of depression and mania on the physiologic, cognitive, psychologic, behavioral, and social spheres. Intervention for clients experiencing depression and mania requires that nurses maintain self-awareness and boundaries regarding their own reactions to clients, because client depression, irritability, anger, negativity, euphoria, and hyperactivity can influence nursing response. It is potentially difficult and exhausting to interact with clients who provoke personal feelings and reactions during highly emotional encounters. Initiating and maintaining a therapeutic connection with clients is accomplished through consistency, caring, concern, empathy, and genuineness on the part of the nurse. Clients with mood disorders may have a difficult time developing a therapeutic alliance and avoid interpersonal connection with others. A knowledgeable, consistent, and matter-of-fact (but genuine and caring) presentation is reassuring to clients and promotes their confidence in the nurse.

Mood Disorders

Nursing Care in the Community

Working with persons experiencing mood disorders can be challenging for the community mental health nurse. The nurse must deal with a wide range of behaviors and may find recommendations to be minimized by the client, if not negated entirely. A person manifesting a manic episode will often be grandiose, express pleasure in his or her increased activity level, and become irritable when confronted about problematic behavior. In contrast, a person suffering from depression will also often reject help, because nothing seems meaningful and change appears impossible. In either case the client may see the process of assessment as intrusive, and efforts toward engagement may be rejected. The nurse must work carefully through the evaluation process to decide whether hospitalization is indicated.

Context and timing are significant when evaluating the mood-disordered individual in the community. The nurse should consider the following questions:

Have situational stressors caused the sadness?

Has a grief process evolved into a depressed state?

Have vegetative signs developed? (Have the person's sleeping and eating patterns changed?)

Are nonverbal signs such as posture and affect consistent with expressed emotion?

Is there a history of suicidal behavior, current suicidality, or a plan for suicide?

Has the person ever been treated for depression successfully?

Is the person willing to accept treatment now?

The nurse must hold an unbiased stance, neither trying to superficially cheer the client nor offering situational advice. The nurse may suggest treatment options and assess the client's response. Screening tests for depression may be used to facilitate diagnosis. Some facilities offer free screening for depression in the community.

Assessing the person experiencing a manic episode is often dramatic and can be frustrating for the nurse. The manic individual reiterates that he or she is fine, does not need help from anyone, and resents the "interrogation." It is best to enlist the help of members of the client's support system, as well as the client, to identify a developing manic episode on the basis of behavioral changes. The client may be experiencing increases in spending patterns, sexual activity, or erratic sleep patterns. It is easier to influence the client to seek help early, rather than waiting until sleep deprivation and increased tension have made the client so irritable or fatigued that he or she experiences psychosis, requiring involuntary hospitalization.

Monitoring medication levels and effectiveness is another critical element for the nurse caring for clients with mood disorders in the community. Antidepressants may cause clients to feel stronger but still depressed enough to be at high risk for suicide. Antimanic medications such as lithium carbonate and carbamazepine (Tegretol) can be life threatening if excesses build up in the client's system. These medications require periodic blood tests to verify medication compliance and discriminate between toxic and therapeutic levels. Symptoms of toxicity may resemble an increasing disease process, and higher doses of medication may be administered if evaluation is not timely and insightful. The nurse must encourage the client to discriminate among feeling states and pathologic or physiologic symptoms so that he or she can seek assistance if out of control.

NURSING INTERVENTIONS

1. Conduct a suicide assessment as necessary *to ensure the client's safety and prevent harm to self or others.*
2. Maintain a safe, harm-free environment through close and frequent observations *to minimize the risk of violence.*
3. Establish rapport and a trusting relationship with the client *to facilitate the client's willingness to communicate thoughts and feelings.*
4. Assist the client in verbalizing feelings *to promote a healthy, expressive form of communication.*
5. Identify the client's social support system and encourage the client to use it *to minimize isolation and loneliness as possible precursors to hopelessness.*
6. Praise the client for attempts at alternate activities and interactions with others *to encourage socialization.*
7. Monitor the client's fluid intake and output, food intake, and weight *to ensure adequate nutrition and hydration and adequate weight for body size and metabolic need.*
8. Promote self-care activities, such as bathing, dressing, feeding, and grooming, *to ascertain the client's level of functioning and increase self-esteem.*
9. Assist the client in establishing daily goals and expectations *to promote structure and minimize confusion/anxiety.*
10. Plan self-care activities around those times when the client may have more energy *to increase activity tolerance and minimize fatigue.*
11. Reduce choices of clothing and tasks *to make decision making easier, increasing choices as the client improves cognitively.*
12. Assess the client's cognitive/perceptual process *to ascertain the existence of hallucinations/delusions that may be troubling or harmful for the client.*
13. Assist the client in identifying negative, self-defeating thoughts and modifying them with realistic thoughts *to promote more accurate, positive thoughts about self* (see Chapter 3).
14. Encourage the client to attend therapeutic groups

▲ NURSING CARE PLAN

Kathy is a 41-year-old mother of two children. Her husband recently divorced her and married another woman. Kathy also just learned that her mother had been diagnosed with advanced breast cancer. Kathy had two previous episodes of manic behavior in her thirties, including grandiosity, hyperactivity, spending sprees, and decreased need for sleep. During those times Kathy believed that she had special abilities for financial matters and would someday manage a major corporation. She also had four previous episodes of depression, the first when she was 20. During the episodes of depression Kathy was unable to work at her job as an accountant, slept 14 to 16 hours a day, lost weight, and considered suicide. For the past 3 weeks Kathy has become increasingly depressed, sleeping 14 to 16 hours a day, losing 16 pounds from her usual weight of 115 pounds, not caring for her personal appearance and looking disheveled, moving and talking more slowly than usual, and missing work. She was taken to the hospital by her ex-husband after she told him she wanted to die. The children went to live with their father on Kathy's hospital admission. She admits that she has not been taking her medications of lithium and fluoxetine (Prozac). She is being treated with albuterol (Proventil) inhaler for her asthma. In the hospital, she was given lithium 300 mg qid and nortriptylene (Pamelor) 25 mg qid.

DSM-IV Diagnoses

Axis I	Bipolar I disorder, current episode depressed
Axis II	Deferred
Axis III	Asthma
Axis IV	Severity of psychosocial stressors: severe (divorce, mother's serious illness, children moved in with husband)
Axis V	GAF = 35 (current)
	GAF = 70 (past year)

Nursing Diagnosis: Violence, risk for: self-directed. Risk factors: depressed mood, hopelessness, and suicidal ideation.

Client Outcomes

- Kathy will remain safe from self-harm.
- Kathy will verbalize any suicidal ideations and contract not to harm self.
- Kathy will be able to discuss feelings about her situation. Kathy will be able to provide reasons to live.
- Kathy will identify resources and options available to her in the community if she begins to feel suicidal.

Nursing Interventions

- Assess suicidal thinking, including frequency, plan, opportunity, and past attempts, *to determine suicidal risk and intent.*
- Provide close observation as indicated *to ensure the client's safety.*
- Monitor the environment for potentially harmful items (e.g., sharp objects, hoarded medications, and belts) *to provide a safe, nonthreatening environment.*
- Observe for behaviors and statements that may be indicators of self-harm intent, such as statements of hopelessness, giving away of possessions, sudden calmness, or a change in behavior, *because such behaviors may be signals of suicidal thoughts and intent.*
- Contract with Kathy to tell someone if her suicidal thinking increases or if she feels as though she might act on a plan. *Contracting establishes an expectation of behavior between nurse and client.*
- Encourage Kathy to express her feelings rather than suppress them *to relieve pent-up feelings and allow them to be validated.*
- Encourage Kathy to focus on people and things that are important to her, such as her children, *to reinforce the client's strengths and positive resources.*
- Encourage Kathy to problem solve about alternatives to self-harm, such as talking with friends, *to promote activation of alternative coping mechanisms that increase self-control.*
- Provide Kathy with information about community resources available if she begins to feel suicidal, including community mental health or a crisis line, *to provide resources available for assistance.*

Evaluation

- Kathy remained safe from self-harm.
- Kathy discussed her suicidal thoughts with staff when they occurred and contracted not to harm herself.
- Kathy reported the absence of suicidal intent on discharge.
- Kathy willingly discussed her feelings with staff.
- Kathy provided reasons important to her for living.
- Kathy identified resources, including people and activities, available to her if she begins to feel suicidal in the community.

NURSING CARE PLAN —*cont'd*

Nursing Diagnosis: Social interaction, impaired, related to low self-esteem, psychomotor retardation, hypersomnia, fatigue, depressed mood, and actual and perceived loss, as evidenced by self-imposed seclusion, failure to initiate interaction, divorce, and concern regarding mother's potential death.

Client Outcomes	Nursing Interventions	Evaluation
• Kathy will participate in unit activities while in the hospital. • Kathy will initiate social interaction with family, friends, and peers.	• Encourage Kathy to attend group and unit activities *to promote social interaction; clients gain support from others.* • Arrange to spend time with Kathy at a regular, prearranged time for interaction *to provide a supportive presence and encourage interaction.* • Help Kathy to identify opportunities for social interaction with family, friends, and peers both in the hospital and after discharge *to strengthen the client's social support network.* • Provide positive reinforcement to Kathy for engaging in social interactions *to reinforce rewarding, supportive interactions.*	• Kathy participated in most unit activities in the hospital. • Kathy initiated contact with family and friends while in the hospital. • Kathy described a plan for continued social interaction with family and friends after discharge.

Nursing Diagnosis: Noncompliance (medications) related to belief that medications were not helpful, as evidenced by self-reported failure to take medications.

Client Outcomes	Nursing Interventions	Evaluation
• Kathy will adhere to her treatment regimen, including taking her medications as prescribed.	• Teach Kathy about her medications, including their value and success in treating depression and mania, their actions, their therapeutic and side effects, and the usual dosage. *Knowledge allows the client to make informed choices about medications and promotes adherence to prescribed medications.* • Review the potential side effects of the medications and develop strategies with Kathy to address these effects *to allow the client a sense of control with medications and enable her to initiate self-care strategies that minimize side effects.* • Discourage Kathy from stopping her medications without input from her mental health provider. The client *may experience withdrawal symptoms and relapse of depression.* • Provide opportunities for Kathy to discuss her feelings about her disorder and the need to be taking medication. *Expression of values and feelings provides validation for the client's experience.*	• Kathy was able to discuss the rationale for her medication therapy and the action, side effects, and dosage of the medications. • Kathy was able to describe self-care strategies to address the side effects of her medications. • Kathy's lithium and nortriptyline levels were within normal therapeutic ranges.

that provide feedback regarding thinking *to reframe thinking with the support of others* (see Chapter 3).

15. Provide simple, clear directives/communication in a low-stimulus environment *to assist with focus, attention, and concentration with minimal distractions.*

16. Teach the client and significant others about the disorder and treatment *to minimize guilt and remorse in clients and families about the disorder.*

17. Gradually increase levels of activity and exercise *to minimize fatigue and increase activity tolerance.*

18. Identify sources of external stress and assist the client in coping with them in a more effective manner *to minimize stressors and promote adaptive coping mechanisms.*

19. Educate the client with depression about the disorder and symptoms as appropriate *to lessen feelings of inadequacy, minimize guilt, and increase the knowledge base about the effects of the illness.*

20. Educate the client with mania about the disorder and symptoms as appropriate *to lessen feelings of inadequacy, minimize guilt, and increase the knowledge base about the effects of the illness.*

CASE STUDY

Anne, a 53-year-old widow, arrived at the internal medicine clinic complaining of "headaches." She appeared tired and sad. She moved slowly and frequently sighed deeply. She reported that she was having difficulty getting out of bed in the morning because of headaches and general malaise. Anne had gained 35 pounds in the past 3 months. She told the nurse that she was worried that she might be dying. She was so distraught that she had stopped attending her weekly movie night with her friends.

Critical Thinking—Assessment

1. Which data suggest that Anne might be experiencing a mood disorder?
2. What other types of information about Anne would be important for the nurse to assess at this point?
3. Which type of mood disorder might Anne be experiencing?
4. What are three relevant assessment criteria for Anne?

ADDITIONAL TREATMENT MODALITIES
Psychopharmacology

Over the past 30 years there have been major advances in the use of medications to treat symptoms of mood disorders. Investigation of the neurobiology of depression and mania has provided directions for development of these new medications. These are discussed in Chapter 23. Because there are multiple types of medications that seem to work with various individuals and their types of depression and mania, selecting the drug and the dosage that is effective for any individual is often a difficult process. Clients who do not respond to one type of medication may do well with another.

Various types of antidepressant medications are used to treat persons with episodes of major depression and some persons with dysthymia. These include tricyclics, heterocyclics, MAOIs, SSRIs, and, most recently, serotonin and norepinephrine reuptake inhibitors. These medications exert powerful effects not only on mood, but also on the entire syndrome of depression symptoms, including the neurovegetative symptoms. Not surprisingly, medications also create side effects that can create discomfort and even danger. Taken in large quantities, many are toxic or even lethal. In addition, these medications usually have a lag period of 1 to 6 weeks for initiation of therapeutic effects, during which time the side effects are often the most pronounced. As the medication begins to exert its therapeutic effect, the side effects often diminish. In view of recent data regarding the recurrent nature of depression and how it impairs functioning over time, many clients are now taking these medications for years, or for an entire lifetime.

Mood stabilizers have been demonstrated to be effective in treating mania in clients with bipolar disorders. The primary, most widely used mood stabilizer is lithium, although anticonvulsants (e.g., carbamazepine, valproate) also appear to promote mood stabilization. Lithium acts as a salt within the body, and its blood levels are closely linked to the client's hydration and sodium intake. The side effects of lithium include neuromuscular and central nervous system effects (tremor, forgetfulness, slowed cognition), gastrointestinal effects (nausea, diarrhea), weight gain and hypothyroidism, and renal effects (polyuria). Blood levels are monitored to ensure an adequate, but not toxic, level. Usually, blood levels of 0.5 to 1.0 mEq/L are appropriate for maintenance therapy, whereas in the treatment of acute mania, levels of up to 1.5 mEq/L are required. The therapeutic-range blood level for lithium is narrow; toxicity can occur quickly and is marked by vomiting, oversedation, ataxia, and, finally, seizures. Lithium blood levels approaching 2.0 are considered toxic. Lithium is excreted through the kidneys and should be used with caution in clients with renal disease. Clients taking lithium should use diuretics only with extreme caution and under close supervision, because diuretics can elevate lithium blood levels quickly.

⚠ CLINICAL ALERT

The nurse must be alert to suicidal ideation and intent with clients with depression and clients with mania who are cycling into depression or whose insight and judgment are impaired. A particularly high-risk time is 1 to 6 weeks after the initiation of antidepressant therapy, before it reaches its full therapeutic effect.

Other medications prescribed for clients during episodes of depression or mania may include benzodiazepines for associated anxiety symptoms, sedative-hypnotics for sleep regulation, and antipsychotics for relief from hallucinations, delusions, and extremely agitated behavior. Although antidepressants and mood stabilizers can assist with minimizing and regulating symptoms related to anxiety and sleep, their therapeutic effects take longer to occur than those of the other medications mentioned here.

Although medications are prescribed by physicians or advanced practice nurses, the nursing care related to administration of psychopharmacologic agents is extensive. The nurse needs to understand the mechanisms of action, dosages (therapeutic), side effects, and self-care considerations of each medication. This enables the nurse to explain the medication to clients and observe for intended and unintended effects. Through teaching clients more about their medications, the nurse promotes and encour-

⚠ CLINICAL ALERT

Foods containing tyramine must be avoided while taking MAOI antidepressants. These include avocados; yogurt; aged cheese; smoked or pickled fish, meat, or poultry; processed meats; yeast; overripe fruit; chicken or beef liver pate; red wine; beer; liqueurs; and fava beans. Foods to use in moderation include caffeine beverages, cottage and cream cheese, soy sauce, chocolate, and sour cream. *Medications* to avoid include over-the-counter cough and cold medicines, appetite suppressants, muscle relaxants, allergy remedies, hay fever remedies, narcotics, analgesics, and several prescription medications. The nurse should ask the client to contact the physician or nurse *before* taking any over-the-counter medication.

ages adherence to the treatment regimen and the minimization of negative effects. Clients are able to discuss their concerns and to make informed decisions about their treatments.

Many of these medications require special considerations that clients must understand to ensure efficacy and safety. Nurses teach clients specific self-care activities associated with medication, such as the required dietary restrictions for MAOIs, precautions regarding hydration and salt intake for lithium, and management of anticholinergic effects of the tricyclics. The Client & Family Teaching Guidelines boxes on this page present teaching plans for clients taking SSRIs and lithium, respectively (also see Chapter 23).

Client & Family TEACHING GUIDELINES

Serotonin Selective Reuptake Inhibitors

Teach the client:

The purpose of SSRIs is to treat depression. The medication alters brain nerve cells, thus increasing the availability of serotonin. A deficiency of serotonin in the brain is believed to be related to the onset of depression.

It is important to take the medication as prescribed; changing the dosage or missing a dose can prevent it from helping the depression.

Common side effects of SSRIs include nausea, increased anxiety, and insomnia. These side effects often diminish once the medication begins to exert its therapeutic effect.

The medication usually does not immediately improve symptoms of depression. It may take 1 to 6 weeks before you feel the effects of the medication. At first, you may still feel depressed but have more energy and look less depressed. These medications often work "from the outside inward."

Biologic Intervention

Electroconvulsive therapy. Electroconvulsive therapy (ECT) involves the use of electrically induced seizures to treat severe depression or, less frequently, intense mania not controlled with lithium or antipsychotics. Research has demonstrated it to be the most effective treatment for

Client & Family TEACHING GUIDELINES

Lithium

Teach the client:

Lithium is a mood stabilizer for persons with mania and depression.

Lithium alters brain neurotransmission, changes cell membrane function, and inhibits release of thyroid hormone. It is not clear how lithium specifically stabilizes mood.

Before lithium is started, laboratory tests are done to ensure adequate functioning of the heart, kidneys, thyroid gland, and electrolytes.

It is important to take lithium daily as prescribed in order to maintain a steady blood level of the medication. Do not take extra doses to make up for missed doses.

Lithium may take a week to begin working and to develop a steady blood level. Your health care provider will have you get your blood drawn to check lithium blood levels. Blood for the lithium level must be drawn about 12 hours after the last dose of lithium (e.g., if you take your dose at 8 PM, your blood level must be drawn at 8 AM).

Common side effects of lithium include increased urine output, increased thirst, fine tremors, muscle weakness, nausea, weight gain, and diarrhea.

Lithium levels can be increased rapidly, leading to toxicity. Signs of toxicity include nausea and vomiting, marked tremors, muscle weakness, muscle twitching, lack of coordination, sluggishness and drowsiness, confusion, seizures, and coma. Toxicity can occur as blood levels approach 2.0.

It is important to maintain a stable blood level of lithium. You should not change the amount of sodium (salt) in your diet, because decreasing salt may increase the amount of lithium in the blood.

Any activity or situation that can affect your fluid and salt intake or output can change the level of lithium in your blood. Exercise, sunbathing, and the flu are examples of situations in which you may perspire and lose salt and fluid, increasing your lithium level. It is important to contact your health care provider if you believe that your lithium level may be changed or if you experience any side effects or early toxic signs.

Other drugs can affect your lithium level. Medications (e.g., diuretics, ibuprofen, verapamil) can raise lithium levels. Be sure to check with your health care provider before taking any new prescribed or over-the-counter medications.

Lithium can cause birth defects if taken during the first trimester of pregnancy. Tell your health care provider if you intend to become pregnant or are pregnant.

psychotic depression (Depression Guideline Panel, 1993). Although ECT was introduced in the 1930s, its use decreased after the discovery of antidepressants and lithium. In recent years procedures have been developed for ECT that make it a safe and effective treatment for many individuals who have not achieved a treatment response with medication or other types of treatment. The exact mechanism by which ECT alleviates depression and mania is unknown, but it is believed to be related to alteration of **neurotransmission**. A complete discussion of ECT is presented in Chapter 23.

Transcranial magnetic stimulation. Transcranial magnetic stimulation (TMS) is an intervention currently being investigated for its antidepressant effects. This is a noninvasive procedure in which an electromagnet is placed on the scalp. Electrical current is generated by rapid oscillations in the magnetic field, causing the cortical neurons to depolarize. Although the specific mechanisms involved in its antidepressant effect remain unclear, this intervention may increase monoamine concentrations in the brain when used repetitively. The initial research has been encouraging with respect to its effects with unipolar depression (George et al, 1997).

Phototherapy. SAD has been identified as a type of mood disorder, and its features are recognized in the DSM-IV classification. Phototherapy is one type of treatment that has effectively lessened symptoms of this recurrent, seasonal disorder. The exact mechanism of action remains unclear, although it is believed that exposure to morning light causes a circadian rhythm shift (phase advance) that regulates the normal relationships between sleep and circadian rhythms.

Clients are referred for phototherapy after a careful and complete psychiatric history that documents the occurrence of SAD. Phototherapy consisting of a minimum of 2500 lux is usually administered on waking in the morning. Clients sit or lie in front of the light box for 30 minutes to several hours, depending on the strength of the light source. An antidepressant effect is usually seen within 2 to 4 days and is complete after 2 weeks. Maintenance therapy consists of sitting in front of the lights for about 30 minutes each day. Side effects are rare, although some clients do report irritability, headaches, or insomnia. Phototherapy is not effective for everyone with a diagnosis of SAD; some fail to respond, and others experience only a partial response. Because phototherapy requires a large amount of time each day, research is in progress that examines alternative methods to acquire the additional light, including the use of light visors and lights that shine onto the bed in early morning before awakening.

Family Intervention
Mood disorders affect the entire family, not just the client who is experiencing the depression or mania. Most often,

the family or significant others become known to the nurse during the client's acute episode of depression or mania. Conflicts and communication problems, which may have existed in the family network before the onset of the episode, become intensified, and the usual role functioning is disrupted.

Nurses in both the hospital and the community interact with the client's family, who often appreciate the opportunity to vent feelings of confusion, anger, concern, or frustration. Teaching family members about the client's disorder, especially the biologic nature of the disorder, allows them to reframe the situation and minimize blame on the client. Many are relieved to hear that their loved one's behavior has an explanation and can be managed. They also find it helpful to know that the client's behavior (e.g., irritability, inability to accept love, and negativity) is not necessarily a personal affront to other family members but may be part of the symptomology of depression or mania. Nurses run family education groups in the hospital and in the community, inviting family and clients to learn more about the disorder and its impact on the family.

Nurses also collaborate with other mental health professionals, including advanced practice nurses, regarding assessing the need for family therapy. Nurses observe client-family interactions, listen to their concerns, and identify potential problem areas. Referrals are made for marital therapy or family therapy that also includes the children.

Interventions that include preparing the family for a client's discharge from the hospital can facilitate the client's return to functioning in the community. Recent data suggest that even after abatement of symptoms, the client who has experienced affective episodes continues to have difficulty in his or her interpersonal and occupational functioning (Klerman and Weissman, 1992).

Group Intervention
Group intervention can provide multiple benefits to clients with mood disorders, including socialization, education about their disorder and more useful coping mechanisms, the opportunity to vent feelings, the establishment of personal goals, and the realization that others have similar problems, thus reducing isolation and hopelessness (see Understanding & Applying Research box.) Nurses assess clients' ability to participate in groups based on their behavior, mental status, psychologic readiness in view of the nature of the particular group, and physiologic status. For example, clients with mania who are hyperactive and extremely agitated are not able to attend to the group discussion and may become overstimulated and disruptive in the group. Clients with severe depression with psychomotor retardation and cognitive impairment may have a difficult time and become overwhelmed by a formal group. Certain types of groups (e.g., a unit community meeting or activities groups) may be less structured and less imposing to clients than formal group therapy.

Understanding & Applying Research

This study examined the number and types of social relationships for 39 women hospitalized for unipolar depression, and the social support and conflict that occur in these relationships. The participants ranged in age from 18 to 65. They were administered the Social Network Questionnaire, the Norbeck Social Support Questionnaire with two additional items measuring conflict, and the Beck Depression Inventory. The participants reported relationships that were similar in amount and diversity to those of nondepressed persons. They also reported higher perceived social support and lower amounts of conflict than expected. Close female relationships appeared to provide the most support without the attached conflict. These findings suggest that depressed women may not be as isolated as presumed and that relationships with close female friends may be an important source of support without the inherent conflict found in relationships with household members.

Pitula CR, Daugherty SR: Sources of social support and conflict in hospitalized depressed women, *Res Nurs Health* 18(2):325, 1995.

In addition to assessing clients' readiness for groups, nurses encourage their attendance at the appropriate functions. Some clients may need to be directed with statements such as, "It's time for group now. I'll walk there with you." Others require only encouragement or reminders.

Nurses who are qualified may conduct groups in conjunction with other nurses or therapists. Nurses may initiate and lead groups, such as social skills training and educational groups. Clients often need to debrief or discuss their experiences and reactions after the completion of a group. Nurses listen, allow ventilation of feelings, and reinforce new insights or perceptions experienced by the clients.

Psychotherapeutic Intervention

Although the effectiveness of antidepressant and mood-stabilizing medications is undisputed, psychotherapeutic interventions are also important in the treatment of mood disorders. Psychopharmacologic agents pose a number of problems for many clients. These medications have major side effects that create discomfort, interfere with usual functioning, and promote noncompliance. Alternative treatment is required for the 20% to 30% of persons with mood disorders who do not respond to medications. Also, although mood disorders represent alterations in neurobiologic functioning, numerous psychologic, social, and interpersonal issues that warrant psychotherapeutic intervention are associated with episodes of depression and mania.

Types of psychotherapy that have been used to treat mood disorders and associated psychosocial issues include cognitive therapy, behavioral therapy, interpersonal relationship therapy, and psychodynamic therapy. Although each of these differs with respect to the underlying theoretic framework, goals, and approach, there are some commonalities. Therapeutic success is related to several factors: the nature of the relationship between the therapist and client; the provision of understanding, support, help, and hope; the establishment of a framework for understanding and interpreting clients' problems; and the provision of an opportunity to explore and try out new coping strategies.

Cognitive therapy. Cognitive therapy, as outlined by Beck (1967), addresses systematic errors in the client's thinking that maintain negative cognitive processing. The goal of the therapy is to identify underlying cognitive schemata and specific cognitive distortions. Schemata are internal models of the self and the world that individuals use to perceive, code, and recall information. Clients are asked to identify their automatic thoughts, silent assumptions, and arbitrary inferences so that negative thoughts and assumptions can be examined logically, challenged against realistic attributes, and subsequently validated or refuted.

Cognitive therapy has been demonstrated to be effective in treating outpatients with unipolar mild to moderate depression. In studies that have investigated the effectiveness of medication versus cognitive therapy, findings indicate that both appear to be equally effective with outpatients with depression and may provide some modest gain when used in combination (Gloaguen et al, 1998; Scott, 1996). In addition, use of cognitive therapy also may increase the rate of symptom improvement in depression, although longer-term follow-up studies fail to find differences over time. The use of cognitive therapy with inpatients experiencing severe depression has not been extensively explored, although there are indications that it may be useful for symptom reduction (Stravynski and Greenberg, 1992).

Behavioral therapy. Behavioral therapy, often used in conjunction with cognitive therapy for treating mild to moderately depressed outpatients, is an effective treatment for depression, comparing favorably with medication and cognitive therapy (Stravynski and Greenberg, 1992). There is less information about its usefulness with persons experiencing mania (Freeman et al, 1990).

The behavioral approach is based on learning theory. Abnormal behaviors such as the symptoms of depression and mania represent behaviors acquired as a result of aversive (negative) environmental events. These are reinforced by positive environmental responses to the maladaptive behaviors or by avoidance of negative consequences. The behavioral therapist works with clients to determine specific behaviors to be modified and to identify the factors that evoke and reinforce these behaviors. Using role modeling, role playing, and situational analysis, clients are assisted in learning and practicing different adaptive behaviors that elicit positive environmental reinforcement. The therapy is not concerned with understanding underlying issues or pathopsychology; it is only concerned with those discrete behaviors that can be modified. Behavioral therapy has several advantages (e.g., shorter treatment duration than other types of therapy, focus on specific behaviors that can be modified) and is applicable to various types of clients.

Interpersonal therapy. The therapist using interpersonal therapy views depression as developing from pathologic, early interpersonal relationship patterns that continue to be repeated in adulthood. The emphasis is on social functioning and interpersonal relationships, with particular emphasis on the milieu. Life events, including change, loss, and relationship conflict, trigger earlier relationship patterns, and the client experiences a sense of failure, decreased importance, and loss. The goal of the therapy is to understand the social context of current problems based on earlier relationships and to provide symptomatic relief by solving or managing current interpersonal problems. The client and the therapist select one or two current interpersonal problems and examine new communication and interpersonal strategies for more effective management of relationships.

Interpersonal therapy has been demonstrated to be effective for clients with mild to moderate depression, although not more so than other types of psychotherapy. Some research suggests that when used in combination with medications, interpersonal therapy may help clients adhere to medication treatment and may lengthen the time between the recovery period and recurrence of a major depression episode (Frank et al, 1991; Klerman, 1990).

CASE STUDY

George, a 48-year-old manager for an insurance company, was admitted to an inpatient psychiatric unit, diagnosed with bipolar I disorder, manic episode. This was his fifth episode of mania since the onset of his disorder 23 years ago. He admitted himself after spending the night in his yard cutting down all of his trees with a chain saw. He had become increasingly active over the past week, driving all over the state to visit insurance colleagues, ordering new office furniture, and announcing that he would be appointed the next president of this national insurance company. George's wife was able to convince him to be hospitalized. George has been pacing in the unit, unable to sit during a meal, intruding in other's conversations, and writing memos to his employees.

Critical Thinking—Outcome Identification

1. What specific information would be assessed by the nurse immediately on George's admission to the unit?
2. Which nursing diagnoses are most relevant for George according to the data?
3. What long- and short-term outcomes might be reasonable to establish with George?

Psychodynamic therapy. Psychodynamic therapy is derived from Freud's psychoanalytic model (see Chapter 3). Depression is viewed as a result of early childhood loss of a love object and ambivalence about the object; introjection of anger onto the ego, resulting in blockage of the libido; and unresolved intrapsychic conflict during the oral or anal stage of psychosexual development. Thus self-esteem is damaged and eroded, with repetition of the primary loss pattern occurring throughout life. Through the relationship with the therapist, the client is helped to uncover repressed experiences, experience catharsis of feelings, confront defenses, interpret current behavior, and work through early loss and cravings for love.

There has been little research on the effect of psychodynamic psychotherapy on depression or mania. Techniques used in this therapy have been modified over time, and there have been problems with standardizing the approach for research purposes. For some clients, psychodynamic psychotherapy assists in developing insights that promote behavioral change. However, many clients, including those with severe depression, may be unable or unmotivated to participate in this type of therapy. For these clients, problems such as self-care deficits, psychomotor retardation, and fatigue assume priority.

EVALUATION

Nurses evaluate clients' progress by measuring their achievement of identified outcomes. Data that support or refute achievement of outcomes are collected from personal observations, clients, clients' family and friends, and other health care providers. Evaluation occurs throughout hospitalization and may be continued by community mental health providers after clients have been discharged. Nurses working in community settings, such as psychiatric home care, may be evaluating outcomes for clients who have never been admitted to an inpatient setting.

With decreasing lengths of stay in hospitals, nurses in inpatient psychiatric units may not see dramatic changes in client's symptoms. However, they must see some clear progress related to priority short-term outcomes, such as absence of imminent suicidal intent, a plan for addressing the potential return of suicidal ideation after discharge, the ability to conduct self-care activities, some alleviation of the neurovegetative symptoms of depression (sleep, loss of appetite, fatigue, psychomotor retardation), alleviation of the severe hyperactive behavior of mania, improvement in cognitive functioning and communication, and initial understanding of the disorder and its treatment, including necessary self-care management. Referrals are made to therapists, psychiatrists, home care and community mental health agencies, and partial hospitalization programs for continued care in the community.

Nurses working with clients in the community see improvement in longer-term outcomes such as improved socialization, return to usual activities, reduction in negative thinking, increased self-esteem, use of new coping strategies, resumption of family/work roles, continued improvement in cognitive processes (e.g., attention and concentration), decreased or absence of fatigue, and adherence to regimens. For some clients, these outcomes become evident within weeks of starting psychotherapy or somatic treatment regimens. For others, improvement may require months before longer-term outcomes are achieved. Recent data suggest that return to previous levels of functioning after an episode of depression takes longer than

previously thought, particularly if clients have had multiple episodes (Klerman and Weissman, 1992).

Clients with mania present a unique evaluative situation, because episodes of mania may be followed by episodes of depression. Therefore, although clients may have returned to a hypomanic or euthymic state at the time of hospital discharge, the nurse should be alert to any indications of depression. Careful follow-up after discharge into the community is imperative for clients with bipolar disorders.

▲ NURSING CARE PLAN

Janice is a 50-year-old woman who has been diagnosed with bipolar disorder since she was 26. She is an English professor at the local university and is on summer break. Three weeks ago, Janice began to stay up all night, writing a novel. Her speech became more rapid and pressured, and she described her thoughts as racing. Her home study was becoming increasingly cluttered, and no one was able to walk into it because of the piles of books, articles, and papers on the floor. She would write for several minutes, pace around the house, then write for several more minutes. She began calling *The New York Times*, telling them that they would want to read the book she was finishing, because it was the best novel ever written. Janice began telling people that she was Louisa May Alcott reincarnated. She spent more than $5000 on new books to build her library. She had not slept more than 2 hours a night for several weeks and had not eaten for 2 days. Janice's husband, Rob, brought her to the psychiatric emergency department for admission. She was angry with him,

insisting that he was interfering with her work. On admission to the unit, she exhibited pacing, flight of ideas, pressured speech, and angry, rude, and intrusive behavior. She was dressed in a short red skirt, pink low-cut blouse, and a yellow straw hat, and she was barefoot. Janice wore heavy, bright makeup and changed her clothes up to 15 times each day. She was given lithium 300 mg qid and haloperidol (Haldol) 5 mg bid. She had been on a regimen of lithium, but stopped taking the medication 4 months ago after becoming concerned about its long-term effects.

DSM-IV Diagnoses

Axis I:	Bipolar I disorder, current episode, manic
Axis II:	Deferred
Axis III:	Rule out dehydration
Axis IV:	Severity of psychosocial stressors: moderate
Axis V:	GAF = 25 (current)
	GAF = 78 (past year)

Nursing Diagnosis: Self-care deficit (dressing/grooming, feeding) related to manic hyperactivity and difficulty concentrating and making decisions, as evidenced by inappropriate dress and dysfunctional eating patterns.

Client Outcomes
- Janice will dress self appropriately for age and status.
- Janice will eat and drink adequately to sustain fluid balance and proper nutrition.

Nursing Interventions
- Offer assistance in selecting clothing and in grooming *to provide input and direction for appropriateness of dress and hygiene to preserve self-esteem and avoid embarrassment.*
- Encourage and remind Janice to drink fluids and eat nutritious food *to focus the client on necessary feeding activities to prevent dehydration and starvation.*
- Offer Janice beverages in easy-to-carry containers and nutritious, high-protein, high-calorie finger foods *to provide important nutrients and fluids in a way that the client is able to eat and drink, because she is unable to sit and complete a meal.*
- Reduce environmental stimulation, such as noise or the presence of other people, during self-care times (e.g., have the client eat meals alone in her room rather than in the dining room). *Decreased stimulation allows for better concentration on tasks.*
- Provide recognition and positive reinforcement for feeding and dressing/grooming accomplishments *to reinforce appropriate behaviors and enhance self-esteem.*

Evaluation
- Janice dresses self appropriately and maintains hygiene.
- Janice eats and drinks fluids necessary to maintain physical health.

Continued

NURSING CARE PLAN —cont'd

Nursing Diagnosis: Coping, defensive, related to impaired self-concept and unrealistic perceptions of self, secondary to manic episode, as evidenced by intrusive and disruptive behavior, grandiosity, anger, impulsivity, and excessive use of makeup and inappropriate clothing.

Client Outcomes

- Janice will refrain from interrupting and disrupting activities and conversations of others.
- Janice will adhere to established limits and expectations.
- Janice will realistically discuss her thoughts, feelings, and behaviors.

Nursing Interventions

- Continue to state the rules and expectations of the unit in a calm, matter-of-fact way. *A nonthreatening manner is better tolerated by a client with mania, and repetition of rules and expectations may be needed as a result of impaired concentration and impulsivity.*
- Praise the client for statements about realistic self-appraisal and adherence to expectations *to provide support, positive reinforcement, and learning.*
- Establish any necessary limits in a calm, matter-of-fact, nonpunitive way *to prevent alienation from the client and assist in regaining control.*
- Provide opportunities for the client to interact with others in ways that are manageable, such as short activities, *to help the client to focus, prevent overstimulation, and provide opportunity for support and reality testing.*
- As the client improves, encourage expression of feelings, beliefs, and actions *to assist the client in gaining insight and appropriately expressing feelings.*

Evaluation

- Janice stated unit rules and expectations.
- Janice stopped intrusive, disruptive behaviors and adhered to expectations and unit rules.
- Janice was able to discuss her self-perceptions in a nongrandiose manner and related feelings she was experiencing.

Nursing Diagnosis: Thought processes, altered, related to psychomotor hyperactivity, ineffective processing of internal and external stimuli, anxiety, and psychosocial stresses, secondary to biologic disruption of neurotransmission, as evidenced by flight of ideas, grandiosity, and impaired judgment and decision making.

Client Outcomes

- Janice will demonstrate logical and coherent flow of thoughts, with the absence of delusion of grandeur.
- Janice will demonstrate appropriate decision making and judgment.

Nursing Interventions

- Demonstrate concern and acceptance of the client's underlying feelings while not overtly agreeing with the client's delusion of grandeur *to promote trust and self-esteem but not reinforce the delusion.*
- Listen for themes, feelings, and meanings behind the client's words and reflect on those *to build trust, demonstrate understanding, and reinforce reality and expression of feelings.*
- Redirect the client to here-and-now activities and topics *to provide a reality-oriented focus.*
- Praise the client for expressing doubt about her delusion and for attempting to focus thoughts in a more logical, relevant manner *to promote self-esteem and reality-based thinking.*
- Relate to the client with simple, concrete, here-and-now words and interactions, avoiding abstractions. *Simple, direct, and clear communication can be better understood.*
- Teach the client about lithium, including its action, therapeutic effects, side effects, dosage, and importance in controlling mood, *because information promotes compliance.*

Evaluation

- Janice was able to express herself logically and clearly, acknowledging that she was not a famous author (e.g., Louisa May Alcott).
- Janice expressed a desire to remain in the hospital until her mania was better controlled and stated that she understood why her husband had brought her to the hospital.

▲ NURSING CARE PLAN —*cont'd*

Nursing Diagnosis: Noncompliance (medication regimen) related to knowledge deficit and belief system, as evidenced by failure to continue lithium as prescribed.

Client Outcomes	Nursing Interventions	Evaluation
• Janice will adhere to the medication regimen, taking medications as prescribed. • Janice will discuss her feelings about lithium and her bipolar disorder.	• Teach the client about bipolar disorder and the need for lifelong management *because information promotes compliance.* • Teach the client about lithium and other medications as needed *because information promotes adherence.* • Discuss with the client her feelings about lithium and having a lifelong disorder requiring medication management *to provide an opportunity to express feelings and beliefs about medication and bipolar disorder.*	• Janice expressed the importance of taking her lithium and agreed to stay on the medication. • Her lithium blood level 2 weeks after discharge was 0.95. • Janice discussed her feelings about lithium and her disorder.

Summary of Key Concepts

1. Mood disorders are a major public health problem, and depression has been identified as the fourth leading cause of "burden," including morbidity and mortality, in the world.
2. Major depression is currently occurring at younger ages, and those most at risk are women with a family history of mood disorders.
3. Mood disorders are usually recurrent and require lifelong management.
4. Two broad types of mood disorders include unipolar depressive and bipolar disorders.
5. Mood disorders are explained by multiple theories, including biologic, cognitive, psychodynamic, and personality theories. Mood disorders are probably caused by the interaction of multiple factors, including a genetic, biologic predisposition for risk.
6. Mania and depression are manifested by symptoms involving the affective, cognitive, physical, social, and spiritual aspects of the individual.
7. The nursing care of persons experiencing depression or mania consists of thorough assessment and subsequent planning and interventions for an array of nursing diagnoses related to physical, psychosocial, and spiritual needs.
8. Nurses collaborate with other mental health care providers for care related to somatic, family, and group interventions.

REFERENCES

Abramson LY, Melalsy GI, Alloy LB: Hopelessness depression: a theory-based type of depression, *Psychol Rev* 93:358, 1989.

Abramson LY, Seligman MEP, Teasdale JD: Learned helplessness in humans: critique and reformulation, *Abnorm Psychol* 87:49, 1978.

Akiskal HS: New insights into the nature and heterogeneity of mood disorders, *J Clin Psychiatry* 50:6, 1989.

American Psychiatric Association: *Diagnostic and statistical manual of mental disorders*, ed 4, Washington, DC, 1994, The Association.

American Psychiatric Association Task Force: The dexamethasone suppression test: an overview of its current status in psychiatry, *Am J Psychiatry* 144:1253, 1987.

Angst J: Clinical course of affective disorders. In Helgason T, Daly R, editors: *Depressive illness: prediction of course and outcome*, Berlin, Germany, 1988, Springer-Verlag.

Barondes S: *Molecules and mental illness*, New York, 1993, Scientific American Library.

Barondes S: *Mood genes: hunting for the origins of mania and depression*, New York, 1998, WH Freeman.

Beck AT: *Depression: clinical, experiential, and theoretical aspects*, New York, 1967, Hober.

Boulby J: *Attachment*, New York, 1969, Basic Books.

Boyce P et al: Personality as a vulnerability factor to depression, *Br J Psychiatry* 159:106, 1991.

Brown GW, Harris T: *Social origins of depression*, New York, 1978, The Free Press.

Consensus Development Panel: Mood disorders: pharmacological prevention of recurrences, *Am J Psychiatry* 142:469, 1985.

Cornelis CM, Ameling EH, Delonghe F: Life events and social network in relation to the onset of depression, *Acta Psychiatr Scand* 80:174, 1989.

Depression Guideline Panel: *Depression in primary care*, vol 1, *Detection and diagnosis*, Washington DC, 1993, U.S. Department of Health and Human Services, Agency for Health Care Policy and Research.

Diehl DJ, Gershon S: The role of dopamine in mental disorders, *Compr Psychiatry* 33:115, 1992.

Ehlers CL, Frank E, Kupfer DJ: Social zeitgebers and biological rhythms: a unified approach to understanding the etiology of depression, *Arch Gen Psychiatry* 45:948, 1988.

Frank E et al: Efficacy of interpersonal psychotherapy as a maintenance treatment of recurrent depression. *Arch Gen Psychiatry* 48:1053, 1991.

Freeman A et al: *Clinical applications of cognitive therapy*, New York, 1990, Plenum Press.

Freud S: Mourning and melancholia. In *The complete psychological works of Sigmund Freud*, London, 1957, Hogarth Press.

Fuller RW: Role of serotonin in therapy of depression and related disorders, *J Clin Psychiatry* 52:52, 1991.

George MS et al: Mood improvement following daily left prefrontal repetitive transcranial magnetic stimulation in patients with depression: a placebo-controlled crossover trial, *Am J Psychiatry* 154:1752, 1997.

Gloaguen V et al: A meta-analysis of the effects of cognitive therapy in depressed patients, *J Affect Disord* 49:59, 1998.

Greden JF: *Recurrent depression*, Indianapolis, 1993, Dista Products.

Hagerty BM et al: Prodromal symptoms of recurrent major depressive episodes: a qualitative analysis, *Am J Orthopsychiatry* 67:308, 1997.

Hirshfeld RMA et al: Premorbid personality assessments of first onset of major depression, *Arch Gen Psychiatry* 46:345, 1989.

Horwath E et al: Depressive symptoms as relative and attributable risk factors for first onset major depression, *Arch Gen Psychiatry* 49:817, 1992.

Keller MB: The course of manic-depressive illness, *Clin Psychiatry* 49:4, 1988.

Kendler KS et al: The identification and validation of distinct depressive syndromes in a population-based sample of female twins, *Arch Gen Psychiatry*:391, 1996.

Kessler RC et al: Lifetime and 12-month prevalence of DSM-IIIR psychiatric disorders in the U.S., *Arch Gen Psychiatry* 51:8, 1994.

Klerman GL: Treatment of recurrent unipolar major depressive disorder, *Arch Gen Psychiatry* 47:1158-1162, 1990.

Klerman GL, Weissman MM: The course, morbidity, and costs of depression, *Arch Gen Psychiatry* 49:831, 1992.

Kraepelin E: *Lectures in clinical psychiatry*, London, 1913, Bailliere, Tindall, & Cox.

Kraepelin E: *Manic-depressive insanity and paranoia*, Edinburgh, UK, 1921, E & S Livingstone.

Leonard BE: Biochemical aspects of treatment-resistant depression, *Br J Psychiatry* 152:453, 1988.

Leonhard K: Aufteilung der endogenen Psychosen. Cited in Buher J: *Depression: theory and research*, New York, 1974, Winston Wiley.

Lewinsohn PM et al: Age cohort changes in the lifetime occurrence of depression and other mental disorders, *J Abnorm Psychiatry* 102:110, 1993.

McGriffin P, Katz R: The genetics of depression: current approaches, *Br J Psychiatry* 155:18, 1989.

McPherson H, Herbison P, Romans S: Life events and relapse in established bipolar affective disorder, *Br J Psychiatry* 157:381, 1993.

Murray CJL, Lopez AD: *The global burden of disease: a comprehensive assessment of mortality and disability from diseases, injuries, and risk factors in 1990 and projected*, Boston, 1996, Harvard University Press.

Nolen-Hoeksema S: Sex differences in unipolar women: evidence and theory, *Psychol Bull* 101(2):259, 1987.

North American Nursing Diagnosis Association: *NANDA nursing diagnoses: definitions and classifications 1999-2000*, Philadelphia, 1999, The Association.

Paykel ES: Recent life events in the development of the depressive disorder. In Depue RA, editor: *The psychobiology of the depressive disorders: implications for the effects of stress*, New York, 1979, Academic Press.

Phillips KA et al: A review of the depressive personality, *Am J Psychiatry* 147:830, 1990.

Pilgrim JA et al: Low blood pressure, low mood? *Br Med J* 304:75, 1992.

Pitula CR, Daugherty SR: Sources of social support and conflict in hospitalized depressed women, *Res Nurs Health* 18(2):325, 1995.

Post RM: Transduction of psychosocial stress in the neurobiology of recurrent affective disorders, *Am J Psychiatry* 149:999, 1992.

Post RM: Molecular biology of behavior, *Arch Gen Psychiatry*, 607, 1997.

Robins CJ, Hayes AM: An appraisal of cognitive therapy, *J Consult Clin Psychol* 61:205, 1993.

Sargeant JK et al: Factors associated with 1-year outcome of major depression in the community, *Arch Gen Psychiatry* 47:519, 1990.

Schmaling K, Becker J: Empirical studies of the interpersonal relations of adult depressives. In Becker J, Kleinman D, editors: *Psychosocial aspects of depression*, Hillsdale, NJ, 1991, Lawrence Erlbaum.

Scott J: Cognitive therapy of affective disorders: a review, *J Affect Disord* 37:1, 1996.

Seligman MEP: *Helplessness: on depression development and death*, New York, 1975, WH Freeman.

Stravynski A, Greenberg D: The psychological management of depression, *Acta Psychiatr Scand* 85:407, 1992.

Thase ME: Long-term treatment of recurrent depressive disorders, *J Clin Psychiatry* 53:32, 1992.

Tweed DL: Depression-related impairment: estimating concurrent and lingering effects, *Psychol Med* 23:373, 1993.

Young EA et al: Dissociation between pituitary and adrenal suppression to dexamethasone in depression, *Arch Gen Psychiatry* 50:395, 1993.

Zimmerman M, Coryell W, Pfohl B: The validity of the DST as a maker for endogenous depression, *Arch Gen Psychiatry* 43:347, 1986.

CHAPTER 14

The Schizophrenias

Katherine M. Fortinash

OBJECTIVES

- Explain the various theories and models that evolved over the years to describe the schizophrenic disorders.

- Discuss the various assessment tools and data currently available for medical and nursing diagnoses of the schizophrenias.

- Apply the nursing process to clients experiencing the negative and positive symptoms of schizophrenia.

- Differentiate the nursing responsibilities in the care of clients with schizophrenia from those of other disciplines, and compare and contrast the approaches.

- Appraise the situation of persons with schizophrenia and their families in the community, developing nursing care plans for prevention, aftercare, and education.

- Compare and contrast the course of illness, symptomatology, and nursing interventions for the subtypes of schizophrenia and for the closely related disorders, such as schizoaffective disorder.

- Describe the major differences between typical and atypical antipsychotic medications, particularly in regard to their effects on the negative symptoms of schizophrenia, such as apathy and impaired social skills.

- Evaluate the effectiveness of the various treatment modalities in the clinical setting.

Affect Outward, bodily expression of emotions, ranging from joy to sorrow to anger. **Blunted affect:** Restricted expression of emotions. **Flat affect:** Lack of outward expression of emotions. **Inappropriate affect:** Affect that is not congruent with the emotion being felt (e.g., laughing when feeling sad). **Labile affect:** Rapid changes in emotional expression.

Agnosia Inability to recognize familiar environmental stimuli such as sounds or objects seen or felt.

Ambivalence Simultaneously holding two different attitudes, emotions, thoughts, or feelings about a person, object, or situation.

Autistic thinking Disturbances in thought due to the intrusion of a private fantasy world that is internally stimulated, resulting in abnormal responses to people and events in the real world.

Delusions False beliefs held by a person that are fixed and resistant to logic or reasoning.

Dereism A loss of connection with reality and logic that occurs just before autistic thinking. Thoughts become private and idiosyncratic. Dereism is seen in schizophrenia.

Double-bind A situation in which contradictory messages are given to one person by another, demanding a response or choice between two opposing alternatives.

Flight of ideas An abrupt change of topics that are expressed in a rapid flow of speech. It may be seen in schizophrenia but is more common in the manic phase of bipolar disorder. It is more reality based than loosening of associations (LOA) and can be a response to stressful stimuli.

Hallucination A subjective disorder of sensory perception in which one of the five senses is involved, in the absence of external stimulation.

Loosening of associations (LOA) Thought disturbance in which the speaker rapidly shifts expression of ideas from one subject to another in an unrelated manner. Most commonly noted in schizophrenia.

Negative symptoms Syndrome that includes flat affect, poverty of speech, poor grooming, withdrawal, and disturbance in volition.

Perseveration A disturbance in thought association in which there is a persistent repetition of the same idea in response to different questions.

Positive symptoms Syndrome that includes hallucinations, increased speech production with loose associations, and bizarre behavior.

Poverty of thought A psychopathologic thought disturbance in schizophrenia. The client's inability to think logically and sequentially is reflected in **poverty of content of speech,** which is vague, repetitious, and disconnected.

Premorbid Period just preceding the onset of a mental illness. Characteristics of the personality may indicate the type of disorder that may occur.

Primary process thinking Prelogical thought that aims for wish fulfillment. It is associated with the pleasure principle characteristic of the *id* portion of the personality.

Prodromal symptoms Early symptoms, such as a deterioration in functioning, that may mark the onset of a mental illness.

Psychosis Inability to recognize reality or bizarre behaviors or to deal with life's demands.

Residual symptoms Minor disturbances that may remain after an episode of schizophrenia but do not include delusions, hallucinations, incoherence, or gross disorganization.

Schizoaffective disorder A disorder closely related to schizophrenia, with a typical age of onset in early adulthood, although it can occur any time from adolescence to late in life. Essential to the diagnosis are an uninterrupted period of illness during which there is an episode of either major depression, mania, or a mixed episode; delusions or hallucinations for at least 2 weeks in the absence of prominent mood symptoms; and mood symptoms throughout most of the illness.

Thought blocking Abrupt interruption in the flow of thoughts or ideas due to a disturbance in the speed of associations.

Schizophrenia is a condition that exists in all cultures and in all socioeconomic groups (Betemps and Ragiel, 1994; Kaplan and Sadock, 1998). Despite their prevalence, the schizophrenias have not had the benefit of a scientific, biologic approach until the midnineteenth century.

Research supporting the relationship of these complex disorders with the structure and function of the brain cautiously offers hope for more effective treatment.

HISTORICAL AND THEORETIC PERSPECTIVES

If space is the last frontier in exploration of the universe, then schizophrenia is the last frontier in medical science discoveries. Until recently, little was known about the cognitive functioning of the brain. The term *schizophrenia* has been used to describe a particular form of mental illness only since the mid-1800s (Arieti, 1974).

Clients with schizophrenia are particularly troubling for society because of their overt **psychosis,** a state in which one's capacity to recognize reality is limited or absent, resulting in an impaired ability to deal with life's demands. The earliest knowledge about recognition and treatment of psychotic disorders comes from artifacts and cave drawings from the Stone Age, a half million years ago. The earliest writings on the subject date to the Sanskrit (an ancient Indo-European language) of 1400 BC. The notion of possession by demons persisted as early civilizations developed, as noted in the early writings of the Hebrews, Egyptians, Chinese, and Greeks.

Two prominent psychiatrists in the nineteenth century made progress related to symptoms now associated with the schizophrenias. The first was Emil Kraepelin (1856-1926), who described *dementia praecox,* a syndrome characterized by **hallucinations** (a subjective disorder of sensory perception involving any one of the five senses in the absence of external stimulation) and **delusions** (false beliefs that are fixed and resistant to logic or reasoning).

The second major psychiatrist, Eugen Bleuler (1857-1939), saw the inconsistency between emotion, thought, and behavior noted in the client with schizophrenia. He introduced the term *schizophrenia,* which means "split minded." The "split," however, refers only to emotion, thought, and behavior, not to personality, and should not be confused with dissociative identity disorder (see Chapter 12). He also further refined the description by calling it a *thought disorder* with fundamental symptoms, known as Bleuler's four *A*'s:

- **Loosening of associations (LOA):** Thought disturbance in which the speaker rapidly changes from one subject to another in an unrelated fragmented manner
- Disturbances of **affect:** Observable, outward, bodily expression of emotions, such as joy, sorrow, and anger.

Blunted affect: Restricted expression of emotions
Flat affect: Lack of expression of emotions
Inappropriate affect: Affect that is not congruent with the emotion being felt (e.g., laughing when sad)
Labile affect: Rapid changes in emotional expression
- **Ambivalence:** Simultaneously holding two different attitudes, emotions, thoughts, or feelings about a person, object, or situation
- **Autistic thinking:** Disturbances in thought due to the intrusion of a private fantasy world that is internally stimulated, resulting in abnormal responses to people and events in the real world

In addition, Bleuler named hallucinations and delusions as accessory symptoms to the syndrome (Kaplan and Sadock, 1994).

Sullivan, a social learning theorist, emphasized the importance of interpersonal relationships and believed that social isolation was the key in schizophrenia. Schneider described various delusional and hallucinatory experiences as first-rank symptoms and less decisive symptoms (such as perceptual disturbances, confusion, mood changes, and emotional impoverishment), as second-rank symptoms (Kaplan and Sadock, 1998).

ETIOLOGY

The foremost etiology of schizophrenia today is the biologic perspective. This includes not only the traditional medical model that stresses chemical management (medication), but also the new discoveries of genetic influences; the role of neuroanatomy, endocrinology, and immunology in producing symptoms; and the issues of trauma and disease in causation. Declaring brain research as one of the truly great frontiers of science, Congress designated the decade beginning January 1, 1990, as the "Decade of the Brain." This designation has renewed interest in schizophrenia as a disease. The research being generated in this decade presents a strong challenge for nurses, who now must integrate the biologic sciences with the caring concepts of the psychosocial models. Box 14-1 lists etiologic factors.

BIOLOGIC FACTORS

Several early twentieth-century theorists favored biologic factors as causes for schizophrenia. Hans Selye (1936) was a successful pioneer with his work on the general adaptation syndrome (GAS). Selye demonstrated that the phases of alarm, resistance, and exhaustion following stress were related in a causal manner to several physiologic disease states (e.g., hypertension and peptic ulcer) (McCain and Smith, 1994). Extensive research on the neuroendocrine mechanisms underlying the stress response also influenced the psychiatrists as a possible explanation of several forms of psychotic states. This foundation remains a part of the theoretic framework explaining psychopathology

| Box 14-1 | Etiologic Factors |

Biologic Factors
Heredity and genetics
Neuroanatomics and neurochemicals
  Structure and function of the nervous system
  Teratogenic drug exposure
  Neuroanatomic differences in the brain
Neurotransmitter function
  Abnormal neurotransmitter-endocrine interactions
Immunologic factors
  Viral exposure in pregnancy
High arousal levels from stress, disease, trauma, and drugs
  Stress such as a bombardment of stimuli from life events
  Diseases such as prenatal virus exposure and encephalitis
  Trauma from obstetric complications, head trauma, and childhood accidents
  Drugs such as cannabis and cocaine

Psychoanalytic and Developmental Factors
Distortions in the mother-child relationship
Ego disorganization
Faulty reality interpretation

Familial Factors
Repressed unhappiness
Double-bind patterns
Marital schism of parents
Destructive, expressed emotion communication patterns

Cultural and Environmental Theories
Low socioeconomic status
Lessened social support of family and community; changes in social roles

Learning Theories and Behavioral Models
Irrational problem-solving methods, distorted thinking, and deficient communication patterns learned from parents
Generalized social interactions

Theories of Psychophysiologic Effects of the Environment
Toxic substances (selenium) in the atmospheric pollution

4. The immunologic model
5. The stress/disease/trauma causation model

Heredity and Genetic Influences
There are two ways of looking at a possible connection between heredity and schizophrenia. One is related to the well-known twin study in 1953, an early example of the epidemiologic potential for the occurrence of schizophrenia among related individuals. The research statistics have been challenged, and later studies have shown a lower incidence of schizophrenia among first-degree relatives than the 86% that was initially predicted. However, the lifetime risk of developing schizophrenia when one has a parent, identical twin, or sibling with schizophrenia is much higher (46% for an identical twin of a person with schizophrenia and 10% for a sibling) than in the population at large (1% for an unrelated person). In Figure 14-1, magnetic resonance imaging (MRI) scans compare the size of brain ventricles in identical twins, one who has schizophrenia and one who does not.

Recent studies in genetic epidemiology support the theme of familial transmission, although how it occurs is not known (Malone, 1990; Shore, 1989). Evidence shows that there are multiple correlated risk factors that are important in susceptibility, although inheritance is regarded as the most important component.

The search for a major gene or gene sites consistent with schizophrenia (Tsuang, 1994) is another area of study. A major goal at the Salk Institute for Biological Studies in La Jolla, California, is to produce a map of the human genetic structure that will isolate and identify all of the genes (50,000 to 100,000) in the human cell nucleus.

Currently, about 5000 genes have been identified, with about 2000 mapped on the chromosomes. Although a linkage to schizophrenia was established by one researcher from a genetic anomaly on chromosome 5, the finding was controversial because further analyses failed to support inheritance of schizophrenic tendencies through a single major gene.

Neuroanatomic and Neurochemical Factors
There have been many recent advances in the study of neuroanatomic and neurochemical factors as they relate to schizophrenia. Starting with the work of Plum (1972), Crow (1980), and others, the field has expanded to include the study of the human nervous system from the perspectives of physiology, chemistry, and endocrinology (Hemsley et al, 1993; Joseph, 1993). Also, the immune system may be involved in schizophrenia (Lieberman and Koreen, 1993; Tsuang, 1994).

Structural and functional factors. The structure of the nervous system may include both gross and microanatomic defects, possibly resulting from a congenital developmental condition (Benes, 1993; Bogerts, 1993; Cannon and Marco, 1994). Other researchers have called attention

even today, and a part of the stress and adaptation theories used in psychiatric nursing (e.g., Roy's adaptation model).

Five biologic models have been expanded or changed as a result of recent research:

1. The heredity/genetic model
2. The neuroanatomic and neurochemical model
3. Neurotransmitters and the dopamine hypothesis

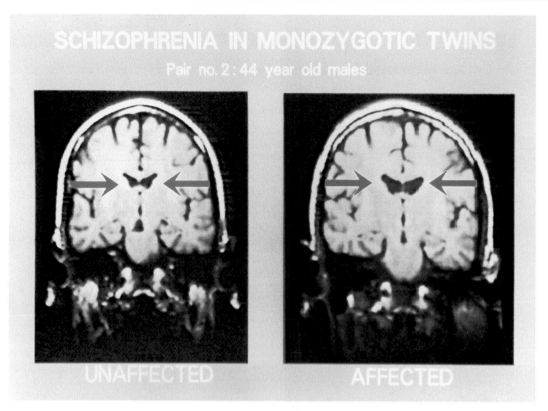

Figure 14-1   Loss of brain volume associated with schizophrenia is clearly shown by magnetic resonance imaging (MRI) scans comparing the size of ventricles (butterfly-shaped, fluid-filled spaces in the midbrain) of identical twins, one of whom has schizophrenia *(right)*. The ventricles of the person with schizophrenia are larger. (Courtesy National Institute of Mental Health, Biological Psychiatry Branch, U.S. Department of Health and Human Services.)

to teratogenic drug exposure in utero or to birth trauma, leading to gradual deteriorative changes that seem to affect many clients with chronic schizophrenia. Both of these notions may be part of a faulty developmental pattern.

With the help of electroencephalograms (EEGs) and the new brain imaging techniques available today, it has been found that ventricular enlargement, prominence of cortical sulci, defects in limbic brain structures, and cortical atrophy occur and are usually more pronounced in the left hemisphere. Smaller cerebrums and frontal lobes are noted in clients with chronic schizophrenia. Specifically, there are subtle neuroanatomic differences in parts of the thalamus, septum, hypothalamus, hippocampus, amygdala, and cingulate gyrus in the brains of these clients when compared with the brains of unaffected persons (Bogerts, 1993; Cannon and Marco, 1994; Joseph, 1993) (see Figure 14-1).

Physiologically, there is a decrease in metabolic activity and slower brain waves in the frontal lobes (Malone, 1990). At the micro level, changes in neurotransmitter activity at the synaptic junctions between the nerve cells lead to abnormalities in the brain circuits (Benes, 1993; Cannon and Marco, 1994). It is difficult to establish the relationship between neuron damage and functional impairment, but Previc (1993) maintains that the visual-perceptual and visual-motor functions of the brain, situated in the posterior parietal lobes, are affected in individuals with schizophrenia. Consequently, they manifest poor audiovisual integration, spatial orientation difficulties, prolonged reaction time responses, accommodation problems, and distortions in perceived body image. Some clients with schizophrenia cannot tell whether another person is looking at them or not, and then always think the person is, as a result of eye tracking dysfunctions (Clementz, McDowell, and Zisook, 1994). To cite another specific relationship, Hemsley et al (1993) believe that hippocampal lesions can cause learning failure and an inability to differentiate between meaningless and meaningful information. These are only two examples of the functional difficulties encountered by clients as a result of damage in neuron structures (see Understanding & Applying Research box).

Neurotransmitters and the Dopamine Hypothesis

Although there are many neurotransmitters involved in brain and body activity, seven are known to be of special importance in schizophrenia: dopamine, serotonin, acetylcholine, norepinephrine, cholecystokinin, glutamate, and γ-aminobutyric acid (GABA). Their types and functions are shown in Table 14-1.

Theories about schizophrenia and the role of neuro-transmitters include:

A serotonin deficiency may be responsible for some forms of schizophrenia.

Norepinephrine may be insufficient in clients with schizophrenia displaying anhedonia.

The dopamine hypothesis, explained in Table 14-1.

The dopamine hypothesis is the major neurotransmitter hypothesis for schizophrenia. Dopamine affects mood, affect, thoughts, and motor behavior. Too much dopamine could result in psychosis, and not enough could cause movement disorders. Recently this theory has been challenged as being limited in scope. There is evidence that other neurotransmitters are also involved, either alone or in interactions with dopamine neural systems (Joseph, 1993; Kaplan and Sadock, 1998; Lieberman and Koreen, 1993; Previc, 1993). The dopamine theory states that there is too much dopamine in schizophrenia. This is supported by postmortem data showing that in schizophrenia the numbers of dopamine receptors are increased by two thirds. Also, the positive effects of the older antipsychotic drugs were due to their action as dopamine antagonists, blocking the dopamine receptors (Figure 14-2) so that less dopamine was available, thus reducing the client's psychosis.

One of the newer antipsychotic drugs, clozapine, is more selective in which receptors it blocks. It also decreases psychosis but does not produce movement disorders as the older drugs do (Lieberman and Koreen, 1993). Other dopamine receptors, have been investigated in recent years but were not found to be associated with the presence of schizophrenia (Macciardi et al, 1994; Sabate et al, 1994). In all studies, there is no clear evidence of do-

Understanding & Applying Research

The purpose of this study was to monitor the brain activity of clients with schizophrenia, through the use of positive emission tomography (PET) scanning of the brain, during episodes of hallucinations (sensory perceptual alterations). The experiment involved six clients who reported hearing "voices" that were relentless and demeaning in nature, which they could not control. Using the PET scan, a picture was taken every 10 seconds until a photo album of the brain during active hallucinations was accomplished. A total of 744 pictures were taken on the first client, with the experiment repeated on the remaining five participants, all yielding dramatic results. Researchers believe that a window on the workings of the diseased mind may be opened, which could eventually lead to better treatments. In an article published in *Nature* magazine, a team of U.S. and British researchers reported that they had pinpointed brain circuits that seemed to control the auditory and visual hallucinations of schizophrenia. Dr. David Silbersweig at New York Hospital–Cornell Medical Center was quoted as saying, "We've identified the areas that are responsible for the brain creating its own reality." The new research suggests that hallucinations are jointly generated by the brain's deep structures that regulate thinking and emotions, and surface regions that process sights and sounds. Dr. Silbersweig says that by integrating fleeting voices and visions with emotion, the schizophrenic brain may give these simulacra an acute sense of reality. This discovery may eventually help to tailor medications. The findings cast doubt on one theory—that hallucinating clients are actually talking to themselves. The brain scans found activity in the areas responsible for hearing but not in those involved in speech.

Mattos J: Science—brain work, pictures shed light on the mystery of schizophrenia, *Time Magazine* 146(21), 1995; reporting on a study by U.S. and British researchers, led by Dr. David Silbersweig, New York Hospital–Cornell Medical Center.

Table 14-1	Neurotransmitters in Schizophrenia: Type and Function	
Neurotransmitter	**Type**	**Function**
Dopamine	Catecholamine	Regulates motor behavior and also transmits in the cortex Increases vigilance; may increase aggressive behavior
Serotonin	Indolamine	Brain stem transmitter Modulates mood, lowers aggressive tendencies
Acetylcholine	Cholinergic	Transmits at nerve-muscle connections (central nervous system and autonomic nervous system) A deficiency may increase confusion and acting-out behavior Controls extrapyramidal symptoms (EPS)
Norepinephrine	Catecholamine	Transmits in the sympathetic nervous system; induces hypervigilance: "fight or flight" syndrome
Cholecystokinin	Peptide	Excites limbic neurons; a deficiency is related to avolition and flat affect
Glutamate	Amino acid	Excitatory neurotransmitter
γ-aminobutyric acid (GABA)	Amino acid	Inhibitory neurotransmitter (predominant brain transmitter)

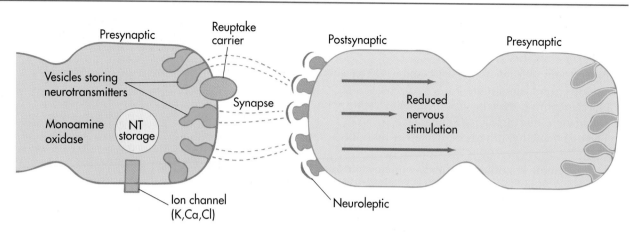

Figure 14-2 Neuroleptic action. Neurotransmitter action at the synapse is modified by neuroleptics, which block postsynaptic receptor sites to reduce nervous stimulation.

pamine abnormalities, but the refined hypothesis continues to generate interest in researching the involvement of the neurotransmitters and neuroendocrine systems in schizophrenia (Joseph, 1993; vanKarmen et al, 1994).

Neurotransmitter-endocrine interactions. Human behavior, thoughts, and feelings are also influenced by a much larger and more complex component, the endocrine system. Schizophrenia has been linked to abnormal neurotransmitter and neuroendocrine interactions (Benes, 1993; Hemsley et al, 1993; Lieberman and Koreen, 1993; Malone, 1990). For example, although direct evidence of serotonal dysfunction has not been obtained, the antipsychotic drugs clozapine and risperidone owe their unique therapeutic effects to their influence on dopamine and the serotonin receptors in the frontal cortex. The role of GABA in schizophrenia promotes a balance of dopamine and glutamate and thus inhibits impulsive behaviors.

Several recent studies have examined not only neurotransmitter interactions in schizophrenia, but also the effect of interactions between hormones and neurotransmitters. Patterns of dopamine-thyroid interactions and dopamine–pituitary hormone secretions were found to be consistent with schizophrenia symptoms. Other patterns involved β-endorphins and other opioid compounds, cholecystokinin and other neuropeptides, in interaction with dopamine. In addition, abnormal composition and structure of neuronal membranes may also contribute to schizophrenic symptoms (Lieberman and Koreen, 1993).

Presently, the studies of neurochemistry and neuroendocrinology are fragmentary but show promise. It is clear that the patterns and balance between the neurotransmitter and neuroendocrine systems in schizophrenia are distinctly different from those of unaffected individuals.

IMMUNOLOGIC FACTORS

Viral exposure, particularly exposure to influenza during pregnancy, is a risk factor for schizophrenia. It is theorized that the influenza virus may create maternal antibodies. In the fetus these become autoantibodies, which are an external source of developmental change (Cannon and Marco, 1994; Malone, 1990; Takei et al, 1994; Tsuang, 1994). There are few immunologic studies of schizophrenia, and they depend on epidemiologic data for their hypotheses.

Stress, Disease, Trauma, and Drug Abuse

In Selye's stress model, the individual was seen as interacting with the environment, being bombarded by various stimuli in the form of life events. This created stress, which differed in magnitude and meaning for each individual.

For clients with chronic schizophrenia, environmental stressors of events and situations are always present. They increase dopaminergic transmission and precipitate a high level of arousal, leading to episodic recurrences of the disease. The high level of arousal results in intense hallucinatory experiences (Hemsley et al, 1993). Several of the nursing theories (King's, Levine's, and Neuman's, for instance) examined the relationship between stress and illness (physical or mental) using this notion.

Some recent studies support the idea that schizophrenia may be developmentally related to disease and trauma occurring during the prenatal period or in early childhood. Takei and his associates (1994) studied the effect of prenatal exposure to the influenza virus. They concluded that exposure in the second trimester of pregnancy was a significant risk for adult schizophrenia, especially for females. Thus there are observed gender differences in the presentation of the disease.

With regard to trauma, a few studies have focused on obstetric complications or childhood accidents that could cause minimal brain damage and hinder development of the cerebral cortex. Obstetric complications studied included preeclampsia, antepartum hemorrhage, premature rupture of the membranes, prolonged labor, umbilical cord prolapse, unusual or uncommon presentations (such as breech births), prematurity, and postmaturity.

Studies of childhood included encephalitis, found to

be a risk factor for schizophrenia. Also, studies of head trauma requiring hospitalization for the child under 10 years of age indicated there was a significant difference in the later occurrence of schizophrenia between persons who had suffered prenatal or childhood head trauma and a comparison group. The injuries included hemorrhage into the ventricles and ischemic damage to the cortex in areas commonly associated with schizophrenia (Gureje et al, 1994).

The relationship between drugs of abuse and schizophrenia has also been studied. Cannabis abuse may be a precipitant of schizophrenia or may promote relapse, according to Linszen et al (1994). Also, the extreme stimulating effect of cocaine, which generates impulsivity, induces relapse in persons with schizophrenia (Stirling et al, 1994). Cocaine initiates neurochemical changes in the brain by substituting for the natural endorphins, creating an intense craving for the drug. Eventually, the long-term user experiences apathy, depression, and anhedonia, as often seen in clients with chronic schizophrenia. In addition, there is accumulating evidence that certain drugs, taken in pregnancy, are linked with later schizotypal illnesses in childhood and adolescence. For example, cocaine used by a pregnant woman is linked to later schizotypal illness in the child victim (Scherling, 1994).

PSYCHODYNAMIC THEORIES

Many biologic factors may predispose one to schizophrenia; however, psychosocial considerations are significant as well. Most causative models postulate that vulnerability interacts with stressful environmental influences to produce the symptoms of schizophrenia (Kaplan and Sadock, 1998). The theories that deal with psychosocial and environmental factors are psychoanalytic, family, and sociocultural/environmental. Systems theory has also been used to explain the reciprocal interactions among the theories.

Psychoanalytic and Developmental Theories

Psychoanalytic theory states that there are distortions in the mother-child relationship, brought on by anxious mothering, so that the child is unable to progress beyond dependence. This affects the ego organization and the interpretation of reality in the developing child. Being unable to interpret reality, the individual is susceptible to a fantasy world in which hallucinations and delusions attempt to create a reality of wishful thinking or to express inner fears. Inner drives, such as sex and aggression, are not brought under the person's control, and self-object differentiation is not achieved. Thus the person's sense of identity is weak, and his or her personality is vulnerable to stress (Kaplan and Sadock, 1998).

Family Theory Model

According to the family theory model, the child is assumed to have been raised in an atmosphere of unhappiness and tension, which may not be apparent to others or even to the family members themselves. Families make great attempts to conceal or repress unhappiness, resulting in psychologic insensitivity. However, no studies have demonstrated that family attributes are *causally* related to schizophrenia. Considering the reciprocal nature of interactions, one cannot say whether stressful relationships would precede or follow an episode of schizophrenia.

Several family patterns have been cited as being particularly damaging to the developing child. The first pattern is the **double-bind,** in which the child is forced to make a choice between two unreasonable perceptions, thus producing confusion, anxiety, and fear in the child's mind. For example, a verbal message may differ from a nonverbal one; a parent may insist that he or she is not angry at the child's behavior but expresses obvious anger in aggressive, hostile, and destructive behavior.

The second family pattern seen as destructive involves marital problems between the parents. This pattern results in the children being asked to support one parent against the other. Such a situation causes guilt feelings in the children because of divided loyalties. Often a power struggle begins between the parents, with one parent emerging as dominant and authoritative. This authoritative stand is likely to suppress the child's drive toward independence. In addition, the spouse forced to submit may displace his or her anger onto the children or make one child in particular a scapegoat.

The third serious family disturbance arises from destructive expressed emotion communication patterns within the family. At times there is a false agreement about family rules that is not communicated directly but produces explosive behavior when violated. There is also an air of pseudohostility that forces some family members into emotional isolation. The constant criticism and hostility destroy the family functions of support and protection.

Cultural and Environmental Theories

Although schizophrenia exists in all socioeconomic groups, it is disproportionately represented in the lower socioeconomic group. Various explanations have been advanced for this condition, one having to do with a "downward drift hypothesis" (Kaplan and Sadock, 1998). According to this hypothesis, the client with schizophrenia who possesses low social skills either moves into a lower socioeconomic group or fails to rise to a higher group.

On the other hand, some social scientists believe that the stress of living in a lower socioeconomic group is often enough to trigger schizophrenia in the vulnerable population (Fortinash and Holoday-Worret, 1999). Individuals with schizophrenia who are under psychologic stress manifest low levels of self-esteem and self-efficacy perception (view of the self as a normally functioning, partially functioning, or a dysfunctioning member of society) and may have limited resources to cope with their situation. In addition, the family networks of mentally ill persons are often not able to be supportive (Bendik, 1992).

Low socioeconomic status affects not only the psychologic, but also the biologic, functioning of an individual, adding to chronic symptom profiles (Cohen, 1993). For example, clients with schizophrenia are more likely than other persons in the lower socioeconomic group to get an infectious disease, particularly tuberculosis. Living in heavily populated rural areas, in poverty, adversity, and fear due to rising crime rates, is conducive to psychopathology (Betemps and Ragiel, 1994).

LEARNING THEORY

According to learning theory, the irrational ways of handling situations, the distorted thinking, and the deficient communication patterns of persons with schizophrenia are a result of poor parental models in early childhood: children learn what they are exposed to on a daily basis, from parents who have their own significant emotional problems. Thus the child does not develop skill in forming good interpersonal relationships (Fortinash and Holoday-Worret, 1999; Kaplan and Sadock, 1998).

Sullivan was a principal proponent of learning theory, believing that the developing individual was shaped by social interactions. Therefore the complex of feelings, thoughts, and behavioral expressions grew out of the individual's experiences with those closest to him or her. For example, if the child's father was perceived as mean and dictatorial, this perception may have generalized to other men in positions of authority, such as teachers, policemen, and employers, and colored the interpersonal relationships with these individuals. Or, if the child's mother coped with problems by projecting blame onto others, the child learned this pattern of behavior and alienated others by putting it into practice.

Theories of Psychophysiologic Effects of the Environment

Recent studies have also looked at the physical environment and its relationship to schizophrenia. Since toxic substances that cause a variety of illnesses may come to people through atmospheric pollution or through the food chain (e.g., lead and mercury), researchers have compared the geographic distribution of selenium and other trace elements with the prevalence of schizophrenia in the same area. The hypotheses were formulated according to an assumption that either an excess or a deficiency of certain substances in the environment can cause the disease (Brown, 1994).

EPIDEMIOLOGY

The incidence of schizophrenia, or the frequency of newly diagnosed cases in a specified population during a certain time period, is between 0.3% and 0.6% per 1000 persons

---

Box 14-2	Epidemiology

New diagnoses of schizophrenia occur between 0.3% and 0.6% per 1000 persons per year in the United States.

1.5% of the U.S. population has been diagnosed with schizophrenia.

The age of onset is greater in females than in males.

Paranoid-type schizophrenia occurs earlier in males than in females.

Disorganized-type schizophrenia occurs earlier in females than in males.

Prevalence is equal for males and females.

The oldest age-of-onset group is between 66 and 77 years old.

A female fetus exposed to influenza has a higher risk for schizophrenia than a male fetus.

Males show significantly more structural brain abnormalities from perinatal or early childhood trauma than females.

50% of persons with schizophrenia attempt suicide.

---

per year in the United States (Box 14-2). The lifetime prevalence, or the total number of cases in the U.S. population, is about 1.5%. The prevalence and prognosis of the disease vary according to socioeconomic, geographic, and cultural factors; schizophrenia presents itself in different ways, depending on the clients' situations and demographic characteristics (Betemps and Ragiel, 1994; Kaplan and Sadock, 1998). Family, twin, and adoption studies have consistently found varying rates of inheritance patterns, according to the closeness of the genetic relationship (Kaplan and Sadock, 1998; Kendler and Diehl, 1993).

AGE AND GENDER

Two demographic characteristics that have been extensively studied with regard to schizophrenia are age and gender. These variables have an interactive effect. For example, the age of onset of the disease in females is significantly greater than the age of onset in males.

Subtypes of schizophrenia tend to appear at different times. In males the paranoid type, in which prominent delusions or auditory hallucinations of a persecutory nature are present, appears earlier than in females. On the other hand, the disorganized type, which features confusion in speech, disorganization in behavior, and inappropriate affect, appears earlier in females (American Psychiatric Association [APA], 1994; Castle and Murray, 1993). Over the course of time, however, there is no difference in the prevalence of schizophrenia between males and females (Kaplan and Sadock, 1998).

In a recent incidence study of the age of onset, the oldest group ranged in age from 66 to 77 years, and composed about one third of the prevalence rate. This is contrary to earlier beliefs that schizophrenia rarely occurs after age 50. Clients in the oldest age-of-onset group tended to be women exhibiting paranoid symptoms (Castle and Murray, 1993).

When the fetus is exposed to the influenza of the mother during the second trimester, it is the female child who is at greatest risk for schizophrenia in her adult years (Takei et al, 1994). Males, on the other hand, show significantly more structural brain abnormalities than females as a result of perinatal or early childhood trauma (Gureje et al, 1994). In all, gender differences in the age of onset, physiologic deficits, prognosis, and response to treatment give evidence of a gender difference in the expression of schizophrenia.

MARITAL STATUS, RATES OF REPRODUCTION, AND MORTALITY

Since the introduction of psychotherapeutic drugs, people with schizophrenia have been freed from continual care in a state mental institution. Free of many of their symptoms and allowed access to rehabilitation programs where available, many with schizophrenia have gone on to live reasonably normal and even productive lives, including marrying and having a family. Thus the marriage and fertility rates among people with schizophrenias, once low, are nearly on a par with the larger population aggregate (Fortinash and Holoday-Worret, 1999; Kaplan and Sadock, 1998).

However, schizophrenia still carries with it the high rates of suicide in those who cannot cope with the demands of society. Despite the relief of some of their symptoms, many people with schizophrenia are prone to episodic decompensation when the disorder is exacerbated. During these times they may attempt suicide, become accident prone, or neglect their health, raising their morbidity rates and accounting for the lifetime 50% suicide attempt figure in the population with schizophrenia.

SOCIOECONOMIC CLASS

The portion of schizophrenia that can be attributed to the social problems endured by the lower class remains controversial (Betemps and Ragiel, 1994; Fortinash and Holoday-Worret, 1999; Kaplan and Sadock, 1998). However, the population density of the slums and the homeless mentally ill persons who receive poor follow-up care add to the stress on this vulnerable population. In economic terms, schizophrenia is the costliest of all mental disorders.

CULTURE, GEOGRAPHY, AND SEASONAL INFLUENCES

The manifestations of schizophrenia and its prognosis vary in different cultures. In less-developed nations, the prognosis for schizophrenia is better than in the technologically advanced cultures. Clients in the developing countries tend to have a more acute onset, fewer episodic occurrences, and less frequent problems with affect. Severe cognitive impairment is rare in Western nations. However, after an acute episode, the person with schizo-phrenia in the developing countries is more readily reintegrated into the family and community (Betemps and Ragiel, 1994; Kaplan and Sadock, 1998).

Variations in the prevalence of schizophrenia in different geographic regions have been studied. In some climates, seasonality of birth is a factor. More babies who later become schizophrenic are born in the winter months. There are two possible explanations for this phenomenon. One is that schizophrenia may be related to prenatal exposure to viral infections. The other is that there is a seasonal release of overripe ova in the winter, which results in consequent anomalies in the fetus at fertilization (Kaplan and Sadock, 1998).

CLINICAL DESCRIPTION

Schizophrenia, according to the DSM-IV classification, has the following criteria: (1) it lasts at least 6 months, at least 1 month of which includes "active-phase symptoms," and (2) the active-phase symptoms include at least two of these manifestations: hallucinations, delusions, disorganized or catatonic behavior, or disorganized speech (see DSM-IV Criteria box on p. 304).

There are five major subtypes of schizophrenia and several closely related disorders. The five subtypes of schizophrenia are:

Paranoid
Disorganized (formerly called hebephrenic)
Catatonic
Undifferentiated
Residual

The closely related disorders are:

Schizophreniform
Schizoaffective
Delusional
Brief psychotic disorder
Shared psychotic disorder
Psychotic disorder due to a general medical condition
Substance-induced psychotic disorder
Pervasive developmental disorder (autism and others)
Simple schizophrenia
Postpsychotic depressive disorder of schizophrenia
Psychotic disorder not otherwise specified (NOS)

PARANOID SCHIZOPHRENIA

Paranoid schizophrenia results in less neurologic and cognitive impairment and a better prognosis for the individual. However, in the active phase of the disorder, the afflicted individual is extremely ill, and the symptoms may constitute a danger to self or others.

Delusions tend to be persecutory or grandiose and have a coherent theme. The persecutory delusions may generate anxiety, suspiciousness, anger, hostility, and vio-

Schizophrenia

A. *Characteristic symptoms:* Two (or more) of the following, each present for a significant portion of time during a 1-month period (or less if successfully treated):
   1. Delusions
   2. Hallucinations
   3. Disorganized speech (e.g., frequent derailment or incoherence)
   4. Grossly disorganized or catatonic behavior
   5. Negative symptoms, (i.e., affective flattening, alogia, or avolition)
   NOTE: Only one Criterion A symptom is required if delusions are bizarre or hallucinations consist of a voice keeping up a running commentary on the person's behavior or thoughts, or two or more voices conversing with each other.

B. *Social/occupational dysfunction:* For a significant portion of the time since the onset of the disturbance, one or more major areas of functioning, such as work, interpersonal relations, or self-care, are markedly below the level achieved prior to the onset (or when the onset is in childhood or adolescence, failure to achieve expected level of interpersonal, academic, or occupational achievement).

C. *Duration:* Continuous signs of the disturbance persist for at least 6 months. This 6-month period must include at least 1 month of symptoms (or less if successfully treated) that meet Criterion A (i.e., active-phase symptoms) and may include periods of prodromal or residual symptoms. During these prodromal or residual periods, the signs of the disturbance may be manifested by only negative symptoms or two or more symptoms listed in Criterion A present in an attenuated form (e.g., odd beliefs, unusual perceptual experiences).

D. *Schizoaffective and mood disorder exclusion:* Schizoaffective disorder and mood disorder with psychotic features have been ruled out because either (1) no major depressive, manic, or mixed episodes have occurred concurrently with the active-phase symptoms; or (2) if mood episodes have occurred during active-phase symptoms, their total duration has been brief relative to the duration of the active and residual periods.

E. *Substance/general medical condition exclusion:* The disturbance is not due to the direct physiologic effects of a substance (e.g., a drug of abuse, a medication) or a general medical condition.

F. *Relationship to a pervasive developmental disorder:* If there is a history of autistic disorder or another pervasive developmental disorder, the additional diagnosis of schizophrenia is made only if prominent delusions or hallucinations are also present for at least a month (or less if successfully treated).

Classification of longitudinal course (can be applied only after at least 1 year has elapsed since the initial onset of active-phase symptoms):

Episodic with interepisode residual symptoms (episodes are defined by the reemergence of prominent psychotic symptoms); *also specify if:* **with prominent negative symptoms**

Episodic with no interepisode residual symptoms

Continuous (prominent psychotic symptoms are present throughout the period of observation); *also specify if:* **with prominent negative symptoms**

Single episode in partial remission; *also specify if:* **with prominent negative symptoms**

Single episode in full remission

Other or unspecified pattern

From American Psychiatric Association: *Diagnostic and statistical manual of mental disorders,* ed 4, Washington, DC, 1994, The Association.

lent behavior. Auditory hallucinations are common and are related to the delusionary theme. Interactions with others are rigid, intense, and controlled (APA, 1994; Fortinash and Holoday-Worret, 1999; Kaplan and Sadock, 1998).

According to the DSM-IV criteria for schizophrenia, a diagnosis of paranoid schizophrenia must meet two of the symptoms in Criterion A: the presence of delusions and hallucinations.

The other diagnostic criteria for paranoid schizophrenia—disorganized speech, behavior, and other negative symptoms—are not prominent. The delusions and hallucinations must be present for a significant portion of the time over a period of 1 month. This period can be shorter if the condition is successfully treated. Also, if delusions are unusually bizarre, or if the hallucinations involve commanding or commenting voices, then only one of the criteria needs to be met. Paranoid schizophrenia often has a sudden onset, sometimes triggered by severe stressors (APA, 1994; Fortinash and Holoday-Worret, 1999). The

individual with paranoid schizophrenia is sometimes referred to as a type I, productive client, with positive symptoms.

Crow (1980) proposed that symptoms in schizophrenia could be classified as **positive symptoms** (the syndrome includes hallucinations, increased speech production with loose associations, and bizarre behavior) or **negative symptoms** (the syndrome includes flat affect, poverty of speech, poor grooming, withdrawal, and disturbance in volition) as a guide to establishing the prognosis (Andreasen and Carpenter, 1993). Table 14-2 defines positive and negative symptoms.

Prognosis

The course of paranoid schizophrenia is varied but tends to be more hopeful than the courses of other subtypes. Of all the schizophrenias, paranoid schizophrenia is the most responsive to proper treatment and the most likely to qualify for the course of a single episode in full remission (APA, 1994; Kaplan and Sadock, 1998).

Table 14-2	Symptoms of Schizophrenia Classified According to Type I (Positive) or Type II (Negative)
Type I	**Type II**
Delusions, persecutory or grandiose	Flat or inappropriate affect
Delusions of being controlled	Poor eye contact
Mind reading or thought insertion ideas	Anhedonic attitude and asocial behavior; withdrawal
Hallucinations, auditory or other sensory modes	Poverty of speech; blocking and lack of inflection
Bizarre dress and behavior	Poor grooming and hygiene
Thought disorganization and tangential speech	Decreased spontaneity in behavior
Aggressive, agitated behavior	Lack of expressive gestures
Pressured speech	Lack of volition; apathy
Suicidal ideation may be present	Severely disturbed relationships with family, friends, peers
Ideas of reference	Inattentiveness

DISORGANIZED SCHIZOPHRENIA

The disorganized type of schizophrenia, formerly known as hebephrenic schizophrenia because of its early, insidious onset and silly, childish affect, is characterized by a severe disintegration of the personality. Speech is disorganized and may include word salad (communication that includes both real and imaginary words, in no logical order), incoherent speech, and clanging (rhyming). Behavior is odd, encompassing grimacing, grunting, sniffing, posturing, rocking, stereotyped behaviors, and uninhibited sexual behaviors such as masturbating in public. Socially, the client with disorganized schizophrenia is withdrawn and inept. There may be many cognitive and psychomotor defects, such as concrete thinking, the literal interpretation and use of language or inability to abstract; **primary process thinking**, prelogical thought that aims for wish fulfillment and is associated with the pleasure principle characteristic of the id portion of the personality; and poor coordination (APA, 1994; Fortinash and Holoday-Worret, 1999).

The client with disorganized schizophrenia has poor personal grooming and is often unable to complete activities of daily living (ADLs) without constant structural reminders, because the behavior is aimless and without goals (Kaplan and Sadock, 1998). Many type II symptoms are present. Development seems to have been impaired and held to about the age of 7 or 8.

Prognosis

Prognosis for the client with disorganized schizophrenia is poor, stemming from an early premorbid history of impaired adjustment that continues after the active phase of the disorder. **Premorbid** refers to the period just preceding the onset of the mental illness. This individual may or may not hallucinate or have delusions, but, if they exist, they are disorganized and fragmented.

Of all the subtypes, paranoid schizophrenia and disorganized schizophrenia have the most clearly defined clinical criteria and have been studied the most. However, according to Andreasen and Carpenter (1993), insufficient attention has been paid to the negative symptoms by both the medical and the pharmacologic communities. It is, after all, the residual negative symptoms that prevent former clients from holding jobs and forming normal relationships.

CATATONIC SCHIZOPHRENIA

Catatonic schizophrenia has, as its predominant feature, intense psychomotor disturbance. This disturbance may take the form of stupor (psychomotor retardation) or excitement (psychomotor excitation). Manifestations of psychomotor disturbance include posturing, immobility, catalepsy (waxy flexibility), mutism, and negativism. There may be automatic obedience on the one hand and excessive and purposeless movement on the other. Other symptoms include echopraxia (imitating the movements of others), echolalia (repeating what was said by another), grimacing, and stereotypic movements. Often there is rapid alteration between these extremes (APA, 1994; Fortinash and Holoday-Worret, 1999; Kaplan and Sadock, 1998).

The onset of catatonic schizophrenia often occurs with dramatic suddenness. Catatonic stupor may be preceded by an earlier withdrawal, carried to the extreme. It reflects the individual's reduced neurologic ability to filter out stimuli. There is no significant difference of age, sex, or education in the incidence of catatonic schizophrenia. To meet the DSM-IV criteria for catatonic schizophrenia, the client must exhibit two of the following behaviors: motor immobility or excessive motor activity; extreme negativism (resistance to all instructions and attempts to be moved); peculiar voluntary movements such as grimacing, stereotyped movements, or posturing; and echolalia or echopraxia (APA, 1994).

The person with catatonic schizophrenia presents a nursing challenge. While in a state of psychomotor excitement, the client may develop hyperpyrexia or collapse from extreme exhaustion. Close watch is indicated to prevent harm to self or others. Conversely, while in a stuporous state, the disease can be life threatening because the person approaches a vegetative condition, will not eat, and is in danger of malnutrition or even starvation. Other complications may include pressure sores from lack of mobility or strange posturing, constipation, or even stasis pneumonia in the older client.

Delusions often persist throughout the withdrawn state. For example, a client may believe that he has to hold his hand out flat in front of him because the forces of good and evil are warring on the palm of his hand and he will upset the balance of good and evil if he moves his hand. Oddly enough, although this individual may seem not to be attending to the environment around him, when he later returns to a normal state of consciousness he will remember in detail what has occurred. Nurses need to be aware of this factor and not say or do anything within the stuporous client's hearing that they would not say or do when the client is in a normal state of consciousness.

Prognosis

The prognosis for catatonic schizophrenia varies, depending on the age of onset, which is often in the early twenties to thirties. It tends to begin with an acute episode having an identifiable precipitating factor. If the client has developed a good support system before the illness, he or she will probably recover from the acute phase and have a partial or complete remission. More research is indicated for this particular type of illness, especially since it seems to have subsided in Western nations but is more prevalent in undeveloped nations, where remission is usually complete.

UNDIFFERENTIATED SCHIZOPHRENIA

Undifferentiated schizophrenia meets Criterion A for schizophrenia but cannot be classified as paranoid, disorganized, or catatonic. It does not clearly meet the criteria necessary for a diagnosis in any of these conditions, but it has some aspects of each type. The psychotic manifestations are extreme, including fragmented delusions, vague hallucinations, bizarre and disorganized behavior, disorientation, and incoherence (Fortinash and Holoday-Worret, 1999; Kaplan and Sadock, 1998). Affect is usually inappropriate rather than flat, and catatonic symptoms are not present. A clinical pathway for a client presenting with psychosis is shown in Figure 14-3.

The onset can be acute, with excited behaviors such as aggressive hitting or biting. Or the client may have chronic schizophrenia, with behavior that no longer fits a specific type but is a mixture of positive and negative symptoms. Usually the **prodromal symptoms** have developed over a period of years. Growth and development milestones may have been delayed. Thought processes are fragmented and have a high fantasy content (primary process thinking). The individual has few or no friends, and family relationships are strained because of odd and restless behaviors. Dress and grooming are careless, and the individual seems bored with life. Sleep patterns are disturbed by nightmares and early morning awakening.

Prognosis

The prognosis for the client with undifferentiated schizophrenia is generally poor, and the course is usually a chronic one. There are periods of exacerbation and remission where many negative symptoms prevent the patient from doing productive work, pursuing normal relationships, or enjoying life (Kaplan and Sadock, 1998).

RESIDUAL SCHIZOPHRENIA

If an individual has had at least one acute episode of schizophrenia and is now free of prominent positive symptoms but has some negative symptoms, he or she is diagnosed as suffering from residual schizophrenia, or **residual symptoms.** In some clients, this pattern may persist for years, with or without exacerbations. In others it seems to taper down to a complete remission. The usual signs of the illness that may persist for the chronic or subchronic individual are mild loosening of associations, illogical thinking, emotional blunting, social withdrawal, and eccentric behavior. Diagnostic criteria for the client with residual schizophrenia are (1) absence of prominent delusions, hallucinations, disorganized speech, and disorganized or catatonic behavior; and (2) continuing evidence of the presence of negative symptoms or attenuated positive symptoms.

Prognosis

Prognosis is varied and unpredictable. It depends largely on premorbid history and the adequacy of support systems (APA, 1994; Kaplan and Sadock, 1998).

SCHIZOPHRENIFORM DISORDER

The defining characteristics of schizophreniform disorder are the same as for schizophrenia, with two exceptions. The first is the duration, and the second is impairment of function. The duration is at least 1 month but less than 6 months. If symptoms persist for 6 months or longer, the diagnosis is changed to schizophrenia. Social or occupational functioning may or may not occur in this disorder, unlike the diagnosis of schizophrenia, where functional disturbance (relationships, school or work, self-care) will be present.

SCHIZOAFFECTIVE DISORDER

Schizoaffective disorder is a closely related disorder of schizophrenia that presents with severe mood swings of either mania or depression and also with some of the psychotic symptoms. Most of the time, mania or depression coexists with the psychotic symptoms, but there must be at least one 2-week period in which there are only psychotic episodes. The onset of illness generally occurs later in life than in schizophrenia, and the disorder often has a better prognosis than schizophrenia but a less positive prognosis than depression.

Text continued on p. 310

Psychosis

Interval / Location	Day of Admit	Day 2	Day 3	Day 4	Day 5	Day 6	Day 7	Day 8
Physiologic	*Takes adequate fluid/nutrition with assistance *Tolerates meds	*Takes adequate fluid/nutrition with assistance *Increased sleep/rest time *Adequate elimination	*Adequate nutrition with reminders *Adequate elimination	*Sleeps 3-6 hours *Adequate elimination	*Takes adequate nutrition/fluids *Drug levels therapeutic range	*Sleeps 5-8 hours *Absence drug toxicity side effects	*Sleeps 5-8 hours	*Sleeps 5-8 hours *Able to manage food/activity requirements independently
Psychologic	*Tolerates orientation to unit within capacity	*Oriented ×2	*Oriented ×3 *Demonstrates reduction in hallucinations and delusions	*Oriented ×4 *Reality testing with staff *Increased trust demonstrated	*Demonstrates more reality-based thoughts	*Able to focus on one topic 5-10 minutes	*Able to complete unit assignments and activities	*Able to complete unit assignment and activities independently *Able to plan/structure day
Functional Status/Role (OUTCOMES)	*Refrains from harming self or others with assistance	*Refrains from harming self *Attends to basic ADLs *Seeks staff when anxious	*Refrains from harming self *Increased trust demonstrated *Increased ADLs *Complies with meds with reminders	*Increased ADLs *Controls impulses with assistance *Utilizing basic stress management techniques with assistance	*Demonstrates less psychosis and intrusive behavior	*Interacts with peers *Able to make decisions	*Able to maintain safety *Demonstrates safe behaviors	*Able to maintain safety *Independently complies with medical regime
Family/Community Reintegration	*Family/significant other aware of treatment program goals *Family/significant other provide history including meds	*Identifies family/significant other to staff	*Attends community meetings/milieu activities with staff supervision. *Identifies family/significant other *Communicates with SW for increased understanding of Treatment goals/DC plans	*Family/significant other included in treatment/DC plans	*Identifies DC needs	*Identifies DC needs	*Identifies DC needs *Able to identify supports and how to use them	*Able to utilize supports and list ways to access them *State specific plans to manage symptoms, comply with meds and aftercare

Note: This Clinical Pathway is a tool to assist health care providers in achieving quality patient outcomes by providing appropriate and timely patient care. It is not intended to establish a community standard of care, replace a clinician's medical judgment, establish a protocol for all patients, or exclude alternative therapies. (See Variances at end of figure.)

Abbreviations: *CBC,* complete blood chemistry; *DC,* discharge; *ELOS,* estimated length of stay; *eval,* evaluation; *H/O,* history of; *I&O,* intake and output; milieu, therapeutic patient environment; *OT,* occupational therapist; *Reiserrit,* hearing to determine if patient is cognitively able to make a decision to refuse psychotropic medication; *S&R,* seclusion and restraint; *SW,* social worker; *UR,* utilization review.

Figure 14-3 Clinical pathway for psychosis.

Continued

Interval / Location	Day of Admit	Day 2	Day 3	Day 4	Day 5	Day 6	Day 7	Day 8
Discharge Planning	*(SW) initiate assessment *Identify DC placement ELOS contact family/significant other (nursing) initiates assessment *Identify H/O med compliance knowledge deficit and chronicity	*Team involved in DC planning *Discussed with MD *UR notify managed care	*SW evaluation completed *Specific DC plan identified *Treatment team meeting #1	*Involve family/significant other in DC plan *Review with patient	*Patient, family/significant other communicate understanding DC plan and follow-up *UR contact manage care	*Reinforce patient, family/significant other understanding DC plan and follow-up	*Transition to day treatment if indicated *Continue to identify/reinforce support system	*DC to least restrictive environment
Education	*Orient to unit *Patient's rights *Assess patient/significant other *Assess knowledge of meds and chronicity	*Assist with symptom recognition and importance of compliance *Include family/significant other as necessary	*Continue with symptom recognition *Continue to assess level of knowledge re: disorder and meds	*Assist in linking symptoms with precipitating event	*Assist in linking symptoms with precipitating events (noncompliance, drug abuse)	*Reinforce med education *Importance of compliance	*Develop aftercare plan to manage symptoms *Contact supports	*Develop aftercare plan to manage symptoms and contact supports
Psychosocial/ Spiritual/Legal	*Assess: Safety issues Mental status Spirituality Voluntary status	*Continue to assess: Safety issues Mental status Spirituality Voluntary status	*Continue to assess: Safety issues Mental status Spirituality Voluntary status	*Complete assessments and confirm: Safety Mental status Spirituality Legal status	*Continue to assess: Safety issues Mental status Spiritual Voluntary status	*Continue to assess: Safety issues Mental status Spiritual Voluntary status	*Continue to assess: Safety issues Mental status Spirituality Voluntary status	*Legal, psychosocial, spiritual eval completed
Consults	*Physical exam within 24 hours ( )	*Other consults as needed	*Other consults as needed	*Other consults as needed	*Other consults as needed	*Other consults as needed	*Arrange aftercare consults as ordered	*Complete all consults
Tests/Procedures	*Med levels ( ) *Drug screen ( ) *CBC ( ) *Thyroid function ( ) *SMAC ( )	*Other test/ procedures as ordered	*Other test/ procedures as ordered	*Other test/ procedures as ordered	*Other test/ procedures as ordered	*Other test/ procedures as ordered *Check drug levels in therapeutic range	*Other test/ procedures as ordered	*Test procedures as ordered outpatient
Treatment	*Monitor I&O *Monitor sleep/rest patterns *Level of observation 1:1 ( ); every 15 min ( ); every 30 min ( ) *Reduce milieu stimulation *Treatment as ordered *S&R ( ) yes ( ) no ( )	*Monitor I&O *Monitor sleep/rest patterns *Level of observation 1:1 ( ); every 15 min ( ); every 30 min ( ) *Treatment as ordered	*Monitor I&O *Monitor sleep/rest patterns *Level of observation 1:1 ( ); every 15 min ( ); every 30 min ( ) *Treatment as ordered	*Monitor I&O *Monitor sleep/rest patterns *Level of observation 1:1 ( ); every 15 min ( ); every 30 min ( ) *Continue treatment plan as ordered	*Level of observation: 1:1 ( ); every 15 min ( ); every 30 min ( ) *Treatment plan as ordered *Monitor sleep/rest pattern	*Level of observation: 1:1 ( ); every 15 min ( ); every 30 min ( ) *Treatment plan as ordered *Monitor sleep/rest pattern	*Level of observation: 1:1 ( ); every 15 min ( ); every 30 min ( ) *Treatment plan as ordered *Monitor sleep/rest pattern	*Discharge with specified treatment confirmed for aftercare

PROCESS

PROCESSES							
Medications (IV & Others)	*Meds as ordered *Protocols for antipsychotic med management *Monitor side effects *Toxicity	*Meds as ordered *Protocols for antipsychotic med management *Monitor side effects *Toxicity	*Meds as ordered *Protocols for antipsychotic med management *Monitor side effects *Toxicity	*Meds as ordered *Contact managed care with med changes *Protocols for antipsychotic med management *Monitor side effects *Toxicity	*Meds as ordered *Protocols for antipsychotic med management *Monitor side effects *Toxicity *Review meds with family/significant other	*Meds as ordered *Protocols for antipsychotic med management *Monitor side effects *Toxicity	*Discharge with meds and instructions as ordered
Activity	*OT assessment *1:1 reality orient/brief contact *Assist with ADLs *Interventions to control self/other harm/impulses	*Continue OT eval *Engage in groups as tolerated *Assist with ADLs *Interventions to control self/other harm/impulses	*OT eval *Engage in groups as tolerated *ADLs with reminders *Interventions to control self/other harm/impulses	*Engage in 2 groups as tolerated *Interventions to control self/other harm/impulses	*Independent ADLs *Engage in 2 groups per day *Provide opportunity for simple decision making	*Independent ADLs *Engage in all unit activities *Provide opportunity for simple decision making	*Independent ADLs *Engage in all unit activities *Encourage independent decision making	*Independent ADLs *Engage in all unit activities *Confirm decision making *Confirm safety
Diet/Nutrition	*Nutritional screening *Elicit food preference *Offer adequate nutrition/fluids *Baseline weight (weekly unless otherwise ordered)	*Offer adequate nutrition/fluids *Provide simple meals: Finger foods Room-temperature drinks	*Offer adequate nutrition/fluids *Encourage meals in milieu as tolerated with staff supervision	*Offer adequate nutrition/fluids *Encourage meals in milieu as tolerated with staff supervision	*Offer adequate nutrition/fluids *Teach family/significant other importance of adequate nutrition/fluids	*Offer adequate nutrition/fluids *Teach family/significant other importance of adequate nutrition/fluids	*Reinforce adequate nutrition/fluids *Weekly weight	*Confirm patient family/significant other knowledge adequate nutrition/fluids *Confirm adequate nutrition/fluids

Pathway Variances: P1. CP completed early   P2. Patient off CP   P3. Pathway Completed & Patient Not Discharged   P4. Initial Interval Not Appropriate

Element Variances:

1. Patient/Family:
1. Patient physiologic status
2. Patient psychologic status
3. Patient/family refusal
4. Patient/family unavailable
5. Patient/family other
6. Patient/family communication barrier
7. Element met early

2. Clinician:
1. Order differs from CP
2. Action differs from CP
3. Response time
4. Clinician other
5. Court/guardianship

3. Operating Unit:
1. Bed/appointment not available
2. Lack of data
3. Supplies/equipment not available
4. Department overbooked/closed
5. Court/guardianship
6. Operating unit other

4. Community:
1. Placement not available
2. Home care not available
3. Ambulance delay
4. Transportation not available
5. Community other

5. Payer:
1. Delayed giving authorization number
2. Payer limitations
3. Payer other

Figure 14-3—cont'd   For legend see p. 307.

Symptoms

Symptoms that may occur during the depressed phase:

> Poor appetite
> Weight loss
> Inability to sleep
> Agitation
> General slowing down
> Loss of interest in usual activities (anhedonia)
> Lack of energy or fatigue
> Feelings of worthlessness
> Self-reproach
> Excessive guilt
> Inability to think or concentrate, or thoughts of death or suicide

Symptoms that may occur during the manic phase:

> Increase in social, work, or sexual activity
> Increased talkativeness
> Rapid or racing thoughts
> Grandiosity
> Decreased need for sleep
> Increased goal-directed activity
> Agitation
> Inflated self-esteem
> Distractibility
> Involvement in self-destructive activities

Symptoms that may occur during psychotic episodes:

> Delusions (fixed beliefs—altered thought processes)
> Hallucinations (sensory/perceptual alterations)
> Incoherence
> Severely disorganized speech or thinking
> Grossly disorganized behavior
> Total immobility
> Lack of facial emotional expression (flattened or blunted affect)
> Lack of speech or motivation

Etiology

The cause of schizoaffective disorder is as yet unknown, but most researchers believe that the etiology is related to a combination of biologic, genetic, and environmental factors.

Course

Schizoaffective disorder is a lifelong illness for most individuals. The precise course of illness differs for each person, but most people have a worsening of symptoms periodically, during times of stress. These relapses may be severe enough to limit functioning and may even require hospitalization. After a relapse, there is generally a gradual return to the previous level of functioning.

Between relapses, most individuals experience mild symptoms.

Treatment

Psychotherapy. It is recommended that the nurse and client work together to establish goals.

Medications, consisting of antipsychotics, antidepressants, lithium, and/or other mood stabilizers. Often several medications are used in combination.

Skills training, which may focus on interpersonal skills, grooming and hygiene, budgeting, grocery shopping, job seeking, cooking, etc.

Self-Management

The following instructions may be given to the client regarding measures that may maximize the prognosis:

> Accept the fact that this is a prolonged illness.
> Identify strengths and limitations.
> Set clear, realistic goals.
> After a relapse, slowly and gradually return to responsibilities.
> Plan a regular, consistent, predictable, daily routine.
> Make home a quiet, calm, relaxed place (as possible).
> Identify and reduce stress (as possible).
> Make only one change in life at a time.
> Work toward an active, trusting relationship with nurses and treatment staff.
> Take medication regularly, as prescribed.
> Identify early signs of relapse and develop an early warning list.
> Become involved with people whom you feel comfortable with.
> Avoid street drugs.
> Discuss intake of alcoholic beverages with your physician.
> Eat a well-balanced diet.
> Get sufficient rest.
> Exercise regularly.
> Check reality with a trusted individual if you are unsure of the nature of your thoughts or feelings.
> Contrast your behavior with others if you are unsure of the nature of your actions.
> Accept that there may be occasional setbacks.

Managing Relapse

The following instructions may be given to the client for managing a relapse:

> Develop a plan of action with your nurse or therapist if relapse signs appear. (This is best done during well periods.)
> Involve a friend, family member, or other trusted individual to help in times of relapse.
> Your plan should include specific warning signs of re-

lapse, an agreement to notify the nurse or therapist as soon as relapse warning signs appear, an agreement to contact those individuals who can help reduce stress and stimulation, and a list of specific ways to decrease stress and stimulation and increase structure.

SYMPTOM PROFILES

Neuropsychiatrists have tried to find common threads that link the schizophrenias or areas of differentiation that separate them. There is a common, underlying dimension in schizophrenic disorder that gives rise to certain symptom profiles of a perceptual, cognitive, emotional, behavioral, or social nature. They are displayed in Table 14-3.

Perceptual Disturbances

Hallucinations can occur in any of the five receptive senses (auditory, visual, tactile, olfactory, or gustatory), but the most common are auditory. It is believed that a left hemisphere brain abnormality may precipitate hallucinations because the left hemisphere contains Broca's area, the language-processing center. From assessment procedures, it was determined that the left hemisphere responded to hallucinations as if it were hearing real voices. There is an indication that the hallucinations are a reflection of the actual delusional thinking of the person with schizophrenia (Green et al, 1994; Lewandowski, 1991).

Another aspect of perception that has been explored in the individual with schizophrenia is self-perception (Fortinash, 1990). One way in which the nurse can assess the severity of perceptual disturbances is by using art forms that indicate how the person with schizophrenia perceives the world or the self. Because of their tendency to generalize, individuals with schizophrenia often report an overall negative self-perception (Evans et al, 1994). However, Dzurec (1990) revealed that clients with schizophrenia who lived in a satisfactory setting saw themselves as mentally well, although they were disabled to the extent that they were not able to live independently.

Cognitive Disturbances

According to D'Angelo (1993), thought disorders can begin in children at risk for schizophrenia because of their heredity. Children of parents with schizophrenia tend to be conceptually disorganized, possibly because they do not correctly categorize information as other children do, in the childhood learning process. Also, children are very distractable (Smothergill and Kraut, 1993). Implications for the psychoeducation of persons with schizophrenia include:

Using times when symptoms are relatively stable
Simplifying instructions and reducing distractions
Providing both visual and verbal information
Using direct, clear terms
Teaching in small segments with frequent reinforcement
Not offering choices, which often confuse

As a result of thought disturbance, speech is affected. Subtle forms of speech disorders are *circumstantiality*, in which the person digresses to unnecessary details, and *tangentiality*, or responding in a manner irrelevant to the topic at hand. If the person is less impaired, listening for themes may help to identify client concerns (Hoffman, 1994; Kaplan and Sadock, 1998).

The process of thought in schizophrenia fluctuates with the clinical status and may venture into the world of fantasy, with autistic thinking, **perseveration** (persistent repetition of the same idea, in response to different questions), or **poverty of thought** (lack of ability to produce thoughts, loose associations) (Gundel and Rudolf, 1993; Kaplan and Sadock, 1998). In the client who is chronic, there is a general decline in intellectual functioning over the years.

Memory in adult-onset schizophrenia is usually intact, but in persons with chronic schizophrenia it is affected by emotion; the client remembers less and forgets rapidly over time. However, negative emotional experiences and concepts are remembered more readily than positive ones, perhaps reflecting a depressed and negative outlook on the world (Calev and Edelist, 1993). Clients with chronic schizophrenia have little insight into their illness and suffer impaired judgment.

Emotional Disturbances

Although emotional disturbance is a primary sign of all forms of schizophrenia, affect flattening and poor eye contact are most associated with undifferentiated schizophrenia. Persons with schizophrenia cannot adapt their thinking to the common reality; they block whatever does not fit into their own inner reality (Gundel and Rudolf, 1993).

Biologically, the individual with schizophrenia may be unable to screen out disruptive stimuli because of an imbalance in neurotransmitters. A deficiency in GABA, for example, may result in a rush of conflicting stimuli and labile or inappropriate emotional expression, whereas a deficiency in cholecystokinin is related to avolition and flat affect (see Table 14-1). Developmentally, it was found that in children at risk for schizophrenia, neuromotor dysfunction due to trauma or other causes indicated the later appearance of flat affect (Dworkin et al, 1993).

Behavioral Disturbances

The behavioral disturbance of greatest concern that is seen in schizophrenia is the possibility of violence. The incidence and type of violence largely depend on certain factors: diagnostic type of schizophrenia, degree of psychopathology, history of violent behavior in the past,

Table 14-3　Clinical Symptoms of Schizophrenia

Perceptual	Cognitive	Emotional	Behavioral	Social
Hallucinations: Auditory: May be commanding; content matches delusions Visual Tactile (e.g., may feel like being surrounded by spiderwebs) Olfactory and gustatory: Client may refuse to eat because food seems to smell or taste bad **Illusions:** False perceptions due to misinterpretations of real objects **Altered internal sensations:** Formication: Sensation of worms crawling around inside one Chill: Feeling of chills in the marrow of one's bones **Agnosia:** Perceptual failure to recognize familiar environmental stimuli, such as sounds or objects seen or felt; sometimes called "negative hallucinations" **Distortion of body image:** With respect to size, facial expression, activity, amount and nature of detail, exaggeration or diminution of body parts **Negative self-perception:** With respect to ability and competence	**Delusions:** Unusual ideas, not reality based: Omnipotence Persecution Controlling or being controlled **Derealization:** Loss of ego boundaries; cannot tell where own body ends and environment begins; feeling that the world around one is not real or distorted **Ideas of reference:** Notion that other people or the media are talking to or about one **Errors in recall of memory:** Due to incorrect categorization **Difficulty sustaining attention:** Unable to complete tasks Errors of omission **Incorrect use of language:** Neologisms (invented words) Incoherence Echolalia and word salad Concrete, restricted vocabulary Comprehension difficulties Looseness of associations **Flight of ideas:** Abrupt change of topic in a rapid flow of speech	**Labile affect: range of emotions:** Apathy, dulled response Flattened affect Reduced responsiveness Exaggerated euphoria Rage **Inappropriate affect:** Laughing at sad events, crying over joyous ones **Disruption in limbic functioning:** Inability to screen out disruptive stimuli and loss of voluntary control of response	**Little impulse control:** Sudden scream as a protest of frustration Self-mutilation, to substitute physical for emotional pain Injury to a body part believed to be offensive Response to command hallucinations **Inability to cope with depression:** Depressed client has a 50% risk for suicide Frequent exacerbations and remissions in one who has insight Lack of social support to help **Inability to manage anger:** Anger and lack of impulse control lead to violence—verbal aggression, destruction of property, injury to others, homicide **Substance abuse as coping:** Dulls painful psychologic symptoms **Noncompliance with medication:** May feel it is not needed or has too many side effects	**Poor peer relationships:** Few friends as a child or adolescent Preference for solitude **Low interest in hobbies and activities:** Daydreamer Not functioning well in social or occupational areas Preoccupied and detached Behavioral autism **Loss of interest in appearance:** Careless grooming Introversion **Not competitive in sports or academics:** Poor adjustment to school Withdrawal from activities **May suffer from:** Attention deficit disorder Somatic symptoms

Table 14-4	Diagnostic Profiles of Bleuler and Schneider
Bleuler	**Schneider**

Characteristics of schizophrenia:
  Incongruence between feelings and thoughts
  Incongruence in the behavioral expression of feelings and
    thoughts
Four primary symptoms of schizophrenia:
  Affect is disturbed
  Autism is present
  Ambivalence is common
  Associations are loosened
Assessory symptoms:
  Hallucinations
  Delusions
	First-rank symptoms of schizophrenia:
	  Hallucinations
	  Thought withdrawal (belief that one's thoughts have been
	    removed from one's head)
	  Thought broadcasting (belief that one's thoughts are broad-
	    cast from one's head)
	  Delusions
	  Somatic experiences
	Second-rank symptoms of schizophrenia:
	  Perceptual disorders
	  Perplexity
	  Mood changes
	  Feelings of emotional impoverishment

abuse of substances, and noncompliance with medications (Kennedy, 1993; Mulvey, 1994). In terms of diagnostic type, there is a significant difference between paranoid schizophrenia and other types of schizophrenia; the client with paranoia is higher in physical aggression toward other people (Kennedy, 1993; Mulvey, 1994).

However, although the *relative risk* for violence is higher in the mentally ill population (of any diagnosis) than in the general population, the *absolute risk* is very small (Mulvey, 1994). Whether or not the inclination for violence is expressed depends on other factors, as indicated above.

Social Competence Profiles

Typically, the individual with schizophrenia has a history of a schizoid or schizotypal personality. According to Dworkin et al (1994), poor social competence may be important in the development of schizophrenia. Once again, the issue of nature versus nurture arises, and there is speculation that children raised by parents with schizophrenia may emulate their parents in socialization behavior (Turner, 1993). There is a detachment from the environment and an autistic relationship to reality (Gundel and Rudolf, 1993; Kaplan and Sadock, 1998).

Of all of the diagnostic profiles, however, the two still most commonly used to describe schizophrenia were derived from the early work of Bleuler and Schneider, as presented in Table 14-4 (Kaplan and Sadock, 1998).

Biologic Profiles

Symptom profiles are supported by neurologic examinations, neuropsychologic tests, and various brain-scanning techniques (neuroimaging) relevant for clients with schizophrenia (see Chapter 3). Some of these examinations are presented in Table 14-5. In general, the tests verify findings that schizophrenia has diffuse, nonlocalizable areas of dysfunction. Evidence of generalized impair-

ment can be found in persons with a first episode, as well as chronic schizophrenia, although the degree of impairment may differ with subtypes. Individuals with schizophrenia seem to have impairments in the stimulus inhibition (gating) circuitry of the brain, sometimes leading to stimulus overload. They are thus handicapped in sorting out and paying attention to the information necessary to solve a problem.

Modern brain-scanning technology has enabled scientists to assemble not only a structural image of the brain, active or inert, but also a functional image that indicates activity in various areas. Figure 14-4 shows a bio-electron activity measure (BEAM) of a client with schizophrenia.

PROGNOSIS

In addition to the general statements about the prognosis to be expected for each subtype of schizophrenia, there is recent evidence for specific relationships between symptom profiles and prognostic predictions. For example, Goldman et al (1993) looked at the interrelationship between neuropsychologic functioning and treatment response and found that the ability to encode, process information, and interact with the environment depends on being able to attend, focus, and remember. When these abilities are compromised by frontal lobe impairment, negative symptoms tend to remain and interfere with daily living.

Unfortunately, although there are many drugs on the market that have helped some clients with schizophrenia, the drugs do not seem to be effective for all. Those clients having positive symptoms are most helped by drugs. However, clozapine, discussed later in this chapter, does seem to relieve some negative symptoms as well (Breier et al, 1994). A better adjustment to the community is thus made possible for more clients with schizophrenia. Specific issues a community nurse faces are discussed in the Nursing Care in the Community box.

Table 14-5   Biologic Profiles in Schizophrenia

Neurologic Examinations

Test	Function
Apgar rating of the newborn	To rate functioning of the newborn nervous system
Physiologic and anatomic testing of the nervous system (general)	To discover infections, lesions, or metabolic problems that may affect the nervous system

Neuropsychologic Tests

Test	Function
Halstead-Reitan Battery	To test higher cortical functioning
	To detect early signs of memory and cognitive dysfunction
	To design and evaluate remediation programs (Osmon, 1991)
Luria-Nebraska Test Battery	To predict behavior by examining neurologic functioning (Meador and Nichols, 1991)
	To assess client progress in various areas
Eye-tracking and auditory tests	To discover information-processing deficits (Perry and Braff, 1994)

Electrical Impulse Testing

Test	Function
Electrodermal activity (EDA) test	To indicate the extent of negative symptomatology present in the client with schizophrenia (Fuentes et al, 1993)
Electroencephalogram (EEG)	To detect electrical activity in seizure disorders, sometimes associated with schizophrenia

Nursing Care in the Community

The Schizophrenias

The community mental health nurse often works with a continuum of clients with schizophrenia. This clientele includes young persons newly diagnosed and mature adults with schizophrenic illnesses who have been functioning adequately for several years with antipsychotic medications.

The nurse must also help older adults, who are often socially isolated because their support systems have been exhausted as friends and family members have withdrawn, moved away, or died. Their most important contacts may be either in mental health agencies or in peripheral support systems, such as board-and-care operators, hotel managers, store owners in the proximate community, or employers. They may need not only monitoring regarding medications but also help with financial management and basic activities of daily living (ADLs), such as those involving nutrition, clothing, and cleanliness. Sometimes planning a periodic special outing promotes increased interest in appearance and behavior.

When a young person who has been hospitalized and received a diagnosis of schizophrenia returns to the community, the family has already been disrupted by bizarre behavior. Parents and siblings may need increased help in adjusting to this disturbing diagnosis. The community mental health nurse is an essential liaison to the medical establishment and may also provide a reality check when family interactions seem out of control. The nurse may make referrals to community service organizations and support groups while serving as the liaison with the hospital.

For the adult client who carries a diagnosis of schizophrenia, the community mental health nurse is also an important contact. The nurse can help with problems of medication management, give support when stressful situations arise, and advise the psychiatrist when the client's behavior indicates that the current medication regimen is not effective. The goal is to maintain the client at an optimal, satisfying level of life activities.

The problem of street drug abuse and homelessness is also a concern of mental health nurses in the community. Many socially isolated individuals with a diagnosis of schizophrenia find the society of the streets to be a tolerant environment and the use of street drugs an acceptable alternative to prescribed medications. The mental health nurse who attempts to intervene in this cycle may encounter immense resistance from the client and the community. Often it requires the support of a trained mental health team, as well as the education and participation of the entire community, to break this destructive cycle. Mental health nurses must be prepared to collaborate with the community to help clients reach their potential.

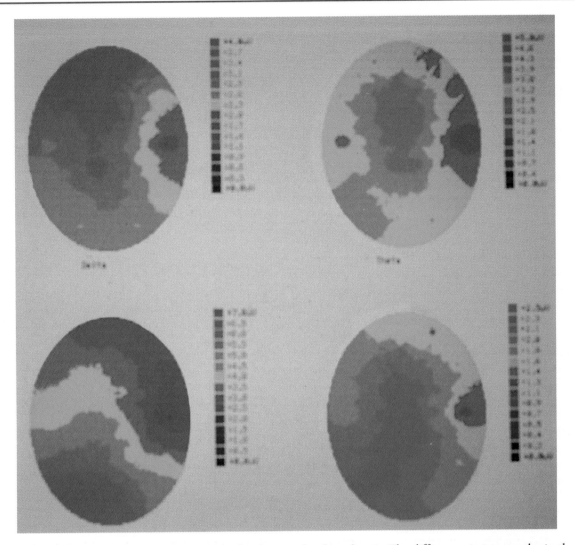

Figure 14-4 Bio-electron activity measure (BEAM) of a client with schizophrenia. The differences in topography in the various brainwave bands indicate differences in metabolism. When compared with BEAMs of individuals without the disorder, variations can confirm symptoms such as hallucinations or emotional withdrawal. (From Orrison WW et al: *Functional brain imaging*, St. Louis, 1995, Mosby.)

DISCHARGE CRITERIA

For the client with schizophrenia to be discharged to the community, the following criteria need to be met.

Client will:

Demonstrate absence of suicidality

Verbalize absence or control of hallucinations.

Identify events or episodes of increased anxiety that promote hallucinations.

Have family or a significant other willing to serve as a support network.

Accept referral of self or a significant other to a physician, therapist, or agency for help and monitoring

Accept responsibility for own actions and self-care

Verbalize ways of coping with anxiety, stress, and problems encountered in the community.

Have access to a safe living environment in the community: own home, board-and-care facility, or halfway house.

Use known community resources, such as support groups, day care centers, and vocational or rehabilitation programs.

Explain the following about medication: importance, expected effects, adverse effects, prescribed dose and time of taking the medication, and effects of the interaction of the medication with other substances such as food or alcohol.

THE NURSING PROCESS

ASSESSMENT

Assessment of the individual with schizophrenia is complicated because of the different symptom profiles for the various subtypes of the condition. Subjective data are obtained through symptom reporting and by the behavioral descriptions of significant others. Objective assessment is done by observation, by using rating scales, and by checking biologic indicators, as described in earlier sections. For psychiatric mental health nurses, it is important not to lose sight of the biologic focus so prevalent in the other specialties. For example, ataxia may indicate extrapyramidal side effects of medication. Also, just as with any patient, vital signs, nutrition, exercise, and sleep assessment are important (Trygstad, 1994).

Although the nursing assessment includes certain biologic indicators, it relies largely on psychologic data and may use the Mental Status Examination rating scale to organize the data (see Chapter 7). The Mental Status Examination considers the categories of appearance, behavior, orientation, memory, thought processes, perceptual processes, intellectual functioning, feelings (mood) and affect, insight, and judgment. Four of these categories are particularly important in schizophrenia: disturbances in perception, thought, feelings, and behavior (see Nursing Assessment Questions box).

For children and adolescents the assessment of positive and negative symptoms must take into consideration the developmental status of the individual. Measures of thought disturbances in children must consider that their normal patterns of thinking are concrete; abstract thought is not a part of normal thinking in the child. Likewise, since impulse control is developmental in the adolescent, the measures of impulse control must be adjusted in consideration of the client's age (Fields et al, 1994).

NURSING DIAGNOSIS

Nursing diagnoses are formulated from the information obtained during the assessment phase of the nursing process. The accuracy of the diagnosis depends on a careful in-depth assessment. The following is a listing of some of the more common diagnoses applicable to schizophrenia (see Collaborative Diagnoses box).

NURSING DIAGNOSES FOR SCHIZOPHRENIA

Communication, impaired verbal
Coping, ineffective individual
Family processes, altered
Self-care deficit (bathing/hygiene, dressing/grooming, feeding, toileting)
Sensory/perceptual alterations

NURSING ASSESSMENT QUESTIONS

The Schizophrenias

1. What problems have you been having recently? How do you feel differently now than before? (To determine the client's perception of the problem.)
2. Do you now or have you ever in the past used alcohol or drugs? If so, when and how often? (To determine the client's use of substances.)
3. Have you heard (sounds, voices, messages), seen (lights, figures), smelled (strange, bad, good odors), tasted (strange, bad, good tastes), or felt (touching, warm, cold sensation) anything that others who were present did not? (To determine if the client is having hallucinations.)
4. What are the voices that you hear like? What do they say? Are they troubling for you? (To determine if they instruct the client to harm self or others.)

Questions to Determine if the Client Is Experiencing Delusions

1. Do you feel that someone or something outside of you is controlling you in some way? Are you able to control other people?

2. Do you feel you are being watched? Followed?
3. Are people talking about you? If yes, explain how you know this.
4. Are you experiencing guilt? Do you have anything to feel guilty about? Do you think you are a bad person? If yes, what makes you believe this?

Things to Observe for During Assessment

Cognitive changes (e.g., concrete thinking, delusions, fantasies, or autistic communication)
Hallucinations
Depersonalization
Somatization
Unusual gestures, posture, tone of voice, mannerisms
Flat affect
Disheveled, unkempt physical appearance
Reaction to the interviewer (receptive, distant, resistant)

Social isolation
Thought processes, altered
Violence, risk for: directed at others
Violence, risk for: self-directed

OUTCOME IDENTIFICATION

Outcome identification is an estimate of the behavioral change anticipated following interventions and is influenced by the severity of the symptoms, the cultural milieu, and the prognosis for the particular diagnosis. Thus the outcomes of schizophrenia may reflect complex interactions.

Client will:

1. Demonstrate significant reduction in hallucinations and delusions.
2. Demonstrate absence of self-mutilating, violent, or aggressive behaviors.
3. Demonstrate reality-based thinking and behavior.
4. Engage in own hygiene, grooming, and ADL skills.
5. Socialize with peers and staff and participate in all groups.
6. Comply with medication regimen and verbalize an understanding of the role of medications in reducing psychotic symptoms.
7. Demonstrate more functional coping and problem-solving methods.
8. Participate in discharge planning with family.

COLLABORATIVE DIAGNOSES

DSM-IV Diagnoses*	**NANDA Diagnoses†**
Schizophrenia, catatonic	Communication, impaired verbal
Schizophrenia, disorganized	Coping, ineffective individual
Schizophrenia, paranoid	Family processes, altered
Schizophrenia, residual	Sensory/perceptual alterations
Schizophrenia, undifferentiated	Thought processes, altered
	Violence, risk for: directed at others
	Violence, risk for: self-directed

*From American Psychiatric Association: *Diagnostic and statistical manual of mental disorders*, ed 4, Washington, DC, 1994, The Association.
†From North American Nursing Diagnosis Association: *NANDA nursing diagnoses: definitions and classifications, 1999-2000*, Philadelphia, 1999, The Association.

PLANNING

Planning nursing interventions and treatment geared to the whole person and his or her social environment, including the family, is challenging. Since behavioral problems come from many sources and may range from less serious to much more serious, interventions at a variety of levels also need to be considered. Medical interventions generally are focused on underlying biologic factors and involve diagnostic procedures such as neuroimaging, somatic strategies, and treatment with medication. The nurse's role at this level is to prepare the client and family by explaining the rationale for the interventions and assisting with compliance. The nurse can also use nursing measures at this level, based on his or her knowledge of basic biologic functioning and needs.

Interpersonally and socially, clients with schizophrenia are disadvantaged by being unable to view things from the perspective of others. Because of the inability to abstract and correctly interpret, the individual with schizophrenia sees others as unpredictable, as being competitors for attention, and as being in control of what is "right" or "wrong" in an absolute sense. Role-playing scenarios, which help clients to see things from another person's perspective, are helpful. Socialization should be a focus of the treatment plan by including the clients in activities that

---

CASE STUDY

Henry, a 40-year-old man living on Social Security payments in a single-room occupancy (SRO) facility, was never quite able to budget his meager income to last the whole month. An individual with chronic schizophrenia, Henry had a fixed delusion that he owned the hotel where he lived but that the manager and the town government were defrauding him of his rental money. When he was short of cash at the end of the month, he became abusive and aggressive. Fearing assault, the manager would call the police, and Henry would be readmitted to the psychiatric hospital. In about 10 days he would be discharged to the same SRO, where he lived quietly for a while, helping the manager with tasks. This was a repetitive pattern.

Critical Thinking—Outcome Identification

1. What is the significance of Henry's delusion, given his low socioeconomic status?
2. Henry received good care at the psychiatric hospital. Standard outcome criteria for discharge were always met. If this continued, what would the chances be that Henry would hold his delusion? Why might a nurse's attempt to challenge the delusion be risky?
3. What are some teaching strategies that nurses could try with this client? In what form would they best be implemented?
4. If you were a community mental health nurse, how would you do follow-up care on Henry? What signs of escalating anxiety would you look for?

are supportive and nonthreatening and that provide helpful feedback on how the client presents to others. Activities that do not include competition are useful in quelling or preventing aggressive tendencies. Nurses must be alert to avoid power struggles.

Family interactions may be particularly difficult for the client with schizophrenia. If the family (or foster family) does not understand what the treatment team is trying to accomplish and how they are structuring the treatment plan, clients who have been discharged from the hospital after an acute psychotic episode are more likely to experience recidivism. The closer the kinship, the stronger the tension created by ambivalent emotions, which often confuse the client whose insight may be poor (McEnvoy et al, 1993).

IMPLEMENTATION

First and most important is the involvement of the client and family in the treatment process, with explanations and rationales given for all interventions. Interventions may be well planned but still be challenging for the nurse if there are misunderstandings about what is expected; resistance from client, family, or others; or financial or environmental constraints. As much as possible, clients should set their own goals and pace for treatment and progress.

In the beginning, a client may be so ill that he or she cannot understand or accept an appropriate effort to help. In that case, the nurse may need to work on establishing a therapeutic relationship first before the well-meaning interventions will be accepted.

An existing therapeutic relationship between the client and nurse will later be expanded to include the client's family or significant others for lasting effectiveness of the proposed interventions. In some cases the interventions will need to be made at yet another level, the level of the school or the workplace. Everyone must be made aware of the what, why, and how of the therapeutic plan so that they can work as a team. The client's cultural background should also be considered when planning interventions.

The family's economic situation also deserves attention. Health care personnel are not usually thinking of the cost of implementing a care plan, which may involve psychotherapy, medication, diet, transportation access to outpatient care, or other factors creating unplanned expenses. It is important to assess for such expenses, problem solve the issues, and include the solutions with the plan.

NURSING INTERVENTIONS

Following are some nursing interventions that have proved to be effective during interactions with clients who have a diagnosis of schizophrenia:

1. Assess and monitor risk factors *to prevent violence and promote safety of the client and others.*
2. Reduce/minimize environmental stimulation *to promote a quiet, soothing milieu that may lessen the client's impulsivity and agitation and prevent accident or injury.*
3. Provide frequent "time-outs" and/or brief, low-key interactions *to calm the client by providing opportunities for rest, relaxation, and ventilation of impulsive feelings, which will reduce the risk of acting-out behavior.*
4. Support and monitor prescribed medical and psychosocial interventions *to encourage the client and family in the treatment plan and prevent the client's behavior from escalating to violence.*
5. Use clear, concrete statements versus abstract, general statements. *The client may not be able to understand complex messages, and, as such, they may exacerbate misperceptions and/or hallucinations. Individuals with schizophrenia generally respond better to concrete messages during the acute phase.*
6. Attempt to determine precipitating factors that may exacerbate the client's hallucinatory experiences (e.g., stressors that may trigger sensory-perceptual disturbances). *Although hallucinations may have a biochemical etiology, they may be exacerbated by outside stressors in a vulnerable client, and identifying such stressors may help to prevent the severity of the hallucinatory experience.*
7. Praise the client for reality-based perceptions, reduction/cessation in aggressive/acting-out behaviors, and appropriate social interaction and group participation. *Warranted praise reinforces repetition of functional behaviors when given at appropriate times during the treatment regimen, such as when medication has begun to take effect.*
8. Educate the client and family/significant others about the client's symptoms, the importance of medication compliance, and continued use of therapeutic support services after discharge *to facilitate the client and family/significant other knowledge base, ensure the client's continued therapeutic support, and possibly prevent relapse after discharge from the hospital.*
9. Distract the client from delusions that tend to exacerbate aggressive or potentially violent episodes. *Engaging the client in more functional, less anxiety-provoking activities increases the reality base and decreases the risk for violent episodes that may be provoked by troubling delusions.*
10. Focus on the meaning or feeling engendered by the client's delusional system rather than focusing on the delusional content itself *to help meet the client's needs, reinforce reality, and discourage the false belief without challenging or threatening the client.*
11. Accompany the client to group activities, beginning with the more structured, less threatening ones first, and gradually incorporating more informal, spontaneous activities, *to increase the client's socialization skills and expand the reality base in a nonthreatening way.*
12. Assist with personal hygiene, appropriate dress, and grooming until the client can function independently

Text continued on p. 321

NURSING CARE PLAN

Brian, a 29-year-old man, was estranged from his family at the age of 20 as a result of a diagnosis of chronic undifferentiated schizophrenia, which resulted in his unpredictable and disruptive behavior at home that became intolerable. He was sent to live-in board-and-care facilities, where he was maintained if he took his medications and complied with the program established at a day treatment center that he attended. The center provided necessary and predictable structure, support and guidance from staff, and some affiliation and socialization with others. Because of his disorder, Brian was easily influenced by others. One day he was persuaded by "pseudo" friends to take the government assistance check he had just received to "go party." He stopped taking his medications, took various street drugs, and failed to return to the board-and-care facility or the day treatment center for a week. He showed up at the center one morning disheveled, dirty, incoherent, and frightened, stating "I am really scared. Everybody left me. I'm hearing voices saying that I'm stupid and hopeless, and no one would help me because I'm not worth saving." Brian was admitted to the acute care unit in a psychiatric hospital.

DSM-IV Diagnoses

Axis I   Schizophrenia, chronic undifferentiated
Axis II   (Personality disorders) No diagnosis
Axis III (Medical diagnosis) None
Axis IV   (Severity of psychosocial stressors)
          Moderate to severe = 6 to 7
          Negative influence of "friends"
          Rejection by peers
          Ingestion of illicit drugs
          Lack of adequate support system (family, friends)
          Economic issues (misuse of government assistance check)
Axis V   GAF = 10 (current)
          GAF = 30 (past year)

Nursing Diagnosis: Sensory/perceptual alterations (auditory hallucinations) related to the fact that client stopped taking medications; substance use; inability to process information (biologic factors) secondary to diagnosis of schizophrenia; rejection by peers; isolation and loneliness; low self-esteem; negative self-image/self-concept; and lack of adequate supports; as evidenced by verbalization that he hears derogatory voices; fear that no one will help; anxiety; frustration; self-depreciation; and self-care deficit.

Client Outcomes	Nursing Intervention	Evaluation
• Brian will demonstrate a reduction in symptoms and an absence of behavior that is harmful to self or others.	• Focus on modification and management of symptoms versus elimination of symptoms. *Hallucinations may not be helped by interventions initially. In the meantime, client needs coping skills.* • Continually assess Brian for risk of harm to self or others, even thought past history is negative. *Frustration, anger, inability to cope, and derogatory hallucinations could result in violence.*	• Brian remains safe on the unit even though the voices are troubling to him.
• Brian will verbalize that voices are under control ("the voices don't bother me" or "I don't hear the voices").	• Assess Brian's hallucinatory activity, and observe for verbal and nonverbal behaviors associated with hallucinations (talking to self; bolting and running out of the room). *The nurse must first recognize disturbance before intervention is possible.* • Identify, whenever possible, the need filled by hallucinations (dependency, loneliness, rejection). *Hallucinations may fill the void created by lack of human contact. Once identified, the client experiences relief/anxiety reduction and the nurse may then use the therapeutic alliance to assist the client with strategies for growth and change.* • Explore auditory hallucinations for violent content (command hallucinations to harm self or others). *Immediate intervention is required if the client is a threat to self or others. Otherwise, discussions of content serve only to fix negative beliefs.*	• Brian continues to respond to voices. • Hallucinations increase when Brian is rejected by peers, but brief, frequent discussions with nursing staff decrease his anxiety. • No threatening content is voiced by Brian.
• Brian will focus on real events and people in the environment.	• Orient the client to actual activities and events *to present reality.* • Address Brian, other clients, and staff by name. *Reinforces reality and orients client.*	• Brian is better able to focus on events when rested and not under stress. • Brian responds to own name when he is addressed.

Continued

NURSING CARE PLAN —cont'd

Client Outcomes	Nursing Intervention	Evaluation
• Brian will participate in relevant conversations with staff and other clients.	• Use simple, concrete, specific language (versus abstract, global language). *The client's misperceptions and altered perceptions may influence the message and interfere with understanding.*	• Brian responds coherently when conversation is simple and undemanding.
	• Use direct verbal responses versus unclear gestures (nodding head yes or no). *May provide distorted perception or misinterpretation of reality.*	• Brian misinterprets any subtle conversations or gestures by staff or peers.
	• Help Brian to speak slowly and clearly, if incoherent. *Encourages organization of thought processes and ability to be understood.*	• Brian can slow down and make himself understood when encouraged.
• Brian will participate in planned treatment to decrease or eliminate hallucinations.	• Assist Brian in stopping or managing hallucinations *to give him some control and increase his self-esteem.*	• Brian continues to practice techniques when staff remind him.
	• Teach techniques that will help control hallucinations: Instruct Brian to sing, whistle, or clap hands over voices; describe disbelief in messages; contact staff when voices are bothersome; engage in an activity, exercise, or a project when voices begin. *Provides alternatives and gives the client control.*	
	• Describe the hallucinatory behavior when the client appears to be hallucinating. "Brian, you seem distracted. Are you hearing voices?" *By reflecting on the client's behavior in an accepting way, the nurse facilitates disclosure and promotes trust.*	• Brian accepts the nurse's observations and attempts techniques.
• Brian will engage in more reality-based dialogue with staff.	• Refrain from arguing or discussing details of content. *When the nurse disagrees, the client will defend the content, which reinforces the importance of the hallucinations.*	• Brian is beginning to discuss real events more often each day, as staff focus on reality and accept him.
	• Voice the nurse's reality about Brian's hallucinations (e.g., "I don't hear the voices you describe, Brian. The only voices I hear are those of the people in this room. I know you hear the voices, but with time they may stop.") Don't deny the client's experience. *Helps the client to distinguish actual voices from internal stimulation.*	• Brian states he hears the voices less when engaged with staff.
	• Refrain from judgmental remarks. *Avoids diminishing self-esteem.*	• Brian says he appreciates not being made fun of.
	• Support the medical regimen, including medications. *Assists in managing biologic factors related to hallucinations.*	• Brian takes all prescribed medications; symptoms are remitting.
	• Discuss with Brian that sometimes voices do not completely go away, but that he can learn to manage them. *Helps the client to tolerate persistent, unremitting hallucinations and continue techniques that relieve them (whistling, singing, clapping).*	• Brian expresses hope that he can continue strategies when discharged.
• Brian will name two precipitating events occurring just before the onset of hallucinations (e.g., frustration, fear).	• Help the client to name precipitants (stressors that trigger hallucinations). *Example:* "What happened just before you heard the voices?" *Anxiety-provoking situations may precede hallucinations. When situations are identified, the client understands the connection and begins to manage, avoid, reduce, or eliminate them.*	• Brian is able to reduce the frequency and intensity of hallucinations by using learned techniques (whistling, singing, clapping).

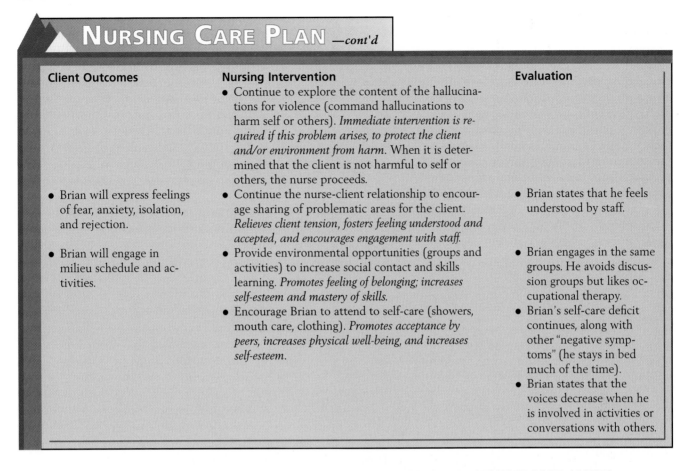

NURSING CARE PLAN —cont'd

Client Outcomes	Nursing Intervention	Evaluation
	• Continue to explore the content of the hallucinations for violence (command hallucinations to harm self or others). *Immediate intervention is required if this problem arises, to protect the client and/or environment from harm.* When it is determined that the client is not harmful to self or others, the nurse proceeds.	
• Brian will express feelings of fear, anxiety, isolation, and rejection.	• Continue the nurse-client relationship to encourage sharing of problematic areas for the client. *Relieves client tension, fosters feeling understood and accepted, and encourages engagement with staff.*	• Brian states that he feels understood by staff.
• Brian will engage in milieu schedule and activities.	• Provide environmental opportunities (groups and activities) to increase social contact and skills learning. *Promotes feeling of belonging; increases self-esteem and mastery of skills.*	• Brian engages in the same groups. He avoids discussion groups but likes occupational therapy.
	• Encourage Brian to attend to self-care (showers, mouth care, clothing). *Promotes acceptance by peers, increases physical well-being, and increases self-esteem.*	• Brian's self-care deficit continues, along with other "negative symptoms" (he stays in bed much of the time).
		• Brian states that the voices decrease when he is involved in activities or conversations with others.

to prevent physical complications and preserve self-esteem.

13. Establish routine times and goals for self-care and add more complex tasks as the client's condition improves. *Routine and structure tend to organize and promote reality in the client's world.*

14. Spend intervals of time with the client each day, engaging in nonchallenging interactions, *to ease the client out into the community by first developing trust, rapport, and respect.*

15. Assess the client's self-concept. *A low self-concept may result from or perpetuate social isolation.*

16. Act as a role model for social behaviors in interactions by maintaining good eye contact, appropriate social distance, and a calm demeanor *to help the client identify appropriate social behaviors.*

17. Keep all appointments for interactions with the client *to promote client trust and self-esteem.*

18. Listen actively to the client's family/significant others, allowing them to express fears and anxieties about mental illness, giving them support and empathy, and emphasizing client's strengths, *to provide ventilation of pent-up emotions and calm irrational fears while acknowledging realistic concerns; to promote hope and bonding between the family/significant others and the client.*

ADDITIONAL TREATMENT MODALITIES

It is very important that the mental health interdisciplinary treatment team work together to manage each client's mental and emotional disorder and symptoms. Consequently, team meetings are common on the psychiatric unit, where psychiatric mental health nurses, psychiatrists, psychologists, social workers, occupational therapists, recreational therapists, pharmacologists, special education teachers (for children and adolescents), and other support staff come together to communicate their expertise regarding the client's diagnosis, problems, and treatment plans. Briefly described below are the various gaols and activities of these collaborative professionals in their respective disciplines.

Psychopharmacology

Psychopharmacology is the somatic treatment of choice today. The pharmacist dispenses medications for psychiatric clients according to the physician's prescription, keeps informed on new developments in psychotropic drugs, and in collaboration with the physician educates the staff regarding the actions and side effects of the newer neuroleptic drugs. The pharmacist also consults with the psychiatrist, regarding chemical properties of the medications and their interactions with food and other drugs. In many institutions the pharmacist also takes some responsibility, along with physicians and nurses, for client education.

For an extensive discussion of the psychotrophic drugs used for the treatment of schizophrenia, refer to Chapter 23.

Psychotrophic drugs often have serious side effects. Two of the most serious are akathisia and neuroleptic malignant syndrome (NMS).

Atypical antipsychotic medications such as clozapine (Clozaril), which has been effective in treating refractory clients; risperidone (Risperdal); olanzapine (Zyprexa); and quetiapine (Seroquel) have successfully improved the negative symptoms of schizophrenia, such as apathy, lack of motivation, and decreased social skills. Although these newer antipsychotics have reduced or in some cases eliminated serious side effects such as extrapyramidal symptoms, tardive dyskinesia, and neuroleptic malignant syn-

drome (NMS), unpredicted toxicities may arise in the future; thus keen nursing observations remain a critical intervention in medication therapy (see Chapter 23).

When a client is discharged to the family and community, one important criterion is that he or she accept responsibility for self-care, particularly with respect to medication. This has important implications for health teaching by nurses (see Client & Family Teaching Guidelines box).

Somatic Therapy

Somatic therapy had its origin in the concept of the sanitarium, a place where persons with mental illness could go for rest and healthy physical treatment. The idea of the sanitarium was to offer the clients fresh air, vitamins, a

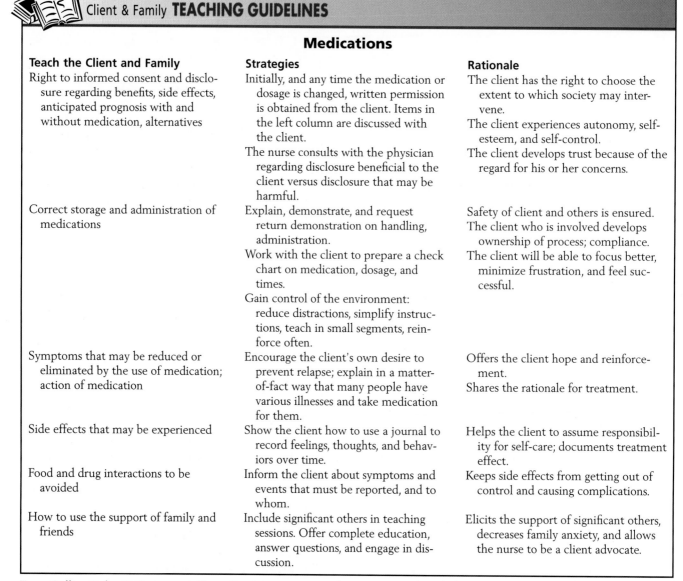

Client & Family TEACHING GUIDELINES

Medications

Teach the Client and Family	Strategies	Rationale
Right to informed consent and disclosure regarding benefits, side effects, anticipated prognosis with and without medication, alternatives	Initially, and any time the medication or dosage is changed, written permission is obtained from the client. Items in the left column are discussed with the client. The nurse consults with the physician regarding disclosure beneficial to the client versus disclosure that may be harmful.	The client has the right to choose the extent to which society may intervene. The client experiences autonomy, self-esteem, and self-control. The client develops trust because of the regard for his or her concerns.
Correct storage and administration of medications	Explain, demonstrate, and request return demonstration on handling, administration. Work with the client to prepare a check chart on medication, dosage, and times. Gain control of the environment: reduce distractions, simplify instructions, teach in small segments, reinforce often.	Safety of client and others is ensured. The client who is involved develops ownership of process; compliance. The client will be able to focus better, minimize frustration, and feel successful.
Symptoms that may be reduced or eliminated by the use of medication; action of medication	Encourage the client's own desire to prevent relapse; explain in a matter-of-fact way that many people have various illnesses and take medication for them.	Offers the client hope and reinforcement. Shares the rationale for treatment.
Side effects that may be experienced	Show the client how to use a journal to record feelings, thoughts, and behaviors over time.	Helps the client to assume responsibility for self-care; documents treatment effect.
Food and drug interactions to be avoided	Inform the client about symptoms and events that must be reported, and to whom.	Keeps side effects from getting out of control and causing complications.
How to use the support of family and friends	Include significant others in teaching sessions. Offer complete education, answer questions, and engage in discussion.	Elicits the support of significant others, decreases family anxiety, and allows the nurse to be a client advocate.

From Collins-Colon T: Do it yourself: medication management for community-based clients, *J Psychosoc Nurs* 28(6):25, 1990; and Weiss F: The right to refuse: informed consent and the psychosocial nurse, *J Psychosoc Nurs* 28(8):25, 1990.

healthy diet, and rest and relaxation. This is still a good idea, although more than palliative treatment is available today.

Somatic therapies are infrequently used today, except for electroconvulsive therapy (ECT), which is used most often for severe depression and for some schizophrenic syndromes that are short term and have affective symptoms (Valente, 1991). ECT is also useful for the client with catatonic schizophrenia. A course of treatment usually consists of 6 to 12 episodes. Nursing implications for the client receiving therapy are explanation, renegotiation of the client's consent, nurturance, monitoring, orientation, support, family teaching, and analgesics for headache following treatment. ECT is discussed in detail in Chapter 23.

Other somatic therapies that have fallen into disuse are psychosurgery (lobotomy), insulin coma therapy, hydrotherapy, and narcotherapy. Therapeutic use of seclusion, restraints, and jackets is a means for the client to gain self-control of escalating aggressive behavior that may pose a danger to self or others (see Table 14-6).

Milieu Therapy

Milieu therapy is a 24-hour environment that shelters, protects, supports, and enhances the client with mental illness. This is the model currently in use on psychiatric units today. It is characterized by individualized treatment programs, self-governance, humanistic attitudes, an enhancing environment, and links to the family and community. The purpose of milieu therapy is to assist the client in learning to manage and cope with stress, as well as to correct maladaptive behaviors.

Psychosocial Rehabilitation

As clients move toward community living, a similar model, the psychosocial rehabilitation model, helps them readjust to community living (Boyd, 1994; Olfson et al, 1993). This model, with the assistance of community services, encourages clients to participate with others in the community. This enables clients to develop skills and talents that have lain dormant during their illnesses. The model differs from the hospital-based program in that there is more emphasis on autonomy and fewer constraints (Harris, 1990). Psychosocial rehabilitation is coordinated by psychiatric mental health nurses who assess physical problems, oversee the functioning of the client in the environment, dispense medications, meet with families, and refer clients to job training and to appropriate service providers in the community. With the loss of hospital beds, future trends point toward case management and psychosocial rehabilitation (Mann et al, 1993; Thompson and Strand, 1994).

Individual Psychotherapy

Individual psychotherapy may be given by a psychiatrist, a psychologist, a psychiatric social worker, a psychiatric clinical nurse specialist, or a specialist in family and child counseling, all of whom are educationally prepared at the master's or doctorate level and work autonomously with their clients. The purpose of psychotherapy is to effect a positive change in the client by helping him or her develop effective coping patterns and overcome the feeling of helplessness most clients experience. There are many types of therapy, as described in Chapter 22. The choice of therapy depends on the client's condition and symptoms, as well as the therapist's area of expertise. The levels of therapy are as follows.

Supportive therapy allows the person to express feelings and reinforces effective coping mechanisms. It is particularly effective for clients with schizophrenia (Olfson et al, 1993).

Re-educative therapy is useful for the higher-functioning client. It is a cognitive technique that uses role-playing to explore new ways of perceiving and behaving.

Reconstructive therapy is not considered helpful for clients with schizophrenia (Olfson et al, 1993). It consists of psychoanalysis or intensive therapy groups and delves into all aspects of the client's life (Weiden and Havens, 1994).

Group Therapy

Group therapy is discussed in detail in Chapter 22. However, the type of group therapy suitable for clients with schizophrenia varies according to their level of functioning. Nurses generally use the Rogerian model, which helps clients to express and clarify feelings and promotes feelings of acceptance. This therapy uses the technique of reflection, is evocative, is not confrontative, and may allow behavioral tryouts.

Family Therapy

For a detailed discussion on family therapy, refer to Chapter 22. For the client with schizophrenia, especially one with paranoia, it may be necessary to begin with individual family therapy in which each family member has a therapist. This type of family therapy is also recommended as a first step for extremely disturbed families. Later, the family may progress to conjoint (nuclear) family therapy, in which communication patterns are emphasized among family members and the integrity of each family member is supported. According to Bellack and Mueser (1993), intervention programs that include educating families through family therapy have helped them cope with the client's illness and show positive effects on the course of the schizophrenia.

Behavior Modification

Behavior modification is a precise approach to bringing about behavioral change. Those types that are used for schizophrenia are listed below.

Operant conditioning is widely used in child and adolescent units and is useful for anyone needing to control the behavior of other individuals. It operates on the principle of reinforcing desirable behaviors so that they will reoccur and ignoring negative behaviors. The techniques used include relaxation and self-control procedures. Results from using this form of therapy indicate that intolerable behaviors such as withdrawal, screaming, incontinence, and incoherence lessen. In some cases it has then been possible to prepare chronically ill, hospitalized persons to live in the community, as both positive and negative symptoms of schizophrenia have improved (Liberman et al, 1994).

Cognitive therapy explores the connection between distorted thinking and negative behavior. For example, the client who engages in all-or-nothing thinking may not be participating in a craft session because "I can never do anything right." For high-functioning patients, "homework" is assigned to separate out negative thoughts from negative feelings. Intensive cognitive behavior therapy has been used in connection with reduction of neuroleptic dosages in clients who have negative symptoms, suffer medication side effects, and are minimally responsive to medication.

Imagery is often combined with relaxation therapy. The client pictures past pleasant memories. Imagery is sometimes combined with role-playing.

Assertiveness training deconditions the anxiety arising from interpersonal relationships, which are usually a problem for the client with schizophrenia. This training promotes expressive, spontaneous, goal-directed, self-enhancing behavior.

Exercise, movement therapy, and dance therapy promote identification of the body image through kinesthetic stimulation, as well as providing a form of coping for stress (see Chapter 26).

ADDITIONAL TREATMENT MODALITIES
For the Client With Schizophrenia

Psychopharmacology
Somatic therapy
Milieu therapy
Psychosocial rehabilitation
Individual psychotherapy
   Supportive therapy
   Re-educative therapy
   Reconstructive therapy
Group therapy
Family therapy
Behavior modification
   Operant conditioning
   Cognitive therapy
   Imagery
   Assertiveness training
   Exercise, movement therapy, and dance therapy
Occupational and recreational therapy
Therapies to prevent acting out or assault

Occupational and Recreational Therapy

Occupational therapy is a diagnostic tool that assesses the functional level and progress of the client with schizophrenia. The occupational therapist uses crafts as a tool to check hand-eye coordination, perception, and fine muscle tone. Some visit the client's home to provide special equipment or needed therapy. In fact, today's psychosocial rehabilitation programs depend on active-directive learning principles designed to help the client regain or improve skills, or to develop alternate, compensatory skills useful for community living (Boyd, 1994).

The recreational therapist's emphasis is on body kinesics, movement therapy, and resocialization through recreation. The emphasis is on cooperation rather than competition, especially for the client with schizophrenia. The therapist works on client motivation, planning trips and outings. For a more detailed description of occupational and recreational therapy, see Chapter 26.

Special Therapies to Prevent Acting Out or Assault

Given that there is a possibility for violent behaviors in seriously ill clients with schizophrenia, clinicians take steps to avoid impending assault. There are two ideas to be considered. The first idea is to predict when violence may occur as a result of the emotional stress, attitude, or behavior of others toward the client with schizophrenia (Vincent and White, 1994). The second idea is to employ de-escalation skills to reduce the threat of violence and/or physical methods to contain it (Turnbull et al, 1990).

De-escalation skills are useful techniques that can be used for interpersonal relationships in any context but are especially important for the psychiatric mental health nurse. The skills range from using nonthreatening verbal and nonverbal messages to safely disengaging and controlling the aggressor physically. The choice to use the techniques set forth in Table 14-6 will depend on the stage of the threat, the speed of escalation of the impending violence, and the feedback received from the client, representing the effectiveness of the technique.

Violence in interpersonal relationships frequently arises as a result of differing expectations regarding therapeutic or social rules and their enforcement; it also may be triggered by substance abuse. Negative reinforcement may play a part, in that violent behavior intimidates people and drives them away from the aggressor, who experiences self-gain in control (Morrison, 1994). Although the expression of aggressive behavior may be influenced by defective functioning of the central nervous system (Harper-Jaques and Reimer, 1992), mental health practitioners need to be aware of the ways that anger, aggression, and violence are reinforced, whatever the inciting event (see Chapters 27 and 28.)

EVALUATION

At its most basic level, evaluation follows specific intervention statements and behavioral objectives incorporating the concepts of quality, quantity, and time. For example, if a goal is to resocialize a client who has been isolating herself while on the unit, an intervention might consist of having the client join the current affairs discussion group along with other clients on the unit. To evaluate the effectiveness of this intervention, specific behavioral client outcomes to be accomplished are stated in measurable terms. For example, a beginning behavioral objective might be: "On her second day on the unit, Mary will accompany the nurse to the current affairs discussion group, and she will remain with the group for 15 minutes."

Note that the outcome is criteria specific as to time (on the second day), quality of experience (going to the discussion group with the nurse), and quantity (for 15 minutes). These criteria can be seen and measured. If all criteria are met, the minimal acceptable level of performance will progress, so that by the third day, the client outcome might read: "Mary will go to the discussion group on her own, remain for a half hour, and make at least one comment."

Nursing process is not a static concept. It is an ongoing design for interaction with the environment and is evaluated as such. If the criteria were evaluated and found not to be met on the second day, for instance, the client outcomes and nursing interventions would have to be reconsidered and perhaps rewritten at a level closer to the client's ability to perform. If outcomes are revised and are still not met, the rest of the nursing process will need to be examined in total. Thus eventual success with the nursing process demands patience and persistence, as gains are made in small increments, especially in clients with chronic schizophrenia.

Table 14-6   De-Escalation of Aggressive Behavior

Concept	Behavior	Rationale
Managing the environment	Persuade the client to move to another area. Enlist help from colleagues to remove other clients, but have one colleague near you.	Prevents anxiety contagion; protects others.
Showing confidence and leadership	(Hold regular drills with staff to practice strategies.) Give clear instructions. Be brief. Be assertive. Negotiate options. If the client has a weapon, instruct him/her to put it on the floor.	Prevents panic when crises occur. Avoids misunderstandings, not knowing what to do. Allows the client to feel that he or she has some room in exercising options.
Encouraging verbalization	Ask questions that are open ended and non-threatening. Use "How?" "What?" "When?" to get details, but *not* "Why?" Keep voice calm and modulated.	Refocuses on the client's problem and not on his or her intent to act out the anger. Stops anger from escalating.
Using nonverbal expression	Allow the client body space; do not stand closer than about 8 feet. Keep your body at a 45-degree angle. Assume an open posture; hands at sides, palms outward.	Conveys nonthreatening message, willingness to listen and accommodate the client.
Personalizing yourself and showing concern	Remind the client who *you* are; the world may be nasty, but *you* haven't done any harm to him or her. Use words such as "we" or "us." Show that you are listening; use encouragers such as "go on . . ." to show empathy.	Encourages and reflects cooperation.
Using disengagement breakaways	Manage hair pulls, strangle holds, grabs, and hugs according to safety instructions, videos, and return demonstrations.	Prevents injury to self, the client, and others.
Using removal, seclusion, and restraints	Rehearse these procedures regularly.	Allows the client to regain self-control.
Accurately documenting the event; holding a debriefing session with staff	Keep a detailed record: time, place, circumstances. Review and discuss the event.	Keeps an accurate account (e.g., for legal aspects). Helps staff to de-escalate and learn.

Modified from Turnbull J et al: Turn it around: short-term management for aggression and anger, *J Psychosoc Nurs* 28(6):6, 1990.

Summary of Key Concepts

1. The schizophrenias are the largest group of mental disorders.
2. Biologic factors are foremost in the research and interest in the etiology of schizophrenia. Five biologic models currently considered are heredity/genetic, neuroanatomic/neurochemical, neurotransmitter function, immunologic, and stress/disease/trauma/drug abuse.
3. The five major subtypes of schizophrenia are paranoid, disorganized, catatonic, undifferentiated, and residual.
4. Diagnostic criteria for schizophrenia include two or more symptoms of hallucinations, delusions, disorganized or catatonic behavior, or disorganized speech that are evident for at least 1 month.
5. Involving the client with schizophrenia and the client's family or significant others in the treatment plan is very important and contributes to more effective treatment.
6. Psychopharmacology is a widely used intervention for symptoms of schizophrenia.
7. Milieu therapy, psychosocial rehabilitation, psychotherapy, and behavior modification techniques are some treatments used with clients with schizophrenia.

REFERENCES

American Psychiatric Association: *Diagnostic and statistical manual of mental disorders*, ed 4, Washington, DC, 1994, The Association.

Andreasen N, Carpenter W: Diagnosis and classification of schizophrenia, *Schizophr Bull* 19(2):199, 1993.

Arieti S: *Interpretation of schizophrenia*, ed 2, New York, 1974, Basic Books.

Arieti S: Schizophrenia: the manifest symptomatology, the psychodynamic and formal mechanisms. In Arieti S, editor: *American handbook of psychiatry*, vol 1, New York, 1959, Basic Books.

Bawden E: Reaching out to the mentally ill homeless, *J Psychosoc Nurs* 28(3):6, 1990.

Bellack A, Mueser K: Psychosocial treatment for schizophrenia, *Schizophr Bull* 19(2):317, 1993.

Bendik M: Reaching the breaking point: dangers of mistreatment in elder caregiving situations, *J Elder Abuse Negl* 4(3):39, 1992.

Benes F: Neurobiological investigations in cingulate cortex of schizophrenic brain, *Schizophr Bull* 19(3):537, 1993.

Betemps E, Ragiel C: Psychiatric epidemiology: facts and myths on mental health and illness, *J Psychosoc Nurs* 32(5):23, 1994.

Bogerts B: Recent advances in the neuropathology of schizophrenia, *Schizophr Bull* 19(2):431, 1993.

Boyd M: Integration of psychosocial rehabilitation into psychiatric nursing practice, *Issues Ment Health Nurs* 15:13, 1994.

Breier A et al: Effects of clozapine on positive and negative symptoms in outpatients with schizophrenia, *Am J Psychiatry* 151(1):20, 1994.

Brown J: Role of selenium and other trace elements in the geography of schizophrenia, *Schizophr Bull* 20(2):387, 1994.

Calev A, Edelist S: Affect and memory in schizophrenia: negative emotion words are forgotten less rapidly than other words by long-hospitalized schizophrenics, *Psychopathology* 26:229, 1993.

Cannon J, Marco E: Structural brain abnormalities as indicators of vulnerability to schizophrenia, *Schizophr Bull* 20(1):89, 1994.

Castle D, Murray R: The epidemiology of late-onset schizophrenia, *Schizophr Bull* 19(4):691, 1993.

Clementz B, McDowell J, Zisook S: Saccadic system fixing among schizophrenic patients and their first-degree biological relatives, *J Abnorm Psychol* 130(2):277, 1994.

Cohen C: Poverty and the course of schizophrenia: implications for research and policy, *Hosp Community Psychiatry* 44(10):951, 1993.

Collins-Colon T: Do it yourself: medication management for community-based clients, *J Psychosoc Nurs* 28(6): 25, 1990.

Crow T: Molecular pathology of schizophrenia: more than one disease process? *BMJ* 12:66, January 1980.

D'Angelo E: Conceptual disorganization in children at risk for schizophrenia, *Psychopathology* 26:195, 1993.

Dauner A, Blair D: Akathisia: when treatment creates a problem, *J Psychosoc Nurs* 28(10):13, 1990.

DeMann J: First person account: the evolution of a person with schizophrenia, *Schizophr Bull* 20(3):579, 1994.

Draine J et al: Predictors of reincarceration among patients who received psychiatric services in jail, *Hosp Community Psychiatry* 45(2):163, 1994.

Dworkin R et al: Childhood precursors of affective vs. social deficits in adolescents at risk for schizophrenia, *Schizophr Bull* 19(3):563, 1993.

Dworkin R et al: Social competence deficits in adolescents at risk for schizophrenia, *J Nerv Ment Dis* 182(2):103, 1994.

Dzurec L: How do they see themselves? Self-perception and functioning for people with chronic schizophrenia, *J Psychosoc Nurs* 28(8):10, 1990.

Elkashef A et al: Basal ganglia pathology in schizophrenia and tardive dyskinesia: an MRI quantitative study, *Am J Psychiatry* 151(5):752, 1994.

Evans D et al: Self-perception and adolescent psychopathology: a clinical-developmental perspective, *Am J Orthopsychiatry* 64(2):293, 1994.

Fields J et al: Assessing positive and negative symptoms in children and adolescents, *Am J Psychiatry* 151(2):249, 1994.

Fortinash KM: Assessment of mental status. In Malasanos L, Barkauskas V, Stoltenberg-Allen K, editors: *Health assessment*, ed 4, St. Louis, 1990, Mosby.

Fortinash KM, Holoday-Worret PA: *Psychiatric nursing care plans*, ed 3, St. Louis, 1999, Mosby.

Fuentes I et al: Relationships between electrodermal activity and symptomatology in schizophrenia, *Psychopathology* 26:47, 1993.

Goldman R et al: Neuropsychological prediction of treatment efficacy and one-year outcome in schizophrenia, *Psychopathology* 26:122, 1993.

Green M et al: Dichotic listening during auditory hallucinations in patients with schizophrenia, *Am J Psychiatry* 151(3):357, 1994.

Gundel H, Rudolf G: Schizophrenic autism: proposal for a nomothetic definition, *Psychopathology* 26:304, 1993.

Gur R et al: Clinical subtypes of schizophrenia: differences in brain and CSF volume, *Am J Psychiatry* 151(3):343, 1994.

Gur R, Pearlson G: Neuroimaging in schizophrenia research, *Schizophr Bull* 19(2):337, 1993.

Gureje O et al: Early brain trauma and schizophrenia in Nigerian patients, *Am J Psychiatry* 151(3):368, 1994.

Harper-Jaques S, Reimer M: Aggressive behavior and the brain: a different perspective for the mental health nurse, *Arch Psychiatr Nurs* 6(5):312, 1992.

Harris J: Self-care actions of chronic schizophrenics associated with meeting solitude and social interaction requisites, *Arch Psychiatr Nurs* 4(5):298, 1990.

Hemsley D et al: The neuropsychology of schizophrenia: act 3, *BBS* 16(1):209, 1993.

Hietala J et al: Striatal D_2 dopamine receptor characteristics in neuroleptic-naive schizophrenic patients studied with positron emission tomography, *Arch Gen Psychiatry* 51:116, 1994.

Hoffman R: Commentary: dissecting psychotic speech, *J Nerv Ment Dis* 182(4):212, 1994.

Janicak P et al: *Principles and practice of psychopharmacotherapy*, Baltimore, 1993, Williams & Wilkins.

Joseph M: The neuropsychology of schizophrenia: beyond the dopamine hypothesis to behavioral function, *BBS* 16(1):203, 1993.

Kaplan HI, Sadock BJ: *Synopsis of psychiatry: behavioral sciences, clinical psychiatry*, ed 8, Baltimore, 1998, Williams & Wilkins.

Keltner N, Folks D: *Psychotropic drugs*, St. Louis, 1993, Mosby.

Kendler K, Diehl S: The genetics of schizophrenia: a current, genetic-epidemiologic perspective, *Schizophr Bull* 19(2):261, 1993.

Kennedy B et al: Hallucinatory experiences of psychiatric patients in seclusion, *Arch Psychiatr Nurs* 8(3):169, 1994.

Kennedy M: Relationship between psychiatric diagnosis and patient aggression, *Issues Ment Health Nurs* 14:263, 1993.

Lenzenweger M: Psychometric high-risk paradigm, perceptual aberrations, and schizotypy: an update, *Schizophr Bull* 20(1):121-135, 1994.

Lewandowski L: Brain-behavior relationships. In Hartlage L et al, editors: *Essentials of neuropsychological assessment*, New York, 1991, Springer.

Lieberman J, Koreen: Neurochemistry and neuroendocrinology of schizophrenia: a selective review, *Schizophr Bull* 19(2), 371, 1993.

Liberman R et al: Optimal drug and behavior therapy for treatment-refractory schizophrenic patients, *Am J Psychiatry* 151(5):756, 1994.

Linszen D et al: Cannabis abuse and the course of recent-onset schizophrenic disorders, *Arch Gen Psychiatry* 51(4):273, 1994.

Macciardi F et al: Analysis of the D_4 dopamine receptor gene in an Italian schizophrenia kindred, *Arch Gen Psychiatry* 51(4):288, 1994.

Malone J: Schizophrenia research update: implications for nursing, *J Psychosoc Nurs* 28(8), 4, 1990.

Mann N et al: Psychosocial rehabilitation in schizophrenia: beginnings in acute hospitalization, *Arch Psychiatr Nurs* 7(3):154, 1993.

Mannion E et al: Designing psychoeducational services for spouses of persons with serious mental illness, *Community Ment Health J* 30(2):177-190, 1994.

Mattos J: Science—brain work, pictures shed light on the mystery of schizophrenia, *Time Magazine* 146(21), 1995.

McCain N, Smith J: Stress and coping in the context of psychoneuroimmunology: a holistic framework for nursing practice and research, *Arch Psychiatr Nurs* 8(4):221, 1994.

McEnvoy J et al: Insight about psychosis among outpatients with schizophrenia, *Hosp Community Psychiatry* 44(9):883, 1993.

Meador K, Nichols F: The neurological examination as it relates to neuropsychological issues. In Hartlage L et al, editors: *Essentials of neuropsychological assessment*, New York, 1991, Springer.

Morrison E: The evolution of a concept: aggression and violence in psychiatric settings, *Arch Psychiatr Nurs* 8(4):245, 1994.

Mulvey E: Assessing the evidence of a link between mental illness and violence, *Hosp Community Psychiatry* 45(7):663, 1994.

Natale A, Barron C: Mothers' causal explanations for their son's schizophrenia: relationship to depression and guilt, *Arch Psychiatr Nurs* 8(4):228, 1994.

North American Nursing Diagnosis Association: *NANDA nursing diagnoses: definitions and classifications: 1999-2000*, Philadelphia, 1999, The Association.

Oke S et al: The contingent negative variation in positive and negative types of schizophrenia, *Am J Psychiatry* 151(3):432, 1994.

Olfson M et al: Inpatient treatment of schizophrenia in general hospitals, *Hosp Community Psychiatry* 44(1):40, 1993.

Orrison WW et al: *Functional brain imaging*, St. Louis, 1995, Mosby.

Osmon D: The neuropsychological examination. In Hartlage L et al, editors: *Essentials of neuropsychological assessment* New York, 1991, Springer.

Peplau H: Future directions in psychiatric nursing from the perspective of history, *J Psychosoc Nurs* 18, 1989.

Peplau H: Principles of psychiatric nursing. In Arieti S, editor: *American handbook of psychiatry*, vol 2, New York, 1959, Basic Books.

Perry W, Braff D: Information-processing deficits and thought disorder in schizophrenia, *Am J Psychiatry* 151(3):363, 1994.

Plum F: Prospects for research on schizophrenia. III. Neuropsychology: neuropathological findings, *Neurosci Res Prog Bull* 10:348, 1972.

Previc F: A neuropsychology of schizophrenia without vision, *BBS* 16(1):207, 1993.

Sabate O et al: Failure to find evidence of linkage or association between dopamine D$_3$ receptor gene and schizophrenia, *Am J Psychiatry* 151(1):107, 1994.

Scherling D: Prenatal cocaine exposure and childhood psychopathology, *Am J Orthopsychiatry* 64(1):9, 1994.

Shore D: *Recent developments in schizophrenia research: relevance for psychiatric nurses*. Plenary session address to American Psychiatric Nurses' Association Convention, Denver, 1989.

Smothergill D, Kraut A: Toward the more direct study of attention in schizophrenia: alertness decrement and encoding facilitation, *BBS* 16(1):208, 1993.

Stirling J et al: Expressed emotion and schizophrenia: the ontogeny of EE during an 18-month follow-up, *Capsules Comments Psychiatr Nurs* 1(1):40, 1994.

Takei N et al: Prenatal exposure to influenza and the development of schizophrenia: is the effect confined to females? *Am J Psychiatry* 151(1):117, 1994.

Thompson J, Strand K: Psychiatric nursing in a psychosocial setting, *J Psychosoc Nurs* 32(2):25, 1994.

Trygstad L: The need to know: biological learning needs identified by practicing psychiatric nurses, *J Psychosoc Nurs* 32(2):13, 1994.

Tsuang M: Genetics, epidemiology, and the search for causes of schizophrenia, *Am J Psychiatry* 151(1):3, 1994.

Turnbull J et al: Turn it around: short-term management for aggression and anger, *J Psychosoc Nurs* 28(6):6, 1990.

Turner B: First person account: the children of madness, *Schizophr Bull* 19(3):649, 1993.

Valente S: Electroconvulsive therapy, *Arch Psychiatr Nurs* 5(4):223, 1991.

vanKarmen D et al: CSF dopamine B-hydroxylase in schizophrenia: associations with premorbid functioning and brain computerized tomography scan measures, *Am J Psychiatry* 151(3):372, 1994.

Vincent M, White K: Patient violence toward a nurse: predictable and preventable? *J Psychosoc Nurs* 32(2):30, 1994.

Weiden P, Havens L: Psychotherapeutic management techniques in the treatment of outpatients with schizophrenia, *Hosp Community Psychiatry* 45(6):549, 1994.

Weiss F: The right to refuse: informed consent and the psychosocial nurse, *J Psychosoc Nurs* 28(8):25, 1990.

Notes

CHAPTER 15

Personality Disorders

Pamela E. Marcus

OBJECTIVES

- Discuss three elements of personality development as described by Freud in the psychosexual stages of development.

- Describe two contributions made by Margaret Mahler and Otto Kernberg to object relations theory.

- Identify two biologic indices that are often abnormal in clients with a personality disorder.

- Describe one behavior, in one or two words, that differentiates between Clusters A, B, and C of Axis II in the DSM-IV.

- Discuss two nursing diagnoses for each cluster of the personality disorders.

- Define splitting behaviors, and list two nursing interventions that effectively challenge the client's "black or white" view of the world.

- Identify a plan of care for two different personality disorders, including two treatment modalities that are collaborative and two outcome criteria relevant to the client's DSM-IV diagnosis.

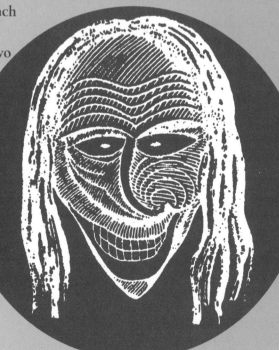

PERSONALITY DISORDERS

DEFINITION OF PERSONALITY DISORDERS

The definition of personality disorders, as classified by the DSM-IV, are long-standing, pervasive, maladaptive patterns of behavior and relating to others that are not caused by Axis I disorders (Kaplan and Sadock, 1990). According to the DSM-IV, a personality disorder is an "enduring pattern of inner experience and behavior that deviates markedly from the expectations of the individual's culture, is pervasive and inflexible, has an onset in adolescence or early adulthood, is stable over time, and leads to distress or impairment" (American Psychiatric Association [APA], 1994). All human beings have a personality made up of one's definition of self, skills used to relate to others, and a defense structure. When studying personality disorders, one has to determine to what degree these qualities are compromised. One can determine these behaviors by observing how individuals relate to others, their perception of surroundings, and their ability to problem solve. According to Manfield (1992):

The term personality disorder, also called a "disorder of the self," refers to a lack of a genuine sense of "self" and a consequent impairment of self-regulating abilities. Instead of looking within themselves to locate feelings or to make decisions, persons with personality disorders look outside themselves for evaluations, directions, rules, or opinions to guide them.

DEFINITION OF AXIS II IN DSM-IV

When reviewing the diagnostic criteria for the various personality disorders (Axis II), it is important to differentiate personality traits from personality disorders. DSM-IV has

Comorbid More than one psychiatric diagnosis occurring at the same time in the same individual.

Devaluation Dealing with emotional conflict or stressors by attributing exaggerated negative qualities to self or others.

Idealization The tendency of a person with borderline personality disorder to idealize persons or groups beyond their capabilities when they are meeting that person's needs.

Milieu therapy
Re-creates a community atmosphere on an inpatient hospital unit, a partial hospitalization unit, and a day treatment setting in order to facilitate interaction between client peers to identify and problem solve issues that occur while relating to others.

Object constancy The ability to maintain a relationship regardless of frustration and changes in the relationship. Also, a stage in growth and development when the toddler can maintain the image of the mother even when she is not within the toddler's sight.

Object relations The stability and depth of an individual's relations with significant others as manifested by warmth, dedication, concern, and tactfulness.

Personality traits
Behaviors and enduring patterns of perceiving, relating to, and thinking about the environment and oneself that are exhibited in a wide range of social and personal contexts.

Projective identification Projecting one's emotional conflicts and stressors to another who does not fully disavow what is projected. The individual remains aware of his or her own affects or impulses but misattributes them as justifiable reactions to the other person.

Splitting Keeping the positive and negative aspects of self and others separate from each other. An individual who uses the unconscious defense mechanism of splitting cannot tolerate ambiguity. Therefore people, events, or ideas are either good or bad, right or wrong, black or white, but not gray.

State disorders
The diagnoses made on Axis I. These diagnoses constitute behavior patterns that are not as pervasive or long lasting as trait disorders.

Trait disorders The diagnoses made on Axis II, which is used exclusively for the description of personality disorders and mental retardation. The symptoms of a personality disorder or mental retardation are not time limited and do not occur only in a time of crisis.

Transitional objects Objects that remind one of a significant person. For example, a man keeps a picture of his wife on his desk, which reminds him of her during work hours.

Personality Disorder

DSM-IV CRITERIA

A. An enduring pattern of inner experience and behavior that deviates markedly from the expectations of the individual's culture. This pattern is manifested in two (or more) of the following areas:
  1. Cognition (i.e., ways of perceiving and interpreting self, other people, and events)
  2. Affectivity (i.e., the range, intensity, lability, and appropriateness of emotional response)
  3. Interpersonal functioning
  4. Impulse control
B. The enduring pattern is inflexible and pervasive across a broad range of personal and social situations.
C. The enduring pattern leads to clinically significant distress or impairment in social, occupational, or other important areas of functioning.
D. The pattern is stable and of long duration, and its onset can be traced back at least to adolescence or early adulthood.
E. The enduring pattern is not better accounted for as a manifestation or consequence of another mental disorder.
F. The enduring pattern is not due to the direct physiologic effects of a substance (e.g., a drug of abuse, a medication) or a general medical condition (e.g., head trauma).

From American Psychiatric Association: *Diagnostic and statistical manual of mental disorders*, ed 4, Washington, DC, 1994, The Association.

defined six general diagnostic criteria for a personality disorder as listed in the DSM-IV Criteria box.

Personality traits are those behaviors, patterns of perceiving, relating to others, and thinking about the environment and oneself that are exhibited in a wide range of social and personal contexts (APA, 1994). These traits may be adaptive or maladaptive **trait disorders,** depending on whether the trait is inflexible or causes significant functional impairment or subjective distress. When this occurs, one is said to have a personality disorder. The symptoms of a personality disorder are neither time limited nor do they occur only in a time of crisis (APA, 1994; Kaplan and Sadock, 1990; Kreisman and Straus, 1989). Behaviors are long-standing, enduring, and not responsive to short-term psychotherapy or pharmacologic measures.

Diagnoses made on Axis I are considered **state disorders.** These diagnoses constitute behavior patterns that are not as long in duration (Kreisman and Straus, 1989). Often the symptoms of these disorders can be alleviated through the use of medication, psychotherapy, and milieu therapy for severe symptoms. Personality disorder diagnoses are classified on Axis II of the DSM-IV in a cluster format as follows:

Cluster A:

Paranoid, schizoid, and schizotypal are described as the odd and/or eccentric cluster.
These diagnoses are more likely to be **comorbid** (i.e., both diagnoses may be present in the same individual with psychotic disorders).

Cluster B:

Antisocial, borderline, histrionic, and narcissistic are described as the dramatic and emotional cluster.
The Cluster B group is often comorbid with affective disorders.

Cluster C:

Avoidant, dependent, and obsessive-compulsive compose the anxious and fearful cluster.
These diagnoses are often affiliated with anxiety disorders (APA, 1994; Oldham and Skodol, 1992; Widiger and Rogers, 1989).

Individuals with personality disorder diagnoses in each cluster may be predisposed to developing a comorbidity with specific Axis I diagnoses. However, this is not a hard-and-fast rule, and there are no consistent research findings that bear this out (APA, 1994; Oldham and Skodol, 1992; Widiger and Rogers, 1989).

THEORIES OF PERSONALITY DEVELOPMENT
FREUDIAN THEORIES

Sigmund Freud was one of the early published students of human development and inner psychologic conflict. The two areas that are covered in this chapter are (1) his structural theory, often referred to as the tripartite model of the hypothetical psychic structures of the id, ego, and superego, and (2) his psychosexual stages of development.

The psychosexual stages of development are described by Freud (1905) in his "Three Essays on the Theory of Sexuality." The first stage described by Freud is the oral stage. The traits associated with successful completion of this stage include the ability to relate to others without excessive dependency or jealously. Trust begins to develop, and with trust comes a sense of self-reliance and trust of self. Individuals who have difficulty with this stage often lack trust and are self-centered, dependent, and jealous (Tyson and Tyson, 1990).

The anal stage is the second stage described by Freud. This stage takes place during the time when the child begins to develop enough sphincter control to be able to control excretion of feces. This takes place approximately from ages 1 to 3 years. Successful completion of this stage is demonstrated in adult functioning by the individual's ability to deal with ambivalence in such a manner that decisions are made without shame or self-doubt; there is a sense of self-autonomy. A person who has difficulty with successful completion of this stage of development is unable to make decisions, withholds friendships or cannot share with others, is rageful, is stubborn, and has sadomasochistic tendencies (Tyson and Tyson, 1990).

The phallic stage is the next stage identified by Freud. It is the period of development when the child becomes interested in his or her genitals. Freud understood this stage in terms of male development; according to his theory, the phallus is the principal organ of concern for both boys and girls. This stage occurs during the ages of 3 through 6 or 7 years. Successful completion of this stage assists the child in achieving mastery over his or her internal processes and impulses, as well as in gaining a beginning sense of relating to other people in the environment. Individuals who are unable to resolve the conflict inherent in the phallic stage have multiple psychiatric disorders, particularly those that involve the superego function of guilt (i.e., the individual with an antisocial personality disorder does not have a well-developed superego).

According to Freud, the antisocial, borderline, histrionic, and narcissistic personality disorders involve individuals who experienced problems identifying with their sexual identity during the critical phallic stage. For example, an individual with a histrionic personality disorder who acts sexually provocative but denies that this behavior is sexually driven may have experienced an internal conflict with his or her sexual identity.

The next stage of psychosexual development is the latency stage. This stage is when the child represses the libidinal (sexual) drives, and attention is turned toward learning and industry. At this time there is further development of the ego in an effort to gain control over instinctual impulses. This stage takes place from the sixth or seventh year of life until puberty.

With this stage comes the exploration of the environment and play, when the child learns how to do things, to enjoy life, and have fun, and continues to develop inner control over instinctive drives and emotions. This stage is important for later adult functioning, because the child with a sense of industry is able to delay gratification, which helps in areas of learning, work, and relating to others. Problems in successful completion of this stage are seen with individuals who either have too much or too little ability to develop inner control. Those who lack inner control have difficulty relating to others, since their emotions rule their interactions and problem-solving abilities. Those individuals who have an excess of inner control have isolated their emotions and are more regulated, using repetition of thoughts or behavior to relate or problem solve.

The genital stage is the last stage described by Freud in an individual's psychosexual development. This stage takes place during puberty. The importance of this stage is that there is an opportunity to rework earlier issues that have not been resolved, in the service of achieving a healthy, mature sense of sexual and adult identity. With the ability to work and learn, individuals can establish goals and values within the context of their own unique personal identities.

If individuals have difficulty during the genital stage, their sense of self and ability to relate to others will be compromised. They will therefore be unable to attain their identified goals or form values. They will also experience difficulty in identifying their strengths and weaknesses, likes and dislikes, and types of skills they want to acquire. Individuals who have difficulty resolving the genital stage can manifest symptoms and behaviors that are described within the whole range of personality disorders.

OBJECT RELATIONS

As theorists studied human behavior further, particularly observing development of personality structure and relatedness, the theory of object relations began to be developed. This theory has many contributors and is being reevaluated and expanded as the study of human relations and personality development and disorders is more clearly understood. Tyson and Tyson (1990) have clarified the difference between interpersonal relations and object relations in the following manner:

The first (interpersonal relations) has to do with the actual interactions between people. **Object relations** (or "internalized" object relations) refers to the intrapsychic dimensions of experiences with others—that is, to the mental representations of the self and of the other and of the role of each in their interactions.

Object relations, then, is the stability and depth of an individual's relations with significant others as manifested by warmth, dedication, concern, and tactfulness.

Separation-Individuation Phase

When studying object relations from a developmental standpoint, Margaret Mahler identified and studied the separation-individuation phase of development occurring between ages 3 and 25 months. Mahler's theory of separation and individuation evolved from a longitudinal study where she observed normal mothers and their babies during the child's first 3 years of life. The term *separation* in this context refers to the child's gradually developing an intrapsychic self-representation that is distinct and separate from the representation of the mother. The term *individuation* is used in this context to recognize the infant's attempts to form a distinctive identity and to develop characteristics that are unique to that individual (Mahler, 1963; Tyson and Tyson, 1990).

Mahler (1963, 1972a) described four stages of the process of separation-individuation: differentiation, practicing, rapprochement, and object constancy. These stages are explained in Box 15-1.

Box 15-1   **Mahler's Stages of Separation-Individuation**

1. *Differentiation.* Occurs when the child is between 3 and 8 months old. During this stage, the child begins to differentiate his or her own image from that of the mother or significant nurturer.
2. *Practicing.* Occurs when the child is between 8 and 15 months old. The task of this stage is for the child to actively explore his or her world in a manner in which the child seems oblivious to the mother. This occurs when the child begins to walk and is able to explore the environment around him or her, as locomotion becomes more stabilized.
3. *Rapprochement.* Occurs when the child is between 15 and 22 months old. The child begins to return to the mother for emotional needs when the exploration of the surroundings (which is done during the practicing phase) is completed. During this time the toddler becomes moody and in distress with temper tantrums, even when the mother is with the child. The child wishes to have things his or her way, which may not be what the mother had planned. The task is for the child to deal with the conflict between his or her wish for independence and individuation, and with wanting to be loved and comforted by the mother.
4. *The beginning of object constancy.* Occurs around 25 months. Object constancy involves the ability to maintain a relationship regardless of frustration and changes in the relationship. The toddler at 25 months can think about the mother even when the mother is not close to the child and can therefore comfort himself or herself by the mother's representation. This comfort may include a blanket or stuffed toy that may remind the child of the mother.

Modified from Mahler MS: Thoughts about development and individuation, *Psychoanal Study Child* 18:307, 1963; and Mahler MS: On the first three subphases of the separation-individuation process, *Int J Psychoanal* 53:333, 1972.

Kernberg's Theories

Otto Kernberg studied individuals with severe personality disorders and formulated some ideas about these disorders and their development, primarily with borderline and narcissistic personality disorders. According to Kernberg (1984), a person who is emotionally healthy has an integrated working structure of the id, superego, and ego. This means that the ego is intact, with sufficient ability to determine reality from fantasy and to separate self from another object. The superego is functional, not too rigid or punishing, but a filter for the ego. The id is integrated and not in conflict with the other two structures.

Kernberg identified two essential tasks that the early ego must accomplish for the internalization of object relations. The first task involves the ability of the child to distinguish between self and other people in order to formulate healthy feelings about self and identification with the other person. This is similar to Mahler's differentiation stage. The second task that Kernberg discussed in relation to the internalization of object relations is that there is an integration of "good" and "bad" self-images, as well as an integration of "good" and "bad" object (the other person's) images. This consolidation of images leads to total self and object representations that are differentiated from one another and realistic in that both structures have good and bad, satisfaction and frustration, in their systems.

In the borderline personality disorder, or what Kernberg has called the "borderline personality organization," this is a particularly important aspect. Kernberg identified splitting as a primary defense of the individual with borderline personality disorder. **Splitting** is the inability to synthesize the positive and negative aspects of self and others. The person with borderline personality disorder exhibits splitting by his or her difficulty in perceiving that he or she and other people have both good and bad aspects. There is a tendency to idealize persons or groups when those persons meet the needs of the individual with borderline personality disorder. This process is called **idealization.** At the other extreme, a person with borderline personality disorder can devalue persons or groups when needs are not perceived to be met. This process is called **devaluation.** The person with borderline personality disorder views self and others as either all good or all bad and is unable to reach a state of **object constancy,** which means that one is unable to hold the memory of significant others in mind. This individual is unable to use **transitional objects** that represent the significant other person and that help the individual remember the other person. For example, an individual with object constancy can think of his or her loved one when experiencing something that may remind him or her of the other person, such as a favorite song or a tangible object. An individual who is unable to obtain object constancy cannot picture his or her loved one when that individual is away from him or her. Therefore the person views the absence of the significant other as an abandonment.

Masterson (1976) identified four defenses that block the client's developmental growth from the stages of individuation-separation to autonomy: projection, clinging, denial, and avoidance. According to Masterson, the client with borderline personality disorder becomes stuck in the subphases of the individuation-separation stage. This leads to the client's failure to achieve object constancy.

A client with borderline personality disorder does not relate to people as wholes but as parts. He or she is unable to sustain a relationship through the frustration of everyday living and tends to experience anger and rage when feeling rejected or ignored. This individual is unable to evoke the image of the other when the other is not present. If a significant person in the client's life dies, the client with borderline personality disorder cannot mourn but may exhibit one or more of the six constituent states:

depression, anger and rage, fear, guilt, passivity and help-lessness, and emptiness and void.

Another defense against the client's anxiety that is important in understanding the individual with a Cluster B personality disorder is **projective identification**. This defense is a primitive type of projection. Kernberg (1984) described this defense as having the following characteristics:

The tendency to continue to experience the impulse that is simultaneously being projected onto the other person

Fear of the other person under influence of that projected impulse

The need to control the other person under the influence of this mechanism

BIOLOGIC CONTRIBUTIONS TO PERSONALITY DISORDERS

As researchers in the biologic aspects of behaviors began to study some of the physiologic markers consistent with the Axis I diagnoses, some of the same studies were used with individuals with personality disorders, with consistent results. There have been family studies, including twin studies, that demonstrate a strong genetic influence, thus suggesting some ties between biologic factors and personality organization (Coryell and Zimmerman, 1989; Kavoussi and Siever, 1991; Marin et al, 1989; Siever, 1992; Siever and Davis, 1991).

One interesting aspect of this research is noted in the studies done on individuals with schizotypal personality disorder who demonstrate impaired eye-tracking behavior. Impaired eye-tracking behavior is described as "the inability to track a smoothly moving target" (Siever, 1992). This is important for cognitive interpretation of information in the environment. Individuals with schizophrenia demonstrate difficulty with smooth-pursuit eye movements, and this is thought to reflect disrupted neurointegrative functioning of the frontal lobes (Siever, 1992). The impaired eye-tracking studies are associated with the "deficit" traits of schizophrenia, namely the social isolation, detachment, and inability to relate to others.

Another biologic test indicative of cognitive-perceptual difficulties that is often seen in clients who have schizotypal personality disorder is *backward masking*. This test of neurointegrative functioning involves a "process in which a visual stimulus is rapidly followed by another visual stimulus and the subject is asked to identify the original stimulus" (Kavoussi and Siever, 1991). Siever (1985) found individuals with this personality disorder to have results similar to those noted in individuals with schizophrenia, but not as severe.

The ability to pay attention to stimuli is a biologic/cognitive marker that can be used to predict schizophrenia. The Continuous Performance Test, Identical Pairs Version,

tests the ability to attend to stimuli. In their study of the schizotypal personality disorder, Roitman et al (1997) reported that individuals demonstrated a verbal and spatial deficit when tested with the Continuous Performance Test, Identical Pairs Version, as compared with normal subjects and individuals who had other types of personality disorders. The test results were similar to the pattern usually seen with individuals with schizophrenia.

There are some neurochemical measures that are important indicators of biologic manifestations of the schizotypal personality disorder. Siever (1992) reported that cerebrospinal fluid homovanillic acid was increased in preliminary studies of schizotypal clients and correlated with positive psychotic-like criteria for schizotypal personality but without the negative or deficit symptoms. He also reported that plasma homovanillic acid was increased in clients with schizotypal personality disorder, as compared with client controls (Kavoussi and Siever, 1991). In 1988 researchers found that clients with borderline personality disorder who also had schizotypal personality disorder demonstrated evidence of a worsening of psychotic-like symptoms in response to an infusion of amphetamines.

In clients who have difficulty with affective regulation, some biologic indices are important to consider. The dexamethasone suppression test (DST), the thyrotropin-releasing hormone test (TRH), and electroencephalographic (EEG) sleep studies have been used in research as biologic markers of affective disorders. Abnormal DST and TRH results were found in clients with borderline personality disorder, prompting researchers to question whether these clients have a variant of mood disorders. However, in studies that separated clients with borderline personality disorder into groups with and without depression, it was reported that the nondepressed subjects had a higher percentage of normal DST and TRH results. Marin et al (1989) have suggested that these results may be related to depression rather than to the personality disorder.

Several studies demonstrate disturbances in central serotonergic neurotransmission, indicating that aggressive and suicidal behaviors in individuals with a personality disorder correlate with reduced levels of the cerebrospinal fluid 5-hydroxyindoleacetic acid, a major metabolite of serotonin, which indicates a reduction in serotonin activity (Brown et al, 1982). Mann et al (1986) found increased postsynaptic serotonergic receptors in suicide victims. Stanley and Stanley (1990) demonstrated information on both presynaptic and postsynaptic serotonergic "markers," which suggests that a reduction in serotonin neurotransmission is an underlying biochemical "risk factor" for suicide. Marin et al (1989) and Kavoussi and Siever (1991) surveyed several studies involving serotonin and its metabolites and found that there seems to be serotonergic reduction in behaviors such as impulsiveness, motor aggression, and suicidal tendencies. Brown and Linnoila (1990) studied the cerebrospinal fluid metabolites of serotonin

(5-HIAA), which indicated a relationship between reduced serotonergic activity and aggressive and impulsive behavior.

There may also be a dysfunction of the brain system's ability to modulate and inhibit aggressive responses to environmental stimuli (Siever and Davis, 1991). There are some data that EEG slow-wave activity and a low threshold for sedation discriminate individuals with antisocial personality disorder from individuals with long-term depression (Siever and Davis, 1991).

That individuals with personality disorders manifest some biologic markers is exciting for researchers and clinicians, since this information provides some suggestions that may be useful when treating this population. There is a need for future research in this area as the functions of the brain and the neurotransmitters become better known and understood.

CLINICAL DESCRIPTION AND EPIDEMIOLOGY
CLUSTER A PERSONALITY DISORDERS

Cluster A, often described as the "odd" or "eccentric" cluster, consists of the following personality disorders: paranoid, schizoid, and schizotypal. The clients in this cluster all have difficulty relating to others, isolate themselves, and are unable to socialize comfortably. The Clinical Symptoms box below and Box 15-2 provide summaries of the key clinical symptoms and epidemiology of each disorder.

CLUSTER B PERSONALITY DISORDERS

Cluster B personality disorders have components of dramatic behavior, a description widely used when describing individuals with a Cluster B personality disorder. The four diagnostic categories that make up this cluster are antisocial, borderline, histrionic, and narcissistic. Each personality disorder has unique features; each shares a dramatic quality in the way the individual lives his or her life. The Clinical Symptoms box on p. 337 and Box 15-3 summarize the key clinical symptoms and epidemiology of each of these disorders.

CLINICAL SYMPTOMS

Cluster A Personality Disorders

Paranoid Personality Disorder

Distrust, suspicion
Difficulty adjusting to change
Sensitivity, argumentation
Feelings of irreversible injury by others—often without evidence
Anxiety, difficulty relaxing
Short temper
Difficulty with problem solving
Lack of tender feelings toward others
Unwillingness to forgive even minor events
Jealousy of spouse or significant other—often without evidence

Schizoid Personality Disorder

Lack of desire to socialize; enjoys solitude
Lacks strong emotions
Detached, self-absorbed affect
Lacks trust in others
Brief psychotic episodes in response to stressful events
Difficulty expressing anger
Passive reactions to crises

Schizotypal Personality Disorder

Incorrect interpretation of external events/belief that all events refer to self
Superstition, preoccupation with paranormal phenomena
Belief in possession of magical control over others
Constricted or inappropriate affect
Anxiety in social situations

Box 15-2   Epidemiology of Cluster A Personality Disorders

Paranoid Personality Disorder

Diagnosed in 0.5% to 2.5% of the general population.
10% to 30% of the paranoid population are in inpatient psychiatric settings.
2% to 10% are in outpatient mental health clinics.
Families who have one or more members already diagnosed with paranoid personality disorder are at increased risk.
Males are diagnosed more often than females.
Substance abuse is common.

Schizoid Personality Disorder

Males are diagnosed slightly more often than females.
Families with members who have schizophrenia or schizotypal personality disorder have increased prevalence.

Schizotypal Personality Disorder

Diagnosed in 3% of the general population.
30% to 50% also have major depression.
Individuals with schizotypal personality disorder seek treatment for anxiety and/or depression, not for the personality disorder features.
First-degree relatives of individuals with schizophrenia are at increased risk.
Males are diagnosed slightly more often than females.

CLUSTER C PERSONALITY DISORDERS

Cluster C personality disorders are described as the anxious or fearful cluster. They include avoidant personality disorder, dependent personality disorder, and obsessive-compulsive personality disorder. The Clinical Symptoms box on p. 338 and Box 15-4 summarize the key clinical symptoms and epidemiology of these disorders.

UNSPECIFIED PERSONALITY DISORDERS

The category of unspecified personality disorders describes individuals whose personality pattern meets the general criteria for a personality disorder but not the criteria for any specific personality disorder. It is also used for an individual whose personality pattern meets the general criteria for a personality disorder, but the person is considered to have a personality disorder that is not included in the current classification, such as passive-aggressive personality disorder.

PROGNOSIS

When providing nursing care to clients with personality disorders, it is important to consider the prognosis for improvement. This is especially important during the planning and evaluating portions of the nursing care plan. By definition, individuals with personality disorders have

---

CLINICAL SYMPTOMS

Cluster B Personality Disorders

Antisocial Personality Disorder

Irresponsibility
Failure to honor financial obligations, plan ahead, provide children with basic needs
Involvement in illegal activities
Lack of guilt
Difficulty learning from mistakes
Initial charm dissolves to coldness, manipulation, blaming others
Lacks empathy
Irritability
Abuse of substances

Borderline Personality Disorder

Intense, stormy relationships
Sees people as "all good" or "all bad"
Impulsivity
Self-mutilation
Difficulty identifying self
Negative or angry affect
Feelings of emptiness and boredom
Difficulty being alone, feeling of abandonment
Engages in impulsive acts (e.g., binging, spending money, reckless driving, unsafe sex)
Suicidal ideations

Histrionic Personality Disorder

Fluctuation in emotions
Attention-seeking, self-centered attitude
Sexual seduction and flamboyance
Attentiveness to own physical appearance
Dramatic, impressionistic speech style
Vague logic—lack of conviction in arguments, often switching sides
Shallow emotional expression
Craving for immediate satisfaction
Complaints of physical illness, somatization
Use of suicidal gestures and threats to get attention

Narcissistic Personality Disorder

Grandiose view of self
Lacks empathy toward others
Need for admiration
Preoccupation with fantasies of success, brilliance, beauty, ideal love

---

Box 15-3   Epidemiology of Cluster B Personality Disorders

Antisocial Personality Disorder

Usually diagnosed by age 18.
Individuals have a history of conduct disorders before age 15.
Males are diagnosed more often than females.
Characteristics are evident by early childhood in males and by puberty in females.
High percentage of diagnosed individuals are in substance abuse treatment settings and prisons.
Incidence is more common in the lower socioeconomic classes.
Substance abuse is common.
Impulsive behavior is common.

Borderline Personality Disorder

Diagnosed in 2% of the general population.
10% of this population are in outpatient mental health clinics.
20% are in inpatient psychiatric settings.
75% of diagnosed individuals are female.
60% of the diagnosed disorder population have borderline personality disorder.
Diagnosed individuals have a history of physical and sexual abuse, neglect, hostile conflict, and early parental losses or separation.

Histrionic Personality Disorder

Females are diagnosed more often than males.
Diagnosed in 2% to 3% of the general population.
10% to 15% of the individuals who seek treatment have this disorder.

Narcissistic Personality Disorder

Diagnosed in less than 1% of the general population.
Diagnosed in 2% to 16% of the clinical population.
50% to 75% of those diagnosed are male.

CLINICAL SYMPTOMS

Cluster C Personality Disorders

Avoidant Personality Disorder

Fearful of criticism, disapproval, or rejection
Avoids social interactions
Withholds thoughts or feelings
Negative sense of self, low self-esteem

Dependent Personality Disorder

Submissive, clinging
Unable to make decisions independently
Cannot express negative emotions
Difficulty following through on tasks

Obsessive-Compulsive Personality Disorder

Preoccupation with perfection, organization, structure, control
Procrastination
Abandonment of projects due to dissatisfaction
Excessive devotion to work
Difficulty relaxing
Rule-conscious behavior
Self-criticism and inability to forgive own errors
Reluctance to delegate
Inability to discard anything
Insistence on others' conforming to own methods
Rejection of praise
Reluctance to spend money
Background of stiff and formal relationships
Preoccupation with logic and intellect

Box 15-4   Epidemiology of Cluster C Personality Disorders

Avoidant Personality Disorder

Diagnosis is equal for males and females.
Diagnosed in 0.5% to 1% of the general population.
10% are diagnosed in outpatient settings.

Dependent Personality Disorder

Most frequently diagnosed personality disorder.
More females are diagnosed than males.
Symptoms are demonstrated early in life.
Children or adolescents with chronic physical illness or separation anxiety disorder may be predisposed.

Obsessive-Compulsive Personality Disorder

Diagnosed in 1% of the general population.
Diagnosed in 3% to 10% of the population who seek treatment.
Males are diagnosed twice as often as females.

---

demonstrated pervasive and inflexible behaviors and thoughts that deviate from their cultural expectations (APA, 1994). These patterns first begin in adolescence or early adulthood and are stable over time. The symptoms lead to distress and functional and relationship impairment in the individual. With this definition in mind, the prognosis for individuals with personality disorders is guarded.

An example of how the manifestations of a personality disorder can be demonstrated in adolescence is made by examining the symptoms of conduct disorder in adolescence and the development of antisocial disorder in adulthood. Pajer (1998) studied the literature to determine if girls who displayed symptoms of conduct disorder continued the symptoms to demonstrate antisocial personality disorder as adults. The conclusion of this research was that the adults had higher mortality rates; a tenfold to fortyfold increase in criminal behavior; many psychiatric comorbid symptoms, such as suicidal behavior; disturbed and sometimes violent significant relationships, with a high rate of divorce and extramarital sexual activity; poor educational achievement; less stable work histories; and a high rate of service utilization, such as welfare systems and child protective agencies. Myers, Stewart, and Brown (1998)

studied the progression of symptoms from those demonstrated in conduct disorder to antisocial personality disorder, in adolescents who were seeking treatment for substance abuse (see Understanding & Applying Research box). These studies conclude that early, structured therapy may decrease the severity of the personality disorder in adult life.

Realistic expectations for improvement include a commitment by the client to explore and evaluate his or her thoughts and behaviors, especially when under stress. The nurse plays a powerful role by providing support, tools for this exploration, and client teaching. If the client can use the knowledge of his or her dysfunctional patterns to predict how he or she will respond when faced with a stressor, innovative options for problem solving can be planned. In this way, the individual learns new responses and can improve functioning. This process often needs to be repeated over time before behavioral and thought patterns change. Therefore long-term treatment aimed at problem solving and cognitive reframing is indicated for these clients.

Linehan (1993) studied behavioral patterns of individuals with borderline personality disorder, identifying repeating behavioral patterns. She then began to study what interventions could decrease the most destructive behavioral patterns, such as parasuicidal behavior, splitting, and intense emotional reactivity. This research yielded a treatment strategy called dialectical behavioral therapy (DBT). The principal assumption is to use the dialogue to assist the client in reworking destructive ways of dealing with crises. DBT teaches the client that there are choices in working through the crisis that can decrease the suicidal thoughts or emotionally reactive patterns. The

Myers and associates studied 137 adolescents who initially received treatment for substance abuse in an inpatient setting. These individuals were followed by the research team for 4 years to determine the correlation between conduct disorder, substance abuse, and the development of antisocial personality disorder. Several tools were used during the study. The Structural Clinical Interview for Adolescents was used to gather data on the subjects' demographic information, as well as academic, social, occupational, family, and health functioning. The Customary Drinking and Drug Use Record was used to determine the substance abuse pattern. The Conduct Disorder/Antisocial Personality Disorder Questionnaire assesses whether an individual has conduct disorder and/or antisocial personality disorder.

The researchers compared the functioning of the subjects in the following domains: schoolwork, interpersonal functioning, emotional well-being, and illegal behavior. Myers and associates found that their results showed a relationship between substance abuse and antisocial behavior. This is reflected in the theoretic models that draw a comparison between adolescents with conduct disorder and substance abuse and those who later develop antisocial personality disorder. The researchers found that individuals with more symptoms of drug and alcohol abuse were more likely to also develop antisocial personality disorder. Adolescents in this study who demonstrated difficulty in functioning in the measured domains of schoolwork, interpersonal functioning, emotional well-being, and illegal behavior also later developed antisocial personality disorder. If there was substance abuse in those individuals who later displayed antisocial personality disorder, there were also more problems in functioning in the domains mentioned above. The researchers concluded that the "prominence of substance use in relation to poorer overall functioning . . . [suggests] that alcohol and drug abuse may be inextricably involved in the progression of antisocial pathology among young people with a history of substance abuse."

This correlation between substance abuse, conduct disorder, and antisocial personality disorder is important in planning treatment. Patients should be carefully assessed for conduct disorder that may occur before, and independent of, substance abuse for treatment considerations. Individuals who have conduct disorder before the substance abuse are at higher risk. These individuals need an intensive treatment program with multisystem therapeutic modalities.

Myers MG, Stewart DG, Brown SA: Progression from conduct disorder to antisocial personality disorder following treatment for adolescent substance abuse, *Am J Psychiatry* 155:479, 1998.

therapy focuses on the client's learning new patterns of thoughts and behaviors.

DISCHARGE CRITERIA

Clients with personality disorders are treated in both inpatient and outpatient settings, such as day treatment facilities, partial hospital units, clinics, and private office practices. To determine when to discharge a client from an inpatient hospital setting, it is important to consider the risk factor of safety for the client and others. Some clients with personality disorders have suicidal ideas that are part of their day-to-day thought process. When evaluating clients with this ongoing theme, it is important to ascertain whether the client has a suicidal plan and if he or she intends to implement that plan (see Chapter 28).

Individuals with a personality disorder who are hospitalized often have more than one psychiatric diagnosis. Their lives can be complex and chaotic. Psychiatric follow-up, whether in a partial hospitalization program, a day treatment center, or with an outpatient psychotherapist, is important in order to assist the client in working through some of the issues that contributed to the crisis that culminated in the hospital stay. Before discharge from the hospital, it is important for the client to have a plan for outpatient follow-up and the first posthospital appointment established.

Client teaching is a powerful tool to help the client understand the psychiatric problems that he or she is experiencing, as well as to help prevent a relapse of symptoms. Before discharge from the hospital, each client should receive education in the following areas:

The need for follow-up in an outpatient setting
The psychiatric symptoms that indicate a need for emergent treatment
An understanding of any medications that the client may be receiving

This client teaching can take place in a group setting or on an individual basis. If one of the milieu activities is a relapse prevention group and/or a medication group, it is helpful for the primary nurse to review the material specific to each client before his or her discharge.

If the client is being treated in an outpatient setting, the following issues must be considered before discharge from treatment:

The client no longer has active thoughts of wanting to harm self or others.
The client controls self-destructive impulses, such as substance abuse when feeling upset or shoplifting when feeling empty.
The client has an understanding of the symptoms that precipitated the need for psychotherapy.
The client understands the types of symptoms that indicate a need for further treatment in the future.
The client can use community 12-step groups if this is relevant to his or her problems, such as Alcoholics Anonymous, Narcotics Anonymous, Co-Dependents Anonymous, Incest Survivors Anonymous, and Overeaters Anonymous.

Personality Disorders

The community mental health nurse often encounters many challenges when working with clients with Axis II diagnoses. The extent of the client's disorder may not be immediately apparent since clients with Axis II disorders may appear in control under certain circumstances. Interactions require constant vigilance, since the nurse's suggestions may be distorted by the client as criticism or blame, and professional attention may be perceived as interest in personal involvement. Helpful attempts by the nurse may be negated or rejected by clients with personality disorders, and their distress and complaints will continue, resulting in frustration for both the nurse and the client. The nurse needs to be cautious when clients attempt to "pit" staff against each other. A client may idealize one staff member while disparaging another, in an effort to meet his or her needs inappropriately. Such behaviors are known as "splitting," and need to be addressed by the nurse in a calm, impassive manner. For example, if a client tells a nurse that the nurse is caring and understanding, but that everyone else misunderstands the client, the nurse should remain unimpressed and remind the client of the consistencies in treatment by all staff.

The client may also attempt to manipulate the nurse emotionally by expressing thoughts of suicide or self-mutilation to justify prolonged attention, including subsequent hospitalization. The nurse's reaction must always remain calm and impassive, no matter how much the client acts out self-threatening behaviors. Clients need to be encouraged to consider the outcomes of these behaviors and think about other options they could pursue. Control of the interaction and self-awareness is especially important for the mental health nurse in the community, since colleagues may not be available for a reality check.

Clients with Axis II disorders may often appear charming, engaging, and possessed of insightful humor, although they seem unable to use their intellectual gifts to help themselves break the cycles of substance abuse and/or self-mutilation. A cohesive, team approach is essential, since the demands of this group of clients tend to frustrate and even "burn out" individual case workers. All decisions concerning care of these clients should be made in consensus with the entire health care team.

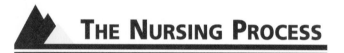

THE NURSING PROCESS

ASSESSMENT

The client being assessed for a personality disorder should be interviewed in a comfortable, quiet, private, safe environment. There should be no interruptions during the assessment. Individuals with these disorders may be withdrawn, defensive, guarded, and impulsive, or they may be charming and friendly.

The nurse should not be judgmental or confrontational during the interview. If the client demonstrates an escalation of anger or makes hostile, threatening comments to the assessment questions, a break may help the client regain composure. The client should not be threatened with seclusion or restraints, because this may provoke him or her to impulsively lose control (see Nursing Care in the Community box).

Box 15-5 represents a comprehensive evaluation that can be used with clients who have a personality disorder. The five domains of human behavior examined are the physical, emotional, cognitive, social, and spiritual domains.

NURSING DIAGNOSIS

The nursing diagnosis is developed based on the in-depth assessment of the client's health status. The nursing diagnosis is a statement that defines the problem, its characteristics and contributing factors, and guides the development of the nursing care plan (Carpenito, 1992) (see Nursing Assessment Questions box). The following are the nursing diagnoses that are most common when caring for clients with a personality disorder.

NURSING DIAGNOSES FOR PARANOID, SCHIZOID, AND SCHIZOTYPAL PERSONALITY DISORDERS (CLUSTER A)

Anxiety
Coping, ineffective individual
Social isolation
Thought processes, altered

NURSING DIAGNOSES FOR ANTISOCIAL, BORDERLINE, HISTRIONIC, AND NARCISSISTIC PERSONALITY DISORDERS (CLUSTER B)

Coping, ineffective individual
Personal identity disturbance
Self-esteem, chronic low
Self-mutilation, risk for
Social interaction, impaired
Violence, risk for: directed at others
Violence, risk for: self-directed

NURSING DIAGNOSES FOR AVOIDANT, DEPENDENT, AND OBSESSIVE-COMPULSIVE PERSONALITY DISORDERS (CLUSTER C)

Anxiety
Coping, ineffective individual
Self-esteem, chronic low
Social interaction, impaired

Box 15-5   Assessment of Individuals With Personality Disorders

Physical Domain

Is there evidence of appropriate activities of daily living?

Is the client neatly groomed?

Is the client dressed appropriately?

Does the client appear adequately nourished?

Is there evidence of a regular exercise program in his or her life?

Is there evidence of any physical illnesses?

Does the client concentrate on somatic concerns?

Is the client able to maintain eye contact?

Is the client experiencing tension?

Does the client demonstrate sympathetic stimulation, cardiovascular excitation, superficial vasoconstriction, and/or pupil dilation?

Does the client report trouble sleeping?

Is the client glancing about?

Is the client demonstrating extraneous movements, such as foot shuffling, or hand and arm movements?

Does the client show facial tension?

Is his or her voice quivering?

Does the client report increased wariness?

Is the client having an increase in perspiration?

Does the client have a history of any of the following physical conditions?

  Temporal lobe epilepsy

  Progressive central nervous system disorder

  Head trauma

  Hormonal imbalance

  Mental retardation

  Abuse of alcohol and/or drugs

  Mania

Is the client dressed inappropriately or in a seductive manner?

Does the client have a high incidence of accidents?

Is the client overly concerned with physical attractiveness?

Emotional Domain

Does the client demonstrate demanding, hostile behavior?

Does the client have a history of aggressive actions?

Is the client emotionally volatile?

Does the client have poor impulse control?

Does the client indicate having thoughts of harming self or others?

Is the client suspicious of others?

Is the client fearful or highly anxious?

Does the client express feelings of helplessness?

Does the client appear apprehensive?

Does the client's thought pattern include feelings of uncertainty?

Does the client discuss concerns about unspecified consequences?

Does the client have persistent worries?

Does the client demonstrate critical behavior toward self and others?

Does the client have low self-esteem?

Is the client concerned about how others will evaluate him or her?

Does the client inflate his or her importance?

Does the client describe feelings of guilt or regret?

Does the client lack remorse and justify hurting another with excuses?

Does the client lack empathy?

Is the client vindictive?

Does the client demonstrate a low frustration tolerance?

Does the client show a lack of motivation?

Is the client dependent on others to meet his or her needs?

Is the client's behavior passive?

Does the client discuss feelings of inadequacy?

Does the client deny strong emotions, such as anger and joy?

Is the client describing feelings of hopelessness?

Does the client demonstrate inappropriate sexually seductive behavior?

Does the client manifest a constricted affect?

Does the client exhibit an inappropriate affect, such as silly or aloof facial expressions?

Does the client display lability of his or her mood?

Cognitive Domain

Does the client demonstrate inaccurate interpretation of stimuli, both internal and external?

Does the client have difficulty understanding abstract ideas?

Is the client able to identify problem areas?

Is the client able to identify options to solve the problems?

Does the client's identification of the problem area involve blaming others or self?

Is the client vindictive in his or her problem solving?

Does the client lie?

Is the client able to identify both good and bad traits in others?

Is the client able to distinguish positive and negative options to problem solving?

Does the client ruminate over issues of concern?

Is the client's thought pattern redundant?

Is the client able to tolerate a delay in gratification?

Is the client able to identify his or her value system?

Does the client have difficulty learning from his or her mistakes?

Is the client impulsive?

Does the client manifest any deficits in long-term or short-term memory?

Is the client preoccupied?

Does the client have a lack of consensual validation?

Does the client describe any delusions?

Does the client experience any hallucinations? What type: auditory, visual, tactile, gustatory, olfactory? What is the content of the hallucinations?

Does the client reveal any perceptual experiences?

Does the client confirm having any ideas of reference?

Does the client discuss any odd beliefs or magical thinking that influence his or her behavior?

Is the client's speech impoverished, digressive, vague, or inappropriately abstract?

Continued

Box 15-5   Assessment of Individuals With Personality Disorders—cont'd

Social Domain

Does the client prefer to be alone?

Does the client express a desire to socialize but have concerns that he or she will not be accepted by others?

Is the client dependent on others for meeting his or her needs?

Does the client participate in family activities?

Does the client have any friends?

Does the client have unstable relationships that consist of conflict and concerns about abandonment?

Is the client able to identify the dynamics of relationship problems?

Is the client using manipulative behavior as a means of getting needs met?

Does the client show evidence of splitting: Does the client place great value on relating with one person while becoming critical and angry with the other? Does the client devalue and complain about one individual to another person with whom the client has a positive relationship?

Does the client identify his or her sense of self by indicating membership in a relationship?

Is the client attention seeking, wanting to be the center of attention?

Is the client preoccupied with how others view him or her?

Is this client extremely sensitive to praise and criticism of others?

Is the client reluctant to give time, gifts, and support to his or her friends unless the client can profit?

Does the client choose solitary activities?

Does the client engage in any social activities?

Does the client feel increasingly anxious when in a social situation?

Does the client express no desire to have a sexual experience with another person?

Does the client have multiple sexual partners?

Is this client indifferent to praise and criticism of others?

Does the client expect others to exploit him or her?

Does the client exploit others to get his or her needs met?

Does the client question the loyalty or trustworthiness of friends or associates? Does the client question the fidelity of his or her spouse or sexual partner?

Does the client read hidden meanings into benign remarks of others?

Does the client bear grudges against others?

Is the client reluctant to confide in others?

Is the client preoccupied with self to the exclusion of others?

Does the client fail to honor financial obligations?

Does the client fail to plan ahead, such as traveling without a clear plan or quitting work without plans to begin another job?

Does the client provide his or her children with the basic needs for health?

Does the client engage in illegal activities?

Does the client abuse drugs or alcohol?

Does the client demonstrate a belief that he or she is owed a sense of entitlement?

Spiritual Domain

Does the client have a belief in a higher power?

Is the client able to state a meaning and purpose to his or her life?

NURSING ASSESSMENT QUESTIONS

Personality Disorders

These questions involve *the nurse's observation of the client's appearance, general nutritional status, and level of observable anxiety manifestations:*

1. Does the client appear appropriately dressed? Is eye contact maintained? Does he or she appear properly nourished? Does the client exhibit signs of anxiety, such as pacing, foot tapping, sighing, or facial tension? Does the client appear hypervigilant? Does the client appear withdrawn?

The following questions are suggestions for the nurse to ask the client *to determine if there are disturbances in the client's relationships, thought processes, and behavior:*

2. How would you describe yourself? What do you like about yourself? What would you like to change about yourself?

3. Describe your relationship with your spouse or significant other, your children, your parents, and other family members. Describe your relationship with your friends. What do you talk about? What types of activities do you do together?

4. How do you feel about your job? Do you get along with your boss and co-workers?

5. If you have a personal problem, who do you trust to help you with it?

6. What are your main worries? How often do you think about them? Do you talk to anyone about these worries? Does that help?

7. Do you ever feel like hurting yourself or anyone else? Have you ever been suicidal? Have you ever hurt yourself by cutting your skin or burning yourself? How often does this occur?

8. Have you ever felt hopeless, helpless, worthless, and a burden? Do you feel this now? Are you getting any support from friends or family?

9. Do you ever use alcohol and/or illegal drugs? Have you ever gone to the doctor to get tranquilizers to reduce your nervousness? What did the doctor give you? What are you taking now?

10. What are your religious beliefs and practices?

OUTCOME IDENTIFICATION

An individual with a personality disorder has disturbances in self-image and relationships throughout life. Identifying outcomes includes the client's ability to demonstrate understanding of problem areas and to display healthy and effective adaptive behaviors. The focus is on helping the individual find patterns of maladaptive behavior, thoughts, and emotions that produce distress. The nurse and the client can work together to explore options to change these maladaptive patterns to more effective coping strategies.

The outcome criteria are derived from the nursing diagnoses and are the expected client responses or behaviors that occur as a result of the plan of care. Outcomes are written in clear, measurable terms.

Client will:

1. Demonstrate absence of suicidal ideation.
2. No longer have any thoughts of harming others.
3. Refrain from self-mutilation.
4. Reach and maintain the highest functioning possible, as demonstrated by the ability to function at home, work, and in the community.
5. Identify two impulsive behavior patterns that take place during times of stress.
6. Recognize when he or she is experiencing cognitive distortions during a stressful period of time.
7. Be able to identify a cognitive distortion used most often during times of stress.
8. Identify one new method of problem solving.
9. Reward self, both with an item (such as some flowers) and a positive thought when able to successfully identify and change a cognitive distortion.
10. Identify some patterns of isolative behavior.
11. Tolerate short interactive periods with the nurse, family members, and peers.
12. Identify with positive role models.
13. Contribute one statement in a group setting directed toward facilitating increased socialization.

PLANNING

When planning interventions with a client with a personality disorder, it is important for the nurse to recognize that changes in behavior or thoughts often occur slowly.

CASE STUDY

James, a 32-year-old single man, was evaluated by a nurse in an outpatient clinic at the recommendation of his father because of an increase in his isolative behavior. James did not want to come in for the interview, since he did not consider "being alone" a problem. He was oriented three times but was not spontaneous with answers to the nurse's assessment questions. His affect was flat, he kept his eyes averted with no eye contact, and his leg was shaking. He was unkempt, with a disheveled appearance and mismatched clothing. He had a vague, wandering, nonspecific way of discussing his problem and his lifestyle.

His mother had been recently hospitalized with pneumonia—however, James did not see that as part of his problem. He perceived his boss as "disliking" him, because the boss thought he was "weird." James said that he had no friends, found socializing difficult, and tended to withdraw further when forced to interact with others. He was suspicious of the interviewer and of his father's motives for asking him to seek psychiatric intervention.

The problem he identified was that he felt he had to "do more around the house" in his mother's absence. That seemed "unfair and like a burden" to James. "She just got sick so she wouldn't have to cook supper or do the laundry," James stated. "The doctors put her in the hospital so they can make more money off of her. Dad is in on it; he sent me here so you could make money."

James had not visited his mother in the hospital because he was afraid he would get "germs" there. Although he saw no reason for this interview, he consented to return to the clinic to "help" his father.

Critical Thinking—Assessment

1. What questions should the nurse ask James to determine symptoms in the physical domain?
2. How could the nurse assess the emotional domain?
3. How could James's problems in the cognitive domain be assessed?
4. What information about James helps to determine his functioning in the social domain?
5. What questions could the nurse ask James to assess how he functions in the spiritual domain?

CASE STUDY

Jean has been working with a nurse for the past 3 years in outpatient psychotherapy. She was recently arrested for stealing some candy and lipstick at a local department store following an argument with her boyfriend. During the session following the arrest, the nurse suggested that Jean explore the dynamics of the incident and how this was related to the argument with her boyfriend. Jean became angry, then scared, expressing concern that she might lose the respect and the therapeutic relationship with the nurse. She ran out of the room, yelling that the nurse did not understand her pain, and slammed the door. Several minutes later, Jean returned, apologized, and asked the nurse to forgive her.

Critical Thinking—Outcome Identification

1. What responses by Jean would indicate to the nurse that Jean had some insight into the dynamics of her impulsive stealing behaviors?
2. What changes in behavior are anticipated as a result of Jean's gaining understanding about her impulsive behavior?
3. Describe two outcomes that would be realistic for Jean.

These changes are a result of the client's perception of the need for that change. Individuals with a personality disorder have disturbed interpersonal relationships and values that do not reflect the views held by the general population. Because of these disturbances, the nurse must collaborate with the client on the goals identified during treatment (see Collaborative Diagnoses box).

IMPLEMENTATION

The implementation of the plan of care for clients with personality disorders includes interventions focused toward modifying lifelong disruptive and dysfunctional behaviors and thoughts, with the promotion of safety.

NURSING INTERVENTIONS

1. Assess the client for suicidal ideation and determine the level of lethality *to prevent harm or injury.*
2. If warranted, place the client on suicidal precaution, depending on his or her level of lethality (e.g., client

---

COLLABORATIVE DIAGNOSES

DSM-IV Diagnoses*	NANDA Diagnoses†
Cluster A	
Paranoid personality disorder	Anxiety
	Coping, ineffective individual
Schizoid personality disorder	Social isolation
	Thought process, altered
Schizotypal personality disorder	
Cluster B	
Antisocial personality disorder	Coping, ineffective individual
	Violence, risk for: directed at others
Borderline personality disorder	Violence, risk for: self-directed
Histrionic personality disorder	Self-mutilation, risk for
	Personal identity disturbance
Narcissistic personality disorder	Coping, ineffective individual
	Self-esteem, chronic low
	Social interaction, impaired
Cluster C	
Avoidant personality disorder	Anxiety
	Coping, ineffective individual
Dependent personality disorder	Self-esteem, chronic low
	Social interaction, impaired
Obsessive-compulsive personality disorder	

*From American Psychiatric Association: *Diagnostic and statistical manual of mental disorders*, ed 4, Washington, DC, 1994, The Association.

†From North American Nursing Diagnosis Association: *NANDA nursing diagnoses: definitions and classifications, 1999-2000*, Philadelphia, 1999, The Association.

---

who has verbalized plans to hang himself or herself while on the unit should be placed on close individual observation as long as those plans are still viable, with no means or provisions to carry out the intent) *to prevent suicide.*

3. Establish a contract for safety with the client by asking the client to write a statement indicating that he or she will not harm himself or herself. If the suicidal impulse becomes too strong, encourage the client to seek out a staff member to discuss the increase in intensity of suicidal ideation *to protect the client from acting on suicidal impulses.*

4. Encourage the client to attend all unit group sessions *to receive support from peers and to provide opportunities for problem solving.*

5. Assess the client for an escalation of anger to rage and possible impulsive actions against others (obtain a history of violence if possible) *to prevent harm or injury to others.*

6. Contract with the client that he or she will no longer threaten staff or peers during hospitalization *to ensure the safety of others.*

7. Teach the client other options to manage the angry, impulsive feelings and behavior (such as leaving the room where the conflict is occurring) or using a quiet area (such as an unlocked seclusion room) until the impulse to do harm passes. *Removing the client from a stimulating, provocative environment may decrease angry impulses.*

8. Discuss angry feelings in a group setting that is focused on exploring alternative options for problem solving. *Alternative actions may distract the client from angry feelings and help to focus his or her energy on constructive activities.*

9. Assess the client for evidence of self-mutilation. *Clients who are self-destructive are likely to repeat such acts and may require further interventions.*

10. Obtain a contract from the client that he or she will approach a staff member when the urge to self-mutilate is present *to ensure the safety of the client.*

11. Place the client on an individual, close watch until the urge to harm self passes or until the client is able to identify another way to obtain emotional relief (e.g., wrapping in a sheet or participating in a movement therapy group) *to protect the client from harmful impulses and redirect the impulses toward alternative, constructive methods.*

12. If self-mutilation occurs, attend to the wounds in a matter-of-fact manner *to provide safe care to the client in a nonjudgmental way.*

13. Encourage the client to keep a journal of thoughts and feelings the client had before experiencing the urge to self-mutilate *to help the client acknowledge feelings and thoughts and help decrease impulsivity.*

14. Medicate the client with an anxiolytic or antipsychotic medication, prn as ordered *to help the client con-*

NURSING CARE PLAN

Sam was admitted to the psychiatric unit directly from the emergency department because he was involved in a fight with another man at a bar. He was under the influence of PCP, as well as alcohol, while at the bar. The emergency department staff assessed him as medically stable but suggested admission because of his potential for violence.

When Sam arrived on the unit, he was angry, loudly stating that he had been treated unfairly in the emergency department and that he did not need admission to the psychiatric unit "with all those nuts!" He demanded a TV in his room and a cigarette. When the staff denied his requests, he became louder and threatening. He told the charge nurse that he would get his way, that he had friends on the hospital board, and that there would be an investigation into the hospital treatment of his case if he was not allowed to smoke or to watch TV in private. He reminded the nurse that he was admitted for fighting in a bar, and he "knows how to get his way."

DSM-IV Diagnosis

Axis I: Substance abuse (alcohol and PCP)
Axis II: Antisocial personality disorder
Axis III: Medically stable, related to withdrawal symptoms
Axis IV: Problems related to the social environment
Axis V: GAF = 40 (current)
             GAF = 60 (past year)

Nursing Diagnosis: Violence, risk for: directed at others. Risk factors: a perception that others are denying him his rights and control over his environment; a history of violence against others; and an increase in verbal demands, a loud voice, and verbally threatening behavior.

Client Outcomes	Nursing Interventions	Evaluation
• Sam will be able to maintain control of his anger so that he will not threaten or harm others.	• Monitor the client for escalation of the anger to rage or impulsive action *to predict any increase in impulsivity and prevent injury to self or others.* • Contract with the client that he will no longer threaten staff or client peers during the hospitalization *to assist Sam in impulse control.*	• Sam was able to discuss his feelings about entering the hospital without threatening or aggressive behavior.
• Sam will use the interactions with the nurse, members of the interdisciplinary team, and groups in the milieu to discuss alternative options to deal with situations that provoke angry, potentially violent responses.	• Teach the client other options to manage the angry feelings, such as leaving the area where the conflict is occurring and using a quiet area such as an unlocked seclusion room until the impulse to do harm passes, *to provide other ways to handle angry feelings, rather than violence.* • Discuss angry feelings in the group setting, how the anger can escalate out of control, and what to do to control violent impulses *to use group input to provide alternative solutions to deal with angry feelings rather than resorting to violence.*	• Sam was able to control angry outbursts and ask for his needs in a calm manner during his hospital stay and shared his feelings with the group.

Nursing Diagnosis: Coping, ineffective individual, related to intoxication from alcohol and PCP, as evidenced by the client's loud and threatening behavior.

Client Outcomes	Nursing Interventions	Evaluation
• Sam will be able to determine his basic needs, make requests in a calm, thoughtful manner, and make some choices about his treatment and care.	• The nurse will observe for symptoms of intoxication and withdrawal from alcohol and PCP, which may require medication, and administer medications as needed. *Symptoms of intoxication and withdrawal of both substances may include irritability and loss of impulse control.* • The nurse will assist Sam in becoming adjusted to the unit by providing a tour, giving statements of support, telling Sam how the hospitalization will help him, and providing Sam with choices in his care when appropriate. *The client will feel in control with an understanding of the environment and expectations, as well as being able to make some decisions regarding his care.*	• Sam was able to decrease his loud and threatening behavior after medication was given to decrease withdrawal symptoms, and he was able to make some decisions regarding his care.

Continued

NURSING CARE PLAN —cont'd

Nursing Diagnosis: Self-esteem, chronic low, related to long-term negative feedback and the belief that he is unable to deal with problems, as evidenced by self-destructive behavior (drinking and physical fighting in the bar), inability to accept constructive limit setting from the nursing staff, and the degradation of others to increase his own feelings of self-worth.

Client Outcomes	Nursing Interventions	Evaluation
• Sam will be able to discuss during a one-to-one session with his primary nurse or in a problem-solving milieu group that his threatening behavior and degradation of others reveal his own feelings of low self-esteem.	• Encourage Sam to attend all verbal milieu groups for problem solving, particularly those that discuss behavior and feelings. *Sam will obtain feedback from other group members about his threatening and degrading behavior toward others, therefore hearing the same feedback from several sources.* • Discuss how threatening behavior and derogatory remarks toward others distance people. *This discussion will help Sam determine his part in the process of others not attending to his needs, therefore reinforcing his low self-esteem.*	• Sam asked for an identified need without threatening another person. He determined other options to meet the identified need if the other person elected not to assist Sam.
• Sam will be able to identify a positive attribute to his personality.	• Assist Sam in listing the strengths and areas needing adjustment as he views himself. *Sam only identifies negative parts of himself. Listing both strengths and weaknesses helps Sam have a more balanced view of himself.* • Provide positive feedback to Sam when he accomplishes something within the unit milieu or in discussion with others. *Positive feedback reinforces functional behavior.*	• Sam was able to identify two strengths in his character that he values, and agreed to recognize these strengths in the future.

trol his or her intense anxiety or rage rather than self-mutilate.

15. Use a time-out period, seclusion room, and physical restraints if all attempts of least restrictive measures have been unsuccessful *to protect the client.*

16. Assist the client in recognizing thought patterns that contribute to impulsive behavior. This can be done by helping the client understand the role that intense feelings (e.g., abandonment, anger, rage, or anxiety) play in precipitating impulsive behavior or distorted thinking. Using a journal to document such feelings and thoughts and receiving feedback during group sessions are helpful, instructive methods. *Clients can be taught to manage impulsive behavior and distorted beliefs through a variety of methods within the milieu.*

17. Suggest alternative behaviors that can be learned to deal with the intense feelings, such as:

    Recognizing the intense emotional state and writing in a journal or thinking about an action that may help to relieve the intensity of the feeling without resorting to impulsive or self-destructive acts.

    Talking about the intense feeling while looking into a mirror, telling the mirror what the client would like to express to the object of anger.

Identifying healthy options to deal with the anger, such as discussing the issue with the person who is involved in the interaction.

Role-playing with the nursing staff different ways to approach the problem that precipitated the intense feelings.

Introducing the issue in the problem-solving milieu group meeting to receive feedback from peers.

Rewarding self with something that is pleasant and healthful, such as buying flowers or reading a novel. *Learning alternative ways to cope with intense feelings can reduce anger/anxiety and provide constructive ways of managing life stressors.*

18. Help the client explore behavior that relates to the community, such as safe driving and responsibilities for the environment, *to help the client focus on changes that he or she can do to live in a more healthy and responsible way.*

19. Evaluate the client's family system by observing the family dynamics and determining the client's role within the family. *How the client interacts within the family system and the role the client takes (e.g., victim, placator) offers the nurse insight into the client's self-perception* (see Client & Family Teaching Guidelines box on p. 348).

NURSING CARE PLAN

Angela is a 29-year-old single woman who became suicidal after her boyfriend, Al, told her their relationship was over. She started to drink and use diazepam (Valium) to calm down after Al told her they were through. The relationship had become stormy, with frequent threats from Al that he would stop seeing her. Angela became vengeful, went to Al's parent's house where he was staying, and threw a rock into their living room window, shouting that she loved Al and could not live without him. She shouted, "I don't want to hurt anyone. I just want to die!" and ran into the street in front of an oncoming car. The driver slammed on the brakes and hit Angela hard enough to knock her down and cause a pelvic fracture. She was admitted to the local hospital, still vowing to harm herself if Al did not return to her.

DSM-IV Diagnoses

Axis I: Substance abuse (alcohol and diazepam)
Axis II: Borderline personality disorder
Axis III: Pelvic fracture
Axis IV: Problems with primary support groups
Axis V: GAF = 30 (current)
            GAF = 60 (past year)

Nursing Diagnosis: Violence, risk for: self-directed. Risk factors: intense feelings of abandonment, increased anxiety level, and a history of suicidal attempts.

Client Outcomes	Nursing Interventions	Evaluation
• Angela will not act on her suicidal thoughts.	• Place the client on suicide watch and assess her level of depressed thoughts *to prevent any further suicide attempts through early intervention.*	• Angela decreased her suicidal ideation within 2 days of hospitalization.
• Angela will honor the terms of her contract for safety.	• Assist Angela in writing contract for safety that states that she will inform the staff if her suicidal ideation increases, *because early preventive measures can be taken to prevent a suicidal gesture.*	• Angela was able to use the contract for safety to assist with impulse control.
• Angela will contact the staff when she experiences suicidal thoughts.	• Teach Angela to inform the staff if there is an increase in her suicidal ideation *to help her become an active participant in her suicide prevention and more aware of how her thoughts and feelings influence her behavior.*	• Angela contacted staff when she had suicidal thoughts, feelings of abandonment, and other troubling feelings.

Nursing Diagnosis: Coping, ineffective individual, related to ending a significant relationship, as evidenced by the client's vengeful behavior, her impulsive behavior to do self-harm, and her use of drugs and alcohol.

Client Outcomes	Nursing Interventions	Evaluation
• Angela will identify impulsive behavior patterns that take place during times of stress, record these feelings in a journal, and share them in appropriate groups.	• Teach Angela to link her feelings and behavior to her response to the events in her relationship with the use of a journal about her thoughts and feelings, one-to-one discussions with her assigned nurse, and the use of the groups in the inpatient milieu. *A journal will help Angela acknowledge her feelings and thoughts, determine her impulsive behavioral patterns, and decrease her reaction to those thoughts and feelings.*	• Angela was able to talk about her intense feelings of loss and emptiness with her assigned nurse and in the verbal groups on the unit. She was able to use her journal as a coping mechanism when the emotions became overwhelming.
• Angela will be able to identify at least one new method of problem solving to manage negative thoughts and impulses.	• Teach the client healthy ways of dealing with intense feelings of anger and sadness, such as expressing these feelings to supportive friends and family members. Teach her to employ a behavior to help cope with the intense emotion, such as listening to music, taking a hot bath, going to an exercise class, buying flowers, or writing in the journal. *These activities will help Angela learn new coping patterns to deal with intense, painful emotions.*	• Angela was able to use her journal by writing poetry to problem solve and calm herself when feelings became intense during the hospitalization.

Continued

NURSING CARE PLAN —cont'd

Nursing Diagnosis: Grieving, dysfunctional, related to ending a significant relationship, as evidenced by the client's use of drugs and alcohol, vengeful behavior, suicidal ideation, and impulsive behavior to do self-harm.

Client Outcomes	Nursing Interventions	Evaluation
• Angela will identify feelings generated by the ending of the relationship with Al, such as anger, fear of being alone, and sadness.	• Discuss Angela's feelings about the end of the relationship with Al in an open manner *to encourage her to be able to discuss her hurt feelings, fear of loneliness, and abandonment issues to facilitate healthy mourning of the loss of the relationship.*	• At the end of the hospitalization, Angela was able to talk about the end of her relationship with Al without suicidal thoughts or cravings for alcohol or diazepam.
• Angela will share her loss with group members who also experienced losses.	• Encourage Angela to attend group problem-solving sessions on the unit to discuss her loss with other peers in the unit *to give Angela a better perspective on how others have dealt with losses.*	• Angela shared her loss with appropriate group members.
• Angela will use healthy methods to deal with her loss and not use alcohol or diazepam to mask her feelings.	• Encourage Angela to write her thoughts and feelings about the end of the relationship in her journal, *because recognizing the thoughts and feelings about the loss of the relationship may help her come to terms with the unresolved issues associated with the loss.*	• Angela developed journal writing as a healthy method of dealing with her loss and working through painful issues.

Client & Family TEACHING GUIDELINES

SET Method

Clients with personality disorders often have difficulties recognizing problem areas and identifying options that could be solutions. The nurse could incorporate teaching clients and family members to problem solve more effectively as part of the care plan. One area of difficulty is communication. Kreisman and Straus (1989) have suggested using the "SET" method of communication. This was originally developed for clients with borderline personality disorder who were in crisis and were unable to communicate effectively. Kreisman and Straus's "SET" is a three-part system of communication. This is a particularly useful tool when the client is impulsive, is having outbursts of rage, is harmful to self or others, or is making unreasonable demands on others for caregiving. In the SET method:

The *S* stands for *support;* the nurse states a personal statement of concern for the client.

The *E* is for *empathy*, in which the nurse acknowledges the individual's chaotic feelings in a neutral way, with the emphasis on the client's painful experience, not the staff member's feelings.

The *T* is a *truth* statement used to highlight the client's responsibility for his or her behavior and life (Kreisman and Straus, 1989).

For example, Charles had become enraged when his wife, Margaret, did not go shopping and cook some meals for him before she went away for a business trip. His anger mounted, and he drank to deal with his intense feelings. He came to his partial hospitalization program, reporting a hangover.

His primary nurse led the following discussion about Charles's response to Margaret's travel on business:

Nurse: I know it is hard for you when Margaret has to go away. *[E]*

Charles: You got that right. It makes me so angry that she can't complete all her work here.

Nurse: Okay, I hear you *[S]*, but in her job, travel is a big part of how business is conducted. *[T]*

Charles: Yeah, I know, and I think she's good at what she does. I just get so lonely, so empty, I then get angry and scared.

Nurse: Can you look at what type of things you can do when she is away that may help your feelings of emptiness? *[T]*

Charles: Like what?

Nurse: Like going to the movies on the night Margaret is out of town and seeing something she isn't interested in. Treat yourself to carryout Chinese or fast-food, so that you can have dinner without a lot of fuss. Does that sound like something that may help? *[T]*

Charles: I'll try.

20. Engage the client in frequent short interactions several times during the shift *to illustrate the value of interacting with others.*
21. Use milieu groups, such as problem-solving groups and groups that concentrate on self-care and community responsibilities, *to help the client understand the value of interacting with others.*
22. Teach the client assertiveness techniques *to improve the client's ability to relate to others.*
23. Provide direct feedback to the client about his or her interaction with others in a nonjudgmental fashion *to facilitate learning new social skills.*

> **ADDITIONAL TREATMENT MODALITIES**
> *For Clients With Personality Disorders*
> Occupational therapy
> Art therapy
> Music therapy
> Movement therapy
> Recreational therapy
> Medication therapy
> Individual therapy
> Group therapy
> Family therapy
> Milieu therapy

CLINICAL ALERT

Clients with personality disorders have difficulty relating to others. A consequence of this is that these individuals have difficulty defining boundaries between self and others. Part of nursing care is to define boundaries within the therapeutic relationship in order to develop safe, client-centered therapeutic relationships. This is particularly important for the nurse to think about when he or she is feeling vulnerable, perhaps because of other personal or professional stressors. Smith et al (1997) have highlighted ways to recognize and prevent sexually inappropriate behavior with a client. It is important that nurses assess their feelings toward the clients that are in their care, as well as the nurses' own current stressors. Nurses need to ask: Are the stressors interfering with functioning on the job? What are ways to deal with these issues without becoming vulnerable to the clients under the nurses' care? If nurses recognize that they are experiencing special feelings for a particular client, they should discuss these feelings with a colleague and/or obtain clinical supervision/assistance from the employee assistance program.

ADDITIONAL TREATMENT MODALITIES

A team approach, involving nursing staff, the psychiatrist, psychologist, advanced practice psychiatric mental health nurse practitioner/clinical specialist, social worker, occupational therapist, art therapist, music therapist, movement therapist, and recreational therapist, provides the most comprehensive interventions for a client with a personality disorder in an inpatient, partial hospitalization, or day treatment setting (see Additional Treatment Modalities box).

Occupational Therapy

The occupational therapist assesses a client's abilities and disabilities and helps the client increase functioning and independent living skills in areas such as self-care, work, or leisure activity. The occupational therapist teaches adaptive skills for home, school, or job functioning. Groups such as stress management, enhancing parenting skills, conflict resolution, time management, money manage-

ment, budgeting, feeling, and self-awareness are often planned and co-led by the occupational therapist.

Art Therapy

The art therapist uses art as a means of helping the client express thoughts and feelings he or she may not be able to verbalize. This intervention helps the client to understand problem areas from a symbolic standpoint. The art therapist also teaches the client an alternative means of expression and self-soothing. For example, a client who is feeling intense rage and has feelings of wanting to self-mutilate may use art to draw these feelings rather than act on them.

Music Therapy

The music therapist uses music to help the client express feelings and thoughts that may not be easily verbalized. Music is used to help the client relax and learn alternative self-soothing strategies.

Movement Therapy

Movement therapy teaches clients how they move their bodies when stressed and helps them learn methods of relaxation. Movement therapy is helpful for clients who become "numb" when feeling intense feelings, such as abandonment or anger, to use methods of self-touching to reestablish a feeling state rather than self-mutilate.

Recreational Therapy

Recreational therapy helps clients with personality disorders explore ways to enjoy themselves without the use of self-destructive behaviors, such as abusing alcohol or drugs. This modality is helpful for clients who have difficulty socializing, because recreation strengthens social skills.

Medication Therapy

Medications can play a major role in helping the client with a personality disorder. Clients who are demonstrating violence against others may require medications to gain emotional and behavioral control over their impulses. Keltner and Folks (1993) have suggested that clients who are able to take an oral anxiolytic or the sedative-hypnotic class may respond well to the use of a benzodiazepine. Clients who are very agitated or psychotic may respond to the use of a neuroleptic or antipsychotic class medication. Clients with extreme violence who are unable to control this impulse may be given intravenous or intermuscular sedative-hypnotics such as barbiturates, benzodiazepines such as diazepam, or antipsychotics such as haloperidol.

Clients who demonstrate depression along with the symptoms of a personality disorder may benefit from antidepressants. Tricyclic antidepressants (TCAs) are helpful in decreasing depression and the neurovegetative signs in clients with both depression and personality disorders. The selective serotonin reuptake inhibitors (SSRIs) demonstrate a reduction in depressed symptoms in clients with both depression and a personality disorder. The SSRIs have some advantages over the TCAs. There is a reduced probability of completed suicide with an overdose, and there are fewer side effects with the SSRIs than with the TCAs. SSRIs are more expensive than TCAs, which may be limiting to clients who are unable to afford the cost. Some physicians may prescribe an SSRI with a TCA for clients who have severe depression. Monitoring side effects is an important nursing function.

Soloff et al (1991) studied the impact of medications on individuals with borderline personality disorder and schizotypal personality disorder. They reported that haloperidol helped clients increase global functioning, decrease schizotypal symptoms, decrease hostility, and increase impulse control. They also reported that amitriptyline (a TCA medication) decreased hostility and increased impulse control for clients with borderline personality disorder who were evaluated as being unstable.

Individual Therapy

Individual therapy helps the client explore problem areas, define new options, and discuss how the new behavior may help solve the original problem. With the emphasis in the health care system on short-term therapy, individual therapy is now problem solving oriented as opposed to explorative based on early trauma.

Group Therapy

Group therapy is also problem solving oriented. The work in group therapy is based on the repeated dynamics of the individuals in the group. This is especially beneficial for clients with a Cluster B personality disorder, who are dramatic and require a lot of attention. The group members will help the client to understand the effect his or her behavior has on each of them so that the client can use this information when relating to significant people in his or her everyday life.

Family Therapy

Family therapy is helpful for clients with a personality disorder, since the dynamics of the family system are often repeated in other relationships in the client's life, such as with his or her boss or spouse. The family sessions consist of an assessment of the family system and an exploration of how the family dynamics are affected by the current problems that caused the client to seek care. Because of the current philosophy of short-term therapy, exploration of earlier dynamics and/or trauma is focused on the current issue.

Milieu Therapy

When a client is hospitalized in an inpatient psychiatric setting or participates in a partial hospitalization program or a day treatment facility, the client becomes part of that milieu (environment). The purpose of **milieu therapy** is to recreate a community setting on these units so that the client can interact with other client peers in order to identify and problem solve issues that occur while relating to others. Such relationship issues may be discussed in community meetings or other problem-solving groups, such as a coping skills group.

The community meetings may be used to delegate tasks of the unit, such as cleaning off the tables at the end of the meal. This meeting can be used to ask each member to think through a daily goal for therapy and discuss how he or she plans to meet that goal. If something happens on the unit (e.g., if someone becomes aggressive or brings drugs or alcohol on the unit), these concerns are discussed in the community meeting.

Problem-solving groups, such as coping skills groups, may pick a common area of concern; the group works together to explore the issues and options necessary to solve the dilemma.

As in any other community, socializing is an important part of the interaction. In an inpatient, partial hospitalization program or day treatment milieu, socialization groups discuss problems with socializing. The socialization group may use a discussion of a movie the group has just seen or current events read from a magazine or a newspaper as a means of enriching the discussion.

EVALUATION

The evaluation stage of the nursing process is ongoing and takes place to ensure accountable nursing practice. There are two steps to the evaluation stage:

1. The nurse compares the client's current functioning with the outcome criteria.
2. The nurse asks questions to determine possible reasons if the outcome criteria were not met (Fortinash and Holoday-Worret, 1999).

Summary of Key Concepts

1. A personality disorder is a long-standing, pervasive, maladaptive pattern of behavior and relating to others that is not caused by an Axis I disorder.

2. There are several theories for the development of a personality disorder. In psychodynamic theory there is a belief that an individual who develops a personality disorder has deficits in his or her psychosexual development or a failure to achieve object constancy. Research has hypothesized biologic considerations as possible causal factors for individuals developing personality disorders.

3. The DSM-IV Axis II is set up in a three-cluster format.

4. Clients with personality disorders have difficulty relating to others at home, at work, and in the community.

5. When working with individuals with personality disorders, it is important to assess each client for the risk of violence toward self and/or others.

6. Clients with personality disorders often exhibit self-destructive behaviors such as self-mutilation, eating disorders, alcohol or substance abuse, and shoplifting.

7. Realistic expectations for improvement include a commitment by the client to explore and evaluate his or her thoughts, relationships, and behaviors, especially when under stress.

REFERENCES

Akhtar S: *Broken structures: severe personality disorders and their treatments*, Northvale, NJ, 1992, Jason Aronson.

Alger I: The dialectical approach to understanding and treating borderline personality disorder, *Psychiatr Serv* 47:927, September 1996.

American Psychiatric Association: *The American Psychiatric Association's psychiatric glossary*, Washington, DC, 1984, American Psychiatric Press.

American Psychiatric Association: *Diagnostic and statistical manual of mental disorders*, ed 4, Washington, DC, 1994, The Association.

Brown GL et al: Aggression, suicide and serotonin relationships to CSF amine metabolites, *Am J Psychiatry* 139:741, 1982.

Brown GL, Linnoila MI: CSF serotonin metabolite (5-HIAA) studies in depression, impulsivity, and violence, *J Clin Psychiatry* 51(suppl):31, April 1990.

Carpenito LJ: *Nursing diagnosis: application to clinical practice*, Philadelphia, 1992, JB Lippincott.

Coryell WH, Zimmerman MBA: Personality disorder in the families of depressed, schizophrenia, and never-ill probands, *Am J Psychiatry* 146:496, April 1989.

Erikson EH: *Childhood and society*, New York, 1950, WW Norton.

Fortinash KM, Holoday-Worret PA: *Psychiatric nursing care plans*, ed 2, St Louis, 1999, Mosby.

Freud S: Three essays on the theory of sexuality, *Standard Edition* 7:125, 1905.

Freud S: The development of the libido and the sexual organizations, *Standard Edition* 16:320, 1917.

Freud S: The ego and the id, *Standard Edition* 19:3, 1923.

Freud S: The dissolution of the Oedipus complex, *Standard Edition* 19:72, 1924.

Gunderson JG: *Borderline personality disorder*, Washington, DC, 1984, American Psychiatric Press.

Horner AJ: *The primacy of structure: psychotherapy of underlying character pathology*, Northvale, NJ, 1990, Jason Arnson.

Houseman C: The paranoid person: a biopsychosocial perspective, *Arch Psychiatr Nurs* 5(6):176, 1990.

Kaplan HI, Sadock BJ: *Pocket handbook of clinical psychiatry*, Baltimore, 1990, Williams & Wilkins.

Kavoussi RJ, Siever LJ: Biologic validators of personality disorders. In Oldham JM, editor: *Personality disorders: new perspectives on diagnostic validity*, Washington, DC, 1991, American Psychiatric Press.

Keltner NL, Folks DG: *Psychotropic drugs*, St Louis, 1993, Mosby.

Kernberg OF: *Severe personality disorders: psychotherapeutic strategies*, New Haven, Conn, 1984, Yale University Press.

Kernberg OF: *Borderline conditions and pathological narcissism*, Northvale, NJ, 1985, Jason Aronson.

Kreisman JJ, Straus H: *I hate you—don't leave me: understanding the borderline personality*, Los Angeles, 1989, Body Press.

Lencz T et al: Impaired eye tracking in undergraduates with schizotypal personality disorder, *Am J Psychiatry* 150(1):152, 1993.

Linehan MM: *Cognitive-behavioral treatment of borderline personality disorder*, New York, 1993, Guilford Press.

Mahler MS: Thoughts about development and individuation, *Psychoanal Study Child* 18:307, 1963.

Mahler MS: A study of the separation-individuation process and its possible application to borderline phenomena in the psychoanalytic situation, *Psychoanal Study Child* 26:403, 1971.

Mahler MS: On the first three subphases of the separation-individuation process, *Int J Psychoanal* 53:333, 1972a.

Mahler MS: Rapprochement subphase of the separation-individuation process, *Psychoanal Q* 41:487, 1972b.

Manfield P: *Split self split object: understanding and treating borderline, narcissistic, and schizoid disorders,* Northvale, NJ, 1992, Jason Aronson.

Mann JJ et al: Increased serotonin-2 and beta-adrenergic receptor binding in the frontal cortices of suicide victims, *Arch Gen Psychiatry* 43:954, 1986.

Marin D et al: Biological models and treatments for personality disorders, *Psychiatr Ann* 19:143, March 1989.

Masterson JF: *Psychotherapy of the borderline adult: a developmental approach,* New York, 1976, Brunner/Mazel.

Myers MG, Stewart DG, Brown SA: Progression from conduct disorder to antisocial personality disorder following treatment for adolescent substance abuse, *Am J Psychiatry* 155:479, 1998.

North American Nursing Diagnosis Association: *NANDA nursing diagnoses: definitions and classification, 1999-2000,* Philadelphia, 1999, The Association.

Oldham JM, Skodol AE: Personality disorders and mood disorders. In Tasman A, Riba MB, editors: *American Psychiatric Press Review of Psychiatry,* vol 11, Washington, DC, 1992, American Psychiatric Press.

Pajer KA: What happens to "bad" girls? A review of the adult outcomes of antisocial adolescent girls, *Am J Psychiatry* 155:862, July 1998.

Roitman SE et al: Attentional functioning in schizoptypal personality disorder, *Am J Psychiatry* 154:655, 1997.

Siever LJ: Biologic markers in schizotypal personality disorder, *Schizophr Bull* 11:564, 1985.

Siever LJ: Schizophrenia spectrum personality disorders. In Tasman A, Riba MB, editors: *American Psychiatric Press Review of Psychiatry,* vol 11, Washington, DC, 1992, American Psychiatric Press.

Siever LJ, Davis KL: A psychobiological perspective on the personality disorders, *Am J Psychiatry* 148(12):1647, 1991.

Smith LL et al: Nurse-patient boundaries crossing the line: how to recognize signs of professional sexual misconduct and intervene effectively, *Am J Nursing* 97:26, December 1997.

Soloff PH et al: Pharmacotherapy and borderline subtypes. In Oldham JM, editor: *Personality disorders: new perspectives on diagnostic validity,* Washington, DC, 1991, American Psychiatric Press.

Stanley M, Stanley B: Postmortem evidence for serotonin's role in suicide, *J Clin Psychiatry* 51(suppl):22, April 1990.

Steele RL: Staff attitudes toward seclusion and restraint: anything new? *Perspect Psychiatr Care* 29:23, July-September 1993.

Townsend MC: *Nursing diagnoses in psychiatric nursing: a pocket guide for care plan construction,* ed 3, Philadelphia, 1994, FA Davis.

Tyson P, Tyson R: *Psychoanalytic theories of development and integration,* New Haven, Conn, 1990, Yale University Press.

Valente SM: Deliberate self-injury management in a psychiatric setting, *J Psychosoc Nurs* 29:19, December 1991.

Widiger TA, Corbitt EM, Millon T: Antisocial personality disorder. In Tasman A, Riba M, editors: *American Psychiatric Press Review of Psychiatry,* vol 11, Washington, DC, 1992, American Psychiatric Press.

Widiger TA, Rogers JH: Prevalence and comorbidity of personality disorders, *Psychiatr Ann* 19:132, March 1989.

Notes

CHAPTER 16

Substance-Related Disorders

Ona Z. Riggin and Barbara A. Redding

Abuse A maladaptive pattern of substance use leading to problems in psychosocial, biologic, cognitive/perceptual, or spiritual/belief dimensions of life.

Alcoholism A chronic, progressive, and potentially fatal biogenic and psychosocial disease characterized by impaired control over drinking, tolerance, and physical dependence that leads to loss of control, distorted thinking, and other social consequences.

Substance-related disorders are a significant health problem in today's society. Problems associated with **abuse** of alcohol, tobacco, and other drugs continue to consume a major proportion of the health care dollar. In addition to treating problems related to substance abuse, secondary complications of drug use account for a large percentage of admissions to emergency departments and inpatient facilities.

Individuals of all age-groups, cultures, and ethnic populations are affected by substance abuse. Health care professionals are uniquely positioned to initiate preventive programs, perform routine screenings, recognize the diagnosis, perform brief interventions, and make appropriate referrals for intense treatment and rehabilitation. Since the age of onset for developing problems with alcohol or other drugs is increasingly occurring at an earlier age, effective prevention programs must be implemented in preschool and early elementary grades. The nurse is in an ideal position to provide preventive education services about substance use to individuals, families, and the community at large.

Blackout Acute anterograde amnesia without recognition formation of long-term memory (e.g., a period of memory loss during which there is no recall of activities, resulting from the ingestion of alcohol and/or other drugs).

Codependency An emotional, psychologic, and behavioral pattern of coping that an individual develops as a result of prolonged exposure to a dysfunctional pattern of behavior within the family of origin. The individual experiences difficulty with identity development and setting of functional boundaries, which leads to taking care of others rather than self.

Cross-tolerance A condition in which tolerance to one drug often results in a tolerance to chemically similar drugs. Tolerance is originally produced by long-term administration of one drug, which is manifested toward a second drug that has not been administered previously (e.g., tolerance to alcohol is accompanied by cross-tolerance to volatile anesthetics or barbiturates).

Detoxification Treatment that assists the individual in withdrawing from the physical effects of alcohol and/or other addictive substances and that helps eliminate severe withdrawal symptoms that can occur with abrupt withdrawal. It can be provided in a hospital, day treatment, or outpatient setting.

Dual diagnosis The simultaneous occurrence of a substance-related disorder and a medical or psychiatric disorder in an individual.

Enmeshed An individual's inability to differentiate or establish a personal identity. Enmeshed individuals have diffuse boundaries within the family and live solely for each other. Member roles are permeable, with a tendency to cut off outside interactions.

Fetal alcohol syndrome (FAS) A condition caused by prenatal exposure to alcohol in which the individual exhibits a combination of irreversible birth disorders, including facial abnormalities, growth deficiency, and central nervous system deficits.

Half-life Time required for the serum concentration of a drug to decrease by 50%. Drugs dosed at intervals less than their half-life will accumulate in the body, often to toxic levels.

Physical dependence A physiologic state of adaptation to a drug or alcohol, usually characterized by the development of tolerance to drug effects and the emergence of a withdrawal syndrome during prolonged abstinence.

Psychologic dependence The compulsive use of substances, leading to a state of craving a drug or alcohol for its positive effect or to avoid negative effects associated with its absence, or the inability to exercise behavioral restraint.

Relapse/relapse prevention Resumption of a pattern of substance use or dependency after a period of sobriety, and/or the process in which indicators or warning signs appear before the individual's actual resumption of the substance. Relapse prevention is a means of helping the chemically dependent individual maintain behavioral changes over a prolonged period of time.

Sobriety The state of complete abstinence from alcohol and/or other drugs of abuse in conjunction with a satisfactory quality of life.

Teratogens Substances that cause developmental malformations in the fetus.

Tolerance Physiologic adaptation to the effect of drugs that diminishes effects with constant dosages or maintains the intensity and duration of effects through increased dosage.

HISTORICAL AND THEORETIC PERSPECTIVES

The use and abuse of alcohol and other substances have been reported for centuries. References to the use of alcohol are reported in the Old Testament. Greek and Roman mythology had gods of wine (Dionysus and Bacchus, respectively). Alcohol was a part of the meal, as well as a staple in many early cultures' diets. In addition, it was used in celebrations of births, deaths, coronations, and religious ceremonies. Cannabis was used as a minor pain reliever, as an additive to beer to produce hallucinogenic effects, and as a component of ritualistic ceremonies.

MEDICAL USE

In early times, alcohol was used as an anesthetic to cleanse wounds and as an ingredient in salves and tonics. Many drugs, specifically elixirs, were alcohol based. In the late 1800s and early 1900s, patent medicines and remedies were sold by traveling medicine men, physicians, and pseudophysicians. A large number of these medicines and remedies contained drugs such as opium, heroin, and alcohol. Since the production of these substances was not governed by law, poisonings (especially of infants), deaths, and addiction occurred in large numbers. In the nineteenth century morphine and codeine were extracted from opium. The production of synthetic narcotics followed. Today the production and use of medications subject to abuse are regulated by federal laws.

ETIOLOGY

The literature of substance abuse indicates that no one theory adequately explains the etiology of substance abuse. Historically, **alcoholism** and abuse of other substances were viewed from a psychologic or moral perspective, with the indication that those who abuse alcohol and other drugs are weak and have the capacity to refrain from use if they desire to do so. Recent research findings indicate that genetic factors may be responsible for alcohol abuse and addiction. Saitz and O'Malley (1997) noted that alcohol affects endogenous opiates and several neurotransmitters in the brain, including γ-amino butyric acid (GABA), glutamate, and dopamine. Major etiologic factors of substance abuse are summarized in Box 16-1.

BIOLOGIC THEORIES

One of the earliest observations that some people have a predisposition to alcoholism was proposed by Jellinek (1946). Jellinek conjectured that the addictive process and the "loss of control" over the use of alcohol may have a biochemical basis. One of the earliest classifications for alcoholism was proposed by Jellinek (1977) when he noted that persons with alcoholism pass through various stages, including the prealcoholic symptomatic phase, the prodromal phase, the crucial phase, and the chronic phase.

Box 16-1   Etiologic Factors Related to Substance-Related Theories

Biologic Theories
Genetic predisposition to alcoholism
Low response to ethanol

Psychologic Theories
Regression and fixation at the pregenital, oral level of psychosexual development
Dependent personality
Low self-esteem
Basic depressive personality organization
Intolerance for frustration and pain
Lack of success
Lack of meaningful relationships
Difficulty with intimacy

Family Theories
Enmeshment
Emotional compensation
Underlying familial problems
Separation/individuation issues

Learning Theories
Positive effect of mood alterations
Media reinforcement
Peer pressures

Jellinek's work was reinforced in the late 1950s by research reports based on Scandinavian twin studies. The longitudinal research focused on twins of alcoholic parents who were reared in three different environments, (i.e., their own parents, alcoholic foster parents, and foster parents who did not consume alcohol). After 25 years, the incidence of alcoholism in all three groups was almost identical. The research strongly suggested that a genetic factor predisposed the twins to alcoholism.

In 1973 and 1974 Goodwin et al studied identical twins of alcoholic and nonalcoholic fathers. All twins in the study were adopted at birth. Fifty percent of the twins were placed in alcoholic homes, and 50% were placed in nonalcoholic homes. The twins of alcoholic biologic fathers developed alcoholism at a significantly higher rate than twins of nonalcoholic biologic fathers, even when they were raised in nonalcoholic homes. Twins of nonalcoholic biologic fathers who were raised in alcoholic homes did not develop alcoholism at a greater rate than that of the general population.

Schuckit (1985) reported that children of alcoholic biologic parents were four times as likely to develop alcoholism, even when they were adopted by nonalcoholic families at birth. Identical twins had a 60% or greater chance of developing alcoholism, whereas fraternal twins had a 30% or less chance. The research further substantiated the finding that when children of nonalcoholic biologic parents are reared by alcoholic parents, they are not at increased risk for developing alcoholism.

In 1994 Schuckit reported on research in which young adults who had a low response to ethanol were followed for approximately a decade. The data revealed that a strong relationship existed between a less intense response to ethanol and the later development of dependence on alcohol and/or alcohol abuse.

PSYCHOLOGIC THEORIES

Various psychologic theories have been proposed to explain substance abuse. The earliest theories focus on a psychoanalytic perspective and view the substance abuser as regressed and fixated at the pregenital, oral level of psychosexual development. The individual seeks need satisfaction through oral behaviors that include smoking and ingestion of substances or food.

Interpersonal theories focus on the individual with a dependent personality who is unable to fulfill gratification needs, or the individual with an inadequate personality or low self-esteem who uses substances to feel a sense of control, reduce anxiety, and thereby feel more competent.

Knott (1994) stated that there is no addictive personality for alcoholism. He identified several psychodynamic factors that are associated with alcoholism, including a basic depressive personality organization, an intolerance for frustration and pain, a lack of success, a lack of affectionate and meaningful relationships in life, low self-esteem, lack of self-regard, and a tendency toward risk behaviors.

Problems with sexual identity, difficulty with intimacy, marked narcissistic trends, and personal insecurity have also been implicated. Generally speaking, theories of psychologic causation are less well accepted at the present time and are considered to be insufficient to adequately explain the need for excessive substance use.

FAMILY THEORIES

Family systems theory (Bowen, 1978) can be used as a conceptual model to describe the interrelated and interdependent concepts that provide an understanding of emotional family functioning. Several of Bowen's concepts exemplify what happens in the family with an individual who abuses substances.

Children from these families have a tendency to be "nondifferentiated" and **enmeshed** in the family system. Enmeshed individuals have an inability to differentiate or establish a personal identity. They have diffuse boundaries within the family and live solely for each other. Family secrets and myths are used as survival measures by family members, with a tendency to cut off outside interactions. The "multigenerational transmission process" can be used to trace the existence of the disease in the extended family.

Crespi and Sabatelli (1997) identified an interconnection between the developmental implications of parental alcoholism and the individuation process. Dysfunctional families have a tendency to restrict the individuation process.

Miller (1997) reported that a relationship exists between family structure and levels of teenage drug use. He noted that a domino effect occurs, which leads to a variety of delinquent behaviors, including drug use when parents spend less time with teenagers.

LEARNING THEORIES

Learning theory based on operant conditioning models and modeling theory provides additional explanations for substance use. In accordance with operant conditioning theories, drug use develops and is reinforced through the positive effect of mood alterations that occur as a result of chemical alterations in the body.

Differential reinforcement of the effects of drugs occurs at many levels. Media portrayals of "good times" with alcohol and drugs serve as powerful reinforcing mechanisms for adolescents and young adults. Peer group pressures and the need to belong to the group also have positive reinforcing powers. Children and adolescents reared in homes where substances are readily available frequently model the behavior of adults and role models who use substances to feel good.

Initially the effects of substances are pleasant physical and emotional sensations. The individual experiences increased feelings of self-confidence; relief from tension, anxiety, and fear; and a general feeling of well-being. Unfortunately, drugs serve as their own reinforcers and become a necessary way of life for the drug user. When negative consequences occur as a result of excessive use, the initial learned or conditioned response remains and the negative response is insufficient to stop use of the substance. At this time other interventions, including conditioning with less dangerous drugs (e.g., methadone or antabuse), may be required.

EPIDEMIOLOGY

Substance abuse is the number one health problem in the United States. As such, it places an undue burden on the health care system and increases the cost of health care. Substance abuse affects every facet of society and places an enormous strain on the quality of life, not only for the abuser but also for the family.

There are more deaths, illnesses, accidents, and disabilities from substance abuse than from any other preventable health problem. The cost of substance abuse has been estimated to be a staggering $238 billion per year. Of this cost, $99 billion is attributed to alcohol, $67 billion to illicit drugs, and $72 billion to smoking (Rice, 1990).

The impact on individuals who abuse substances, as well as the impact on their families and on society, varies for each substance. Productivity losses, illness, accidents, and premature deaths account for the major cost for alcohol, whereas crime and juvenile detention play a major

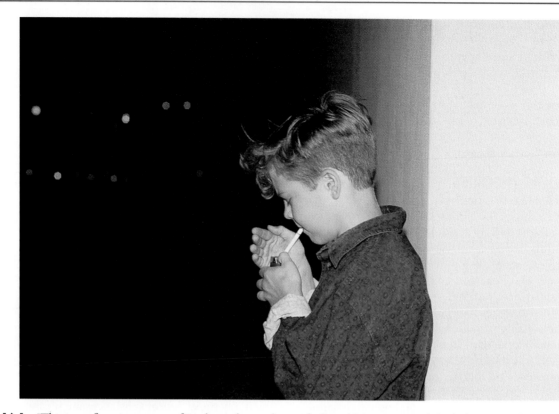

Figure 16-1   "This is my first cigarette; my friends say they make you feel good." Cigarettes and alcohol are considered "gateway drugs" because they usually lead to the use of other drugs. (Copyright Cathy Lander-Goldberg, Lander Photographics)

role for illicit drug-related costs. With regard to smoking, more than 63% of the cost is attributed to premature deaths due to lung cancer, coronary heart disease, and chronic bronchitis, emphysema, and other smoke-related chronic lung diseases (Horgan et al, 1990).

Many elementary schoolchildren begin to experiment with alcohol, tobacco, and illicit drugs in the fifth and sixth grades (Figure 16-1). Since alcohol and cigarettes usually precede the use of illicit drugs, they are referred to as "gateway drugs." It is estimated that by the eighth grade, 70% of young persons have tried alcohol, 44% have smoked cigarettes, 10% have tried marijuana, and 2% have used cocaine. By the twelfth grade these percentages have increased as follows: 80% have used alcohol, 63% have used tobacco, 37% have used marijuana, and 8% have used cocaine (Horgan et al, 1990). The age at which an individual first uses drugs is a strong predictor of heavy use throughout his or her lifetime. Use at an early age also subjects the individual to the probability of early dependence and addiction.

DEMOGRAPHIC VARIABLES

In 1996 the number of Americans who used illicit drugs was estimated at 13 million (6.1% of the population age 12 years and older), based on statistics published by the National Institute on Drug Abuse (NIDA) in 1997. This figure did not differ substantially from the 1995 statistics, when the estimated prevalence was 12.8 million. Rates of drug use varied considerably by age: 2.2% of 12- to 13-year-olds, 15.6% of 16- to 17-year-olds, and 20% of individuals ages 18 to 20 were reported to be current drug users. Fifty percent of individuals ages 21 to 25 had tried illicit drugs, and 13% were current users. In adults ages 26 to 34, 8.4% were current users, and in adults ages 35 to 49, 5.2% were current users.

According to the NIDA statistics, demographic variables, including ethnicity, race, gender, level of education, and place of residence, affect the prevalence of drug use. In 1996, 74% (9.7 million) of all current drug users were white, 14% (1.8 million) were African-American, and 8% (1.1 million) were Hispanic. Men continued to use drugs at a higher percentage than women (8.1% versus 4.2%). Illicit drug use remained highly correlated with educational status. Among young adults ages 18 to 34, high school graduates had the highest rate of current drug use—16.8% as compared with 6.9% for college graduates. This occurred despite the fact that both groups had tried illicit drugs in their lifetime (49.0% for high school graduates and 48.6% for college graduates).

The highest rate of current illicit drug use occurred in metropolitan areas. Variability of use according to the region of the country was as follows: 7.3% in the West, 6.9%

in the North Central region, 5.5% in the South, and 4.8% in the Northeast.

Employment status was also highly correlated with current rates of illicit drug use. Nonemployed adults consistently manifested a higher rate of illicit drug use (12.5% versus 6.2% of employed adults). Seventy-three percent of current illicit drug users 18 years and older (8.1 million) were employed (6.2 million full time and 1.9 million part time).

SUBSTANCE ABUSE IN SPECIAL POPULATIONS
PERINATAL CONCERNS

The use and abuse of chemical substances by pregnant women are on the increase. Although some mothers stop using chemical substances during the first 3 or 4 months of pregnancy, 75% resume substance use following pregnancy. Tobacco (in the form of cigarettes) continues to be the most common drug that pregnant women use. Approximately 25% to 30% of women expose their children to nicotine in utero. Smoking during pregnancy results in an increase in miscarriages, low-birth-weight infants, and early infant death from sudden infant death syndrome (SIDS). In the older child there is an increased incidence of respiratory illnesses and delayed cognitive development.

Prenatal alcohol consumption continues to be a major concern. According to the NIDA 1996 National Pregnancy and Health Survey, more than 18% of pregnant women and 3 out of every 5 women of childbearing age drink alcohol. One in every 10 American women consumes 2 or more drinks daily, 14 or more drinks weekly, or up to 60 drinks monthly and is classified as a moderate drinker. Approximately 6% to 8% of pregnant women have serious alcohol problems (Ewing, 1992). Sixteen percent of women of childbearing age acknowledged using an illicit drug within 30 days of being questioned in the 1996 NIDA National Pregnancy and Health Survey. This survey also revealed a strong link between cigarette and alcohol use and the use of illicit drugs, specifically marijuana and cocaine. An estimated 5% of infants born in the United States each year have been exposed to illicit substances in utero. Actually, this number would be much larger if the maternal use of nicotine and alcohol were included.

Many of the substances abused by pregnant women are **teratogens** to the offspring, causing developmental malformations in the fetus. However, since many pregnant women are polydrug users, it is difficult in most instances to predict the outcome in their offspring. The effect of substances on fetuses is dependent on a number of factors, including the amount and pattern of maternal consumption, the properties of the chemical substance/drug, and the timing of exposure. A critical period for vital organ development occurs during the embryonic phase, from the second through the eighth week after conception. Drug exposure after this period is more likely to result in intrauterine growth retardation and more subtle mental and behavioral deficits (Cook et al, 1990).

Generally, intrauterine drug exposure has been associated with:

Low birth weight (small for gestational age), decreased length, and small head circumference
Specific congenital physical malformations
Mild to severe withdrawal effects that include irritability, tremors, seizures, hypertonia, abdominal distention, increased respiratory rate, and vomiting
Central nervous system damage that may delay or impair neurobehavioral development

These neurobehavioral effects may include subtle behavioral abnormalities or latent developmental deficits and/or delays that are frequently not obvious at birth (Cook et al, 1990).

Fetal Alcohol Syndrome/Alcohol-Related Effects

In 1996 the Institute of Medicine defined criteria for diagnosing **fetal alcohol syndrome (FAS)** and described the effects on the infant exposed to alcohol during the prenatal period. Children with FAS demonstrate a low birth weight, certain facial characteristics, and neurologic abnormalities, including developmental and/or intellectual delays. The facial characteristics include microcephaly (head circumference below the third percentile), microthalmia (small eyes) and/or short palpebral fissures, a poorly developed philtrum (median groove between the upper lip and the nose), a thin upper lip, a short nose, a small chin, and flattening of the maxillary area (Figure 16-2).

Children with alcohol-related effects may be identified as those with alcohol-related birth defects (ARBDs) or alcohol-related neurodevelopmental disorders (ARNDs). Those with ARBDs have a variety of defects affecting other organ systems, including cardiac defects, visual problems, hearing defects, dental malalignments, and minor genital anomalies. Children with ARNDs may exhibit mental retardation, impaired fine motor skills, hyperactivity that evolves into problems of easy distractibility, inability to attend to relevant data, and the inability to ignore irrelevant information. In addition, these individuals show poor coordination and attention, dependence, stubbornness or sullenness, social withdrawal, teasing or bullying, crying or laughing too easily, impulsivity, and periods of high anxiety.

Whether working with an adolescent or an adult client, one must recognize that some of these individuals may have or develop other medical or psychologic problems; therefore it is important to consider the existence of comorbidity, the presence of two or more disorders in the same person.

Those who have awareness of the etiology of the syndrome manifest a high incidence of depression, anger, sui-

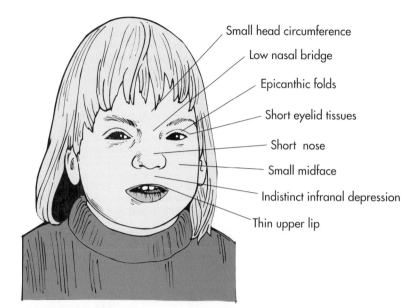

- Small head circumference
- Low nasal bridge
- Epicanthic folds
- Short eyelid tissues
- Short nose
- Small midface
- Indistinct infranal depression
- Thin upper lip

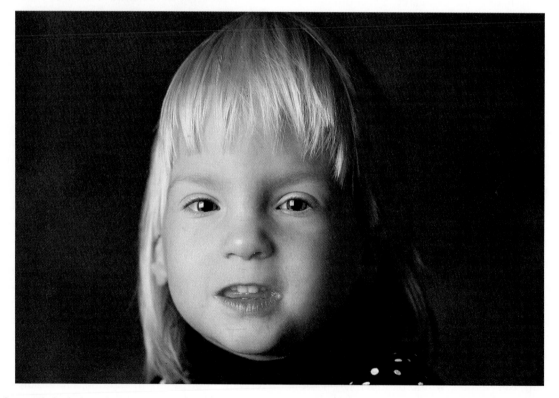

Figure 16-2   Fetal alcohol syndrome (FAS). Milder forms of alcohol-induced effects on the fetus and the infant are known as fetal alcohol effects.

cidal ideation, antisocial behavior, and drug and alcohol use. Many of these men and women are unable to lead normal, independent lives. Their family or caregivers must make plans for long-term community support and care.

Cocaine Use

Cocaine use by the pregnant mother and the effect on her child show great variability. Some of the infants have severe effects (e.g., missing digits, cerebral stroke, and malformations of major body systems), whereas other children appear to compensate for or show no effects of cocaine exposure. As more of these children enter the school system, an increase in learning and behavioral problems may be documented. When a child experiences such problems, the exposure during fetal life to alcohol and other drugs, including cocaine, should be explored.

ADOLESCENT SUBSTANCE ABUSE

Adolescent substance abuse is a major health and social problem. Rates of substance use and abuse among American high school students and college students remain the highest in the industrialized world (Johnson et al, 1988). The true measure of the problem is further complicated by the fact that substance abuse in adolescence is an illicit behavior with potential legal complications. Adolescent peers are reluctant to volunteer information about drinking behaviors or other drug use (Kozel and Adams, 1986).

Another problem related to adolescent drug use concerns the DSM-IV classification for substance abuse. The labels of dependence and abuse as described in the DSM-IV classification do not adequately describe the problem in adolescence; nor are they helpful in treating adolescents. It is more appropriate to use the term *problematic use*, because adolescents drink in response to specific events, emotional crisis, or peer group pressure (Flynn, 1992). They may not develop the usual signs of psychologic or physical dependence because they have not used alcohol or other drugs for a sufficient period of time. **Psychologic dependence** is the compulsive use of substances leading to a state of craving a drug or alcohol for its positive effect or to avoid negative effects associated with its absence or the ability to exercise behavioral restraint. **Physical dependence** is a physiologic state of adaptation to a drug or alcohol, usually characterized by the development of tolerance to drug effects and the emergence of a withdrawal syndrome during prolonged abstinence. Adolescents who have continuing problems with drinking alcohol and using other drugs develop dependence and manifest a pervasive, recurrent pattern that has serious consequences in several areas of their lives, including family, school, social relationships, and job performance. Legal consequences frequently occur as a result of drug use in adolescence.

The following are significant factors that place the adolescent at risk for substance use/abuse:

> School dropout
> Emotionally disadvantaged background
> Children of drug abusers
> Victims of abuse—child/parental, sexual
> Experienced trouble with law
> History of mental problems
> Suicide attempts
> Long-term physical pain
> Dysfunctional families; divorce
> Feelings of inferiority—emotional, physical, academic

The Client & Family Teaching Guidelines box lists signs of substance abuse and strategies to prevent substance abuse. These are especially useful guidelines for parents.

IMPAIRED PROFESSIONALS

Substance dependence in health care professionals has received increasing attention from professional groups. Statistics concerning substance dependence in nurses vary greatly from one study to another. An early study by the American Nurses Association (ANA) (1984) indicated that 5% of 2.4 million nurses were chemical abusers and 8% to 10% were chemically dependent.

Sullivan and Handley (1992) concluded that the prevalence of alcohol and drug problems in nurses and student nurses does not exceed that of others in society. The authors identified that published research is limited in scope because results are based on small, nonrandom selected samples. Several studies examine risk factors and characteristics of impaired nurses. Mynatt (1996) reported that impaired nurses live chaotic lives, start drug use at an early age, frequently suffer from low self-esteem, and use denial.

Trinkoff and Storr (1998) explored the association between nursing specialty and past year substance use. Results indicate that rate of use by specialty varied even when sociodemographics were controlled. When specialties were compared with nurses in women's health, pediatrics, and general practice, emergency room nurses were 3.5 times as likely to use marijuana or cocaine. Oncology nurses and nurses in administration engaged in binge drinking twice as often, and psychiatric nurses had higher rates of substance use and were most likely to smoke cigarettes.

Several states have established intervention programs

Client & Family TEACHING GUIDELINES

Signs of Adolescent Drug Use/Abuse

Sudden behavioral changes
Sweating, especially at night
Needle marks
Inebriation
Change in nutritional intake
Nasal congestion
Rhinorrhea with cocaine use
School problems

Prevention of Adolescent Substance Use/Abuse

Provide positive role modeling by parents and adults in the adolescent's world.
Reinforce positive behaviors and the dangers of substance use.
Support the adolescent in coping with the social pressure exerted by peers.
Establish normative expectations for the adolescent's behavior.
Help the adolescent anticipate pressures and reinforce behaviors to cope with realities.
Encourage involvement in life skills training programs where the emphasis is on positive skills training, resistance training, and group support.
Monitor the adolescent's television viewing, since media may portray legal and illegal substance use as a part of daily life.

for impaired nurses based on the model that is used in Florida. Impaired nurses who participate in the program and seek treatment do not lose their license to practice. Following a period of acute treatment, they must submit to random drug testing and participate in a 12-step group for impaired nurses for 2 to 3 years.

DUAL DIAGNOSIS
PERSONS WITH DUAL DIAGNOSIS

Comorbidity is the presence of two or more disorders in the same person that may occur simultaneously or sequentially. If the disorders occur simultaneously, the comorbidity is also known as **dual diagnosis,** which indicates that an individual has two initially unrelated disorders that interact and cause increased manifestations of the other disorder (Lehman et al, 1987).

Individuals with a dual diagnosis have two separate chronic disorders that influence each other. This group of individuals, who represent a minimum of 50% of individuals with substance abuse and mental disorders, have higher levels of physical, social, and psychologic impairment than individuals with either disorder by itself (Gafoor and Rassool, 1998).

El-Mallakh (1998) reported on studies conducted by the National Comorbidity Survey, which indicated that up to 51% of individuals with serious mental illness are also dependent on substances. He noted that too few of these individuals receive treatment for both conditions at the same time and emphasized the importance of an "integrated model" of treatment.

Dual diagnosis that focuses on individuals with specific psychiatric diagnoses include the following. Landry et al (1991) reported on individuals with depression and anxiety disorders who abuse alcohol. Dulit et al (1990) found that borderline personality and substance abuse disorders were interrelated in two thirds of the population they studied. Mueser et al (1990) and Cuffel (1992) focused their research on individuals with schizophrenia and the prevalence of stimulant and hallucinogen use.

Recent research that focused on prevalence rates of dual diagnosis in low-income, inner-city populations determined that two thirds of patients being treated in outpatient inner-city clinics met lifetime criteria for a dual diagnosis (Zimberg et al, 1997).

PERSONS WITH HIV DISEASE

The transmission of human immunodeficiency virus (HIV) occurs through infected blood or blood products and through sexual contact. Sexual contact is considered the major route of transmission. In the United States the incidence of heterosexual transmission continues to rise. The use of alcohol and other drugs is one of the major causes that contributes to "sexual risk-taking behavior" such as failure to use a condom, multiple partners, or engagement in alternative sexual acts. A second major cause

is drug abuse that includes intravenous, intradermal (skin popping), or intramuscular (steroid abuse route) injection. Many injection drug users also use noninjection drugs. Grella, Anglin, and Wagalter (1995) reported that many clients at high risk for HIV were crack and cocaine users.

Alcohol is known to have immunosuppressive effects that may increase an individual's susceptibility to the HIV virus or, if the individual has been exposed, increase the onset of symptoms of HIV disease. It is also believed that the effects of alcohol on the immune system and on the HIV infection may be influenced by the individual's drinking habits. Persons with chronic alcoholism who have a history of liver disease may be at greater risk for HIV infection.

CLINICAL DESCRIPTION

The DSM-IV includes the diagnostic classification substance-related disorders. Subcategories exist in each of these classes. Most of the categories include dependence, abuse, intoxication, withdrawal, delirium, psychotic disorders with delusions, psychotic disorders with hallucinations, mood disorders, anxiety disorders, sexual dysfunction, sleep disorders, and disorder not otherwise specified (NOS). The DSM-IV criteria for substance abuse and substance dependence are found in the DSM-IV Criteria boxes on p. 362 and 363, respectively.

DSM-IV CRITERIA

Substance Abuse

A. A maladaptive pattern of substance use leading to clinically significant impairment or distress, as manifested by one (or more) of the following, occurring within a 12-month period:
 1. Recurrent substance use resulting in a failure to fulfill major role obligations at work, school, or home (e.g., repeated absences or poor job performance related to substance use; substance-related absences, suspensions, or expulsions from school; neglect of children or household)
 2. Recurrent substance use in situations in which it is physically hazardous (e.g., driving an automobile or operating a machine when impaired by substance use)
 3. Recurrent substance-related legal problems (e.g., arrests for substance-related disorderly conduct)
 4. Continued substance use despite having persistent or recurrent social or interpersonal problems caused or exacerbated by the effects of the substance (e.g., arguments with spouse about consequences of intoxication; physical fights)
B. The symptoms have never met the criteria for substance dependence for this class of substance.

From American Psychiatric Association: *Diagnostic and statistical manual of mental disorders,* ed 4, Washington, DC, 1994, The Association.

Although alcohol is the most frequently abused drug, a variety of other psychoactive drugs are abused, including barbiturates, benzodiazepines, opioids, cocaine, stimulants, and nicotine. A brief description of each type of drug follows (see Chapter 23).

ALCOHOL ABUSE

Alcohol is one of the earliest substances of abuse. As noted earlier in the chapter, historically alcohol was used for medicinal purposes before the use of other anesthetics and

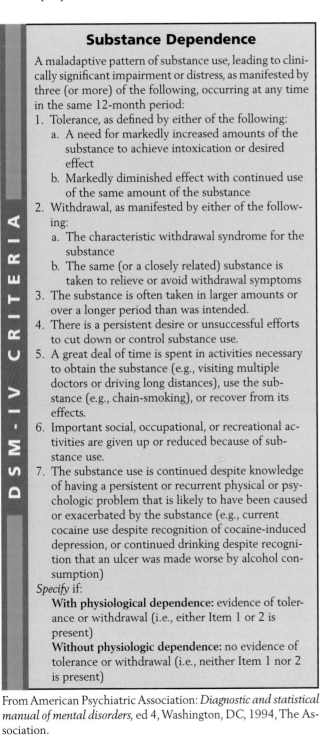

Substance Dependence

A maladaptive pattern of substance use, leading to clinically significant impairment or distress, as manifested by three (or more) of the following, occurring at any time in the same 12-month period:

1. Tolerance, as defined by either of the following:
   a. A need for markedly increased amounts of the substance to achieve intoxication or desired effect
   b. Markedly diminished effect with continued use of the same amount of the substance
2. Withdrawal, as manifested by either of the following:
   a. The characteristic withdrawal syndrome for the substance
   b. The same (or a closely related) substance is taken to relieve or avoid withdrawal symptoms
3. The substance is often taken in larger amounts or over a longer period than was intended.
4. There is a persistent desire or unsuccessful efforts to cut down or control substance use.
5. A great deal of time is spent in activities necessary to obtain the substance (e.g., visiting multiple doctors or driving long distances), use the substance (e.g., chain-smoking), or recover from its effects.
6. Important social, occupational, or recreational activities are given up or reduced because of substance use.
7. The substance use is continued despite knowledge of having a persistent or recurrent physical or psychologic problem that is likely to have been caused or exacerbated by the substance (e.g., current cocaine use despite recognition of cocaine-induced depression, or continued drinking despite recognition that an ulcer was made worse by alcohol consumption)

Specify if:

With physiological dependence: evidence of tolerance or withdrawal (i.e., either Item 1 or 2 is present)

Without physiologic dependence: no evidence of tolerance or withdrawal (i.e., neither Item 1 nor 2 is present)

DSM-IV CRITERIA

From American Psychiatric Association: *Diagnostic and statistical manual of mental disorders*, ed 4, Washington, DC, 1994, The Association.

disinfectants. Alcohol is derived from a number of fruits and vegetables in the form of wine and is distilled into other forms of alcohol, including liquor, whiskey, brandy, and liqueur.

Alcohol abuse and dependence have many physiologic complications affecting several body systems. These complications are discussed in the following section along with signs and symptoms of alcohol withdrawal.

Effects on the Neurologic System

Excessive use of alcohol produces several changes in the neurologic system that result from damage to brain cells. The following discussion describes common resulting syndromes.

Blackouts occur most frequently with excessive use of alcohol and present as an early sign of alcoholism. Individuals who experience blackouts enter a fuguelike amnestic state during which recollection of activities are lost from conscious recall. These individuals remain conscious and appear to function normally to those in their environment. Blackouts may last for a relatively short period of time, 24 to 48 hours, or they may last for a week or longer.

Idiosyncratic intoxification usually has a sudden onset manifested by agitation, altered consciousness, aggressiveness, fear, and anxiety. It may be accompanied by mental confusion, disorientation, delusions, and hallucinations. Suicide attempts may occur as a result of hallucinations or the heightened state of anxiety and agitation. The attacks last from a few moments to a day or more and usually end with a long period of sleep. The next day a "hangover" occurs, which is commonly characterized by headache, gastrointestinal upsets, and general malaise. Most often, the individual has very little if any recollection of what transpired during the time of idiosyncratic intoxification.

Substance withdrawal delirium (delirium tremens [DTs]) is the most severe form of alcohol withdrawal. It occurs approximately 24 to 72 hours after the individual has had the last drink. DTs occur in heavy drinkers and are manifested by an acute psychotic state. Approximately 5% of all alcoholics hospitalized for alcohol withdrawal develop DTs. Confusion and disorientation regarding time and place are common. Other symptoms include vivid visual and auditory hallucinations that are accusatory and threatening to the patient, illusions (light cords appearing as snakes), severe agitation, profuse sweating, tachycardia, tachypnea, and possible grand mal seizure activity (Box 16-2). The condition may be life threatening if immediate medical intervention does not occur.

Several protocols exist to treat alcohol withdrawal and DTs. Benzodiazepines are the drugs of choice for the management of alcohol withdrawal and prevention of seizures and DTs. Clonidine (Catapres) and carbamazepine (Tegretol) may be used to reduce symptoms (Saitz and O'Malley, 1997).

Acute alcoholic hallucinosis occurs after a prolonged period of drinking. The syndrome is characterized by threat-

---

Box 16-2   Alcohol Withdrawal Symptoms and Treatment

Withdrawal Symptoms

Tremulousness ("the shakes"); onset 3 to 36 hours after the last drink

Increased psychomotor hyperactivity with tremors

Insomnia

Acute anxiety and hyperalertness

Tachycardia (120 to 140 beats/min)

Hypertension

Anorexia

Agitation

Possible nausea, abdominal cramps, vomiting

Weakness

Craving for alcohol or sedative drug

Acute hallucinosis

    Auditory or visual hallucinations assume prominence; this may indicate that alcohol withdrawal delirium is impending

Alcohol withdrawal delirium (the horrors, delirium tremens, DTs); onset 24 to 72 hours after last drink; most serious of withdrawal phases (5% to 36% mortality)

    Disorientation

    Hallucinations

    Delusions

    Delirium

    Severe agitation

Treatment of Withdrawal

Impending withdrawal

Monitor vital signs every 3 hours; notify physician of any abnormal readings

Provide a quiet, nonstimulating environment, yet keep a light on in room

Administer sedating medications promptly as ordered (do not undersedate); ensure that medications are taken

Frequently orient client to place, person, time; quietly and simply explain all procedures, routines, and expected components of treatment process

Accurately record intake and output (including emesis, diarrhea, estimated loss from diaphoresis)

Do not force fluids until it has been established that client is dehydrated; however, ensure that client takes estimated minimum of fluids per 24-hour period

Allow ambulation ad lib if ordered and *if client is stable*, since this channels excess agitation

Allow client to express fears regarding withdrawal; provide nonjudgmental, caring concern

Institute seizure precautions (oral airway, upright side rails, remove potentially harmful objects)

Assist client with activities of daily living (bathing, eating, mouth care) without overstimulating client (e.g., no shaving or nail care)

Provide small, frequent, high-carbohydrate feedings that are easily digested; administer antiemetic prn before meals (offer patient flavored fluids, gelatins); administer vitamins as ordered, such as multivitamin, vitamin B-complex including thiamine, and vitamin C

Test urine for specific gravity and stools for guaiac to detect gastrointestinal dysfunction

Be there; spend time with client and family

Alcohol withdrawal delirium

Monitor vital signs qh

Assess neurologic status qh

Stimulate patient to cough and deep breathe q2h

Carefully evaluate bladder and bowel functions

Inspect skin for signs of breakdown or traumatic injury

IVs, tube feedings, catheter if ordered

Restrain client to prevent injury if needed

Check client at least every 15 minutes

Administer anticonvulsant medications as ordered

From Beare PG, Myers JL: *Adult health nursing,* ed 2, St. Louis, 1998, Mosby.

---

ening auditory hallucinations. This condition is differentiated from DTs in that the individual remains oriented to time and place; during lucid periods, the person usually can recall occurrences after recovery. Some individuals incorporate the auditory hallucinations into an elaborate delusional system that may be threatening to those in the immediate environment.

Wernicke's syndrome and Korsakoff's syndrome occur after many years of excessive alcohol intake. The syndromes affect the entire neurologic system. Korsakoff's syndrome is an amnestic syndrome caused by deficiency in the B vitamins, including thiamine, riboflavin, and folic acid. It is characterized by amnesia, disorientation to time and place, falsification of memory, and severe peripheral neuropathy (i.e., tingling; muscle weakness; sore, burning muscles; parathesias; and extreme pain on movement).

The extremities, especially the lower extremities, are affected. Precaution must be taken in moving clients because of the severe pain they experience. An important nursing care requirement is to prevent footdrop.

Wernicke's syndrome, also referred to as *alcoholic encephalopathy,* most frequently occurs simultaneously with Korsakoff's syndrome but may occur as an isolated condition. It is a neurologic disease characterized by ataxia, ophthalmoplegia (particularly involving the sixth cranial nerve), nystagmus, and confusion. It is caused by severe deficiency in vitamin B_1 due to the lack of adequate food intake. The early stage responds rapidly to large doses of parenteral thiamine. If the condition is not adequately treated at an early point, it progresses to a chronic, severe lifetime condition that requires custodial care. The chronic condition is becoming more rare in recent years as a result of the rapid use of thiamine as a treatment modality (Kaplan and Sadock, 1994).

Effects on the Liver

The liver is characteristically the body organ most affected by excessive use of alcohol. Alcohol passes directly into the bloodstream through the stomach and intestinal walls. It is processed by the liver, where enzymes change alcohol into acetaldehyde, which is further metabolized into acetate, carbon dioxide, and water. Alcohol metabolism releases excessive amounts of hydrogen into the liver; this inhibits certain metabolic processes, including metabolism of fats. As a result, the unburned fat becomes deposited into the liver and causes hepatic steatosis, or "fatty liver" (Lieber and Leo, 1982).

Alcoholic hepatitis occurs after a prolonged period (usually several years) of alcohol abuse. It is an inflammatory condition of the liver characterized by fever, chills, nausea, pain in the upper abdomen, and jaundice. Treatment consists of abstinence with nutritional support. Early treatment of fatty liver and alcoholic hepatitis can reverse the progression of the disease. Cirrhosis, which occurs in 10% to 20% of individuals who consume 120 to 180 g/day over a period of 15 years, is not reversible (Stein, 1997).

Effects on the Gastrointestinal Tract

Gastrointestinal complaints manifested by bloating, nausea, and vomiting are frequent complications of heavy alcohol intake. Alcohol stimulates gastric secretions, slows gastric emptying, and causes injury to gastric mucosa, causing gastric ulcers. Acute and chronic pancreatitis result from heavy chronic alcohol intake and must be differentiated from gastritis and gastric ulcers (Stein, 1997).

Effects on the Cardiovascular System

Chronic alcoholism may also affect the cardiovascular system. Alcoholic cardiomyopathy with congestive failure and atrial fibrillation may occur. Other manifestations include narrow pulse pressure, tachycardia, elevated diastolic pressure, hypertension, and peripheral edema. According to Donahue et al (1986), the risk of hemorrhagic stroke is doubled for light consumers of alcohol and tripled for heavy drinkers. Elective surgery for individuals who consume excessive amounts of alcohol is frequently delayed because of the negative effects of alcohol on the cardiovascular system.

Effects on Other Systems

Excessive alcohol intake may affect any system in the body. Men with alcoholism may experience impotence. Effects on the reproductive system are substantiated for mothers and their unborn infants, as discussed under FAS. Women with alcoholism frequently experience infertility and decreased menstruation, a process called "telescoping," which occurs as a result of more rapid development of dependence.

Acute myopathy is another common sequelae of long-term alcohol abuse, characterized by sudden leg cramps. If alcohol abuse continues, chronic myopathy may occur, resulting in weakness and atrophy of the leg muscles. Persons with alcoholism are also at risk for metabolic bone disease (Bikle, 1980).

Effects of alcohol on the endocrine system are less well documented. It is believed that alcohol affects the hypothalamic-pituitary adrenal system, causing hypoglycemia, which, in turn, causes the person to drink.

ABUSE OF OTHER DRUGS
Barbiturates

First introduced in 1903, barbiturates are used as hypnotics, sedatives, and anticonvulsants. Phenobarbital and barbital are long-acting drugs with a **half-life** (the time required for the serum concentration of a drug to decrease by 50%) of 12 to 24 hours. Amobarbital (Amytal) has an intermediate active half-life of 6 to 12 hours; pentobarbital (Nembutal) and secobarbital (Seconal) are short-acting drugs with a half-life of 3 to 6 hours (Kaplan and Sadock, 1994).

Barbiturates are frequently abused drugs because they are legitimately manufactured in large quantities and available in many forms. Secobarbital, pentobarbital, and amobarbital are the three most frequently abused barbiturates. When they are available through the black market, the strength of the drug is unknown because most of it has been replaced with sugar and other substances (Kaplan and Sadock, 1994). Abuse of barbiturates, as well as prescriptions for barbiturates, have been reduced since they have been classified as controlled substances and are under federal legal control with the implementation of the Harrison Narcotic Act in 1914.

Barbiturate abuse occurs most frequently among young users or among middle-age individuals who abuse prescription drugs. Consumption is through oral or intravenous routes. Young abusers may substitute barbiturates for heroin or morphine because they are cheaper and more readily available. Barbiturates have a **cross-tolerance** to other chemically similar drugs, including alcohol, benzodiazepines, and heroin. Intravenous users experience a sudden warm "rush" followed by a prolonged drowsy feeling.

Individuals who present with mild barbiturate intoxication experience the following symptoms: sluggishness in coordination, emotional lability, aggressive impulses, slowness of speech, thought disorders, and faulty judgment. Neurologic signs include nystagmus (involuntary eye oscillations), diplopia (double vision), strabismus (deviation of the eye), ataxic gait, positive Romberg's sign (swaying of the body when standing with the feet close together and eyes closed), hypotonia, dysmetria (disturbance to control range of movement in muscular acts), and decreased superficial reflexes. The diagnosis of barbiturate intoxication is confirmed by blood tests (Kaplan and Sadock, 1994).

Barbiturates are especially dangerous because all patterns of overuse have potentially deleterious effects on the individual's health. They are a common cause of lethal accidents and are frequently used in suicide attempts. Barbiturates found in home medicine cabinets may be consumed by children and may result in fatal drug overdoses. Death occurs as a result of deep coma, which progresses to respiratory arrest and cardiovascular failure. Lethal doses vary widely from individual to individual. There is a narrow therapeutic index for sedative effects, with the therapeutic dose being very close to the lethal dose (Kaplan and Sadock, 1994).

Benzodiazepines

Benzodiazepines, introduced in the early 1960s, have largely supplanted barbiturates and barbiturate-like substances in clinical practice. Two patterns of benzodiazepine abuse and addiction that are most prominent are chronic use and use with multiple drugs or alcohol (Juergens, 1997). Benzodiazepines taken in combination with alcohol and/or barbiturates lead to central nervous system depression and may cause death (Paul, 1988).

Benzodiazepines have a wide range of pharmacologic differences, including their rapidity of onset of action, their half-life, and the ways in which they are metabolized in the body (Scharf et al, 1988).

Benzodiazepines that have a rapid onset of action are more likely to have abuse potential. Diazepam (Valium) is the most rapidly absorbed of the group and produces an affective euphoria. It is the most widely abused benzodiazepine and one of the most widely abused prescription drugs. The scientific community lacks agreement on the abuse potential of diazepam when prescribed for medical reasons.

The benzodiazepines, including diazepam, are not likely to produce abuse in clients who do not have a history of substance dependence. Although the specific mechanisms are unknown, individuals with a chemical dependence react differently to diazepam than do individuals with no chemical dependence. **Tolerance** in individuals with a substance dependence is rapid for sedative and euphoric effects and negligible for antianxiety effects (Francis and Miller, 1991).

Opioids

Included in this classification of drugs are opium alkaloids derived from opium (juice of the opium poppy *Pavaver somniferum*), of which morphine is the best known. Other opiate alkaloids are heroin, codeine, and hydromorphine (Dilaudid). Synthetic opioids made in the laboratory include meperidine (Demerol), methadone, and propoxyphene (Darvon).

The most widely abused opiate is heroin. There are an estimated 400,000 to 600,000 heroin addicts in the United States. Male heroin addicts outnumber female addicts 3 to 1. Most heroin addicts have a long history of substance dependence, starting with substance abuse at an early age and progressing to heroin in their late twenties and early thirties. Most heroin addicts spend more than $200 a day to support their habit. Many obtain money through engaging in criminal activity, including pushing and selling drugs (Kaplan and Sadock, 1994).

Tolerance to opiates develops rapidly; however, tolerance to the respiratory depressant effect of opiates does not. Most deaths occur as a result of respiratory arrest. An overdose of morphine is life threatening. In addition to marked analgesic effects, the triad of coma, pinpoint pupils, and respiratory depression signal opiate overdose.

Emergency medical intervention with an opiate antagonist is necessary in the case of an overdose. Naloxone (Narcan) is administered intravenously, beginning with an initial dose of 0.4 mg. The dose may be repeated up to four or five times in the initial 30 to 45 minutes, depending on vital signs and the client's level of responsiveness. It is imperative to ensure an open airway and provide continuous monitoring of vital signs until the client is fully responsive and out of danger. Naloxone has a short duration of action (4 to 5 hours); therefore, continuous monitoring is imperative to prevent recurrence of toxic symptoms from the opiate effects (Kaplan and Sadock, 1994).

Withdrawal From Opiates

Morphine and heroin addicts consume huge amounts (up to 5000 mg) of the drug. Withdrawal symptoms begin 6 to 8 hours after the last dose and reach their peak intensity within 48 to 72 hours. Withdrawal symptoms include myalgia, nausea, vomiting, diarrhea, diaphoresis, rhinorrhea, lacrimation, pupillary dilation, hypertension, tachycardia, and temperature irregularities, including chills and fever (Slaby, 1997). The term *cold turkey*, which denotes the abstinence syndrome, comes from another common symptom, the appearance of "gooseflesh." A single dose of morphine can alleviate all symptoms.

Methadone Treatment

Methadone treatment is the treatment of choice for morphine and heroin addicts. Methadone is a synthetic opioid given to addicts to suppress withdrawal symptoms. A methadone dose of 20 to 80 mg/day is usually sufficient to stabilize a client. Methadone maintenance is continued until the client can be withdrawn from methadone. Methadone itself is addicting, but clients can be withdrawn by gradually decreasing the total daily dose until the client is methadone free. Special precautions need to be exercised in maintaining and withdrawing pregnant clients from opiates. Usually smaller doses of methadone are indicated (10 to 40 mg/day) (Kaplan and Sadock, 1994).

Cocaine

Cocaine ("snow," "coke," "girl," "lady") is a highly addictive alkaloid derived from *Erythroxylon coca*, a plant indigenous to Bolivia and Peru. The addictive properties of cocaine were not fully recognized until the 1980s when both the general public and physicians became aware of the problem. Cocaine use peaked in 1985 when 12 million used the drug and decreased significantly to 8 million users in 1988 (Adams et al, 1989).

Pharmacologic effects of cocaine that block reuptake of serotonin and the catecholamine neurotransmitters, particularly dopamine, produce an intense feeling of euphoria. This makes cocaine a highly addictive drug. A single dose of cocaine, especially in the form of "crack," may cause psychologic dependence. The main effect of cocaine is relatively brief (30 to 60 minutes) when used intravenously or sniffed. However, cocaine remains in the brain for approximately 10 days. After the acute drug effect, there is usually a period of depression that may be sufficiently severe to precipitate suicidal ideation (Kaplan and Sadock, 1994).

Individuals who inhale while they smoke cocaine may experience swelling and inflammation of the nasal passages and ulceration of the nose. Those who are sensitive to crack may experience sudden cardiac arrest. As with all intravenous use, the risk of sharing needles may cause infection and emboli at the injection site and predispose the individual to the risk of contracting HIV disease.

Cocaine intoxication is characterized by extreme irritability, agitation, aggressiveness, impulsive sexual activity, and manic excitement. The course of intoxication is usually self-limiting to approximately 24 hours, after which time withdrawal symptoms occur. These withdrawal symptoms are often referred to as the "crash."

Cocaine withdrawal in the DSM IV classification is defined as a characteristic withdrawal syndrome that develops within hours to days after cessation of cocaine use.

Abrupt withdrawal creates an intense craving for the drug. Clients experience severe depression with suicidal ideation. They become hypersomnolent and complain of fatigue, anhedonia, and general malaise. Symptoms usually subside in a number of weeks. An inherent danger is that clients will seek other mood-altering substances, including alcohol and benzodiazepines, to fill the void they experience from giving up cocaine.

The treatment for cocaine users is varied and requires cooperation by the family, employer, and health professionals. Many individuals require hospitalization to ensure separation from the drug and other substances. Urine testing for toxicologic analysis should be a part of the continuing treatment program. Psychotherapy is helpful in addressing underlying psychologic problems, and family support for the individual should be sought. Support groups such as Cocaine Anonymous (CA) are critical in helping the individual remain abstinent. The underlying depression and possible psychosis require medical treatment with antidepressant and antipsychotic medications.

Stimulants

Stimulant drugs include caffeine, ephidrine, propanolamine (PPA), and amphetamine. Amphetamines have the greatest abuse potential. Amphetamine was first synthesized in 1887; however, it was not marketed until 1932, when it was marketed under the name Benzedrine. The Benzedrine inhaler is available as a nonprescription drug for nasal congestion and asthma. Amphetamines and amphetamine congeners (drugs that have a similar action on muscle groups) compose a large group of central nervous system stimulant drugs. Among the best known are dextroamphetamine (Dexedrine), methamphetamine (Methedrine), and methylphenidine (Ritalin) (Kaplan and Sadock, 1994).

Amphetamine is a highly addictive drug. Although it is not as addictive as cocaine, occasional users soon begin to abuse the drug and use it intravenously, which leads to physical and psychosocial morbidity. In the United States, amphetamine abuse reached epidemic proportions in the 1970s.

The therapeutic use of the drug according to the Food and Drug Administration (FDA) is restricted to attention-deficit/hyperactivity disorder in children and adults, narcolepsy, and obesity. Black market use of the drug continues. It is particularly popular with students, athletes, entertainers, and truck drivers because it produces a sense of well-being and reduces fatigue. The amphetamine that has been called the drug of the 1990s is "ice," a pure form of methamphetamine. "Ice" is inhaled or used intravenously. Of greatest concern is the fact that "ice" is a synthetic drug that can be easily synthesized in illicit domestic laboratories (Kaplan and Sadock, 1994).

Since tolerance develops rapidly for amphetamines, some abusers may consume up to 1 g/day. Death may occur with doses of 120 mg in nonusers. Life-threatening, adverse effects include cardiac arrest, stroke, and neurologic involvement, including twitching, tetany, convulsions, coma, and death.

Amphetamines also have severe psychologic effects that include restlessness, dysphoria, insomnia, irritability, confusion, and panic. Intoxication of high doses of amphetamines may lead to induced paranoia and ideas of reference. Homicidal behavior also has been reported. Diagnosis of amphetamine intoxication is made on the basis of symptoms and history. Specific laboratory tests to detect amphetamines in the urine are the most reliable tests to diagnose "intoxication"; however, urine testing is ineffective if more than 48 hours have elapsed since the last dose. Withdrawal symptoms usually peak in 48 to 72 hours after the drug is discontinued; symptoms may last for several weeks. The most frequent and dangerous symptom is depression with suicidal ideation (Kaplan and Sadock, 1994).

Phencyclidine

Phencyclidine (PCP), known as "angel dust," is a powerful hallucinogen that has cholinergic, dopaminergic, and opioid properties. It is a dangerous drug that can cause death, if consumed in large doses, from status epilepticus, adrenergic crisis, and respiratory failure. The drug can be consumed orally, intravenously, snorted, or smoked. PCP intoxification is a true medical emergency and may require treatment in a medical unit (Slaby, 1997).

Nicotine

Nicotine dependence is classified under nicotine use disorder and nicotine withdrawal is classified under nicotine-induced disorder in the DSM-IV classification. More than one third of the world's population uses nicotine. The most frequent form of ingestion is through cigarette smoking. Although nicotine use in the United States has declined in recent years, it continues to be heavily used by certain groups and populations, including women, adolescents, African-Americans, the elderly, and psychiatric clients. Nicotine use has increased in other countries, especially Japan and some European countries. Individuals with other substance-abuse problems, especially alcohol abuse, are generally heavy smokers. Many, in fact, "chain-smoke" (i.e., they light their next cigarette from the one they are currently smoking).

Dependence on nicotine occurs in a relatively short period of time. The average smoker uses 20 to 30 cigarettes a day. Individuals who chain-smoke may use several packs a day. Withdrawal of nicotine causes marked withdrawal symptoms, including irritability, restlessness, difficulty concentrating, insomnia, and depression. Many individuals gain weight as a result of increased appetite. Without medical assistance 80% of smokers who quit will relapse within the first 2 years. In recent years nicotine gum, nicotine nasal sprays, and nicotine patches have been used to decrease withdrawal symptoms and craving. Medical supervision is advised when these methods are used to monitor the amount of nicotine that the client is receiving.

PROGNOSIS

Sobriety, abstinence from use of alcohol or drugs, together with a satisfactory quality of life, is the goal for complete recovery from substance abuse or dependence. Many clients relapse several times before achieving sobriety. The course of the disorders varies with the class of substance, route of administration, and other factors (APA, 1994). A diagnosis of substance abuse is more likely in persons who have begun using substances only recently. For many, substance abuse with particular substances can evolve into

substance dependence for the same substances, particularly for substances that have a high potential for development of tolerance, withdrawal, and patterns of compulsive use (APA, 1994).

The course of substance dependence is variable. The course is usually chronic, lasting years, with periods of heavy intake and partial or full remission. During the first 10 months after the onset of remission, one is particularly vulnerable to relapse.

DISCHARGE CRITERIA

Client will:

Maintain abstinence.

Admit to lifelong dependence on psychoactive substances.

Express knowledge of the continual process of recovery ("one day at a time").

Verbalize realistic goals.

Maintain attendance in a support group (Alcoholics Anonymous, Narcotics Anonymous).

Express increased self-esteem.

Verbalize decreased guilt, loneliness, shame, despair, and anger.

Demonstrate new coping mechanisms and strategies to manage anxiety, frustration, and anger.

List tangible substitutes to replace drug-seeking, drug-taking behaviors (hobbies, school, employment, volunteer work, social functions).

Express the feeling of being in control of own life.

Express hope for the future.

Attend a self-help group (client and family).

Abandon people and situations that influence and contribute to drug-taking behaviors.

State consequences of psychoactive substances on biopsychosocial/cultural/spiritual well-being.

State names and phone numbers of resources to contact when unable to cope or feel a need to revert to substance-taking behaviors.

Investigate substance abuse assistance programs such as the Employee Assistance Program (EAP).

Encourage family and/or significant others to attend Al-anon/Alateen support groups.

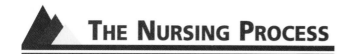

THE NURSING PROCESS

ASSESSMENT

In gathering information about drug use, the nurse uses a systematic approach by integrating questions into the general history regarding legal substances, including over-the-counter drugs, inhalants, and prescription drugs. Specific

questions are asked about the use of nicotine, caffeine, and alcohol, including first use, patterns of use, frequency, and quantity. In addition, information should be asked about other drug categories listed in Box 16-3.

A client's positive response regarding the use of any of

Box 16-3   Drug Categories Considered in an Assessment

Nicotine: cigarettes, chewing tobacco, pipe smoking, snuff, etc.

Alcohol: beer, wine, whiskey, gin, etc.

Cannabis: marijuana, "pot," "hashish"

Cocaine: "crack," etc.

Central nervous system depressants: barbiturates, benzodiazepines, methaqualone (quaaludes, "sopers")

Central nervous system stimulants: caffeine, amphetamines, diet pills, benzedrine inhalers

Opioids: heroin, codeine, methadone

Hallucinogens: lysergic acid diethylamide (LSD), mescaline, phencyclidine (PCP), mushrooms, peyote

Inhalants: glue, paint, aromatic hydrocarbons

Anabolic steroids

Synthetics: meperidine hydrochloride (Demerol), propoxyphene hydrochloride (Darvon)

Over-the-counter (OTC) drugs: antihistamines, cough syrups, sleeping pills, etc.

Designer drugs: methylenedioxylmethamphetamine (Ecstasy), fentanyl analogues ("China white," synthetic heroin), painkillers, mood elevators

---

these drugs should alert the interviewer to obtain further information about the specific drug, including the age of first use, the period of heaviest lifetime use, patterns of use, the presence or absence of binges, and any occurrence of blackouts. It is important to ascertain use during the immediate past to determine the possibility of withdrawal symptoms and/or toxicity. In many instances, such as when the client is a poor historian because of the effects of drug use/abuse, it is important to corroborate the history with a family member, significant others, and previous treatment facilities. If the client is taking methadone, it is essential for the nurse to ascertain when the last dose was administered. It is also important to ascertain whether the client has obtained methadone on the street before admission.

The other components of a complete health history include a psychosocial history, family history, risk for suicide or violence (toward self or others), and a mental status examination. See Understanding & Applying Research box for a discussion of recommendations for assessment of elderly clients with alcoholism.

Collaboration among the nurse, the client, the family, and the treatment team is essential in the development and revision of the plan of care. For the client who abuses substances, the road to abstinence and recovery requires realistic outcome criteria and a consistent plan of care.

PHYSICAL EXAMINATION

Physical assessment of the client may alert the nurse to the physical indicators of substance abuse. Particular attention is given to the areas of assessment listed in Table 16-1. During the assessment process the nurse observes for and questions the client regarding the incidence of accidents and injuries. Clients who have a history of trauma and repeat hospital admissions may abuse substances, ruling out other possible causes for accidents or injury incidents. The nurse should also assess the client for alterations or disturbances in cognition, sensory perception, emotion, or behavior.

SCREENING INSTRUMENTS

In addition to a complete history and physical examination, screening instruments are useful in identifying potential drug use. The instrument most frequently incorporated into the interview is the CAGE test (Box 16-4). A

Understanding & Applying Research

Nurses, more than any other professionals, have the ability to conduct assessments covering many facets, because of their educational backgrounds and the quantity and quality of time that they spend with the elderly. This study conducted functional assessments on older persons with alcoholism in a home setting to provide data that would assist nurses in better assessing and intervening with them.

Fifteen individuals participated in the study, all of whom were 55 years of age or older. All of the participants were surveyed in the home to assess their levels of functioning in five areas: physical, mental, social, economic, and self-care capacity.

The data from this study suggest that a comprehensive functional assessment of the older person with alcoholism is much more appropriate than a symptom-oriented approach. Symptoms of alcohol abuse, such as confusion, self-neglect, or repeated falls, can sometimes be attributed to the effects of aging, rather than suspected as signs of alcoholism. A functional assessment in the home setting allows the nurse to make an accurate evaluation of the older person with alcoholism and to develop an effective treatment plan.

The following interventions were suggested to be effective when working with an older person with alcoholism in a home setting:

Establish rapport to gain the individual's confidence.

Avoid use of terminology such as *alcoholic* or *alcoholism.*

Use whatever is important in the person's life as a possible motivating force for change.

Include significant others in the treatment plan.

Build on strengths; remember that you are working with survivors.

Nurses must successfully work with elderly clients with alcoholism by exploring personal attitudes toward aging and alcoholism and by developing an understanding of the aging process and alcoholism to differentiate alcohol-related changes from those related to normal aging.

Krach P: Discovering the secret: nursing assessment of elderly alcoholics in the home, *J Gerontol Nurs* 16(11):32, 1992.

Table 16-1	Significant Areas for Physical Assessment of the Client With Substance Abuse
Area of Assessment	**Observable Signs**
Temperature	Elevated
Pulse	Rapid; regular; irregular
Respirations	Rapid; shallow; depressed
Height	
Weight	Weight loss; malnourished appearance
Eyes	Conjunctivitis; red/bloodshot; pupils dilated or pinpoint; teariness; nystagmus
Nose	Congested; red; rhinorrhea
Skin	Cool; clammy; bruises; abrasions; sweating; petechiae (small hemorrhagic spots on the skin); telangiectasis (vascular lesions formed by dilation of a group of small blood vessels); erythematous palms; gooseflesh; needle marks
Oral cavity	Mucosa red, irritated; edematous, coated tongue
Abdomen	Epigastric tenderness; distended abdomen; vomiting; diarrhea; hepatomegaly (enlargement of the liver)
Speech	Slurred; incoherent; deviations in volume and sound
Cognition	Impaired; memory disturbance; thought blockage
Neuromuscular coordination	Motor incoordination; fine muscle tremor; unsteady, weaving, shuffling gait; clumsiness
Sensorium	Distortion in orientation, time, place, and person

positive response to two of the four items of the CAGE indicates a potential problem for alcoholism.

Other frequently used instruments are:

Short Michigan Alcohol Screening Test (SMAST) (Seltzer, 1975)
Alcohol Use Disorders Identification Test (AUDIT) (Babor et al, 1989)
Brief Trauma Scale (Skinner et al, 1984)

LABORATORY TESTS

In addition to the history and physical examination, part of the assessment process includes laboratory testing for drug use. Ethical issues continue to be a concern with drug testing, such as potential infringement of civil rights and the issue of obtaining the client's informed consent (see Chapter 5).

Box 16-4	CAGE Screening Test for Alcoholism

1. Have you ever felt you ought to Cut down on your drinking?
2. Have people Annoyed you by criticizing your drinking?
3. Have you ever felt Guilty about your drinking?
4. Have you ever had a drink first thing in the morning to steady your nerves or get rid of a hangover (Eye-opener)?

From Ewing JA: Detecting alcoholism: the CAGE questionnaire. *JAMA* 252:1905, 1984.

A comprehensive urine screen is an important part of early detection, treatment, and follow-up. A significant number of false-positive and false-negative findings are reported, so it is important to be familiar with the values reported by a specific laboratory.

The use of laboratory tests for diagnosing substance abuse continues to become more complex and sophisticated. A large number of variables may affect the results, including the uniqueness of the drug, the dosage taken, the frequency of use, the type of body fluid tested (urine, blood, stool), differences in drug metabolism, the half-life of the drug, the sample collection time and its relationship to the time of use, and the sensitivity of the test itself.

Several laboratory tests may be ordered while the diagnosis of alcohol or other drug use is being considered. The most commonly used laboratory tests are the blood alcohol level (BAL), the γ-glutamyl transferase (GGT), and the mean corpuscle value (MCV). In most states, the BAL is used to determine legal intoxication. The serum GGT levels rise in response to ingestion of alcohol. About 60% to 80% of individuals with chronic alcohol abuse will have an increased GGT, whether or not other signs of liver damage are present. The MCV is elevated in 35% of individuals who are heavy or chronic alcohol abusers. An additional test that may be performed is the aspartate aminotransferase (AST). An elevation of the AST level indicates liver damage in 35% of heavy alcohol users.

NURSING DIAGNOSIS

Nursing diagnoses are made from the information obtained during the assessment phase. The accuracy of diag-

Table 16-2	Alcohol Intoxication*
Blood Alcohol Levels	**Consequences**
20-50 mg/dl blood (0.02-0.05)	No legal consequences; some loss of sensory function; potential changes in behavior
80-100 mg alcohol/dl blood (0.08-0.1)	Legal intoxication in most states; impaired ability to drive; balance incoordination; staggered gait; slurred speech; impaired sensory function
100-150 mg alcohol/dl blood (0.1-0.15)	Marked balance incoordination; grossly distorted cognition and judgment
Levels above 200 mg/dl blood (0.2-0.3)	Marked impairment in all sensory and motor functions
Levels above 300 mg/dl blood (0.3 and above)	Potential cardiovascular and respiratory collapse; coma and death occur if immediate lifesaving measures are not initiated

Data from Fleming MF, Barry KL: *Addictive disorders*, St. Louis, 1992, Mosby; and Mendelson JH, Mello NK: Diagnostic criteria for alcoholism and alcohol abuse. In Mendelson JH, Mello NK, editors: *The diagnosis and treatment of alcoholism*, New York, 1985, McGraw-Hill.

*NOTE: As tolerance develops, these figures are no longer accurate. Levels may also be affected by the individual's gender, weight, and health status.

noses depends on a careful, in-depth assessment. Table 16-2 provides information on alcohol intoxication.

NURSING DIAGNOSES FOR SUBSTANCE-RELATED DISORDERS

Coping, ineffective individual
Denial, ineffective
Family processes, altered
Family processes, altered: alcoholism
Nutrition, altered
Thought processes, altered
Trauma, risk for
Violence, risk for

See also Collaborative Diagnoses box.

OUTCOME IDENTIFICATION

Outcome criteria are derived from nursing diagnoses and are the expected client responses to be achieved.
    Client will:

1. Maintain vital signs within normal range.
2. Verbalize a reduction in delusional thinking, absence of hallucinations, absence of suicidal or homicidal ideation.
3. Maintain normal fluid hydration.
4. Remain free of seizure activity.
5. Verbalize, "I feel safe in my environment."
6. Verbalize a desire to stop drinking/drug use.
7. State that there is a reduction in the symptoms of withdrawal (which may occur weeks after last use).
8. Participate in the therapeutic activities of the treatment plan (individual/group).

9. Ingest a well-balanced diet of sufficient calories to meet prescribed nutritional needs.
10. Express a need to contact family members/significant others regarding support.
11. Explore factors that may interfere with the treatment plan (e.g., lack of social or family support, lack of financial resources, seeking old "drinking buddies").
12. Develop realistic goals for rehabilitation (e.g., continue with the twelve-step program).
13. Verbalize that recovery is a lifelong process that occurs one day at a time.
14. Verbalize the ability to sleep without sedation.
15. Express the desire to establish relationships with nondrinking friends and avoid situations that previously invoked alcohol intake.

PLANNING

Because the client frequently has a long history of alcohol and other drug abuse, the nurse must develop a plan of care that meets the individual's ongoing needs. Client care is based on the data gathered during the assessment process and the immediate needs, as well as the long-range goals of treatment and aftercare (See the clinical pathway on p. 372-373).

Collaboration among the nurse, the client, the family, and the treatment team is essential in the development and revision of the plan of care. For the client who abuses substances, the road to abstinence and recovery requires realistic outcome criteria and a consistent plan of care.

IMPLEMENTATION

The nurse providing care for a client who abuses alcohol and other drugs will consider a plan of care that meets the

DRG#/DIAGNOSIS/DESCRIPTION: Alcohol Dependence-Requiring inpatient detox due to #1–(Alcohol withdrawal delirium ICD 291.0) #2–(Severe comorbid medical condition requiring hospitalization for safe withdrawal or treatment of comorbid condition DSM 303.90, ICD 303)

ALLOWABLE LENGTH OF STAY (LOS): _____

DAY OUTLIER:	☐ NO ☐ YES	DATE: _____
COST OUTLIER:	☐ NO ☐ YES	DATE: _____
PHYSICIAN: _____	ADMITTING: _____	SURGEON: _____

ADDRESSOGRAPH

* = OUTCOME

TIMING SEQUENCE	DAY 1	DAY 2	DAY 3	DAY 4 (DISCHARGE)
PREDICTED LOCATION	OPEN DETOX UNIT	OPEN DETOX UNIT	OPEN DETOX UNIT	OPEN DETOX UNIT
PROCEDURES (LABS, DIAGNOSTIC TESTS)	• Routine labs, EKG • Chest x-ray if indicated • Toxicology screens, alcohol blood level • Labs for comorbid conditions • Studies obtained if delirium with head injury (MRI) or GI bleed.	• Labs in chart • Neuro/GI tests complete if ordered • Additional labs/studies as indicated	• Anticonvulsant level if on med	
	☐ Yes ☐ No	☐ Yes ☐ No	☐ Yes ☐ No	☐ Yes ☐ No
PHYSIOLOGIC	• On I.V. • Seizure precautions • Nursing assessment, initial V.S. q 4 hours • P.E. by attending or consultant • I&O if indicated • Adjunctive medical tx. as needed (P.T., etc.)	• On I.V., seizure precautions • V.S. q 4 hours • I&O as needed • Adjunctive medical treatments as needed	• I.V. discontinued	• Specific medical treatments confirmed for aftercare (CPT, Resp. Therapy, etc.)
	☐ Yes ☐ No	☐ Yes ☐ No	☐ Yes ☐ No	☐ Yes ☐ No
PSYCHOSOCIAL	• S.W. assessment completed following contacts with significant others • Discharge options identified • S.W. and nursing assessment of supports	• S.W. assessment in chart • Specific discharge plan formulated • Socialization/safety assess q shift	• D/C living situation and medical aftercare confirmed with all parties • Discharge transportation confirmed	• Discharge to least restrictive environment (nursing home, residential program, home with day treatment, or visiting nurses)
	☐ Yes ☐ No	☐ Yes ☐ No	☐ Yes ☐ No	☐ Yes ☐ No
MEDICATIONS	• Liberal anxiolytic sedatives routine and prn's to titrate • Routine symptomatic prn's • Meds for comorbid conditions as needed • Anticonvulsants considered • Meds. parenteral or oral	• Sedative antidylics on qid schedule reflecting baseline requirement in 1st 24 hours	• Qid sedatives dropped 25% • Meds oral • Routine meds for comorbid conditions • Anticonvulsants stabilized if indicated	• Rx written for 1–2 days for close follow-up • Qid sedatives dropped to 50% of baseline • Specific aftercare plan formulated to complete detox in 2–10 days
	* ☐ Yes ☐ No	* ☐ Yes ☐ No	* ☐ Yes ☐ No	* ☐ Yes ☐ No

ACTIVITY	• Bed rest, OOB to bathroom only • Q 15 minute checks • Restraints if needed • Special precautions as needed (suicide, violence, escape, etc.) * ☐ Yes ☐ No	• Per M.D. orders and nursing assessment • Restraints discontinued * ☐ Yes ☐ No	• OOB but unit restricted • Continue 15 minute checks • Discontinue special precautions * ☐ Yes ☐ No	• Special needs for discharge finalized (exercise restrictions, appliances, etc.) * ☐ Yes ☐ No
NUTRITION	• Assess appetite and GI tolerance • Check weight • Clear fluids, bland diet as indicated * ☐ Yes ☐ No	• Dietary consult considered * ☐ Yes ☐ No	• Special dietary instructions as needed and tolerated * ☐ Yes ☐ No	• Routine aftercare diet achieved • Recheck weight • Patient sign-off on special instructions * ☐ Yes ☐ No
PATIENT/FAMILY EDUCATION	• Patient/family oriented to unit and MAP • Meds and patient rights reviewed • Aftercare plan devised with family • 12-Step/codependency materials introduced as needed. * ☐ Yes ☐ No	• Family session to address discharge contingencies, codependency factors (SW or nursing directed) * ☐ Yes ☐ No	• Family understands: 1) Aftercare plans and meds for patient 2) Supports and phone numbers • Family meeting to review finalized aftercare plans * ☐ Yes ☐ No	• Check off aftercare plans with patient and family * ☐ Yes ☐ No
M.D. CONSULTS	• Ordered as indicated by attending • Neuro consult begun if mentative changes with head injury • GI consult begun question GI bleed * ☐ Yes ☐ No	• Neuro/GI consults completed if ordered • Others ordered as appropriate * ☐ Yes ☐ No	• Plans/Appointments made for outpatient completion of incomplete consults * ☐ Yes ☐ No	• Follow-up appointments and consults confirmed with patient and family * ☐ Yes ☐ No
COMORBIDITY	• Medical conditions noted in M.D. admit note and nursing plans • Adjunctive medical therapies as needed (P.T., Resp therapy) * ☐ Yes ☐ No	• Other specialists follow patient every day as needed * ☐ Yes ☐ No	• Follow-up outpatient appointments scheduled with other specialists * ☐ Yes ☐ No	• Follow-up appointments confirmed with patient family * ☐ Yes ☐ No
THERAPIES	• After mentation clear, staff confirms that patient has had basic orientation to 12-Step approach, aftercare program, and patient has 12-Step literature * ☐ Yes ☐ No	• Attending sees qd for ongoing assessment and D/C planning * ☐ Yes ☐ No	* ☐ Yes ☐ No	• Attending reviews discharge plan in detail with patient * ☐ Yes ☐ No
LEGAL	• Involuntary process considered, if necessary • Patient rights orientation * ☐ Yes ☐ No	• Guardianship process initiated if legally justified and likely necessary for aftercare compliance * ☐ Yes ☐ No	* ☐ Yes ☐ No	• Discharge voluntary or per guardian or court • Discharge order in chart • Discharge diagnosis in chart * ☐ Yes ☐ No

Notes: 1) Routine alcohol withdrawal defined as outpatient procedure (e.g., residential setting, day program, home health program, nursing home). 2) Open unit assumed, with detox capability defined as appropriate access to acute nursing. May be on an open mental health unit. 3) Involuntary patient due to delirium may be treated in restraints initially, on open unit. Developed by and reprinted with permission of Dr. Marshall Lewis, M.D., La Mesa, California

CASE STUDY

Nancy Smith is a 28-year-old, married woman who, when out to dinner with her husband, had four margaritas and became intoxicated. When she left the restaurant, she experienced difficulty walking and fell. She became verbally abusive with her husband. As he attempted to put her into the car, she became combative. He transported her to the emergency department, where she told the admitting nurse, "I am going home. There's nothing wrong with me."

Critical Thinking—Assessment

1. What is Nancy's most immediate problem?
2. Is Nancy a danger to herself or others? Why or why not?
3. What symptoms displayed by Nancy are typical of an individual with a suspected diagnosis of alcoholism?
4. Given Nancy's behavior, how would you assess her for alcoholism?
5. What laboratory tests could be used to assess her involvement with alcohol?

COLLABORATIVE DIAGNOSES

DSM-IV Diagnoses*	NANDA Diagnoses†
Alcohol use disorders	Adjustment, impaired
Alcohol-induced disorders	Aspiration, risk for
Amphetamine use disorders	Body image disturbance
Amphetamine-induced disorders	Breathing pattern, ineffective
Caffeine use disorders	Cardiac output, decreased
Caffeine-induced disorders	Coping, ineffective family: disabling
Cannabis use disorders	Coping, ineffective individual
Cannabis-induced disorders	Decisional conflict (specify)
Cocaine use disorders	Denial, ineffective
Cocaine-induced disorders	Diarrhea
Hallucinogen use disorders	Family processes, altered
Hallucinogen-induced disorders	Fluid volume deficit
Inhalant use disorders	Gas exchange, impaired
Inhalant-induced disorders	Health maintenance, altered
Nicotine use disorders	Hypothermia
Nicotine-induced disorders	Infection, risk for
Opioid use disorders	Noncompliance (specify)
Opioid-induced disorders	Nutrition, altered: less than body requirements
Phencyclidine use disorders	Parenting, altered
Phencyclidine-induced disorders	Role performance, altered
Sedative, hypnotic, or anxiolytic use disorders	Self-esteem disturbance
Sedative, hypnotic, or anxiolytic-induced disorders	Self-mutilation, risk for
	Sexual dysfunction
	Sleep pattern disturbance
Other (or unknown) substance use disorders	Social interaction, impaired
	Thought processes, altered
Other (or unknown) substance-induced disorders	Trauma, risk for
	Violence, risk for: directed at others
	Violence, risk for: self-directed

*From American Psychiatric Association: *Diagnostic and statistical manual of mental disorders*, ed 4, Washington, DC, 1994, The Association.
†From North American Nursing Diagnosis Association: *NANDA nursing diagnoses: definitions and classifications, 1999-2000*, Philadelphia, 1999, The Association.

client's needs in relation to an identified stage in the recovery process. Recovery from a substance abuse problem is a long-term process often interrupted by periods of relapse. The nurse realistically recognizes this problem and develops a plan that meets the client's individual needs.

The plan includes helping the client with withdrawal symptoms/complications of substance use, providing nutritional support as needed, helping the client resolve anger/potential violence toward self or others, providing support to increase the client's self-worth, helping the client set realistic short-term/long-term goals, reintegrating the client with the family/significant others, providing resources for vocational rehabilitation, and monitoring the client's progress postdischarge.

NURSING INTERVENTIONS

1. Monitor the client's vital signs, while observing for signs and symptoms of substance overdose, withdrawal, and drug-to-drug interactions *to establish baseline information about the client's condition.*
2. Assess the physiologic and psychologic symptoms of withdrawal and the effects of medications prescribed during the withdrawal process *to provide safe, effective treatment during withdrawal.*
3. Initiate therapeutic interventions to treat withdrawal symptoms, including anxiety and other complications, *to help the client safely withdraw from the addictive substance.*
4. Provide psychologic support to the client/family/significant others *to include the family in the client's treatment process.*
5. Provide a safe, calm, nonthreatening environment for the client who is in withdrawal *because of possible illusions, delusions, or hallucinations experienced during*

withdrawal, the potential danger to self or others, and grand mal seizures.
6. Support the client in meeting nutritional/metabolic needs either orally or intravenously, depending on the client's ability to take and retain fluids, *to provide adequate hydration as needed.*
7. Refer to a nutritionist as needed, considering the client's personal, cultural, or spiritual preferences, *to offer holistic and interdisciplinary care.*
8. Increase carbohydrate intake as needed (e.g., hard candies and other such snacks) *to decrease some of the client's cravings for illicit substances and satisfy the client's oral needs.*

Mr. J. is a 36-year-old African-American veteran who has been homeless for the last 6 months. He has been admitted to the psychiatric acute care unit of the Veteran's Administration hospital with a diagnosis of polysubstance abuse that includes heavy use of alcohol and nicotine. He has no other illnesses, but he appears malnourished. He has been separated from his wife of 10 years for the last 8 months. He is the father of two boys, ages 4 and 6. Mrs. J. has returned to work as a computer technician at a local data-processing company.

Previous to his drug use, Mr. J. owned a small electrical shop. On admission he indicated a desire to get his life together so that he can be rehabilitated and reunited with his wife and children. The wife states that she loves her husband and will do whatever she can to assist with treatment and rehabilitation.

Since admission to the unit. Mr. J. has reported that he has not been able to sleep at night. He has been visited by his minister and his wife, who reports that the children "are eager to have Daddy well and home."

DSM-IV Diagnoses

Axis I	Alcohol dependence
	Nicotine dependence
	Cocaine dependence
Axis II	No diagnosis
Axis III	Medical diagnoses: malnourished; sleep disturbance
Axis IV	Severity of psychosocial stressors (Extreme = 5)
	Homeless; financial: loss of job; interpersonal: loss of family
Axis V	Global assessment of functioning: current GAF = 40 (current)
	GAF = 70 (past year)

Nursing Diagnosis: Coping, ineffective individual, related to personal vulnerability and inadequate coping methods, as evidenced by dependence on alcohol and nicotine, being separated from wife and family, and homelessness.

Client Outcomes	Nursing Interventions	Evaluation
• Mr. J. will verbalize that he is "powerless" over alcohol and other drugs.	• Support Mr. J.'s statement that he is powerless over alcohol *to begin breaking through denial. Additional support by the nurse can help him to replace his dependence on alcohol.*	• Mr. J. verbalizes that he is powerless over alcohol.
• Mr. J. will use effective coping skills that were previously successful and newly acquired skills to manage problems related to substance abuse.	• Assess Mr. J.'s usual coping style through interview/counseling techniques and help him explore strengths and weaknesses *because, to build new coping skills, previous effective coping methods must be explored.*	• Mr. J. is effectively integrating existing coping skills with newly acquired coping methods at the time of discharge.

Nursing Diagnosis: Self-esteem disturbance related to negative thoughts and feelings about self, as evidenced by failure of marriage, failure as a father and in business, and alcohol use/abuse.

Client Outcomes	Nursing Interventions	Evaluation
• Mr. J. will begin to verbalize positive comments about self to nursing staff.	• Reinforce Mr. J.'s statements of self-worth *to build self-esteem with continuing support from the nurse and others.*	• Mr. J. shares his feelings of self-worth with his wife and children at the time of discharge.
• Mr. J. will express hope for a drug-free future.	• Support Mr. J.'s expressed plan for the future *because clients need the opportunity to discuss future plans while in a therapeutic environment.*	• Mr. J. has a concrete plan for action, including a new job and continuation in a 12-step treatment plan.

Nursing Diagnosis: Family processes, altered, related to the effects of chronic use of alcohol and cocaine, as evidenced by separation from wife and children for 8 months.

Client Outcomes	Nursing Interventions	Evaluation
• Mr. J. will initiate contact with family through phone call and request for family visits.	• Provide Mr. J. with encouragement to initiate contact with wife and children *to provide a solid family support system to help reintegrate him back into the family and stop substance use/abuse.*	• Mr. J. returned home with his family at the time of discharge.
• Mr. J. will attend family counseling sessions with Mrs. J.	• Teach Mr. and Mrs. J about the benefits of family therapy *because both adult family members need support with resolution of disabling effects of substance-abuse problems.*	• Mr. and Mrs. J. are attending family therapy sessions at discharge.
• Mrs. J. will attend weekly Al-Anon meetings.	• Support Mrs. J. in her decision to attend Al-Anon meetings *to help her learn new ways to effectively deal with partner.*	• Mrs. J. is attending Al-Anon at the time of Mr. J.'s discharge.

Continued

NURSING CARE PLAN —cont'd

Nursing Diagnosis: Nutrition, altered: less than body requirements, related to lack of interest in food and/or substitution of alcohol or drug for nutrients, as evidenced by malnourishment and vitamin and mineral deficiencies.

Client Outcomes	Nursing Interventions	Evaluation
• Mr. J. will eat a minimum of 50% of provided nutrients at each meal.	• Provide preferred foods high in proteins, carbohydrates, and vitamins, especially the B vitamins, *so Mr. J will eat more of favored foods and become better nourished in accordance with metabolic needs.*	• Mr. J. ate 100% of well-balanced meals at the time of discharge.
• Mr. J. will select a diet including "desired" foods.	• Offer encouragement with dietary choices until Mr. J feels secure *to help him realize he is able to make appropriate choices for himself.*	• Mr. J. selected a balanced diet based on the food pyramid at the time of discharge.

Nursing Diagnosis: Sleep pattern disturbance related to the effects of psychologic stress, as evidenced by irritability, restlessness, depression, and the inability to fall asleep and stay asleep during the night without a sedative.

Client Outcomes	Nursing Interventions	Evaluation
• Mr. J. will sleep soundly through the entire night without sedation for 1 week.	• Provide information regarding supportive measures to induce sleep, such as the use of relaxation techniques, white noise, and a soothing back rub *to help him relax and use these techniques as a substitute for alcohol use.*	• Mr. J. was sleeping throughout the night without sedation at the time of discharge.

9. Initiate the necessary vitamin and mineral replacement therapeutic regimen (see Box 6-2). *Low levels of vitamin B can occur even in the absence of dietary deficiencies and malabsorption. Other vitamins affected are A, C, D, E, and K. Iron, magnesium, and zinc levels may also be affected by the ingestion of alcohol.*

10. Provide support to the client in working through denial. Establish a therapeutic, caring relationship when working with the client who denies that a substance abuse problem exists. A variety of techniques may be used with the client, including psychotherapeutic techniques, confrontation, and behavioral approaches as described in this chapter. Family therapy may also be indicated (see Chapter 22). *Providing support and empathy, yet not enabling the client, assists the client in working through the denial process and helps develop awareness that many of his or her life problems are related to substance-abuse* (see Chapter 22).

11. Intervene with secondary complications exhibited by the client as a result of substance abuse (Table 16-3; see also Table 16-1). *The prolonged use/abuse of alcohol or other drugs may cause a variety of complications or damage to all major body systems.*

12. Establish a caring, empathic relationship through individual and group interactions *to help the client improve self-esteem and deal with thoughts of guilt and remorse. Clients who abuse substances have a tendency to feel inadequate and unwanted.*

13. Encourage client's efforts to establish/reestablish/ strengthen family and significant other supports through a variety of measures such as role-playing; providing a quiet, congenial environment for the client to meet with family; and possibly remaining with the client and family during the first visit. Inform the family of the client's needs before their meeting. *Clients who abuse substances frequently have lost meaningful contact with their family/significant others.*

14. Teach the client, family, and significant others about substance abuse, symptoms, management, and treatment outcomes individually, as a group, or with written material. *Client, family, and significant others need opportunities to learn about substance abuse. Information about substance abuse, especially taught in a group, provides a common base for understanding and provides opportunities for client and family to interact with and learn from others.*

15. Support the client and family members in maintaining active involvement with 12-step support groups, such as AA, Al-Anon, Al-a-Teen, ACoA, NA, and CA. *Past experience in working with substance abuse clients indicates that lifelong membership in a 12-step program is essential, to remain drug free.*

16. Encourage the family to be flexible and patient regarding the client's participation in support groups. *Establishing a new lifestyle, such as engaging in a support group network, takes time, effort, and motivation.*

Table 16-3	Disorders Related to Excessive Alcohol Intake and Abuse of Other Substances
Problem	**Suspected Cause**
Hypoglycemia	Limited food intake, depletion of glycogen stores, inhibition of gluconeogenesis
Lactic acidosis	Excessive production of lactic acid by hepatocytes
Hyperuricemia	Reduced renal clearance of uric acid associated with lactic acid accumulation in the body and the need to eliminate it
Esophagitis	Direct toxic effect, vomiting
Gastritis	Direct toxic effect, increased secretin and histamine production
Duodenal ulceration	Increased secretin and histamine production
Malabsorption	Pancreatic insufficiency, mucosal damage associated with reduced transport activity and disaccharidase production, hyperperistalsis
Fatty liver	Triglyceride accumulation in hepatocytes
Hyperlipidemia	Increased lipoprotein production, increased lipoprotein clearance, mobilization of nonhepatic fat stores
Hyperketonemia	Excessive fat metabolism
Alcoholic hepatitis	Hepatocyte inflammation and necrosis related to alcohol and its metabolism
Cirrhosis	Scarification of liver tissue associated with long-term fatty infiltration or hepatitis
Pancreatitis	Alcohol-induced inflammation of the pancreas leading to increased secretin production
Anemias	Direct toxic effect, malabsorption of nutrients, malnutrition, decreased transferrin synthesis
Beriberi heart disease	Thiamine deficiency
Cardiomyopathy	Direct toxic effect, malnutrition
Skeletal myopathies	Direct toxic effect
Reduced bone density with increased fracture risk	Excessive excretion of calcium in the urine, poor diet, malabsorption of vitamin D, reduced liver hydroxylation of vitamin D
Impaired immune response	Malnutrition, direct toxic effect
Hemorrhagic displays	Impaired production of blood-clotting proteins
Wernicke-Korsakoff syndrome	Thiamine deficiency
Tuberculosis/pneumonia	Reduced resistance to infection, atelectasis
Cancer of the gastrointestinal system (neck, throat, stomach, pancreas)	Indirect toxic effects
Impotency	Neuropathy and CNS depressant
Peripheral neuritis	Malnutrition, especially vitamin deficiencies (B complex)
Malnutrition	Alcohol is high in calories and acts as appetite suppressant

From Beare PG, Myers JL: *Adult health nursing*, ed 2, St. Louis, 1998, Mosby.

17. Teach the client, family/significant others about substance abuse and the preventive aspects by providing factual information and suggestions for preventing the use of alcohol and other drugs. *The nurse should be available as an advocate and a resource regarding the dangers of substance abuse and the need for a healthy lifestyle.*

18. Support the client in establishing a social support system by putting him or her in touch with community organizations where the client may find alternative housing, make new friends, and build inner strength that will assist in the recovery process. *The client is faced with the enormous task of establishing new social support systems and cannot do it without support and guidance.*

ADDITIONAL TREATMENT MODALITIES

Collaborative interventions include the entire team involved with the client's treatment and rehabilitation. These interventions include, but are not limited to, medications for the treatment of withdrawal symptoms and vitamin and mineral deficiencies, conditioning therapy, psychotherapy, vocational rehabilitation counseling, and relapse prevention. Additional modalities used in the treatment of substance-related disorders include behavioral therapy and techniques, group therapy, and family therapy. The various other modalities and collaborative interventions are summarized in the Additional Treatment Modalities box.

Withdrawal/Detoxification

Sudden withdrawal of a drug in a physically dependent individual requires immediate medical intervention. If severe withdrawal symptoms occur, the client must undergo **detoxification.** Gradual weaning from the drug or the use of an alternative drug that blocks the occurrence or minimizes withdrawal symptoms is required. Early symptoms of withdrawal include tremors, diaphoresis, rapid pulse

---

ADDITIONAL TREATMENT MODALITIES
For the Client With a
Substance-Related Disorder

Withdrawal/Detoxification
Medical interventions
Vitamin therapy

Psychotherapy
Individual therapy
Group therapy
Family therapy

Behavior Therapy
Aversive conditioning with disulfiram (Antabuse)

Twelve-Step Support Groups
Alcoholics Anonymous (AA)
Narcotics Anonymous (NA)
Al-Anon
Al-a-Teen
Adult Children of Alcoholics (ACoA)

Halfway Houses

Day or Night Hospitalization

(120 to 140 beats/min), elevated blood pressure (150/90 or above), and insomnia. In addition, clients experience hyperalertness and a feeling of internal jitters. Auditory and visual hallucinations and grand mal seizures may occur when and if treatment strategies are unsuccessful. Adequate and rapid medical intervention in clients who are withdrawing from alcohol should eliminate more severe symptoms, including delirium tremens.

Most detoxification units have an established drug protocol managed and monitored by the nurse. A typical protocol provides for 25 to 50 mg of chlordiazepoxide every 2 to 4 hours. The client's vital signs are monitored every 15 minutes until vital signs are stable. Close monitoring of vital signs is indicated for 48 to 72 hours or longer. If the client does not respond to the medication, larger doses of the medication are indicated. It is not unusual to give 50 to 100 mg of chlordiazepoxide at 2- to 4-hour intervals. As much as 10 to 20 times the normal dose may be needed to prevent withdrawal symptoms. Higher doses of medication require close monitoring by the nurse and physician to guard against drug overdose. Adequate treatment and careful monitoring prevent grand mal seizures and possible cardiovascular collapse and death.

Clients experiencing severe withdrawal symptoms from alcohol usually require B vitamins, including thiamine (vitamin B_1), folic acid, and vitamin B_{12}, as a result of inadequate dietary intake and malabsorption. Thiamine replacement helps in preventing Wernicke's syndrome (Francis and Franklin, 1988).

It is necessary to monitor the client's fluid and electro-

lytes. Replacement therapy may be indicated as a result of vomiting, diarrhea, and diaphoresis. Caution should be taken not to overhydrate the client. Alcohol intake with elevated blood alcohol levels causes diureses. But as the blood alcohol level drops, fluid retention occurs and the individual becomes overhydrated. The sequence may result in congestive heart failure. Monitoring the client for signs of overhydration is essential. Other medications indicated include anticonvulsants to prevent seizures and magnesium sulfate to raise the seizure threshold. If indicated, potassium replacement is used to restore electrolyte balance and vitamin B replacement therapy.

Detoxification from other drugs requires similar precautions to those mentioned above. Individuals who are addicted to heroin and are receiving methadone therapy require careful monitoring of methadone levels in addition to vital signs. Overdose of methadone may lead to cardiovascular collapse and death.

Individuals who are heavy users of hallucinogens may present with toxic psychosis. It is important to ascertain the specific drug, because nursing care approaches differ. Individuals experiencing psychosis due to PCP are belligerent and strike out. They do not respond well to interpersonal approaches. Conversely, individuals experiencing a "bad trip" from LSD respond to verbal reassurance and reorientation (Vourakis and Bennett, 1979).

Psychotherapy

Psychotherapy with clients who abuse alcohol or other drugs may take many forms, including individual, group, and family therapy.

Individual therapy. Individual psychotherapy is indicated for clients with substance-related disorders who have a high level of anxiety, inadequate coping mechanisms, and low tolerance for frustration.

Communication during the initial contact with the therapist is crucial. The therapist must be empathic, supportive, and assume an active role in therapy. Clients with alcoholism are conditioned to experience rejection. Reticence in overtly addressing the problem of alcoholism and the client's psychologic defenses may be interpreted by the client as rejection. Removal of intellectual and emotional barriers between the client and the therapist should be an early goal.

Psychotherapy with clients who abuse alcohol has many attendant problems. Clients continue to test the therapeutic bond between client and therapist throughout the period of therapy. Therapists must be aware of several occurrences during the process of therapy, including the possibility of **relapse** (resumption of a pattern of substance abuse or dependence), the onset of depression, and the refusal to continue in therapy. Many clients with alcoholism become depressed when they give up alcohol and are forced to learn new ways of coping because previous coping patterns and defenses are no longer adequate.

Spouse and family understanding of the problem is essential. Involving the spouse in conjoint couples therapy and the family in family therapy can aid the psychotherapeutic process. Referral of the spouse and teens to 12-step support groups provides support for them and helps family members gain a better understanding of the disease process, the client's defense patterns, and the client's need for support.

Group therapy. Group therapy has certain advantages for clients with alcoholism that are difficult to achieve in individual therapy. In a group setting clients with similar experiences and problems can confront and support each other in a relatively safe environment (Figure 16-3). The therapist's role is to facilitate group members' participation and to assist in clarifying interpersonal interactions within the group. Clients in recovery who have maintained sobriety can share experiences and serve as role models for newly admitted clients.

Group discussions are best facilitated when ground rules and goals are established with clients early in the group therapy experience. Sobriety, regular attendance, willingness to share experiences and confront defenses, and confidentiality are common ground rules. Goals include sobriety; a desire to change and learn new ways of coping with problems; and a willingness to recognize and identify feelings and thoughts, such as guilt, depression, inadequacy, anxiety, and fear.

Family therapy. In recent years family therapy has gained credibility with clients with alcoholism. Family therapy is a treatment modality based on family systems theory. The genogram (Bowen, 1978) is a useful instrument to trace intergenerational use of substances. The recognition and acceptance of alcoholism as an illness that affects all members of the family indicates the need for family therapy. Often when the family member who abuses alcohol suddenly attains sobriety, the dynamics of the entire family change. It is a well-known fact that some clients relapse because the family does not know how to relate to the person when he or she is sober. For instance, the spouse of a client with alcoholism experiences difficulty giving up the power position in the family that was assumed while the client was abusing alcohol.

Family members in alcoholic families have a tendency to lack trust for one another, feel unloved and unwanted, and carry a heavy burden of guilt. Family myths and fam-

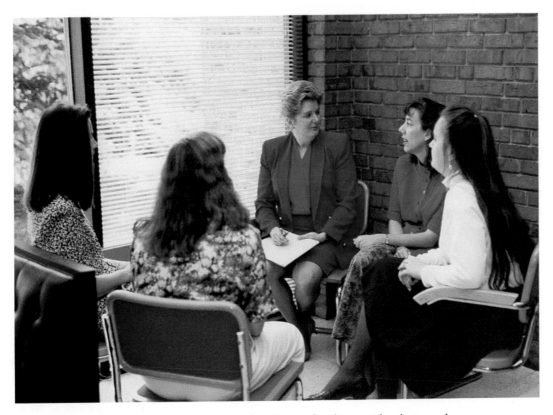

Figure 16-3 Group therapy can be effective for clients with substance abuse.

ily secrets are coveted. Family therapy provides opportunities to learn healthy ways of interacting with one another and of solving problems. Hope and trust can be instilled, and children can be relieved of the heavy burdens that they carry, not the least of which is the guilt they experience in relation to the belief that they are responsible for the parent's drinking problem.

Family therapy provides a structure in which the entire family can be educated about alcoholism as a disease. Children who are at high risk for developing problems with alcohol because of a genetic predisposition and environmental circumstances can be helped to understand the importance of refraining from alcohol use. Family members can be enlisted to support the client's attendance at AA meetings, even if attendance conflicts with planned family activities.

Behavioral Therapy

Aversive conditioning with disulfiram (Antabuse) is the most frequently used technique of behavior therapy. The client is conditioned by pairing the sight, smell, and taste of alcohol with an emetic. Induced nausea and vomiting act as aversions to alcohol. Following the conditioning experience, the client is given disulfiram (Antabuse). Disulfiram inhibits the enzyme aldehyde dehydrogenase; even a small amount of alcohol can cause a toxic reaction because of acetaldehyde accumulation in the blood.

Clients must be in good health, highly motivated, and cooperative. They are warned about the consequences of using the drug disulfiram if and when even small amounts of alcohol are ingested. Clients experience flushing and feelings of heat in the face, chest, and upper limbs. Other symptoms include pallor, hypotension, nausea, general malaise, dizziness, blurred vision, palpitations, air hunger, and numbness of the upper extremities. The most serious consequence is severe hypotension.

Most clients receive 250 mg of disulfiram daily. If larger doses are prescribed, toxic psychoses may occur, with memory impairment and confusion (Kaplan and Sadock, 1994). Clients taking disulfiram (Antabuse) should carry a card similar to that given to clients with diabetes. The card states that they are taking Antabuse and require medical treatment instead of incarceration if found in a debilitated state.

Other behavioral therapy techniques employed with clients with alcoholism include skills training to assist them in refusing drinks, assertiveness training, relaxation training, and **relapse prevention** therapy (a means of helping the chemically dependent individual maintain behavioral changes over a prolonged period of time). Most clients relapse a minimum of 3 to 4 times before they attain sobriety (complete abstinence from alcohol or other drugs of abuse in conjunction with a satisfactory quality of life).

Twelve-Step Support Groups

Alcoholics Anonymous (AA) is the original self-help group for recovering alcoholics. AA was founded in 1935 by two individuals with alcoholism: a stockbroker and a surgeon. It is built on the premise that support and encouragement from others with alcoholism can aid persons on the road to recovery. New members are assigned a sponsor (a recovering alcoholic who provides 24-hour assistance as needed). AA meetings are built on a 12-step program that allows individuals with alcoholism to restructure their

---

CLINICAL ALERT

All clients taking disulfiram (Antabuse) should carry a card similar to that carried by clients with diabetes, stating that they are taking Antabuse and should be taken to an emergency department if found in a debilitated state, which may include nausea, vomiting, headache, difficulty breathing, and a rapid or irregular heartbeat.

Box 16-5 The Twelve Steps of Alcoholics Anonymous

1. We admitted we were powerless over alcohol, that our lives had become unmanageable.
2. Came to believe that a Power greater than ourselves could restore us to sanity.
3. Made a decision to turn our will and our lives over to the care of God as we understood Him.
4. Made a searching and fearless moral inventory of ourselves.
5. Admitted to God, to ourselves, and to another human being the exact nature of our wrongs.
6. Were entirely ready to have God remove all these defects of character.
7. Humbly asked him to remove our shortcomings.
8. Made a list of all persons we had harmed, and became willing to make amends to them all.
9. Made direct amends to such people wherever possible, except when to do so would injure them or others.
10. Continued to take personal inventory, and when we were wrong promptly admitted it.
11. Sought through prayer and meditation to improve our conscious contact with God as we understood Him, praying only for knowledge of His will for us and the power to carry that out.
12. Having had a spiritual awakening as the result of these steps, we tried to carry this message to alcoholics and to practice these principles in all our affairs.

The Twelve Steps are reprinted with permission of Alcoholics Anonymous World Services, Inc. Permission to reprint this material does not mean that AA has reviewed or approved the contents of this publication. AA is a program of recovery from alcoholism *only*—use of the Twelve Steps in connection with programs and activities that are patterned after AA, but which address other problems, does not imply otherwise.

lives and make the necessary changes. The 12 steps of Alcoholics Anonymous are listed in Box 16-5.

A variety of AA groups are available in each community. Meetings may be open or closed. During open meetings, spouses, friends, and significant others are invited to attend; they are also open to observers such as nursing and other health professional students. Closed meetings are restricted to individuals in the recovery process. Some groups are identified for special populations such as women, nonsmokers, identified business interests, and specialized professional groups.

Narcotics Anonymous (NA) embraces a similar philosophy to AA. It is a support group for individuals addicted to narcotics, especially opiates. Since many substance abusers are polysubstance abusers, attendees may have problems with one or more substances.

Al-Anon and Al-a-Teen self-help groups operate independent of AA groups. They are formed to help family members of people with alcoholism cope with common problems.

Al-Anon is a support group for spouses and friends of individuals with alcoholism. Opportunities are provided to learn about alcohol as a disease and to share common problems and solutions with other spouses. Behaviors and issues common to the disease process are dealt with, such as avoidance, enabling, self-inflicted guilt, and shame.

Al-a-Teen is a nationwide support group for teens (children over 10 years of age) who have alcoholic parents. Similar to Al-Anon, the group helps remove self-guilt as the cause of the parent's drinking and restore feelings of self-worth. The group meetings are beneficial and therapeutic.

Adult Children of Alcoholics (ACoA) is a support group for adults who were reared in alcoholic homes. Children of alcoholic parents are frequently deprived of nurturing and loving parents. They enter adulthood with poor self-concepts and experience interpersonal difficulties. The support groups provide opportunities to discuss problems and feel acceptance from others who have had similar experiences.

Adult children of alcoholics may manifest **codependency,** which focuses on control, enabling, making excuses for others' behaviors (especially the behavior of alcoholic individuals), inability to trust self, and feelings of inadequacy and insecurity. Codependent individuals have a constant need to assume responsibility and take care of others' needs.

Many codependent behaviors (e.g., caring, nurturing, assisting and supporting others, and self-denial) are often associated with women and especially nurses. Individuals who were reared in alcoholic homes may experience a higher degree of codependency; however, recent findings indicate that individuals from nonalcoholic homes may have similar behaviors. The overresponsible behaviors, especially of codependent spouses, may be more easily explained on the basis of stress rather than on inadequate or disturbed personalities (Montgomery and Johnson, 1992).

Halfway Houses

Clients who are discharged from acute treatment settings often need additional time to begin the rehabilitation process. Halfway houses provide shelter as well as support, group therapy, and direct access to AA meetings. An opportunity is provided for gradual reentrance into the family and progressive reentry into the work world and society. Halfway house placement is highly recommended for clients who have been alienated from their families or have no place to live.

Day or Night Hospitalization

Partial hospitalization is recommended for clients who need additional therapeutic support from professionals. Some clients resume employment and spend the night in the hospital, whereas others spend the day at the treatment center and go home at night. As with the halfway house, partial hospitalization provides additional therapeutic support during early or difficult phases of rehabilitation.

EVALUATION

The purpose of evaluation is to ascertain changes that occur as a result of nursing and other interdisciplinary interventions. The nurse observes for changes in the client's behaviors and responses to treatment and interventions using the outcome criteria. It is important to recognize that resolution of the acute phase is merely the first step in treatment. Success for the recovery process and rehabilitation depends on many factors, including access to twelve-step support groups, continuing health care, support of family/significant others, vocational rehabilitation and community support (see Nursing Care in the Community box).

It is recognized that many clients relapse several times during the rehabilitation process. For this reason, it is difficult to predict the time when clients finally achieve acceptance of the fact that they are powerless over alcohol and/or drugs. As they attain sobriety, they develop a commitment to change their lifestyle, which often affects their relationships with family, significant others, and co-workers. Many clients develop a lifetime commitment to their twelve-step program.

Substance-Related Disorders

Nursing Care in the Community

The nurse working with chemically dependent clients in the community may experience judgmental reactions toward chronic relapse. Resumption of substance abuse is a common occurrence that causes frustration for both the client and the nurse, who may both feel hopeless in the face of this self-destructive behavior. Allowance must be made for impaired thought processes as a result of chronic alcohol or drug use. It is crucial to understand that in some cases relapse is a part of the process and that continual reinforcement of positive interactive and coping skills will ultimately make a difference in the client's behavior.

Resilience is perhaps the most essential quality the nurse can cultivate when treating this client population. Repeatedly offering help and support when nothing seems to be working requires tenacity and endurance. A knowledge of the predictable stages experienced by these clients throughout treatment can help the nurse in accepting clients while encouraging positive behavioral changes. It is important to evaluate the client's acceptance of dependence on alcohol/drugs and the detrimental impact this dependence has had on the quality of life. The client who is denying the existence of a problem is in need of a strong reality check rather than referrals to community programs.

The developmental level of the client must be considered in encouraging the client to admit dependence on an illicit substance. Teenagers, for example, will listen to a peer counselor more readily than to an adult. The client's prior level of functioning should also be assessed, since many clients present with dual diagnoses and may be impaired in their ability to function even when sober. Depression is a consistent comorbid finding in clients with substance-related disorders, and monitoring for suicidal thoughts is crucial for the psychiatric mental health nurse, especially with the client who would "rather be dead than drunk."

The nurse must continually recommend contact with Alcoholics Anonymous or other support groups, give encouragement and counseling to family members, enlist the help of other professionals such as social workers, and investigate the opportunity to enroll the client in some sort of community service group to increase a sense of involvement and self-worth. Interaction between the nurse and the client in the community setting is based on choice; thus the cultivation of the relationship is essential. This does not mean, however, that the nurse should ignore the client's problems. The relationship requires a rigorous and nonaccusatory honesty, suggesting that both parties aspire to high standards of behavior and responsibility.

At times the community nurse must venture into stressful situations. There may be blatant drug use, visible paraphernalia, and/or groups of people who are obviously "under the influence" of some substance, whether controlled or not. This may seem threatening to or at least be distinctly uncomfortable for the visiting nurse. The best way to handle this situation is through a professional, "matter-of-fact" attitude, including identifying oneself clearly to everyone and stating the purpose of the visit. This is the time to carefully monitor one's own emotional responses and leave the situation if it is perceived to be unsafe.

Summary of Key Concepts

1. Assessment for substance abuse should be a part of every client history and physical examination.
2. Alcohol is the number one drug of abuse in American society today at all age levels.
3. Nicotine use is a major health problem and, along with alcohol, serves as a "gateway" to illicit drug use.
4. Fetal alcohol syndrome is 100% preventable if the pregnant woman abstains from alcohol use throughout her pregnancy.
5. A positive family history of alcoholism is the number one risk factor for developing alcoholism.
6. The incidence of substance abuse varies with cultural groups. Native Americans have the highest incidence of alcohol abuse.
7. Dual diagnosis/comorbidity requires in-depth assessment followed by treatment of both the substance abuse and the psychiatric diagnosis.
8. Current DSM-IV diagnoses of abuse and dependency do not adequately describe substance use in the adolescent population. It is preferable to use terms such as "problematic" drinking or excessive substance use.
9. An individual who uses drugs indiscriminately is identified as a polydrug user.
10. Secondary complications of alcoholism may be causative factors for disease conditions in any of the major organs or body systems.
11. Commitment to long-term treatment and rehabilitation programs, including 12-step groups, is essential for recovery from substance abuse.

REFERENCES

Adams EH et al: *Overview of selected drug trends* (NIDA Publ No. RP0731), Rockville, Md, 1989, National Institute on Drug Abuse.

American Nurses Association: *Addictions and psychological dysfunction in nursing*, New York, 1984, The Association.

American Psychiatric Association: *Diagnostic and statistical manual of mental disorders*, ed 4, Washington, DC, 1994, The Association.

Babor TF et al: *AUDIT: the alcohol use disorders identification test: guidelines for use in primary care*, Geneva, 1989, World Health Organization.

Beare PG, Myers JL: *Adult health nursing*, ed 3, St. Louis, 1998, Mosby.

Bikle D: Effects of alcohol disease on bone, *Compr Ther* 14(2):16, 1980.

Bowen M: *Family therapy in clinical practice*, New York, 1978, Jason Aronson.

Cigarette smoking among adults, *MMWR* 41(20), 1990.

Cook P et al: *Alcohol, tobacco, and other drugs may harm the unborn*, Rockville, Md, 1990, U.S. Department of Health and Human Services, Office for Substance Abuse Prevention.

Cooper ML: Alcohol and increased behavioral risks for AIDS, *Alcohol Health Res World* 16:64, 1990.

Crespi TM, Sabatelli RM: Children of alcoholics and adolescence: individuation development and family systems, *Adolesence* 32:407, 1997.

Cuffel BJ: Prevalence estimates of substance abuse in schizophrenia and their correlates, *J Nerv Dis* 180(9):589, 1992.

Donahue RP et al: Alcohol and hemorrhagic stroke, *JAMA* 255:2311, 1986.

Drake RE et al: Diagnosis of alcohol use disorders in schizophrenia, *Schizophr Bull* 16(1):57, 1990.

Dupont RL, Saylor KE: Sedatives/hypnotics and benzodiazepines. In Francis RJ, Miller SI: *Clinical textbook of addictive disorders*, New York, 1991, Guilford Press.

Dulit RA et al: Substance use in borderline personality disorder, *Am J Psychiatry* 147(8):1002, 1990.

El-Mallakh P: Treatment models for clients with co-occurring addictive and mental disorders, *Arch Psychiatr Nurs* 12(2):71, 1998.

Ewing H: Care of women and children in the prenatal period. In Fleming MF, Barry KL, editors: *Addictive disorders*, St. Louis, 1992, Mosby.

Ewing JA: Detecting alcoholism: the CAGE questionnaire, *JAMA* 252:1905, 1984.

Fleming MF, Barry KL: *Addictive disorders*, St. Louis, 1992, Mosby.

Flynn S: Adolescent substance abuse. In Fleming MF, Barry KL, editors: *Addictive disorders*, St. Louis, 1992, Mosby.

Francis RI, Franklin IE: Alcohol and other psychoactive substance use disorders. In Talbott IA et al, editors: *Textbook of psychiatry*, Washington, DC, 1988, American Psychiatric Association.

Francis RJ, Miller SI: Addiction treatment: the widening scope. In Francis RJ, Miller SI, editors: *Clinical textbook of addictive disorders*, New York, 1991, Guilford Press.

Gafoor M, Rassool GH: The coexistence of psychiatric disorders and substance abuse: working with dual diagnosis patients, *J Adv Nurs* 27:497, 1998.

Galamos JT: Alcoholic liver disease: fatty liver, hepatitis and cirrhosis. In Berk JE, editor: *Gastroenterology*, Philadelphia, 1985, WB Saunders.

Goodwin DW et al: Alcohol problems in four adoptees raised apart from biological parents, *Arch Gen Psychiatry* 28:228, 1973.

Goodwin DW et al: Drinking problems in adopted and nonadopted sons of alcoholics, *Arch Gen Psychiatry* 31:164, 1974.

Grella CE, Anglin MD, Wagalter SE: Cocaine and crack use and HIV risk behaviors among high-risk methadone maintenance clients, *Drug Alcohol Depend* 37:15, 1995.

High school senior survey. Unpublished data, Institute for Health and Aging, University of California at San Francisco (1990). In Horgan et al: *Substance abuse: the nation's number one health problem*, Princeton, NJ, 1990, Institute for Health Policy, Brandeis University, The Robert Wood Johnson Foundation.

Horgan et al: Substance abuse: the nation's number one health problem, Princeton, NJ, 1990, Institute for Health Policy, Brandeis University, The Robert Wood Johnson Foundation.

Jellinek EM: *Phases in drinking history of alcoholics*, New Haven, Conn, 1946, Hillhouse Press.

Jellinek EM: *The disease concept of alcoholism*, New Haven, Conn, 1960, Hillhouse Press.

Jellinek EM: Phases of alcohol addiction, *Q J Stud Alcohol* 38:114, 1977.

Johnson L et al: *Details of annual survey*, Ann Arbor, 1988, University of Michigan News and Information Services.

Juergens MS: Benzodiazepines, other sedatives, hypnotics, and anxiolytic drugs, and addiction. In Miller NS, editor: *The principles and practice of addictions in psychiatry*, Philadelphia, 1997, WB Saunders.

Kaplan HI, Sadock BJ: *Synopsis of psychiatry: behavioral sciences, clinic psychiatry*, ed 7, Baltimore, Md, 1994, Williams & Wilkins.

Kelly SJ et al: Birth outcomes, health problems, and neglect with prenatal exposure to cocaine, *J Pediatr Nurs* 17:130, 1991.

Knott DH: The addictive process. Lecture presented June 1987 at the University of Utah Summer School on Alcoholism and Other Drug Dependencies, Salt Lake City. In Varcarolis EM, editor: *Foundations of psychiatric mental health nursing*, ed 2, Philadelphia, 1994, WB Saunders.

Kozel NJ, Adams EH: Epidemiology of drug abuse: an overview, *Science* 234:970, 1986.

Krach P: Discovering the secret: nursing assessment of elderly alcoholics in the home, *J Geronol Nurs* 16(11):32, 1992.

Landry MJ et al: Anxiety, depression and substance use disorder: diagnosis, treatment and prescribing practices, *J Psychoactive Drugs* 23(4):397, 1991.

Lehman A et al: Assessment and classification of patients with psychiatric and substance abuse syndromes, *Hosp Community Psychiatry* 40(10):1019, 1987.

Lieber CS, Leo MA: Alcohol and the liver. In Lieber CS, editor: *Medical disorders of alcoholism: pathogenesis and treatment*, Philadelphia, 1982, WB Saunders.

McDonald DI: *Drugs, drinking and adolescents*, St Louis, 1989, Mosby.

Mendelson JH, Mello NK: Diagnostic criteria for alcoholism and alcohol abuse. In Mendelson JH, Mello NK, editors: *The diagnosis and treatment of alcoholism*, New York, 1985, McGraw-Hill.

Miller P: Family structure, personality, drinking, smoking and illicit drug use: a study of UK teenagers, *Drug Alcohol Depend* 45:121, 1997.

Montgomery P, Johnson B: The stress of marriage to an alcoholic, *J Psychosoc Nurs* 30(10):12, 1992.

Mueser PR et al: Prevalence of substance abuse in schizophrenics: demographic and clinical correlates, *Schizophr Bull* 16(1):31, 1990.

Mynatt S: A model of contributing risk factors to chemical dependency in nurses, *J Psychosoc Nurs* 34:13, 1996.

National Institute on Drug Abuse: *National household survey on drug abuse: preliminary results from 1996 national survey on drug abuse*, Washington, DC, 1997, U.S. Department of Health and Human Services.

North American Nursing Diagnosis Association: *NANDA nursing diagnoses: definitions and classifications, 1999-2000*, Philadelphia, 1999, The Association.

Nurses: help your patients stop smoking, Washington, DC, 1992, U.S. Department of Health and Human Services.

Office of National Drug Control Policy: *National drug control strategy, part 1 (September 1989)*, Washington, DC, 1989, U.S. Government Printing Office.

Office of National Drug Control Policy: *National drug control strategy: reclaiming our community from drugs and violence (February 1994)*, Washington, DC, 1994, U.S. Government Printing Office.

Paul SM: Anxiety and depression: a common neurobiological substrate? *J Clin Psychiatry* 49:13, 1988.

Rice DP: Unpublished data, Institute for Health and Aging, University of California at San Francisco (1990). In Horgan C et al: *Substance abuse: the nation's number one health problem*, Princeton, NJ, 1990, Institute for Health Policy, Brandeis University, The Robert Wood Johnson Foundation.

Robins LN et al: Lifetime prevalence of specific psychiatric disorders in three sites, *Arch Gen Psychiatry* 41:949, 1984.

Ross HE et al: The prevalence of psychiatric disorders in patients with alcohol and other drug problems, *Arch Gen Psychiatry* 17(3):321, 1988.

Saitz R, O'Malley SS: Alcohol and other substance abuse: pharmacotherapeutics for alcohol abuse, *Med Clin North Am* 18(4):881, 1997.

Scharf MB et al: Therapeutic substitution: clinical differences among benzodiazepine compounds, *US Pharmacist* H1, December 1988.

Scheitlin K: Identifying and helping children of alcoholics, *Nurse Pract* 15(2):34, 1990.

Schuckit MA: Low level response to alcohol as a predictor of future alcoholism, *Am J Psychiatry* 15:184, 1994.

Schuckit M: Genetics and the risk of alcoholism, *JAMA* 254:2614, 1985.

Seltzer MS et al: A self administered Short Michigan Alcoholism Screening Test (SMAST), *J Stud Alcohol* 36(1):117, 1975.

Skinner HA et al: Identification of alcohol abuse using laboratory tests and a history of trauma, *Ann Intern Med* 101:847, 1984.

Slaby A: Treatment of addictive disorders in emergency populations. In Miller NS, editor: *The principles and practice of addictions in psychiatry*, Philadelphia, 1997, WB Saunders.

Stanton MD et al: *The family therapy of drug abuse and addiction*, New York, 1982, Guilford Press.

Stein M: Medical disorders in addicted patients. In Miller NS, editor: *The principles and practice of addictions in psychiatry*, Philadelphia, 1997, WB Saunders.

Stratton K, Howe C, Battaglia F, editors: *Fetal alcohol syndrome: diagnosis, epidemiology prevention, and treatment*, Washington, DC, 1996, National Academy Press.

Sullivan EJ: Comparison of chemically dependent and nondependent nurses on familial, personal and professional characteristics, *J Stud Alcohol* 48:563, 1987.

Sullivan EJ, Handley SM: Alcohol and drug abuse in nurses, *Annu Rev Nurs Res* 10:113, 1992.

Trinkoff A, Storr C: Substance use among nurses: difference between specialty, *Am J Public Health* 88(4):581, 1998.

Vourakis C, Bennett G: Angel dust: not heaven sent, *Am J Nurs* 79:649, 1979.

Zimberg S et al: Dual diagnosis in urban substance abuse and mental health clinics, *Psychiatr Serv* 48(8):1058, 1997.

Notes

CHAPTER 17

Delirium, Dementia, and Amnestic and Other Cognitive Disorders

Kathleen Pace-Murphy, Carmel Bitondo Dyer, and Mary S. Gleason

OBJECTIVES

- Discuss the various theories of the nature and development of Alzheimer's disease and rationale of the most currently accepted theories.

- Describe the pathophysiologic changes in the brain related to Alzheimer's disease.

- Classify the progressive symptoms of Alzheimer's disease into three stages (onset/mild, middle/moderate, terminal/severe).

- Compare the different types of dementia (reversible/irreversible).

- Describe and plan therapeutic activities for clients experiencing dementia.

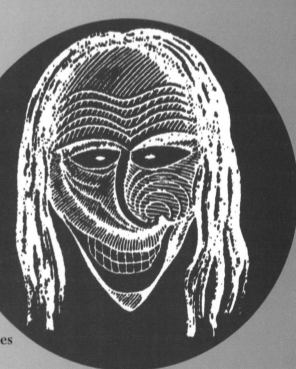

DELIRIUM, DEMENTIA, AND AMNESTIC AND OTHER COGNITIVE DISORDERS

Dementia is a global impairment of intellectual (cognitive) functions that is usually progressive and of sufficient severity to interfere with a person's normal social and occupational functioning. Many diseases and pathologic processes are categorized under this medical syndrome, of which Alzheimer's disease is the most prevalent. Dementia is often confused with the lay term *senility*, which refers to the deterioration of both cognitive abilities and body function with advancing age. This confusion has obscured the significance and incidence of dementia until the past decade.

Alzheimer's disease affects short-term memory first and then a whole range of intellectual abilities, such as speech, reading, writing, and comprehension. These clients grow confused and unaware of their surroundings and later become progressively incapable of caring for their basic activities of daily living (ADL) such as feeding, grooming, and toileting (Figure 17-1). Morbidity increases and death follows.

HISTORICAL AND THEORETIC PERSPECTIVES

Dementia in individuals over 65 years of age (late-onset type) has been well known since the time of Hippocrates, the father of medicine (460-375 BC), and Galen, the father of experimental physiology (130-200 AD). Early-onset dementia was first described by Griesinger in his

Agnosia The loss of comprehension of auditory, visual, or other sensations, although the senses are intact.

Agraphia The loss of the ability to write.

Alexia The loss of the ability to understand and interpret the written word.

Alzheimer's disease A neurodegenerative disease characterized by progressive, irreversible, and lethal structural damage to the brain due to the presence of β-amyloid proteins and leading to loss of cognitive functions and symptoms of progressive dementia.

Aphasia
Expressive The inability to speak or write (also known as Broca's aphasia).
Receptive The inability to comprehend what is being said or written (also known as Wernicke's aphasia).

Apraxia The loss of the ability to carry out purposeful, complex movements and to use objects properly.

Catastrophic reaction A sudden or gradual negative change in the behavior of clients with dementia, caused by their inability to understand and cope with stimuli in the environment.

Delirium A disturbance of consciousness and change in cognition that develops over a short period of time and tends to fluctuate during the course of the day, characterized by disorientation to time and place; reduced ability to focus, sustain, or shift attention; incoherent speech; continual aimless physical activity.

Dementia A global impairment of intellectual (cognitive) functions (e.g., thinking, remembering, reasoning) that usually is progressive and of sufficient severity to interfere with a person's normal social and occupational functioning.

Dysarthria Difficulty in articulating words; this is especially frustrating, because the client knows what words to use but has trouble forming them (more commonly found in vascular dementias and strokes).

Neologism Invention of words to which meanings are attached.

Neuritic plaques Maltese cross–appearing clumps composed of amyloid fibers found in the brains of persons with Alzheimer's disease.

Neurofibrillary tangle The accumulation of twisted filaments inside brain cells, which is one of the characteristic structural abnormalities found on autopsy that confirms the diagnosis of Alzheimer's disease.

Perseveration Repetitive motions or repetitive verbalization.

Sundowning A behavioral disorder associated with an increase in confusion and agitation that occurs in the evening hours.

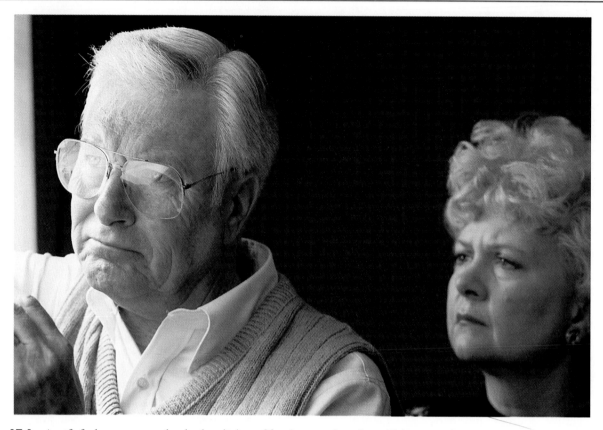

Figure 17-1   A wife feels sorrow over her husband's loss of faculties resulting from Alzheimer's disease. (Copyright Cathy Lander-Goldberg, Lander Photographics)

textbook on psychiatric pathology. He differentiated this condition from arterial disease and neurosyphilis, stressing gross brain atrophy, which was found at autopsy.

Alois Alzheimer (1864-1915), a German-trained neurologist, was inspired by the neurologist Franz Nissl (1860-1919) to study neuropathology. In 1895 Nissl moved to Germany to work with the psychiatrist Emil Kraepelin (1856-1926) on the structural basis of psychiatric disease. Kraepelin transferred his operations to Munich in 1903, taking Nissl and Alzheimer with him. At about the same time, a revolution in histologic techniques was taking place in both microscope technology and the advent of metallic stains for nervous tissue. In 1899 Ramón y Cajal demonstrated the usefulness of this new staining technique in studying the structure and form of nervous tissue. Nissl produced his stain for neuronal cell bodies in 1892, and in 1902 Max Bielschowsky, a German neuropathologist (1869-1940), produced the silver-based stain that allowed Alzheimer to demonstrate the now-familiar neuritic (senile) plaques and neurofibrillary tangles in the brain. In 1906 Alzheimer announced his findings of these lesions in the brain of a 51-year-old woman suffering from dementia and paranoia, and he published them in 1907.

In 1910 Kraepelin referred to cases similar to that of Dr. Alzheimer's as Alzheimer's disease or "presenile" dementia (now called early-onset dementia in the DSM-IV

classification), the frequency of which we now know to be much less than that of "senile" dementia (or late-onset dementia in the DSM-IV classification). The incorporation of Alzheimer's disease in Kraepelin's classic text categorized Alzheimer's disease as a psychiatric process rather than a neurologic one, and thus for many decades designated it as the responsibility of specialists in psychiatry.

Early descriptions of Alzheimer's lesions affecting individuals with Down syndrome over the age of 40 were described initially by Jervis in 1948 and tended to relate Alzheimer's disease to an accelerated aging process (which at that time Down syndrome was thought to be).

It was not until the publication in 1968 to 1970 of an important series of papers by the team of British clinical pathologists, Tomlinson, Blessed, and Roth, that Alzheimer's disease moved into its modern era. These authors compared the brains of individuals over age 65 without dementia to an age-matched group with dementia. Much to their surprise, they found that 62% of cases with dementia had the tangles and plaques described by Alzheimer. Using a neuropsychologic test, they showed that the severity of dementia correlated with the number of cerebral plaques. Only 22% of these cases had evidence of arteriosclerosis and brain softening, indicative of cerebrovascular disease.

The application of the electron microscope magnified

images up to 400,000 diameters, which further defined the lesions of Alzheimer's disease. The tangles revealed by the microscope were composed of parts of two twisted ribbon-like structures, known as paired helical filaments. The senile plaques and vascular lesions were made of bundles of twisted, nonbranching structures—the fibers of amyloid.

The major recent advance in the knowledge of the development of Alzheimer's disease is derived from the discovery of the chemical nature of the amyloid deposits making up the plaques and vascular lesions. Glenner and Wong (1984a, 1984b) defined these as being composed of a unique protein, the β-amyloid protein. This discovery has led to other studies and implications of the nature and treatment of Alzheimer's disease.

ETIOLOGY

Alzheimer's disease is the most common form of dementing illness. There are, however, many other types of dementia, and some are reversible. A simple way to approach the problem of memory loss is to think of two types of disorders: (1) those that are reversible and (2) those that are irreversible. Table 17-1 lists several types of irreversible dementias. Table 17-2 lists the reversible dementing illnesses. Approximately 10% of clients with dementia have reversible disease that can be improved, and in a small percentage of cases cured, with proper treatment (see DSM-IV Criteria box on p. 390).

THE IRREVERSIBLE DEMENTIAS

Alzheimer's disease has been called the disease of the century. It is an insidious, irreversible progressive disease that ultimately leads to death. Several theories are currently being investigated. Among these are the following:

Infectious agents
Neurotoxic agents
Angiopathy and blood-brain barrier incompetence
Neurotransmitter and receptor deficiencies
Abnormal proteins and their products
Genetic defects

Table 17-1	Etiologic Factors in Primary Dementia (Irreversible Dementia)
Diseases That Cause Primary Dementia	Incidence at Autopsy (%)
Alzheimer's disease (AD)	62.6
Vascular dementia (formerly called multiinfarct dementia [MID])	21.4
Mixed Alzheimer's disease and vascular dementia (MIX)	6.3
Parkinson's disease	5.7
Pick's disease	3.0
Creutzfeldt-Jakob (including Gerstmann-Sträussler-Sheinker) disease	0.5
Other cases: Diffuse Lewy body disease Progressive supranuclear palsy Binswanger's disease Down's syndrome	0.5

From Glenner GG: Alzheimer's disease. In *Encyclopedia of human biology* 1:103, 1994.

Infectious Agents

A fibrillar protein, or prion, is associated with the infectious process in Creutzfeldt-Jakob disease. The prion has the characteristics of amyloid fibrils and is found in the gray matter of the brain (the cortex). This finding suggested a relationship with Alzheimer's disease (Prusiner, 1984, 1991). However, the order in which the amino acids occur in the amyloid fibrils of Alzheimer's disease deposits was found to be distinctly different from that of the prion. This negated a chemical identity between these two types of dementia.

Neurotoxic Agents

McNiel (1995) reported that aluminum had been found in the brains of some patients with Alzheimer's disease. The research has not been able to confirm these study results. Because of research study findings inconsistencies, it

Table 17-2	Etiologic Factors in Secondary Dementia (Reversible Dementia)		
Toxic Causes	Other Electrolyte Disturbances	Infective Causes	Cerebral Disease
Barbiturate intoxication	Hepatic disease	Chronic respiratory infection with cardiac decompensation	Slow-growing cerebral tumor (e.g., frontal meningioma)
Alcoholism	Porphyria	Pulmonary tuberculosis	Multiple cerebral emboli
Polypharmacy	Nutritional	Bacterial endocarditis	Normal-pressure hydrocephalus*
Metabolic disorders	Undernutrition by prolonged neglect or self-isolation	Endocrine disease	
Potassium loss from self-purgation	Chronic malabsorption syndrome	Myxedema	
	Vitamin B_{12} deficiency	Pituitary insufficiency	
	Nicotinic acid encephalopathy	Addison's disease	

*Normal-pressure hydrocephalus is a disorder characterized by dementia, gait disorder, and urinary incontinence. Dilation of the ventricles in the absence of increased cerebrospinal fluid is a prominent manifestation. A shunt is usually effective treatment.

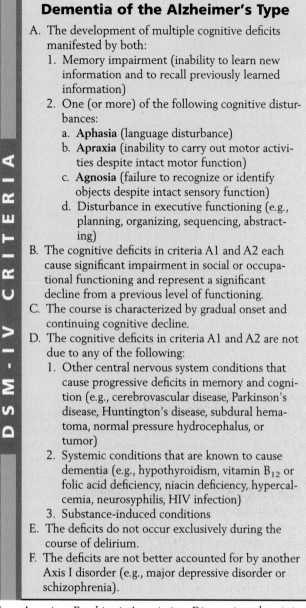

DSM-IV CRITERIA

Dementia of the Alzheimer's Type

A. The development of multiple cognitive deficits manifested by both:
  1. Memory impairment (inability to learn new information and to recall previously learned information)
  2. One (or more) of the following cognitive disturbances:
    a. **Aphasia** (language disturbance)
    b. **Apraxia** (inability to carry out motor activities despite intact motor function)
    c. **Agnosia** (failure to recognize or identify objects despite intact sensory function)
    d. Disturbance in executive functioning (e.g., planning, organizing, sequencing, abstracting)
B. The cognitive deficits in criteria A1 and A2 each cause significant impairment in social or occupational functioning and represent a significant decline from a previous level of functioning.
C. The course is characterized by gradual onset and continuing cognitive decline.
D. The cognitive deficits in criteria A1 and A2 are not due to any of the following:
  1. Other central nervous system conditions that cause progressive deficits in memory and cognition (e.g., cerebrovascular disease, Parkinson's disease, Huntington's disease, subdural hematoma, normal pressure hydrocephalus, or tumor)
  2. Systemic conditions that are known to cause dementia (e.g., hypothyroidism, vitamin B_{12} or folic acid deficiency, niacin deficiency, hypercalcemia, neurosyphilis, HIV infection)
  3. Substance-induced conditions
E. The deficits do not occur exclusively during the course of delirium.
F. The deficits are not better accounted for by another Axis I disorder (e.g., major depressive disorder or schizophrenia).

From American Psychiatric Association: *Diagnostic and statistical manual of mental disorders*, ed 4, Washington, DC, 1994, The Association.

is uncertain whether aluminum is a contributing factor in Alzheimer's disease.

The presence of zinc in the development of Alzheimer's disease is currently being studied. Low levels of zinc in the hippocampal area on autopsy has been found; however, other research has demonstrated toxic zinc levels. The role of zinc will need to be further defined.

Angiopathy and Blood-Brain Barrier Incompetence

Physical alterations of capillary walls have been noted in studies of the brains of persons with Alzheimer's disease. These changes include lumpy thickening and nodular ves-

sels and loss of the fine network of nerve fibers normally investing the blood-contacting surfaces. It has been suggested that these lesions, and the resulting devastation of nerves, destroy the barrier that prevents many blood serum components from entering the brain (the blood-brain barrier). The fact that amyloid deposition in the walls of blood vessels and in capillaries in the cerebral cortex almost always accompanies Alzheimer's disease was recently demonstrated. This has reaffirmed that these vascular lesions result in blood-brain barrier incompetence (Scheibel et al, 1987). Thus serum proteins leak into the gray matter (cortex) of the brain. Evidence that a serum protein, sphingolipid activator protein (SAP), can be identified and isolated from the amyloid core of neuritic plaques (Scheibel et al, 1987) strongly suggests that blood-brain barrier incompetence exists in Alzheimer's disease.

Neurotransmitter Deficiencies

Choline acetyl transferase is an enzyme responsible for the production of acetylcholine. Acetylcholine is a neurotransmitter whose role is to conduct impulses between neurons. Research findings have demonstrated diminished activity of choline acetyl transferase in the brains of patients with Alzheimer's disease. This decrease in available acetylcholine is directly associated with memory and cognitive impairment.

Abnormal Proteins and Their Products

Two proteins have been identified as playing a role in Alzheimer's disease. β-Amyloid and tau proteins interact within the hippocampal and cerebral cortex of the brain. It is believed that they act as part of a communication system that is responsible for memory, cognition, and behavior.

The discovery of the major protein that makes up the amyloid fibrillar deposits, the β-amyloid protein, in both Alzheimer's disease and Down syndrome, has initiated biochemical and molecular biologic studies. This protein was first isolated and purified, and its amino acid sequence determined, from amyloid-laden cerebral vessels of clients with Alzheimer's disease and Down syndrome (Wong et al, 1985). Based on its presence as amyloid fibrils in 100% of individuals with Down syndrome, it was suggested that the β-amyloid protein was a chemical marker for Down syndrome and that the gene encoding for its precursor would be found on chromosome 21, the abnormally tripled chromosome found in Down syndrome (Glenner and Wong, 1984a, 1984b).

Current knowledge suggests that there are complex genetic sequences of events leading to cerebrovascular amyloidosis, plaques, and tangles.

The identification of abnormal enzyme(s) responsible for amyloid formation in the brain could result in the development of specific inhibitors and thus a treatment for Alzheimer's disease. Such findings could also lead to a true diagnostic test for Alzheimer's disease that could be applied without requiring autopsy or brain biopsy.

Genetic Defects

Defects on chromosomes 14 and 21 have been shown to be associated with a small percentage of cases of familial Alzheimer's disease. However, chromosome 19, which codes for apolipoprotein E (apo E), may be associated with late-onset Alzheimer's disease. There are three alleles of APOE: E_2, E_3, and E_4. The E_4 allele is the one that imparts the increased risk. A single E_4 allele carries a 47% risk, and two E_4 alleles carry a 91% risk for Alzheimer's disease. Since only 40% of those with late-onset Alzheimer's disease carry one or more apo E_4 alleles, this test is being used by researchers and is *not* yet recommended for clinical use.

NATURE OF ALZHEIMER'S DISEASE

Alzheimer's disease is a neurodegenerative disorder in which, predominantly, the cortex of the brain containing nerve cells involved in memory and cognition is destroyed. The loss of gray matter causes a separation of the brain from the skull, widening of crevices that produce its convoluted appearance (sulci), and dilation of the cisterns that collect waste fluid and substances from the brain (ventricles).

The degradation of the gray matter is caused by the accumulation of destructive lesions, which are the hallmarks of the disease. These are the senile **neuritic plaques,** which are composed of amyloid fibers, and **neurofibrillary tangles,** which are composed of paired helical filaments that destroy nerve cells and amyloid deposits in the walls of cerebral blood vessels. Although the exact process of gray matter destruction by these lesions is not completely known, certain assumptions can be made. In Alzheimer's disease an abnormal βPP circulates in the blood and forms amyloid fibrils in blood vessel walls. The amyloid fibrils disrupt the vessel, causing it to leak. This abnormal βPP then enters the brain tissue, where it blocks receptors that are necessary for the proper metabolism of nerve cells. This leads to an interference in nerve function and the formation of tangles that destroy the nerve cells. The precursor also seeps into brain areas, where digestive enzymes cleave it to release the β-protein that accumulates to form senile plaques. Where they contact nerve fibers, these plaques envelop the nerve fibers and cause their destruction.

OTHER DEMENTIAS

Vascular Dementia (Multiinfarct Dementia)

Vascular dementia, formerly called multiinfarct dementia, results from the occlusion or obstruction of small arteries or arterioles in the cortex of the brain by the increased number of cells of the vessel so that nutrients cannot enter the brain. Occasionally, rupture of these vessels may occur, producing hemorrhage into the brain substance or vessel blockage, causing "softening" (strokes) and open spaces (lacunae). Paralysis rarely occurs, since the damage tends to be

---

DSM-IV CRITERIA

Vascular Dementia

A. The development of multiple cognitive deficits manifested by both:
   1. Memory impairment (impaired ability to learn new information or to recall previously learned information)
   2. One (or more) of the following cognitive disturbances:
      a. Aphasia
      b. Apraxia
      c. Agnosia
      d. Disturbance in executive functioning
B. The cognitive deficits in criteria A1 and A2 each cause significant impairment of occupational functioning and represent a significant decline from a previous level of functioning.
C. Focal neurological signs and symptoms (e.g., exaggeration of deep tendon reflexes, extensor plantar response, pseudobulbar palsy, gait abnormalities, weakness of an extremity) or laboratory (MRI) evidence indicative of cerebrovascular disease (e.g., multiple infarctions involving cortex and underlying white matter) that is judged to be etiologically related to the disturbance.
D. The deficits do not occur exclusively during the course of delirium.

From American Psychiatric Association: *Diagnostic and statistical manual of mental disorders*, ed 4, Washington, DC, 1994, The Association.

---

limited to the gray matter. Computed tomography (CT), magnetic resonance imaging (MRI), or positron emission tomography (PET) scans often reveal otherwise undetectable strokes. The DSM-IV criteria for vascular dementia are listed in the DSM-IV criteria box above.

Parkinson's Dementia

Parkinson's dementia is associated with Parkinson's disease, which was first described in 1817 by Parkinson in his *Essay on the Shaking Palsy* as "involuntary tremulous motion, with lessened muscular power, in parts not in action and even when supported; with a propensity to bend the trunk forwards, and to pass from a walking to a running pace; the senses and intellects being uninjured." The muscular stiffness, the immobile face, and the mumbling speech were later emphasized clinically. These characteristic motor signs are still diagnostic criteria. Nerve cells in the substantia nigra (brain stem), where dopamine is produced, develop pigmented lesions within them that are a sign of the disease. These were first described by Lewy in 1913 and are called Lewy bodies. In about 30% of cases of Parkinson's disease the amyloid lesions of Alzheimer's disease can be seen, whereas, conversely, about 50% of clients with Alzheimer's disease demonstrate typical symptoms of Parkinson's disease.

Pick's Disease

Pick's disease, named after the Czechoslovakian physician Arnold Pick (1851-1924), is a degenerative process of nerve cells, usually localized to the frontal and temporal lobe of the brain. It is distinguished clinically by changes in personality early in the course of the disease, deterioration of social skills, emotional blunting, behavioral disinhibition, and prominent language abnormalities.

Creutzfeldt-Jakob Disease

Creutzfeldt-Jakob disease, first described by Jakob in 1921, is an infectious (but not contagious) process that can be transmitted by corneal grafts, infected electrodes, and injected crude growth hormone derived from human pituitaries. It is believed to be caused by an infectious agent, called a prion, and produces a spongy appearance to the brain (spongiform encephalopathy) with vacuolization of nerve cells (the creation of a clear space in cell protoplasm filled with fluid or air). Its course is more rapid than that of Alzheimer's disease. Creutzfeldt-Jakob disease begins with the insidious onset of confusion, depression, and altered sensation, progressing in weeks or months to dementia, ataxia, palsy, and sometimes cortical blindness. Even though Creutzfeldt-Jakob disease constitutes only 0.5% of primary dementia cases, it is advisable to remove a client with chronic dementia from any donor list, because there is a risk of transmitting the disease.

Gerstmann-Sträussler-Sheinker Disease

Gerstmann-Sträussler-Sheinker disease is, like Creutzfeld-Jakob disease, an infectious process, but it has a genetic component, a mutation in the prion protein, that results in a familial disease.

Diffuse Lewy Body Disease

Diffuse Lewy Body disease is a late-life primary degenerative dementia noted predominantly in men in which Lewy bodies, as seen in Parkinson's disease, are present in neurons in the gray matter. Early ataxic gait, psychiatric symptoms (hallucinations, delusions, and violent or aggressive behavior) are not uncommon. It is associated with Alzheimer's disease lesions, as well as those of Parkinson's disease.

Progressive Supranuclear Palsy

Progressive supranuclear palsy is a degenerative disease that particularly affects the nucleus of the neuron and presents clinically with dementia, progressive paralysis of downward (vertical) gaze, difficulty in articulation of joints (dysarthria), muscular rigidity (most marked in the neck), and ataxic gait. Males are affected more than twice as often as females.

Binswanger's Disease

Binswanger's disease affects small arteries and arterioles in the brain, producing moderate to severe narrowing defects such as those seen in multiinfarct dementia. Lesions appear in the white and gray matter. Dementia is a common but not constant symptom, with dizziness, ataxic gait, and hemiparesis occurring.

Down Syndrome Dementia

Down syndrome dementia is difficult to diagnose, despite the extensive Alzheimer's disease-type lesions seen in the cortex of the brain on autopsy. Only about 50% of individuals with Down syndrome over age 40 can be determined as having dementia, which is usually first manifested as memory loss. This is probably due to the difficulty in ascertaining dementia in the face of mental deficiency.

CEREBROVASCULAR ACCIDENTS

Cerebrovascular accidents (CVAs) are strokelike episodes that occur in approximately 20% of clients with Alzheimer's disease and are due to the effects of cerebrovascular amyloid deposits either blocking the vessel or causing it to rupture to produce a cerebral hemorrhage. This lesion occurs predominantly in the gray matter and therefore does not result in paralysis. However, if the vessel ruptures in the leptomeninges (i.e., on the brain surface), severe hemorrhage can result in paralysis and death.

THE REVERSIBLE DEMENTIAS

Reversible dementias are a group of processes that represent about 20% of dementia cases. The vast majority of these are treatable. For example, metabolic disease, vitamin B_{12} deficiency, mimics most of the Alzheimer's disease symptoms. When the client is treated by a physician with injections of vitamin B_{12} before irreversible damage occurs, the dementia symptoms can be eliminated and the well-being of the client readily restored. This is the case with certain superficial benign tumors (meningiomas), which, when completely removed by the surgeon, will eliminate the dementia symptoms. Etiologic factors in secondary dementia are discussed in Table 17-2.

Depression is a very common reversible dementia seen in the elderly. Elderly clients may not have the usual signs and symptoms of depression and may present with only memory loss. Depression is easily treated with the newer antidepressant medications available. Sometimes clients have both depression and dementia, which makes diagnosis more difficult.

DISORDERS OFTEN CONFUSED WITH DEMENTIA

It is easy to mistake disorders such as delirium or amnestic disorder with dementia, since clients may have some of the same symptoms. The treatment for each of these disorders varies widely, making recognition and diagnosis very important.

DELIRIUM

Delirium is a state of mental confusion and excitement characterized by disorientation for time and place, usually with illusions and hallucinations. The mind wanders, speech is incoherent, and the client is often in a state of continual, aimless physical activity.

Delirium is characterized by a clouding of consciousness with a reduced capacity to shift focus and sustain attention. The client may or may not be agitated or sleepy and may or may not display hallucinations. The duration of onset ranges from hours to days, and symptoms fluctuate over the course of a day (Rockwell, 1991). There may be periods of lucidity or a change in cognition such as memory deficit, language disturbance, or perceptual impairment. Clients may be agitated or withdrawn, tearful, and even sad. As such, they can appear depressed. Delirium always has an organic basis that needs to be carefully assessed.

Delirium is usually seen in clients with Alzheimer's disease when a severe infection or other medical condition is superimposed on the preexisting conditions. At least 22% of elderly clients become delirious at some point during hospitalization (Lyness, 1990). Delirium can also be the first or only indicator of illnesses ranging from pneumonia to myocardial infarction to drug toxicity. Failure to recognize delirium can lead to significant morbidity and mortality, both from the underlying illness and from inadvertently self-inflicted injuries. When delirium overlies dementia of the Alzheimer's type, differentiating becomes more difficult yet more vital to positive client outcomes. The DSM-IV criteria for delirium are listed in the DSM-IV criteria box on p. 394). A comparison of delirium, depression, and dementia is found in Table 17-3.

AMNESTIC DISORDERS

Amnestic disorders are characterized by a disturbance in memory that is due to either the direct physiologic effects of a general medical condition or the persisting effects of a substance use/abuse or toxin exposure. The main focus is memory disturbance and can be specified as transient

Table 17-3	Delirium, Depression, and Dementia Comparison		
	Delirium	**Depression**	**Dementia**
Onset	Rapid (hours to days)	Rapid (weeks to months)	Gradual (years)
Course	Wide fluctuations; may continue for weeks if cause not found	May be self-limited or may become chronic without treatment	Chronic; slow but continuous decline
Level of consciousness	Fluctuates from hyperalert to difficult to arouse	Normal	Normal
Orientation	Client is disoriented, confused	Client may seem disoriented	Client is disoriented, confused
Affect	Fluctuating	Sad, depressed, worried, guilty	Labile; apathy in later stages
Attention	Always impaired	Difficulty concentrating; client may check and recheck all actions	May be intact; client may focus on one thing for long periods
Sleep	Always disturbed	Disturbed; excess sleeping or insomnia, especially early-morning waking	Usually normal
Behavior	Agitated, restless	Client may be fatigued, apathetic; may occasionally be agitated	Client may be agitated or apathetic; may wander
Speech	Sparse or rapid; client may be incoherent	Flat, sparse, may have outbursts; understandable	Sparse or rapid; repetitive; client may be incoherent
Memory	Impaired, especially for recent events	Varies from day to day; slow recall; often short-term deficit	Impaired, especially for recent events
Cognition	Disordered reasoning	May seem impaired	Disordered reasoning and calculation
Thought content	Incoherent, confused, delusions, stereotyped	Negative, hypochondriac, thoughts of death, paranoid	Disorganized, rich content, delusional, paranoid
Perception	Misinterpretations, illusions, hallucinations	Distorted; client may have auditory hallucinations; negative interpretation of people and events	No change
Judgment	Poor	Poor	Poor; socially inappropriate behavior
Insight	May be present in lucid moments	May be impaired	Absent
Performance on mental status exams	Poor but variable; improves during lucid moments and with recovery	Memory impaired; calculation, drawing, following directions usually not impaired; frequent "I don't know" answers	Consistently poor; progressively worsens; client attempts to answer all questions

From Holt J: How to help confused patients, *Am J Nurs* 93:32-36, 1993.

Delirium

A. Disturbances of consciousness (i.e., reduced clarity of awareness of the environment) with reduced ability to focus, sustain, or shift attention.
B. Change in cognition (such as memory deficit, disorientation, language disturbance, perceptual disturbance) that is not better accounted for by a preexisting, established, or evolving dementia.
C. The disturbance develops over a short period (usually hours to days) and tends to fluctuate during the course of the day.
D. There is evidence from the history, physical examination, or laboratory findings that the disturbance is caused by the direct physiologic consequences of a general medical condition or intoxication or withdrawal from substance abuse.

From American Psychiatric Association: *Diagnostic and statistical manual of mental disorders*, ed 4, Washington, DC, 1994, The Association.

Amnestic Disorders

A. The development of memory impairment as manifested by impairment in the ability to learn new information or the inability to recall previously learned information.
B. The memory disturbance causes significant impairment in social or occupational functioning and represents a significant decline from a previous level of functioning.
C. The memory disturbance does not occur exclusively during the course of a delirium or a dementia.
D. There is evidence from the history, physical examination, or laboratory findings that the disturbance is the direct physiologic consequence of a general medical condition (including physical trauma).

From American Psychiatric Association: *Diagnostic and statistical manual of mental disorders*, ed 4, Washington, DC, 1994, The Association.

Box 17-1   **Dementia Mortality in the United States**

374 deaths per 100,000 men
302 deaths per 100,000 women
Death certificates underestimate mortality
35% of persons with dementia spend time in a long-term care facility during the last year of life

Data from *Neurology* 1998.

(duration of hours or days but less than one month) or chronic (duration of more than 1 month). The DSM-IV criteria for amnestic disorders are listed in the DSM-IV criteria box at left.

EPIDEMIOLOGY

The prevalence of dementing illness between ages 65 to 70 years of age is less than 5%. The prevalence increases with age. Fifty percent of all dementias are a result of Alzheimer's disease.

It is estimated that 4 million people in the United States have Alzheimer's disease, of which 120,000 die each year (Box 17-1). One out of three families with a member age 65 or older will include a person with Alzheimer's disease. More than 50% of nursing home clients have been diagnosed with probable or possible Alzheimer's disease. The age of the youngest autopsy-diagnosed case was 38, whereas the average age of clients with Alzheimer's disease is about 75. The percentage of cases under age 60 is only 0.1%. The remaining life span of a client with Alzheimer's disease is halved, with death ranging from 5 to 15 years after symptoms are first noted. A few cases of 20 to 30 years' duration are on record. Generally, the younger the client, the more rapidly the disease progresses and the more likely it is to be familial.

Death resulting from Alzheimer's disease can be caused by many factors, the most common being aspiration pneumonia, because the client's inability to swallow properly causes regurgitation of food into the lungs. Other causes may be thrombophlebitis and emboli, urinary tract infection, and infected decubitus ulcers.

CLINICAL DESCRIPTION
ALZHEIMER'S DISEASE

Alzheimer's disease is described as a "global" disease affecting all regions of the gray matter (cortex) of the brain. This is the outer surface in which the intellectual processes arise. However, two characteristics make diagnosis difficult in its earliest stage. Initially the hippocampus is attacked by neurofibrillary tangles, producing recent memory loss. This is usually followed by nonsymmetric, or uneven, deterioration of the temporoparietal regions, producing cognitive deficits in learning, attention, judgment, orientation, and/or speech and language use. To further complicate matters, occasionally other regions of the brain may be affected. Thus a panorama of symptoms results. The situation is compounded by the insidious onset of the disease, which to the untrained observer may be perceived as inattention, restlessness, mild forgetfulness, and depression.

Therefore a client with Alzheimer's disease does not present a uniform or coherent history, nor can the time of onset be clearly defined. This can present a serious problem in differential diagnosis. Frequently, family members who have not seen the person for a while fail to notice the subtle changes that have occurred. Rash judgments based on a short visit often lead to conflict between the family caregiver and relatives of the client, particularly when institutionalization comes into question. The loss of a job or a serious auto accident may, unfortunately, be the most convincing evidence of serious cognitive loss and usually motivates the family members to act on behalf of their loved one.

Frequently the first symptoms of dementia are noted following a surgical procedure in which general anesthesia is used. Since the reserve of neurons is markedly depleted by the Alzheimer's disease process, a transient loss of oxygen during anesthesia further depletes the number of functioning nerve cells, thus making the initial symptoms of Alzheimer's disease apparent for the first time.

Caregivers may seek medical care for a loved one when specific behavioral difficulties have been observed, such as the following:

- Trouble with shopping, which requires performing tasks sequentially, correlating lists, planning, remembering, and calculating money
- Problems in the areas of driving, involving accidents or episodes of getting lost
- Missing social engagements and appointments
- Difficulty with financial tasks, particularly balancing a checkbook, getting bills paid, or understanding financial statements
- Aimless pacing or wandering away from home
- Inability to recognize people they should know or misidentifying friends and family members
- Inability to do common household tasks (e.g., cooking and cleaning)

Although clients themselves may notice early signs of cognitive impairment, many will employ one or more of the defense mechanisms of denial, repression, projection, aggression, regression, or rationalization. Some will succeed in deceiving family, friends, and employers for a time. Distinguishing these behaviors from cognitive deficits further complicates the diagnostic process.

A careful history may reveal many or all of the following symptoms:

Altered thought processes (paranoia)
Confused or disoriented state
Impaired intellect and memory (especially short-term memory in the early stage)
Sensory/perceptual alterations (hallucinations)
Decreased sensorium
Loss of body functions
Self-care deficit
Fear, anxiety, depression
Panic/rage reactions (catastrophic reactions)
Self-concept disturbance/powerlessness
Compromised physical ability
Social isolation, apathy
Impaired verbal communication
Emotional lability
Sleep disturbances

STAGES OF ALZHEIMER'S DISEASE

Although up to 15 different stages in the progression of Alzheimer's disease have been proposed by various sources, it is both effective and practical to reduce these to three major categories. These three categories are detailed below and summarized in Table 17-4. Each stage brings with it additional physical and psychoemotive losses, as well as increasing dependency needs.

Stage 1: Onset or Mild

The most distinguishing characteristic of stage 1 is memory loss. Often memory impairment is so mild that the client, family, and caregivers attribute it to "normal aging." But as this insidious disease progresses, the client often recognizes that there is a problem. Recent memory regarding yesterday's events are lost, yet the client may

Table 17-4	**Stages of Alzheimer's Disease**	
Stage 1: **Onset or Mild**	**Stage 2:** **Middle or Moderate**	**Stage 3:** **Terminal or Severe**
Recent memory loss	Stage 1 symptoms increase	Stage 2 symptoms increase
Cognitive loss in:	Behavior problems increase, which may	Incontinence, total
Communicating	include the following:	Choking
Calculating	Catastrophic reactions	Emaciation
Recognition	Sundowning	Total care needed
Anxiety and confusion	Perseveration	Progressive gait disturbances leading to
Mild behavior problems such as the	Aimless pacing	nonambulatory status
inability to initiate and complete a	Wandering	
task	Confusion	
	Incontinence, mild	
	Hypertonia	

articulate in detail events from long ago. Inability to find words or using inappropriate words when unable to remember is common. **Neologisms** (invented words with attached meanings) are also common. It is during this time of self-awareness of loss that many patients suffer profound depression.

Stage 2: Middle or Moderate

Signs from stage 1 continue to increase. Memory and cognitive impairment impede ADL. Clients are often disoriented to time and place. Signs of aphasia are apparent. Clients have difficulty making decisions as a result of decreased concentration and lack of cognitive skills to make appropriate judgments. Clients may develop delusions that are fixed false beliefs that may be paranoid in nature.

As the disease progresses toward the terminal stages, both short- and long-term memory is affected. The client

displays agnosia, apraxia, and **perseveration.** It is not uncommon for clients to experience **sundowning** or **catastrophic reactions** during this time.

Stage 3: Terminal or Severe

The client becomes totally dependent on caregivers for all needs. The client needs assistance with all ADL. There is loss of communication with the client in a meaningful way. All decisions regarding medical and social needs must be made by the caregiver.

PROGNOSIS

There is no known medical treatment that can prevent, arrest, or modify the course of Alzheimer's disease, but methods to modify and lessen some of its symptoms exist. Also, several treatments show promise: vitamin E coupled with donepezil was demonstrated to arrest dementia

---

 Understanding & Applying Research

Behavioral problems are estimated to occur in at least half of community-dwelling elderly clients diagnosed with dementia. This study attempted to test effective nursing interventions between caregivers and clients in a home setting. Fifty-four community-dwelling clients diagnosed with cognitive impairment (probable Alzheimer's disease/multiinfarct dementia) and their primary caregivers made up the study group. The clients had moderate to severe dementia (Mini-Mental Status Examination [MMSE] mean score of 8.9 out of a possible 30).

There were two components to the intervention: an educational program intended to enhance caregiver knowledge and comprehension of dementia and related issues and a behavioral intervention program teaching caregivers techniques to calm clients, enhance functional behaviors, and increase the client's activities of daily living (ADL) independent activities.

The teaching was conducted in the home setting, with both one-to-one instruction and a videotape reinforcing the instruction. The behavioral modification program also was one to one, but included role modeling, as well as printed information. Common problems such as wandering were addressed, as were ADL.

The measurements used to assess change included the MMSE, instrumental activities of daily living (IADL), Dementia Behavior Disturbance Scale, Alzheimer's Disease Knowledge Test, and Caregiver (Relative) Stress Scale. Before beginning, the client and caregiver were randomized into one of four groups. Group 1 received both Alzheimer's and behavioral education; group 2 received Alzheimer's education only; group 3 received the behavioral education only; and, group 4 served as a control comparison group, receiving no educational intervention. Assessments were conducted at baseline and in 6 months.

Although this study did not achieve statistical significance because of its small sample size, important clinical information was attained. Caregiver scores for knowledge increased for

groups 1 and 2. The caregivers rated the following caring tasks and behavioral approaches as effective based on a 5-point Likert scale (5 indicating the highest level of effectiveness):
Bathing:
Be careful not to use physical force. Touching in a forceful way may result in agitation (4.22).
Use visual cues, such as hand motions, to show the patient what you want him or her to do (4.22).
Dressing:
Use touch cautiously. Forcing the patient to dress through use of physical touch may increase resistance and agitation (4.56).
Use praise in an adult tone of voice to let the client know he or she is doing well (4.56).
Toileting:
Be flexible. Do not use physical force to assist the patient to the bathroom. A personal, gentle touch while walking may be helpful (4.43).
If urine leakage occurs, do not scold the client. A negative or tense response may increase frustration (4.43).
Eating:
Keep mealtimes pleasant and relaxed. Do not rush the patient while eating (4.83).
Remove unsafe objects, such as sharp knives, from open areas or easily accessible drawers (4.60).
Repeated behaviors:
If the client needs to manipulate objects with his or her hands, find a useful activity using the same motion (e.g., folding clothes or newspapers). These activities allow the client a positive outlet for behavior (5.00).
This study suggests that education and behavioral intervention instructions may be helpful to caregivers in the community setting. This study will be replicated with a larger sample size and a few other minor methodology revisions.

Burgener SC et al: Effective caregiving approaches for patients with Alzheimer's disease, *Geriatr Nurs* 19(3):121, 1998.

symptoms in a trial with clients with Alzheimer's disease.

Positive interventions by the caregiver can result in behavioral modification and reduce anxiety, avoid incontinence, and eliminate sleep disturbances and depression (see Understanding & Applying Research box). A planned therapeutic activity program can increase the client's awareness, verbal and physical response, and level of function. Drug intervention may be necessary (specifics are addressed later).

DISCHARGE CRITERIA

The characteristics of Alzheimer's disease and other primary dementias do not fall into categories of final discharge. The client and the caregivers will be flowing from one level of need to another. Before adjustments in care are made, the following indications of success in specific areas should be considered.

Client is:

Absent from risk of self-harm or caregiver abuse.

Accomplishing ADL and instrumental activities of daily living (IADL) with minimal possible assistance.

Free from catastrophic reactions and is able to communicate needs and wants.

Is participating in a therapeutic activity program tailored to assessed needs.

Primary caregiver(s) has:

Integrated correct knowledge of Alzheimer's disease or the related disease into daily routines of caregiving.

Used positive behavior interactions at all times.

Instituted plans and developed resources for self-care.

Appropriate legal and financial plans for the client and self in place.

Appropriate backup systems in place in case of emergencies (e.g., sudden illness or death of the client or of the caregiver[s]).

CAREGIVERS

The family deserves special attention, because without support the burdens of caring for someone with Alzheimer's disease can be overwhelming. Placement in a long-term care facility is usually the final step in the family caregiver's commitment. Many years of concern precede this decision for out-of-home care. Emotional stresses as well as financial expenses become significant. Health care and in-home services, special equipment and foods, and loss of income for the client and the caregiver are only a few of the cost factors encountered. More than 50% of nursing home care cost is paid from the private funds of clients and their families. Family education and counseling can ease the demands of caring for a client with Alzheimer's disease.

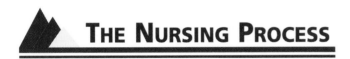

THE NURSING PROCESS

ASSESSMENT

Assessment of clients with dementia is difficult and must rely, to a great degree, on information from several sources. This is especially true of clients with Alzheimer's disease, since often the first symptom reported is recent memory loss, and even remote memory may be adversely affected by the concurrent symptoms of disorientation, depression, delusions, or hallucinations. A comprehensive assessment should include a thorough history, physical assessment, functional assessment, and mental status evaluation.

ASSESSMENT ENVIRONMENT

When interviewing the client or administering an assessment test, it is critical to have a positive physical and emotional environment. The room should be free from distractions, quiet, and away from the noise of any activity. Visual and auditory deficits may be present in the client, and the

evaluator must establish eye contact, speak directly to the client in a low-frequency range (since high tones are usually less discernible), and enunciate clearly. Hearing aids or glasses, if usually worn by the client, should be in clean, working condition. Any printed material that requires a client response should be presented in large, heavy type that is easily read. If English is a second language, someone who speaks the client's primary language should administer the test and/or translate for the client and interviewer to yield valid results. Paraphrasing questions is permissible to clarify an item. Sufficient time needs to be allotted, since the client may take longer to process the information and form a correct response. In general, the attitude of the evaluator must be friendly, nonthreatening, and nonjudgmental. Giving positive feedback to the client by saying, "You're doing fine," "That was good," or "This is a really hard one," can help relieve the stress of testing. Avoid indications that a response is correct or incorrect.

Delirium, Dementia, and Amnestic and Other Cognitive Disorders

As the elderly population increases, both in numbers and in longevity, more community attention should be focused on the support of families whose aging members are behaving in unusual and troubling ways as a result of cognitive disorders or other physical or emotional problems.

The mental health nurse may be asked to evaluate a person who resides at home but is no longer able to provide self-care and is resistant to help from caregivers. The nurse will need to assess the reports of caregivers, observe the behavior of the client, evaluate the client's medication regimen/compliance, and attempt an individual interaction, including a mental status examination. It is essential that this personal contact be deferential and exercised with patience.

The identified behaviors may simply be "acting out" demands in an attempt to meet a basic need that may be rectified by a brief intervention, such as providing a more comfortable environment in terms of temperature or level of stimulation. Pain is a critical factor that may be managed or controlled with medication. Apparent confusion may be a result of a hearing loss that can be treated with a hearing aide or with replacement of a malfunctioning one. The older person may have a urinary tract infection, which can lead to restlessness and agitation. Some prescribed or over-the-counter medications may have paradoxical effects of stimulation or disinhibition, rather than sedation, which might induce the untrained caregiver to increase the dosage, thereby compounding the problem. Taking multiple medications or a conventional dose that is too much for the person's age may also have adverse effects and lead to delirium. It is crucial that the agitated client be protected from falls or other accidental self-injury. Although one of the goals of community nursing is to empower clients to maintain themselves in the home as long as possible, if the nurse cannot discover a causative agent, the decision to hospitalize the client must be considered.

After delirium from physiologic problems has been ruled out, the two most common mental health disorders for elderly clients are dementia and depression. Both dementia and depression have a more gradual onset than delirium, and a thorough mental status examination can often assist the nurse in problem identification and treatment recommendations. Apathy is usually found in both depression and dementia, but the cognitive processes are intact in a depressed individual. The disorders may be combined as well; therefore treating for depression can stabilize a person, so that an underlying cognitive difficulty is more apparent.

Effective medications for the treatment of Alzheimer's dementia have recently become standards of treatment, although they gradually lose their effectiveness over time and only offer a window of improved function. These medications have few side effects and are quite beneficial for containing the early stages of the disease, although they do not appear to have much benefit for clients with later stages of dementia.

The caregiver's need for support should also be carefully appraised, with consideration given to establishing a pattern of respite care that would afford the family needed time for themselves. The community nurse should be aware of facilities in the area that provide day treatment or visiting assistants. If such services are not available in a given community, the nurse may suggest their initiation to city governments and nonprofit agencies.

A relatively recent development has been the proliferation of assisted living facilities. Unlike actual nursing homes, many of these homelike facilities are staffed by unlicensed persons with minimal medical training and experience. Services provided by a visiting mental health nurse can effectively improve the quality of care while providing onsite evaluations of the residents' mental status and response to or need for medication.

COGNITIVE ASSESSMENT TOOLS

A variety of tools can lend insight into a person's cognitive status. Administering a test in sections is permissible if the client has become too fatigued, has too short an attention span, or shows signs of anxiety. It is best to test the client alone, without an informant/caregiver, so that responses are entirely the client's own and not colored by hints or responses from someone else.

Interviews with the caregiver also should include the same courtesies as used with the client and should be conducted separately and in private. This will ensure honest responses and avoid the danger of talking about the client in front of him or her.

There are cognitive assessment tools that assess orientation, intellectual functioning, memory, and reading and math skills. Among the most common are:

Mini-Mental Status Examination (MMSE)
NIMH Dementia Mood Assessment Scale (DMAS)
Blessed Dementia Rating Scale (Blessed DRS)

Mini-Mental Status Examination

The MMSE, developed by Folstein, appears to be the most useful and popular tool. It can be administered in as short a time as 5 to 10 minutes and provides standardized methods of data collection, scoring, and interpretation in specific areas of cognitive impairment (see Figure 11-2).

NIMH Dementia Mood Assessment Scale

Increased precision is possible with the DMAS, but the test itself is quite lengthy. Data are collected through a clinical interview. Objective information from the family or professional caregiver is also obtained. Scoring is more complicated than with the MMSE; however, it can give a detailed baseline for future comparison and differential diagnosis.

Blessed Dementia Rating Scale

The Blessed DRS is short, practical, and easy to use and has been used as a standardized assessment scale. It begins to determine loss of function ability as it measures loss of ability to perform ADL. Scoring is easy yet informative.

NEUROLOGIC DEFICITS

The previously discussed pathologic changes in the brain (neuritic plaques, neurofibrillary tangles, and fibrillar deposits in cerebral vessels) result in neurologic deficits with ensuing behavioral changes. Determining the status of a client with Alzheimer's disease or another related dementia must involve assessment of neurologic deficits such as the following (Zgola, 1987). (The mnemonic *PALMER* may help you to remember these areas.)

Perception and Organization

How well does the client interpret:

Sensory cues?

Relationships between objects and between self and environment?

How well does the client organize:

Movement such as sitting, standing, and transferring?

Tasks such as dressing in proper sequence?

Solutions to simple puzzles?

Attention Span

How well does the client:

Initiate an activity?

Sustain an activity (shortened attention span or loss of interest)?

Terminate an activity when completed or in an established pattern (perseveration)?

Language

How well does the client:

Express thoughts verbally? (Inability—expressive **aphasia**)

Comprehend the spoken word? (Inability—receptive aphasia)

Read and comprehend the written word? (Inability—**alexia**)

Express thoughts in writing? (Inability—**agraphia**)

Memory

How well does the client remember:

Recent events immediately following their occurrence (immediate recall)?

Recent events within a matter of minutes (recent memory)?

Events from past events of months or years ago (remote or long-term memory)?

Emotional Control

Is the client's emotional control:

Consistent with and appropriate to the situation?

Sustained for an appropriate length of time?

Changed from previous behavior?

Reasoning and Judgment

How well has the client:

Made appropriate decisions based on good advice or facts?

Conformed to social conventions?

Reacted appropriately in an emergency situation?

EMOTIONAL STATUS

Mood and State of Mind

Each time a nurse approaches a client, an informal assessment of mood and state of mind is done. The Omnibus Budget Reconciliation Act (OBRA) of 1987 requires a more formal psychiatric assessment of a client before ad-

---

NURSING ASSESSMENT QUESTIONS

Delirium, Dementia, and Amnestic and Other Cognitive Disorders

The following questions may be helpful in attaining a thorough nursing history:

1. Has onset been rapid or insidious?
2. Has the progression of cognitive decline fluctuated (delirium) or been a continuous decline (dementia)?
3. What is the duration of the following symptoms?
   a. Difficulty learning and retaining new information
   b. Difficulty with multiple-step tasks (e.g., driving, cooking, financial management)
   c. Problem-solving difficulties
   d. Disorientation
   e. Word-finding problems
   f. Difficulty participating in conversation
   g. Changes in baseline behaviors (irritability, passivity, suspicious)

4. Does the client have a history of the following:
   a. Known psychiatric disorders (depression)
   b. Neurologic disorder (head injury, stroke, Parkinson's disease)
   c. Alcohol or drug use
   d. Endocrine disorder (diabetes mellitus, hypothyroidism)
   e. Renal disorders
   f. Infection (pneumonia, urinary tract infections)
5. Ask the client, family, or caregiver to tell you all of the medications the client is taking (prescribed, over-the-counter, and herbal preparations).
6. Inquire if there is a family history of dementia, Down syndrome, or any familial diseases that may lead to dementia (e.g., Huntington's chorea).

CASE STUDY

Henry has been brought to the emergency department by his wife, Ann, for treatment of a large skin tear on his right forearm, which is bleeding and wrapped in a large gauze roller bandage. While the wound is being treated, the nurse interviews Ann and notes that her appearance is disheveled, grooming is poor, and there are dark circles under her eyes. Henry is 68 and has been retired for 7 years, and Ann is 64 and still trying to work part time as a clerk to supplement their income. Ann relates that Henry has been "acting crazy," "never sits still," "has accidents in the bathroom," and has kept her up for the last three nights. She states that she is exhausted and says, "If I don't get some sleep, I'm going to hit him or something." Further questioning reveals that Henry lost his job as a clerk because of low production and errors in mathematics. Henry's affect is flat and he states, "I can't remember how I hurt myself." His hygiene and grooming are poor, which is evidenced by his untidy appearance, soiled clothing, and offensive body odor. Ann confirms that neither has seen a physician "in a long time," since Henry decided that physicians "are all useless."

Critical Thinking—Assessment

1. What are the primary immediate and long-term needs of Henry and Ann?
2. What approach should be used to gain their confidence?
3. Which assessment tools might be used to determine their psychosocial status?
4. What questions might elicit information about Ann's knowledge regarding Henry's behavior?
5. What approaches might be successful in getting this couple to seek future help?

CLINICAL ALERT

Signs of silent aspiration (choking):
  Watering eyes
  Reddening of the face
  Rhonchi on pulmonary auscultation
  Variable rates of respiration
  Grimacing
  Coughing
  Gagging
  Throat clearing
  Pocketing of food in oral cavity

ness and helplessness. Clients may also display changes in sleep patterns and appetite, as well as increased fatigue. The Geriatric Depression Scale can be used as an assessment tool in the mild stage of Alzheimer's disease, while language ability is present, and the client may communicate feelings of sadness, guilt, and suicidal ideation.

Functional Ability

Determination of a client's functional ability is essential as nursing diagnoses are formulated. Excess disability can occur when the caregiver responds verbally or physically with more assistance than is necessary and diminishes the client's speaking or activity skills. Maintaining independence in ADL and IADL is vital if clients with Alzheimer's disease are to retain their self-esteem and engage in worthwhile activities.

Behavior

Behaviors often found in clients with Alzheimer's disease and other cognitive disorders can be grouped in the following manner:
  Behaviors that are related to mood:

  Pacing, wandering, and rummaging (may indicate anxiety)
  Decreased or inappropriate socialization (may signify apathy)
  Refusal to eat, bathe, or groom (may mean depression)
  Hoarding or accusations of thievery (may manifest paranoia)

  Behaviors that result from perceptual/cognitive deficits:

  Day/night reversal
  Inappropriate eating (eating too rapidly or too much; eating nonfood items)
  Falls/accidents (walking into walls or furniture, not being aware of hazards)
  Delusions, hallucinations, paranoia

mission to a Skilled Nursing Facility (SNF) and before the administration of any psychotropic medications or physical restraints. Consistent use of the following two guidelines to assess clients' symptoms and behaviors will ensure a reliable data assessment tool: (1) significant quoted statements from the client should be noted to increase the objectivity and usefulness of the report and (2) regular documented mental status examinations (MSEs) further assist the professional staff in communicating information in a systematic way.

DEPRESSION

Secondary depression can be a concomitant condition with the client with dementia or Alzheimer's disease, and signs and symptoms should be thoroughly assessed and treatment plans developed (see Chapter 13 and Table 17-3). Foreman et al (1996) distinguished depression from delirium and dementia by the following signs and symptoms: (1) variable onset that is abrupt and reversible with treatment; (2) clear sensorium; (3) normal attention span, but client is easily distracted; (4) selective memory impairment; and (5) intact thinking, but client displays hopeless-

Behaviors that result from the destruction of impulse control:

Inappropriate toilet activities

Inappropriate sexual behavior (masturbating in public, display of penis or breasts, sexually explicit comments or language, inordinate sexual drive)

Inappropriate social behavior (undressing in public, being offensive, rude, or aggressive)

When any change in behavior from previous observations occurs, the client must be reassessed. The client often cannot communicate to others about distressing signs or symptoms of an illness. Determining how a client feels involves use of honed observation skills, especially in the area of assessing body language.

PHYSICAL MANIFESTATIONS

Alteration in nutritional status can be a multifactorial problem. Related reasons could include functional inability to purchase and prepare the food, lack of financial resources to buy food, medical conditions decreasing the elderly client's appetite, or cognitive dysfunction preventing the client from remembering to eat. *Weight changes* of 3 to 5 pounds or more should be noted, and an assessment made for treatable problems unrelated to the dementing illness. If no other clinical signs or symptoms are noted, the client's immediate environment must be examined next. The nurse should observe and correct distracting lighting, seating arrangements (groups should be homogenous and compatible), the noise level, and the physical comfort of table and chairs.

The family/caregiver should be instructed to keep a food diary and to monitor food intake, being alert for dehydration. Often, elderly persons significantly decrease oral intake to prevent incontinence. *Dehydration and malnutrition* lead to multiple medical diagnoses, including hypoalbuminuria, hypoproteinemia, anemia, hypoglycemia, and other vitamin and mineral deficits.

Aspiration is a risk during stage 3 of Alzheimer's disease, and the resulting aspiration pneumonia is frequently the immediate cause of death. The caregiver monitoring feeding should watch for a swallow after each bite, indicated by the larynx rising and returning to the resting position. If possible, clients should sit at a 90-degree angle and be encouraged to keep the chin toward the chest when swallowing, rather than hyperextending the chin. Thickened liquids are often easier to swallow. As clients become more dependent, they should be left in a sitting position for 30 minutes following the meal; the oral cavity should be checked for "pocketed" food, and any found should be removed. These nursing activities will prevent silent aspiration when the client is placed in a lying position.

Changes in gait are often noted, and again nurses must be alert to other disease processes such as vision problems; inner ear disturbances; pain from osteoarthritis or an in-

jury, which the client may not be able to identify; neuropathy resulting from vascular or diabetic problems; and general decrease of the "righting reflex" (the reflexes that enable any animal to maintain the body in a definite relationship to the head and thus maintain its body right side up). Treating underlying problems usually will result in better gait in the client in the early stages of Alzheimer's disease, but as the disease progresses, decrease in sensory interpretation, neurologic deficits, and hypertonia will require increased awareness and interventions by the caregiver to prevent falls.

Clients may complain of *feeling cold*, even on the warmest summer days. The level of activity and the amount of body fat present are among several factors that influence body comfort with regard to heat or cold. The best way to judge a client's response to environmental temperature is to actually feel the skin; if perspiration is present, the amount of clothing should be reduced. Conversely, if the skin feels cold to the touch, the client needs the additional layers of clothing, even though they might appear to be excessive.

Incontinence usually occurs in the later stages of Alzheimer's disease. Because of physical and cognitive changes, the client no longer has the ability to maintain bowel and bladder control. Functional incontinence is associated with cognitive impairment. The loss of urinary control is directly related to physical and cognitive functioning or barriers on the environment. Incontinence may also be a physical sign of a urinary tract infection or benign prostatic hypertrophy in elderly men. A thorough assessment of premorbid bladder and bowel function is essential, as well as continuous assessment of medications, fluid and food intake, and potential environmental constraints (side rails, poor lighting, wheelchair seat belts).

PHYSICAL AND LABORATORY EXAMINATION

Physical examination must be careful and thorough to rule out neoplasia (e.g., brain tumors), metabolic disorders, systemic illnesses (e.g., hypertension, HIV infection), and polypharmacy. Physical examination, mental status assessment and functional assessment are imperative to begin to develop a differential diagnoses list.

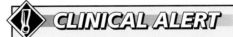

CLINICAL ALERT

Types of urinary incontinence:

Stress: Involuntary loss of small amounts of urine associated with coughing, sneezing, laughing, etc.

Urge: Loss of larger amounts of urine due to inability to delay voiding after feeling the sensation of a full bladder.

Overflow: Loss of small amounts of urine due to stresses on an overly full bladder.

Functional: Loss of large amounts of urine due to cognitive deficits that lead to not recognizing cues from the bladder, inability to find the bathroom, or increasing apraxia.

Diagnostic evaluation is conducted to rule out causes for cognitive changes. Blood studies include a complete blood count (CBC), erythrocyte sedimentation rate (ESR), serum blood chemistries (electrolytes and glucose), vitamin B_{12} and folate, liver function studies, thyroid studies, serology, HIV, and rapid plasma reagin (RPR)/micro hemagglutination for *Treponema pallidum* (MHAT-P) (to rule out neurosyphilis). Other diagnostic studies include a chest x-ray study, electrocardiogram, CT scan (brain), MRI, and urinalysis.

NURSING DIAGNOSIS

Nursing diagnoses are made from the information obtained during the assessment phase of the nursing process. The accuracy of diagnosis depends on a careful, in-depth assessment (see Collaborative Diagnoses box).

NURSING DIAGNOSES FOR DELIRIUM, DEMENTIA, AND AMNESTIC AND OTHER COGNITIVE DISORDERS

Safety and/or health risks:

> Aspiration, risk for
> Body temperature, altered, risk for
> Constipation
> Diarrhea
> Health maintenance, altered

COLLABORATIVE DIAGNOSES

DSM-IV Diagnoses*

Amnestic Disorders

Amnestic disorder due to a general medical condition (e.g., physical trauma or vitamin deficiency)
Amnestic disorder not otherwise specified
Substance-induced persisting amnestic disorder (not separately coded; includes medication side effects)

Delirium Disorders

Delirium due to a general medical condition (e.g., hepatic encephalopathy, electrolyte imbalance, etc.; general medical conditions may also be coded on Axis III)
Delirium not otherwise specified
Substance-induced delirium (not separately coded)
Delirium due to multiple etiologies (not separately coded)

Dementia

Dementia of the Alzheimer's type (early or late onset)
Vascular dementia (formerly called multiinfarct dementia [MID])
Dementia due to HIV disease
Dementia due to head trauma
Dementia due to Parkinson's disease
Dementia due to Huntington's disease
Dementia due to Creutzfeldt-Jakob disease
Dementia due to other general medical conditions (e.g., normal-pressure hydrocephalus, hypothyroidism, brain tumor, vitamin B_{12} deficiency)
Dementia not otherwise specified
Substance-induced persisting dementia (not separately coded)
Dementia due to multiple etiologies (not separately coded)

Other Cognitive Disorders

Cognitive disorders not otherwise specified (e.g., mild neurocognitive disorder or postconcussional disorder following head trauma)

NANDA Diagnoses†

Adjustment, impaired
Anxiety
Aspiration, risk for
Caregiver role strain
Communication, impaired verbal
Community coping, ineffective
Confusion, acute
Confusion, chronic
Constipation
Coping, ineffective family: compromised and/or disabling
Coping, ineffective individual
Denial, ineffective
Environmental interpretation syndrome, impaired
Family processes, altered
Fatigue
Grieving, anticipatory
Health maintenance, altered
Home maintenance management, impaired
Hopelessness
Injury, risk for
Knowledge deficit (pathology, neurology, therapy, medication)
Memory, impaired
Mobility, impaired physical
Nutrition, altered, less than body requirements
Powerlessness
Self-care deficit, bathing/hygiene, dressing, grooming, feeding, toileting
Self-esteem disturbance
Sensory/perceptual alterations
Sexual dysfunction
Sexuality patterns, altered
Sleep pattern disturbance
Social interaction, impaired
Social isolation (client and family)
Thought processes, altered
Violence, risk for: directed at others

*From American Psychiatric Association: *Diagnostic and statistical manual of mental disorders*, ed 4, Washington, DC, 1994, The Association.
†From North America Nursing Diagnosis Association: *NANDA nursing diagnoses: definitions and classifications, 1999-2000*, Philadelphia, 1999, The Association.

Home maintenance management, impaired
Injury, risk for
Nutrition, altered, less than body requirements
Mobility, impaired physical
Pain
Poisoning, risk for
Protection, altered
Self-care deficit, bathing/hygiene
Self-care deficit, dressing/grooming
Self-care deficit, feeding
Self-care deficit, toileting
Suffocation, risk for
Swallowing, impaired
Trauma, risk for
Urinary elimination, altered
Urinary retention
Violence, risk for: directed at others

Perceptual/cognitive disturbances:

Anxiety
Body image disturbance
Bowel incontinence
Confusion: acute
Confusion: chronic
Diversional activity deficit
Environmental interpretation syndrome, impaired
Hopelessness
Incontinence, stress
Incontinence, total
Incontinence, urge
Incontinence, urinary, functional
Incontinence, urinary, reflex
Memory, impaired
Powerlessness
Relocation stress syndrome
Sensory/perceptual alterations (visual, kinesthetic, gustatory, tactile, olfactory)
Sleep pattern disturbances
Thought processes, altered

Problems in communicating and relating to others:

Communication, impaired verbal
Decisional conflict
Fatigue
Self-esteem disturbance
Sexual dysfunction
Sexuality patterns, altered

Disruption in coping abilities (client and/or family):

Adjustment, impaired
Caregiver role strain
Caregiver role strain, risk for
Coping, ineffective individual

Coping, ineffective family: compromised
Coping, ineffective family: disabling
Denial, ineffective
Family processes, altered
Fear
Grieving, anticipatory
Management of therapeutic regimen, individuals: ineffective
Social isolation (client and family)

Client and family teaching needs:

Caregiver role strain

OUTCOME IDENTIFICATION

Outcome criteria are derived from nursing diagnoses and are the expected client responses to be achieved.
Client will:

1. Reach and maintain the highest functional level possible within capacity.
2. Maintain optimal physical status.
3. Participate in a therapeutic activity program for cognitive stimulation and socialization and to meet other psychosocial needs.
4. Participate in planning for care as able, especially making legal/financial decisions while capacity for decision making is still intact.

Caregiver will:

1. Maintain optimum personal physical and mental health status.
2. Initiate contacts with support services for legal and financial planning, support groups or individual counseling, case management, and respite services.
3. Increase knowledge base regarding the disease process, positive behavior interactions, and therapeutic activities.

PLANNING

A few common issues need to be specifically addressed to achieve appropriate planning for the client with a cognitive disorder:

SHORT-TERM AND LONG-TERM GOALS

Nurses in diverse roles will have contact with a client and family for varying lengths of time. Acute care nurses may have only hours or days to formulate and implement a treatment plan, so their opportunities to assess, diagnose, identify outcomes, plan, implement, and evaluate will therefore be focused on resolution of immediate problems (e.g., trauma crisis; preoperative or postoperative care; and stabilization of medical, health, and safety needs).

NURSING CARE PLAN

Gail, a 63-year-old woman, has been referred to a home health nurse by her primary physician for evaluation for home care. The diagnosis given is probable Alzheimer's disease with a secondary diagnosis of controlled hypertension. After an interview with Hal, Gail's husband, who is 64 and still working as a sales representative, the following is determined:

   Two-year history of recent memory loss

   History of being well groomed but now refuses to bathe and change clothes and dresses inappropriately, putting on clothes in the wrong sequence

   Appears to understand spoken language, if thoughts are stated slowly and simply

   Expressive language lacks correct grammar with evidence of word searching and parroting words used by the interviewer

   Gail's widowed sister, Ann, comes to stay with her during the day and stays overnight if the husband has to be out of town

   Recent episodes of crying, negativity, and angry verbal outbursts have caused the sister concern and fear

   Hal is staying away more often and leaving care to the sister, who is losing weight and dropping out of her personal social activities

DSM-IV Diagnoses

Axis I	Dementia of the Alzheimer's type with perceptual disturbances
	Dementia of the Alzheimer's type with behavioral disturbances
Axis II	Rule out dependent personality disorder
Axis III	Hypertension
Axis IV	Problems with access to health care services Other psychosocial problems
Axis V	GAF = 35 (current)
	GAF = 45 (past year)

Nursing Diagnosis: Self-care deficit related to perceptual and cognitive alterations secondary to neurologic damage in the brain as evidenced by inability to recognize the need for self-care (bathing, changing), inability to dress in the right order, and inability to reason and judge (inappropriate choice of clothing).

Client Outcomes	Nursing Interventions	Evaluation
• Gail will bathe three times a week.	• Determine habitual time and manner of bathing. *Establishing a pattern based on Gail's previous habits will use her retained remote memory.* • Ensure privacy *to preserve dignity and self-esteem.* • Determine room and water temperature. *Comfort and safety will encourage positive client response.* • Reduce sensory stimulation (e.g., noise from TV, radio, other people) to enable client to attend to the task at hand). Mirrors may need to be covered if the reflection is incorrectly interpreted by the client to be an observer. *Limiting the number of responses required by Gail will facilitate her cooperation and independence.* • Provide a home health aide (HHA) three times a week for 2 weeks. *Caregivers, Ann and Hal, will increase their knowledge and skills and thus enhance their confidence and ease in assisting Gail. The HHA will teach the caregivers ways in which to maintain skin integrity and general health. The supervising nurse will check on Gail's general health status and hypertension.*	• Gail was successfully bathed by the home health aide twice in the first week with the help of Ann. During the second week Ann was successful on two occasions with the HHA assisting. Extend HHA assistance for 1 more week and reevaluate.
• Gail will be well groomed.	• Determine areas of dysfunction in grooming. • Set adequate routines of visual and verbal cues to assist in grooming routines. • Assist directly only as necessary to complete task. • Employ positive reinforcement. • Refer for dental prophylaxis and assist the family in preplanning with the dentist and hygienist for a successful visit. • Assist Hal and Ann in formulating follow-up plan for daily oral hygiene. *These interventions will reduce stress for client and caregivers, avoid excess disability, provide a positive environment, and avoid unnecessary physical disabilities.*	• Ann and Hal were successful on 5 out of 7 successive days in cuing Gail to complete her dental hygiene and in helping with combing her hair. An appointment has been made with the dentist who previously cared for her, and Hal has informed the dentist of the present situation. Evaluate success of visit later.

Client Outcomes
- Gail will dress herself appropriately.

Nursing Interventions
- Assess clothing supply.
- Simplify dressing choices for Gail by the following:
  Remove clothes not currently being worn.
  Assemble coordinated outfits on one hanger and limit these to six to eight choices.
  Stack clothes in the order in which they are to be put on.
- Assess clothes and assist family in choosing those that are appropriate yet easy for Gail to put on (e.g., eliminate buttons, buckles, pantyhose, etc., and replace with elastic waists, snaps, velcro fasteners, knee- or thigh-high hose). *The client will retain control and independence by making some simple decisions and will be socially acceptable, thus increasing self-esteem and reducing stress for all.*

Evaluation
- Family/nurse/HHA see the improvement in Gail's appearance, and Gail is responding with smiles at the compliments about her appearance. Hal is having some adjustment problems in changing her dress style (not putting on hose and heels as she had) and in moving some of his favorite outfits out of the closet. Ann comments favorably on the ease of dressing Gail now and on Gail's increased comfort, evidenced by her willingness to participate in activities and calmer interactions.

Nursing Diagnosis: Thought processes, altered, related to inability to process and synthesize information as evidenced by recent memory loss; decreased ability to analyze, reason, and form judgments; and interruption in logical stream of thought.

Client Outcomes
- Gail will use her intellect and judgment to the best of her ability.

Nursing Interventions
- Develop a stimulating therapeutic activities program. *Cognitive stimulation in deficit areas and positive reinforcement will promote self-esteem and encourage Gail to attain the highest functional level possible.*

Evaluation
- Hal and Ann have found that Gail enjoys walks, and they have established routines. Gail has recognized some previously familiar birds and indicated she wanted bird seed to feed them. She also enjoys simple puzzles and assisting Ann in laundry tasks.

Client Outcomes
- Gail will retain some control in her life by exercising her right to choose.

- Gail will be oriented to place, time of day, scheduled activities, and family members.

Nursing Interventions
- Assess environment and activities and collaborate with all caregivers to:
  Simplify choices in food, clothes, colors, and activities.
  Use multiple sensory cues, especially auditory, visual, and tactile senses, to indicate choices. *Choices, even simple ones, give control back to Gail and improve her self-esteem, making her more willing to try to participate in daily activities.*
- Develop simple calendars with daily routines and easy-to-read clocks.
- Encourage family members to repeat their names and relationships often in conversations. *These actions will assist in overcoming recent memory loss. Establishing routine decreases the stress of making decisions; verbal cues reinforce recognition and eliminate the need to chat.*

Evaluation
- Gail is responding to the use of multiple cues by increasingly exercising her right to choose. (During the first week Gail made an independent choice five times. During the second week she made seven choices.)
- After 2 weeks, Gail knows the time for her walks with Hal and indicates that she wants her supply of bird seed. She is less frequently confused regarding the identification of persons and never fails to recognize Hal and Ann.

Continued

NURSING CARE PLAN —cont'd

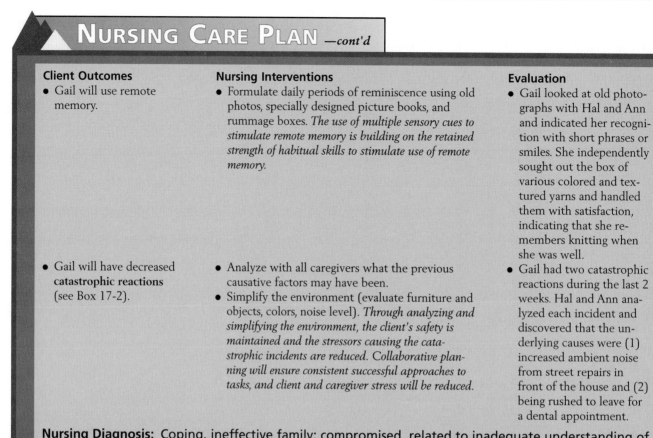

Client Outcomes	Nursing Interventions	Evaluation
• Gail will use remote memory.	• Formulate daily periods of reminiscence using old photos, specially designed picture books, and rummage boxes. *The use of multiple sensory cues to stimulate remote memory is building on the retained strength of habitual skills to stimulate use of remote memory.*	• Gail looked at old photographs with Hal and Ann and indicated her recognition with short phrases or smiles. She independently sought out the box of various colored and textured yarns and handled them with satisfaction, indicating that she remembers knitting when she was well.
• Gail will have decreased **catastrophic reactions** (see Box 17-2).	• Analyze with all caregivers what the previous causative factors may have been. • Simplify the environment (evaluate furniture and objects, colors, noise level). *Through analyzing and simplifying the environment, the client's safety is maintained and the stressors causing the catastrophic incidents are reduced. Collaborative planning will ensure consistent successful approaches to tasks, and client and caregiver stress will be reduced.*	• Gail had two catastrophic reactions during the last 2 weeks. Hal and Ann analyzed each incident and discovered that the underlying causes were (1) increased ambient noise from street repairs in front of the house and (2) being rushed to leave for a dental appointment.

Nursing Diagnosis: Coping, ineffective family: compromised, related to inadequate understanding of the process of Alzheimer's disease by the caregivers, inability of the spouse to adequately manage the emotional conflicts, role changes, temporary abandonment, weak support systems, and ineffective communication/relationship with the secondary caregiver, as evidenced by Hal's being away from home more and Ann's loss of weight and social withdrawal.

Family Outcomes	Nursing Interventions	Evaluation
• Hal and Ann will verbalize realistic perception of their roles and responsibilities in caring for Gail.	• Facilitate meeting with all family members. *Sharing knowledge of status and prognosis will establish the core of a support system based on mutual respect and understanding.* • Address knowledge deficits and obtain feedback from participants. *Understanding allays fears and promotes rational planning; each person retains knowledge in unique ways and, common understandings are vital to successful planning and implementation.* • Collaborate in developing roles for each caregiver. *Understanding each one's role, including expectations and limitations, will reduce behaviors that might lead to abuse or abandonment and elicit positive care outcomes for the client.*	• Hal and Ann met with other family members who live in the area, and these family members expressed gratitude for being included and enlightened; they offered assistance with outings and evening care. On two consecutive nursing visits Hal and Ann successfully reviewed information on the pathologic and neurologic deficits of Alzheimer's disease and are coping with Gail's behavior manifestations. Interventions have been successful on four occasions. They have congratulated each other.

NURSING CARE PLAN —cont'd

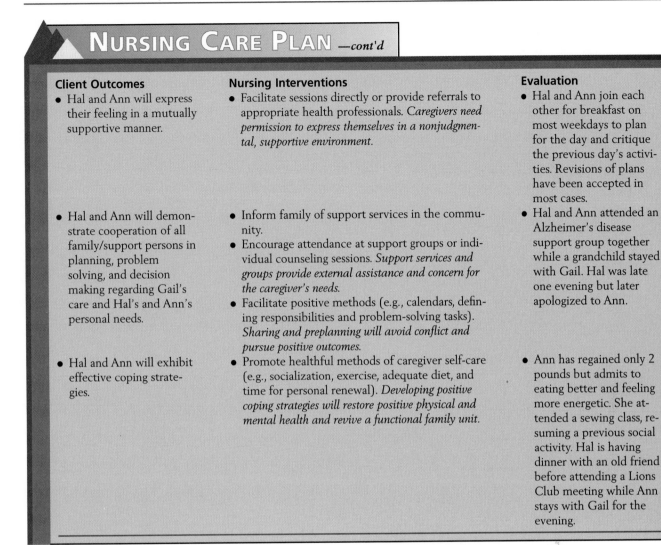

Client Outcomes	Nursing Interventions	Evaluation
• Hal and Ann will express their feeling in a mutually supportive manner.	• Facilitate sessions directly or provide referrals to appropriate health professionals. *Caregivers need permission to express themselves in a nonjudgmental, supportive environment.*	• Hal and Ann join each other for breakfast on most weekdays to plan for the day and critique the previous day's activities. Revisions of plans have been accepted in most cases.
• Hal and Ann will demonstrate cooperation of all family/support persons in planning, problem solving, and decision making regarding Gail's care and Hal's and Ann's personal needs.	• Inform family of support services in the community. • Encourage attendance at support groups or individual counseling sessions. *Support services and groups provide external assistance and concern for the caregiver's needs.* • Facilitate positive methods (e.g., calendars, defining responsibilities and problem-solving tasks). *Sharing and preplanning will avoid conflict and pursue positive outcomes.*	• Hal and Ann attended an Alzheimer's disease support group together while a grandchild stayed with Gail. Hal was late one evening but later apologized to Ann.
• Hal and Ann will exhibit effective coping strategies.	• Promote healthful methods of caregiver self-care (e.g., socialization, exercise, adequate diet, and time for personal renewal). *Developing positive coping strategies will restore positive physical and mental health and revive a functional family unit.*	• Ann has regained only 2 pounds but admits to eating better and feeling more energetic. She attended a sewing class, resuming a previous social activity. Hal is having dinner with an old friend before attending a Lions Club meeting while Ann stays with Gail for the evening.

Nurses specializing in chronic care and geriatrics focus on maintaining the client's highest functional level, educating the caregiver about effective and realistic outcomes and interventions, and referring to available options for care in the home and in the community.

FLEXIBILITY AND CHANGE

Care plan documentation is not permanent because care plans are changed as often as assessment indicates. Acute care nurses may need to adapt the care plan to fit the client's needs as each shift changes, whereas nurses in long-term care need to set routine times (e.g., every 3 months) to closely examine the client's needs and adjust care accordingly.

COLLABORATION

Cooperation by both acute care and long-term care nurses, as well as other members of the health care team, is critical; the collective knowledge and experience at all levels ensure more effective, realistic client outcomes and caregiver gratification (see the clinical pathway on pp. 408-409).

IMPLEMENTATION

The care and treatment of clients with cognitive disorders present the nurse/caregivers with a variety of situations that can be both challenging and gratifying. Each plan of care should reflect the unique qualities of the individual, and special consideration should be given to the family, as well as the client. It is the nurse who keeps the health care team focused on both short-term and long-term goals that address the problems arising from dementia and delirium.

Caregiver and support system integrity must be maintained by involving the family and significant others in planning, intervention, and evaluation. The Client & Family Teaching Guidelines on p. 410 lists issues that need to be addressed in their involvement. Advanced directives, living wills, and treatment options need to be addressed early. The client needs a realistic knowledge base regarding the diagnosis, treatment, and prognosis. As the therapeutic relationship between the nurse, client, and family/caregivers develops, the nurse will be able to introduce these delicate and often painful topics while preserving hopefulness and family integrity. Types and levels of care are detailed in Box 17-2.

DEMENTIA CRITICAL PATH
NORTON HOSPITAL
DRG 429 PATH # N0024

Patient label:

Admit date: _____
Expected LOS: _____14_____
Treatment date: _____

Disch. date: _____
Actual LOS: _____

Suicide attempts #
Psychotic features
Patient falls #
Readmits within 31 days
Readmits within 1 year
Transfer to _____ /from _____
a medical/surgical unit
Treatment of concurrent medical problems/
Dx: _____

	DAY 1 (admit)	DAY 2	DAY 3	DAY 4	DAY 5	DAYS 6–10	DAYS 11–14
ASSESSMENTS/ EVALUATIONS	H&P MMSE nrsg assess VS lifestyle questionnaire continent care evaluation elimination pattern evaluation	SW contact with family dietary evaluation	audiology appt scheduled PT evaluation continent care re-evaluation elimination pattern re-evaluation	Reevaluate privilege level	SW evaluation psych testing OT evaluation Tolerates Meds Free from falls	SW contact with family continent care re-evaluation elimination pattern re-evaluation Leisure Assessment	stabilization of meds SW family conference continent care re-evaluation
TESTS	EKG	routine labs CRX	BDI	CT scan EEG	PPD	BDI - day 9	BDI - day
CONSULTS		MD consults notified				MD consults complete	
DIET/FLUID BALANCE	calorie count I&O weigh (2x/wk - Tues. & Fri.)			nutrition/hydration assessment		nutrition/hydration stable	
ACTIVITY/ SAFETY	unit privilege falls protocol	ambulation asst guidelines AM exercise	sleep disturbance assessment AM exercise	AM exercise OT Group Therapy Group	AM exercise Restraints utilized -passive -posy vest -leather waist -wheelchair	Sleep pattern stable AM exercise daily	AM exercise daily
EDUCATION				Tuesday Nite family Nite referral		"The 36-Hour Day" given educational film shown ADRDA referral Family Nite	d/c instructions given

NOO24.XLS 2/6/92 ngv

1 of 2

©1991 Alliant Health System

Treatment date:

	DAY 1 (admit)			DAY 2			DAY 3			DAY 4			DAY 5			DAYS 6–10			DAYS 11–14		
	N	M	U	N	M	U	N	M	U	N	M	U	N	M	U	N	M	U	N	M	U
TREATMENT TEAM PLANNING/ DISCHARGE PLANNING																multi-disciplinary team mtg ☐ D/C plans complete ☐			multi-disciplinary team mtg ☐☐ O.P. f/u scheduled ☐☐ living arrangements finalized transfer form ☐☐		
VARIANCE ANALYSIS																					
FACTS RE: VARIANCE																					
STEPS TO CORRECT VARIANCE																					

Developed by and reprinted with permission from Connie Anton and David A. Casey, M.D., Norton Psychiatric Clinic, Alliant Health System, Louisville, Kentucky

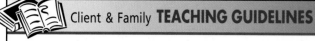

Client & Family TEACHING GUIDELINES

Cognitive Disorders

1. A strong professional and family support network is important for the caregiver who must carry out exhausting tasks.
2. Psychiatric intervention for the caregiver may aid in adjusting and coping with difficulties that arise.
3. The caregiver must be allowed the time and opportunity to mourn and complete the grieving process.
4. Verbalizing concerns and feelings is important for coping.
5. Action regarding finances must be taken while the client still retains the capacity to make decisions.

NURSING INTERVENTIONS

1. Inform all caregivers (family/nursing) of the nursing care plan *to maintain a consistent physical and cognitive approach.*
2. Identify the client's current functional state and encourage him or her to use his or her skills *to promote independence as long as possible.*
3. Keep all interactions with the client pleasant, calm,

and reassuring *to decrease anxiety, because clients with cognitive disorders mirror the emotional climate around them.*

4. Do not ask the client to participate in ADL when agitated *because it will only increase the client's frustration.*
5. Attempt to understand the client's feelings *to decrease frustration and meet client needs.*
6. Respond to the client's feelings and validate them with words, body language, and actions *to make the client feel understood and increase feelings of self-worth.*
7. Help the client maintain self-esteem by keeping interactions on an adult level. Use proper names *to avoid infantilizing or patronizing the client.*
8. If errors or failures occur, assure the client that no harm has been done and avoid any criticism. Avoid negative responses and commands. Avoid "why" questions. *Clients with dementia are often aware that there is something wrong with their performance, and they do not totally comprehend their environment. They are sensitive to criticism and may not be able to respond to "why" questions, which may provoke a sense of failure.*
9. Provide the client with an opportunity to make simple choices. *Choosing offers some control to the client and aids in maintaining a sense of independence.*
10. Set up fairly structured routines. *This helps overcome*

Box 17-2   Types and Levels of Care for Cognitive Disorders

Acute Care

Nurses working in clinics, physicians' offices, emergency department/urgent care units, or acute care facilities must be alert to the signs and symptoms of cognitive impairment. It is critical that nurses understand the differences between dementia, delirium, and depression and plan accordingly. Nursing care must be holistic, assessing and intervening in the needs of the caregiver, as well.

Day Care

Adult day health care licensing regulations throughout the country vary, but in general the focus of these centers is on education, rehabilitation, training, and maintenance of physical functions, as well as mental status.

Dementia day care provides specialized respite, education, and support for the caregivers of clients with dementia. The programs offer therapeutic activity programs and appropriate behavior management approaches for the client with dementia.

In-Home Care

As the disease progresses, an increasing amount of physical and emotional support will be necessary in the home. The role of nurse case managers is to coordinate and provide appropriate care for the client and the caregiver in the home. This enables the client to stay at home longer, thus increasing the quality of life, conserving financial and emotional resources, and postponing institutionalization.

Residential Care Facility

There are many residential care options, and state regulations vary. The services offered may include housekeeping and communal meals, which could be sufficient in the early stages of Alzheimer's disease, but as deficits in memory and decision making increase, more supervision will be necessary. A residential care facility (RCF) is an appropriate placement in the moderate stage of the dementia, since, physically, the client may be very active and otherwise well. Staff involved in residential care usually are specially trained in dementia care and are trained to interact positively for the successful outcome achievement.

Skilled Nursing Facility

Skilled nursing facilities (SNFs) provide 24-hour professional nursing care. Clients in late-stage Alzheimer's dementia are admitted as a result of the extensive physical care needs. Financing this phase of the long-term care continuum is becoming increasingly problematic. The financial resources of the client, family, and state and federal government all become involved.

Hospice Care

Clients in late-stage Alzheimer's disease are considered to be terminally ill and eligible for hospice care services. Hospice care for both the client and the family focuses on quality-of-life issues. Lifesaving measures are not used. Instead, clients are made comfortable, and families are supported during the final stage.

Box 17-3   Catastrophic Reactions

Catastrophic reactions are overexaggerated emotional responses initiated as a result of a perceived failure at a task or change in the environment (Webster and Grossberg, 1996).

Often clients with dementia are unjustly labeled as noncompliant, disruptive, uncooperative, or threatening. Clients are not trying to annoy, get attention, or hurt the caregiver but are trying their best to understand a world they can no longer comprehend. A catastrophic reaction can be displayed as verbal or physical aggression, verbal outbursts, worry, anger, tension expressed in body language, labile mood swings, pacing, paranoia, crying, or hysterical laughter.

Analysis of a Catastrophic Reaction
Was the person:

Trying unsuccessfully to comprehend more than one or two sensory messages at once?

Feeling insecure (e.g., being in new surroundings or surrounded by unfamiliar staff)?

Having a minor mishap (e.g., spilling a drink or dropping something) or failing at a task?

Asked to reason, make a judgment, or perform a multiple step or complex task?

Experiencing negative interactions such as scolding, arguing, anger, frustration, or irritation?

Experiencing an hallucination, delusion, or illusion?

Interventions for a Catastrophic Reaction
Reassure the client that he or she is safe.

Use positive behavior interactions.

Maintain the client's "personal space." Do not touch the person without asking permission.

Eliminate or reduce all outside stimulation.

Identify and remove either the source of the problem or the person.

Redirect the client to a less demanding activity.

Be patient and allow sufficient time for the client to calm down. This may take only a few minutes or hours, varying with each client and situation.

If the nurse cannot stop or minimize the reaction:

Leave the client alone for a while in a quiet, *safe* place within view of staff or family.

When the nurse readdresses the client, act as if nothing has happened. Redirect conversations to familiar topics.

Have one person address the client. Minimize hand gestures and be aware of facial expressions. Speak in a soft nonthreatening voice while redirecting the conversation or task.

---

short-term memory losses, promotes independence, and reduces anxiety.

11. Praise successes and facilitate the use of remaining strengths *to increase self-esteem and reduce a sense of failure.*

12. Simplify the verbal message using no more than five or six words at a time. Accompany words with visual and/or tactile clues *to decrease confusion and increase clarity of the message.*

13. Repeat the message if needed, allowing time for responses. Use the same words. Do not go on to another message until you are sure that the first one has been grasped, or leave and return to explain it in a different way. *Using these techniques may avoid or lessen such common behavior problems as* catastrophic reactions (Box 17-3) *and* sundowning *and deter the development of excess disability.*

14. Break down each task into separate components *to avoid confusion and frustration.*

15. Involve the client in activities that he or she wants to participate in. Arrange the activity to be a one-to-one or small-group activity for a short period *to decrease resistance and promote success.*

16. Allow the client time to himself or herself. Do not overstimulate and fatigue the client *to ensure the client's privacy, demonstrate respect, and conserve the client's energy.*

17. Remain flexible with the daily schedule *to promote the client's feelings of security and reduce frustration.*

AVAILABLE TREATMENT MODALITIES
Interdisciplinary Team
The purpose of the interdisciplinary team is to provide comprehensive holistic care to a client with measurable outcomes. Elderly clients, especially those with cognitive disorders, have complex health, social, and economic problems that necessitate a comprehensive approach. The most important member of the interdisciplinary team is the client, and, if appropriate, the family. The following professionals are part of the team: nurse practitioner, clinical nurse specialist, gerontologist, geropsychiatrist, social worker, dietitian, pharmacist, and rehabilitation specialists (e.g., speech, physical, occupational), each with a special knowledge of gerontology. A clinical pathway for dementia is presented in Appendix D. It details the collaborative treatment interventions for this condition.

ADDITIONAL TREATMENT MODALITIES
For the Client With Dementia/Alzheimer's Disease

Interdisciplinary team
Pharmacologic interventions
    Drugs used to modify behavior and increase function
    Drugs used in the therapy of Alzheimer's disease
Therapeutic activity program

Pharmacologic Interventions

Pharmacologic interventions with cognitive disorders can be successful in two areas:

1. Those medications that aim at modifying behavior to enhance the client's functional level
2. Experimental and Food and Drug Administration (FDA)–approved drugs used for therapy of Alzheimer's disease

Multiple drug administration can cause delirium; therefore medications are used singly at the lowest possible dosage to produce optimal functioning while eliminating adverse symptoms. Medications can then be slowly titrated to higher doses to achieve an optimal effect.

Decisions about pharmacologic management should be based on the extent of signs and symptoms associated with impaired behavior and functional status. Trazodone (Desyrel) is used in behavioral problems of dementia when sedation at night is needed. Clients who have depression-like symptoms may also use trazodone or a specific serotonin reuptake inhibitor. Patients with mild to moderate anxiety or irritability may be prescribed alprazolam (Xanax) or buspirone (BuSpar). Neuroleptics (haloperidol [Haldol] and risperidone [Risperdal]) are used when delusions, hallucinations, paranoia, or agitation (severe) is present. Certain anticonvulsants such as valproic acid (Depakene), divalproex (Sodium Depakote), and carbamazepine (Tegretol) are used with patients demonstrating impulsivity, aggression, and assaultive behavior. Lithium is used in cases of mania. The therapeutic regimen is very individualized and is based on presenting behavioral problems.

Before pharmacologic management is initiated for behavioral problems, it is important to exhaust all behavioral management techniques, as well as environmental and social strategies. If all of these measures fail, then medication should be used to modify behavior. The drugs used to modify behavior and increase function are discussed in detail in Chapter 23.

Experimental drugs in the therapy of Alzheimer's disease.

Many pharmaceutical research studies are currently underway to find a drug that will slow or reverse the cognitive decline in persons with Alzheimer's disease. Cholinergic replacement therapy is available with tacrine (Cognex). The hypothesis for this medication is based on the decrease in acetylcholine in persons with Alzheimer's disease. This drug suppresses cholinesterase so that acetylcholine will not break down as quickly. Another drug called donepezil (Aricept), a cholinesterace inhibitor, is being used to treat primarily mild cases of Alzheimer's disease with some success. Currently, nonsteroidal antiinflammatory drugs are being evaluated for their role. An enzyme, cyclooxygenease, may play a role in delaying the onset of symptoms.

Other clinical trials with estrogen, nerve growth factor, and calcium channel blockers are ongoing. Vitamin E and deprenyl, drugs that inhibit oxidation, have been discussed previously (see Additional Treatment Modalities).

Therapeutic Activity Program

An activity is described as any project a person enjoys and that produces a positive feeling. A *therapeutic activity program* is a total plan of care based on assessment of the client's needs and a history of previous endeavors. It is specifically designed to meet the identified needs and to keep the person functioning at the highest possible level (Stehman et al, 1991).

Building on retained strengths (e.g., retained remote memory, use of habitual skills, preserved large and fine motor skills, and intact emotional responses) is the basis of success. It is exceedingly difficult, if not impossible, for the person with Alzheimer's disease to learn new skills. "Use it or lose it!" is a truism, especially when working with clients with dementia. Once a skill is lost, it is virtually gone forever and not able to be relearned.

For persons with dementia a therapeutic program is considered a primary treatment, since often the first neurologic losses result in the inability to plan, initiate, carry out in ordered steps (sequence), or remember activities by themselves. It is therefore the role of the caregiver to assist the client throughout the activity, from beginning to end. Positive reinforcement should be used at each step of the way.

Success of a therapeutic activity program can be measured on some objective terms by addressing the following questions:

Has the number of times per day or week that the client is actively involved increased or decreased?
Have incidents of catastrophic reactions or sundowning decreased?
Have incidents of the client aimlessly pacing or wandering and getting lost decreased?
Has the level of functioning in ADL and IADL remained stable, or is it decreasing at a slower pace than before the program was initiated?
Are caregivers feeling less stress, which might be indicated by fewer incidents of anger or crying, improved sleep patterns, or enhanced feelings of physical and mental well-being?

EVALUATION

Evaluating the client's progress and the degree to which nurses have achieved satisfactory client and caregiver outcomes is especially challenging when Alzheimer's disease and other dementias are involved. Factors that may influence success vary greatly with each situation and must be carefully considered in this process. Below are some questions that need to be clearly answered and understood before specific topics are addressed.

Is the cognitive impairment reversible or irreversible?

Is the client experiencing delirium, depression, dementia, or a combination of these?

What is the setting (i.e., acute care, long-term care, home)?

What is the caregiving situation?

What medical and psychiatric problems have been identified in the nursing history?

What is the current medication profile?

Is medication compliance a problem?

What behavioral problems have been identified?

What is the client's functional status?

What is the interdisciplinary plan of care?

When the answers to these questions have been agreed on, the nurse and the interdisciplinary team will be better able to determine the degree to which specifics in the outcome identification have been realized.

Summary of Key Concepts

1. Dementia, one of the most pervasive health care problems for older persons, is an age-related disorder affecting approximately 40% of Americans age 75 years and older (Selkoe, 1992).

2. Seventy percent of the 4 million Americans diagnosed with probable Alzheimer's disease are cared for at home (Boyd and Vernon, 1998).

3. The five current theories regarding the cause of Alzheimer's disease state that it is a result of infectious agents, neurotoxic agents, angiopathy and blood-brain incompetency, neurotransmitter and receptor deficiencies, and abnormal proteins and their products.

4. Regardless of the biologic cause, the effect of these diseases is altered neurochemistry or neurophysiology that disrupts metabolism in the brain.

5. The pathologic process of cognitive disorders results in neurologic deficits, such as reduced ability to perceive the environment and organize appropriate responses, decreased attention span, language deficits, memory loss, changes in emotional responses, and a decline in the ability to reason and form judgments.

6. Alzheimer's disease is considered to have three stages: mild, moderate, and severe.

7. A variety of cognitive assessment tools can be used to determine medical and nursing diagnoses.

8. The nurse should plan and supervise therapeutic activity programs to achieve the highest possible functional status for the client and prevent excess disability.

9. Caring for a person with a cognitive disorder is a significant physical and emotional burden for the caregivers.

10. All nursing care for clients with cognitive disorders should be done in collaboration with the client's caregivers.

11. Care plans should be formulated that are based on assessment of both the client's needs and the caregiver's needs.

12. The success of care plans should be based on successful functional status and not on a curative basis.

REFERENCES

Agency for Health Care Policy and Research: *Depression in primary care*, vol 1, *Detection and diagnosis*, Rockville, Md, 1996, U.S. Department of Health and Human Services.

Alzheimer A: Über eine eigenartige Erkrankung der Kirnrinde, *Allgemeine Z Psychiatrie* 64:146, 1907.

American Psychiatric Association: *Diagnostic and statistical manual of mental disorders*, ed 4, Washington DC, 1994, The Association.

Boyd CO, Vernon GM: Primary care of the older adult with end stage Alzheimer's disease, *Nurse Pract* 23(4):63, 1998.

Burgener SC et al: Effective caregiving approaches for patients with Alzheimer's disease, *Geriatr Nurs* 19(3):121, 1998.

Corder EH et al: Gene dose of apolipoprotein E type e4 allele and the risk of Alzheimer's disease in late-onset families, *Science* 261:921, 1993.

Foreman M et al: Assessing cognitive function, *Geriatr Nurs* 5:228, 1996.

Gage FH et al: Gene therapy in the CNS: intracerebral grafting of genetically modified cells, *Prog Brain Res* 86:205, 1990.

Glenner, GG: Alzheimer's disease. In *Encyclopedia of human biology* 1:108, 1994.

Glenner GG, Wong CW: Alzheimer's disease and Down's syndrome: sharing of a unique cerebrovascular amyloid fibril protein, *Biochem Biophys Res Commun* 122:1131, 1984a.

Glenner GG, Wong CW: Alzheimer's disease: initial report of the purification and characterization of a novel cerebrovascular amyloid protein, *Biochem Biophys Res Commun* 120:885, 1984b.

Holt J: How to help confused patients, *Am J Nurs* 93:32, 1993.

Ikeda S et al: Gerstmann-Sträussler-Scheinker disease showing β-protein amyloid deposits in the peripheral regions of PrP-Immunoreactive amyloid plaques, *Neurodegeneration* 1:281, 1992.

Kidd M: Paired helical filaments in electron microscopy of Alzheimer's disease, *Nature* 197:192, 1963.

Lyness JM: Delirium: masquerades and misdiagnosis in elderly patients, *J Am Geriatr Soc* 38(11):1235, 1990.

Mangeno M, Middemiss C: Alzheimer's disease: preventing and recognizing misdiagnoses, *Nurse Pract* 22(10):58, 1997.

McNiel C: *Alzheimer's disease: unraveling the mysteries*, Rockville, Md, 1995, National Institutes of Health.

Needham J: Alzheimer's disease: diagnosis and management, *Contin Med Educ Resources*, p 15, 1998.

North America Nursing Diagnosis Association: *NANDA nursing diagnoses: definitions and classifications, 1999-2000*, Philadelphia, 1999, The Association.

Prusiner SB: Some speculations about prions, amyloid, and Alzheimer's disease, *N Engl J Med* 310:661, 1984.

Prusiner SB: Molecular biology of prion diseases, *Science* 252:1515, 1991.

Rockwell E: *Behavior problems in Alzheimer's disease* (accompanies the video "Speaking for Them"), Silver Spring, Md., 1991, Alzheimer's Disease Education and Referral Center (ADEAR).

Scheibel AB et al: Denervation microangiopathy in senile dementia, Alzheimer type, *Alzheimer Dis Assoc Disord* 1:19, 1987.

Selkoe DJ: Aging brain, aging mind, *Sci Am* 267(3):134, 1992.

Stehman J et al: *Training manual for Alzheimer's care specialists*, Manuscript submitted for publication, 1991.

Tomlinson BE et al: Observations on the brains of demented old people, *J Neurol Sci* 11:205, 1972.

U.S. Department of Health and Human Services: *Depression is a treatable illness: a patient guide*, Rockville, Md, 1993, The Department.

U.S. Department of Health and Human Services: Quick reference guide for clinicians: early identification of Alzheimer's disease and related dementias, *J Am Acad Nurse Pract* 9(2):85, 1997.

Webster J, Grossberg GT: Strategies for treating dementing disorders, *Nurs Home Med* (6):161, 1996.

Wong CW et al: Neuritic plaques and cerebrovascular amyloid in Alzheimer's disease are antigenically related, *Proc Nat Acad Sci USA* 82:8729, 1985.

Zgola J: *Doing things: a guide to programming activities for persons with Alzheimer's disease and related disorders*, Baltimore, 1987, Johns Hopkins University Press.

CHAPTER 18

Disorders of Childhood and Adolescence

Richard C. Lucas

OBJECTIVES

- Describe child/adolescent developmental disorders such as autism, Rett's syndrome, pervasive developmental disorder, Asperger's syndrome, and mental retardation.

- Identify attention-deficit/hyperactivity disorders in children and adolescents.

- Distinguish between oppositional defiant disorder and conduct disorder.

- Describe tic disorders, separation anxiety, and elimination disorders.

- Learn the components of a thorough nursing assessment and application of the nursing process for children or adolescents.

DISORDERS OF CHILDHOOD AND ADOLESCENCE

The nurse will have the opportunity to assess and treat children and adolescents in diverse health care settings. Children and adolescents frequently present for medical problems when in fact the underlying problem may be a mental disorder in need of treatment. The nurse's assessment must be comprehensive to identify those children and adolescents and their families in need of mental health referrals and early intervention. The earlier the identification is made, the sooner the client and family can receive necessary treatment and community resources.

Children and adolescents are treated within the context of the family system. One cannot be separated from the other. It is important for the nurse to understand the mental health issues facing children and adolescents and the impact these issues will have on their growth and development. This chapter discusses the major mental disorders affecting children and adolescents and provides a direction for applying the nursing process with this population.

HISTORICAL AND THEORETIC PERSPECTIVES

History tells a story of a lack of concern for and little attention paid to understanding or treating children. Despert (1967) documented indifference and even cruelty to children through time. DeMause (1995) found that the further back one goes, the lower the level of child care that was present and the less effective the parenting. Children tended to be seen as miniature adults, with no understanding of development.

Acting out The expression of internal affective states through external activities and behaviors that are often destructive and/or maladaptive.

Assent To think or feel; to consent; to give concurrence, acquiescence, or compliance.

Autism A pervasive developmental disorder characterized by marked impairment of social and cognitive abilities.

Behavior modification A systematic, structured, positive reinforcement program that rewards behavioral gains.

Contraband A term used to identify prohibited objects, such as cigarettes, matches, lighters, knives, weapons, drugs, or alcohol.

Encopresis The repeated involuntary or intentional passage of feces into inappropriate places.

Enuresis Repeated involuntary or intentional voiding of urine into bed or clothes.

Pervasive developmental disorders A collection of disorders in which the child experiences deficits in a broad range of developmental areas.

Somatic complaints The manifestation or perception of physical symptoms in the absence of clinically significant organic disease.

Therapeutic play Age-appropriate play activities used purposefully by the nurse for assessment, intervention, and promotion of normal growth and development in children.

Tic A sudden, rapid, recurrent, nonrhythmic, stereotyped movement or vocalization considered irresistible but often suppressible for short periods of time.

Children traditionally had little standing with adults. Not until 1889 did children and adolescents get their own juvenile justice system. They were finally recognized with their own mental health clinics when William Healy started the Juvenile Psychopathic Institute in Chicago and Ernest Southard was assigned director of an outpatient clinic in Boston in the early 1900s (Hirshberg, 1980).

Developmental theories tell us how children respond to multiple biopsychosocial influences. When problems develop, these theories show us how treatment can help. Recently the biologic understanding of psychopathology has added another dimension to treatment.

Reactive theories maintain that the child's mind starts as a blank slate and that environmental influences promote healthy or pathologic development. The major reactive theories include stimulus-response, learning, classical conditioning, and operant conditioning. These theories imply that symptoms are learned behavior and that improvement comes through relearning and environmental change.

Structural theories start with the belief that the child has a genetically determined ability for developing behavior and acts on the environment. Major structural theorists include Bowlby (attachment), Freud (psychosexual developmental lines), Erickson (psychosocial development), and Piaget (cognitive development). Treatment under a structural theory involves a reorganization within the child or adolescent (e.g., resolution of intrapsychic conflicts, alteration of family patterns of interaction, or acquiring a new schema) (Lewis, 1980).

MENTAL RETARDATION
ETIOLOGY AND EPIDEMIOLOGY

Despite extensive evaluations, no clear etiology can be found in 30% to 40% of individuals with mental retardation. When found, the etiology may be primarily biologic or primarily psychosocial, or a combination of the two. Major factors include the following:

- Heredity accounts for approximately 5% of cases and includes Tay-Sachs disease, tuberous sclerosis, Down syndrome, and fragile X syndrome.
- Early problems in embryonic development account for approximately 30% of cases and include chromosomal changes such as trisomy 21 or prenatal exposure to toxins (e.g., maternal alcohol consumption, infections).
- Pregnancy and perinatal problems make up about 10% of cases and include fetal malnutrition, prematurity, hypoxia, viral and other infections, and trauma.
- General medical conditions acquired during infancy or childhood contribute to approximately 5% of cases and include infections, traumas, and poisoning (e.g., lead).
- Environmental influences and other mental disorders contribute to about 15% to 20% of cases. Factors include deprivation of nurturance and social, linguistic, and other stimulation, and severe mental disorders (e.g., autistic disorder) (American Psychiatric Association [APA], 1994).

Although studies vary, the prevalence of mental retardation is estimated at 1% to 3% of the population in developed countries (King et al, 1997) (see DSM-IV Criteria box below).

DSM-IV CRITERIA

Mental Retardation

A. Significant subaverage intellectual functioning: an IQ of approximately 70 or below on an individual administered IQ test, severity determined as follows:

   Mild—IQ 50-55 to approximately 70
   Moderate—IQ 35-40 to 50-55
   Severe—IQ 20-25 to 50-55
   Profound—IQ below 20-25

B. Concurrent deficits or impairments in present adaptive function (i.e., the person's effectiveness in meeting the standards expected for his or her age by his or her cultural group) in at least two of the following areas: communication, self-care, home living, social/interpersonal skills, use of community resources, self-direction, functional academic skills, work, leisure, health, and safety

C. Onset before age 18

From American Psychiatric Association: *Diagnostic and statistical manual of mental disorders*, ed 4, Washington, DC, 1994, The Association.

CLINICAL DESCRIPTION AND PROGNOSIS
General

Individuals typically present with problems in adaptive functioning, defined as "how effectively individuals cope with common life demands and how well they meet the standards of personal independence expected of someone in their particular age-group, sociocultural background, and community setting" (APA, 1994). Several factors may influence adaptive functioning: education, motivation, personality characteristics, social and vocational opportunities, and other coexisting mental and physical conditions (APA, 1994).

Subtypes

Approximately 85% of individuals with mental retardation have mild retardation. These children typically develop social and communication skills during the preschool years, suffer only minimal sensorimotor problems, and often are not identified until a later age. They can generally acquire academic skills up to approximately the sixth grade level. In adulthood they generally achieve social and vocational skills adequate for minimum self-support. They usually require supervision, guidance, and assistance. But, in most cases, they live successfully in the community—some independently, some in supervised settings.

About 10% of the entire population with mental retardation have moderate retardation. Most individuals with moderate mental retardation acquire some communication skills during early childhood and may benefit from vocational training, but they seldom advance academically beyond the second grade level. With moderate supervision, they can usually provide for their own personal care and learn to travel in familiar areas. Peer relationships often deteriorate in adolescence because of problems in recognizing socially correct interactions. During adulthood they generally can perform unskilled or semiskilled work and live in the community in supervised setting.

About 3% to 4% of individuals with mental retardation have severe retardation. They typically acquire little if any communicative speech during early childhood but may learn to talk and develop elementary self-care skills in the school-age period. They may profit from learning to sight-read some "survival" words. As adults they may be able to perform simple skills in tightly supervised settings. They can generally live in the community in group homes or with their families unless some other handicap requires specialized nursing or other care.

Only 1% to 2% of mentally retarded individuals suffer from profound retardation. Most also have an identified neurologic condition causing their retardation. They have considerable sensorimotor problems recognized in early childhood and require a highly structured setting with constant monitoring and assistance in an individualized relationship for optimal development. Under this sort of care, they may develop enough motor skills, self-care skills, and communication to perform simple tasks in a closely supervised and sheltered setting (APA, 1994).

Associated Features

Individuals with mental retardation demonstrate no consistent or specific personality or behavioral features that are generalized to this population. Individual traits range from passive, placid, and dependent styles to aggressive and impulsive styles. Individuals with more severe retardation and associated communication deficits demonstrate more aggression and impulsivity resulting from frustration and lack of ability to interact with their environment adequately. Some medical conditions that cause mental retardation have specific problems associated with them, such as the self-injurious behavior found in Lesch-Nyhan syndrome. Individuals with mental retardation are subjected to exploitation as a result of their vulnerability. They may have rights and opportunities denied or suffer outright physical or sexual abuse.

Individuals with mental retardation have a comorbid mental disorder an estimated three to four times more often than the general population. Any mental disorder may present in retarded individuals, and no evidence indicates any difference in the nature of the mental disorder. However, problems frequently occur in diagnosing mental disorders because of communication skills deficits and other handicaps. The most commonly diagnosed mental disorders include attention-deficit/hyperactivity disorder, mood disorder, pervasive developmental disorder, stereotypic movement disorder, and mental disorders due to a general medical condition (e.g., dementia due to head trauma) (APA, 1994).

PERVASIVE DEVELOPMENTAL DISORDER: AUTISTIC DISORDER

Pervasive developmental disorders are a collection of disorders in which the child experiences deficits in a broad range of developmental areas. Autism, characterized by marked impairment of social and cognitive abilities, is the most common of these disorders (see DSM-IV Criteria box below).

EPIDEMIOLOGY

Studies suggest that the rate of autistic disorder is 2 to 5 cases per 10,000. Rates are four to five times higher in males than in females. Females, however, tend to have more severe mental retardation. Siblings of individuals with the disorder have an increased risk of developing autistic disorder (APA, 1994).

DSM-IV CRITERIA

Autistic Disorder

A. A total of six (or more) items from the following three areas:
   1. Qualitative impairment in social interaction, as manifested by at least two of the following:
      a. Marked impairment in the use of multiple nonverbal behaviors such as eye-to-eye gaze, facial expression, body postures, and gestures to regulate social interaction
      b. Failure to develop peer relationships appropriate to developmental level
      c. A lack of spontaneous seeking to share enjoyment, interests, or achievements with other people (e.g., by a lack of showing, bringing, or pointing out objects of interests)
      d. Lack of social or emotional reciprocity
   2. Qualitative impairments in communication as manifested by at least one of the following:
      a. Delay in, or total lack of, the development of spoken language (not accompanied by an attempt to compensate through alternative modes of communication such as gesture or mime)
      b. In individuals with adequate speech, marked impairment in the ability to initiate or sustain a conversation with others

   c. Stereotyped and repetitive use of language or idiosyncratic language
   d. Lack of varied, spontaneous make-believe play or social imitative play appropriate to developmental level
   3. Restricted repetitive and stereotyped patterns of behavior, interests, and activities, as manifested by at least one of the following:
      a. Encompassing preoccupation with one or more stereotyped and restricted patterns of interest that is abnormal either in intensity or focus
      b. Apparently inflexible adherence to specific, nonfunctional routines or rituals
      c. Stereotyped and repetitive motor mannerisms (e.g., hand or finger flapping or twisting, or complex whole-body movements)
      d. Persistent preoccupation with parts of objects
B. Delays or abnormal functioning in at least one of the following areas with onset before 3 years: (1) social interaction, (2) language as used in social communication, (3) symbolic or imaginative play
C. The disturbance not better accounted for by Rett's disorder or childhood disintegrative disorder

From American Psychiatric Association: *Diagnostic and statistical manual of mental disorders*, ed 4, Washington, DC, 1994, The Association.

CLINICAL DESCRIPTION
Behavioral Manifestations

A variety of behavioral symptoms may present, including any of the following: hyperactivity, short attention span, impulsivity, aggressiveness, self-injurious behaviors, and temper tantrums. Abnormalities of eating (e.g., limiting intake to a few foods or eating nonnutritious objects) or sleeping (e.g., recurrent awakenings with rocking) may be found. Individuals often have restricted, repetitive, and stereotyped patterns of behavior, interest, and activity. They become preoccupied in a way that is abnormal, either in intensity or focus, with an inflexible adherence to specific, nonfunctional routines or rituals; or they use stereotypic and repetitive mannerisms or become persistently preoccupied with parts of objects.

They may demonstrate an obsessive need to maintain sameness and orderliness by insisting on lining up objects over and over again. They may be unable to tolerate even minor changes in the environment and have a catastrophic reaction to minor changes such as a new chair or new seating arrangement at dinner. They may demand maintaining nonfunctional and unreasonable adherence to rituals and routines.

They often demonstrate stereotypic motor activities (e.g., clapping hands, spinning, rocking, swaying) and posture (e.g., walking on tiptoes, odd postures, or strange hand movements). Play cannot be disrupted from preoccupation with objects such as buttons. They frequently show a fascination with movement of such things as fans, revolving objects, or the opening and closing of doors or drawers. They may become highly attached to some unusually inanimate object such as a piece of string or rubber band and ignore typical items such as a blanket or teddy bear.

Emotional Manifestations

Individuals with autistic disorder typically lack emotional reciprocity (e.g., not actively participating in simple social play or games, instead preferring solitary activities or only attempting to involve others as tools or "mechanical" aids). Mood or affective abnormalities can be present, such as giggling or weeping for no apparent reason or no emotional reaction when a reaction is expected. There may be an inappropriate response to danger, with no fear exhibited to real danger or excessive fear exhibited to harmless objects. Self-injurious behavior can include head banging or biting of various body parts. If, during development, the patient acquires sufficient cognitive ability, they may have an awareness of the seriousness of their limitations. This type of insight may result in depression compounded by mental retardation.

Cognitive Manifestations

Approximately 75% of individuals with autistic disorder have some degree of mental retardation, most commonly in the moderate range (IQ 35 to 50). Other cognitive skills may also be impaired. Communication problems usually present so severely in both verbal and nonverbal areas that spoken language may be absent. Individuals who do speak may not be able to begin or sustain a conversation with others, or they use such stereotyped and repetitive or idiosyncratic language that others find it difficult to continue a conversation with them. Speech may often contain abnormalities of pitch, intonation, rate, and rhythm (e.g., monotonous or inappropriate sing-song pitch and rhythm or questionlike raises of tone at the end of declarative sentences). Grammar is often immature, stereotyped, and repetitive (e.g., inappropriate repetition of jingles or commercials, regardless of meaning) or metaphorical (for example, the grammar can only be understood by those familiar with the individual's idiosyncratic use of language). Individuals may not be able to understand simple questions, directions, or jokes. Other children may develop excellent long-term memory of insignificant items such as train schedules, baseball statistics, or songs.

Perceptual Manifestations

Individuals may respond oddly to sensory stimuli (e.g., they have a high pain threshold, oversensitivity to sound or touch, exaggerated response to light or color, or a fascination with a particular sensory stimulation).

Social Manifestations

Autistic disorder presentation depends on the developmental stage and chronologic age, but autism at any age is a severely limiting disorder. Markedly abnormal or impaired development in social interaction and communication, in addition to a markedly restricted range of activity and interest, severely impairs the individual's ability to function in society without a significant amount of persistent family and professional intervention.

Social interaction problems are major and sustained. Individuals typically cannot recognize and use nonverbal social clues and behaviors to regulate social interaction and communication. Peer relationships produce varied difficulties, depending on the individual's developmental level. Young individuals may have little or no interest in friendship, whereas older individuals may have an interest but experience serious problems understanding and dealing with expected and accepted social conventions. Individuals with autistic disorder often fail to demonstrate spontaneous efforts to seek shared enjoyments in interests or achievements (e.g., they may not show or discuss with others the things or ideas they find interesting). They often appear oblivious to others, have no concept of their needs, and do not notice their distress or joy. They often appear to lack the ability to express themselves and have blunted expressions of joy or distress.

Individuals with autism often lack the developmental skills to use varied, spontaneous, make-believe play activity or to use social imitation appropriate for their age. Play becomes mechanical, out of context with others, and lacks the imagination generally expected.

The nature of impairments in social interaction may change over time, depending on developmental levels. Infants may refuse to cuddle, may show an indifference or aversion for affection or physical contact, may fail to demonstrate eye contact or facial responsiveness, or may not smile socially or respond to parents' voices. Young children may treat adults as interchangeable or cling mechanically to one specific person. Even if the child becomes willing to engage in social interactions, the interactions demonstrate unusual behavior (e.g., expecting others to answer ritualized questions in specific ways, showing little sense of personal space boundaries, and being inappropriate in social interactions) (APA, 1994).

PROGNOSIS

Language skills and overall intellectual level are the strongest factors related to the ultimate prognosis. Available studies that have followed the course of this disorder suggest that only a small percentage of individuals with the disorder go on to live and work independently as adults. In about one third of cases, some degree of partial independence is possible. The highest-functioning adults with autistic disorder typically continue to exhibit problems in social interaction and communication together with restricted interests and activities.

OTHER PERVASIVE DEVELOPMENTAL DISORDERS
RETT'S DISORDER

The essential feature of Rett's disorder is development of multiple specific deficits following normal prenatal and perinatal periods and apparent normal development for the first 5 months of life. Between 5 and 48 months, head growth decelerates with a loss of prior purposeful hand skills, and subsequent characteristic stereotyped hand movements resembling hand-wringing or hand washing develop. Interest diminishes in social activities, and problems in coordination of gait and trunk movement develop. An associated impairment in language develops with severe psychomotor retardation. Rett's disorder appears much less frequently than autistic disorder and has been seen only in females. The duration of the disorder is lifelong, and the loss of skills is generally persistent and progressive. Recovery is usually limited. Communication and behavioral difficulties usually remain constant throughout life (APA, 1994).

CHILDHOOD DISINTEGRATIVE DISORDER

Childhood disintegrative disorder is a very rare disorder that is slightly more prevalent in males than in females and is distinguished by marked regression in multiple areas of functioning following at least 2 years of apparently normal development. Before 10 years of age, clinically significant loss of previously acquired skills appears in at least 2 of the following areas: expressive or receptive language, social skills or adaptive behavior, bowel or bladder control, play, or motor skills. Individuals demonstrate social, communicative, and behavioral problems generally seen in autistic disorder. Qualitative problems in social and communicative skills and restricted, repetitive, and stereotyped patterns of behavior and interests develop. The typical clinical presentation demonstrates a loss of skills reaching a plateau, with limited potential for improvement. In some clinical cases the loss of skills is progressive. The disorder follows a continuous course, and usually the duration is lifelong (APA, 1994).

ASPERGER'S DISORDER

Asperger's disorder contains many similar features of autistic disorder: severe and sustained impairment in social interaction and restricted, repetitive patterns of behavior, interests, and activities that produce significant impairment in social, occupational, or other important areas of functioning. However, in contrast to autistic disorder, no clinically significant delays in language, cognitive development, age-appropriate self-help skills, adaptive behavior, or curiosity about the environment occur (APA, 1994). This disorder follows a continuous course, and usually duration is lifelong.

ATTENTION-DEFICIT/ HYPERACTIVITY DISORDER
EPIDEMIOLOGY

Attention-deficit/hyperactivity disorder (ADHD) has been identified in numerous countries throughout the world. Western countries report variations in prevalence that likely arise from varying diagnostic practices rather than from differences in actual clinical presentation. Rates in school-age children approach 10% in boys and 5% in girls. Up to 65% of hyperactive children remain symptomatic as adults. Rates in adults are estimated at 2% to 7%. In elementary school–age children the ratio of boys to girls is 9:1 in clinical settings and 4:1 in epidemiologic studies. In the school setting the male-female ratio ranges from 4:1 in the predominately hyperactive-impulsive type to 2:1 in the inattentive type. As many as two thirds of those diagnosed with ADHD also meet the criteria for another mental disorder, including up to 50% for oppositional defiant disorder, 30% to 50% for conduct disorder, 15% to 20% for mood disorders, and 20% to 25% for anxiety disorders (see DSM-IV Criteria box on p. 422). Other common disorders include Tourette's and chronic tic disorders, substance abuse, speech and language delays, and learning disorders.

Families likely have more stress, feelings of parental incompetence, marital discord, marital disruption, and social isolation. Mothers may display more commanding and

Attention-Deficit/Hyperactivity Disorder

A. Either (1) or (2):

1. Six or more of the following symptoms of inattention have persisted for at least 6 months to a degree that is maladaptive and inconsistent with developmental level:

Inattention

a. Often fails to give close attention to details or makes careless mistakes in schoolwork, work, or other activities

b. Often has difficulty sustaining attention in tasks or play activities

c. Often does not seem to listen when spoken to directly

d. Often does not follow through on instructions and fails to finish schoolwork, chores, or duties in the workplace (not due to oppositional behavior or failure to understand instructions)

e. Often has difficulty organizing tasks and activities

f. Often avoids, dislikes, or is reluctant to engage in tasks that require sustained mental effort (such as schoolwork or homework)

g. Often loses things necessary for tasks or activities (e.g., toys, school assignments, pencils, books, or tools)

h. Is often easily distracted by extraneous stimuli

i. Is often forgetful in daily activities

2. Six or more of the following symptoms of hyperactivity-impulsivity have persisted for at least 6 months to a degree that is maladaptive and inconsistent with developmental level:

Hyperactivity

a. Often fidgets with hands or feet or squirms in seat

b. Often leaves seat in classroom or in other situations in which remaining seated is expected

c. Often runs about or climbs excessively in situations in which it is inappropriate (in adolescents or adults, may be limited to subjective feelings or restlessness)

d. Often has difficulty playing or engaging in leisure activities quietly

e. Is often "on the go" or often acts as if "driven by a motor"

f. Often talks excessively

Impulsivity

a. Often blurts out answers before questions have been completed

b. Often has difficulty awaiting turn

c. Often interrupts or intrudes on others (e.g., butts into conversations or games)

B. Some hyperactive-impulsive or inattentive symptoms that caused impairment were present before age 7 years.

C. Some impairment from the symptoms is present in two or more settings (e.g., at school [or work] and at home).

D. There must be clear evidence of clinically significant impairment in social, academic, or occupational functioning.

E. The symptoms do not occur exclusively during the course of a pervasive developmental disorder, schizophrenia, or other psychotic disorder and are not better accounted for by another mental disorder (e.g., mood disorder, anxiety disorder, dissociative disorder, or personality disorder).

From American Psychiatric Association: *Diagnostic and statistical manual of mental disorders,* ed 4, Washington, DC, 1994, The Association.

controlling behavior and less positive affect, which resolve with treatment (Dulcan et al, 1997).

Genetic factors likely play a role in ADHD. Concordance is 51% in monozygotic twins and 33% in dizygotic twins. Adoption studies support genetics over environment as well (Cantwell, 1996).

ETIOLOGY

Although not necessarily a cause, the following histories have been noted when the diagnosis has been made: child abuse or neglect, multiple foster placements, neurotoxin exposure (e.g., lead poisoning), infections (e.g., encephalitis), drug exposure in utero, low birth weight, and mental retardation. ADHD also has been found more often in the first-degree relatives of children with ADHD (APA, 1994).

CLINICAL DESCRIPTION

Behavioral Manifestations

Behavioral manifestations usually occur in several environments within the child's life, such as the school, home, church, or recreational activities. The level of problems typically varies from time to time in the same or different settings. Symptoms generally worsen in situations that require sustained attention and lack appeal or variety to the child or adolescent, such as listening to teachers, performing repetitive or tedious tasks, or reading lengthy materials. Symptoms may actually disappear or become minimal when under strict control, such as during a diagnostic interview or when receiving frequent rewards for appropriate behavior. Symptoms tend to worsen in unstructured, group situations such as the typical classroom and playground.

Hyperactivity presents in many forms: fidgeting or squirming in one's seat, getting up when one is expected to remain seated, excessive running or climbing when it is dangerous or inappropriate, or loud and disruptive play during quiet activities, demonstrating a driven verbal or motor quality. Even though toddlers developmentally present with a lot of activity and inquisitiveness, toddlers with ADHD present differently qualitatively; they are always on the go, darting back and forth, unable to remain still for completion of simple tasks such as putting on a coat or listening to a simple story, or running, jumping, and climbing on furniture.

School-age children may settle down somewhat but still display excessive overactivity; they demonstrate difficulty remaining seated by hanging onto the edge of their seats, squirming as if they need to shed their skin, playing with objects, or tapping their hands and feet. At home they frequently do not finish meals or even finish activities that they have begun. They make excessive noise, interrupting others during quiet times and talking constantly, such as giving a running commentary on a television show. Adolescents often can express a subjective feeling of restlessness and report a preference to engage in active rather than sedentary activities.

Impulsivity manifests itself in the following ways: impatience, failing to delay responses, blurting out answers before the question has been finished, difficulty waiting for one's turn or problems waiting in line without pushing and shoving, and frequently interrupting others to the point of social, academic, or occupational problems. In addition, they may also make comments out of turn; fail to listen to directions; initiate inappropriate contact with others by interrupting conversations; grab others by their clothing, limbs, or belongings; touch things that are off limits to them; and clown around at times of expected quiet. Accidents may result from their knocking over objects, running into people, grabbing dangerous objects such as a hot pan, or taking dangerous risks without consideration of the consequences, such as riding a bicycle at night without reflective lights. They often exhibit temper outbursts, bossiness, stubbornness, and excessive and frequent insistence that their requests be met.

Emotional Manifestations
Individuals with this disorder may develop a number of other problems as a result of the underlying attention and hyperactive-impulsive problems, including any of the following: low frustration tolerance, mood lability, demoralization, dysphoria, and poor self-esteem.

Cognitive Manifestations
Inattention can take place in one or several settings. Schoolwork or other activities may contain careless errors showing lack of close attention to details. Work may be messy, with evidence of not thinking through the project or schoolwork or of not persisting to adequate comple-

tion. Often it appears that the child is daydreaming and not listening to what is being said or asked. Shifts may occur from one unfinished task to another, with a growing clutter surrounding the child's path. Although chores or schoolwork often do not get completed, care must be taken in attributing this symptom to ADHD, because other problems such as oppositional behavior often occur and would be considered a normal developmental task during early childhood. These individuals often have problems with organizational skills, find tasks that require sustained mental effort unpleasant, and become aversive to such tasks (especially homework). Materials needed for such tasks typically become scattered, lost, or carelessly handled and damaged. Trivial stimuli such as household noises often distract these individuals, who then leave their assigned task to attend to the interrupting stimuli. They often forget and miss appointments, fail to meet schoolwork deadlines, or forget lunch money. As a result, academic achievement is often impaired.

Perceptual Manifestations
Perceptual problems are not usually a problem in ADHD.

Social Manifestations
Social problems may occur as a result of losing the train of conversation and changing topics inappropriately, not following expected rules of games or activities, and appearing uninterested in others. Family members frequently develop resentment and antagonism, particularly when the variability of symptoms leads parents to believe that their children's troublesome behavior is willful. ADHD can cause rejection by peers and conflicts with family and school authorities. Others often interpret inadequate self-application as laziness, irresponsibility, and oppositional behavior (APA, 1994).

PROGNOSIS
ADHD features persist into adolescence in 30% to 80% of children diagnosed as hyperactive and persist into adulthood in up to 65% of cases. A family history of ADHD, psychosocial adversity, and comorbidity with conduct, mood, and anxiety disorders increase the risk of persistence. Delinquent or antisocial behavior is seen in 25% to 40% of clinically referred ADHD children. Specific predictors of poor outcome include oppositional and aggressive behavior directed at adults, low IQ, poor peer relations, and continuing ADHD symptoms. Comorbid oppositional defiant disorder raises the risk of conduct disorder.

CONDUCT DISORDER
ETIOLOGY
Conduct disorder represents the most common reason for referral for psychiatric evaluation and represents 30% to 50% of all referrals in some clinics. The ratio of boys to girls is between 5:1 and 3:1.

Understanding & Applying Research

The overall purpose of this study was to test the prediction of young adult disturbance from adolescent assessment data collected during 1986 to 1992. A national sample included (n = 743) 366 men and 377 women who were 19 through 22 years old in 1992. Ethnicity was 75% non-Latino white, 15% African-American, and 11% other.

The research was reviewed using case-control analysis looking at family variables, cross-informant syndromes, competency scales, stressful experiences, and previous signs of disturbance. Predictive factors for school dropout, unwed pregnancy, mental health services, suicidal behavior, police contacts, being fired from jobs, alcohol abuse, drug use, and a total disturbance scale were assessed.

Study findings did determine that parents remain an important source of information about their children's difficulties, especially regarding anxious/depressed syndromes strongly associated with suicidal behaviors. Delinquent behaviors and poor school functioning predicted the worst outcomes, whereas good school performance was a protective factor. Multiple significant predictors indicate that signs of disturbance are most likely to be multidetermined rather than a direct result of a single event. Delinquent behavior and school functioning may be a good focus area to prevent multiple signs of disturbance among young adults. Further research will be ongoing to develop testing models that will be more precise in predicting signs of disturbance.

Achenback TM et al: Six-year predictors of problems in a national sample: IV. Young adult signs of disturbance, *J Am Acad Child Adolesc Psychiatry* 37:7, 1998.

The following factors have been identified as predisposing the child to conduct disorder: parental rejection and neglect, difficult infant temperament, inconsistent child-rearing practices with harsh discipline, physical or sexual abuse, lack of supervision, early institutional living, frequent changes of caregivers, large family size, association with a delinquent peer group, and certain family psychopathology (see Understanding & Applying Research box). Conduct disorder occurs more frequently when a biologic or adoptive parent has antisocial personality disorder; a biologic parent has alcohol dependence, a mood disorder, schizophrenia, or a history of ADHD or conduct disorder; or a sibling has conduct disorder (APA, 1994).

A definitive model of conduct disorder has not been developed. One possible model proposes a genetic liability triggered by environmental risk and mediated by factors such as poor coping skills (Steiner et al, 1997).

Rogeness (1994) reviewed biologic issues in conduct disorder. Findings indicate that clients with decreased noradrenergic activity and conduct disorder respond poorly to signs of impending punishment and therefore tend to have trouble internalizing societal rules. Studies tend to show that serotonin inhibits aggression, which leads to theories that low serotonin levels play a role in aggressive

acting-out behaviors (the expression of internal affective states through external activities and behaviors that are often destructive and/or maladaptive). The source of these neurotransmitter changes remains unclear, although some studies support psychosocial stress, such as parental neglect, as well as genetic factors.

At least some biologic alterations may be explained by the typical long-term and pronounced maltreatment and emotional trauma that most children with conduct disorder suffer. Other identified risk factors include birth complications, hyperactivity, cognitive deficits, speech and language problems, chronic illness and disability, a combination of early aggression with shyness or peer rejection, inadequate housing, crowding, poverty, and "training in noncompliance" by parental capitulation or inconsistent responses to the child's coercive behavior. Abusive and injurious parenting practices are the most influential risk factors, and child maltreatment is the most specific risk factor (Steiner et al, 1997).

Comorbid conditions frequently include ADHD, oppositional defiant disorder, mood and anxiety disorders, borderline personality disorder in girls, antisocial personality disorder in boys, mental retardation, and specific developmental disabilities (Steiner et al, 1997).

EPIDEMIOLOGY

According to DSM-IV, rates appear higher in urban than in rural settings and vary depending on the nature of the population sampled and methods of ascertainment used; for males under 18, rates vary from 6% to 16%; for females, rates vary from 2% to 9% (APA, 1994) (see DSM-IV Criteria box on p. 425). Bauermeister et al (1994) found the pattern of conduct disorder to be highest in 13- to 16-year-olds, with a sharp decline thereafter. In boys the prevalence reached a high point from 10 to 13 years of age, with a gradual decline from ages 13 to 20. In girls a gradual increase occurred in late childhood and early adolescence, peaking at age 16 and followed by a sharp decline.

CLINICAL DESCRIPTION
Behavioral Manifestations

Conduct disorder presents mainly with a repetitive and persistent pattern of behavior that violates the basic rights of others or major age-appropriate societal norms or rules. The behavior typically presents in a variety of settings, including home, school, and the community. But it can be difficult to detect because the child or adolescent tends to minimize the problems, and adults may not have full knowledge because of their inability to adequately supervise the child or adolescent.

Clients with conduct disorder manifest aggressive behavior and react aggressively toward others. They bully, threaten, and intimidate; initiate physical fights; use weapons in ways that could lead to injury; act cruelly to people

Conduct Disorder

DSM-IV CRITERIA

A. A repetitive and persistent pattern of behavior in which the basic rights of others or major age-appropriate norms or rules are violated, as manifested by the presence of three or more of the following criteria in the past 12 months, with at least one criterion present in the past 6 months:

Aggression to People or Animals
1. Often bullies, threatens, or intimidates others
2. Often initiates physical fights
3. Has used a weapon that can cause serious physical harm to others (e.g., a bat, brick, broken bottle, knife, gun)
4. Has been physically cruel to people
5. Has been physically cruel to animals
6. Has stolen while confronting a victim (e.g., mugging, purse snatching, extortion, armed robbery)
7. Has forced someone into sexual activity

Destruction of Property
8. Has deliberately engaged in fire setting with the intention of causing serious damage
9. Has deliberately destroyed others' property (other than by fire setting)

Deceitfulness or Theft
10. Has broken into someone else's house, building, or car
11. Often lies to obtain goods or favors or to avoid obligations (i.e., "cons" others)
12. Has stolen items of nontrivial value without confronting a victim (e.g., shoplifting, but without breaking and entering; forgery)

Serious Violations of Rules
13. Often stays out at night despite parental prohibitions, beginning before age 13 years
14. Has run away from home overnight at least twice while living in parental or parental surrogate home (or once without returning for a lengthy period)
15. Is often truant from school, beginning before age 13 years

B. The disturbance in behavior causes clinically significant impairment in social, academic, or occupational functioning.

C. If the individual is age 18 years or older, criteria are not met for antisocial personality disorder.

From American Psychiatric Association: *Diagnostic and statistical manual of mental disorders*, ed 4, Washington, DC, 1994, The Association.

or animals; steal; and force sexual activity. The severity of these behaviors may involve rape, assault, or (rarely) homicide. Deliberate destruction of property may result in fire damage, vandalism, and destruction of others' property for simple vengeance. In addition to theft or robbery, the child or adolescent may be deceitful, demonstrating frequent lying or breaking promises to obtain goods or favors or to avoid obligations or responsibility. Running away for safety in order to avoid physical or sexual abuse does not meet the criteria; the running away typically occurs in conjunction with violation of other norms and rules.

These clients also frequently attempt to avoid consequences by attempting to blame others. Early onset of behavior usually includes sexual activity, drinking, smoking, use of illegal substances, and other high-risk–taking acts. Behaviors usually persist into adulthood. These behaviors frequently lead to school suspensions, unplanned pregnancy, physical injury, sexually transmitted diseases, legal problems, dismissals from work or other activities, and the inability to attend regular schools.

Children or adolescents with conduct disorder generally exhibit callous behavior but may express guilt or remorse because they have learned that it may reduce or prevent punishment. This stated sense of remorse is often insincere and fabricated.

Although they may project an image of "toughness," they often experience low self-esteem with resulting poor frustration tolerance, irritability, temper outbursts, and reckless behavior.

Emotional Manifestations
Individuals with conduct disorders usually have little empathy or concern for the feelings, wishes, and well-being of others. Suicide ideation, attempts, and completions occur at a higher rate than expected.

Perceptual Manifestations
Clients with conduct disorder often have misconceptions about the intentions of others, especially in ambiguous situations. They typically perceive others as threatening and hostile and therefore feel justified in responding aggressively.

Cognitive Manifestations
Individuals with conduct disorder may have various learning disorders or impairments in cognitive functioning, such as borderline intelligence, but none appears specific to conduct disorder.

Social Manifestations
Accident rates appear higher. Peer relationships often are impaired as a result of the behaviors associated with conduct disorder (APA, 1994).

PROGNOSIS

Less severe symptoms tend to emerge initially. Males dominate in the childhood-onset group and tend to exhibit more fighting, stealing, vandalism, and school discipline problems. Females tend to have symptoms of lying, running away, substance use, and prostitution. Males tend to use more confrontational aggression; females tend to use more nonconfrontational behaviors. An onset of conduct disorder before age 10 (childhood-onset type) generally indicates a more severe and persistent type that often develops into adult antisocial personality disorder. These individuals typically are male, display more physical aggression, are more likely have oppositional defiant disorder during childhood, and meet full criteria for conduct disorder before puberty. Individuals in the adolescent-onset group (no symptoms of conduct disorder before age 10) display less aggression, are likely to have better peer relationships, and display conduct problems in groups (APA, 1994).

Delinquent behavior driven by peer pressure may respond better to attempts to limit negative peer contacts. Delinquent behavior resulting from an inability or unwillingness to change would not likely change by limiting peer contacts (Steiner et al, 1997).

OPPOSITIONAL DEFIANT DISORDER

ETIOLOGY

Oppositional defiant disorder occurs more often in families where child care has been disrupted by a succession of different caregivers, or where harsh, inconsistent, or neglectful child-rearing practices occur. The disorder occurs more commonly when serious marital problems are present (APA, 1994) (see DSM-IV Criteria box at right).

EPIDEMIOLOGY

Rates vary considerably from 2% to 16%, based on the nature of the population sample and method of assessment. Oppositional defiant disorder occurs more frequently in males before puberty and with approximately equal frequency after puberty. The disorder also occurs more commonly when at least one parent has a history of one of the following: mood disorder, oppositional defiant disorder, conduct disorder, ADHD, antisocial personality disorder, or a substance-related disorder. ADHD commonly occurs, and learning disorders and communication disorders tend to be associated with oppositional defiant disorder (APA, 1994).

CLINICAL DESCRIPTION

Behavioral Manifestations

The essential features of negativism, defiance, disobedience, and hostility toward authority figures typically present with persistent stubbornness, resistance to direc-

DSM-IV CRITERIA

Oppositional Defiant Disorder

A. A pattern of negativistic, hostile, and defiant behavior lasting at least 6 months, during which four or more of the following are present:
   1. Often loses temper
   2. Often argues with adults
   3. Often actively defies or refuses to comply with adults' requests or rules
   4. Often deliberately annoys people
   5. Often blames others for his or her mistakes or misbehavior
   6. Is often touchy or easily annoyed by others
   7. Is often angry and resentful
   8. Is often spiteful or vindictive
   NOTE: Consider a criterion met only if the behavior occurs more frequently than is typically observed in individuals of comparable age and developmental level.
B. The disturbance in behavior causes clinically significant impairment in social, academic, or occupational functioning.
C. The behaviors do not occur exclusively during the course of a psychotic or mood disorder.
D. Criteria are not met for conduct disorder, and, if the individual is age 18 years or older, criteria are not met for antisocial personality disorder.

From American Psychiatric Association: *Diagnostic and statistical manual of mental disorders*, ed 4, Washington, DC, 1994, The Association.

tions, and unwillingness to compromise, give in, or negotiate with adults. Evidence of defiance can also present as deliberate or persistent testing of limits, typically by ignoring directions, arguing, and refusing to accept responsibility for misbehavior. Hostility may be directed at adults or peers and includes deliberately annoying others verbally. Symptoms invariably present at home but may be absent or minimal at school and are generally directed toward those the child knows best. Individuals with oppositional defiant disorder do not tend to regard themselves as troublesome but blame others for making unreasonable demands or blame the circumstances.

Emotional Manifestations

During school years the following problems may be seen: low self-esteem, mood lability, and low frustration tolerance.

Cognitive and Perceptual Manifestations

Cognitive and perceptual symptoms do not usually present as significant symptoms in oppositional defiant disorder.

Social Manifestations

During early childhood, evidence of difficult temperament (e.g., high reactivity, difficulty in being soothed) or high motor activity has been noted. There may be swearing and precocious use of alcohol, tobacco, or illicit drugs. A negativistic cycle of parent and child bringing out the worst characteristics in each other frequently exists (APA, 1994).

PROGNOSIS

The onset is typically gradual, usually occurring over the course of months or years. In a significant number of cases, oppositional defiant disorder develops into conduct disorder.

TIC DISORDER: TOURETTE'S DISORDER

ETIOLOGY AND EPIDEMIOLOGY

Although genetically transmitted in an autosomal dominant pattern, penetrance of Tourette's disorder is only about 70% in females but reaches 99% in males (APA, 1994).

Tourette's disorder occurs in approximately 4 to 5 persons per 10,000. It is approximately 1.5 to 3 times more common in males than in females. Other disorders associated with Tourette's disorder include ADHD, obsessive-compulsive disorder, and learning disorders (APA, 1994) (see DSM IV Criteria box below).

CLINICAL DESCRIPTION

Behavioral Manifestations

Tics present as a physical symptom seen as behavior. A **tic** is defined as a sudden, rapid, recurrent, nonrhythmic, stereotyped motor movement or vocalization. Although experienced as irresistible, it can often be suppressed for a varying length of time. Stress typically exacerbates tics,

and absorbing activities such as reading or sewing may reduce them. Sleep markedly decreases tics.

Simple motor tics include eye blinking, neck jerking, shoulder shrugging, facial grimacing, and coughing. Simple vocal tics include throat clearing, grunting, sniffing, snorting, and barking. Complex motor tics include facial gestures, grooming behaviors, jumping, touching, stamping, smelling an object, and echokinesis (imitation of another's movements). Complex vocal tics include repeating words or phrases out of context, coprolalia (repeating socially unacceptable words, typically obscene or swear words), palilalia (repeating one's own sounds or words), and echolalia (repeating the last-heard word, sound, or phrase).

In Tourette's disorder the number, type, frequency, complexity, and severity of the tics vary over time. Most common tics in Tourette's disorder involve the head and parts of the body such as the torso and limbs. Common vocal tics include clicks, grunts, barks, sniffs, snorts, and coughs. Coprolalia occurs in less than 10% of the cases. Complex motor tics reported in Tourette's disorder include touching, squatting, deep knee bends, retracing steps, and twirling during walking. The most frequent initial tic is blinking. Other initial tics reported include tongue protrusion, squatting, sniffing, hopping, skipping, throat clearing, stuttering, uttering sounds or words, and coprolalia. Other relatively common issues include hyperactivity, distractibility, and impulsivity. Retinal detachment can occur from head banging; orthopedic problems can occur from knee bending, neck jerking, or head turning; and skin problems can result from picking.

Emotional Manifestations

Shame, self-consciousness, and depressed mood may occur as a secondary result of problems stemming from Tourette's disorder.

Cognitive Manifestations

Obsessions and compulsions make up the most common cognitive features seen in a client with Tourette's disorder.

Perceptual Manifestations

Perceptual problems are not a typical problem area in Tourette's disorder.

Social Manifestations

Frequently reported associated symptoms include social discomfort and rejection by others that interfere with social, academic, and occupational functioning. In severe cases tics may interfere with activities of daily living, such as reading or eating, or cause medical complications (APA, 1994).

PROGNOSIS

Tourette's disorder may begin as early as 2 years of age but typically presents during childhood or early adolescence. Although it is almost always a lifelong disorder, in most

---

DSM-IV CRITERIA

Tourette's Disorder

A. Both multiple motor and one or more vocal tics have been present at some time during the illness, although not necessarily concurrently.
B. The tics occur many times a day (usually in bouts) nearly every day or intermittently throughout a period of more than 1 year, and during this period there was never a tic-free period of more than 3 consecutive months.
C. The disturbance causes marked distress or significant impairment in social, occupational, or other important areas of functioning.
D. The onset is before age 18.
E. The disturbance is not due to the direct physiologic effects of a substance (e.g., stimulants) or a general medical condition (e.g., Huntington's disease or postviral encephalitis).

From American Psychiatric Association: *Diagnostic and statistical manual of mental disorders*, ed 4, Washington, DC, 1994, The Association.

cases symptoms diminish during adolescence and adulthood (APA, 1994).

OTHER TIC DISORDERS
CHRONIC MOTOR OR VOCAL TIC DISORDER

Chronic motor or vocal tic disorder resembles Tourette's disorder, except the tics may be either motor or vocal and need not be multiple. It also tends to be less severe (APA, 1994).

TRANSIENT TIC DISORDER

The diagnosis of transient tic disorder is made if the tics last more than 1 year. Otherwise, the criteria are the same as for Tourette's disorder but symptoms typically occur with less severity (APA, 1994).

TIC DISORDER NOT OTHERWISE SPECIFIED

The diagnosis of tic disorder not otherwise specified is used when other, more specific diagnoses cannot be made. Examples include tics lasting less than 4 weeks or tics with an onset after 18 years of age (APA, 1994).

SEPARATION ANXIETY DISORDER
ETIOLOGY AND EPIDEMIOLOGY

Separation anxiety disorder appears to be more common in first-degree relatives and may be more common in children whose mothers have panic disorder. It may develop after some life stress (e.g., death of a relative or pet, illness in the child or parent, or a change in the environment) (APA, 1994).

This disorder occurs in approximately 4% of children and adolescents and is more common in females. It typically presents before late adolescence (APA, 1994) (see DSM-IV Criteria box below).

CLINICAL DESCRIPTION
Behavioral Manifestations

With a need to know the whereabouts of their parents or others, individuals with separation anxiety often display attempts to stay in touch with frequent telephone calls. Because of significant discomfort in being away from home, they may become resistant to traveling alone and reluctant to attend activities that other peers enjoy and look forward to, such as camp, school, and sleepovers at friends' houses. They may not stay in a room alone. Children with separation anxiety disorder may demonstrate clinging behavior; they may attempt to shadow their parents around the home and, with increasing frequency and intensity, attempt to shadow their parents outside the home. Bedtime can be quite difficult, with the child or adolescent insisting that the parent remain with him or her until he or she falls asleep. During the night these individuals may attempt to get in bed with the parents or another significant figure; if their way is obstructed, they may sleep outside the parents' or other's door.

Physical complaints often appear during actual or anticipated separation and frequently include stomachaches,

---

DSM-IV CRITERIA

Separation Anxiety

A. Developmentally inappropriate and excessive anxiety concerning separation from home or from those to whom the individual is attached, as evidenced by three or more of the following:
1. Recurrent excessive distress when separation from home or major attachment figures occurs or is anticipated
2. Persistent and excessive worry about losing or possible harm befalling major attachment figures
3. Persistent and excessive worry that an untoward event will lead to separation from a major attachment figure (e.g., getting lost or being kidnapped)
4. Persistent reluctance or refusal to go to school or elsewhere because of fear of separation
5. Persistent and excessive fear or reluctance to be alone or without major attachment figures at home, or without significant adults in other settings
6. Persistent reluctance or refusal to go to sleep without being near a major attachment figure or to sleep away from home
7. Repeated nightmares with the theme of separation
8. Repeated complaints of physical symptoms (such as headaches, stomachaches, nausea, or vomiting) when separation from major attachment figures occurs or is anticipated
B. The duration of the disturbance is at least 4 weeks.
C. The onset is before age 18.
D. The disturbance causes clinically significant distress or impairment in social, academic (occupational), or other important areas of functioning.
E. The disturbance does not occur exclusively during the course of a pervasive developmental disorder, schizophrenia, or other psychotic disorder and, in adolescents and adults, is not better accounted for by panic disorder with agoraphobia.

From American Psychiatric Association: *Diagnostic and statistical manual of mental disorders*, ed 4, Washington, DC, 1994, The Association.

headaches, nausea, and vomiting. Older children and adolescents may experience a racing or pounding heart, dizziness, and faintness. The somatic complaints often lead to numerous trips to physicians and subsequent medical procedures.

Emotional Manifestations

Individuals with this disorder may experience recurrent, excessive distress when they are away from home or major attachment figures. Some become extremely distraught and miserable away from home and become preoccupied with reunion fantasies. They may become extremely fearful that some imagined harm will happen to the significant other(s). Fears about danger to themselves or their families may present as fear of animals, monsters, the dark, muggers, burglars, kidnappers, accidents, or plane or train travel. Fears may also present as concerns about death and dying. They may show various moods, such as excessive worry that no one loves them and they therefore want to die, or unusual anger when someone tries to separate them from their parent or significant other. The depressed mood may at times justify a diagnosis of depression. As adulthood is reached, some of these individuals may develop panic disorder with agoraphobia.

Cognitive Manifestations

Nightmares often contain elements of the individual's fears, such as family death through fire, murder, or other catastrophe. Academic difficulties may result from refusal to attend school and thus increase the problem with social avoidance.

Perceptual Manifestations

When alone, young children may experience perceptual problems such as seeing people peering into their room, scary creatures reaching for them, and eyes staring at them.

Social Manifestations

With a typically close-knit family, clients with separation anxiety disorder may exhibit social withdrawal, apathy, sadness, or concentration difficulties at work or play when away from the parents or significant others. Families frequently experience significant conflict, with parental resentment and frustration. At times, however, these children may also become unusually conscientious, compliant, and eager to please. Parents often describe these children as demanding, intrusive, and in need of constant attention; the children may physically strike out (APA, 1994).

PROGNOSIS

Typically there are periods of severity and reduction of symptoms. Both the anxiety about possible separation and the avoidance of situations involving separation may persist for many years.

ELIMINATION DISORDERS: ENCOPRESIS

ETIOLOGY AND EPIDEMIOLOGY

Certain conditions such as inadequate, inconsistent toilet training and psychosocial stress (e.g., entering school or the birth of a sibling) may predispose the child to **encopresis** (APA, 1994), which is the repeated passage of feces into inappropriate places, whether involuntary or intentional.

Approximately 1% of 5-year-olds have encopresis. It is more common in males (APA, 1994) (see DSM-IV Criteria box below).

CLINICAL DESCRIPTION

Most often the fecal soiling is involuntary, but at times it may be intentional. Fecal soiling often is the result of a power struggle between the child or adolescent and an authority figure. It is not due to the direct physiologic effects of a substance such as laxatives or a medical condition except through a mechanism involving constipation. Involuntary soiling often involves constipation, impaction, and retention with leakage around the hardened stool. The underlying reason for constipation typically involves a psychologic reason such as anxiety specific to a place or a more general pattern of oppositional or anxious behavior.

ASSOCIATED FEATURES

Individuals with encopresis often feel ashamed about the condition and attempt to avoid situations that would lead to further embarrassment, such as camp, school, and sleepovers. Impairment generally relates to the effects of social ostracism, as well as anger, punishment, and rejection by caregivers, on the child's self-esteem. Smearing as an associated feature may be due to an attempt to clean or hide feces or may be more clearly deliberate. When deliberate, the individual often exhibits features of oppositional defiant disorder or conduct disorder (APA, 1994).

DSM-IV CRITERIA

Encopresis

A. Repeated passage of feces into inappropriate places (e.g., clothing or floor) whether involuntary or intentional.
B. At least one such event a month for at least 3 months.
C. Chronologic age is at least 4 years (or equivalent developmental level).
D. The behavior is not due exclusively to the direct physiologic effects of a substance (e.g., laxatives) or a general medical condition except through a mechanism involving constipation.

From American Psychiatric Association: *Diagnostic and statistical manual of mental disorders*, ed 4, Washington, DC, 1994, The Association.

PROGNOSIS

Encopresis can persist for years with remissions and exacerbations but rarely becomes chronic (APA, 1994).

ELIMINATION DISORDERS: ENURESIS

ETIOLOGY AND EPIDEMIOLOGY

Enuresis is the repeated voiding of urine into the bed or clothes, whether involuntary or intentional. Some possible predisposing factors include delayed or lax toilet training, psychosocial stress, a dysfunction in the ability to concentrate urine, and a lower bladder volume threshold for involuntary voiding (APA, 1994).

At 5 years of age, 7% of boys and 3% of girls experience enuresis. At 10 years of age, 3% of boys and 2% of girls experience it (APA, 1994) (see DSM-IV Criteria box below).

CLINICAL DESCRIPTION AND ASSOCIATED FEATURES

The diagnostic criteria for enuresis present the typical problem of voiding in inappropriate places during the day or night when control is expected. Impairment usually comes from interference with social activities or the effects of social ostracism and caregiver anger, rejection, and punishment on the child's self-esteem. Other disorders sometimes seen with enuresis include encopresis, sleepwalking disorder, and sleep terror disorder (APA, 1994).

PROGNOSIS

Enuresis persists at age 18 in only 1% of boys and less for girls. Only about 1% of cases continue into adulthood. About 75% of all children with enuresis have a first-degree relative who had the disorder (APA, 1994).

DSM-IV CRITERIA

Enuresis

A. Repeated voiding of urine into bed or clothes (whether involuntary or intentional).
B. The behavior is clinically significant as manifested by either a frequency of twice a week for at least 3 consecutive months or the presence of clinically significant distress or impairment in social, academic (occupational), or other important areas of functioning.
C. Chronologic age is at least 5 years (or equivalent developmental level).
D. The behavior is not due exclusively to the direct physiologic effect of a substance (e.g., a diuretic) or a general medical condition (e.g., diabetes, spina bifida, or a seizure disorder).

From American Psychiatric Association: *Diagnostic and statistical manual of mental disorders*, ed 4, Washington, DC, 1994, The Association.

DEVELOPMENTAL DISORDERS: LEARNING DISORDER, COORDINATION DISORDER, COMMUNICATION DISORDER

ETIOLOGY

Learning disorders are associated with a number of factors, such as genetic predisposition, perinatal injury, and various neurologic or medical conditions. However, these conditions do not inevitably predict learning disorders. Certain medical conditions have a strong association with learning disorders: lead poisoning, fetal alcohol syndrome, and fragile X syndrome. A number of factors must be ruled out when evaluating for a learning disorder: normal variations in academic attainment, lack of opportunity, inadequate teaching, cultural factors, and impaired hearing or vision (APA, 1994).

EPIDEMIOLOGY

A growing consensus supports the theory that genetic factors play a significant role in the determination of reading ability and disability. Two distinct reading problems have been linked to chromosome 6 (phonologic awareness) and chromosome 15 (single-word reading) (Breitchman and Yound, 1997).

Learning disorders are found in about 2% to 10% of children, depending on the nature of assessment and the definitions applied. Approximately 5% of public school students have an identified learning disorder. Reading disorder affects an estimated 4% of school-age children in the United States, and approximately 1% of school-age children have mathematics disorder. Prevalence has not been clearly established for disorder of written expression, but it is rare when not associated with other learning disorders. Motor coordination disorder may affect as many as 6% of 5- to 11-year-old children. Developmental expressive language disorder occurs in approximately 3% to 5% of children and is acquired in fewer children. The developmental type of mixed receptive-expressive language disorder is estimated at up to 3% of school-age children. About 2% to 3% of 6- and 7-year-olds show phonologic disorder, which falls to 0.5% by age 17. Stuttering occurs in 1% of prepubertal children and drops to 0.8% in adolescence. Males predominate with a ratio of 3 : 1 over females (APA, 1994).

CLINICAL DESCRIPTION

Learning Disorders

The National Joint Committee on Learning Disabilities defines learning disabilities as follows (Breitchman and Yound, 1997).

Learning disabilities is a general term that refers to a heterogeneous group of disorders manifested by significant difficulties in the acquisition and use of listening, speaking, reading, writing, reasoning, or mathematic abilities. These disorders are intrinsic to the individual, presumed to be due to central nervous system dysfunction, and may occur across the life span. Problems in self-regulatory behaviors, social perception, and social interaction may exist with learning disabilities but do not by themselves constitute a learning disability.

Learning disorders encompass problems with reading, writing, math, and a not-otherwise-specified category. The disorders are diagnosed through individually administered, standardized tests when performance is substantially below expected (generally defined as 1 to 2 standard deviations below the average) and when there is significant interference with academic achievement or activities of daily living. Many problems can result from learning disorders, including demoralization, low self-esteem, and deficits in social skills. Children and adolescents with learning disorders drop out of school at a rate of nearly 40% (approximately 1.5 the average rate). Ten percent to 25% of individuals with conduct disorder, oppositional defiant disorder, ADHD, major depression, or dysthymic disorders have learning disorders as well. Language delay may occur in learning disorders, and learning disorders may be associated with a higher rate of developmental coordination disorder. Underlying abnormalities in cognitive abilities may exist (e.g., deficits in visual perception, linguistic processes, attention, memory, or a combination) that often precede or are associated with learning disorders.

Coordination Disorders

Developmental coordination disorder is only diagnosed if motor coordination significantly interferes with academic achievement or activities of daily living and is not due to a medical condition (e.g., cerebral palsy or muscular dystrophy). Specific activities or tasks that may be impaired or altered include walking, crawling, sitting, tying shoelaces, buttoning shirts, or zipping pants. Communication disorders also may be associated (APA, 1994).

Communication Disorders

Expressive language disorder features vary but may include a limited amount of speech, limited range of vocabulary, difficulty acquiring new words, word-finding or vocabulary errors, shortened sentences, simplified grammar use, omissions of critical parts of a sentence, use of unusual word order, and slow rate of language development. Intelligence measured by performance tests is usually normal. Expressive language disorder may be acquired as a result of a neurologic or medical condition (e.g., encephalitis, head trauma, or irradiation) or developmental (i.e., no known neurologic condition). Mixed receptive-expressive language disorder symptoms include receptive difficulties (e.g., markedly limited vocabulary, errors in tense, difficulty recalling words or producing developmentally appropriate sentences, and general difficulty expressing ideas) and language development problems (e.g., difficulty understanding words, sentences, or specific types

of words). As with expressive language disorder, mixed receptive-expressive language disorder may be developmental or acquired. A child may initially appear confused or inattentive, follow commands incorrectly, and give inappropriate responses to questions. The child may appear quiet or unusually talkative. Other communication disorders include phonologic disorder (problems using expected speech sounds) and stuttering (a disturbance in normal fluency and time patterns of speech) (APA, 1994).

PROGNOSIS

The prognosis for reading disorder is good with early identification and intervention, but the disorder may persist into adult life. The degree of impairment usually depends on the overall intelligence level in mathematics disorder. Brighter children may be able to function at or near grade level in early grades, but by the fifth grade the reading disorder almost always becomes apparent. The course of written expression disorder has not been clearly defined. Motor coordination disorder has a variable course and may last into adolescence or adulthood. Approximately one half of children with developmental expressive language disorder outgrow it, whereas the other half have long-lasting difficulties. In the acquired type, recovery depends on the severity and location of the injury, as well as the child's age at the time of occurrence. Recovery may be rapid and complete, or the injury may get progressively worse. The prognosis for mixed receptive-expressive language disorder of the acquired type is worse than for expressive language disorder. The acquired type has a variable prognosis-like expressive language disorder. The prognosis for phonologic disorder varies according to the cause and severity. In severe cases speech may not be recognizable and the disorder may persist, whereas mild cases may remit spontaneously. Stuttering typically occurs insidiously and, when noticed, has a waxing and waning course. Recovery occurs in up to 80%, of cases and spontaneously in 60%. Recovery typically occurs at age 16 (APA, 1994).

DISCHARGE CRITERIA

Client will:

Engage in self-care within level of capability.

Demonstrate emotional control within capacity.

Attend to tasks, schoolwork, and performance without undue anger or frustration.

Exhibit healthy self-concept and self-esteem.

Demonstrate functional eating habits and behaviors appropriate for age and stature.

Use cognitive, communication, and language skills to make self understood and to get needs met.

Demonstrate interactive skills appropriate for level of development.

Verbalize satisfaction with gender identity and sexual preference.

Interact meaningfully with staff, peers, and family within capability.

Seek attention and assistance appropriately from significant persons and refrain from undue or unnecessary interactions with strangers.

Adhere to treatment regimen, including medication as needed.

Play appropriately with peers.

Engage in educational and vocational programs within capacity.

Use adaptive coping techniques and stress-reducing strategies.

Respond satisfactorily to others' attentions and requests.

Use community resources to enhance quality of life.

Engage in ongoing individual and family therapy.

CHILD ABUSE

Child abuse, which may include physical or sexual abuse, neglect, or being a witness to violence, produces many problems that need to be addressed in childhood and adolescence. There is a significant increase in rates of physical aggression and antisocial acts by victims of child abuse. Aggressive behavior and inappropriate sexual behavior make up the single most common symptom in sexually abused children. Other problems include delinquency, violence, running away, substance abuse, and teen pregnancy (Bellis and Putnam, 1994).

In 1993 the National Research Council reported that 9.4 to 107 cases of child abuse occurred per 1000 children per year (Bellis and Putnam, 1994). In 1990 the U.S. Advisory Board on Child Abuse reported 1.5 million cases of child abuse and 3.3 million cases of children being exposed to violence. It gave rates of 5.7 cases of physical abuse per 1000 children per year and 2.5 cases of sexual abuse per 1000 children per year (Lewis, 1994) (see Chapter 27).

ADOLESCENT SUICIDE

Adolescent suicide does not neatly fall under any diagnostic category. Adolescent suicides have quadrupled since 1950 from 2.5 to 11.2 per 100,000 and currently represent 12% of all deaths in this age-group. It ranks second only to accidents as the leading cause of death in adolescents. Reported predisposing factors include anxiety, disruptive disorder, bipolar disorder, substance abuse and personality disorders, a family history of mood disorders, a family history of suicidal behavior, exposure to family violence, impulsivity, and availability of methods.

Shaffer (1974) found two groups at risk for completed suicide in a late childhood/early adolescent sample: (1) intelligent and isolated individuals with mothers who had a psychiatric disorder and (2) aggressive, suspicious individuals with school problems who were vulnerable to criticism. Both groups displayed antisocial behavior. The suicide was most often precipitated by a disciplinary crisis.

Thompson (1987) found that those younger than 15 tended to be more angry and nervous and less depressed than the older adolescents. Hanging was the most common method in the 10- to 15-year age-group, and firearms were the most common method in later adolescence. Fewer warning signs and fewer precipitating events preceded the suicide in children and young adolescents. Intoxication and romantic failure did not appear to constitute a risk in those younger than 15, as so often occurs in older adolescents.

ADULT DISORDERS IN CHILDREN AND ADOLESCENTS
SUBSTANCE ABUSE

Although a large number of adolescents try drugs or alcohol, the majority do not progress to abuse or dependence. In 1996 the annual Monitoring the Future Study found that nearly one third of high school seniors reported having been drunk in the past month and one fifth reported marijuana use. Nearly 5% reported daily marijuana use (Weinberg et al, 1998).

By the end of high school approximately 90% of students have tried alcohol and 40% have tried an illicit drug, typically marijuana (Bukstein et al, 1997).

It is believed that drug use appears to be more a function of social and peer factors, whereas abuse and dependence are more related to biologic and psychologic processes. Risk factors include the following: executive cognitive dysfunction; disorders of behavioral self-regulation; difficulties with planning, attention, abstract reasoning, foresight, judgment, self-monitoring, and motor control; need for sensation seeking; difficulties with affect regulation; drug-abusing parents; maternal depression; and anxiety. Factors that are thought to protect against use include the following: intelligence, problem-solving ability, social facility, positive self-esteem, supportive family relationships, positive role models, and affect regulation (Weinberg et al, 1998).

DEPRESSION

Population studies report a prevalence between 0.4% and 2.5% in children and 0.4% and 8.3% in adolescents, with a lifetime prevalence of major depression in adolescents of 15% to 20%. Developmentally, symptoms of melancholia, psychosis, suicide attempts, lethality of attempts, and impairment of functioning increase with age. Symptoms of separation anxiety, phobias, **somatic complaints,** and behavioral problems occur more frequently in children. Psychotic depression manifests in children as auditory hallucinations instead of delusions, as seen in adolescents and adults. Children and adolescents with depression have a comorbid diagnosis in 40% to 70% of cases; those with dysthymic disorder or anxiety have a comorbid diagnosis in 30% to 80% of cases; those with disruptive disorders have comorbidity in 10% to 80% of cases; and those with substance abuse have comorbidity in 20% to 30% of cases (Birmaher et al, 1996).

BIPOLAR DISORDER

Children frequently present with atypical symptoms. They are often markedly labile and erratic rather than persistent and are irritable, belligerent, or mixed rather than euphoric. Reckless behavior often leads to school failure, fighting, dangerous play, and inappropriate sexual activity. These symptoms must be differentiated from common childhood phenomena of boasting, imaginary play, overactivity, and youthful indiscretions (McClellan et al, 1997).

A child may appear amusing and show misleading infectious cheerfulness in the midst of significant problems such as school suspensions and family fights. The thinking of these children frequently defies logic. These children or adolescents often harass teachers about how to teach the class. They may fail intentionally because they believe they are being taught incorrectly. They may hold a belief that they will achieve in a prominent profession despite failing grades. They may believe that stealing is legal for them. In contrast, conduct-disordered children and adolescents know that stealing is wrong but believe they are above the law.

They often overreact to minor perturbations in the environment, behave inappropriately sexually by propositioning teachers and making overt comments to peers, call sex (1-900) lines, become overly interested in money and purchase items from (1-800) lines with others' credit cards, and take more dangerous dares, believing that they are above the possibility of danger.

PSYCHOSIS

Schizophrenia rarely presents before 12 years of age, although cases have been documented as young as 3 and 5 years of age. An onset before age 13 usually has an insidious nature and includes withdrawal, odd behavior, and isolation. Other developmental delays have been noted, including lags in cognitive, motor, sensory, and social functioning (McClellan et al, 1997).

The presence of psychosis in preschool-age children presents an extremely difficult problem. Transient hallucinations under stress, imaginary friends, and fantasy figures are common. By the school-age years, persistent hallucinations are associated with serious disorders. Delusional content and hallucinations usually reflect developmental concerns. Hallucinations often include monsters, pets, or toys, and delusions typically revolve around identity issues and are less complex and systemic. After age 7, loose and illogical thinking does not usually occur in normal children.

ANXIETY DISORDERS

A pediatric primary care sample revealed a 1-year prevalence of 15.4% in 7- to 11-year-olds. Epidemiologic studies in nonreferred 11-year-olds documented the following prevalences: separation anxiety, 3.5%; overanxious disorder, 2.9%; simple phobia, 2.4%; social phobia, 1%. Risk factors for development of anxiety disorders in children include behavioral inhibition, insecure attachment, cognitive factors, developmental events, traumatic events, and access to support systems (Bernstein, Borchardt, and Perwien, 1996).

Developmental differences exist in the symptoms of anxiety. Children ages 5 to 8 most commonly report unrealistic worry about harm to parents and attachment figures and school refusal. From ages 9 to 12, children report excessive distress at times of separation. Adolescents typically report somatic complaints and school refusal. At any age, unrealistic worry about future events is key in overanxious disorder in children and adolescents. School refusal is present in three quarters of those identified with separation anxiety disorder.

In a community sample, more than two fifths of youths met criteria for exposure to at least one major trauma by age 18. Six percent met the criteria for a lifetime diagnosis of posttraumatic stress disorder. Avoidance symptoms were more common in younger children. They were more likely to have spontaneous intrusive phenomena. Older children reported more reexperiencing and arousal, particularly with specific reminders. After a natural disaster, separation from parents, ongoing maternal preoccupation with the event, and altered family functioning were greater predictors of symptom development than exposure alone.

Obsessive-compulsive disorder has a 6-month prevalence of 1 in 200 children and adolescents. Children typically demonstrate normal age-dependent obsessive-compulsive behaviors such as wanting things done "just so" and may insist on elaborate bedtime rituals. These behaviors are usually gone by middle childhood and are replaced by collections, hobbies, and focused interest. These can be reliably discriminated on the basis of timing, content, and severity. Frequently observed symptoms in children and adolescents include the following: obsessions (contamination fears); worry about harm to self or others; aggressive themes; sexual ideas; scrupulosity/religiosity; forbidden thoughts; symmetry urges; need to tell, ask, or confess; and compulsions (washing, repeating, checking, touching, counting, ordering/arranging, hoarding, praying).

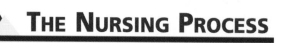

THE NURSING PROCESS

The nursing process (assessment, nursing diagnosis, outcome identification, planning, implementation, and evaluation) is applicable to children and adolescents in the psychiatric setting. Working with children and adolescents can be a very rewarding job opportunity for nurses. When working within the mental health setting, this population can be a major challenge to even the most skilled nurse. Knowledge of growth and development is essential, as is the ability to do a thorough clinical assessment, including both medical and psychosocial aspects. The child or adolescent must be assessed within the context of the entire family structure and dynamics, including the cultural and socioeconomic situation.

Parents often seek treatment for the child or adolescent after being referred by the school system or after their own multiple attempts to change the child or adolescent have been unsuccessful. Parents may present a medical concern (e.g., a stomachache) as the primary identified problem, when the underlying primary problem is often one of a psychiatric nature. It can be very difficult for adults to comprehend that children, especially young children, have mental disorders. As a result, treatment may be delayed for years in the hope that the child will "grow out of it."

Although it is common for a family to present a child or adolescent as the "identified client" (family member with the problem), it is very important to remember that children will often act out the underlying family dynamics or family psychopathology. In addition, families may be in denial that the child may have a disorder that has been identified in other family members, such as tic disorders, obsessive-compulsive disorders, mood disorders, or psychosis.

In addition to the nursing process, the nurse will focus on educating the entire family about the disorder and family system dynamics, since most children and adolescents will continue to live with their families.

Families may be eager for increased positive behaviors from the child but fail to change previous verbal and nonverbal patterns of interaction that may be punitive or negative.

Families can be skeptical of proposed treatment recommendations and discredit the therapeutic interventions. They may continue to use unhealthy multigenerational parenting techniques. Families may see initial improvement from a child or adolescent in treatment and then discontinue newly adopted interventions. This will inevitably result in the relapse of the child or adolescent's condition and family dysfunction. The child or adolescent may suffer academically and socially because of lack of implementation of treatment. With time and continuing growth of the child or adolescent, months or years of progress and development may be lost if the family does not continue with recommended treatment.

Treatment success and outcome depend on family commitment to learning new skills and consistently applying them. Early assessment and intervention from all caregivers and educators is the most ideal treatment goal.

Setting realistic and achievable goals within the family system may be one of the biggest challenges in the nursing process. Treatment may be very short term and result in only one or two target behaviors as the focus of treatment.

ASSESSMENT

As the nurse assesses children and adolescents, it is critical to have thorough understanding of growth and development. In addition, the nurse will have taken a thorough history, which will reveal the child or adolescent's baseline level of functioning for the past year and the current level of functioning. As the nurse obtains the history, it is significant to identify and ask caretakers about the child or adolescent's strengths and positive characteristics. Caretakers can be so exasperated with the child or adolescent at the onset of treatment that it may be difficult for them to identify strengths. It is common for children and adolescents to not demonstrate the negative behaviors for several weeks, in both inpatient and outpatient settings. Once the child or adolescent begins to act out his or her true behavioral problems, knowing and using the child's strengths can enhance the nurse-client relationship.

As the child or adolescent challenges the nurse in the treatment process, it will be of great value to maximize treatment goals based on strengths identified during the assessment phase. Children and adolescents have the potential and often the desire to obtain help and improve. It can be very rewarding for the nurse to see the client's improvement and know that the nursing process can result in a major life-changing outcome for the client and the family.

DEVELOPMENTAL STAGE

Each child and adolescent attempts to progress along the course of growth and development in all aspects of his or her life. Some, however, struggle in areas such as social skills, language, cognition, or moral, psychologic, cultural, or behavioral development. Because each child and adolescent has unique strengths and weaknesses, the nurse is challenged to assess the patient in the context of the family culture and socioeconomic circumstances throughout the developmental phases of normal growth and development. Children and adolescents may experience developmental delays as a result of family traumas, social deprivation, abuse, neglect, or complications from a major mental disorder. Children and adolescents may be advanced in developmental phases in some aspects of their life, such as cognition, but may be retarded in other aspects, such as social skills, at the same time.

CLINICAL ALERT

The nurse must be acutely observant of the ADHD child or adolescent taking medications. Children or adolescents taking stimulant medications such as methylphenidate hydrochloride (Ritalin) may demonstrate adverse changes in appetite, sleep, and levels of restlessness. In addition, children or adolescents may develop new tics or have an exacerbation of previously existent mild tics. It is imperative that the nurse hold the medication, document the findings, and notify the provider of the clinical observations. Often changes in dosage or discontinuance of the medication is required.

PHYSICAL ASSESSMENT

A thorough physical assessment involving all body systems and history is important in providing a comprehensive mental health evaluation. The nurse plays a key role in identifying potential health conditions that may contribute to the overall health and well-being of the child or adolescent. The nurse usually assesses the child or adolescent's immunization history, nutrition, grooming, and dental hygiene status. In addition, the nurse may assess other health care information such as allergies, otitis media, sinusitis, asthma, gastrointestinal and gastrourinary functioning, diabetes, scoliosis, or other preexisting conditions. It is important to be alert for undiagnosed health care conditions such as abnormal neurologic signs that may have a direct impact on the well-being of the child or adolescent's optimal level of functioning.

FAMILY LIFE

The child or adolescent's family life and home environment are crucial during assessment for comprehensive understanding of the presenting mental health problems. Many of today's families are blended and diverse, with mixed races, cultures, religions, and beliefs. An increasing number of families are affected by separation and divorce. The traditional family unit is no longer the only model. Our society has families where children and adolescents are being raised by homosexual parents or parents who elect to live with significant others without marriage. Other families may have the grandparents assuming the role of the primary caregivers as a result of financial problems, drug abuse, HIV or AIDS, death, or other situations where the biologic parents are unable to raise the child or adolescent.

The nurse must gain an understanding of the types of interactions within the family relationships and each member's perception of the issues. It is important for the nurse to understand characteristics of the home environment, including cleanliness and the size of the home, where and with whom the child or adolescent sleeps, patterns for meals, pet care, chores, homework, times and frequencies of recreational activities, and bedtime rituals.

CASE STUDY

Cody, an intelligent 9-year-old boy, is reported by his parents to be argumentative, irritable, and not able to follow through on simple instructions, needing constant reminders. It takes him hours to complete his homework every evening. He becomes easily frustrated and is not able to finish his assignments. At school, his teacher reports that he is restless, talks out of turn, interrupts, and frequently leaves his seat to disturb other students in the classroom. During recess he is constantly fighting with peers and is unable to make friends at school. In his neighborhood, none of the children want him on their team because he is a poor sport and argues about all the rules.

Critical Thinking—Assessment

1. What is an appropriate level of adult supervision for a 9-year-old? Why?
2. What effect will punishment have on Cody's school progress?
3. Is Cody's self-esteem positive or negative, based on his peer interactions?
4. Are Cody's frustrations a result of being a bad child or being a child in need of therapeutic intervention?

CLINICAL ALERT

When working with children, the nurse must remember that the child or adolescent is a minor and that the primary caregiver/guardian has legal rights in addition to the child's rights. Children and adolescents can give **assent,** and caregivers/guardians give informed consent. This applies to all forms of treatment such as medications and research studied and, in the inpatient setting, to all client rights, including admission to the mental health units, and seclusion and restraint.

Whenever possible, the nurse should obtain the child or adolescent's signature on all assent and consent forms in addition to the caregiver/guardian's signature.

ACTIVITIES OF DAILY LIVING

The child or adolescent's activities of daily living (ADL) reveal much about the child or adolescent's level of independence or dependence and current level of developmental functioning. Many families struggle with their children or adolescents over ADL, and a thorough assessment may reveal family dynamics with expectations that are either too high or too low for the child or adolescent. Children and adolescents often act out family power struggles over the expectations of ADL. These power struggles may occur daily in the morning in getting the child or adolescent up and off to school, on return from school, and at bedtime. Excessive consequences or punishments, and even negative rituals, may develop within the family structure centered around the ADL. The nurse may have a powerful impact in the role of establishing age-appropriate expectations and in teaching successful behavioral techniques to the child or adolescent and the caregivers, which promotes positive family interactions centered around ADL.

NURSING DIAGNOSIS

The nursing diagnosis process for children and adolescents is similar to that for adult clients. Accurate diagnosis always follows a thorough and astute assessment. As has been stated, the key to working effectively with children and adolescents is the accurate assessment of growth and development issues. This allows for an accurate, realistic diagnostic process. The family must be taken into consideration in this process as well.

All currently used NANDA nursing diagnoses are applicable to children and adolescents. However, because of the tendency for children and adolescents to act out the many issues they struggle with, some diagnoses may be more important. Safety issues are significant with any client in the mental health setting. It is even more crucial for children and adolescents, because even children who are developing normally may have little impulse control. Thus diagnoses such as violence, risk for: directed at others; violence, risk for: self-directed; and injury, risk for, are important for the nurse to consider. This is especially true in some of the pervasive developmental disorders where autistic behaviors can lead to self-mutilating activities and, in the case of attention-deficit/hyperactivity disorder, where extreme impulsivity and hyperactive behavior can result in injury.

Communication and relationship issues present a challenge for the diagnostic process. Children, especially young children, often do not have adequate verbal skills with which to communicate needs and feelings to the nurse. In some developmental disorders this may be even more of a complicating factor. For adolescents, mistrust of authority and power may cause difficulty in the development of the nurse-client relationship and hinder care. Thus diagnoses related to difficulties in communication may be indicated. In addition, the diagnosis of growth and development, altered, should be considered when there is a series of deficits that affect nursing care and discharge planning.

Finally, family issues may be more pertinent for the nurse to consider than in other client care situations. Role performance, altered; parenting, altered; and family processes, altered, are all important diagnoses for the nurse to consider. The needs of the family should always be considered in the process of assigning a nursing diagnosis.

OUTCOME IDENTIFICATION

Outcome criteria flow from the nursing diagnosis in the nursing process and are stated in simple terms. The out-

---

COLLABORATIVE DIAGNOSES

DSM-IV Diagnoses*	NANDA Diagnoses†
Autistic disorder	Social isolation
	Self-care deficit
	Self-mutilation, risk for
Conduct disorder	Violence, risk for: directed at others
	Violence, risk for: self-directed
	Social interaction, impaired
Separation anxiety disorder	Anxiety
	Coping, ineffective individual

*From American Psychiatric Association: *Diagnostic and statistical manual of mental disorders*, ed 4, Washington, DC, 1994, The Association.
†From North American Nursing Diagnosis Association: *NANDA nursing diagnoses: definitions and classifications, 1999-2000*, Philadelphia, 1999, The Association.

---

come criteria for children and adolescents will focus on promotion of normal growth and development in an effort to improve areas of current developmental deficits. The outcome criteria will integrate the treatment goals of the interdisciplinary team, the caregivers, and the child or adolescent. Children and adolescents are more motivated to actively participate in the treatment process when they have had an opportunity to express their opinions about the treatment goals.

Clients will:

1. Demonstrate age-appropriate relationships with adults.
2. Demonstrate age-appropriate relationships with peers.
3. Demonstrate a decrease or elimination of aggressive behaviors toward self and others.
4. Use age-appropriate play and recreational activities to express self.
5. Identify triggers that may provoke negative behavioral responses.
6. Seek assistance and support from adults before losing self-control.

PLANNING

In the beginning phases of the nursing process, the nurse sets realistic expectations based on the child or adolescent's developmental level of ability and function. The nurse is aware that negative behavioral patterns have been an integral part of the family dynamics and often have been established for very long periods of time. Children and adolescents want the world to be fair, and they resist treatment plans that are set too high, too suddenly. They also resist insincerity from adult authority figures. Ideally, the nurse plans for small, incremental changes in behavior, with obtainable goals. The nurse's effort for mutual goal setting will demonstrate respect and trust with the child or adolescent. The nurse may explain the plan to the child or adolescent in simple terms, requesting their active participation and best effort, with the understanding that the nurse will work in a cooperative effort with the patient to obtain these treatment goals.

IMPLEMENTATION

As the nursing plan is implemented, the nurse's role is to support the child or adolescent through the behavioral change process. The child or adolescent will be tempted to continue to use previously established behaviors, many of which may be negative. The nurse can demonstrate clear, consistent, and realistic expectations using role-modeling and communication skills. The nurse will need to set consistent boundaries and limits as the child or adolescent questions authority and struggles to learn adaptive developmental functioning.

The nurse-client relationship is essential in the implementation phase. The child or adolescent will look to the nurse for the trust and respect that was set forth in the planning phase. However, the implementation phase is often the most challenging as the child or adolescent tests limits, acts out, and may become manipulative, deviant, defiant, or aggressive in an effort to revert to preexisting family dynamics and behaviors. Maintaining the safety of the child or adolescent may be a target goal in the implementation phase. It is common for the adolescent to be increasingly aggressive, often resulting in seclusion and restraint. The child or adolescent may fail repeatedly in the initial phases of treatment. The nurse will be the catalyst to promote the change process, and the child or adolescent will look for reassurance, encouragement, and support from the nurse. The nurse constantly reassesses the expectations throughout the implementation phase to ensure realistic and obtainable goals for the child or adolescent. It may be necessary to reset the expectations if they are either too easy or too difficult to achieve.

THERAPEUTIC PLAY

For the younger child, nursing interventions take place in activities of **therapeutic play.** Play is the work of children. The child can use recreational and creative play activities in relationships with peers and adults as they work to master new developmental tasks. Children may express their thoughts, feelings, frustrations, fears, and hopes through therapeutic play. The astute nurse will keenly observe the child in play and interact to modify distortions and reestablish healthy boundaries and safe parameters as the child redefines behaviors through play.

Group play and recreational activities are another means to assist the child or adolescent in developing positive peer communication and improve interpersonal relationships. Group play can be an excellent opportunity for the nurse to role model and teach new age-appropriate skills, reinforce positive behaviors, and promote nurturing peer relationships. The nurse will set limits in group play

to promote a safe environment and to demonstrate showing cooperation and respect to peers. Children and adolescents often have learned to tease and provoke peers in group settings. The nurse can assist them in redefining successful relationships.

Interventions with adolescents are often more difficult than with children, depending on the clinical presentation. It is normal growth and development behavior for adolescents to question authority and test limits and rules. The nurse must establish rapport and establish a therapeutic alliance with the adolescent early in the course of treatment. Nursing interventions that promote the development of a trusting nurse-client relationship are fundamental to working with adolescents. The nurse sincerely communicates empathy and understanding regarding the difficult developmental issues the adolescent encounters at this stage. Adolescents will resist efforts of the nurse to exercise authoritative power over their point of view. The nurse works to integrate the caregiver's perspective with the adolescent's perspective.

Adolescents are looking for role models, so it is imperative that the nurse maintain appropriate boundaries and not seek to behave as an adolescent to gain their acceptance. Adolescents may attempt to be flirtatious with nursing personnel of both genders, and the nurse has the opportunity to demonstrate self-control, respect, and mature modeling of healthy interpersonal relationships. The nurse will continue to demonstrate empathy, understanding, sincerity, and caring, while at the same time role modeling consistent adult interactions and boundaries.

Group activities provide an excellent opportunity for the nurse to interact with adolescents during treatment. Group activities enable the adolescent to develop interpersonal skills, give and accept feedback and communicate with peers, attempt to implement more adultlike relationships, and listen and learn success and appropriate ways to interact with the world.

BEHAVIOR MODIFICATION PROGRAMS

For the child approximately 3 to 11 years old, a behavior modification program is frequently used in treatment plans. **Behavior modification** involves a systematic and structured program that is extremely effective. A behavior modification program establishes developmental and age-appropriate goals that are observable and measurable within an established time frame. The goals are often geared toward ADL and peer and sibling relationships. The child is rewarded for the accomplishment of each goal. There often is a chart that correlates with each goal, and the child is rewarded with stars, stickers, or colors to signify progress. Many school systems use colored charts, and a behavior program can be implemented in the home to correlate with the school program. This provides increased consistency and a stabilized structured program for the child and the family to use.

Preadolescents and adolescents are less likely to use a

▲ NURSING CARE PLAN

Kenny is a 12-year-old boy who presents to the clinic with a diagnosis of conduct disorder. He has a history of poor peer and sibling relationships. At school he has had numerous detentions in the past year and was suspended last month for fighting in the gym locker room. He threatened bodily harm to the teacher who intervened in the fight. He has been physically assaultive at home with his 14-year-old and 9-year-old male siblings. He verbally provokes his 16-year-old sister daily. At the age of 8 years, he burned down the family toolshed while playing with matches. The family has had money, coin collections, and tools stolen from the home, and on one occasion he and a peer were caught attempting to steal his brother's bicycle. He has never been convicted of a crime. Kenny kicks the family dog and was discovered torturing the family cat in the past 3 months. He teases younger children on the way to school.

The nursing assessment reveals a well-groomed boy with acne. He is angry, profane, and denies any problems at home or school. He denies lying, stealing, or cruelty to children and animals. He states that his siblings are jealous of him and trying to get him into trouble and says that is why he is here to-

day. The family history is significant for major depression with a suicide by a maternal uncle, completed by gun shot, when Kenny was 8 years old. The family history also includes alcoholism for the biologic father. Kenny has received C's and D's in his grades during the past schoolyear, but previously he was an A and B student. Kenny refuses to participate in treatment and blames his parents for everything. He promises revenge on his teacher for getting him into trouble.

DSM-IV Diagnoses

Axis I   Conduct disorder
              Rule out learning disability
Axis II   None
Axis III   Acne
Axis IV   Severity of stressors = 3 (moderate): school detentions—suspension; completed suicide by maternal uncle; alcoholism of biologic father; financial problems (father recently laid off)
Axis V   GAF = 45 (current)
              GAF = 5 (past year)

Nursing Diagnosis: Violence, risk for: directed at others. Risk factors: a positive history of aggression toward peers and siblings, detentions and school suspensions, threatening a teacher, history of cruelty to children and animals, and history of fire setting.

Client Outcomes	Nursing Interventions	Evaluation
Kenny will refrain from threatening others	• Monitor all peer/adult interactions and conversations. • Set firm limits on any provocation to others, both passive and overt. *Structure and clear expectations clarify boundaries for improved self-control.*	• Kenny continues to verbally provoke peers in a subtle, passive/aggressive manner two times daily.
Kenny will identify precipitating events preceding his acting-out, aggressive actions.	• Have a daily one-to-one conversation with Kenny to discuss situations that have occurred and correlate his feelings before and during the situation with his behavioral reaction *to connect negative feelings with aggressive actions.* • Promote active participation in all structured activities.	• Kenny is able to identify precipitating events and feelings and their relationship 50% of the time per day. • Kenny participates in 90% of group activities daily.
Kenny will maintain a behavioral contract to establish self-control.	• When angry, Kenny will remove himself from the person or situation immediately (to aid self-control). • Kenny will write in his journal one time per day *to express his hostile feelings in a safe manner.* • Kenny will request recreational time to express his hostilities (e.g., basketball, skate boarding) *to promote socially acceptable and safe ventilation of negative feelings.* • Kenny will immediately go to an adult for support when his angry impulses are present *to promote social support during times of lack of self-control.*	• Kenny walks away when provoked in 100% of stressful situations. • Kenny writes in his journal every evening. • Kenny shoots basketball hoops when angry one time per day. He prefers solitary play versus group play at times of intense anger. • Kenny continues to need adult intervention when he is extremely angry to promote self-control and safety.

▲ NURSING CARE PLAN —cont'd

Nursing Diagnosis: Social interaction, impaired, related to lack of positive peer and sibling relationships, as evidenced by threatening and provoking peers and siblings.

Client Outcomes	Nursing Interventions	Evaluation
Kenny will interact in age-appropriate social activities with peers and siblings in a constructive manner.	• Engage Kenny in age-appropriate activities *to increase self-esteem and to facilitate positive peer and sibling relationships.* • Immediately praise and give positive reinforcement to Kenny for all socially appropriate peer interactions. Set firm and consistent limits on negative interactions *to encourage clear parameters for what is acceptable social interactions.*	• Kenny engages in peer activities 75% of the time without evidence of threatening behavior.
Kenny will engage in a therapeutic relationship with his primary nurse.	• Meet with Kenny one time per day for a one-to-one interaction to discuss his journal and feelings about current peer, sibling, or family interactions *to promote constructive and positive ventilation of feelings and to role model appropriate adult-client interactions.*	• Kenny meets once per day with his primary nurse to discuss feelings and thoughts constructively.
Kenny will identify, establish, and use support systems.	• Demonstrate to Kenny the accessibility of systems support *to promote a safe and secure resource for him to approach during times of intense stress, anger, or feelings of aggressiveness* and *to role model a positive client relationship with authority figures.*	• Kenny is able to approach staff and adult figures one time per day to request discussion and to discuss feelings in a positive manner.

structured behavior modification program with a chart that uses rewards such as stars and stickers. This may be perceived as insulting in their efforts to strive for independence and autonomy. Preadolescents and adolescents are often given behavioral contracts. These contracts may emphasize only one to three goals, and the goals are more psychodynamic in nature (e.g., will speak to others with respect; will actively participate in group activities). Instead of giving such things as stars and stickers when goals are accomplished by the preadolescent or adolescent, a checkmark can be placed after each goal to signify that the adolescent has accomplished that goal.

NURSING INTERVENTIONS

Maintain a safe environment at all times. Assess for potential dangers, **contraband,** the presence of suicidal ideation, and plans or access to a method (pills, weapons, etc.) *to provide safety.*

1. Monitor and continually assess for behavioral changes and signals that may indicate increasing irritation, frustration, anger, hostility, or distorted thinking that may result in assaultive behaviors *to prevent violence.*
2. Communicate respect and trust, both verbally and nonverbally, *to promote a therapeutic alliance with the child or adolescent.*
3. Maintain a therapeutic environment by setting simple,

fair, and consistent limits *to promote healthy boundaries and expectations.*
4. Use positive reinforcement and praise with genuine sincerity *to promote and increase self-esteem and confidence.*
5. Communicate effectively with the family and child or adolescent *to reinforce treatment gains and application of new skills in the home.*

ADDITIONAL TREATMENT MODALITIES

A variety of collaborative interventions are used with children and adolescents in the mental health setting. Medications have been used for decades, often with great success. The classifications and dosages are changing rapidly with the emphasis on biologic psychiatry in the twenty-first century. Many medications used with adults can be used with children and adolescents. The predominant classifications remain stimulants, antidepressants, antianxiety agents, anticonvulsants, and antipsychotics. The nurse plays a crucial role in administration of the medication, monitoring for clinical effectiveness, monitoring for adverse reactions, assessing for titration of dose and times of medication administration, and promotion of optimal health functioning. The nurse plays a key role in the communication of these findings to the multidisciplinary treatment team and to the primary care provider. The nurse must continually be educated regarding current and newly developed medications and their clinical impact on this population.

Recreational, occupational, music, and art therapies, in addition to school, group, family, and individual therapies, are treatment modalities that also play a significant role in this population to promote overall health and well-being for the child and adolescent. Close coordination and communication by the entire multidisciplinary team enhances developmental gains and reinforces newly established therapeutic skills. The nurse involved in these modalities can assess the patient in various settings while at the same time promoting development of growth and fine motor skills and interpersonal development.

Most individuals with moderate mental retardation acquire some communication skills during early childhood and may benefit from vocational training, but they seldom advance academically beyond the second grade level.

They can generally live in the community in group homes or with their families unless some other physical or mental challenge requires specialized care.

EVALUATION

The evaluation phase of the nursing process documents the treatment progress, as evidenced by actual outcomes. The observant nurse objectively reviews the evaluation phase to determine the effectiveness of the treatment plan. In addition to outcomes, the nurse examines other factors. For instance, were the treatment goals cognitively and developmentally appropriate for the child or adolescent? Are there other stressors within the family or social support system that may be compounding the presenting problems, thus contributing to unrealistic expectations of the child or adolescent (e.g., health, financial, or placement problems).

It is possible to have the correct treatment goals but overestimate or underestimate the potential for the child. This may be easily corrected by modifying the measurable component. For example, if the nurse stated that Johnny would decrease negative peer interactions by 90% in 1 week and at the end of 1 week Johnny has made no progress whatsoever, it would be unrealistic to continue to expect a 90% decrease. Modification of the percent (e.g., decreased to 60%) and/or the time frame (e.g., increased to 3 weeks) would result in a more realistic expected outcome for the child to accomplish.

It is wise to use the expertise of the multidisciplinary team to coordinate any care plan modifications in an effort to maintain cohesiveness within the treatment implementation. It is also important to continually communicate the treatment evaluation with the caregivers. This helps to reinforce treatment gains, reinforce new methods of parental interventions, and assist the caregivers in monitoring and reestablishing new realistic expectations. As stated earlier, many of the behavior problems have been longstanding, so it will take an increased amount of time to see marked change.

Inpatient hospitalization time has been severely shortened as a result of pressures from the insurance and the health care industries. Therefore it is critical that the nurse assist the caregivers in comprehending the treatment goals and teach them to implement and evaluate the care plan in the home setting. It is recommended that the nurse begin early in the course of treatment with the family, to prepare them for the potential and pending discharge. Work that is initially begun in an inpatient setting will be transitioned to home or other placement such as foster care, residential care, or a group home. In more severe and chronic cases, state hospitals for the mentally ill may be where the discharged child or adolescent is placed. These placements are becoming severely limited as states and counties throughout the country privatize mental health services. More and more often, children with severe and chronic mental disorders are returning to the home setting, with the responsibility and burden of care falling on the family.

When working with children and adolescents, the nurse is aware of the significance of the nurse-client relationship and permits appropriate time for healthy termination. Children and adolescents frequently act out with increasing negativity at the time of the termination (see Chapter 1).

It can be a challenge for the nurse to continue to be nurturing and therapeutic while role modeling the termination process in a manner that maintains the integrity, respect, and trust established in the treatment process. This role modeling may set a lifelong impression for healthy termination, and its significance to the child and adolescent in the mental health setting must not be underestimated.

In the evaluation phase, the nurse encourages the child or adolescent, and the family to make healthy transitions to the ongoing therapeutic relationship that will be maintained with the next primary mental health provider (i.e., nurse specialist, social worker, psychologist, or psychiatrist). The nurse's role is fundamental for the child or adolescent during the therapeutic treatment process, even if much work lies ahead in the future treatment for the client and the family.

Summary of Key Concepts

1. Of mentally retarded individuals, 85% are mildly retarded, 10% are moderately retarded; 3% to 4% are severely retarded, and 1% to 2% are profoundly retarded.

2. The most commonly diagnosed mental disorders are attention-deficit/hyperactivity disorder (ADHD), mood disorder, pervasive development disorder, stereotype movement disorder, and mental disorders due to a general medical condition.

3. Children with autistic disorder present with repetitive movements, no emotional reciprocity, impaired communication (both verbal and nonverbal), and an indifference to affection. Seventy-five percent have some degree of mental retardation.

4. Children with ADHD may have the following histories: child abuse or neglect, multiple foster placements, neurotoxin exposure, infections, drug exposure in utero, low birth weight, and mental retardation.

5. ADHD causes problems in academics, social relationships, self-esteem, and occupation due to its demanding, impulsive, and seemingly lazy manifestations.

6. One of the main characteristics of conduct disorder is the client's violent and/or aggressive behavior with little concern for those his or her actions affect.

7. Like autistic disorder, Tourette's disorder involves repetitive movements, sounds, and actions; however, unlike autistic disorder, these symptoms diminish during adolescence and adulthood.

8. Separation anxiety is a disruptive disorder that prevents children from engaging in normal activities because of incessant fear that their loved ones will be harmed in their absence.

9. Encopresis often is the result of a major power struggle between the child/adolescent and an authority figure.

10. Behavior modification programs are systematic structured plans with specific goals and time frames. The client is rewarded for goal attainment.

11. Early identification and treatment of the child and adolescent may assist the client in the home, school, and social setting for both the long and short term.

12. Nursing interventions with children and adolescents are intense and challenging. The nurse must work closely with the family and the multidisciplinary team.

REFERENCES

Achenback TM et al: Six-year predictors of problems in a national sample. IV. Young adult signs of disturbance, *J Am Acad Child Adolesc Psychiatry* 37:7, 1998.

American Psychiatric Association: *Diagnostic and statistical manual of mental disorders*, ed 4, Washington DC, 1994, The Association.

Bauermeister J et al: Epidemiology of disruptive behavior disorders, *Child Adolesc Psychiatr Clin North Am* 3(2) 1994.

Beitchman J, Yound A: Learning disorders with emphasis on reading disorders: a review of the past 10 years, *J Am Acad Child Adolesc Psychiatry* 36:8, 1997.

Bellis M, Putnam F: The psychobiology of childhood maltreatment, *Child Adolesc Psychiatr Clin North Am* 3(4), 1994.

Bernstein GA, Borchardt CM, Perwien AR: Anxiety disorder in children and adolescents: a review of the past 10 years, *J Am Acad Child Adolesc Psychiatry* 35:9, 1996.

Birmaher B et al: Childhood and adolescent depression: a review of the past 10 years, part I, *J Am Acad Child Adolesc Psychiatry* 35:11, 1996.

Bukstein O et al: Practice parameters for the assessment and treatment of children and adolescents with substance use disorders, *J Am Acad Child Adolesc Psychiatry* 36:10, 1997.

Cantwell DP: Attention deficit disorder: a review of the past 10 years, *J Am Acad Child Adolesc Psychiatry* 35:8, 1996.

DeMause L: The evolution of childhood. In DeMause, editor: *History of childhood*, Psychohistory Press, New York, 1974. Northvale, NJ, 1995, Jason Aronson.

Despert J: *The emotionally disturbed child: then and now*, New York, 1967, Vantage Press.

Dulcan M et al: Practice parameters for the assessment and treatment of children, adolescents, and adults with ADHA, *J Am Acad Child Adolesc Psychiatry* 36:10, 1997.

Fortinash KM, Holoday-Worret PA: *Psychiatric nursing care plans*, ed 3, St. Louis, 1999, Mosby.

Geller B, Luby J: Child and adolescent bipolar disorder: a review of the past 10 years, *J Am Acad Child Adolesc Psychiatry* 36:9, 1997.

Grøholt B et al: Suicide among children and younger and older adolescents in Norway: a comparative study, *J Am Acad Child Adolesc Psychiatry* 37:5, 1998.

Hirshberg JC: Child psychiatry: introduction. In Kaplan H et al, editors: *Comprehensive textbook of psychiatry/III*, ed 3, vol 3, Baltimore, 1980, Williams & Wilkins.

King BH et al: Mental retardation: a review of the past 10 years, part I, *J Am Acad Child Adolesc Psychiatry* 36:12, 1997.

Lewis M: A structural overview of psychopathology in childhood and adolescence. In Kaplan H et al, editors: *Comprehensive textbook of psychiatry/III*, ed 3, vol 3, Baltimore, 1980, Williams & Wilkins.

March JS, Leonard HL: Obsessive-compulsive disorder in children and adolescents: a review of the past 10 years, *J Am Acad Child Adolesc Psychiatry* 34:10, 1996.

McClellan J et al: Practice parameters for the assessment and treatment of children and adolescents with bipolar disorder, *J Am Acad Child Adolesc Psychiatry* 36:10, 1997.

North American Nursing Diagnosis Association: *NANDA nursing diagnoses: definitions and classifications, 1999-2000*, Philadelphia, 1999, The Association.

Otnow LD: Etiology of aggressive conduct disorders: neuropsychiatric and family contributions, *Child Adolesc Psychiatr Clin North Am* 3(2), 1994.

Pfefferbaum B: Posttraumatic stress disorder in children: a review of the past 10 years, *J Am Acad Child Adolesc Psychiatry* 36:11, 1997.

Rogeness G: Biologic findings in conduct disorder, *Child Adolesc Psychiatr Clin North Am* 3(2), 1994.

Shaffer D: Suicide in children and early adolescence, *J Child Psychol Psychiatry* 15(4): 275, 1974.

Steiner H et al: Practice parameters for assessment and treatment of children and adolescents with conduct disorder, *J Am Acad Child Adolesc Psychiatry* 36:10, 1997.

Sulik LR, Garfinkel BD: Adolescent suicidal behavior: understanding the breadth of the problem, *Child Adolesc Psychiatr Clin North Am* 1(1), 1992.

Thompson T: Childhood and adolescent suicide in Manitoba: a demographic study *Can J Psychiatry* 32(4): 264, 1987.

Volkmar FR: Childhood and adolescent psychosis: a review of the past 10 years, *J Am Acad Child Adolesc Psychiatry* 35:7, 1996.

Weinberg NZ et al: Adolescent substance abuse: a review of the past 10 years, *J Am Acad Child Adolesc Psychiatry* 37:3, 1998.

Notes

CHAPTER 19

Eating Disorders

Anne Clarkin-Watts

OBJECTIVES

- Identify the behavioral and psychologic symptoms of anorexia nervosa and bulimia nervosa.

- Compare and contrast the medical complications of anorexic and bulimic behavior.

- Analyze the complex interplay of biologic, sociocultural, familial, and psychologic factors that contribute to the etiology of eating disorders.

- Explain the "vicious cycle" of eating disorder behavior.

- Discuss the psychologic issues that underlie eating disorder behavior.

- Describe the type of therapeutic relationship that is most effective with clients with eating disorders, including the approach and attitude the nurse should demonstrate to achieve this relationship.

- Apply the nursing process—assessment, diagnosis, outcome identification, planning, implementation, and evaluation—for clients with eating disorders.

Eating disorders have many facets and many causes. Although they have become quite common and are seen in a wide variety of clinical settings, eating disorders are considered to be a relatively new phenomenon. Self-starvation, gorging, and purging behaviors have existed for centuries but, historically, have been rare and poorly understood conditions. The incidence of **anorexia nervosa,** characterized primarily by self-starvation and distorted body image, and **bulimia nervosa,** characterized primarily by binge eating and purging behavior, has increased dramatically in the past quarter-century. With this increase has come a rapidly growing body of literature, including medical research, psychiatric research, psychologic literature, and popular press, as well as enormous media attention. This information has helped educate us about eating disorders, but many controversies and conflicts have ensued.

Throughout history it appears that women have used food as a symbol to express a variety of issues in a variety of contexts. Because food has always been a compelling cultural symbol (of wealth, of nurturing, and of survival), the rejection of food and denial of appetite are always attention-getters. Although most individuals with eating disorders are female, there are some males who suffer from anorexia nervosa and bulimia nervosa.

The increase in eating disorders in the late twentieth century has coincided with three major cultural trends: the fashion industry, the diet and fitness industry, and the women's movement. A trend toward thinness in fashion, the creation of the diet and fitness industry, and the changes in the women's movement have all contributed to the current epidemic of eating disorders. Box 19-1 summarizes these cultural trends.

Affective instability Rapidly fluctuating moods in which the individual is emotionally reactive to external events and lacks coping skills to manage feeling states.

Alexithymia A condition in which individuals have difficulty recognizing and describing their emotions. The term literally means "no words for feelings." Individuals with eating disorders often have a restricted emotional life.

Anorexia nervosa An eating disorder classified in DSM-IV, characterized by self-starvation, weight loss below minimum normal weight, intense fear of being fat even when emaciated, distorted body image, and amenorrhea in females.

Binge eating disorder (BED) (proposed) A pattern of binge eating without the purging characteristic of bulimia nervosa. BED is commonly known as compulsive overeating. It is classified in DSM-IV as a proposed diagnosis for further study.

Body image disturbance A perceptual disturbance in the way an individual's body shape, size, weight, and proportions are subjectively perceived and experienced. Typically, persons with anorexia complain of feeling "fat" or see their stomach, hips, and thighs as fat when they are clearly underweight.

Bulimia nervosa An eating disorder classified in DSM-IV, characterized by recurrent episodes of binge eating subjectively experienced as out of control, followed by inappropriate compensatory behavior to prevent weight gain, such as self-induced vomiting, overuse of laxatives, diuretics, diet pills, fasting, or excessive exercise, and excessive preoccupation with body shape and weight.

Comorbidity The co-occurrence of two or more psychiatric or other disorders, which may be due to a causal relationship between the two, an underlying predisposition to both, or the disorders may be unrelated. Depression is a common comorbid disorder in clients with eating disorders. Different theories exist about the association between eating disorders and mood disorders.

Dichotomous thinking A cognitive distortion common to people with eating disorders, in which an individual views a situation as all or nothing, black or white, all good or all bad. If a situation is less than perfect, it is perceived as a failure.

Enmeshed families A pattern of family relationships in which children are pressured to conform to parental expectations rather than express their individuality. Overinvolvement among family members, discouragement of outside relationships, and blurring of boundaries occur (e.g., a mother will "feel" her daughter's emotions).

Interoceptive deficits Inability to correctly identify and respond to bodily sensations. Individuals with eating disorders are often out of touch with their bodies and either fail to recognize or mistrust physical sensations such as hunger, satiety, fatigue, or pain, as well as emotional states.

Purging The use of self-induced vomiting, the abuse of laxatives, diuretics, syrup of ipecac, diet pills, or enemas to avoid weight gain following a binge. One or more of these behaviors, as well as periods of fasting and excessive exercise during an episode of bulimia nervosa, may be used.

Secondary gain Any benefit, such as personal attention or sympathy from others, or escape from unwanted responsibilities, as a result of illness. Individuals with eating disorders may experience secondary gain when family or friends pay a great deal of attention to their eating behavior (e.g., preparing special meals or making special arrangements in an attempt to encourage them to eat).

Box 19-1   Cultural Trends and Eating Disorders

Fashion Industry

Cultural ideals of beauty have always been reflected in the fashion of the day. The trend in fashion since the 1960s has been more and more toward thinness. In the late twentieth century, fashion has become a huge industry, fueled by advertising dollars and exerting great influence on women. With the media as the vehicle, women are bombarded with images of the thin, fit, "perfect" woman, an ideal unattainable for most women (Figure 19-1). Epidemiologic studies show that 0.1% of women have a natural body type that matches the ideal, leading most to believe that their normal, healthy shape is too fat. The pervasiveness of this trend is reflected in the dieting behavior and body dissatisfaction among not only high school but also elementary and middle school children.

Diet and Fitness Industry

The second trend is the birth of the diet and fitness industry. Since the 1950s, weight management has moved out of the doctor's office into multibillion-dollar businesses, which are run by opportunistic entrepreneurs who are not part of the health professions. Women are deluged by the media with an array of products, such as pills, powders, packaged food, diet books, videos, and a variety of health club and diet program memberships designed to help them attain the "perfect body."

Women's Movement

A third trend is the ongoing women's movement. Although women's struggles for equality are not new, women's roles have changed dramatically during the past 20 to 25 years. Pressure to be "superwoman"—to balance motherhood, marriage, and career—is new and has influenced women of all generations. The need for women to achieve academically and professionally while still fulfilling their traditional female roles creates conflicts, even as it affords women greater societal rights and freedom.

Professional women need to be assertive and even aggressive to successfully compete in the business world, yet women are still socialized to be passive and accommodating. Some feminist writers such as Susie Orbach and Susan Wooley view the drive for thinness as possibly symbolizing a woman's attempt to destroy her femininity in order to compete in a man's world or as male society's backlash against the women's movement. Pressuring women to strive for an impossible ideal of thinness may promote feelings of inadequacy that drive women to constantly diet and exercise to please men (Orbach, 1978; Wooley and Wooley, 1985).

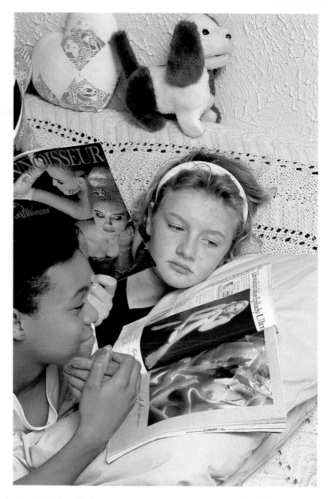

Figure 19-1 Fashion magazines are one example of the media's influence on women's perceptions of themselves. (Copyright Cathy Lander-Goldberg, Lander Photographics.)

HISTORICAL AND THEORETIC PERSPECTIVES

Eating disorders are not just a late twentieth-century fad of young, fashion-conscious American women; they have existed in various forms for hundreds of years. The explosion of written material on eating disorders includes some careful and thorough research into the history of both anorexia nervosa and bulimia nervosa (Bell, 1987; Brumberg, 1989).

INCIDENCE IN HISTORY

Brumberg, in *Fasting Girls* (1989), and Bell, in *Holy Anorexia* (1987), note that medieval women commonly starved themselves in devotion to Christ. These women were canonized as miracles of female holiness for their refusal of food, sustaining themselves only on the Christian Eucharist and prayer. Both authors detail the case of Saint Catherine of Siena, Italy (1347-1380), who kept an extensive diary of her fasting and self-induced vomiting. Her piety also included self-flagellation and other self-punishing behavior, not very different from the self-destructive behavior common today among clients with anorexia and bulimia. Medieval physicians called this phenomenon "anorexia mirabilis" (miraculously inspired loss of appetite). Like Catherine, many "holy anorectics" occasionally binged and purged. This demonstrates the intertwining of anorexic and bulimic behaviors from the beginning of their known existence.

Fasting continued in the ensuing centuries in Europe as a demonstration of piety but also of mysticism and magic. Skeptics accused persons with anorexia of Satanism, of witchcraft, and of malingering (Brumberg, 1989).

Many persons with anorexia nervosa binged and purged, but few clinical accounts of normal-weight bulimia nervosa existed until the twentieth century, when case histories began to appear in psychoanalytic literature. In "The Case of Ellen West," American psychoanalyst Binswanger (1958) describes a woman he treated in approximately 1915. She dieted from 165 to 92 pounds, but she also binged and purged with excessive exercise, laxative abuse, and self-induced vomiting. She was obsessed with food and clinically depressed, and she committed suicide 13 years later (Binswanger, 1958). In *The Fifty Minute Hour*, psychiatrist Robert Lindner (1955) describes the case of "Laura," a client with bulimia nervosa.

Since these were psychoanalytic case studies, the writings do not include any discussion of sociocultural or biologic influences but instead focus on the bulimic symptom complex as a manifestation of oral impregnation fears, oral eroticism, rejection of femininity, and unconscious hatred of the mother. A few less well-known case studies noted bulimic behavior among young girls in boarding schools and refugee children (Johnson and Connors, 1987). These cases were clearly related to separation issues, which are a primary factor in the development of bulimia nervosa among college women today.

In the 1950s, binge eating among the overweight and obese population was described as another form of an eating disorder (Hamburger, 1951; Stunkard, 1959). This common condition was compared with alcoholism, with its similar cravings and secret binges, followed by shame and guilt. The term *compulsive overeating* has been used most commonly to describe this disorder.

In the mid-1970s, psychologist Marlene Boskind-Lodahl coined the term *bulimarexia* to describe a group of women of normal and low-normal weight she saw at Cornell University's mental health clinic, who shared the anorectic individual's fear of fat and drive for thinness but were not emaciated and who regularly binged and purged. In her 1983 book, she describes her extensive clinical experience and groundbreaking research with this group, who represented the first wave of the current outbreak of eating disorders. Bulimarexia has never been formally used as a diagnosis. The DSM-III-R and DSM-IV chose *bulimia nervosa*, the term coined by Russell (1979) linking bulimia to

anorexia nervosa, for its formal nomenclature (Boskind-Lodahl, 1976; Boskind-Lodahl and White, 1983).

Box 19-2   Etiologic Factors Related to Eating Disorders

Biologic Factors
Family history of depression
Tendency to be overweight

Sociocultural Factors
Diet and fitness industry
Fashion industry
Women's movement
Developmental peer pressure

Psychologic Factors
Low self-esteem
Perfectionism
Affective instability
Interoceptive deficits
Ineffectiveness
Compliance—a "people pleaser"

Familial Factors
Enmeshment
Poor conflict resolution
Separation/individuation issues
Some incidence of alcoholism or physical or sexual abuse

ETIOLOGY

A wide variety of etiologic theories regarding eating disorders have been explored. Except for a few extremists, there has been a convergence among many disparate etiologic views from biology, sociology, psychoanalysis, and other models to form a new model of eating disorders as multifaceted, multidetermined syndromes. Most of the current literature describes eating disorders as complex, with biologic, sociocultural, and psychodynamic variables (Box 19-2).

BIOLOGIC FACTORS

Most research into a biologic basis for eating disorders finds a connection between eating disorders and depression. There is a high incidence of comorbid affective disorders among those with eating disorders and a high incidence of depression among their family members. Since biogenetic factors are believed to predispose individuals to affective illness, the same factors may contribute to the development of eating disorders. The efficacy of antidepressant medication in treating comorbid depression and decreasing some eating disorder symptoms further suggests a link.

Recent studies show evidence of serotonin dysregulation in eating disorders (Brewerton, 1995). Other studies show abnormally high levels of stress hormones and low levels of satiety-controlling gut hormones (U.S. Department of Health and Human Services, 1993). Whether these neuroendocrinologic markers are a cause or an effect of eating disorders is not known.

A biologic tendency to be overweight increases the likelihood of body dissatisfaction and dieting behavior, which is a major factor in triggering an eating disorder.

SOCIOCULTURAL FACTORS

By adolescence the preanorexic or prebulimic woman has been exposed to countless advertisements, fueled by the diet and fashion industries, that encourage her to eat, dress, and exercise to look beautiful. She has learned from an early age to idealize an unrealistically thin shape (Vernon-Guidry, Williamson, and Netemeyer, 1997). She has equated food with pleasure, comfort, and love and may have been nurtured, punished, or rewarded with food within her family.

Frequently the person with anorexia nervosa or bulimia nervosa may also have been observing her grandmother's and mother's often unsuccessful struggles to balance all of society's expectations. These include the need to maintain a feminine image and still achieve the superwoman role. Food plays a significant role in this dichotomy. Such conflicting dynamics influence the woman's eating patterns.

PSYCHOLOGIC FACTORS

Although the same sociocultural pressures challenge all adolescents, only a few, approximately 8%, develop eating disorders. Some teens seem to cope more effectively than others, based on their personalities and support systems. Personality traits common among those with eating disorders include the following:

Perfectionism
Social insecurity
Affective instability (rapidly fluctuating moods)
Interoceptive deficits (inability to correctly identify and respond to bodily sensations)
Alexithymia (difficulty naming and expressing emotions)
Immaturity
Compliance
A sense of ineffectiveness in dealing with the world

These traits increase vulnerability to eating disorders. Self-esteem is another important factor. Studies show that individuals diagnosed with eating disorders have lower self-esteem than other diagnostic groups.

Cognitive therapy literature describes certain distorted thinking patterns as characteristic of eating disorders (Bauer and Anderson, 1989). They include **dichoto-**

mous thinking (individuals view situations as either all good or all bad), erroneous control issues (individuals feel solely responsible for the happiness and failure of others), and personalization (individuals compare themselves endlessly with others and believe everything other people do is a reaction to them).

FAMILIAL FACTORS

Personality characteristics can be partially influenced by family environment. Despite early stereotypes of "eating disorder families" described by Minuchin, Rosman, and Baker (1978), a clear picture of a "type" of family that has a member with an eating disorder is difficult to portray. They come from all socioeconomic levels, races, and cultures. Some common characteristics do exist in their interactional patterns. The family environments of persons with eating disorders are often tense, rigid, and enmeshed. **Enmeshed families** have poor boundaries, overinvolvement among members, and a pattern of relating in which individuality is discouraged and conformity is expected. These families discourage the direct expression of feeling. They tend to demonstrate poor conflict resolution skills, in which disagreement may be displayed as denial of conflicts, conflict avoidance, repetitive and unproductive arguments, or escalation to violence. The result is ongoing tension, fear of conflict, and a belief that conflict is bad and dangerous. These families often put a great deal of importance on outward appearance, social acceptance, and achievement. Many family environments include substance abuse, severe mood disorders, and even sexual abuse.

In extremely dysfunctional families the damage can be severe. Sexual abuse has devastating effects. But even in families without physical or sexual abuse, the child may not feel encouraged to be independent, to develop self-trust, or to have confidence in the child's own individual abilities. The child may learn to avoid conflict, to please others, and to fear adult responsibilities. Because the child did not learn to be autonomous or independent, adolescence is a crisis. The sense of self never fully developed, and the pressures to separate and be an individual in adolescence can be terrifying, not only to the child but also to the parents.

Confronted with this crisis, it is not surprising that a young woman feels overwhelmed. She perceives her life as out of control and desperately wants to feel in control. The myth of thinness as the key to confidence and success portrayed in the diet program advertisement may be very compelling and be perceived as a good way to "get control of my life." The young woman, then, begins dieting, loses weight, and begins to feel better about herself. Consequently, she continues dieting and losing weight, focusing on this as an accomplishment, and feels more in control. Unfortunately, this behavior is often reinforced by **secondary gains** such as attention and envy from her peers. Later, when people tell her she is getting too thin and should eat more, she feels a sense of power and control she has never felt before. By losing weight, she not only has gotten attention, but also has been able to cause envy and frustrate those who try to make her eat normally. These secondary gains can be very rewarding, especially to an individual with low self-esteem. The diet has thus distracted her from her actual conflicts and given her a sense of mastery, albeit false, which she does not want to give up.

Sometimes a young woman in this situation cannot stick to the diet. Binging often begins as a reaction to the deprivation of dieting. Binge eating not only relieves hunger but also numbs pain and distracts from actual conflicts. It may also represent an angry rebellion against the pressure to be thin. The binge is temporary, however, and the problems soon come back. With them comes guilt about eating, and panic about loss of control and weight gain. So, the young woman purges to undo the binge—and the guilt. Figure 19-2 illustrates the interrelationship of all the etiologic factors in the cycle of eating disorders.

EPIDEMIOLOGY

Studies report wide discrepancies in estimates of prevalence of bulimia nervosa. Methodologic problems, particularly the criteria used to define bulimia, the low response rate of samples, and the use of self-report questionnaires, are probably responsible for the discrepancies. Studies using strict DSM-IV criteria estimate that 5% to 8% of adolescent and college-age women and 2% of all adolescent males are bulimic. The rate drops to 2% among the general population. However, disturbed eating patterns, including dieting with occasional use of diet pills, laxatives, or vomiting, occurs in 13% of young women. Binge eating without purging at least once a week occurs in approximately 5% to 20% of all women and slightly fewer men.

The studies of prevalence of anorexia nervosa are less methodologically flawed. A rate of 0.5% to 1% in adolescent and college-age women is more consistently reported. Anorexia nervosa is much less common in males.

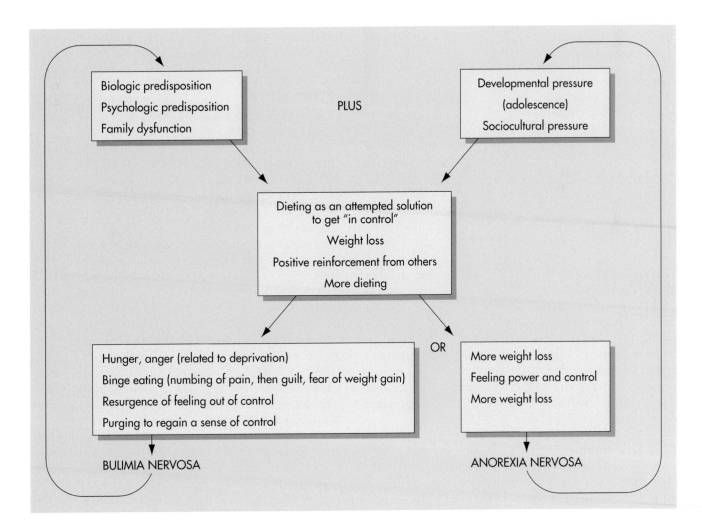

Figure 19-2 The cycle of eating disorders.

Box 19-3   **Epidemiology for Eating Disorders**

8 million people suffer from eating disorders in the United States.

Average age of onset is 14-18 for anorexia nervosa; 18 for bulimia nervosa.

5%-8% of adolescent and college-age women and 2% of adolescent men have bulimia nervosa.

2% of women and less than 1% of men in the general population have bulimia nervosa.

Less than 1% of the general population has anorexia nervosa

10% of adolescent and college-age women have subclinical anorexia nervosa; 15% have subclinical bulimia nervosa.

5%-20% of the general population (male and female) binge regularly (but do not purge).

1% of adolescent and college-age women have anorexia nervosa. Anorexia nervosa is much less common in males.

95%-99% of clients with eating disorders are female.

Mortality rates for bulimia nervosa are 0%-19%; for anorexia nervosa, mortality rates are 6%-20%.

Similar incidence and prevalence rates are found among Western countries where food is abundant and dieting is common; eating disorders are not found in underdeveloped countries.

Comorbidity:

Axis I   Mood disorders
          Anxiety disorders
          Dissociative disorders
          Substance-related disorders
Axis II   Borderline personality disorder
          Avoidant personality disorder
          Obsessive-compulsive personality disorder

The incidence and prevalence of eating disorders are summarized in Box 19-3.

SEX RATIO

Eating disorders are predominantly female disorders. Some researchers believe eating disorders are underreported in men and that men are not encouraged to seek help for what is labeled a "female" problem. Most samples report that 95% to 99% of clients with eating disorders are female.

AGE OF ONSET

The average age of onset of bulimia nervosa is age 18, with 80% of cases reported with an onset between ages 15 and 30. In anorexia nervosa the peak ages of onset are ages 14 and 18. The range of onset ages for both disorders is 9 to 50 years of age.

CROSS-CULTURAL STUDIES

The incidence and prevalence of eating disorders around the world show similar rates among European countries, the United States, Canada, Mexico, Japan, Australia, and other westernized countries with plentiful food supplies.

Underdeveloped countries do not show any cases of eating disorders. It is generally believed that abundance of food is necessary for an outbreak of eating disorders; when dieting becomes common, eating disorders begin to appear.

In the United States there is no evidence of any significant differences among racial, ethnic, or socioeconomic groups. There was a gap in past decades, with clients with eating disorders being predominantly white, upper-middle-class women, but this gap has disappeared in more recent studies.

MORTALITY

In anorexia nervosa the mortality rate after 10 years is 6% to 7%. After 20 to 30 years it rises to somewhere between 18% and 20%. In bulimia nervosa, estimates of mortality range from 0% to 19%. The lower rates in some studies is likely due to the fact that many deaths from purging are recorded as cardiac arrest or cardiomyopathy and are never connected directly to bulimia nervosa.

Suicide is frequently the cause of death in persons with eating disorders, occurring in 2% of cases.

COMORBIDITY

Comorbidity is the concurrent existence of two or more disorders. Eating disorders are often accompanied by other Axis I and Axis II disorders. The previous section on etiology mentioned the high incidence of depression in eating disorders (50% to 80%). Depression seems to occur more frequently with bulimia nervosa than with anorexia nervosa. Less common than depression but also frequently seen in clients with bulimia are generalized anxiety disorders, panic, or substance abuse disorders.

In anorexia nervosa, depressive disorders are also the most frequent Axis I diagnosis, followed by anxiety disorders, especially panic disorder, agoraphobia, social phobia, and obsessive-compulsive disorder (Halmi et al, 1991). In one study 37% of clients with anorexia nervosa met DSM criteria for obsessive-compulsive disorder, compared with 3% of clients with bulimia nervosa (Thornton & Russell, 1997). In anorexia nervosa weight loss and malnutrition tend to exacerbate depressive, anxiety, and obsessive-compulsive symptomatology. These symptoms improve but do not disappear with weight restoration (Pollice et al, 1997). Recent studies have begun to look at the incidence of dissociative disorders in clients with eating disorders (Vanderlinden et al, 1993). This is discussed later in this chapter.

Numerous studies have investigated the phenomenon of *comorbid personality* disorders, which is well known to clinicians dealing with eating disorders. Varying rates of prevalence of comorbid personality disorders have been reported, with one third to three fourths of clients with eating disorders having an Axis II diagnosis (Gartner, Marcus, and Halmi, 1989; Herzog et al, 1992).

Borderline personality disorder is the Axis II diagnosis most commonly associated with eating disorders, with avoidant and obsessive-compulsive personality disorders also prevalent (Herzog et al, 1992).

In the discussion of eating disorders, borderline personality disorder, and dissociative disorders, the issue of sexual abuse must be raised. Many researchers have investigated a possible link between a history of sexual abuse and the development of eating disorders, borderline personality disorder, and dissociative identity disorder. Well-controlled research studies report a high incidence (25% to 30%) of childhood sexual abuse among clients with eating disorders. However, this is not a significantly higher incidence than is reported in females in the general psychiatric population. Thus childhood sexual abuse is a risk factor for the development of a psychiatric disorder but not specifically for an eating disorder. However, those clients with eating disorders who had been sexually abused had a higher incidence of comorbid dissociative disorders, obsessive-compulsive disorders, and phobias (Connors and Morse, 1993; Folsom et al, 1993; Moyer et al, 1997; Waller, 1993).

The phenomenon of dissociative disorders, especially dissociative identity disorder (formerly multiple personality disorder), in clients with eating disorders is a new, quite compelling area of research. Studies are beginning to investigate how a history of sexual (and physical) abuse contributes to the development of an eating disorder, and the ramifications of this phenomenon on treatment (see Understanding & Applying Research box).

Understanding & Applying Research

The researchers describe two cases of individuals who presented for inpatient treatment for eating disorders and were subsequently found to have Dissociative Identity Disorder, formerly known as Multiple Personality Disorder in DSM-III-R. The intertwining of the eating disorder symptoms and the dissociative phenomena resulted in an atypical clinical picture for an eating disorder. The authors describe how the diagnosis of Dissociative Identity Disorder (which was the primary Axis I diagnosis) was crucial for the successful treatment of these clients. They also propose that undiagnosed comorbid Dissociative Identity Disorder may be responsible for the refractory course seen in some clients with eating disorders. The authors encourage clinicians to assess for Dissociative Identity Disorder in clients with eating disorders who are resistant to treatment.

Levin A et al: Multiple personality in eating disorder patients, *Int J Eat Disord* 13(2):235, 1993.

CLINICAL DESCRIPTION

Eating disorders are an easily recognizable group of psychiatric diagnoses. Refusal to eat, severe weight loss, and self-induced vomiting are unmistakable indicators of an eating disorder. However, making a precise DSM-IV diagnosis and determining specific nursing diagnoses to reflect a particular client's case can be confusing and complicated tasks.

Eating disorders make up a relatively new diagnostic category in DSM. This reflects the recent rapid increase in prevalence from obscurity to a common phenomenon seen by most clinicians in most health care settings. Although there is extensive literature on eating disorders, clinicians and researchers are still learning about the phenomenon. Evolving knowledge is reflected in each revision of DSM criteria. DSM-IV has brought new refinements in eating disorder diagnoses.

Anorexia nervosa and bulimia nervosa are the two specific eating disorder diagnoses in the DSM-IV classification. The category of eating disorder not otherwise specified is provided to diagnose those individuals with eating disorder symptoms who do not meet the criteria for anorexia nervosa or bulimia nervosa. The DSM-IV Criteria box details the DSM-IV criteria for these three diagnoses. The clinical symptoms of anorexia nervosa and bulimia nervosa are listed in the Clinical Symptoms boxes on pp. 453 and 454, respectively.

Obesity is not included as an eating disorder in the DSM-IV classification because it has not been established that all cases of obesity involve underlying psychiatric illness. In cases where psychologic factors are directly affecting an individual's obesity, this can be classified within the DSM-IV as psychologic factors affecting the medical condition. Obesity itself is classified in the International Classification of Diseases (ICD-10) as a general medical condition (APA, 1994).

Inclusion or exclusion of **binge eating disorder (BED)** in the DSM-IV classification has been a controversial issue. Although it was not included as a separate diagnosis, it is cited as an example of an eating disorder not otherwise specified and is included in the DSM-IV classification as a proposed diagnosis for further study. Further research may lead to its inclusion as a separate eating disorder diagnosis in the next revision of the DSM. BED is described specifically as recurrent episodes of binge eating, in which the individual eats more than most people would during a similar period of time and feels out of control while eating. Specific behavioral indicators for loss of control are included, such as eating when not hungry, eating until uncomfortably full, eating alone due to embarrassment, etc. Other criteria include distress, guilt, and disgust regarding the behavior. A frequency of two binge episodes a week for 6 months is required (APA, 1994; Spitzer et al, 1992, 1993).

Eating Disorders

Anorexia Nervosa

A. Refusal to maintain body weight at or above a minimally normal weight for age and height (e.g., weight loss leading to maintenance of body weight less than 85% of that expected; or failure to make expected weight gain during period of growth, leading to body weight less than 85% of that expected).

B. Intense fear of gaining weight or becoming fat, even though underweight.

C. Disturbance in the way in which one's body weight or shape is experienced, undue influence of body weight or shape on self-evaluation, or denial of the seriousness of the current low body weight.

D. In postmenarcheal females, amenorrhea, i.e., the absence of at least three consecutive menstrual cycles. (A woman is considered to have amenorrhea if her periods occur only following hormone, e.g., estrogen, administration.)

Specify type:

Restricting type: During the current episode of anorexia nervosa the person has not regularly engaged in binge eating or **purging** behavior (i.e., self-induced vomiting or the misuse of laxatives, diuretics, or enemas).

Binge-eating/purging type: During the current episode of anorexia nervosa, the person has regularly engaged in binge-eating or purging behavior (i.e., self-induced vomiting or the misuse of laxatives, diuretics, or enemas).

Bulimia Nervosa

A. Recurrent episodes of binge eating. An episode of binge eating is characterized by both of the following:

   1. Eating, in a discrete period of time (e.g., within any 2-hour period), an amount of food that is definitely larger than most people would eat during a similar period of time and under similar circumstances

   2. A sense of lack of control over eating during the episode (e.g., a feeling that one cannot stop eating or control what or how much one is eating)

B. Recurrent inappropriate compensatory behavior in order to prevent weight gain, such as self-induced vomiting; misuse of laxatives, diuretics, enemas, or other medications; fasting; or excessive exercise.

C. The binge eating and inappropriate compensatory behaviors both occur, on average, at least twice a week for 3 months.

D. Self-evaluation is unduly influenced by body shape and weight.

E. The disturbance does not occur exclusively during episodes of anorexia nervosa.

Specify type:

Purging type: During the current episode of bulimia nervosa, the person has regularly engaged in self-induced vomiting or the misuse of laxatives, diuretics, or enemas.

Nonpurging type: During the current episode of bulimia nervosa, the person has used other inappropriate compensatory behaviors, such as fasting or excessive exercise, but has not regularly engaged in self-induced vomiting or the misuse of laxatives, diuretics, or enemas.

Eating Disorder Not Otherwise Specified

Disorders of eating that do not meet the criteria for a specific eating disorder. Examples include the following:

1. For females, all of the criteria for anorexia nervosa are met except amenorrhea.

2. All of the criteria for anorexia nervosa are met except that, despite significant weight loss, the individual's current weight is in the normal range.

3. All of the criteria for bulimia nervosa are met except that the frequency of binge eating is less than twice a week, or the duration has been less than 3 months.

4. Average-weight individual who regularly uses inappropriate compensatory behavior but does not binge eat.

5. Repeatedly chewing and spitting out but not swallowing large amounts of food.

6. Binge eating disorder: recurrent episodes of binge eating in the absence of the regular use of inappropriate compensatory behaviors characteristic of bulimia nervosa.

(DSM-IV CRITERIA)

From American Psychiatric Association: *Diagnostic and statistical manual of mental disorders*, ed 4, Washington, DC, 1994, The Association.

Anorexia nervosa and bulimia nervosa are classified as distinct diagnoses but have many overlapping features. In clinical practice many low-weight persons with anorexia binge and purge occasionally, and many purge small amounts of food but never binge. The subtypes assist the clinician in making the most precise diagnosis. For example, if an individual meets the criteria for both bulimia nervosa and anorexia nervosa, the diagnosis of anorexia nervosa, binge eating/purging type is made, because it is the only category that includes *all* of the symptoms (neither subtype of bulimia nervosa deals with weight loss).

PROGNOSIS

The prognosis for eating disorders is considered to be poor as compared with other diagnostic groups. However, eating disorders are very treatable, and many individuals recover completely. The course of the illness is variable. A few individuals recover fully from a single, time-limited episode of anorexia nervosa or bulimia nervosa (usually less than a year). Some teenagers who become anorexic recover their normal weight within a year but later develop bulimia nervosa. Others with anorexia nervosa follow a chronic course over many years, either remaining

CLINICAL SYMPTOMS

Anorexia Nervosa

Behavioral Symptoms

Self-starvation—reported intake restriction and refusal to eat

Rituals or compulsive behaviors regarding food, eating, and/or weight loss

May engage in self-induced vomiting, laxatives, diuretics, or excessive exercise to lose weight

May wear baggy or inappropriate layers of clothing

Physical Symptoms

Weight loss 15% below ideal weight

Amenorrhea—absence of three or more menstrual cycles when expected to occur (primary or secondary)

Slow pulse, decreased body temperature

Cachexia, sunken eyes, protruding bones, dry skin

Growth of lanugo on face

Constipation

Cold sensitivity

Psychologic Symptoms

Denial of the seriousness of current low weight

Body image disturbance—claiming to see self as fat when emaciated or to experience parts of the body (such as stomach, buttocks, hips, and thighs) as unrealistically large, as depicted in Figure 19-3

Intense and irrational fear of weight gain that does not diminish as weight is lost

Constant striving for "perfect" body

Self-concept unduly influenced by shape and weight

Preoccupation with food, cooking, nutritional information, and feeding others

May exhibit delayed psychosexual development or lack age-appropriate interest in sex and relationships

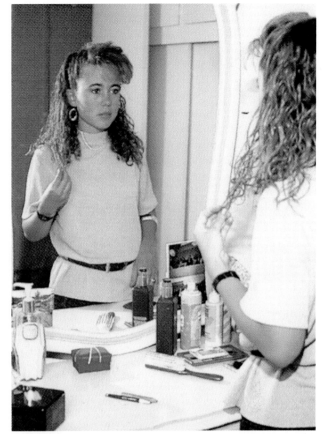

A

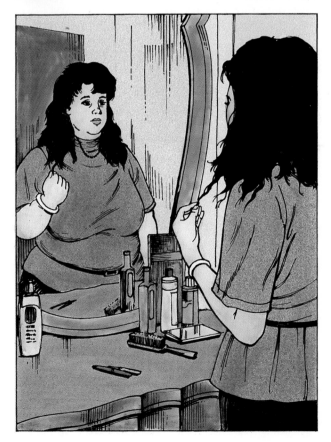

B

Figure 19-3   Clients with eating disorders have a distorted view of their physical appearance, perceiving themselves as unrealistically large. **A,** A girl views herself in the mirror. **B,** The unrealistically large image the girl sees of herself in the mirror.

at a consistent low weight or slowly deteriorating to lower and lower weights. Others demonstrate pattern of weight restoration followed by episodes of relapse. Bulimia nervosa is commonly episodic, with periods of remission free of binging and purging followed by relapse. A chronic, unremitting course of bulimia nervosa is possible as well.

Since long-term, methodologically sound outcome studies with large samples and good control groups are few, it is difficult to accurately assess the prognosis. The existing outcome studies suggest that most individuals with bulimia nervosa do improve symptomatically with treatment and that 40% to 50% of clients with anorexia nervosa regain normal weight (Herzog et al, 1996; Mehler 1996). Most studies credit multidisciplinary treatment, using cognitive techniques, behavioral techniques, pharmacology, and individual and group therapy, as most effectively reducing binge/purge episodes and restoring normal weight for the long term (Halmi, 1992; Wilson and Fairburn, 1993).

The discussion of comorbidity indicates that the presence of personality disorders and/or dissociative disorders suggests a much poorer prognosis (Glassman et al, 1990; Levin et al, 1993). Severe depression increases the risk of suicide. Lower weight in both anorexia nervosa and bulimia nervosa and later onset have been associated with a poorer prognosis (Glassman et al, 1990).

DISCHARGE CRITERIA
Client will:

Be free from self-harm.

Achieve minimum (within 15%) normal weight as determined by the treatment team.

Consume adequate calories to maintain a minimum normal weight.

CLINICAL SYMPTOMS

Bulimia Nervosa

Behavioral Symptoms
Recurrent episodes of binge eating (rapid consumption of a large amount of food in a discrete period of time) (Figure 19-4)

Engages in purging behavior such as self-induced vomiting, use of laxatives, diuretics, diet pills, ipecac, enemas, excessive exercise, or periods of fasting to compensate for the binge

Physical Symptoms
May experience fluid and electrolyte imbalances from purging:
  Hypokalemia
  Alkalosis
  Dehydration
  Idiopathic edema
Cardiovascular:
  Hypotension
  Cardiac arrhythmia/dysrhythmia
  Cardiomyopathy
Endocrine:
  Hypoglycemia
  May experience menstrual dysfunction
Gastrointestinal:
  Constipation, diarrhea
  Gastroparesis (delayed gastric emptying)
  Esophageal reflux, esophagitis
  Mallory-Weiss tears (in esophagus)
Dental:
  Enamel erosion
Parotid gland enlargement

Psychologic Symptoms
Body image disturbance, seeing self as unrealistically fat when at or near ideal weight or experiencing parts of the body as unrealistically fat or out of proportion
Persistent overconcern with weight, shape, and proportions
Mood swings and irritability
Self-concept unduly influenced by body weight and shape

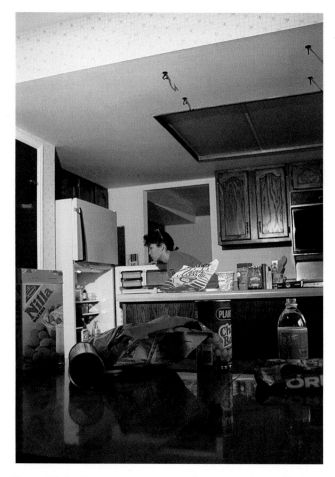

Figure 19-4   Binge eating is a significant symptom of bulimia nervosa. (Copyright Cathy Lander-Goldberg, Lander Photographics.)

Demonstrate ability to comply with the treatment regimen recommended for postdischarge (i.e., compliance with medication, food plan, control over binge/purge behavior, plan for follow-up care).

Verbalize awareness and understanding of the psychologic issues related to the eating disorder behavior and the maladaptive use of food and weight control to try to cope with these issues.

Demonstrate the use of improved coping abilities to respond to stress and to manage emotional issues.

Exhibit more functional behaviors within the family system.

Demonstrate decreased enmeshment with family members.

Attend group therapy sessions that encourage healthy eating patterns and positive self-image and self-concept.

Interact with peers who assist the client in maintaining healthy coping patterns.

Keep appointments to monitor behaviors and medications.

◢ THE NURSING PROCESS

ASSESSMENT

Nursing assessment of clients with eating disorders involves sensitivity, thoroughness, and keen observation skills (Figure 19-5). The first few minutes of the interview are crucial, since first impressions set the tone for the entire treatment experience. Clients with eating disorders are very sensitive to others and are quick to judge them as trustworthy or not. If a therapeutic alliance can be forged immediately, much of the power struggles can be avoided.

Because many clients with eating disorders have one or more coexisting disorders, it is critical for the nurse to assess for the disorders listed in Box 19-4.

NURSING DIAGNOSIS

Nursing diagnoses are made from the information obtained during the assessment phase of the nursing process. The accuracy of diagnosis depends on a careful, in-depth assessment.

NURSING DIAGNOSES FOR ANOREXIA NERVOSA

Safety and/or health risks:

Body temperature, altered, risk for
Constipation
Constipation, perceived
Fluid volume deficit
Growth and development, altered
Nutrition, altered: less than body requirements
Self-mutilation, risk for

Perceptual/cognitive/emotional disturbances:

Anxiety
Body image disturbance
Hopelessness
Powerlessness
Self-esteem disturbance

Problems in communicating and relating to others:

Sexual dysfunction
Social interaction, impaired
Social isolation

Disruptions in coping abilities:

Coping, ineffective family: compromised
Coping, ineffective family: disabling
Coping, ineffective individual
Denial, ineffective

Box 19-4   **Comorbid Disorders Commonly Found in Eating Disorders**

Mood disorders
  Dysthymic disorder
  Major depressive disorder
Anxiety disorders
  Generalized anxiety disorder
  Agoraphobia
  Panic disorder
  Social phobia
  Obsessive-compulsive disorder
  Posttraumatic stress disorder
Dissociative disorders
  Dissociative identity disorder
Substance-related disorders
Personality disorders
  Borderline personality disorder
  Obsessive-compulsive personality disorder
  Avoidant personality disorder

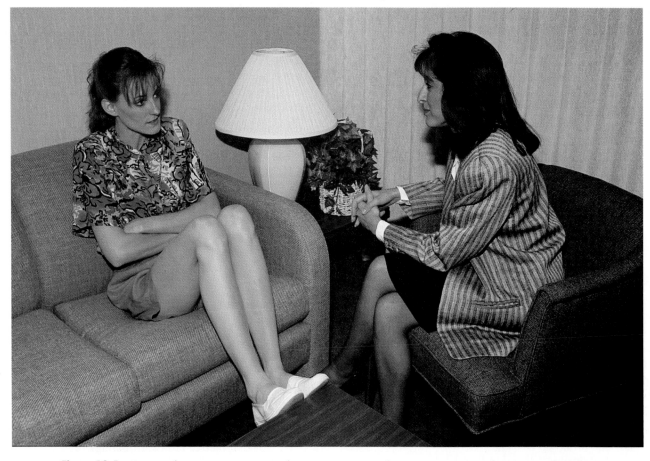

Figure 19-5   An initial assessment interview between a nurse and a young woman with an eating disorder.

CASE STUDY

Sarah is a 20-year-old college student who was brought to the emergency department by her boyfriend after she fainted in the shower. The boyfriend took the nurse aside and confided that Sarah was bulimic and that he was concerned that her eating disorder was related to the fainting episode. He went on to say that Sarah was very secretive and somewhat defensive about the bulimia. The initial physical examination of Sarah showed no injuries from the fall, and her vital signs were normal. Her parotid glands appeared enlarged. Her weight appeared within a normal range. Her affect was tense and anxious. She avoided eye contact with the nurse and mumbled that she had been up late recently, studying, and had not been getting enough sleep.

Critical Thinking—Assessment
1. How should the nurse approach Sarah? How can the subject of bulimia nervosa be brought up?
2. If Sarah responds defensively or with denial, how should the nurse respond?
3. What further physical assessments should be done?
4. What other information is needed to complete the nursing assessment?

Client and family teaching needs:

Knowledge deficit regarding nutrition and medical side effects of anorexic behavior
Noncompliance with refeeding process

NURSING DIAGNOSES FOR BULIMIA NERVOSA
Safety and/or health risks:

Constipation
Constipation, perceived
Fluid volume deficit
Nutrition, altered: less than body requirements
Self-mutilation, risk for

Perceptual/cognitive/emotional disturbances:

Anxiety
Body image disturbance
Hopelessness
Powerlessness
Self-esteem disturbance

NURSING ASSESSMENT QUESTIONS

Eating Disorders

1. "How do you feel about being here today?"
   (To determine if self-referred or forced into treatment and to assess willingness to engage in treatment)
2. "Have you ever talked with anyone before about your eating disorder?"
   (To assess level of self-disclosure and to reduce anxiety and feelings of shame)
3. "Have you been in therapy before?"
   (To assess treatment history and get details of previous treatment, including the name of clinician, dates of treatment, outcomes, and client's experience of the treatment)
4. "Describe your weight throughout your life."
   (To determine patterns and perceptions regarding weight)
   Include the following:
   Current weight, including fluctuations during past 6 months
   Desired weight
   Lowest and highest adult weight (excluding pregnancy)
   Lowest and highest adolescent weight
   Perception of childhood weight
   Perception of adolescent weight
   Perception of present weight
   Childhood experiences related to weight
5. "How do you feel about the way your body looks?"
   (To assess body dissatisfaction and body image distortion)

6. Assess dieting history:
   "When did you first diet?"
   "What started it?"
   "What happened?"
   "Did you lose/gain?"
   "Has anyone encouraged you to lose weight?"
   "What dieting behaviors have you used?"
   (To determine use of fasting, structured diet, restriction, diet products/programs)
7. Assess binge eating:
   "Do you binge eat?"
   "When was the first time?"
   Get details about typical binge eating, including when, where, duration, frequency, type and amount of food, any rituals or patterns involved.
   Ask if secrecy, hiding, stealing, or lying is involved.
   (To determine use of fasting, structured diet, restriction, diet products/programs)
   Assess control (i.e., can client interrupt a binge once it has begun?).
8. Help client identify feeling states associated with the binge: before binging, in the planning stages, and during and after the binge.
   Ask client to focus on past binge episodes to answer this question: "Did you feel angry? Anxious?"
   (To determine client's feelings regarding binge behaviors)
9. Assess food cravings (time of day, weekends, where in menstrual cycle, associated with places (car, work, home, store).
   (To determine if client can associate cravings with specific times/situations)

10. Assess purging behavior:
    (To identify client's usual methods of purging)

Type:	Frequency: (Times/week)	Amount:	First used: (Age)	Last used: (Date)
Vomiting				
Diuretics				
Laxatives				
Diet pills				
Ipecac				
Thyroid pills				
Amphetamines				
Cocaine				
Exercise (type)				

11. Assess menstrual history (onset of menses, regularity, premenstrual syndrome, menstrual dysfunction, any hormone therapy).
    (To determine effect of dysfunctional behaviors on menses)

12. Assess medical side effects of eating disorder.
    (To identify any concomitant medical problems)
13. Assess comorbidity (mood disorders, anxiety, substance abuse).

Problems in communicating and relating to others:

Sexual dysfunction
Social interaction, impaired
Social isolation

Disruptions in coping abilities:

Coping, ineffective family: compromised
Coping, ineffective family: disabling
Coping, ineffective individual

Client and family teaching:

Knowledge deficit regarding nutrition, side effects of bulimic behavior
Noncompliance with treatment program

OUTCOME IDENTIFICATION

Outcome criteria are derived from nursing diagnoses and are the expected client responses to be achieved.

OUTCOME IDENTIFICATION FOR ANOREXIA NERVOSA

Client will:

1. Participate in therapeutic contact with staff.
2. Consume adequate calories for age, height, and metabolic need.
3. Achieve minimum normal weight.
4. Maintain normal fluid and electrolyte levels.
5. Resume normal menstrual cycle.
6. Demonstrate improvement in body image with a more realistic view of body shape and size.
7. Demonstrate more effective coping skills to deal with conflicts.
8. Manage family dysfunction more effectively.
9. Verbalize awareness of underlying psychologic issues.
10. Achieve ideal body weight for age, height, and metabolic need.
11. Perceive body weight and shape as normal and acceptable.
12. Resume sexual interest and age-appropriate sexual behavior.
13. Demonstrate absence of food rituals, preoccupation with food, or fears of food.
14. Resolve family issues.

OUTCOME IDENTIFICATION FOR BULIMIA NERVOSA

Client will:

1. Participate in therapeutic contact with staff.
2. Maintain normal fluid and electrolyte levels.
3. Consume adequate calories for age, height, and metabolic need.

COLLABORATIVE DIAGNOSES

DSM-IV Diagnoses*	NANDA Diagnoses†
Anorexia nervosa	Anxiety
	Body image disturbance
	Nutrition, altered: less than body requirements
	Social isolation
Bulimia nervosa	Coping, ineffective individual
	Fluid volume deficit
	Self-esteem disturbance

*From American Psychiatric Association: *Diagnostic and statistical manual of mental disorders*, ed 4, Washington, DC, 1994, The Association.

†From North American Nursing Diagnosis Association: *NANDA nursing diagnoses: definitions and classifications, 1999-2000*, Philadelphia, 1994, The Association.

4. Cease binge/purge episodes while in inpatient setting.
5. Demonstrate more effective coping skills to deal with conflicts.
6. Manage family dysfunction more effectively.
7. Verbalize awareness of underlying psychologic issues.
8. Cease binge/purge episodes completely; cease dieting behavior.
9. Perceive body shape and weight as normal and acceptable.
10. Resolve family and other underlying issues.

PLANNING

The nurse's attitude toward the client with an eating disorder is as critical in the plan of care as any specific therapeutic intervention. Clients with eating disorders appear fragile, and although they are vulnerable, they can also be quite rigid and frustrating. If a good working alliance is not formed, with the nurse taking a firm, yet compassionate approach, client care quickly turns into a series of power struggles, and the treatment is doomed to fail. Therefore the plan of care will include consistent, collaborative efforts by the client, family, and interdisciplinary staff.

IMPLEMENTATION

For the client with an eating disorder, the nurse needs to implement a balanced plan of action that includes behavioral interventions to interrupt the cycle of eating disorder behavior. Psychologic interventions are used to improve coping skills, communication skills, and insight into underlying issues. Implementation of the plan will provide a safe, structured environment to prevent self-harm; promote weight gain and/or nutritional restoration; help the client express in words what the client is acting out with the behavior; teach more effective coping skills; monitor the use of medications; and coordinate the multidisci-

---

CASE STUDY

Laura is a 27-year-old married mother of a 3-year-old child. Laura has been hospitalized following a suicide attempt, in which she overdosed on a combination of 100 laxatives and a full bottle of her antidepressant medication. She is currently seeing a psychiatrist for depression and bulimia nervosa. The nursing assessment reveals that Laura currently binges and purges up to three times per day. Purging consists of self-induced vomiting, as well as the use of laxatives (usually 5 or 6 pills every day). She is within normal weight range at 140 pounds at 5 feet 9 inches. Laura is participating in milieu activities willingly, although her affect is depressed. She is eating very little at meals and has agreed not to purge while in the hospital.

Critical Thinking—Outcome Identification

1. How will the nurse determine Laura's therapeutic involvement with staff and peers?
2. What are realistic expectations of Laura for eating regular meals? What data should be monitored to track her improvement in nutritional status?
3. How will the nurse recognize improvements in eating behavior and cessation of purging?
4. How will Laura demonstrate awareness of the psychologic issues underlying her bulimia?

---

plinary efforts of the treatment team. Specific issues faced by a community nurse working with a client with eating disorders are discussed in the Nursing Care in the Community box.

NURSING INTERVENTIONS

1. Provide a safe environment *to ensure safety and prevent violence.*
2. Assess any risk of suicide (suicidal ideation, gesture, plan) *to prevent self-harm* (see Chapter 28).
3. Engage the client in a therapeutic alliance *to encourage expression of a wide range of thoughts and feelings, including any self-destructive urges.*
4. Restore minimum weight and nutritional balance through a behavioral program *to promote health and wellness.*

> Anorexia includes refeeding with food, food supplements, and tube feeding when necessary.
> Bulimia includes eating meals prescribed by a dietitian and avoidance of purging by the nurse remaining with the client for at least 1 hour after each meal.

5. Create a structured, supportive environment with clear, consistent, firm limits *to help establish a predictable routine and promote an internal locus of control that the client now lacks.*
6. Construct a behavioral plan that includes weight-gain goals (approximately 3 pounds per week) specific eat-

Nursing Care in the Community

Eating Disorders

The most overt problem encountered by community mental health nurses in assisting clients with a pattern of eating disorders involves the potential power struggle over participation in a treatment regimen. It is impossible for the community mental health nurse to continually observe the client's eating patterns, including self-starvation and self-induced vomiting. Clients with eating disorders are often evasive about their actual intent or emotions. Clients may say the "right" thing (i.e., what the nurse wants to hear), thereby confusing the nurse's assessment. Only when the client's physical state deteriorates can the counselor obtain a clear picture of what is actually occurring.

The nurse must frequently use the observations of family, friends, and other professionals to validate the reports of the client. This may be achieved by offering support groups not only for the clients, but also for their families and significant others. Nurses treating clients with eating disorders must be knowledgeable in the area of reality testing and other cognitive/behavioral therapies. They must also be educated about the signs and symptoms of the disorder, potential problems, and suggestions for positive changes in communication dynamics, including communication among family members. They must be certain to offer support rather than criticism throughout treatment.

The community nurse must plan interventions to empower the client and family to participate effectively in treatment. Written contracts may be engaging tools that offer the client a feeling of involvement and accountability. Clients are encouraged to identify situations that have been problematic for them in the past. They are assured that help is readily available and are encouraged to ask for help in curtailing their habitual dysfunctional patterns. The nurse helps individual clients and groups to use effective coping skills. Bonding techniques are employed to extend and expand support groups, especially those clients who are in their teens or early twenties and in need of a comforting peer support group.

The nurse should be aware of community support groups for clients with anorexia and bulimia. Overeaters Anonymous (OA) often has affiliated groups for persons with other eating disorders and can serve as a resource for those experiencing other eating disorders. Clients may also require antidepressant medication, which must be monitored for effectiveness and side effects. As in any prolonged illness, hospitalization must always be an option if the client's behaviors become life threatening.

ing goals (eating 75% of all meals), and consequences for compliance (preferably increased privileges for compliance rather than punishment for noncompliance). *Structure helps the client gain self-control and reduces the anxiety generated by noncompliance and an unpredictable routine.*
7. Encourage the client to express thoughts, feelings, and concerns about body and body image. *Verbalization*

helps to solidify concerns, helps the client to transform a pervasive sense of shame, guilt, and fear into specific areas of conflict, and clarifies the underlying issues (intimacy, sex, adult responsibility, identity).

8. Continue to help the client increase understanding of body image distortion. *The goal is for the client to recognize that preoccupation with breasts, hips, stomach, legs, etc., actually symbolizes underlying issues that will not resolve by changing the client's body.*

9. Assist the client in recalling positive eating experiences, such as a time when the client was able to eat a small portion of sweets and stop without binging, *to emphasize the fact that the client is capable of engaging in successful episodes of eating and to promote hope.*

10. Assume a caring, yet matter-of-fact approach without being overly sympathetic or overly confrontive and authoritarian *to assist the client in maintaining clear boundaries and to avoid power struggles.*

11. Intervene with the client's anxiety by helping the client associate feelings of anxiety with unmet needs and expectations that may represent threats to the self-system. *The client's recognition that anxiety can be a result of unconscious conflicts can in itself bring relief and start the process of problem solving.*

12. Offer positive feedback and praise when the client adheres to the treatment plan and strives to maintain the goals of the individual contract. *Praise increases self-esteem, promotes compliance, and encourages repetition of positive behaviors.*

    Examples:
    "You have eaten three new foods this week."
    "You listen attentively in group."

13. Engage the client in therapeutic interactions and groups (i.e., individual therapy, group therapy, family therapy, occupational/recreational therapy) *to express feelings and conflicts engendered by eating disorder behaviors in a supportive environment and reduce/rechannel anxiety in a more structured and meaningful way.*

14. Assist the client in identifying issues of low self-esteem, identity disturbance, separation, family dysfunction, and fear of maturity *to uncover and process the psychologic conflicts that underlie the eating disorder.*

15. Discuss with the client how obsession with food and weight helps the client avoid more difficult life problems and challenges *to help the client increase awareness and gain insight about the dynamics of the disorder.*

16. Collaborate with the dietitian to teach the client about adequate nutrition for the client's height and body type *to counter erroneous information about ideal weight and size and provide education regarding cultural pressures to be unrealistically thin.*

17. Collaborate with the social worker, family therapist, physician, and other members of the interdisciplinary team *to promote consistency in implementing the treatment plan.*

18. Teach adaptive therapeutic strategies (cognitive, behavioral, assertive) *to promote realistic thoughts, feelings, and coping behaviors and help the client to realize that it is irrational to believe that losing weight will solve his or her problems.*

19. Teach the client, family, and significant others about the disorder, symptom management, and prevention. *Knowledge promotes power and control and reduces fear and anxiety.*

20. Educate the family about healthy boundaries and normal separation and individuation versus overprotectiveness and family enmeshment *to help the family*

Client & Family TEACHING GUIDELINES

Teach the client's family members:

1. To not focus exclusively on the client's weight and food intake as indicators of progress. Help them to understand that eating disorder behaviors are symptomatic of underlying psychologic issues. Specify and explain common underlying issues such as low self-esteem, separation/individuation conflicts, interoceptive deficits, fear of maturity, and conflict avoidance.

2. To encourage the client to share what the client has learned in group and individual therapy regarding the particular psychologic issues underlying the eating disorder.

3. To encourage the client to verbalize thoughts and feelings about family interactions that the client may previously have been fearful or reluctant to disclose directly.

4. To relinquish control over the client's behavior; to stop monitoring what, when, and/or how much the client eats and what the client weighs.

5. To understand how their monitoring and controlling behaviors serve to reinforce the eating disorder behavior by setting up a power struggle in which the client feels controlled and rebels against this indirectly by worsening the behavior.

6. To decrease enmeshment; to stop behaviors such as preparing separate meals, not setting age-appropriate limits, or not expecting the client to follow family rules.

7. To understand that their well-intentioned attempts to be supportive backfire by sending the message that their child is helpless and exempt from age-appropriate responsibilities.

Teach the client:

1. To stop acting out conflicts and feelings with the eating disorder behavior. To stop trying to get needs met indirectly through behaviors, but rather to identify and verbalize conflicts, needs, and feelings.

2. To express thoughts and feelings verbally in group and one-to-one interactions. To transform diffuse feelings of guilt, anxiety, fear, emptiness, and sadness into concrete concerns. These feelings are expressed as experiences related to the body and about being fat. Ask the client to be very specific about the feeling: "What specifically are you afraid will happen?" or "When you say, 'I'm freaking out,' what thoughts are going through your head?"

relinquish unnecessary controls and promote mutually satisfying interpersonal relationships among family members (see Client & Family Teaching Guidelines box).

21. Collaborate with the occupational therapist to teach the client about appropriate exercise *to reduce compulsive behavior and promote moderation.*

ADDITIONAL TREATMENT MODALITIES
Biologic Modalities
Clients with anorexia who are more than 15% below ideal body weight should be closely monitored medically. After the initial assessment and treatment for effects of starvation, such as amenorrhea, osteoporosis, and vitamin and mineral deficiencies, the client should be closely monitored while refeeding takes place. The risk of refeeding syndrome, a possibly life-threatening complication, is high in the early phase of treating a severely malnourished client with total parenteral nutrition. Refeeding syndrome can be prevented by carefully monitoring electrolyte levels while slowly increasing parenteral nutrition by no more than 200 to 300 calories every 3 to 4 days (Mehler, 1996).

Clients with bulimia need to be initially assessed for acute fluid and electrolyte imbalance and for any of the dangerous side effects related to their individual purging behaviors. If purging is not completely stopped during treatment, the electrolytes need to be continually monitored.

There are many other accepted modalities of treatment for eating disorders. These are listed in the Additional Treatment Modalities box and are discussed in the following section.

Pharmacologic Modalities
Tricyclic antidepressants and, more recently, selective serotonin reuptake inhibitors (SSRIs) such as fluoxetine (Prozac), sertraline (Zoloft), and paroxetine (Paxil) have been effective in treating the comorbid eating disorder/affective disorder (Pope and Hudson, 1984). SSRIs have been shown to help prevent relapse after weight restoration in anorexia nervosa and to significantly decrease binge urges in bulimia nervosa. The dosage of SSRIs needed to obtain decreased binge urges, known as the "antibulimic" effect, is usually 60 mg or more (Devlin and Walsh, 1989; Jimerson et al, 1996). Buproprion (Wellbutrin) is contraindicated with bulimia nervosa because of a high incidence of seizures during clinical trials. MAOI antidepressants are not popular because of the strict dietary restrictions they require.

Antipsychotics may be used for extreme agitation or in clients exhibiting psychotic symptoms. Antianxiety medications are avoided because of their addictive qualities and also because clients with eating disorders need to learn to tolerate and cope with their anxiety rather than avoid it.

Often the medical side effects of eating disorders require the use of medication. Hypokalemia may be treated with potassium supplements, either orally or intravenously. Nutritional anemia may be treated with iron supplements. Gastroparesis, or delayed gastric emptying, may be treated with metoclopramide (Reglan). Infected parotid glands may be treated with antibiotics. Laxative dependence is often treated with a combination of stool softeners, bran, fiber, fluids, and decreasing doses of laxatives (if taking very high doses, such as 50 to 100 laxatives at a time, abrupt withdrawal is quite dangerous and gradual withdrawal is done under close supervision.)

Psychotherapeutic Modalities
Individual psychotherapy.   Some type of individual psychotherapy is generally recommended as the preferred treatment for eating disorders. Psychodynamically oriented therapists recommend long-term, insight-oriented therapy to repair early developmental failures or traumas, which are seen as primary etiologic factors. All but the most conservative psychoanalytic therapists, however, do recommend an active therapeutic stance and encourage the use of behavioral techniques for symptom management and cognitive restructuring to alter distorted thinking patterns.

ADDITIONAL TREATMENT MODALITIES
For the Client With an Eating Disorder

Biologic
Pharmacologic
Psychotherapeutic
   Individual psychotherapy
   Behavioral therapy
   Cognitive therapy
   Family therapy
   Group therapy
   Expressive therapies
Adjunctive therapy
   Occupational therapy
   Nutrition education and counseling
Social work
   Interdisciplinary treatment team
   Community support groups

⚠ CLINICAL ALERT

If the client is compliant with the contract but does not make the expected weight gain, the nurse may suspect that the client is purging and report this to the treatment team, who may recommend that the nurse confront the client with the purging behavior. Increased supervision after meals and during administration of supplements to prevent purging will follow. The nurse remains in the room with the client for an hour following eating or has the client sit at the nursing station for that time period. The contract may be amended to include these changes. If weight gain does not occur in a few days, tube feeding may be initiated.

NURSING CARE PLAN

Melissa is a 19-year-old college freshman who is hospitalized for severe cachexia (95 pounds at 5 feet 7 inches) with hypokalemia, nutritional anemia, and cardiac dysrhythmia. She had arrived home after flunking out of her first semester at college, and her parents, who had not seen her in several months, immediately took her to the family physician, who hospitalized her. Melissa's physician reports that she has been dieting and excessively exercising for the past 2 years but that she had always kept her weight within 10% of ideal body weight and that she had been in individual psychotherapy for a year before going to college. Melissa now states that she did not continue with therapy in college, as she had promised. Melissa minimizes her weight loss, complains of feeling fat, is sullen and angry, and wants to be discharged.

DSM-IV Diagnoses

Axis I   Anorexia nervosa, binge eating/purging type
Axis II   Rule out borderline personality disorder
Axis III Deferred
Axis IV   Moderate—3 (moving away from home to college)
Axis V   GAF = 50 (current)
          GAF = 65 (past year)

Nursing Diagnosis: Nutrition, altered: less than body requirements, related to self-starvation and possible purging behavior, as evidenced by severe weight loss, hypokalemia, and cardiac dysrhythmia.

Client Outcomes	Nursing Interventions	Evaluation
• Melissa will consume adequate calories for age, height, and metabolic need (e.g., 75% of each meal will be consumed by the end of the hospital stay).	• Initiate refeeding in collaboration with treatment team (Box 19-5). *Starving behavior is out of control, and Melissa cannot begin eating again on her own.*	• Melissa ate only 25% of meals on day 1, but on day 2, she ate 50% and drank all three dietary supplements. After 7 days, she was eating 75% of all meals and the supplements were discontinued.
	• Encourage Melissa to choose her own menu. *Melissa may be more cooperative if she feels she has some control over the refeeding process.*	• Melissa selected her own meals on day 3.
• Melissa will achieve minimum normal weight (less than 15% below ideal weight: for 5 feet, 7 inches, approximately 115 pounds).	• Weigh daily with the client's back facing the scale. *Melissa's obsession with weight may be reinforced by her knowledge of daily weight changes. Not knowing may help her tolerate weight gain and help her to let go of her overcontrol of her body.*	• Melissa achieved her goal weight by discharge.
• Melissa will gain an average of 4 pounds per week.	• Continue to implement the refeeding plan and contract as needed *to maintain the client's expected weight.*	

Nursing Diagnosis: Body image disturbance related to underlying psychologic conflicts (fear of growing up, fear of sexuality), as evidenced by complaints of body dissatisfaction, fear of weight gain, and minimizing weight loss when more than 15% below minimal normal weight (e.g., 95 pounds at 5 feet 7 inches).

Client Outcomes	Nursing Interventions	Evaluation
• Melissa will demonstrate realistic perceptions of body shape and size.	• Encourage expression of thoughts and feelings regarding body. *Verbalizing specific concerns may help Melissa uncover psychologic issues related to her body image.*	• Client verbalized awareness that she is underweight and that her dissatisfaction with her body has to do more with psychologic issues than with her weight.
• Melissa will demonstrate increased insight into body image distortion.	• Collaborate with dietitian to give fact-based information to counter irrational beliefs about body size and shape (e.g., "You are 20 pounds below minimum healthy weight for your age and height,") *to provide reality orientation of discrepancy between ideal weight and current weight.*	• Melissa verbalized that she perceives herself as heavier than her actual weight.

NURSING CARE PLAN —cont'd

Client Outcomes	Nursing Interventions	Evaluation
• Melissa will demonstrate an enhanced self-concept based on positive attributes, rather than totally based on her body shape.	• Give Melissa feedback regarding positive qualities that she demonstrates in the milieu. *Melissa's self-concept is overly defined by her body, and she needs to view herself more realistically.*	• Melissa verbalized positive qualities about herself that were unrelated to her body.

Nursing Diagnosis: Noncompliance with the treatment plan related to underlying psychologic conflicts (control issues or separation issues), as evidenced by anger, refusal to self-disclose to the staff, and requests to be discharged.

Client Outcomes	Nursing Interventions	Evaluation
• Melissa will participate in therapeutic contacts with staff.	• Engage Melissa in therapeutic alliance (e.g., using Melissa's input to develop a collaborative treatment plan). *Including Melissa as a part of the treatment team increases her power base and decreases power struggles, strengthening the therapeutic alliance.*	• Melissa participated as part of the treatment team.
• Melissa will comply with the interdisciplinary treatment plan. • Melissa will acknowledge her condition and the need for treatment.	• Use interdisciplinary-designed contracts, with clear expectations and consequences, *to increase client compliance and further reduce power struggles.* • Use reality orientation to challenge Melissa's minimization of the seriousness of her condition. Give information about laboratory results, medical status, etc. *Melissa's denial will decrease when challenged with concrete information.*	• Melissa complied with the expectations of her behavioral contract. • Melissa verbalized awareness of the need for hospitalization and treatment.

Cognitive therapists are more likely to recommend structured, short-term individual therapy with less insight orientation and more focus on thought patterns.

Most therapists, whatever their orientation, use hospitalization as a means to manage acute exacerbations of either the eating disorder symptoms or concomitant affective disorder symptoms.

Behavioral therapy. Either within the context of individual outpatient therapy or in a hospital setting, behavioral therapy is used for symptom management. Behavioral contracts for weight gain, for regulating eating and exercise behavior, and for diminishing binge/purge behaviors are commonly used tools in inpatient and outpatient treatment. Exposure plus response prevention, in which clients eat "scary" or binge foods and are then prevented from purging, is an effective intervention for bulimia nervosa.

Cognitive therapy. Most treatment programs and therapists mention the use of cognitive therapy in the treatment of eating disorders. Most clients demonstrate distorted thoughts and beliefs related to food and weight, as well as to self-concept. Techniques such as reframing, cognitive restructuring, and rational-emotive therapy are commonly used to alter these cognitive distortions.

Family therapy. Adolescents with eating disorders almost always participate in family therapy as part of their treatment. Educating the family about eating disorders is very important, since the eating disorder behavior often becomes the focal point of the family, leading to overinvolvement and constant power struggles that inadvertently reinforce the behavior. Decreasing these secondary gains and uncovering any underlying family dysfunction are the initial goals of family therapy. Improving family interactions and interrelationships are goals for the longer term.

Group therapy. Group psychotherapy is widely used in both inpatient and outpatient settings for the treatment

---

Box 19-5   Refeeding Procedure

If Melissa does not eat 75% of her meals on day 1, she will receive three dietary supplements on day 2. Supplements will continue daily until she eats 75% of her meals. If she does not finish her supplements on day 2, she will be tube fed on day 3. Tube feeding will continue until she eats 75% of all meals for 1 day. If she refuses tube feeding, she will be discharged.

of eating disorders. The rationale is twofold. Clients with anorexia and bulimia often set themselves apart from others with their unusual stance toward food and eating, resulting in secretiveness, feeling misunderstood, and secondary gains related to feeling "special." Being in a group with others with eating disorders allows them a safe place to self-disclose and be accepted/understood, while preventing manipulation and secondary gains related to being "different."

Expressive therapies.   Art therapy, music therapy, dance/movement therapy, journal writing, and poetry are often used as part of a multidisciplinary approach to eating disorders. Because the eating disorder symptoms are an indirect expression, on a physical level, of emotional pain, many clients have great difficulty translating their pain into the words needed for "talking" therapy. The use of nonverbal techniques may allow for greater self-disclosure and exploration of underlying issues.

Adjunctive Therapy

Occupational therapy.   Many clients with eating disorders need assistance in learning how to plan meals, shop, and cook for themselves, especially if they have not eaten properly for many years. Although the dietitian will do the actual meal planning, occupational therapy can help the client carry out the plan. Education concerning healthy moderate exercise is also necessary to alter compulsive exercise patterns.

Nutrition education and counseling.   Although clients with eating disorders are obsessed with food, most have inaccurate, outdated, or distorted information about nutrition. Consultation with a registered dietitian in both inpatient and outpatient settings is an important part of treatment. The dietitian should be the one to calculate the client's ideal weight range, plan a refeeding program, and supervise meal planning. The dietitian can provide nutritional counseling and assist the client with meal planning on an ongoing basis.

Social Work

Clients with chronic eating disorders often do not function well in society. Hospital social workers can be helpful in finding community resources for those clients needing help with day treatment services, alternative living situations such as board-and-care homes, group homes, residential treatment facilities, or vocational rehabilitation. Social workers are also often used to provide family therapy.

Interdisciplinary Treatment Team

An interdisciplinary approach to treatment is recommended for eating disorders. In both inpatient and outpatient settings, a successful treatment outcome depends on the collaboration of nursing, medical, psychiatric, psycho-

---

CASE STUDY

Eileen is a 16-year-old young woman admitted to the hospital for increasingly out-of-control bulimic symptoms, including binging and purging up to 10 times a day and abuse of laxatives.

During her first week of hospitalization, the primary focus was to correct Eileen's fluid and electrolyte balance and monitor her to prevent purging. Eileen slept a great deal her first week. She participated superficially in group sessions, complaining mainly of physical discomfort related to stopping purging and laxatives. During the second week of treatment, the team set goals to help Eileen become "more involved" in the psychologic issues related to her bulimia. The interventions included encouraging Eileen to work on underlying issues of self-esteem and family dysfunction.

Critical Thinking—Evaluation

1. How will the nurse evaluate Eileen's progress in working on underlying issues? What are three specific client outcomes that would indicate such progress?
2. What specific observations should the nurse make during group sessions to evaluate Eileen's progress?
3. What verbalizations made by Eileen would indicate progress in her work on "underlying issues"?

---

logic, dietary, social work, counseling, and occupational therapy professionals.

Interdisciplinary treatment team meetings are the recommended forum for sharing assessment information and developing the multidisciplinary treatment plan. Nurses are usually the ones who coordinate this plan and see that it is implemented. As the health care system changes and managed care takes over more of the mental health care industry, hospital stays become shorter and specialty units such as eating disorder units may disappear. Clients with eating disorders are more likely to be admitted to general psychiatric units or even medical units. Nursing is thus taking more of a leadership role in the coordination of the treatment team.

Community Support Groups

Community-based support and self-help groups are available in some areas. Overeaters Anonymous, a 12-step program, can be very useful for individuals with binge eating disorder. National nonprofit organizations such as Anorexia Nervosa and Associated Disorders (ANAD) provide support groups for people with anorexia nervosa and bulimia nervosa. Names and addresses of other organizations providing help for eating disorders can be found in Appendix C.

EVALUATION

The nurse will evaluate the progress of the client with an eating disorder in an organized, timely manner in accordance with the outcomes delineated in the care plan. For the client with an eating disorder, the evaluation will include physiologic, behavioral, psychologic, social, and cultural spheres. Monitoring laboratory values, vital signs, weight, and food/fluid intake will provide the data to evaluate physiologic responses to treatment. Observing and recording the client's affect, level of program participation, specific eating behaviors, peer interactions, and responses to staff provide evaluative data to track behavioral responses to treatment. Listening to and interacting with the client in group therapy, in milieu activities, and during individual interactions regarding specific issues, the treatment plan, or the contract provides more data to evaluate the client's psychologic and behavioral responses to treatment.

Summary of Key Concepts

1. Eating disorders are syndromes with physiologic, behavioral, and psychologic features.

2. Self-starvation, binge eating, and purging behaviors have existed for many centuries, having various psychologic meanings in different cultural eras. Until recently, eating disorders were a rare occurrence.

3. The recent outbreak of eating disorders is related to current cultural trends in the fashion industry, the diet industry, and the women's movement.

4. Eating disorders have a multidetermined etiology, including biologic, sociocultural, psychologic, and familial factors.

5. There is a high incidence of depression among clients with eating disorders and their families. It is believed that some biologic link may exist between the two disorders.

6. Personality traits common among those with eating disorders include low self-esteem, perfectionism, affective instability, interoceptive deficits, ineffectiveness, and people pleasing.

7. Common dynamics of families of origin of persons with eating disorders include enmeshment, poor conflict resolution, and incomplete separation and may include alcoholism and physical or sexual abuse.

8. Most individuals with eating disorders are female (95% to 99%). Bulimia nervosa is more common than anorexia nervosa. Eating disorders are most common among high school and college students.

9. Clients with eating disorders often have other psychiatric diagnoses. Common Axis I diagnoses are depressive, anxiety, and dissociative disorders. Common Axis II diagnoses are borderline, avoidant, and obsessive-compulsive personality disorders.

10. Anorexia nervosa and bulimia nervosa are distinct diagnoses in the DSM-IV classification but have many overlapping features.

11. The course of the illness may be chronic or episodic, requiring long-term or repeated treatment episodes.

12. Interdisciplinary treatment is indicated to deal with the multifaceted nature of eating disorders.

13. Medical complications from eating disorders can be life threatening. Self-induced vomiting and abuse of laxatives and diuretics can cause serious electrolyte imbalances that may lead to cardiac dysrhythmias and cardiac arrest.

14. The nurse must take a firm, professional, yet compassionate approach to avoid the power struggles that commonly undermine treatment of individuals with eating disorders.

15. The plan of care must balance behavioral interventions that interrupt the cycle of behavior with psychologic interventions that deal with underlying issues.

16. A safe, structured environment must be provided to prevent self-harm, promote nutritional restoration, help the client understand the meaning of his or her behavior, and learn more effective coping skills.

17. Refeeding must be done in a structured manner with clear expectations and consequences. Positive reinforcement is more effective than punishment. Consistency is crucial.

18. The client must understand how he or she is using the eating disorder to avoid psychologic issues. The nurse assists the client in refocusing attention from gaining weight to underlying issues and conflicts.

19. Antidepressants are used to treat the comorbid depression in clients with eating disorders and may help decrease binge urges in clients with bulimia. The mechanism is unknown.

20. Long-term individual psychotherapy of various modalities is generally recommended for all clients with eating disorders. Group and family psychotherapies are also widely used.

REFERENCES

American Psychiatric Association: *Diagnostic and statistical manual of mental disorders*, ed 4, Washington, DC, 1994, The Association.

Bauer B, Anderson W: Bulimic beliefs: food for thought, *J Coun Dev* 67:416, 1989.

Bell R: *Holy anorexia*, Chicago, 1987, University of Chicago Press.

Binswanger L: The case of Ellen West. In May R, Angel E, Ellenburger H, editors: *Existence*, New York, 1958, Basic Books.

Boskind-Lodahl M: Cinderella's stepsisters: a feminist perspective on anorexia nervosa and bulimia, *Signs* 343, 1976.

Boskind-Lodahl M, White W: *Bulimarexia: the binge/purge cycle*, New York, 1983, WW Norton.

Brewerton T: Toward a unified theory of serotonin dysregulation in eating and related disorders, *Psychoneuroendocrinology* 20(6):561, 1995.

Brumberg J: *Fasting girls*, New York, 1989, New American Library.

Connors M, Morse W: Sexual abuse and eating disorders: a review, *Int J Eat Disord* 13(1):1, 1993.

Devlin M, Walsh B: Eating disorders and depression, *Psych Ann* 19(9):473, 1989.

Folsom V et al: The impact of sexual and physical abuse on eating disordered and psychiatric symptoms, *Int J Eat Disord* 13:249, 1993.

Gartner A, Marcus R, Halmi K: DSM-IIIR personality disorders in patients with eating disorders, *Am J Psychiatry* 146:1585, 1989.

Glassman JN et al: Some correlates of treatment response to a multicomponent psychotherapy program in outpatients with eating disorders, *Ann Clin Psychiatry* 2:33, 1990.

Halmi K: *A clinical overview of anorexia nervosa*, Presentation at conference: Eating Disorders: a practical clinical update, San Francisco, 1992.

Halmi K et al: Comorbidity of psychiatric diagnoses in anorexia nervosa, *Arch Gen Psychiatry* 48:712, 1991.

Hamburger W: Emotional aspects of obesity, *Med Clin North Am* 35:483, 1951.

Herzog D et al: The prevalence of personality disorders in 210 women with eating disorders, *J Clin Psychiatry* 53:147, 1992.

Herzog D et al: Comorbidity and outcome in eating disorders, *Psychiatr Clin North Am* 19(4):843, 1996.

Jimerson D et al: Medications in the treatment of eating disorders, *Psychiatr Clin North Am* 19(4):739, 1996.

Johnson C, Connors M: *The etiology and treatment of bulimia nervosa*, New York, 1987, Basic Books.

Levin A et al: Multiple personality in eating disorder patients, *Int J Eat Disord* 13(2):235, 1993.

Lindner R: The case of Laura. In *The fifty minute hour*, New York, 1955, Holt, Rinehart & Winston.

Mehler P: Eating disorders: (1) anorexia nervosa; (2) bulimia nervosa, *Hosp Pract*, 1996.

Minuchin S, Rosman B, Baker L: *Psychosomatic families: anorexia nervosa in context*, Cambridge, Mass., 1978, Harvard University Press.

Moyer D et al: Childhood sexual abuse and precursors of binge eating in an adolescent female population, *Int J Eat Disord* 21(1):23, 1997.

From North American Nursing Diagnosis Association: *NANDA nursing diagnoses: definitions and classifications, 1999-2000*, Philadelphia, 1999, The Association.

Orbach S: *Fat is a feminist issue*, New York, 1978, Berkeley Books.

Pollice C et al: Relationship of depression, anxiety and obsessionality to state of illness in anorexia nervosa, *Int J Eat Disord* 21:367, 1997.

Pope H, Hudson J: *New hope for binge eaters*, New York, 1984, Harper & Row.

Russell G: Bulimia nervosa: an ominous variant of anorexia nervosa, *Psychol Med* 9:429, 1979.

Spitzer R et al: Binge eating disorder: a multisite field trial of the diagnostic criteria, *Int J Eat Disord* 11:191, 1992.

Spitzer R et al: Binge eating disorder: its further validation in a multisite study, *Int J Eat Disord* 13:137, 1993.

Stunkard A: Eating patterns and obesity, *Psychiatry Q* 33:284, 1959.

Thornton C, Russell J: Obsessive compulsive comorbidity in the dieting disorders, *Int J Eat Disord* 21(1):83, 1997.

US Department of Health and Human Services, Public Health Service, NIH pub No. 94-3477, 1993.

Vanderlinden J et al: Dissociative experiences and trauma in eating disorders, *Int J Eat Disord* 13:187, 1993.

Vernon-Guidry, S, Williamson D, Netemeyer R: Structural modeling analysis of body dysphoria and eating disorder symptoms in pre-adolescent girls, *Eat Disord* 5(1):15, 1997.

Waller G: Association of sexual abuse and borderline personality disorder in eating disordered women, *Int J Eat Disord* 13:259, 1993.

Walsh B, Devlin M: The pharmacologic treatment of eating disorders, *Psychiatr Clin North Am* 15:149, 1992.

Wilson G, Fairburn C: Cognitive treatments for eating disorders, *J Consult Clin Psychol* 61:261, 1993.

Wooley S, Wooley O: Intensive outpatient and residential treatment for bulimia. In Garner D, Garfinkel P, editors: *Handbook of psychotherapy for anorexia nervosa and bulimia*, New York, 1985, Guilford Press.

Notes

CHAPTER 20

Sexual Disorders

Kathryn Thomas and Shelly F. Lurie

OBJECTIVES

- Discuss possible etiologies for the origins of sexual dysfunctions.
- Describe various sexual dysfunction diagnoses.
- Examine techniques used in diagnosing various sexual dysfunctions.
- Compare and contrast various treatment modalities.
- Apply the nursing process in caring for clients with sexual dysfunctions.
- Describe the different diagnoses of the sex offender (paraphilic) population.
- Discuss the focus of treatment for paraphilic disorders.
- Explain at least two types of treatment and effects on illness symptomatology.
- Analyze the relationship between treatment and recidivism.
- Apply the nursing process in caring for clients with sexual (paraphilic) disorders.

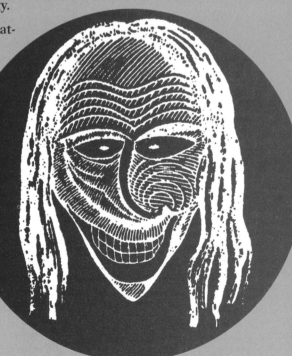

This chapter discusses the two categories of sexual disorders: sexual dysfunctions and paraphilias. Sexual dysfunctions are covered in the first part of the chapter, and paraphilias are covered in the second.

SEXUAL DYSFUNCTIONS: HISTORICAL AND THEORETIC PERSPECTIVES

In 1966 William Masters and Virginia Johnson published their classic work, *Human Sexual Response*. As a result they became famous, practically overnight. Their work was based on the direct laboratory observation of more than 10,000 male and female volunteers (Masters and Johnson, 1966). From this research, they were able to determine exactly what happens to the body during erotic stimulation, from excitement to plateau to orgasm and, finally, to resolution. In 1970 they published a second text, *Human Sexual Inadequacy*, in which they discussed their work in helping others overcome sexual dysfunction. In this book Masters and Johnson outline the probable causes for dysfunction and give detailed prescriptions for treatment.

Masters and Johnson were not the first people to explore the area of sexual dysfunction. Many prominent sexologists—Henry Havelock Ellis, Sigmund Freud, Niles Newton, and Theodoor van de Velde—addressed these issues in earlier eras (Brecher, 1971). However, these works were more theoretic and were not based on scientific data.

For the early pioneers, the treatment focus for sexual dysfunction was psychoanalytic. Childhood experiences were believed to exert a subconscious influence on sexual behavior as an adult. Such infantile feelings as fear of castration and penis envy, coupled with fantasies,

Depo-Provera (medroxyprogesterone acetate) A medication used in the adjunctive treatment of sexual disorders; a sexual appetite suppressant; lowers testosterone level to a prepubescent level.

Ego dystonic pedophile A person who is cognitively aware that his or her behavior is inappropriate and is affected by this, which may lead to seeking treatment.

Ego syntonic pedophile A person who is cognitively aware that his or her behavior is inappropriate but is not troubled by this so will not seek treatment.

Estradiol Increases synthesis of DNA, RNA, and protein in responsive tissues and reduces the release of follicle-stimulating hormone and luteinizing hormone from the pituitary gland.

External vacuum pump A cylindrical vacuum pump applied to the penis that brings blood into the penis and traps it there, thus improving erection.

Intracorporal injections Injections of various medications into the right and left corpus cavernosum to improve erection.

Lupron-Depot (leuprolide) A synthetic analog of naturally occurring gonadotropin-releasing hormone. It inhibits gonadotropin secretion, thus suppressing testicular testosterone.

Nocturnal penile tumescence A test that uses a strain gauge around the penis to depict the pattern of arousal while the client sleeps.

Paraphilias Sexual deviations/disorders presenting with inappropriate sexual fantasies involving deviant sexual acts, inappropriate sexual urges, and acting out of these fantasies and urges.

Penile-brachial index (PBI) A test that determines the difference between the penile and the brachial blood pressure to assess vascularization to the penis.

Plethysmography A diagnostic test for males and females that may help determine arousal patterns and level of arousal and assesses blood flow to the genitals.

Psychoeducation A type of therapy that educates the client with a paraphilic disorder to identify situations/objects that may trigger inappropriate sexual activity and develop awareness of relapse prevention strategies and the importance of treatment compliance.

Recidivisim Chronic, repetitive acting out of sexual behaviors considered to be unacceptable that have or have not resulted in criminal conviction.

Sensate focus A learned exercise developed by Masters and Johnson that involves concentrating on the sensations produced by touching.

Triggers Stimuli that heighten unacceptable sexual cravings.

Vaginal dilators A graduated series of cylindrical dilators introduced into the vagina to decrease involuntary spasm.

Viagra A drug that blocks the enzyme that breaks down cyclic guanosine monophosphate (cGMP), boosting the chemical's relaxing effect on penile smooth muscle cells and creating an erection.

Victimizer Another term used to define a sex offender; may be used when discussing familial transmissions of the paraphilia.

Yohimbine An alpha$_2$ adrenoreceptor blocker that may facilitate blood flow to the genitalia (especially in men) and therefore may improve arousal.

fears, and experiences, combined to create sexual dysfunctions. The treatment was aimed at uncovering these old traumas.

Masters and Johnson radically moved the theoretic perspective to the behavioral sphere. They postulated that sex therapy should be a series of specifically directed exercises guided by a therapist. Their original treatment program consisted of couples therapy in which the clients worked with a male/female treatment team. Couples came to St. Louis and lived in a hotel for 13 days. Treatment consisted of careful assessment, roundtable discussions, and homework assignments. In addition, Masters and Johnson developed many specific techniques, such as sensate focus and the squeeze technique (discussed later in the chapter).

Since the late 1960s, much has been learned about sexual dysfunctions and about sexuality in general. Though they have their benefits, structured treatment programs such as Masters and Johnson's have not proved to be a panacea. Sexuality is too complex to be reduced to a sex manual solution. In recent years, approaches that combine behavioral, cognitive, and communication methods, as well as psychodynamic techniques, have been readily employed. Helen Singer Kaplan (1974) identified the need for behavioral techniques to be reintegrated with psychoanalysis in treatment.

Many others have researched other approaches. Hartman and Fithian (1972) outlined a treatment approach based on careful observational research. Others such as Anon (1976), Leiblum and Rosen (1989), and LoPiccolo and Friedman (1988) have developed other strategies and therapeutic perspectives. The latest treatments involve biologic techniques such as oral preparations, injection, prosthesis, and surgical interventions.

ETIOLOGY

Etiologic possibilities for sexual dysfunctions fall in several different categories: biologic, psychologic, and couple oriented (Box 20-1).

BIOLOGIC FACTORS

Biologic factors that may contribute to sexual dysfunction include vascular, neurologic, and endocrine, as well as a range of diseases such as cancer, degenerative diseases, and genital infections (Wagner and Kaplan, 1993). Vascular factors include cardiac disease and disease of the blood vessels. Neurologic factors may be stroke, head injuries, spinal cord disorders, epilepsy, or peripheral nerve disorders. Endocrine factors include diabetes and altered hormonal levels. The effects of medications should be considered. It is well known that antipsychotics and antihypertensives, as well as sedatives, tranquilizers, narcotics, and alcohol, can all adversely affect sexual functioning. Serotonin reuptake inhibitors have gained increased notoriety for their role in sexual dysfunction. (Labbate et al, 1998).

PSYCHOLOGIC FACTORS

As previously noted, early childhood experiences formed the hallmark of beliefs about causation. Indeed, many still believe that psychosocial factors are more important in the etiology of sexual dysfunctions than other reasons. There is currently much literature and discussion about the impact of childhood sexual trauma on later sexual functioning (Beitchman et al, 1992). Repressive childhood environments that include religious, familial, or cultural restrictions have also been implicated (Money, 1986b).

Other issues such as anxiety and stress may also contribute to changes in sexual functioning. Masters and Johnson (1970) coined the term *spectatoring*. This psychologic factor refers to the tendency to monitor one's own sexual activity, thus detracting from the actual experience. Stress from any source has been noted to lower sexual drive and to decrease both testosterone and luteinizing hormone levels (Morokoff and Gilliland, 1993).

Misinformation and a lack of sex education may account for some degree of sexual dysfunction. One example is ignorance about the placement and function of the clitoris, which may severely affect obtaining sexual pleasure. Myths, such as those that assert that men are always ready for sex and women are never interested, have also influenced attitudes toward sex.

COUPLE-ORIENTED FACTORS

Couple-oriented factors involve differences in sexual drives and interests. Money (1986a) used the term

Box 20-1	Etiologic Factors for Sexual Dysfunctions
Biologic Factors	
Vascular	Cardiac disease
	Diseases of the blood vessels
Neurologic	Stroke
	Head injuries
	Spinal cord disorders
	Epilepsy
	Peripheral nerve disorders
Endocrine	Diabetes
	Altered hormonal levels, especially testosterone
Psychologic Factors	
Childhood experiences	
Anxiety and stress	
Misinformation and lack of sex education	
Couple-Oriented Factors	
Differences in sexual desire or interests	
Lack of communication	
Lack of trust	

lovemap to describe one's idealized picture of who and what make up one's sexual arousal pattern. Lovemaps vary from individual to individual. Thus a couple may not be well matched in the types of behaviors that interest them. Communication is another couple-oriented factor that may affect sexual functioning. Couples often do not discuss what they do or don't enjoy sexually or share their feelings about the experience. Trust between partners is also a crucial factor.

EPIDEMIOLOGY

The prevalence of sexual dysfunction disorders is difficult to determine. This is partially due to a lack of research but also to a lack of such problems being reported. Masters and Johnson (1970) suggest that 50% of all couples have a sexual dysfunction. Spector and Carey (1990) believe that sexual problems are quite common in our society.

Forty-six percent of couples presenting for sex therapy at one treatment center complained of low sexual desire (LoPiccolo and Friedman, 1988). Kaplan (1974) estimates that 50% of all males will experience erectile problems sometime in their lives. Spector and Carey (1990) say that erectile dysfunction is the most common cause of why males seek therapy.

In relationship to orgasmic disorder, Renshaw (1988) found that females with primary orgasmic dysfunction constituted 32% and females with secondary orgasmic dysfunction constituted 37% of all clients seen at a sex clinic. Kinsey et al (1953) notes that 10% of women interviewed reported lifelong anorgasmia. By contrast, Masters and Johnson (1970) find inhibited male orgasm rare. They report only 17 cases in an 11-year period.

Kaplan (1974) cites premature ejaculation as the most common of all sexual dysfunctions. For pain disorders, Renshaw (1988) reports 8% for dyspareunia and 5% for vaginismus, but other investigators cite higher averages. There appears to be a relatively high incidence of sexual dissatisfaction in the population yet a serious lack of research and understanding of the issues.

CLINICAL DESCRIPTION

The DSM-IV divides the sexual dysfunctions into sexual desire disorders, sexual arousal disorders, orgasmic disorders, sexual pain disorders, sexual dysfunction resulting from a general medical condition, substance-induced sexual dysfunction, and sexual dysfunction not otherwise specified (see DSM-IV Criteria box). The first three cat-

Understanding & Applying Research

This study involved a retrospective chart review of 167 men and 429 women treated with serotonin-reuptake inhibitors (SRIs) in an outpatient setting. The participants were asked if they had new-onset sexual dysfunction after beginning on SRIs. The study indicated that 16.3% of these participants reported sexual symptoms while taking SRIs. The mean age for the men was 47.2, and the mean age for women was 37.5. Of those participating in the study, 55% were married, 33.8% had the diagnosis of dysthymic disorder, and 10.2% had the diagnosis of major depression. The majority of individuals studied (50.1%) took fluoxotene. Three other SRIs were represented.

Charts were reviewed by a psychiatric resident. Demographic data, psychiatric diagnosis, medication use, type and duration of sexual side effects, and the use of medication to treat the side effects were noted. Three groups were identified from this chart review. Group 1 contained individuals who reported SRI-induced sexual dysfunction and who tried a pharmacologic antidote; group 2 consisted of those who experienced dysfunction from the SRI but did not take the antidote or stopped taking the SRI, and group 3 was composed of individuals who did not report sexual dysfunction. Of those who reported sexual side effects, there were more men than women and more individuals who were married and who were older. There was no significant difference found between various types of SRIs with respect to sexual dysfunction. The most common problems reported were anorgasmia and orgasmic delay.

After determination of specific symptoms, group 1 was treated with three different pharmacologic antidotes; yohimbine, amantadine, and cyproheptadine. Of these clients, 81% responded positively to yohimbine, 42% to amantandine, and 48% to cyproheptadine. Using a X^2-test, researchers found that those taking yohimbine had a significantly greater improvement in sexual functioning. None of the antidotes caused a depression relapse.

Researchers noted that their finding of 16.3% who reported sexual dysfunction was lower than that reported in other studies. They also noted that underreporting of sexual side effects may have resulted from embarrassment or reluctance to discuss sexual issues. They were of the opinion that the reason why more married individuals, males, and older people reported may have been due to their increased comfort level and not to actual incidence. A number of participants said that they would stop SRI therapy if no treatment for their sexual dysfunction was found. This suggests that sexual side effects may be a significant reason for medication noncompliance. This study relied on retrospective data and participant self-report, both of which limit the usefulness of the study. However, it did rely on a large sample, which increases the study's usefulness. This research clearly adds to the body of knowledge on sexual dysfunction, use of SRIs, and possible treatment approaches for the sexual side effects of these medications.

Data from Ashton A, Hamer R, Rosen R: Serotonin-reuptake inhibitor-induced sexual dysfunction and its treatment: a large scale retrospective study of 596 psychiatric outpatients, *J Sex Marital Ther* 23(3):165, 1997.

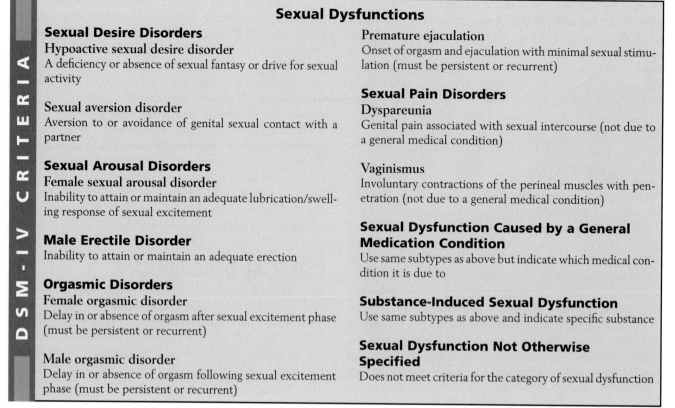

Sexual Dysfunctions

Sexual Desire Disorders

Hypoactive sexual desire disorder
A deficiency or absence of sexual fantasy or drive for sexual activity

Sexual aversion disorder
Aversion to or avoidance of genital sexual contact with a partner

Sexual Arousal Disorders

Female sexual arousal disorder
Inability to attain or maintain an adequate lubrication/swelling response of sexual excitement

Male Erectile Disorder

Inability to attain or maintain an adequate erection

Orgasmic Disorders

Female orgasmic disorder
Delay in or absence of orgasm after sexual excitement phase (must be persistent or recurrent)

Male orgasmic disorder
Delay in or absence of orgasm following sexual excitement phase (must be persistent or recurrent)

Premature ejaculation
Onset of orgasm and ejaculation with minimal sexual stimulation (must be persistent or recurrent)

Sexual Pain Disorders

Dyspareunia
Genital pain associated with sexual intercourse (not due to a general medical condition)

Vaginismus
Involuntary contractions of the perineal muscles with penetration (not due to a general medical condition)

Sexual Dysfunction Caused by a General Medication Condition

Use same subtypes as above but indicate which medical condition it is due to

Substance-Induced Sexual Dysfunction

Use same subtypes as above and indicate specific substance

Sexual Dysfunction Not Otherwise Specified

Does not meet criteria for the category of sexual dysfunction

Modified from American Psychiatric Association: *Diagnostic and statistical manual of mental disorders,* ed 4, Washington, DC, 1994, The Association.

egories are based on Kaplan's (1974) stages of the sexual response cycle.

PROGNOSIS

To guide and properly educate their clients, nurses must understand how successful therapy can be for the individual or for the couple. There are some prognostic data available for sexual dysfunctions in general. However, these data cannot be used specifically for each dysfunction. For example, sexual desire disorders tend to have a more negative prognosis than do orgasmic disorders.

Masters and Johnson (1970) found that primary impotence treatment had a 40.6% failure rate, whereas the failure rate for secondary impotence treatment was 26.2%. Premature ejaculation treatment failed only 2.2% of the time. Concerning intervention rates for orgasmic dysfunction, the failure rate was 19.7% for males and 19.3% for females. When Masters and Johnson did a follow-up study 5 years later, they found that in males and females combined, only 5.1% had relapsed. More recently, sex therapists have suggested that approximately two thirds of all treatment is successful. Zilbergeld and Evans (1980) noted a relapse rate of 54%. This may not be due to a lessening of therapeutic effectiveness but rather to different criteria for data collection. Many professionals believe

that desire phase disorders are the least easily treated. This is perhaps due to the variety of origins of desire.

DISCHARGE CRITERIA

Client will:

1. Express satisfaction with one's sexuality.
2. Develop insight into the disorder, etiology of the disorder, and the symptoms.
3. Develop appropriate strategies to effect the specific disorder.
4. Communicate effectively with significant other regarding sexuality.
5. Demonstrate ability to communicate needs and desires sexually.
6. Develop appropriate coping strategies.

Sexuality is an essential aspect of every human being. All nurses should have the goal of helping their clients achieve positive sexual expressions. Facilitating this goal is a rewarding albeit difficult task.

For any given client or couple, it is difficult to predict how long interventions and treatment must last. Some disorders are more difficult to treat (e.g., sexual desire disorders); some are relatively simple (e.g., orgasmic disorders, premature ejaculation). However, the assumption that this will be true in any given case is shortsighted. Individual factors will speed or complicate the recovery period, thus flexibility must be built in. The astute nurse is consistently aware of this. Additionally, it is not up to the nurse alone to know when goals are met. Individuals vary in the outcomes they expect. Sexual expression and satisfaction are for the individual alone to decide. As long as the expression and satisfaction are not harmful to another, they should not be determined by anyone else except the client.

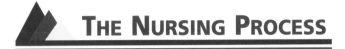

THE NURSING PROCESS

ASSESSMENT

For many reasons, sexuality is a sensitive topic for most people. When discussing sexuality with clients, the nurse should consider these sensitivities. Nurses are not immune to the feelings, beliefs, values, and attitudes that affect others. Therefore when the nurse is dealing with client-related sexual dysfunction issues, it may be uncomfortable for both parties. Yet, a holistic nursing assessment must consider sexuality as important as other functions. An important step in decreasing discomfort is to have the nurse examine his or her own feelings and comfort level with the topic.

The nurse will be better equipped to deal with others in the important area of human sexuality by combining self-understanding, a firm knowledge base, expert use of the nursing process, and nonjudgment.

Assessment is a crucial phase in working with clients with sexual dysfunction. A clear understanding of the complexity of the symptoms and what areas of functioning are affected is needed. Sexual dysfunctions may arise throughout various phases of the sexual response cycle.

Dysfunctions may reflect individual functioning or may be couple related. Sexual assessment must be seen in the context of overall assessment factors such as background, physical health, religious and cultural beliefs, education, occupation, significant relationships, and social relationships. In addition to the assessment of the specific complaint, the nurse must also consider the individual's or couple's perspective of the problem and desire to change.

Box 20-2 presents a sample sexual history form. The following guidelines should apply when doing a sexual assessment:

1. Before beginning a sexual assessment, examine one's own feelings, attitudes, values, and level of comfort.
2. Ensure a private, quiet space for assessment, ample time, and an unhurried attitude.
3. Questions on sexuality should not be the first asked. Begin with background information and fit the sexual assessment into the context of the overall assessment.
4. Questions asked about sexuality should begin with the least sensitive areas and move to areas of greater sensi-

---

Box 20-2   Sample Sexual History Form

Identifying Information
    Age
    Gender
    Other pertinent information
What brings the person for treatment?
Informants for the history
Family history
    Parents
    Siblings
    Extended family
    Family health history
    Social history
    Cultural history
Personal history
    Date, place, and circumstances of birth
    Childhood health history
    Social history
    Educational history
    Occupational history
    Habits (tobacco, alcohol, drugs)

Religious/spiritual history
Adult health history
Psychiatric history
Legal history
Sexual history
    Early childhood sexual history (doctor play, sexual experiences with adults)
    Masturbation history
    Teenage experiences
    Same sex and opposite sex experiences
    History of significant relationships
    Current sexual partner/activities
    Fantasies
    Use of erotica
    Contraception/protection from sexually transmitted diseases
    Satisfaction
    Questions and concerns

tivity. For example, begin by asking when client(s) first learned about sex.

5. Maintain appropriate eye contact and a relaxed, interested manner.
6. Be professional and matter-of-fact about information asked or obtained. Avoid extreme reactions.
7. Use language that is professional but understood by the client(s) being interviewed.
8. Remember, the nurse's tone of voice and manner reflect trust. If clients feel they can trust the nurse, they will be more open.

NURSING DIAGNOSIS

After a thorough gathering of assessment data, the nurse is in a position to analyze the findings and arrive at diagnoses. Diagnoses of sexual dysfunctions should be viewed in relation to the psychiatric diagnoses, DSM-IV, as well as nursing diagnoses that reflect the specific problems. A combination of both helps to ensure that adequate plans for intervention will be developed. Determination of diagnoses is done on an individual basis and carefully selected from all that is known.

NURSING DIAGNOSES FOR SEXUAL DYSFUNCTIONS

Anxiety
Communication, impaired verbal
Fear
Knowledge deficit, human sexuality
Pain
Role performance, altered
Self-esteem disturbance

CASE STUDY

Kelly is a 28-year-old, never-married female who tells the nurse that she has never had an orgasm. On assessment the nurse learns that Kelly has had a total of three male sexual partners. Her first intercourse experience was at age 19. She said she has never masturbated but sometimes fantasizes about sex and can get aroused by reading a sexually explicit story or seeing a movie with sex scenes. She has been in a 3-year monogamous, committed relationship to a man whom she is considering marrying. She said that they have sex 2 to 3 times per week. She generally enjoys sex, but she is unable to achieve orgasm. Lately this has become a problem for her and her partner. He fears that he is unable to please her.

Critical Thinking—Assessment
1. What symptoms exhibited by Kelly pertain to sexual dysfunction?
2. What about Kelly's background leads the nurse to believe that she has sexual problems?
3. How could Kelly's sexual problems affect other areas of her relationship?

Sexual dysfunction
Social isolation

OUTCOME IDENTIFICATION

In this phase the nurse determines clear outcome criteria or expected client outcomes from the nursing diagnosis. Client will:

1. Verbalize specific problem in the sexual area by the time of the second visit with nurse.
2. Write a list of feelings associated with sexual problem by the time of the second visit with nurse.
3. Seek a physical examination (if appropriate) by the time of the third visit with nurse.
4. Participate in sex therapy sessions (if appropriate) by the time of the fourth visit with nurse.
5. Practice recommended strategies learned in sex therapy by the sixth week in therapy.
6. Describe two strategies learned to enhance sexual functioning after the sixth week in therapy.
7. Incorporate strategies learned in sex therapy into routine sexual activity by the time of discharge.

PLANNING

Planning for client care comes about as the result of thorough assessment and analysis. Following formulation of

---

COLLABORATIVE DIAGNOSES

DSM-IV Diagnoses*	NANDA Diagnoses†
Sexual desire disorder	Sexual dysfunction
Hypoactive sexual desire	Fear
Sexual aversion disorder	Anxiety
	Role performance, altered
	Self-esteem disturbance
Sexual arousal disorders	Communication, impaired
Female sexual arousal	verbal
disorder	
Male erectile disorder	
Orgasmic disorders	Knowledge deficit, human
Female orgasmic disorder	sexuality
Male orgasmic disorder	Social isolation
Premature ejaculation	
Sexual pain disorder	Pain
Dyspareunia	
Vaginismus	
Sexual dysfunction due to general medical condition	
Substance-induced sexual dysfunction	
Sexual dysfunction not otherwise specified	

*From American Psychiatric Association: *Diagnostic and statistical manual of mental disorders*, ed 4, Washington, DC, 1994, The Association.

†From North American Nursing Diagnosis Association: *NANDA nursing diagnoses: definitions and classifications, 1999-2000*, Philadelphia, 1999, The Association.

DSM-IV diagnoses and nursing diagnoses that reflect client status, the nurse is ready to begin an individualized plan of care that will address all of the issues. Client care will be based on realistic, mutually agreed on goals.

In working with clients and couples with sexual dysfunction, the nurse must carefully consider the long-term goals and what each participant is willing to do to work toward those goals. These may differ in each situation, based on each person's values and attitudes and how each perceives the problem. For example, the client with a primary orgasmic dysfunction may have difficulty with masturbatory exercises that form one basis for treatment because he or she believes that touching one's own genitals is unacceptable and that orgasmic release must come only from partnered sexuality. Obviously, such individually held beliefs will influence implementation of a care plan.

IMPLEMENTATION

Development of an individualized plan of care is crucial. To do so, one must be aware of the specific nature of the problem and possible etiologies. Implementation includes education, counseling, and assistance in identifying specific strategies and support. The nurse must be aware of various treatment modalities and prognosis of recovery with treatment. The importance of following through on a plan of care, including physical examination and treatments, and on specific sex therapy needs for the individual or the couple must be stressed. The nurse will help the client(s) express concerns about sexual functioning; express feelings about the impact of this; and help enhance client knowledge base, self-esteem, and communication skills. The nurse will also recommend a physical examination and/or treatment and sex therapy, will monitor client compliance and success in treatment, and will help develop appropriate discharge planning.

Sexuality is a sensitive area of intervention. Having a trusting, open, and comfortable relationship with clients is essential. Without this, many sexual problems will go unrecognized and untreated.

The nature of sexuality is partially one of relationships with others. Therefore the nurse must be aware of clients' significant others and how they are affected. Implementation of any plan of care often involves a couple relationship and must be seen in this context. Thus it is often helpful to view the problem as couple oriented instead of placing the blame on either partner. Interventions that are aimed at the couple, in these instances, are the most effective.

NURSING INTERVENTIONS

1. Help client(s) understand human sexual functioning. Teach them about the human sexual response cycle. Recommend appropriate reading materials, such as Masters and Johnson's *Human Sexual Response. This knowledge forms a foundation for understanding other issues related to sexual disorders.*

2. Educate client(s) about sexual dysfunctions, including possible etiologies, symptoms, and treatment options. Various methods of assessment should be included: physical, urologic, gynecologic, and laboratory examinations, as well as a psychosocial sexual assessment. *Education helps to ensure that client(s) understand why changes in sexuality are happening to them and symptoms that may signal a problem.*

3. Help client(s) enhance communication skills around intimacy/sexuality. Teach and reinforce positive communication skills. *The inability to communicate is often the root of a sexual dysfunction problem.*

4. Support client(s) in exploring fears/anxieties related to anxiety in a private, trusting, open atmosphere. Encourage client's recall of early learning about sexuality, possibly through journal writing. *An open forum for discussing sexuality will help the client(s) overcome some of the repressions they have felt and be more open to satisfying sexual experiences.*

5. Help client(s) enhance self-esteem related to sexuality. Encourage positive self-talk and body image exercises. Discuss variations of sexual expression techniques. *Lack of self-esteem is often a contributing factor in sexual dysfunction.*

6. Refer client(s) to physical treatment modalities or sex therapy as applicable *to maximize the client's(s') success in dealing with sexual dysfunction.*

Additional Treatment Modalities

Once careful assessment is done to determine the specific diagnosis of sexual dysfunction, a range of treatment modalities can be instituted.

Psychophysiologic. Physiologic causation must be ruled out in advance of deciding on one or more forms of treatment. Various medical specialties have produced new di-

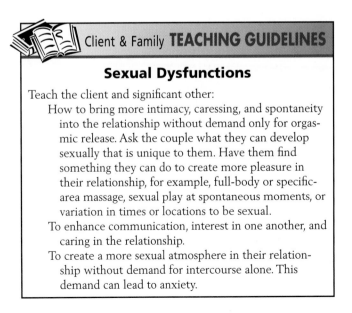

Client & Family **TEACHING GUIDELINES**

Sexual Dysfunctions

Teach the client and significant other:

How to bring more intimacy, caressing, and spontaneity into the relationship without demand only for orgasmic release. Ask the couple what they can develop sexually that is unique to them. Have them find something they can do to create more pleasure in their relationship, for example, full-body or specific-area massage, sexual play at spontaneous moments, or variation in times or locations to be sexual.

To enhance communication, interest in one another, and caring in the relationship.

To create a more sexual atmosphere in their relationship without demand for intercourse alone. This demand can lead to anxiety.

NURSING CARE PLAN

Lisa and Victor are a married couple who talk with the nurse about problems in their sexual relationship. Lisa is 34 years of age; Victor is 35. Both say they are in good physical health, and neither takes any medication routinely. They have two children: Amanda, age 4, and Brandon, age 2. The couple met 6½ years ago and became sexually involved shortly afterward. They lived together for approximately 8 months and married 5½ years ago.

They say that their sexual relationship was good before marriage and the birth of their children. They had sexual intercourse about two to four times per week, and both enjoyed it. Lisa says she occasionally has masturbated and continues to do so. Victor says that as an adolescent he masturbated once a day but that this has gradually decreased. He says that he is not masturbating currently and has no interest in doing so.

Lisa says that Victor's interest in sex has gradually declined and that now he rarely wants to be sexual. She feels he sometimes will have sex just to please her. Victor agrees that his interest in sex has declined. He says he is currently busy and preoccupied with fears and worries. According to Victor, he and a partner started their own business 3 years ago, and it has been a constant struggle. He admits that his sexual drive is down but says he can get an erection with adequate stimulation. Lisa complains that they have not been able to talk about the problem; she says they fight whenever sex is mentioned.

DSM-IV Diagnosis (Victor)

Axis I	Hypoactive sexual desire disorder
Axis II	Deferred
Axis III	None known
Axis IV	Severity of psychosexual stressors (moderate = 3), job stress, and anxiety
Axis V	GAF = 65 (current)
	GAF = 70 (past year)

Nursing Diagnosis: Sexual dysfunction, related to fear, anxiety, and lack of communication, as evidenced by the couple's lack of sexual intimacy and decrease in sexual interest and in masturbation in the husband.

Client Outcomes	Nursing Interventions	Evaluation
• Both Lisa and Victor will discuss how they perceive the problem with each other in the presence of the nurse at the first visit.	• Assess for perception of problem through taking sexual and couple history *to clearly delineate problem in sexual functioning and how couple perceives it.* • Ask each client to discuss how he or she perceives the problem. Allow each an equal amount of time *to help understand the problem thoroughly and to open communication between the partners.*	• Lisa and Victor both identified problem as decrease in sexual interest on Victor's part.
• Lisa and Victor will identify one way to be intimate with each other after the first visit.	• Discuss with couple alternative methods of intimacy they may practice, such as massage or partnered bath taking. *Couple will experience decreased pressure for genital sex that will help with relaxation.* • Give couple suggestions for readings on sexuality. *Sexual books in the market outline alternative ways to be sexual.*	• Lisa and Victor agreed to give each other a half-hour massage this week.
• Victor will have a physical examination by his primary care physician by the end of the second week.	• Discuss with clients need to rule out any physical disorder that may have relationship to sexual change. *Sexual dysfunction may be the result of a medical disorder, which should be determined before further treatment is planned.* • *Refer client to primary care physician if necessary to rule out physical problems.*	• Victor sought out physical examination and was given a clean bill of health.
• Lisa and Victor will agree to enter sex therapy with a qualified therapist after they obtain the results of the physical examination.	• Encourage client to receive treatment for sexual problems. *Sex therapy may be helpful in overcoming sexual difficulty and anxiety.* Educate couple about techniques of sexual therapy. *They may be better informed to make appropriate choices.* • Refer couple to qualified sex therapist *for continued professional help.*	• Lisa and Victor begin work with a sex therapist.

NURSING CARE PLAN —cont'd

Nursing Diagnosis: Anxiety related to job stress, performance anxiety, and lack of communication, as evidenced by Victor's statements that he is anxious and distracted from sexual interaction.

Client Outcomes	Nursing Interventions	Evaluation
• Victor will describe nature of anxiety by the second visit.	• Encourage Victor to be aware of anxiety and how it affects his sexuality. *Knowing what anxieties are will help alleviate need to worry when involved in other activities.* • Ask Victor to discuss what type of issues create anxiety. *Members of the couple are aware of them and create a strategy to overcome them.*	• Victor is able to discuss worries, success of business, and financial security.
• Victor will practice sensate focus exercises with wife during intimacy after the first visit.	• Educate Victor on sensate focus exercises. *This will train Victor to focus on body feeling and not on anxiety during intimacy with wife.* • Recommend reading materials for couple that describe sensate focus exercises as part of education *to enhance learned skills.*	• Victor reports he is able to focus on body sensations during intimacy.

Nursing Diagnosis: Communication, impaired verbal related to anxiety, self-esteem disturbance, and embarrassment as evidenced by Lisa's statement that they could not discuss sexual issues without fighting.

Client Outcomes	Nursing Interventions	Evaluation
• Lisa and Victor will discuss sexual concerns in first session with nurse.	• Encourage couple to be more open verbally about sexual needs and concerns. *Open discussion facilitates mutual understanding and decreases blame.* • Ask direct questions about sexuality and keep focused on this during sessions. *Help decrease anxiety and open up couple communication about sex.*	• Both Lisa and Victor are able to discuss sexual concerns at first session.
• Lisa and Victor will discuss sex with each other 1 hour each week after first session.	• Encourage couple to set aside time to discuss sexual needs *to be able to express needs and thus facilitate sexuality.*	• Lisa and Victor say they are able to discuss needs with each other. Lisa says she would like more time together, and Victor says he would like Lisa to initiate planning times to discuss sexual issues.

agnostic and therapeutic procedures that have quickly changed the practice of sex therapy/clinical sexology.

For men, various psychophysiologic methods are employed in both diagnosis and treatment. **Nocturnal penile tumescence** involves the determination of erectile response during the sleep cycle. The client is generally seen in a sleep lab where plethysmography is used to monitor erection. **Plethysmography** involves the use of a strain gauge that fits around the penis and detects erection. This information, processed through mechanical and computerized equipment, provides a graphic portrayal of the erectile pattern. This testing is time consuming and relatively expensive, but it clearly detects whether erection is possible without competing psychologic stimuli. Determination of erectile potential can also be done by daytime evaluation using visual erotic stimuli and the plethysmograph. Wineze et al (1988) found that laboratory exposure to erotic pictures produced erection in dysfunctional men.

Medical testing for males may include endocrine measures, particularly testosterone and prolactin. Testosterone is the predominantly male sex hormone produced in the testes that is responsible for the male sex drive. In general, a higher level of testosterone in males is associated with greater sexual desire; a higher level of prolactin is associated with decreased sexual interest. The **penile-brachial index (PBI)** is also a useful measure. This monitors the difference between penile and brachial blood pressures. There are other invasive and noninvasive tests for evaluation of arterial and venous blood flow to the penis, including pulse-wave assessments, intracorporal pharmacologic

ADDITIONAL TREATMENT MODALITIES

Psychophysiologic Modalities

Aphrodisiacs
External vacuum devices
Hormonal replacement (testosterone and estrogen)
Intracavernosal injections
Penile prosthesis
Vascular surgery
Viagra
Vibrators
Yohimbine

Psychosocial Modalities

Body therapies (massage, chakra balancing, tantric yoga)
Communication therapy
Education
Erotic stimuli training
Gradual dilation of the vagina
Masturbation training
Semans' stop-start technique
Sensate focus

⚠️ CLINICAL ALERT

Peyronie's Disease

Peyronie's disease is seen in only 1% of men and is more common in men between the ages of 45 and 60 (Ducharme and Gill, 1997). It is a disease that is characterized by lesion formation in the tunica of the corpora cavernosa. This lesion leads to curvature and shortening of the penis with erection. The cause is not well understood but may be due to overly vigorous sexual activity or blunt trauma to the penis. The result can be pain during erection and difficult or impossible intercourse because of the curvature. Men with diabetes also are at risk of developing Peyronie's disease, as well as erectile dysfunction. Surgery, placement of a penile prosthesis, and vitamin E are all used in treatment.

Vaginismus

In one study by Spector and Carey (1990), 12% to 17% of women reporting to a sexual dysfunction clinic had complaints of vaginismus. This condition is best defined as involuntary contractions of the lower third of the vagina. To arrive at a diagnosis, a history of recurrent and involuntary spasms of the pubococcogeal muscles must be noted. The spasms of the vagina may be triggered by anticipated penetration. The cause is unknown, but many factors may contribute, including vaginal surgery, complicated episiotomies, rape, abortion, painful gynecologic examinations, and vaginal infections. These contractions are not under voluntary control, and attempts at penetration result in pain. Medical problems need to be ruled out and treated as needed. In the absence of known medical problems, treatment involves relaxation and dilation techniques, using gradually larger dilatories to relax the vaginal muscles. Psychotherapy is helpful to allay the woman's fears and her partner's frustration. Antianxiety medications sometimes prove useful.

testing, ultrasound (the use of sound waves to evaluate structures and functions within the male genitalia), and cavernosography. Neurologic assessments that carefully evaluate various minute components of neural control of erection are also available.

In women, there is a noticeable lack of assessment and treatment in the psychophysiologic realm. Plethysmography is used to determine blood flow to the vagina, which is an indicator of arousal. However, this procedure is inconsistent and invasive. Endocrine studies can be used, but the hormonal control of female sexuality is more complex and is affected by the menstrual cycle. Thus the findings may not be very useful in diagnosis. **Estradiol** measurement is sometimes done, which determines the level of estradiol in the bloodstream, possibly reflecting levels of desire.

At present, practitioners have several methods of treatment. Drug and hormonal therapies often are used as adjuncts. Sildenafil **(Viagra)** was approved for use in the spring of 1998 and showed immediate worldwide interest. The mechanism of action is to block the enzyme that breaks down cyclic guanosine monophosphate (cGMP) to boost the chemical's relaxing effect on penile muscles. Combined with stimulation, the drug produces erection 1 hour after ingestion. It is currently being tested on women. Early clinical trials suggest that it will increase blood flow to female genitalia, thus increasing arousal. The use of **yohimbine,** an alpha$_2$ adrenoreceptor blocker, is believed to facilitate blood flow to the genitalia (Piletz et al, 1998). Hormonal replacement may also prove useful. This may involve testosterone in males (Wagner, Rabkin, and Rabkin, 1997) and estrogen or testosterone replacement

in females. Anxiolytics have been used successfully in the treatment of vaginismus (Plaut and RachBeisel, 1997).

Intracorporal injections of vasodilators such as prostaglandins, papaverine, or combinations of these and other drugs are made directly into the corpus cavernosa and produce erection. In males, surgery can be done to alter penile arterial blood flow or to implant prosthetic devices. Prosthetic devices come in two different general forms and have been developed over time with more satisfactory results. There is a semirigid rod that can be made of silicone or metal, and there are inflatable pumps of varying degrees of sophistication.

External vacuum pumps improve erection and orgasmic function in males. The vacuum draws blood into the corpus cavernosa of the penis and traps it there. In China a system has been developed that uses herbal tonics, an electronic pumping device, a vagina-like container filled with warm fluid, and a self-control apparatus for the client. Although the system has proved useful in China, it is not used in the United States.

Elaborate physiologic methods of treatment are not available for women but clearly need to be developed. Currently, various types of vibrators are available that can be useful therapeutically for females. However, they are marketed as toys or relaxation devices instead of biomedical instruments and therefore do not have the sanction or the quality of medical instruments.

Psychosocial. There are effective sex therapy techniques for both males and females, as well as couples. These techniques were first developed by Masters and Johnson and have become more effective and comprehensive over the years. Masters and Johnson (1970) developed the **sensate focus** technique, which involves focusing on body sensations, especially those in the breasts and genitals, while shutting out other stimuli.

Body therapies have been used in the field for several decades, including hands-on healing, massage, spiritual energizing techniques, chakra balancing, and the adaptation of Eastern principles of sexuality such as tantric yoga. Couples massage is often utilized to enhance pleasure and provide nonverbal communication. Often couples are instructed to give one another weekly hour-long massages that are nondemand; in other words, the partner being massaged must only receive the sensations without feeling the need to reciprocate. Nondemand also implies that there is no demand for sexual arousal or sexual desire completion.

Sex therapy practitioners and clinical sexologists have a wide range of other psychosocial techniques. In general, homework assignments and supportive counseling form the basis of therapy. Often sex therapy involves weekly or bimonthly visits to the therapists during which clients have the opportunity to discuss symptoms, progress, feelings, and observations (McCarthy, 1997).

Education provides a first-line technique for sex therapy. Cognitive restructuring, involving replacing negative thoughts about sexuality with positive thoughts, can be helpful as well. Communication training is also beneficial. For desire phase disorders, erotic materials may be used to help train the individual to be more sexually focused. Clients are often asked to include sexual thinking and feelings into their daily schedule. Masturbation training can be done for males and females to help them be more sensitive to sexual stimulation. It may then train males and females to become orgasmic or improve orgasmic potential. Becoming orgasmic may also entail the use of cognitive restructuring of beliefs about sexuality and techniques to reduce the fear of losing control. Hypnotherapy has been utilized for a variety of sexual dysfunctions. It focuses specifically on the abatement of symptomatology.

For males, the stop-start technique helps overcome premature ejaculation. This technique, developed in 1956 by Semans, has the couple practice foreplay and stimulation until the point of ejaculation. Then direct stimulation is stopped until the feeling subsides. The couple resumes the procedure a total of three times. This technique trains the male to be more aware of the sensation of impending ejaculation and to better control the timing.

Once medical causations for the sexual pain disorders of dyspareunia and vaginismus have been ruled out, appropriate strategies can be used. Insertions of a finger or **vaginal dilator** in the vagina are begun slowly. The gradual introduction of larger inserters, coupled with relaxation techniques, will help the woman overcome her fear and pain and help decrease involuntary spasm. Sets of dilators may be purchased from medical supply firms for this purpose.

The tools and methods of sex therapy have been important developments in the field. But without the sensitivity and attention to other factors in the client's sexual realm, they may not provide satisfactory results. Some other factors include cultural and religious values, other psychologic disorders, poor sexual learning, and body image issues.

Anon (1976) created what is known as the PLISSIT model of sexual intervention. This is an excellent model for the collaborative care of clients with sexual dysfunctions. The P stands for giving *permission*, that is, giving permission for people to be sexual and to have sexual feelings. If the problem persists, go to LI, giving *limited information*, that is, information and education concerning specific sexual problem(s). If the problem persists, go to SS, making *specific suggestions*, that is, calling on the specific treatments for various dysfunctions. If the problem persists, refer the client to a sex therapist/clinical sexologist for IT, *intensive therapy*.

EVALUATION

Evaluation of the effectiveness of intervention is an ongoing process and involves many levels. If the outcome criteria are thorough and carefully defined, evaluation is a relatively simple process of determining whether these outcomes were met. The nursing process is cyclical; if the nurse determines that outcome criteria were not met, he or she must go back to the assessment phase to determine if some key underlying factors were overlooked.

To better understand this cyclical nature in the area of sexual dysfunction, refer to the nursing care plan on pp. 476-477 concerning Lisa and Victor. During assess-

Sexual Dysfunction

Many people find sexual dysfunctions difficult to discuss because of the traditional reticence regarding the subject of sex. The sources of sexual problems may be found in a variety of factors including the natural changes of the aging process, side effects of various medications or disease processes, rape, or a history of abuse. Some clients may have kept their problems a secret for extended periods or may not have been aware of the original precipitant.

Some individuals may experience gender-related conflict or desire for types of sexual experience that are not condoned by society. Any of these dilemmas may be presented to the community mental health nurse with the expectation that nurses have the knowledge and experience to "fix" the problem. The nurse should respond in a nonjudgmental way no matter how different the client's sexual problem seems from the nurse's view or experience. The nurse should not attempt to condone or excuse hurtful behavior related to sexual activity or abuse and should exert patience as the client attempts to express feelings that may never have been shared with anyone else. The nurse also should acknowledge that there are no easy answers to the client's questions and should emphasize readiness to explore individualized options. It is important to remind the client that thoughts are not harmful to others, that he or she is able to make a choice about turning ideas into actions, and that individual or group support is available.

Sexual issues and problems associated with the maturing process are increasingly common because the population that embraced the birth control pill now must cope with the complexities of acquired immunodeficiency syndrome (AIDS), menopause, and "viripause," as some have dubbed the male version of hormonal changes. Women may experience depression and a lack of sexual desire resulting from diminished hormone levels and related painful intercourse. Men may feel trapped in their jobs/careers and/or in their relationships. Sexually active adults who are not in secure monogamous relationships must always have concerns about sexually transmitted diseases (STDs), even though there are protective methods to reduce risk.

Clients in the community may also include those who have already contracted STDs such as gonorrhea, human immunodeficiency virus (HIV), genital herpes, or full-blown AIDS. These clients can be helped individually and in support groups to allay their guilt and to evaluate their situations with regard to what sort of relationships are possible for them. They must be encouraged to be scrupulously honest with prospective partners and to explore safer forms of intimacy in their relationships.

The mental health nurse in the community must have up-to-date information about medications, especially antidepressants, which may evoke side effects that affect a client's sexual activity, including impaired desire, delayed orgasm, and impotence. Many persons tolerate these departures from their normal patterns in silence and believe that they are still suffering from depression or that they have developed some other abnormality to add to their problems. They will need assurance that their problems are physiologic and not emotional. At present, there are also recent innovations in drug therapy that support the mechanical bodily response during sexual stimulation. These new medications offer relief from certain types of sexual difficulty and show promise in alleviating the side effects of certain therapies and debilitating diseases.

The difference that the mental health nurse will note between working in the community versus a hospital setting is that relationships with clients are more sustained, holistic, and balanced. A partnership is easier to establish with the client in the community, and there may be more interactions and fewer power struggles between nurse and client, than there are in the hospital. For sensitive topics such as sexual disorders, this collaboration can lead to very effective consensual treatment strategies.

Nursing Care in the Community

---

ment, the nurse learned that Victor had decreased sexual desire over the past few years. One of the nursing diagnoses identified was anxiety that may be due to job stress, performance anxiety, and lack of communication. One of the outcome criteria that the nurse determined with Victor was that he would practice sensate focus exercises during intimacy with his wife. The nurse then taught Victor how to do sensate focus. If, on evaluation, Victor says he still cannot focus on his body and is easily distracted, what should the nurse do next?

The answer is that the nurse should go back to assessment. Was something missed? Perhaps something was overlooked in Victor's history, perhaps he put on weight that has affected his body image, or perhaps he has a fear of being touched. Couple issues may have been missed. Lisa may have rejected Victor in the past, and he may still be angry. If any of these or additional issues are found in assessment, the nurse must revamp the care plan to include them. Nursing diagnosis, outcome criteria, and interventions will then change. If nothing was missed in assessment, perhaps the outcome criteria were unrealistic. The issue of Victor's anxiety may be complex and deep, and it may be unrealistic to assume that he will develop insight by the second visit. The need for ongoing evaluation can be seen in this example.

PARAPHILIAS

HISTORICAL AND THEORETIC PERSPECTIVES

The **paraphilias** are a group of behaviors commonly accepted by the clinical description of sexual deviations. Paraphilias present inappropriate sexual fantasies involv-

Understanding & Applying Research

The purpose of this study was to investigate familial patterns of pedophilia. This was done by a double-blind–chart review of 33 male clients with paraphilic disorders and 33 male clients with depression as the control group. Information obtained included demographic data, paraphilic diagnoses according to DSM-III criteria, age of onset, and family history for both groups of patients.

The authors identified that the age of risk for developing a paraphilic disorder was between 15 and 40 years. Results were statistically significant in that 18.5% of the families of patients with a paraphilic disorder had family members (mostly males) with a sexual disorder.

This study identified that perhaps pedophilia, as well as other paraphilic disorders, may indeed run in families across generations. Further studies have been done to determine how this transmission occurs.

Data from Gaffney GR, Lurie SF, Berlin FB: Is there familial transmission of pedophilia? *J Nerv Ment Dis* 172(9):546, 1984.

Box 20-3   **Etiologic Factors for Paraphilias**

Biologic factors
 Chromosomal functioning
 Hormonal levels
Experiential factors
 History of sexual abuse
Environmental factors
Hereditary predisposition

ing deviant sexual acts, inappropriate sexual urges, and acting out of these fantasies and urges.

Once a psychiatric syndrome is described clinically, several steps, including laboratory studies, delimitation from other disorders, follow-up studies, and family studies are necessary to establish diagnostic validity. It is generally acknowledged that no psychiatric syndrome has yet to be fully validated by the complete series of these steps. However, many syndromes have had a substantial body of data published in most phases of the validation.

Little is known, however, about the data in the other areas establishing clinical validity. For instance, there are some laboratory tests and follow-up studies of sexual deviance; however, there are few family studies of paraphilias.

ETIOLOGY

It is also unclear as to what may predispose an individual to developing a paraphilic disorder. Several studies have attempted to suggest etiologic factors and the prevalence of sexual deviancies. Research has not concluded cause-and-effect etiology of the paraphilias.

BIOLOGIC FACTORS

It is important to acknowledge that people do not voluntarily decide what types of sexual arousal patterns they will have. Researchers suggest possible etiologies (Box 20-3). In the biologic domain, two areas will be addressed: chromosomal functioning and hormonal levels.

In 1942, Klinefelter and his colleagues described Klinefelter's syndrome as a condition characterized by (1) the development of gynecomastia (enlarged breasts) at the time of puberty, (2) aspermatogenesis (low sperm pro-

duction), and (3) an increased secretion of follicle stimulating-hormone (FSH) by the pituitary gland in the brain.

In this particular syndrome, the client presents with 47 chromosomes instead of the normal 46. There is an extra X chromosome present. The client may be thought of as a male (XY) with an extra X chromosome or as a female (XX) with an extra Y chromosome. Clients with this syndrome look like a male at birth. Hence, parents will naturally raise them as males and assign them a male sex role. Money (1957) described an otherwise normal 8-year-old boy with Klinefelter's syndrome who insisted he felt more comfortable dressed in girl's clothing. Klinefelter's clients have very small testes and produce little testosterone and virtually no sperm. They also experience problems with sexual orientation and the nature of their erotic desires.

Some theorists suggest that biologic factors may be etiologic considerations in the development of sexual disorders and that early life experiences may contribute to the development of a paraphilic disorder.

HEREDITARY/ENVIRONMENTAL FACTORS

Gaffney et al (1984) found evidence that suggests familial transmission of paraphilic disorders. Groth (1979) has identified children who were sexually active with adults during childhood as being environmentally influenced and therefore potentially predisposed for developing a pedophilic disorder. This is an example of victim turned **victimizer,** or sex offender.

EPIDEMIOLOGY

According to the DSM-IV, although paraphilias are not generally diagnosed in clinical facilities, the sizeable commercial market in paraphiliac pornography and paraphernalia suggests that its prevalence in the community is "likely to be higher" (American Psychiatric Association [APA], 1994). The paraphilias that most commonly present problems are pedophilia, voyeurism, and exhibitionism. About one half of the clients with paraphilias seen clinically are married (APA, 1994).

CLINICAL DESCRIPTION

The essential diagnostic features of a paraphilia are "recurrent, intense sexually arousing fantasies, sexual urges, or behaviors generally involving (1) nonhuman objects, (2) the suffering or humiliation of oneself or one's partner, or (3) children or other nonconsenting persons that occur over a period of at least 6 months" (APA, 1994). Another criterion is that "the behavior, sexual urges, or fantasies cause clinically significant distress in social, occupational, or other important areas of functioning" (APA, 1994). The DSM-IV box summarizes the criteria and description of the paraphilias.

PROGNOSIS

Nurses should be cautioned in attempting to predict **recidivism** (the chronic, repetitive inappropriate acting out of sexual behaviors considered to be unacceptable that have or have not resulted in criminal conviction). Clients currently undergoing treatment for a sexual disorder may have a lower level of sexual recidivism (Berlin et al, 1991). The Berlin et al (1991) study revealed a higher reoffense rate for those clients who do not receive (or who have never received) treatment than for those engaged in treatment. Treatment compliance is a therapeutic issue that nurses treating this population must address.

DSM-IV CRITERIA

DESCRIPTION OF PARAPHILIAS

Exhibitionism

The exposure of one's genitals to an unsuspecting person(s) followed by sexual arousal.

Fetishism

Utilization of objects (e.g., panties, rubber sheeting) for the purpose of becoming sexually aroused.

Frotteurism

Rubbing up against a nonconsenting person to heighten sexual arousal.

Pedophilia

Fondling and/or other types of sexual activities with a prepubescent child (usually under the age of 13 having not yet developed secondary sex characteristics). Heterosexual pedophiles are sexually attracted to female children under the age of 13. Homosexual pedophiles are sexually attracted to male children under the age of 13. **Ego syntonic pedophiles** do not view this type of behavior as troublesome and will not voluntarily seek treatment for it. **Ego dystonic pedophiles** are concerned and troubled with this type of behavior and might voluntarily seek treatment to deal with it.

  Types of pedophiles:
  Homosexual
  Heterosexual
  Bisexual (sexual attraction to both males and females)
  Limited to incest (sexual attraction to a child in one's immediate family)
  Exclusive type (sexually attracted to children only)
  Nonexclusive type (may also be sexually attracted to adults of either sex)

Sexual Masochism

Being the receiver of pain (either physical or emotional), humiliation, or being made to suffer for the purpose of becoming sexually aroused.

Sexual Sadism

The infliction of pain (either physical or emotional) or humiliation onto another person followed by sexual arousal.

Transvestic Fetishism

The act of cross-dressing (heterosexual males wearing female clothing) for the purpose of becoming sexually aroused.

Voyeurism

Observing unsuspecting persons who are naked, in the act of disrobing, or engaging in sexual activity ("peeping tom") followed by sexual arousal.

Paraphilia Not Otherwise Specified

Disorders that do not meet the criteria for the aforementioned categories:

  Telephone scatologia: Obscene phone calling; "900" sex lines
  Necrophilia: Sexual activity with corpses
  Partialism: Exclusive focus on a particular body part for sexual arousal
  Zoophilia: Sexual activity involving participation with animals (bestiality)
  Coprophilia: Sexual arousal by contact with feces
  Klismaphilia: Sexual arousal generated by use of enemas
  Urophilia: Sexual arousal by contact with urine
  Ephebophilia: Fondling and/or other types of sexual activities with pubescent children (usually between the ages of 13 to 18) who are developing secondary sex characteristics (e.g., pubic hair, breasts)
  Paraphilic coercive disorder: Rape; aggressive sexual assault involving an act of sexual intercourse against one's will and without consent

Modified from American Psychiatric Association: *Diagnostic and statistical manual of mental disorders*, ed 4, Washington, DC, 1994, The Association.

It is important for nurses to also acknowledge that treatment efficacy cannot be proven at this time. Further studies are warranted in this area.

DISCHARGE CRITERIA
Client will:

1. State nature of specific paraphilic disorder and its impact on self and others (breakdown/absence of cognitive distortions).

2. Identify **triggers**—stimuli that heighten unacceptable sexual cravings and provoke inappropriate sexual behaviors.
3. Develop appropriate relapse prevention strategies.
4. Communicate and problem solve effectively.
5. Practice appropriate coping strategies.
6. Identify support systems.

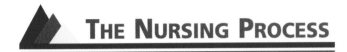

THE NURSING PROCESS

ASSESSMENT
The client with a sexual disorder may exhibit a variety of behavioral symptoms, depending on the nature of the disorder. Some symptoms are more difficult to assess than others. The client with a pedophilic disorder may exhibit perceptual disturbances. It is not uncommon to hear such a client state, for example, "The child looked older than he was." This may also be perceived as a cognitive distortion (an unconscious defense mechanism).

Cognitive distortions may be present in the client with a sexual disorder. Two cognitive distortions most often present in this client population are denial and rationalization. *Denial* is a defense mechanism used to avoid dealing with problems and responsibilities related to one's behaviors. *Rationalization* is a defense mechanism used to justify upsetting behaviors by creating reasons (rationale) that would allow the individual to believe that the behaviors were warranted or appropriate. These are the most critical issues that the nurse must address early in the therapeutic process. A client making a statement such as, "Well, the child didn't fight me and agreed to have sex with me" is a good indication that such cognitive distortions are present.

Another symptom that requires assessment is a disturbance in feeling. Clients with paraphilic disorders com-

monly lack remorse for their victims. If they do experience remorse, they may be unable to acknowledge it as a result of cognitive distortions. Occasionally, clients with a pedophilic disorder may claim to experience feelings of "being loved" by the child with whom they have had inappropriate sexual activity.

Clients with a paraphilic disorder should also be assessed for the presence of behavioral and relating disturbances. These are assessed in the client's inability to develop age-appropriate relationships, altered relationships with others, and social withdrawal that may occur secondary to embarrassment or media attention.

NURSING DIAGNOSIS
After collecting client assessment data, the nurse is ready to begin formulating diagnoses. In doing so, the nurse may find that the client has symptoms indicative of more than one diagnosis, such as a paraphilic disorder, a psychoactive substance disorder, and/or a personality disorder. Multiple diagnoses will not be addressed in this chapter. However, it is important for the nurse to be aware of this possibility.

When addressing nursing diagnoses for the client with a paraphilic disorder, the nurse has many diagnoses from which to choose and will select those that are specific and

---

NURSING ASSESSMENT QUESTIONS
Paraphilias

1. What brings you here for treatment? (To assess client's level of insight)
2. Do you think you have a sexual disorder? (To determine if cognitive distortions are present)

3. Do you think you've caused any physical or emotional harm to your victims? (To determine if there are disturbances of feelings present)
4. How has this problem affected your lifestyle and relationships? (To determine the presence of disturbances in relationships)

COLLABORATIVE DIAGNOSES

DSM-IV Diagnoses*	NANDA Diagnoses†
Exhibitionism	Anxiety
Fetishism	Coping, ineffective individual
Frotteurism	Denial, ineffective
Pedophilia	Family processes, altered
Sexual masochism	Knowledge deficit
Sexual sadism	Personal identity disturbance
Transvestic fetishism	Role performance, altered
Voyeurism	Self-esteem disturbance
	Self-mutilation, risk for
	Sexuality patterns, altered
	Social interaction, impaired
	Violence, risk for: directed at others

(These nursing diagnoses may be applied to all medical diagnoses for the client with a paraphilic disorder.)

*From American Psychiatric Association: *Diagnostic and statistic manual of mental disorders*, ed 4, Washington, DC, 1994, The Association.
†From North American Nursing Diagnosis Association: *NANDA nursing diagnoses: definitions and classifications, 1999-2000*, Philadelphia, 1999, The Association.

appropriate to each individual, based on an analysis of comprehensive data collected during assessment.

NURSING DIAGNOSES FOR PARAPHILIAS

Coping, ineffective individual
Denial, ineffective
Knowledge deficit (of illness and aspects of treatment)
Noncompliance (with therapeutic regimen)
Sexuality patterns, altered
Social interaction, impaired
Violence, risk for: directed at others

OUTCOME IDENTIFICATION

Client-centered outcomes should relate to the client's nursing diagnoses and be the opposite of the defining characteristics. Outcomes should be stated in clear, measurable, behavioral terms and include a time frame, when feasible, in which the client is expected to achieve them. Outcomes may be described as expected or anticipated and are viewed as specific goals to be achieved through the implementation of the plan of care. Examples of behavioral terms the nurse may want to use in developing client-centered outcomes include words such as "Client will . . . state, list, perform, and participate."

OUTCOME IDENTIFICATION FOR PARAPHILIAS
Client will:

1. State two sexually inappropriate behaviors within 3 days of admission.

2. Write a list of triggers that provoke inappropriate sexual acting out within the first week of admission.
3. Describe two appropriate coping strategies within 1 week of admission.
4. List several relapse prevention strategies that are appropriate to his or her disorder within the second week of admission.
5. Actively participate in weekly group psychotherapy sessions for clients with sexual disorders.
6. Verbalize two appropriate methods to meet sexual needs by the time of discharge.
7. Explain the importance of medication compliance and follow-up with outpatient group psychotherapy by time of discharge.

PLANNING

Once diagnoses have been established and client problem identification has occurred, the nurse is ready to begin developing a plan of care specific to the individual client. Client care should be based on mutually agreed on, realistic, client-centered outcomes. The nurse should involve the client in the development of an individualized plan of care, with the expectation that the client will participate in the planning process.

In the population of clients with paraphilic disorders, it is not uncommon to find the presence of cognitive distortions. Nurses must be aware of this as they obtain client input into the development of the plan of care. For example, a client who is in denial of a paraphilic disorder may not be able to fully cooperate with the planning of care or view client-centered outcomes as realistic.

IMPLEMENTATION

The nurse should work with the client to develop an individualized plan of care that will help the client identify the presence of cognitive distortions (if appropriate), prevent reoffending by identifying triggers that provoke inappropriate sexual activity, and develop effective relapse prevention strategies. The nurse should also explain the significance of treatment on recidivism and stress the importance of medication compliance and follow-up with outpatient group psychotherapy.

Providing nursing care to such a client may be difficult because of the sensitive nature of this disorder. Nurses must recognize this and be aware of their own comfort level when discussing sexual issues with these clients. Identifying the presence of a paraphilic disorder may have devastating effects on clients and their significant others. It is important for nurses to include significant others in the interventions to the extent that they can participate.

NURSING INTERVENTIONS

1. Help the client confront cognitive distortions through direct questioning methods that promote reality orien-

Robert is a 50-year-old vice president of a major corporation who has been diagnosed as having voyeurism. He intermittently acted-out by engaging in voyeuristic activities at his country club in the ladies locker room. He would secretly masturbate while "peeping." His wife is currently unaware of his behavior but suspects something is wrong. When she confronted Robert regarding her suspicions, he denied any problems.

Robert voluntarily came for treatment primarily out of concern that his wife would discover his disorder. He also began to recognize that he spends a great deal of time on the job fantasizing and/or engaging in voyeuristic and masturbatory activities. Robert has been lying to his wife about his whereabouts for approximately 10 years.

The treatment team focused on assisting Robert in developing appropriate coping strategies. Treatment also included psychoeducation regarding trigger identification and appropriate relapse prevention strategies. The need for couples counseling to disclose the "secret" of Robert's behavior was also addressed. Robert was given Depo-Provera 500 mg IM q wk to help him control his inappropriate sexual acting-out.

DSM-IV Diagnoses

Axis I	Voyeurism
Axis II	Deferred—compulsive traits noted
Axis III	Medical diagnoses (None)
Axis IV	Severity of psychosocial stressors (moderate = 3), marital conflict, job stress, anxiety
Axis V	GAF = 61 (current) GAF = 61 (past year)

Nursing Diagnosis: Sexuality patterns, altered, related to use of cognitive distortions (denial) and sexual behaviors in a socially unacceptable manner, as evidenced by engaging in sexual behavior without regard for others and public masturbation.

Client Outcomes	Nursing Interventions	Evaluation
• Robert will identify two sexual behaviors that are socially unacceptable within first week of admission.	• Assess for presence of cognitive distortions via a thorough sexual history. *If cognitive distortions are present, Robert may not be able to identify socially unacceptable behaviors and further treatment is warranted.* • Discuss with Robert what are socially unacceptable sexual behaviors and why *to educate the client about problematic sexual behaviors and their implications on society.* • Encourage Robert's participation in a group for clients with sexual disorders. *These clients frequently believe that they are the only ones who experience inappropriate sexual behaviors, which may lead to feelings of hopelessness, embarrassment, and isolation. Group therapy provides confrontation, support, and hope.*	• Robert readily identified his voyeuristic and public masturbatory behaviors as inappropriate, after 1 week of admission.

Nursing Diagnosis: Coping, ineffective individual, related to inability to trust wife with his secret and inadequate problem-solving skills, as evidenced by use of maladaptive coping methods such as lying, ineffective communication with wife (unable to discuss thoughts and feelings regarding disorder), anxiety, and fear of discovery by wife.

Client Outcomes	Nursing Interventions	Evaluation
• Robert will effectively communicate his thoughts and feelings about his disorder and behaviors with his wife and selected staff within 1 week of admission. • Robert will identify two concerns he has about disclosing his disorder and behaviors to his wife by the time of discharge.	• Encourage Robert to verbalize his thoughts and feelings concerning his current coping methods (lying, nondisclosure) *to illustrate to Robert the impact of his present coping strategies on himself and his wife.* • Educate Robert and his wife about his disorder, its implications, and treatment. *Educating Robert and his wife about his disorder and aspects of treatment will alleviate their fears and anxiety, develop trust, and establish an effective, supportive relationship.*	• Robert verbalized many thoughts and feelings about the impact this could have on his marriage. • At the time of discharge, Robert was able to share his "secret" with his wife, who was very supportive and eager to learn more about how she could help her husband cope with his disorder.

Continued

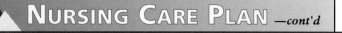

NURSING CARE PLAN —cont'd

Client Outcomes	Nursing Interventions	Evaluation
• Robert will formulate two relapse prevention strategies by the time of discharge, such as calling his wife before leaving work so that she will expect him at a certain time to avoid reoffending.	Help Robert formulate appropriate strategies to use at significant times during his vulnerability *to prevent him from reoffending.*	• Robert discussed two relapse prevention strategies with the staff. He will call his wife before leaving work, and he will discuss inappropriate thoughts with his wife or therapist.

Nursing Diagnosis: Knowledge deficit of illness and aspects of treatment, related to cognitive distortions, anxiety, and uncertainty, as evidenced by failure to seek prior treatment for his disorder and behaviors.

Client Outcomes	Nursing Interventions	Evaluation
• Robert will verbalize an understanding of his illness within 1 week of admission.	• Assess Robert's current level of knowledge regarding his illness and readiness to learn by asking direct questions. *A client must exhibit readiness to learn for learning to occur.* • Create a climate conducive to learning, such as a quiet, private, safe environment. *Learning may occur when the nurse has the client's complete attention and distractions are avoided.*	• Robert has successfully identified triggers that provoke sexual thoughts/ feelings and has developed appropriate relapse prevention strategies at the time of discharge.
• Robert will identify triggers, such as unstructured time, that provoke inappropriate thoughts and feelings within 1 week of admission.	• Teach the importance of trigger identification and development of relapse prevention strategies as critical steps in treatment *to help Robert gain more effective control of inappropriate behaviors.* • Suggest that Robert write a list of triggers that provoke sexually inappropriate activity and review this list with him *to assess Robert's insight into his disorder and symptom occurrence.*	
• Robert will formulate two relapse prevention strategies, such as opening lines of communication with wife, to avoid reoffending by the time of discharge.	• Help Robert develop appropriate relapse prevention strategies for his identified triggers *to construct a realistic plan to avoid reoffending.* • Encourage Robert's participation in a support group for clients with sexual disorders *to receive feedback from peers regarding realistic qualities of trigger identification and relapse prevention strategies.*	

⚠ CLINICAL ALERT

The nurse should be alert for signs of noncompliance with treatment or signs indicative of potential relapse, as evidenced by such things as the client's refusal to take medications and/or attend therapy sessions. Client statements such as "I don't know why I need this, I'm just here because the courts sent me," social withdrawal, presence of cognitive distortions, and lack of candidness may all be viewed as risk factors for noncompliance.

tation as to the client's offending behavior. Open confrontation by the nurse may be needed, including an explanation of the impact of these distortions on treatment outcomes. Journaling may assist in the breakdown of cognitive distortions and help the client track inappropriate sexual fantasies. *Client must be aware of the problem and acknowledge it before treatment can begin.*

2. Educate the client and significant others about paraphilic disorders and aspects of treatment, such as identifying triggers that provoke inappropriate sexual activity and methods that help avoid relapse. Encourage active participation in the educational process by com-

piling lists in a journal for review by the client and the nurse. Copies of these lists should be placed in the client's medical record to inform other team members about the client's progress. *This knowledge forms a foundation for treatment.*

3. Enhance the client's compliance with treatment by openly discussing with him or her the effect of inappropriate sexual behaviors on others. Provide research studies regarding the effects of treatment on recidivism rates and handouts about the scope of treatment and how compliance can assist in regaining control of sexual behaviors. *Compliance with treatment reduces the risk of relapse.*

4. Teach the client appropriate coping strategies, assertiveness skills, and problem-solving techniques *to promote follow-through of the treatment plan and to facilitate appropriate sexual behaviors.*

5. Promote the client's development of appropriate social skills and provide support and encouragement to the client for efforts at control of the disorder. Peer-to-peer mentorship may be appropriate to enhance appropriate social skills and feelings of acceptance. *The client may feel guilty over his or her behavior and become socially isolated. Support and encouragement of the client will signify that there are healthy, functional, acceptable aspects of his or her personality.*

Additional Treatment Modalities

Pharmacologic. The need for medications is based on the collaborative efforts of the multidisciplinary team to assess the intensity and impulsivity of the client's disorder and symptoms.

Depo-Provera (medroxyprogesterone acetate) 500 mg IM q wk has been prescribed with some success for clients with a paraphilic disorder (Berlin and Meineke, 1981). This form of external control helps clients develop their own internal controls to avoid relapse. Clients have reported that this medication lowers the frequency and intensity of inappropriate sexual thoughts and fantasies.

There are several side effects that the nurse needs to be aware of. Because this type of medication decreases testosterone levels and sperm production, the client who is receiving Depo-Provera may not be able to father a child. Common side effects include weight gain, increased blood pressure, and fatigue. The nurse may suggest a dietary consultation to help the client maintain weight and decrease the possibility of weight gain. Blood pressures must be taken before each dose. In general, if the diastolic is 100 mm Hg or greater, the medication should be withheld. The nurse must communicate with the physician regarding blood pressure readings and whether to administer the medication.

The medication is viscous and should be given in no more than 500 mg per muscle. The gluteal muscle may also be used in administering Depo-Provera. It is not necessary to administer this medication via Z track because there is no conclusive evidence that this method of injection increases absorption. Clients may complain of pain in the injection sites and need to be reassured that the pain will subside within a day. If given in the deltoid, the nurse may want to instruct the client to engage in range-of-motion exercises (moving the shoulder and arm in a circular motion).

Depo-Provera should not be administered without informed consent and the client's signature on a consent form that explains about the medication and its therapeutic and nontherapeutic effects. The nurse may review this with the client after a decision has been made by the physician to include this as part of the client's individualized plan of care.

Lupron-Depot (leuprolide) is a relatively new form of treatment, and there is not much experience with its use in the paraphilic population. This medication may be a more powerful antiandrogenic drug. It acts similarly to Depo-Provera by lowering testosterone levels in the client with a paraphilic disorder. This medication is usually prescribed as 7.5 mg IM once a month. It is also available in a nondepo form; the usual prescribed dosage is 1 mg subcutaneous daily.

Side effects include a decrease in libido (the desired result), bone pain, gynecomastia, hair growth, weight gain, high blood pressure, dizziness, headaches, mood swings,

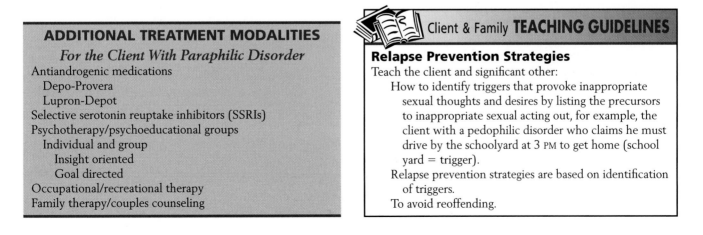

ADDITIONAL TREATMENT MODALITIES
For the Client With Paraphilic Disorder
Antiandrogenic medications
  Depo-Provera
  Lupron-Depot
Selective serotonin reuptake inhibitors (SSRIs)
Psychotherapy/psychoeducational groups
  Individual and group
    Insight oriented
    Goal directed
Occupational/recreational therapy
Family therapy/couples counseling

Client & Family **TEACHING GUIDELINES**

Relapse Prevention Strategies
Teach the client and significant other:
  How to identify triggers that provoke inappropriate sexual thoughts and desires by listing the precursors to inappropriate sexual acting out, for example, the client with a pedophilic disorder who claims he must drive by the schoolyard at 3 PM to get home (school yard = trigger).
  Relapse prevention strategies are based on identification of triggers.
  To avoid reoffending.

and phlebitis. The nurse must have the knowledge to assess for the presence of any and all nontherapeutic effects.

In the beginning of treatment with Lupron-Depot, clients should be prescribed flutamide (Eulexin) 250 mg PO tid to enhance the testosterone-suppressing aspects of Lupron-Depot by blocking testosterone receptors. This should be prescribed secondary to the increase in testosterone production within the first 2 to 4 weeks after having started treatment with Lupron-Depot.

Again, it is important for the nurse to monitor the client's blood pressure before administering Lupron-Depot. The same criteria should apply to Depo-Provera.

Selective serotonin reuptake inhibitors.   Current literature contains several case reports regarding the treatment of paraphilic disorders with selective serotonin reuptake inhibitors (SSRIs), such as Prozac or Zoloft. These medications have fewer side effects than the antiandrogenic medications. Single case reports address the efficacy of paraphilic treatment with SSRIs by increasing serotonin activity, thereby decreasing sexual appetite. It is impor-

tant to note that further research is warranted because of the absence of double-blind–chart studies in this area (Kafka, 1997).

Psychotherapy/psychoeducation groups.   Nurses may lead or co-lead psychotherapy/psychoeducation groups with the physician or another member of the treatment team if they have the appropriate group psychotherapy credentials.

The purpose of group psychotherapy/**psychoeducation** are (1) to address cognitive distortions and (2) to provide education to this client population regarding identification of triggers, relapse prevention strategies, importance of treatment compliance, self-esteem issues, appropriate coping strategies, and problem-solving skills.

Recreational and occupational therapy may also be provided to assist the client in time structuring, which may be viewed as a relapse prevention strategy. (See Chapter 26 for further information.)

Family/couples therapy may also be recommended, depending on the individual client care needs. This form of therapy is usually provided by the social worker and may also be provided by a masters-prepared nurse or physician.

CASE STUDY

Martin is a 24-year-old college student who attends the local university and lives at home with his parents and two older sisters. He was referred for treatment after conviction for raping a 22-year-old female. Martin has been an active participant in an eight-member outpatient sex offender group for the last 5 years. The Department of Parole and Probation is about to release him back into the community without any further legal requirements. The nurse group leader finds herself feeling uncomfortable with Martin's desire to be discharged outright from group. Her discomfort is related to the seriousness of the disorder, not to the amount of progress he has made. Martin has been compliant with treatment within the last 5 years. His treatment consisted of weekly group attendance with participation, compliance with medications when prescribed, development and implementation of appropriate relapse prevention strategies, and sound understanding of the nature of his disorder.

Critical Thinking—Evaluation
1. What criteria does the nurse use to effectively evaluate Martin's readiness for discharge from therapy?
2. What concerns might the nurse have regarding Martin's prognosis after discharge?
3. With whom might the nurse consult in rendering her decision regarding Martin's discharge from the therapy group?
4. Would family therapy be indicated on discharge from the group therapy session? Discuss the rationale for this intervention.
5. How could the nurse be responsible if Martin relapses after discharge from the group?

EVALUATION
Nurses must continually evaluate the effectiveness of their interventions on the behavior to successfully treat this population. If identified nursing interventions are not helping the client achieve his or her outcomes, revisions must be made in the nursing care plan. The nurse may want to discuss the plan with the client and obtain his or her assistance in revising it. The areas in which client outcomes have been successfully achieved should be identified as "resolved." If newly identified problems arise, these should also be addressed in the client's plan of care.

In treating the client with a paraphilic disorder, it is not unrealistic to expect the client to acknowledge the presence of the paraphilic disorder, identify triggers, develop relapse prevention strategies, and state the importance of treatment compliance postdischarge. If these outcomes are not met by the time of discharge, the client would be at a greater risk for reoffending. The need to protect both the client and society from possible relapse or recidivism is critical.

The minimal expected period for outpatient treatment is 2 years, although actual time for treatment may be considerably longer. These clients need to be carefully monitored for any changes in their status that could lead to relapse. Monitoring may occur through weekly outpatient group therapy or, if group is not indicated, by periodic visits with the client's therapist.

A client is formally discharged from outpatient treatment based on the level of progress and current status regarding the paraphilic behaviors.

Summary of Key Concepts

1. The nurse must have an understanding of human sexuality, be aware of his or her feelings and values regarding sexuality, and be committed to incorporating sexuality into client care in a nonjudgmental manner.

2. Sexual dysfunctions are the most common of all sexual problems that come to the attention of health care practitioners. Estimates of the prevalence of sexual dysfunctions are as high as 50%.

3. The lack of sex education and the high rate of sexual repression may contribute to the high incidence of sexual dysfunctions.

4. Establishment of a plan of care should include the significant other. In a couple situation, blame should not be placed on either person.

5. Specific, realistic outcome criteria developed by the client (or client and significant other) are necessary for implementing the plan of care.

6. Nursing interventions should include client education about human sexual functioning, sexual response, and sexual dysfunctions; helping clients improve their communication; support for the clients' fears and anxieties; support for enhancement of the client's self-esteem; and referral for professional help.

7. Many complex diagnostic and treatment modalities have been developed for sexual dysfunctions in the past few decades. These include psychophysiologic methods and psychosocial methods. They include neurologic, endocrine, and vascular treatments, as well as specific sex therapy techniques. Therapeutic modalities are currently more developed for males than for females.

8. Giving permission for sexual feelings and behaviors may be the single most important intervention.

9. Paraphilia is defined as sexual deviations/disorders presenting with inappropriate sexual fantasies involving deviant sexual acts, inappropriate sexual urges, and acting out of these fantasies and urges.

10. Family history positive for the presence of a paraphilic disorder and/or history of victimization may predispose other family members to developing a similar or different paraphilic disorder.

11. Establishing a plan of care should include the client to the extent that he or she is able to participate, and goals should reflect mutual agreement between the nurse and the client.

12. Interventions should be based on the client's individual needs. The plan of care should include confrontation of cognitive distortions, exploration of the effects of inappropriate sexual behaviors on others, psychoeducational group therapy to teach the client how to identify triggers that provoke inappropriate sexual thoughts, development of relapse prevention strategies and the effects of treatment on illness symptomatology, the importance of treatment compliance during the hospital stay and postdischarge, and development of appropriate coping strategies and problem-solving skills.

13. The client with a paraphilic disorder who is compliant with treatment has a lesser risk of recidivism.

REFERENCES

Abel GG et al: Sexually aggressive behavior. In Curran WJ et al, editors: *Forensic psychiatry and psychology*, Philadelphia, 1986, FA Davis.

Abel GG et al: Self-reported sex crimes of nonincarcerated paraphiliacs, *J Interpersonal Violence* 2(1):3, 1987.

Abel GG, Osborn C: Stopping sexual violence, *Psychiatr Ann* 22(6):301, 1992.

American Psychiatric Association: *Diagnostic and statistical manual of mental disorders*, ed 4, Washington, DC, 1994, The Association.

Anon J: The PLISSIT model, *J Sex Educ Ther* 2(1):1, 1976.

Arndt WB Jr: *Gender disorders and the paraphilias*, Madison, Conn, 1991, International Universities Press.

Ashton A, Hamer R, Rosen R: Serotonin-reuptake inhibitor-induced sexual dysfunction and its treatment: a large scale retrospective study of 596 psychiatric outpatients, *J Sex Marital Ther* 23(3):165, 1997.

Baker HJ, Stoller J: Can a biological force contribute to gender identity? *Am J Psychiatry* 124(12):1653, 1968.

Beitchman J et al: A review of the long-term effects of child sexual abuse, *Child Abuse Negl* 16:101, 1992.

Bergner RM: Money's "lovemap" account of the paraphilias: a critique and reformulation, *Am J Psychother* 42(2):254, 1988.

Berlin FS: Special considerations in the psychiatric evaluation of sexual offenders against minors. In Rosner R, Schwartz H, editors: *Juvenile psychiatry and the law: critical issues in American psychiatry and the law*, vol 4, New York, 1989, Plenum Press.

Berlin FS: The paraphilias and Depo-Provera: some medical, ethical and legal considerations, *Bull Am Acad Psychiatry Law* 17(3):233, 1989.

Berlin FS et al: A five-year plus follow-up survey of criminal recidivism within a treated cohort of 406 pedophiles, 111 exhibitionists and 109 sexual aggressives: issues and outcomes, *Am J Forensic Psychiatry* 12(3):5, 1991.

Berlin FS, Malin HM: Media distortion of the public's perception of recidivism and psychiatric rehabilitation, *Am J Psychiatry* 148(11):1572, 1991.

Berlin FS, Meineke CF: Treatment of sex offenders with antiandrogen medication: conceptualization, review of treatment modalities and preliminary findings, *Am J Psychiatry* 138:601, 1981.

Bradford JM, Gratzner TG: A treatment for impulse control disorders and paraphilia, *Can J Psychiatry* 40:4, 1995.

Brecher E: *The sex researchers*, New York, 1971, New American Library.

Ducharme S, Gill K: Management of the male sexual dysfunctions. In Sipski M, Alexander C: *Sexual function in people with disability and chronic illness: a health professionals guide*, Gaithersburg, Md, 1997, Aspen.

Gaffney GS et al: Is there familial transmission of pedophilia? *J Nerv Ment Dis* 172:546, 1984.

Groth AN: *Men who rape*, New York, 1979, Plenum Press.

Hartman W, Fithian M: *Treatment of sexual dysfunction: a bio-psycho-social approach*, Long Beach, Calif, 1972, Center for Marital and Sexual Studies.

Kafka MP: Sertraline pharmacotherapy for paraphilias and paraphilia-related disorders: an open trial, *Ann Clin Psychiatry* 6:189, 1994.

Kafka MP: How are drugs used in the treatment of paraphuilic disorders? *Harvard Ment Health Letter* 13(9):8, 1997.

Kaplan H: *The new sex therapy*, New York, 1974, Brunner/Mazel.

Kaplan HI, Sadock BJ: Paraphilias. In Kaplan HI, Sadock, BJ, editors: *Synopsis of psychiatry, behavioral sciences, clinical psychiatry*, ed 6, Baltimore, 1991, Williams & Wilkins.

Kiersch TA: Treatment of sex offenders with Depo-Provera, *Bull Am Acad Psychiatry Law* 18(2):179, 1990.

Kim MJ et al: *Pocket guide to nursing diagnoses*, ed 5, St. Louis, 1993, Mosby.

Kinsey A et al: *Sexual behavior in the human female*, Philadelphia, 1953, WB Saunders.

Klinefelter HF et al: Syndrome characterized by gynecomastia, aspermatogenesis without A-Leydigism, and increased excretion of FSH, *J Clin Endocrinol Metab* 2(2):615, 1994.

Labbate LL et al: Sexual dysfunction induced by serotonin reuptake antidepressants, *J Sex Marital Ther* 24(1):3, 1998.

Leiblum S, Rosen R: *Principles and practice of sex therapy*, New York, 1989, Guilford Press.

LeMone P: Human sexuality in adults with insulin-dependent diabetes mellitus, *Image: J Nurs Sch* 25(2):101, 1993.

LoPiccolo J, Friedman J: Broad spectrum treatment of low sexual desire: integration of cognitive, behavioral and systematic therapy. In Leiblum S, Rosen R, editors: *Sexual desire disorders*, New York, 1988, Guilford Press.

Masters W, Johnson V: *Human sexual inadequacy*, Boston, 1970, Little, Brown.

Masters W, Johnson V: *Human sexual response*, Boston, 1966, Little, Brown.

McCarthy B: Chronic sexual dysfunction: assessment, intervention and realistic expectations, *J Sex Educ Therapy* 22(2):51, 1997.

Meyer WJ et al: Depo-Provera treatment for sex offending behavior: an evaluation of outcome, *Bull Am Acad Psychiatry Law* 20(3):249, 1992.

Money J et al: Imprinting and the establishment of gender role, *Arch Neurol Psychiatry* 77:333, 1957.

Money J: *Lovemaps*, Buffalo, NY, 1986a, Prometheus Books.

Money J: *Lovemaps: clinical concepts of sexual/erotic health and pathology, paraphilia, and gender transposition in childhood, adolescence, and maturity*, New York, 1986b, Irvington.

Money J: *Venuses penuses: sexology, sexosophy and exigency theory*, Buffalo, NY, 1986c, Prometheus Books.

Money J: Treatment guidelines: antiandrogen and counseling of paraphilic sex offenders, *J Sex Marital Ther* 13(3):219, 1987.

Morokoff P, Gillilland R: Stress, sexual functioning and marital satisfaction, *J Sex Res* 30:43, 1993.

North American Nursing Diagnosis Association: *NANDA nursing diagnoses: definitions and classifications, 1999-2000*, Philadelphia, 1999, The Association.

Piletz J et al: Plasma MHPG response to yohimbine treatment in women with hypoactive sexual desire, *J Sex Marital Ther* 24(1):43, 1998.

Plaut M, RachBeisel J: Use of anxiolytic medication in the treatment of vaginismis and severe aversion to penetration, case report, *J Sex Educ Ther* 22(3):43, 1997.

Renshaw D: Profile of 2376 patients treated at Loyola Sex Clinic between 1972 and 1978, *J Sex Marital Ther* 3:111, 1988.

Schiavi R et al: Erectile function and penile blood pressure in diabetes mellitus, *J Sex Marital Ther* 20(2):119, 1994.

Semans R: Premature ejaculation: a new approach, *South Med J* 49:353, 1956.

Simon WT, Schouten PG: Plethysmography in the assessment of sexual deviance: an overview, *Arch Sex Behav* 20(1):75, 1991.

Spector I, Carey M: Incidence and prevalence of the sexual dysfunctions: a critical review of the literature, *Arch Sex Behav* 19:389, 1990.

Wagner G, Kaplan, HS: *The new injection treatment for impotence*, New York, 1993, Brunner/Mazel.

Wagner G, Rabkin J, Rabkin R: Effects of testosterone replacement therapy on sexual interest, function and behavior in HIV+ men, *J Sex Res* 34(1):27, 1997.

Whipple B, McGreer KB: Management of sexual dysfunction in women. In Sipski M, Alexander C: *Sexual function in people with disability and chronic illness: a health professionals guide*, Gaithersburg, Md, 1997, Aspen.

Wilson GD: An ethological approach to sexual deviation. In Wilson GD, editor: *Variant sexuality: research and theory*, Baltimore, 1987, The Johns Hopkins University Press.

Wincze J et al: Comparison of nocturnal penile tumescence response and penile response to erotic stimulation during waking states in comprehensively diagnosed groups of males experiencing erectile difficulties, *Arch Sex Behav* 17:333, 1988.

Zilbergeld B, Evans M: The inadequacy of Masters and Johnson, *Psych Today* 14:29, 1980.

CHAPTER 21

Adjustment Disorders

Merry A. Armstrong

OBJECTIVES

- Describe five major criteria for an adjustment disorder.

- Analyze the relationship of life events to adjustment disorders.

- Discuss the implications of the diagnosis of adjustment disorder with depressed mood for the nonpsychiatric hospitalized client.

- Apply the nursing process to clients who exhibit symptoms of adjustment disorders.

- Explain the major therapeutic goals for clients who have a diagnosis of adjustment disorder.

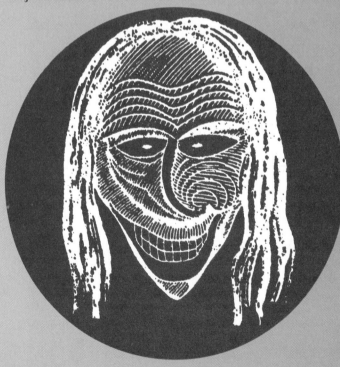

ADJUSTMENT DISORDERS

Adjustment disorders are problematic responses to life events. Problematic responses are behaviors, feelings, or thoughts that interfere with an individual's functioning or sense of well-being. Some of the symptoms of adjustment disorders are similar to those in other diagnostic groups, such as affective mood disorders or anxiety disorders. Adjustment disorders, however, are considered less serious and often represent transient episodes in the lives of otherwise mentally healthy individuals.

People experiencing life transitions such as divorce, relocation, adolescence, or other psychologically challenging events may be diagnosed with an adjustment disorder. Depending on the intensity of their symptoms, such as anxiety or lack of concentration, and the temporal relation of their symptoms to life events, many of these clients are diagnosed with an adjustment disorder. Individuals seeking outpatient therapy for assistance in dealing with responses to such things as specific problematic life events may also be diagnosed as having an adjustment disorder. After obtaining an appropriate developmental history, completing a mental status assessment, and systematically eliminating other potential diagnoses, the mental health practitioner may decide that the client has an adjustment disorder. The term *mental health practitioner* is used because in some states advanced practice nurses (APN), licensed clinical social workers (LCSW), or other licensed, qualified personnel determine DSM-IV pathology. The diagnosis of adjustment disorder suggests the probability that the client possesses or can rally sufficient resources to resolve his or her problematic response within an appropriate time, in this case by responding to therapeutic intervention as a primary treatment modality.

In these situations the diagnosis implies that the mental health practitioner has reason to believe that the client's problematic symptoms will abate when the life event or transitional experience is resolved as a central issue. Like all clients, the client diagnosed with an adjustment disorder would be continually assessed for new or intensifying symptoms that might indicate a developing major depressive disorder or other mental illness.

HISTORICAL AND THEORETIC PERSPECTIVES

Problematic responses to either developmental or situational stressors have been discussed in psychiatric literature for many years. However, adjustment disorders were first professionally categorized and described in 1968 in the second edition of the *Diagnostic and Statistical Manual of Mental Disorders* (DSM-II) as "transient situational disturbance" (American Psychiatric Association [APA], 1968). The DSM-III (APA, 1980) grouped adjustment disorders by clinical presentation. If the client described symptoms of depression without symptoms of major depression, he or she was diagnosed as having an adjustment disorder with depressed mood.

The DSM-III-Revised (APA, 1987) used adjustment disorders as a classification for conditions that did not fulfill criteria for a major psychiatric disorder. Nine types of adjustment disorder were identified.

The DSM-IV (APA, 1994) considers adjustment disorders transient episodes of dysfunction in response to specific stressors. To be diagnosed as having an adjustment disorder, the client must demonstrate criteria for one of six classifications: adjustment disorder with depressed mood, with anxiety, with mixed anxiety and depressed mood, with disturbance of conduct, with mixed disturbance of emotions and conduct, and unspecified. Adjustment disorders may be acute (symptoms last 6 months or less) or chronic (symptoms persist

for more than 6 months) or when the precipitating stressor had long-lasting effects. Examples of these disorders are presented later in the chapter.

As a part of their role, many mental health practitioners are required to arrive at conclusions (diagnoses) about the mental condition of their clients. Without the immediacy or specificity of laboratory tests such as blood values or radiologic studies to rely on, the practitioner initiates a relationship with the client. The developing therapeutic relationship is the forum in which dialogue, discussion, observation, and professional assessment converge to provide material supporting a mental health diagnosis. As the therapeutic relationship continues, diagnoses (medical or nursing) may change depending on the client's symptoms and behaviors, or as other new information becomes known to the professional staff. The diagnosis of adjustment disorder suggests that troublesome symptoms may abate with time and therapeutic intervention. Conversely, adjustment disorders may be precursors to more serious mental health problems. In either case, continual reassessment of the client's symptoms, condition, and situation is required.

ETIOLOGY

The interaction of personality, crisis, stress, developmental factors, and cultural influences must be considered when investigating the formation of adjustment disorders.

CRISIS AND STRESS MODELS

Situational events requiring major physical and/or psychologic adjustment occur normally during a person's lifetime. Most people develop a repertoire of skills to manage difficult situations. However, because of the intensity, timing, or repetition of the stressor or situation, prior methods are sometimes not sufficient to mitigate the problem. Using the model suggested by the crisis theory, one might say that an adjustment disorder results from an individual's inability to use existing coping methods or create new methods in response to a situation. This inability to use former methods or formulate new strategies results in a situation in which the client feels overwhelmed, confused, and helpless, further depleting his or her ability to rally resources. These feelings may be manifested as depression, anxiety, or other combinations of emotional experience.

Stress-adaptation theory, originally formulated by Selye, (1956, 1978) suggested a biologic response to stress called the *general adaptation syndrome (GAS)*. Stress was defined as a situation that required a physiologic response or change. It was noted that people may respond to the same stressful situation in different ways. For example, one individual might experience a headache in response to an argument, whereas another might experience physical or psychologic sensations of relief. An experience might be labeled pleasant or unpleasant, but if a biologic adjustment is required, the GAS is activated and the stress response is present. The stress-adaptation and crisis models are similar in that the client feels overwhelmed and without resources to respond to a situation.

Precipitating Factors

Adjustment disorders can be triggered by a stressor or series of stressors that may be developmental (adolescence, menopause), situational (job change, divorce, hospitalization), or adventitious (earthquake, war, flood). Life events requiring major adjustments can be developmental, situ-

ational, adventitious, or a combination of all three.

For example, serious developmental and situational challenges occur in early adulthood when adolescents graduate from high school and must decide their life direction. Accomplishing the developmental tasks of establishing personal identity, as well as negotiating situational stressors (e.g., decisions after graduation from high school to explore career, school, surfing, peace corps, military) that determine one's life course are complex endeavors (Figure 21-1).

Likewise, people in their middle and older years have significant developmental challenges that may result in transient situational adjustment problems. For example, retirement is often referred to as a benefit and goal of late adulthood, yet it is sometimes experienced as a loss of identity and purpose. Other life events related to individual physical or psychologic development may include the loss of a significant other or the diagnosis of a major disease process. Changes in employment, marital status,

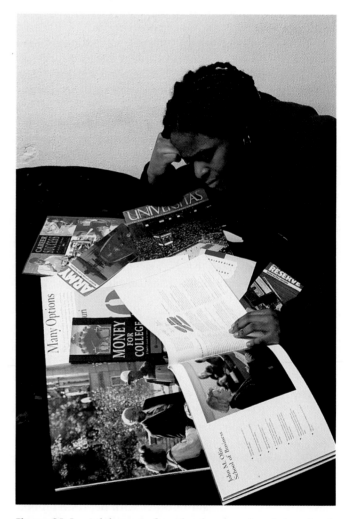

Figure 21-1   Adolescents face developmental and situational challenges as they contemplate decisions for their future, such as options for employment or college.

childbearing, and other life occurrences may also present individuals with significant responsibilities to manage. Illness, major family changes, and/or developmental crises are not uncommon occurrences, and often occur simultaneously.

Review of recent literature indicates that adjustment disorder is a diagnosis frequently used with difficulties of adolescence. Adjustment disorders among adult patients who are hospitalized are associated with shorter lengths of stay and with more concurrent substance abuse disorders (Greenberg, Rosenfeld, and Ortega, 1995; Kovacs et al, 1994).

Loss

A key theme underlying life change is that of **loss,** as described by Kubler-Ross (1969) and since explored and refined by others (Levine, 1987; Walsh and McGoldrick, 1991). Loss is a process characterized by a series of overlapping stages that include common psychologic and behavioral manifestations of recognition, adjustment, and resolution. Numerous examples of loss have been articulated in this chapter, and all change includes loss. Managing a desired change such as retirement, marriage, or establishing a family requires loss of previous status, freedom, or identity. Walsh and McGoldrick (1991) stated that losses require movement through a process of mourning in order to get what is needed from the experience or relationship to continue on with one's life. How persons get what they need from the experience is often contextually determined and influenced by culture and socialization. The nurse plays an instrumental role in educating the client about the loss process and in helping the client mourn loss.

Grief, mourning, and bereavement are other expressions of loss and are discussed in Chapter 29. According to DSM-IV criteria, persons experiencing severe or prolonged difficulties with grief and bereavement would not be diagnosed with adjustment disorders, which are transient in nature.

DEVELOPMENTAL INFLUENCES

Erikson (1963) proposed a developmental theory of the personality through achievement of specific tasks at different stages of the life cycle. Erikson postulated that difficulties in adjustment occurred when age-appropriate behaviors or tasks were not completed, resulting in an inability to move forward with developmental tasks. The **adult developmental theory** suggests that individuals continue to evolve as maturity progresses.

Colarusso and Nemiroff (1981) contended that individuals continue to refine their sense of identity and self and that adulthood is characterized by normative crises based on adult developmental tasks. According to these authors, themes of adult developmental tasks are intimacy, love, and sex; issues related to the body; time and death; relationship to children; relationship to parents;

mentor relationships; relationship to society; work; play; and finances. As people mature, themes of adult development are continuous and important sources of information for the therapist in the process of identifying the dynamics of the client problem or symptoms.

Colarusso and Nemiroff (1981) used the developmental concept of Erikson's model (1963) and suggested that adulthood is divided into rough age groupings: early adulthood (ages 20 to 40), middle adulthood (ages 40 to 60), late adulthood (ages 60 to 80), and late-late adulthood (ages 80 and beyond). These authors further suggested that adult developmental strands existed on a continuum and were experienced differently, depending on issues active in each age category.

For example, the strand, or theme, of adult development, "time and death," might likely be applied as an active developmental task for a person in middle adulthood rather than for someone in early adulthood. So a person in

CASE STUDY

P.R., a 16-year-old high school student, was brought to the counseling center by his parents, who stated that he looked distracted, was not doing well in school, and had developed irregular eating and sleeping patterns. Recent stressors known to his parents included breaking up with his girlfriend of 6 months and being required to lose 15 pounds for the wrestling team. After completion of a thorough medical assessment, the nurse talked with the client about recent events in his life.

P.R. expressed regret about breaking up with his girlfriend but had a positive attitude about this change, feeling that perhaps he was too young for a steady girlfriend, anyway. However, P.R. expressed feeling hopeless about losing the 15 pounds and worried that he would fail to make the wrestling team. He confided to the nurse that in order to lose weight, he had taken pills that another student had given him to ensure weight loss. P.R. found himself unable to sleep or concentrate, so he had started drinking liquor in order to get to sleep. He had hidden this from his parents and was embarrassed to tell them. He was afraid that if he stopped taking the pills, he would gain weight and not make the team. He felt trapped and also knew that his thinking was affected by his lack of sleep and drug use, and he had occasional, fleeting thoughts that he might be better off dead. He did not know who to talk to and was afraid to talk to his wrestling coach. Although he resisted coming to the clinic, he expressed relief to the nurse that his parents had insisted that he talk to a counselor.

Critical Thinking—Assessment

1. P.R. is experiencing several problematic life events. What are they?
2. What is P.R.'s risk for suicide?
3. What implications does the use of drugs have for suicide and/or mental illness?
4. Do you think P.R. is addicted to drugs and/or alcohol?

middle adulthood may, at the same time, be diagnosed with a chronic health problem, have substantial financial and work responsibilities, be involved in parenting teenagers, and experience the death of a parent.

If adults experience developmental challenges unique to their age and situation, as Colarusso and Nemiroff (1981, 1987) contended, how can mental health professionals help clients to identify, attain, and use new skills? A common precipitating event that stimulates adult development is the personal experience of an illness, or the illness of a loved one. Clients at risk for, or who have, adjustment disorders are commonly cared for by nurses in general hospitals, long-term care facilities, rehabilitation centers, or in the home. Nurses have unique opportunities for long-term assessment and subsequent intervention regarding clients' emotional and psychologic difficulties. For example, one of the activities in a mental health assessment is the determination of the meaning of the situation for the client. Being briefly hospitalized for a hernia repair probably does not have the same meaning for a client of the same age who is hospitalized for stabilization of newly diagnosed diabetes.

CULTURAL, SOCIAL, AND PSYCHOLOGIC INFLUENCES

Growth and development must be examined with consideration of contextual aspects of sociocultural influences. This chapter would not be complete without mentioning the scope and volume of currently debated issues of psychologic and personality development. Extending beyond historic disputes of nature versus nurture theories, scholars question classification systems of mental illness (Kirk and Kutchins, 1992) and traditional scientific research methods (Blier, 1986).

In addition, debate continues in the human sciences regarding differences in development and experience according to one's gender and socialization (Gilligan, 1982; Jordan et al, 1991; Lerner, 1988; Lewis, 1986; Meth and Pasick, 1990; Napier, 1991; Pittman, 1991). Gender, culture, and social factors influence the results of measurements such as the intelligence quotient (IQ). If gender, culture, and social factors partially determine a person's reality, how do we give nursing care using standard nursing diagnoses that may not reflect the reality of our clients?

For example, a nurse caring for a client identifies that the client has problems related to the death of a spouse and applies the nursing diagnosis of dysfunctional grieving. However, behaviors that the nurse perceives as problems may be appropriate in the client's culture. If that is the case, the nurse may be missing identification of important facts. Instead of identifying the client's problems, the nurse might have demonstrated cultural bias in expecting all people to resolve issues in the same way. The nurse must be aware that clients may resolve their grief in a culturally and socially appropriate manner and include assessment activities that reveal this information. This sounds like a simple solution, but different cultures also proscribe speaking to persons outside the family about intimate details. Therefore the nurse must also be aware of communication patterns of the culture and other social customs.

Lowenberg (1989), a nurse researcher, explored the practices of consumers and practitioners of American health care, using the framework of an evolving paradigm of health care, **holism.** Historically, illness was thought to represent social deviance (Davis, 1972; Parsons, 1951), and stigma and labeling were applied to a variety of problems culturally interpreted as illness. The author observed that emerging concepts of holism and health suggested that people's physical, mental, emotional, spiritual, and social aspects were interrelated and interdependent. Using this concept, some people have redefined the illness experience from biologic deterioration to a more positive interpretation of illness as a warning sign that adjustments in living are needed. Lowenberg (1989) observed that the emerging health paradigm (holism) considers illness as an opportunity for growth and development.

CONTRIBUTIONS OF NURSING RESEARCH

Nursing research has contributed information leading to a greater understanding of individual experience. Although nursing research has not addressed the diagnosis of adjustment disorders specifically, it has explored meanings of many life events for individual clients and caregivers, using

Understanding & Applying Research

A case study approach was used in this qualitative retrospective study of the experience of 10 residents who had received psychotherapy for treatment of depression, dysthymic disorder, or adjustment disorder. Six men and four women with an average age of 87.2 (**the old old** are defined as those over age 85 years) who lived semiindependently or in the nursing home facility in the same geriatric center were seen by one of several therapists for individual psychotherapy. Each patient was interviewed for his or her understanding about the content and process of therapy and whether it was thought of as helpful. Interview data were combined with chart information and therapist notes to produce case histories for each patient. Patients had positive recollections of their relationship with the therapist, and the perceived benefit of treatment was related to the positive value of the therapeutic relationship rather than to specific techniques or interventions. The researcher concluded that psychotherapy was a positive experience that provided palliative treatment for these clients and that further research is needed to explore the benefits of psychotherapy for the old old. Little is known about the value of psychotherapy among this age-group or with residents of nursing homes in general.

Ruckdeschel H: *Psychotherapy for the old old: ten patients' report on their treatment for depression.* Unpublished doctoral dissertation, 1993, University of Pennsylvania.

qualitative research techniques (Armstrong, 1992; Beck, 1992; Bergum, 1989; Heifner, 1993; Lowenberg, 1989; Main et al, 1993; Mickley et al, 1992; Murphy, 1993; Tanner et al, 1993). Understanding the process of an illness experience can help nurses and other professionals develop effective assessment techniques, methods for intervention, and models for evaluation of treatment (see Understanding & Applying Research box).

EPIDEMIOLOGY

Adult adjustment disorders are thought to be common, although data to support this opinion are scarce (Popkin, 1989). A factor contributing to difficulty in gathering statistics regarding adjustment disorder treatment is that the clinical or symptomatic findings in adjustment disorder vary widely, thus making the diagnosis difficult. The DSM-IV (APA, 1994) cites prevalence rates between 5% and 20% in outpatient populations.

Studies were conducted on the findings of psychiatric consultation/liaison personnel who assessed clients in acute care hospitals. Adjustment disorders in medically ill inpatient clients (Popkin et al, 1990; Razavi et al, 1990; Snyder et al, 1990) were commonly identified. Many clients with terminal diagnoses or severe chronic illness displayed symptoms of either major depression or adjustment disorder.

CLINICAL DESCRIPTION

Six subtypes of adjustment disorder are noted in the DSM-IV. They are coded on Axis IV according to symptom type and with stressor(s) noted. Because adjustment disorder can present with various combinations of symptomatology, it is difficult to categorize discrete symptoms. General clusters of symptoms are provided in Box 21-1.

DSM-IV CRITERIA

Adjustment Disorders

A. A reaction to an identifiable psychosocial stressor (or multiple stressors) that occurs within 3 months of onset of the stressor(s).

B. Symptoms of distress are marked and in excess of a normal and expectable reaction to the stressor(s), *or* the client experiences significant social or occupational impairment.

C. The disturbance does not meet criteria for Axis I or II disorder. A diagnosis of adjustment disorder may be made in the presence of an Axis I or II disorder if the pattern of symptoms is not attributable to these disorders and an identified stressor exists.

D. This diagnosis is not used when symptoms represent bereavement.

E. Symptoms of the disorder must resolve within 6 months of the cessation of the stressor.

However, symptoms persisting longer than 6 months because of the chronicity of the stressor (a chronic physical disease) or as the result of enduring consequences of a stressor (divorce, loss of employment) may be considered chronic adjustment disorders.

From American Psychiatric Association: *Diagnostic and statistical manual of mental disorders*, ed 4, Washington, DC, 1994, The Association.

Box 21-1   Types of Adjustment Disorders

Adjustment Disorder With Depressed Mood
Used when the predominant symptomatology are depressed mood, tearfulness, and feelings of hopelessness.

Adjustment Disorder With Anxious Mood
Used when the predominant symptomatology are nervousness, worry, and jitteriness.

Adjustment Disorder With Mixed Anxiety and Depressed Mood
Used when the predominant manifestation is a combination of depression and anxiety.

Adjustment Disorder With Disturbance of Conduct
Used when the client's conduct violates the rights of others or major age-appropriate societal norms and rules (e.g., vandalism, fighting, defaulting on legal responsibilities).

Adjustment Disorder With Mixed Disturbance of Emotions and Conduct
Used when predominant symptomatology are combinations of emotions (e.g., depression or anxiety) and a disturbance of conduct.

Unspecified
Used for maladaptive reactions (such as physical complaints, social withdrawal, or work or academic inhibition) to psychosocial stressors not classifiable in other specific subtypes.

From American Psychiatric Association: *Diagnostic and statistical manual of mental disorders*, ed 4, Washington, DC, 1994, The Association.

THE NURSING PROCESS

ASSESSMENT

Because clients are not often hospitalized for treatment of adjustment disorder, nurses are more likely to assess clients with an adjustment disorder in an outpatient or home setting (see Nursing Care in the Community box). Out-

---

Nursing Care in the Community

Adjustment Disorders

Adjustment disorders are common in the community mental health field. Some are the long-term results of predictable crises of maturation and development, such as the death of a loved one, employment problems, and financial issues. In such cases therapeutic pathways have been fairly well established and the nurse can follow through with standard crisis intervention strategies to reassure the client that the situation should improve with time. Clients can be introduced to support groups focused on similar issues and, if necessary, be prescribed medication to help mitigate the process until the individual has established functional coping patterns. Most clients will respond well to education and exposure to peers who have had similar experiences, but prolonged adjustment difficulties may be cause for more intensive interventions. The nurse may consider longer-term work with the client, focusing on changes in the client's living situation, and perhaps even lifestyle, to reduce stress, occupy free time, and increase coping abilities.

Unpredictable and sometimes catastrophic crises are much more difficult to manage, requiring active and decisive action on the part of the psychiatric mental health nurse in the community. Assault or other catastrophic events would be examples of such overwhelming trauma, first managed by crisis intervention, but also requiring extremely careful supervision to avoid excessive emotional reactions such as homicidal or suicidal feelings. Nonjudgmental debriefing must be continued to put the situation in perspective and allow the client to both ventilate and distance himself or herself from the trauma.

Prolonged difficulties (e.g., enduring marital problems, adjustment to chronic ill health, or continuing financial problems) require a new level of coping ability. Adjustment should be achieved within 3 to 6 months without attendant anxiety, depression, or changes in typical behavior. The community mental health nurse is in a good position to monitor how well the client has reconciled to the current situation and how positive he or she is about the future.

Finally, if the symptoms of adjustment difficulties continue for more than 6 months, the long-term needs of the client are addressed by giving referrals to an appropriate therapist and a support group for ongoing treatment. Adjustment disorders often require prolonged psychosocial and practical interventions to promote future safety and functionality.

---

patient clients may request treatment based on the symptoms of one or more adjustment disorders. Adjustment disorder subtypes with anxious or depressed mood are the most frequently diagnosed in adult clients (Popkin, 1989).

Nurses need to assess for precipitating stressors that preceded the onset of symptoms of adjustment disorder. Assessment of behavioral symptoms and mood and affect congruity are key to initial nursing assessment. Symptoms depend on the type of adjustment disorder and might include the following:

- *Sensory-perceptual:* Nervousness, worry, and jitteriness; other symptoms congruent with feeling anxious and/or depressed, such as headache, backache, or lethargy
- *Thought disturbances:* Preoccupation with thoughts of death (not suicidal thoughts), inability to attend to tasks, decreased concentration, inattention to external environment, inability to attend to detail, inability to concentrate, and short attention span leading to learning impairment; feelings of ambivalence and inability to make decisions; denial of physical illness and noncompliance with treatment recommendations
- *Feeling disturbances:* Feelings of sadness and sorrow, feelings of emptiness and worthlessness, decreased self-esteem, inability to articulate feelings, excessive worry about life events
- *Behavioral and relating disturbances:* Lack of interest in external events, disruption in relationships, social withdrawal, loss of interest in hobbies, withdrawal from work or academic endeavors, spiritual distress, increased or decreased psychomotor activity, hyperverbal patterns, difficulty continuing conversations, becoming easily distracted, insomnia, violation of age-appropriate norms or rules, violation of rights of others

NURSING DIAGNOSIS

In adjustment disorders, nursing diagnoses are prioritized based on symptoms. Data gathered in the assessment phase of the nursing process provide information about the client's history, symptoms, and (especially in the case of adjustment disorder) behavior and responses to life stressors. The collaborative and multidisciplinary effort in adjustment disorders is appropriately directed toward helping the client rally resources to achieve a functional level of daily living.

NURSING DIAGNOSES FOR ADJUSTMENT DISORDERS

Adjustment, impaired
Anxiety
Coping, ineffective individual
Grieving, dysfunctional
Self-esteem disturbance

NURSING ASSESSMENT QUESTIONS

Adjustment Disorders

1. What has happened in your life in the recent past? (To determine if the client can identify a stressor or stressors preceding an adjustment disorder)
2. In the overall picture of your life, how did that event affect you? (To determine the meaning of the event to the person)
3. What have you done in the past when such events occurred? (To determine whether the client has adequate coping skills and potential resources)
4. Tell me about your family and friends and their roles in this event. (To determine current support networks and obtain information about family/significant others)

Social interaction, impaired
Spiritual distress (distress of the human spirit)
Violence, risk for: directed at others
Violence, risk for: self-directed

OUTCOME IDENTIFICATION

Based on symptoms related to the specific adjustment disorder, outcome criteria may vary. However, regardless of the symptoms, client safety is a prime concern. Client outcomes, which are derived from nursing diagnoses, are the expected and anticipated client behaviors or responses to be achieved.

Client will:

1. Discuss plans for goal achievement.
2. Analyze coping resources and plans for using resources.
3. Describe stressors and effective ways of managing stressful situations in the past.
4. Evaluate any planned life changes in advance for potential sources of distress.

PLANNING

Data from nursing assessment and collaboration with the health care team provide direction for treatment of clients with adjustment disorder. Because clients have different needs, depending on the symptoms of adjustment disorder, nursing care will be (as always) individualized. Symptoms of adjustment disorder are presumed to be short term, so continuing care may be planned once the client is discharged from an inpatient unit. Continuing care is appropriate if the client's symptoms are active at the time of discharge and provide the opportunity to monitor the client's progress after discharge. The nurse must be alert to detect differences in symptoms or their intensity while caring for the client. For example, a client with adjustment disorder with depressed mood may begin to express thoughts of suicide.

IMPLEMENTATION

For the client diagnosed with an adjustment disorder, nursing interventions will be individualized, depending on the symptoms the client exhibits. Any plan of care should include ongoing assessment of symptoms.

COLLABORATIVE DIAGNOSES

DSM-IV Diagnoses*	NANDA Diagnoses†
Adjustment disorder with anxious mood	Anxiety
	Coping, ineffective individual
	Sleep pattern disturbance
Adjustment disorder with depressed mood	Coping, ineffective individual
	Denial, ineffective
	Social isolation
	Spiritual distress (distress of the human spirit)
Adjustment disorder with disturbance of conduct	Adjustment, impaired
	Anxiety
	Coping, defensive
	Coping, ineffective individual
	Role performance, altered
Adjustment disorder with mixed disturbance of emotions and conduct	Adjustment, impaired
	Anxiety
	Coping, defensive
	Coping, ineffective individual
	Denial, ineffective
	Sleep pattern disturbance
	Social isolation
	Spiritual distress (distress of the human spirit)
	Violence, risk for: directed at others
	Violence, risk for: self-directed

*From American Psychiatric Association: *Diagnostic and statistical manual of mental disorders*, ed 4, Washington, DC, 1994, The Association.
†From North American Nursing Diagnosis Association: *NANDA nursing diagnoses: definitions and classifications, 1999-2000*, Philadelphia, 1999, The Association.

▲ NURSING CARE PLAN

Mr. Y., a 57-year-old client in a general medical unit, is well known to the nursing staff. He has been hospitalized many times during the past few years for stabilization of diabetes mellitus, which is difficult to control. During his most recent admission, his involvement with plans for his care has not been typical, because his interest is minimal. Also, he has eaten foods high in sugar content that belong to his roommate. He denies this behavior, is difficult to engage in client education, and is increasingly withdrawn. He says he does his blood glucose testing at home and administers his insulin appropriately.

Mr. Y. has recently retired from his job at a manufacturing plant because of his diabetes, and his retirement benefits are adequate to support his lifestyle. When asked if he feels sad or depressed about his retirement, he denies it in an angry tone of voice. His wife of 10 years died about 8 months ago. He says he has grieved for his wife, acknowledges feeling less sad about her death, and states that he is more at peace with his situation as time goes by. He is able to talk about the good times they had together. At the same time, he acknowledges disappointment at spending his retirement alone and says he feels depressed that his retirement is not as he hoped it would be.

He denies suicidal ideation. Visiting friends told the nurses that he has been reluctant to attend social activities. They say he has told them that he prefers to spend his time alone and just does not feel like being with people. Mr. Y.'s inpatient nurse knows that he will be discharged soon and initiates home health follow-up.

DSM-IV Diagnoses

Axis I	Adjustment disorder with depressed mood
Axis II	None
Axis III	Diabetes mellitus
Axis IV	Extreme = 4 (diabetes, death of spouse)
Axis V	GAF = 60 (current)
	GAF = 80 (past year)

Nursing Diagnosis: Violence, risk for: self-directed. Risk factors: chronic illness, feeling depressed about his retirement, change in marital status (multiple losses).

Client Outcomes	Nursing Intervention	Evaluation
• Mr. Y. will not harm self while in hospital.	• Observe Mr. Y.'s behavior frequently during routine client care. *Close observation is necessary to protect the client from self-harm.*	• Mr. Y. remained safe, unharmed.
• Mr. Y. will refrain from verbal suicidal threats or behavioral gestures.	• Listen closely for suicidal statements and observe nonverbal indications of suicidal intent, such as giving away possessions. *Such behaviors are critical clues regarding risk for self-harm. Clues regarding potential behavior are verbal and nonverbal.*	• Absence of verbalized or behavioral indications of suicidal intent by Mr. Y.
• Mr. Y. will deny any plans for suicide.	• Ask direct questions to determine suicidal intent, plans for suicide, and means to commit suicide. *Suicide risk increases if plans and means exist.*	• Mr. Y. denied active suicidal plan.
• Mr. Y. will agree to terms of a no-harm contract and will seek staff when feeling suicidal.	• Obtain verbal or written agreement from Mr. Y. not to harm self and to seek staff if suicidal feelings and impulses emerge *to confirm that help is available if the client loses control.*	• Mr. Y. agreed to terms of contract, and sought staff to help maintain control.

Nursing Diagnosis: Coping, ineffective individual, related to response to situational crisis (retirement), as evidenced by isolative behavior, changes in mood, and decreased sense of well-being.

Client Outcomes	Nursing Interventions	Evaluation
• Mr. Y. will identify positive coping strategies, such as structuring leisure time.	• Develop trusting relationship with Mr. Y. *to demonstrate caring and encourage Mr. Y to practice new coping skills in a safe therapeutic setting.*	• Mr. Y. voiced trust in nurse-client relationship.
• Mr. Y. will combine past effective coping methods with newly acquired coping strategies.	• Praise Mr. Y. for adaptive coping. *Positive feedback encourages repetition of effective coping by Mr. Y.*	• Mr. Y. discussed plans for use of past and newly learned coping methods.

NURSING CARE PLAN —cont'd

Client Outcomes	Nursing Interventions	Evaluation
• Mr. Y. will cope adaptively by putting anger into words versus actions.	• Assist Mr. Y. in expressing anger and exploring angry feelings. *Verbalization of feelings in a non-threatening relationship may help the client resolve conflicts and provide opportunity to vent feelings.*	• Mr. Y. verbalized feelings of anger and loneliness appropriately.
• Mr. Y. will verbalize understanding of loss as a process that needs to be worked through over time.	• Determine the stage of loss. *Interventions vary with the stage of the loss process. Identification of the stage is necessary for effective interventions.* • Explain to Mr. Y. the feelings and behaviors associated with each stage of loss *to help Mr. Y. understand that feelings such as anger are appropriate and acceptable to resolve loss at this stage.*	• Mr. Y. verbalized knowledge that loss is a natural process and will resolve in time. • Mr. Y. verbalized his understanding of loss stages and identified his own loss process.

Nursing Diagnosis: Social interaction, impaired, related to alteration in role (Mr. Y. is now retired), as evidenced by disruption in usual social activities and isolating behaviors.

Client Outcomes	Nursing Intervention	Evaluation
• Mr. Y. will increase socialization and involvement in activities according to capabilities. • Mr. Y will effectively use social support systems inside and outside the hospital.	• Review Mr. Y.'s resources and identify positive activities that he enjoys and can resume *to encourage Mr. Y. to focus on positive aspects of himself and his situation.* • Explore Mr. Y.'s social support system and his desire to seek help. Identify role changes now that he lives alone. *Opportunity to discuss socialization and preferences for activities helps Mr. Y. identify his own socialization patterns and demonstrates therapeutic alliance.*	• Mr. Y. spent more time socializing with client peers than being alone • Mr. Y socialized with select client peers and identified aftercare social network and activities.

NURSING INTERVENTIONS

1. Assess any risk of suicidal ideation, gesture, or plan *to provide for the client's safety and prevent violence to self.*
2. Help the client identify coping strategies *to encourage use of internal resources.*
3. Support activities that increase socialization *to decrease isolation and foster growth of social support networks.*
4. Help the client name thoughts, feelings, and concerns *to help the client identify patterns of thought and provide opportunities for validation of feeling, reflection, and problem solving.*
5. Teach the client, family, and significant others about the disorder including symptom management *to provide control and reduce fear and anxiety* (see Client & Family Teaching Guidelines box).
6. Engage client in a therapeutic alliance *to encourage discussion of thoughts and feelings, particularly noting any suicidal ideation or increase in symptoms of depression.*
7. Support client's progress toward goals *to foster self-esteem and encourage repetition of positive behaviors.*

Client & Family TEACHING GUIDELINES

Teach the client, family, and/or significant other:
1. To identify the symptoms of adjustment disorders and that:
   Symptoms usually resolve completely.
   Symptoms can be managed using a variety of techniques (e.g., relaxation exercises can be taught to mitigate anxiety).
   Symptoms should be reported to their care provider.
   Thoughts of self-harm or suicide need to be reported immediately to their care provider.
   Their response to a life event is normal because individual people have unique responses to life events.
   They have dealt with difficult life situations in the past using particular coping methods. Reinforce prior successes.
2. Dosage, frequency, and effects of medication. Include information about common side effects of medication and when to call the physician with questions or concerns regarding medication management.

8. Collaborate with multidisciplinary treatment team *to promote consistency in implementing the treatment plan. Consistency provides structure and communicates involvement of the entire team in the treatment of the client; expectations of the client are agreed on and articulated.*

9. Help the client identify symptoms of anxiety and predisposing situational stressors *to promote problem solving and increased feelings of control.*

10. Help the client recall prior instances of success *to foster self-esteem, support creative problem solving, and instill hope for the future.*

ADDITIONAL TREATMENT MODALITIES

The nurse is an integral part of the multidisciplinary team that identifies key (or target) symptoms or behaviors, designs interventions to address key symptoms, and decides on evaluative methods to measure client movement toward or away from desired outcomes. Before the team meeting, representatives from each discipline should complete their own assessment activities and bring pertinent information to the planning session. In this way, primary functions of the individual disciplines within the team are identified, clarified, and maximized toward resolving the client's problems. Because each discipline has a unique perspective on the treatment issues of each client and focuses collective energy on resolving problems, the resulting team plan is greater than the sum of its parts. For example, the nonverbal client may respond to therapies designed by occupational or art therapists while being relatively nonresponsive to verbal interventional techniques.

Medications

Medications are used sparingly for clients with adjustment disorders because the disorders are expected to resolve after their immediate causes are identified and processed. Also, because symptoms of adjustment disorder may in some cases progress to include symptoms of major mental disorders, psychiatric mental health nurses may prefer to observe the client without the effects of medication. Benzodiazepines are often prescribed for brief periods of time to treat symptoms of anxiety. Antidepressants may be prescribed if symptoms are problematic and interfere with the client's ability to mobilize resources.

Adjunctive Therapies

Collaborative approaches to client care frequently include the use of adjunctive therapies. For example, recreational therapies may be used with the client diagnosed with an adjustment disorder. Discovering the client's preference in leisure activities and providing appropriate resource materials may help the client become more comfortable socially and inspire him or her to become self-directed in pursuing recreational activities. If the client is able to exercise, physical exercise and/or movement can be a constructive outlet for tension and anxiety while enhancing self-esteem.

Supportive Therapies

Clinical nurse specialists, physicians, social workers, and psychologists are prepared to provide therapeutic support for clients diagnosed with an adjustment disorder. Since clients with adjustment disorders are typically treated on an outpatient basis, they have a variety of treatment options and referral sources. Depending on professional preference, assessment of the client's problems, and identification of desired outcomes, therapists may employ a variety of interventional methods. Cognitive behavior therapy, interpersonal or psychodynamic psychotherapy, and brief strategic therapeutic techniques may all be effectively used. Family therapy may be indicated when the stressor triggering the adjustment disorder occurs within a family system and the client and family require assistance in resolving the problem. Other therapeutic intervention techniques include biofeedback, relaxation exercises, hypnosis, meditation, journaling, and visual imaging activities.

EVALUATION

Evaluation of outcomes for adjustment disorders depends on the original features of the particular disorder. For the client with depressed or anxious mood, the absence of original problematic symptoms signifies resolution. For most clients, resolution of symptoms signifies a successful outcome to the treatment.

If the client is hospitalized, the nurse is expected to evaluate the client's plan of care and response to interventions at least once every 24 hours. Thoughtful discharge planning with attention to follow-up home health care or a visit to the primary physician's office can allay potential problems once the client is discharged. If the client is not completely free of symptoms before discharge, the treatment team should examine options for placement following the need for acute hospitalization.

PROGNOSIS

Data are not currently available related to specific prognoses for adjustment disorders. Most practitioners believe that because the diagnosis of adjustment disorder ordinarily precludes a major psychiatric problem, there is hope that the client can resolve problems by developing coping methods and mobilizing resources.

DISCHARGE CRITERIA

Client will:

Verbalize absence of thoughts of self-harm.

Identify goals for continuing care after discharge, if indicated.

Identify and analyze coping resources and plans for using resources.

Summary of Key Concepts

1. Adjustment disorders are transient episodes of clinically significant emotional or behavioral nonpsychotic symptoms in response to identifiable psychosocial stress or stressors. Symptoms develop within 3 months after the stressful event.

2. The diagnosis of adjustment disorder is considered if the client's behaviors or symptoms are different from usual patterns of response and if the symptoms have persisted for less than 6 months (acute), unless symptoms are in response to an ongoing stressor or stressors (chronic).

3. The severity of the reaction to the stressor is not predictable from the stressor and is unique to the individual.

4. In an adult population, the most commonly diagnosed adjustment disorders are adjustment disorder with depressed mood and adjustment disorder with anxious mood.

5. Clients with adjustment disorder are often treated as outpatients because the severity of their symptoms or subjective distress does not warrant inpatient hospitalization.

6. Supportive psychotherapy is the most frequently used treatment modality with clients with adjustment disorders.

7. Clients diagnosed with adjustment disorder may experience a resolution of symptoms or an exacerbation and increase of symptoms, supporting the diagnosis of a major psychiatric disorder such as major depression.

8. Research is needed to establish the frequency and incidence of adjustment disorders and to measure outcomes of specific therapeutic interventions.

9. Attempting to understand the client's experience from his or her point of view fosters the therapeutic process. Application of clinical models are of little value unless anticipated outcomes of care are meaningful to the client.

10. Clients know more than anyone else about their lives and must be considered the resident experts in determining the meaning of life events, mobilizing inner strengths, and determining preferences for care.

REFERENCES

American Nurses Association: *Statement on psychiatric-mental health clinical nursing practice and standards of psychiatric-mental health clinical nursing practice*, Washington, DC, 1994, American Nurses Publishing.

American Psychiatric Association: *Diagnostic and statistical manual of mental disorders*, ed 2, Washington, DC, 1968, The Association.

American Psychiatric Association: *Diagnostic and statistical manual of mental disorders*, ed 3, Washington, DC, 1980, The Association.

American Psychiatric Association: *Diagnostic and statistical manual of mental disorders*, ed 3 revised, Washington, DC, 1987, The Association.

American Psychiatric Association: *Diagnostic and statistical manual of mental disorders*, ed 4, Washington, DC, 1994, The Association.

Armstrong M: *Being pregnant and using drugs: a retrospective phenomenological inquiry*. Unpublished doctoral dissertation. San Diego, Calif., 1992, University of San Diego.

Beck C: The lived experience of postpartum depression: a phenomenological study, *Nurs Research* 41(3):166, 1992.

Bergum V: *Woman to mother: a transformation*, Boston, 1989, Bergin & Garvey.

Blier R: *Science and gender*, New York, 1986, Pergamon Press.

Colarusso C, Nemiroff R: *Adult development: a new dimension in psychodynamic theory and practice*, New York, 1981, Plenum Press.

Colarusso C, Nemiroff R: Clinical implications of adult development, *Am J Psychiatry* 144(10):1263, 1987.

Coward D: The lived experience of self-trancendence in women with advanced breast cancer, *Nurs Sci Q* 3(4):162, 1990.

Davis F: Deviance disavowal: the management of strained interaction by the visibly handicapped. In Davis F, editor: *Illness, interaction and the self*, Belmont, Calif, 1972, Wadsworth.

Erikson EH: *Childhood and society*, ed 2, New York, 1963, WW Norton.

Gilligan C: *In a different voice: psychological theory and women's development*, Cambridge, Mass., 1982, Harvard University Press.

Greenberg W, Rosenfeld D, Ortega E: Adjustment disorder as an admission diagnosis, *Am J Psychiatry* 152(3):459, 1995.

Heifner C: Positive connectedness in the psychiatric nurse-patient relationship, *Arch Psychiatr Nurs* 7(1):11, 1993.

Jordan J et al: *Women's growth in connection: writings from the stone center*, New York, 1991, Guilford Press.

Kirk S, Kutchins H: *The selling of DSM: the rhetoric of science in psychiatry*, New York, 1992, Aldine de Gruyter.

Kovacs M et al: A controlled prospective study of DSM-III adjustment disorder in childhood: short-term prognosis and long-term predictive validity, *Arch Gen Psychiatry* 51(4):535, 1994.

Kubler-Ross E: *On death and dying*, New York, 1969, Macmillan.

Lerner H: *Women in therapy*, Northvale, NJ, 1988, Jason Aronson Press.

Levine S: *Healing into life and death,* New York, 1987, Doubleday.

Lewis H: Is Freud an enemy of women's liberation? Some historical considerations. In Bernay T, Cantor D, editors: *The psychology of today's woman: new psychoanalytic visions,* Cambridge, Mass, 1986, Harvard University Press.

Lowenberg J: *Caring and responsibility: the crossroads between holistic practice and traditional medicine,* Pittsburgh, 1989, University of Pennsylvania Press.

Main M et al: Information sharing concerning schizophrenia in a family member: adult siblings' perspectives, *Arch Psychiatr Nurs* 7(3):147, 1993.

Meth R, Pasick R: *Men in therapy: the challenge of change,* New York, 1990, Guilford Press.

Mickley J et al: Spiritual well-being, religiousness and hope among women with breast cancer, *Image J Nurs Sch* 24(4):267, 1992.

Murphy S: Coping strategies of abstainers from alcohol up to three years post-treatment, *Image J Nurs Sch* 25(1):29, 1993.

Napier A: Heroism, men, and marriage, *J Marital Fam Ther* 17(1):9, 1991.

Nemiroff R, Colarusso C: *Psychotherapy and psychoanalysis in the second half of life,* New York, 1985, Plenum Press.

North American Nursing Diagnosis Association: *NANDA nursing diagnoses: definitions and classifications, 1999-2000,* Philadelphia, 1999, The Association.

Parsons T: *The social system,* New York, 1951, The Free Press.

Pittman F: The secret passions of men, *J Marital Fam Ther* 17(1):17, 1991.

Popkin M: Adjustment disorder and impulse control. In Kaplan H, Saddock B, editors: *Comprehensive textbook of psychiatry/V,* Baltimore, 1989, Williams & Wilkins.

Popkin M: Adjustment disorders in medically ill inpatients referred for consultation in a university hospital, *Psychosomatics* 31(4):410, 1990.

Razavi D et al: Screening for adjustment disorders and major depressive disorders in cancer inpatients, *Br J Psychiatry* 156:79, 1990.

Ruckdeschel H: *Psychotherapy for the old old: ten patients' report on their treatment for depression.* Unpublished doctoral dissertation, 1993, University of Pennsylvania.

Selye H: *Stress without distress,* New York, 1956, New American Library.

Selye H: *The stress of life,* New York, 1978, McGraw-Hill.

Snyder S, Strain J, Wolf D: Differentiating major depression from adjustment disorder with depressed mood in the medical setting, *Gen Hosp Psychiatry* 12:159, 1990.

Spector R: *Cultural diversity in health and illness,* ed 3, Norwalk, Conn, 1991, Appleton & Lange.

Tanner C et al: The phenomenology of knowing the patient, *Image J Nurs Sch* 25(4):273, 1993.

Walsh F, McGoldrick M: *Living beyond loss,* New York, 1991, WW Norton.

PART • FIVE

Therapeutic Modalities

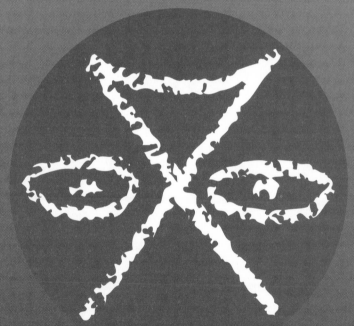

Safe Camp
Hobo

Communication symbols are used by modern "knights of the road," the hobos, and by the homeless. This "safe camp" symbol portrays relief from worldly stressors for individuals in crisis and in need of respite. The chapters in Part Five discuss the various modalities of treatment used to relieve stressors and treat mental disorders.

505

CHAPTER 22

Interactive Therapies and Methods of Implementation

Mary Magenheimer Webster

OBJECTIVES

- Compare the concepts of boundary, safety, and trust development as they relate to individual, milieu, family, and group therapy.

- Discuss the processes that support the various phases of therapy.

- Identify personal characteristics and attitudes that affect one's ability to function as a psychiatric mental health nurse.

- Describe the appropriate tasks for individual, milieu, family, and group therapy and discuss ways in which the nurse promotes these tasks.

- Explain transference and countertransference and their impact on the therapeutic relationship.

Interactive therapy implies one's therapeutic interaction with an individual, a family, or a group. This is not a new concept for nurses. Much of nursing's work involves interacting with the client to promote healing. The nurse changes a dressing on one client to assist wound healing or provides antibiotics to help another client fight an infection. The nurse also manages the many types of equipment required for the client's treatments. All this can be viewed as one individual providing treatment (or therapy) for another. This work, however, reveals the nurse doing something very visible for the client. Nurses use their hands and actively do something that the client can see. Much of the nurse's speech is used for teaching, assessing the client's status, or exchanging pleasantries.

In contrast, much of the work of psychiatric mental health nursing is initially "invisible." Beginning students often complain that there is "nothing to do" in a psychiatric setting, since hands-on treatments are few. Some individuals become confused and frustrated with their roles as psychiatric mental health nurses, or with the delivery of psychiatric mental health nursing care.

The beauty, as well as the challenge, of psychiatric mental health nursing is that the nurse uses the self as the therapeutic agent. The nurse's words and interactions are designed to help the client heal psychically and emotionally. Just as it took time and experience to learn to change dressings, give medications, and manage equipment, it also takes time to use oneself and one's words as healers.

Nurses can be therapeutically interactive without being licensed psychotherapists. A psychotherapist is generally an advanced clinical practitioner with specialized credentials in the area of psychotherapy.

It is essential to examine assumptions regarding the nurse-client relationship in psychiatric mental health

Attending Paying attention to what a client is saying by using words and behaviors that illustrate that the nurse is listening.

Boundary The definition and separation of the self from others through the clarification of limits and extent of responsibilities and duties of oneself in relationship to others.

Countertransference Feelings the nurse has toward the client as a natural part of the therapeutic relationship. The nurse needs to be aware of countertransference and manage it.

Identified client In family therapy the member of the family (or group) whose behavior is seen as causing the problem for the family (or group).

Norms The standards of behavior, attitudes, and, at times, perceptions that a group has for its members; norms represent the shared expectations of appropriateness in behavior.

Roles The socially expected behavior patterns usually determined by an individual's status in a particular group. Peplau (1952) identified four roles for the psychiatric mental health nurse: (1) resource person, (2) counselor, (3) surrogate, and (4) technical expert.

Safety The sense of security developed within the therapeutic relationship when the responsibilities and expectations of each party are clearly defined. Safety develops from knowing the boundaries of a relationship and acting within them.

Themes The recurring patterns of interactions the client experiences in relationships with self and/or others.

Therapeutic milieu
An environment designed to promote emotional health that is based on the assumption that clients are active participants in their own lives and therefore need to be involved in the management of their behavior and environment.

Therapeutic relationship
A personal relationship that is established to help one of the participants deal more effectively and maturely with some difficulty in life. It is a goal-directed, client-centered, and objective relationship.

Transference Feelings the client has toward the therapist and the helping relationship, which truly belong to significant people in the client's life and are transferred to the therapeutic relationship. The nurse needs to be aware of transference and manage it.

Trust The reliance on the truthfulness or accuracy of the therapeutic relationship developed through a congruency between the therapist's words and actions.

nursing. This chapter discusses the role of the nurse with clients in a therapeutic psychiatric environment.

THE THERAPEUTIC RELATIONSHIP

The goal of nursing has always been to promote health. Mental health is defined as the "forward movement of personality and other ongoing human processes in the direction of creative, constructive, productive, personal, and community living" (Peplau, 1952). The psychiatric mental health nurse needs to recognize that every interaction has the potential to promote the health of the client. Psychiatric mental health nurses have an obligation to use their skills within a therapeutic relationship to promote and maintain health.

SOCIAL VERSUS THERAPEUTIC RELATIONSHIPS

The therapeutic relationship is unique in the world of human interactions. It stands apart from other types of relationships in its focus, purpose, and enactment. Beginning practitioners frequently act in ways that are associated more with a social relationship than with a therapeutic one. A social relationship is with friends and acquaintances and exists for the mutual satisfaction of those involved. Its duration, focus, and intensity vary according to the participant's wishes; it is a subjective relationship.

In contrast to the social relationship, the **therapeutic relationship** exists to help one of the participants, the client, deal more effectively and maturely with some difficulty. It is viewed as a personal relationship where "two people come to know each other well enough to face the problem at hand in a cooperative way" (Peplau, 1952). The nursing functions in a therapeutic relationship are (1) to assist the client in identifying emotionally felt difficulties and (2) to apply knowledge of the principles of human relations to the problems or issues that arise at all levels of experiences (Peplau, 1952). This requires nurses to understand themselves and their behavior well enough to be objective and capable of focusing on their clients' needs; this is discussed further in the section on self-development.

ROLES IN THE THERAPEUTIC RELATIONSHIP

Roles are the socially expected behavior patterns determined by an individual's position or status in a particular group or relationship. The psychiatric mental health nurse enacts several educational and therapeutic roles during various phases of the therapeutic relationship. Peplau (1952) has identified four roles: (1) *resource person*, who gives specific information to clients, thus allowing them to understand situations or procedures; (2) *counselor*, who listens to the client's experience and assists in clarifying feelings associated with it; (3) *surrogate*, whom the client casts into roles of past relationships (parent, sibling, spouse, teacher), perhaps needing clarification of feelings; and (4) *technical expert*, who can navigate the complexities of the health care system.

ASPECTS OF THE THERAPEUTIC RELATIONSHIP

The therapeutic relationship is goal-directed, client-centered, and objective (Fortinash and Holoday-Worret, 1999) and involves transference and countertransference.

Goal direction in a relationship implies a purpose for the relationship's existence. The overall goal of any therapeutic relationship is to help the client move toward health by becoming more self-responsible (Kennedy, 1977). Each individual is unique, however, and specific goals need to be defined for each person. Most people desire the relief of uncomfortable symptoms (i.e., anxiety, depression, suicidal thoughts, outbursts of anger, feelings of unworthiness). The therapeutic relationship is initiated to help the individual deal with offending symptoms in a way that is more conducive to health. It is a highly focused relationship, with both participants agreeing to direct their energies toward achieving the identified goal. This also implies that the relationship has limits: it exists to meet certain defined goals, not to meet all of the client's needs. This concept of boundaries is discussed in a later section of this chapter.

Client-centered implies that the relationship is focused on the client; it is the client's goals, reactions, coping strategies, and growth that are at the center of the relationship. The therapeutic relationship requires that nurses turn their attention to another for a while and suspend their preoccupations with events in their own lives, in order to experience a client's sense of being (Kennedy, 1977). This does not mean that the nurse's reactions and sense of self are not important; it means that they are not the focus of the relationship. The nurse's sense of self and reactions to the client are crucial to the work of a psychiatric mental health nurse. By paying attention to one's own reactions and being able to sort them out, the nurse will gain knowledge of the client's interpersonal dynamics. This is some of the most difficult work in psychiatric mental health nursing: to recognize one's own reactions and to use this information in a way that will assist the client in growing toward emotional health.

Objectivity is required on the part of the nurse. Objectivity implies an analytic approach to the subjective experience (i.e., it requires nurses to be aware of their feelings and reactions to being with clients rather than to just responding to clients on a personal level). For example, perhaps a client is acting in a way that makes the nurse increasingly angry. It would not benefit anyone if the nurse snapped back at the client in anger, because this would simply mirror similar experiences the client has had with others in the past; it would not bring the client any closer to the goal of more healthful interactions. Instead, nurses should deal with their own reactions in a way that allows them to be useful therapeutically.

Transference refers to the feelings the client has toward the nurse and the helping relationship. These feelings actually belong to the significant people in the client's life before the therapeutic relationship with the nurse, and they are transferred and replayed in the therapeutic relationship. Nurses must avoid responding as if the client's feelings are directed at them personally; such feelings are evoked by what the nurse represents to the client. This is the surrogate role described by Peplau. For instance, clients who behave in ways that make the nurse angry in the previous example may be responding to the nurse as they would to an overintrusive parent figure. Perhaps the only way the client can attain any separateness is to push the "parent" away with anger. Thus nurses who behave as if the feelings are actually directed toward them personalize the situation and miss an opportunity to be therapeutic. By responding more objectively, nurses can help clients begin to recognize a pattern. Instead of responding in anger, nurses can make open-ended comments, opening the door for clients to explore their feelings. By being objective, the nurse allows the client to take a step beyond the act itself and begin to talk objectively about it rather than continually responding in the same way.

Countertransference is defined as the feelings the nurse has toward the client. These feelings may be positive or negative and are a natural part of a therapeutic relationship. Problems arise only when the feeling is discounted because it upsets, surprises, or embarrasses the nurse in some way. Nurses need to recognize, identify, and accept these feelings; otherwise these feelings will influence their responses to clients, whether or not this is apparent (Kennedy, 1977). For example, nurses who are attracted to, or feel contempt for, their clients may be horrified about having these feelings, knowing that the relationship is a professional one. Nurses may respond by keeping their distance from clients and treating them superficially to distance themselves from their feelings. Thus no work is accomplished in the therapeutic relationship because it is dominated by the nurse's personal concerns. The success of the relationship depends on the nurse's ability to manage transference and countertransference.

PERSONAL QUALITIES OF EFFECTIVE HELPERS

There is growing recognition that the personal qualities of effective helpers are as important in promoting growth in others as the methods they use (Brammer, 1993). Effective helpers express a positive view of people's ability to solve their own problems and manage their own lives. Also, they tend to view people as dependable, friendly, and worthy. Effective helpers tend to identify with people rather than things, demonstrate a capacity to cope, and are willing to reveal their thoughts (to the extent that it is therapeutic) rather than conceal them (Brammer, 1993). Helpers care for themselves and others. A helper must balance a sense of strength and maturity with the humility and vulnerability that come from experiencing life's problems. It is this vulnerability that assists in the building of trust (Brammer, 1993).

PREPARATION FOR INTERACTIVE THERAPY
SELF-AWARENESS

It is clear from the preceding discussion that the psychiatric mental health nurse needs a strong sense of self or at least the willingness to develop one. The term *sense of self* refers to self-awareness or self-knowledge. This is necessary because nurses must be able to separate their own subjective beliefs from the facts. Self-awareness implies a recognition of one's thinking, values, conflicts, interaction styles and attitudes, and an awareness of how these can influence interactions with clients. The nurse need not be perfect—obviously such a goal cannot be achieved even over a lifetime. It is necessary, however, that the nurse be committed and open to self-exploration.

There are many ways for the nurse to do this work. Many schools of therapy require therapists to undergo ongoing personal therapy. This assists developing therapists with resolving issues/conflicts in their own lives and also makes them sensitive to what their clients are experiencing. Other avenues for self-exploration are support groups, values clarification work, role-playing, and individual supervision. The staff at one state hospital participated in a simulation game in which they shared the common experience of temporarily being inpatients as a way to influence their attitudes toward those with mental illness (Cosgray et al, 1990). After the simulation experience, postgame discussion reflected recurring feelings among the staff of powerlessness/helplessness and anger/hostility. The staff "reached consensus about the need to treat patients with respect and dignity" (Cosgray et al, 1990).

Self-reflection is an appropriate first step. Nurses can assess their values, attitudes, and orientation by asking themselves some general questions. Again, the point of this is not to conform to any preconceived therapist role. This self-assessment will increase the nurse's self-awareness and help develop more effective therapeutic interactive skills.

AREAS FOR SELF-ASSESSMENT
Need to Be Liked

It is important to assess the need to be liked, accepted, and valued, which can paralyze the nurse in interactions. For example, the nurse is at risk for becoming hurt or angry if the client acts in an angry or hostile manner. Or the nurse may hesitate to comment, for fear that the client would be offended in some way and consequently think less of the nurse. With time and experience the nurse learns that the key to an effective approach is simply to be comfortable with the other person. This arises out of a sincere effort to attend to the client's words and listen carefully to the experience. Rapport develops best when nurses focus on their clients and forget their own need to be liked (Kennedy, 1977).

Being Judgmental

Another area to evaluate is being judgmental. Judgments are the quick stereotyping of people to fit them into categories to ease one's own interactive experience. Forming judgments is also a survival skill that allows one to decide issues of emotional safety quickly. Often these judgments are based on a few life experiences and tend to be generalized in others. Thus someone who reminds the client in some way of a favorite aunt would tend to be judged favorably even before the client gets to know the person as an individual. Culture also influences the ways in which people are viewed. The portrayals of individuals or groups in the media, for instance, affect one's judgment of them. The end result of this is stereotyping, in which individuals lose a personal identity and are clumped into a collective group. Such judgments have no place in a therapeutic relationship that focuses on the individual. Judgments produce labels that only serve to distance people. Although it is unrealistic to expect anyone to rid themselves of their judgments completely, psychiatric nurses should at least be aware of their judgments and how they affect relationships. Nurses must be able to suspend judgments of clients so that they can focus on their clients' individuality and experiences and remain open to learning (Kennedy, 1977). "Nursing symbolizes the acceptance of people as they are and assistance in their times of stress" (Peplau, 1952).

Responsibility

Another critical area is assuming responsibility. It is necessary for psychiatric mental health nurses to clarify their own understanding of who is responsible for what in the therapeutic relationship. There are areas of nursing where the outcomes depend solely on nursing performance (e.g., the absence of sepsis around a surgical wound, the administration of medication, or the proper rate of fluid replacement via an intravenous infusion). All of these administrations involve the nurse *doing* something for the client. As noted before, many novices in psychiatric mental health nursing feel the need to *do* something visible. Consequently, they tend to ask too many questions rather than listen to clients and to give advice rather than assist clients with their own problem solving. Many nurses are impatient and want or expect to see rapid results rather than wait for the work of therapy to progress. When impatience is a problem, the nurse may take over by becoming overly bossy or judgmental, both of which are nontherapeutic and potentially destructive.

Thus it is important that psychiatric mental health nurses be clear about their responsibility to their clients. It is not up to the nurse to define the area, direction, or time frame of the client's growth, but rather to support the client's own work in the therapeutic process. "Real support arises from entering into the experience of other persons, being able to stand there with them as they explore themselves, and not in backing away when the experience threatens to become hard on us" (Kennedy, 1977).

Potential for Human Growth

The psychiatric mental health nurse needs to have some confidence in the client's ability to grow, learn, and make changes. Nurses need to assess their own assumptions about the potential for human growth. One way is to evaluate their own personal needs for sympathy and protection (Fortinash and Holoday-Worret, 1999). If nurses believe that they need to be protected from life experiences, they may also assume that they are not capable of coping with life stressors. Nurses who believe this about themselves may attribute the same qualities to their clients and then try to protect them from the work of psychologic growth rather than help them move through the challenges to achieve growth.

These areas of self-assessment are not meant to be a complete list. Psychiatric mental health nurses will find themselves examining their values and attitudes anew with each client. They will examine their assumptions about dependence, responsibility, competence, and intimacy (or closeness), to name a few. Self-examination (autodiagnosis) is an ongoing process because each phase of life and each situation is unique.

CONCERNS EXPERIENCED BY THE NURSE

It has been noted that student nurses generally have three concerns: self-consciousness about enacting the role, fears and fantasies about what constitutes professional behavior, and uncertainty about how to proceed technically with clients (Denton, 1987). Novice psychiatric mental health nurses generally demonstrate these anxieties by worrying about their choice of words. They often fear saying "the wrong thing" that may damage the client permanently. They may become awkward about using words and fret over finding the right word or correct way to speak. This heightened self-consciousness is often part of learning to use the self in a therapeutic manner.

This attention to words also extends to the nurse's perception of the client. Students tend to focus solely on the content (or words). By focusing on words only, nurses can miss the richness of the nonverbal information presented by the client and may neglect to follow up on a tone of voice or special look on the client's face.

Psychiatric mental health nursing is not only about words. It is about therapeutic relationships and focusing on another individual. When nurses are aware of the work occurring at each phase of the relationship, they can consciously use a variety of skills to promote the desired change in the client. When the focus is on the work, words can be used more fluidly as a tool. This does not diminish the use of language as an important tool. More experienced practitioners will use sentence structure and word choice as a way of analyzing the client's thought processes.

An important aspect in the development of trust and safety is the nurse's manner or behavior. Nurses must outwardly model or demonstrate their attention to the client. This counseling skill is called **attending** and includes all of

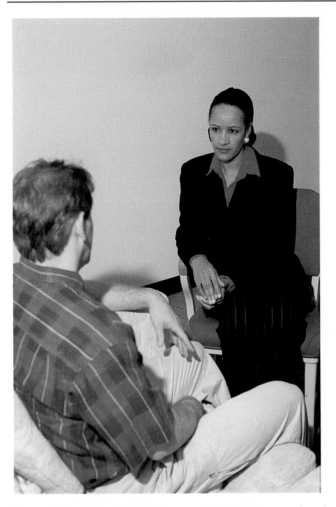

Figure 22-1 This therapist's nonverbal behaviors—relaxed posture, slight forward lean, and good eye contact—indicate openness, acceptance, and interest in the client. (Copyright 1995, Cathy Lander-Goldberg, Lander Photographics.)

the ways in which therapists demonstrate to clients that they are heard; clients are thus encouraged to express feelings and experiences.

The nurse shows this attention nonverbally and verbally. *Nonverbal behaviors* include a relaxed posture (indicating openness and acceptance) with a slightly forward lean (demonstrating interest) (Figure 22-1). The nurse maintains good eye contact, "seeing" the client. It is important not to simply stare or glare at the client, since this is an aggressive behavior, but rather to meet the client's eyes in a relaxed, comfortable manner, occasionally looking away. *Verbal behaviors* associated with attending demonstrate careful listening and include open-ended questions, paraphrasing, reflection of feelings, summarization, and allowing clients to set their own pace (see Chapter 8).

An effective way for nurses to demonstrate attending skills toward clients while earning their trust is for them to enact the qualities of genuineness, respect, and empathy. *Genuineness* has been defined as verbal and behavioral

congruence and authenticity. *Respect* is defined as unconditional positive regard and is noted to be conveyed through consistency and active listening. *Empathy* implies seeing the situation from the client's point of view, yet remaining objective. The empathic nurse can intervene to assist clients in their understanding of a situation and suggest appropriate avenues for change (Fortinash and Holoday-Worret, 1999).

DEVELOPMENT OF A THERAPEUTIC RELATIONSHIP

Establishing a therapeutic relationship is not magic; it requires hard work and the skillful application of knowledge. Beginners in interactive therapy are often so concerned with the content of the session that they overlook the basic concepts at work in every therapeutic relationship. These concepts are boundary development and maintenance, safety development, and trust development. The concepts apply to the individual therapeutic relationship, as well as the family and group processes, although they are expressed in different ways. These three concepts are tightly interwoven, each affecting the other.

BOUNDARY DEVELOPMENT AND MAINTENANCE

The term **boundary** refers to the definition of an entity. The boundaries of a country define its shape, size, and location in relationship to other countries. Each country negotiates for itself in various kinds of social interactions. Boundaries serve to separate and define entities at the point where the entity interacts with others.

In psychologic terms, boundaries refer to the definition and separation of the self from others. They serve to define the responsibilities and duties of one's self in relationship to others. This is an extremely important concept in working with psychiatric clients whose sense of self is often unclear in some way. Often, psychiatric clients do not have a sense of what constitutes their own responsibility and will ask nurses to do things that are not the nurse's responsibility. Consequently, nurses must have a clear sense of self and of their role to prevent collusion with clients in this way. For example, consider the following: A nurse and client have been engaged in an interaction, trying to identify the source of the client's agitation. They finally arrive at a point where the client identifies feeling angry with someone else about an earlier incident. To resolve this, the client suggests that the nurse discuss the incident with the other person so that the person becomes aware of the effect of his or her action. A nurse complying with this request would be in the middle of a confusing situation, that of conveying another person's emotional reaction (or speaking for another person). If, however, nurses in such a situation are aware of their role of furthering the client's sense of self (and its attendant responsibilities), they decline to shuttle information and instead assist the client in finding a way to accomplish this task.

Nurses may be concerned about use of touch when relating to clients. Boundaries can be maintained if touch is used therapeutically to demonstrate caring. An example is when the nurse gently places a hand on the client's forearm. It is best to use touch when trust has been established and when it is appropriate for the client and situation.

SAFETY DEVELOPMENT

Safety is the sense of security within the therapeutic relationship. Well-defined boundaries are essential to developing safety. Safety comes from knowing the expectations of the relationship and the responsibilities of the parties involved (nurse and client). By defining the structure of the therapeutic relationship, clients are safe to experiment within these boundaries while knowing that there are definable limits. All individuals need to feel safe when experimenting with new ways of being; this is especially true of psychiatric clients.

Consequently, part of the nurse's role in a therapeutic relationship is to enhance safety by acting consistently within the defined boundaries. It is confusing and dangerous for clients if a nurse introduces social elements into a therapeutic relationship in an attempt to be "friendly." Nurses should act within the boundaries of their role by assisting the client in focusing on the assigned task and exploring new options for growth, healing, and understanding.

TRUST DEVELOPMENT

Trust is the reliance on the truthfulness or accuracy of the relationship. As the nurse exercises the concepts of boundary and safety, trust develops within the nurse-client relationship. Congruence between words and actions is essential for trust to grow. If nurses consistently do what they say they will, the client is free to focus on the work and tasks of therapy. For many clients the relationship with the caregivers may be the most trusting one in their lives. As nurses continue to model their responsibilities in maintaining a trusting relationship, clients can begin to trust themselves and their reactions more. Trust is essential to the development of a sense of self.

Acting in a trustworthy manner does not imply that conflicts will not occur. Trust does not imply agreement, only consistency. If the client makes an inappropriate demand, the nurse is not expected to meet it to maintain trust. (In fact, trust could be damaged when a nurse meets a demand that is inappropriate for the relationship.) Trust does not develop from doing everything the client asks; trust develops from doing what one said one would do.

• • •

These three concepts of *boundary development and maintenance, safety development,* and *trust development* are the foundations of every therapeutic relationship. The nurse constantly works to develop these in each relationship; it is the "invisible work" of psychiatric nursing. Within these three concepts, the nurse works with the client in a goal-directed, objective, and client-centered way, using a variety of skills such as listening and reflecting.

PHASES OF THE THERAPEUTIC RELATIONSHIP
ORIENTATION PHASE

The *orientation phase* is the first phase of the therapeutic relationship. It occurs when clients enter the system and are experiencing the tension and anxiety associated with their own needs, as well as those generated by exposure to a new and uncertain situation. Successful orientation is essential in helping the client to combine these experiences (rather than split them away in some manner—repression or dissociation) so as to be able to participate fully in the therapeutic relationship (Peplau, 1952). Orientation serves to define and clarify the relationship: the formulation of the client's issue or conflict, the purpose or goal of the work, and the relationship between the client and the nurse. The major "invisible work" of the orientation phase is boundary formation. The nurse works to assist clients in clarifying their impression of the problem, thus defining the scope or boundary of the work. In addition, the nurse helps the client to function within the relationship, to have questions answered, needs expressed, and sincerity developed (Peplau, 1952), thus defining the scope or boundaries of the relationship itself.

Boundary development is done in specific ways. Nurses initially approach clients as strangers (Peplau, 1952) and must work to define themselves as allies and helpers. In introducing themselves to clients, nurses must state their purposes clearly. It is important that when speaking with new clients (strangers), nurses say whatever is appropriate for clients to hear, without using slang terms or incomplete remarks (Peplau, 1952). For example, if meeting a depressed client on an inpatient unit, the nurse could say, "Hello, I'm Mary Webster. I'm your nurse. I'll be working with you while you're here, to help you get used to the hospital and to look at the areas in your life that are troubling you." This introduction serves to identify the relationship as therapeutic and defines the nurse's role as a helping professional. Student psychiatric mental health nurses are frequently vague in their introductions to the client (Sayre, 1978). They may say, "I'd like to help you," or "You're interesting to me." Vague introductions do not work because they do not address the formation of the boundary. The purpose of the introduction is to begin to define the scope of the work and of the relationship.

The next step of the introduction builds on boundary development by defining when the work can be done. This may be as formal as a contract for a scheduled outpatient appointment or as simple as an agreement. The nurse on an inpatient unit might say, "Usually, I'll be able to meet with you individually for 20 minutes a day after lunch. Since we're just getting started, I'd like to spend more time with you now to get acquainted. Would that be all right with you?" This serves to further define the time boundaries. Now the nurse has defined the purpose of the relationship (i.e., orientation to the hospital and work on the troubling issues) and the time frame (i.e., "now" and "20 minutes a day"). The specifics will vary with different clients and in different settings; the words will vary with the nurse's personality. These variances are to be expected and encouraged. For instance, when first meeting a frightened, psychotic client, it is important to speak simply and briefly. The nurse could say, "My name is Mary. I'm your nurse. I will be here today to help keep you safe." This also defines the nurse's role and time frame. However it is done or said, each introduction must define the boundaries for the nurse's role, the scope of the work, and the time frame for doing the work.

Application to Short-Term Psychiatric Hospitalization

With the advent of managed care and concomitant payer systems, many inpatient settings may function as short-term assessment and crisis intervention units, with clients referred to other areas of care, such as day treatment centers, long-term care facilities, or the community. Staff need to accommodate the fluctuating changes in census by rotating assignments on a regular basis. Therefore the nurse may have only 1 to 3 days to work with the client and needs to incorporate the important work of boundary development, trust building, and safety development within that limited time frame. Box 22-1 describes some specific skills that may help the nurse fulfill these critical relationship components within the shorter time frame.

Work of the Orientation Phase

The work of the orientation phase is to help the client become a full participant in the therapeutic process by developing safety and trust. It has been noted that trust and security (or safety) are the first level of any interpersonal experience (Fortinash and Holoday-Worret, 1999). To do this, the nurse must follow through on the agreements made in the introduction. As Peplau (1952) has noted, "A relationship that is useful to the client is one in which what is expected of him is made clear and adhered to consistently, . . . one in which he is treated with understanding and respect as a person."

This is done in specific ways. The nurse demonstrates dependability by being punctual and willing to discuss with the client the length of meetings, location, confidentiality of information; roles of the nurse and the client; and other specifics such as the reason for the hospitalization, the source of the client's problem, or which alternative choices may help the client. (Fortinash and Holoday-Worret, 1999). The nurse's remarks should be simple and clear to orient the client to the situation. It is not a matter of specific words as much as the direction of the nurse's focus on the client that determines the effectiveness of the therapeutic relationship.

In addition, the nurse focuses on clients and their concerns to help them identify and formulate goals. Nurses should listen very carefully to what clients say about their own lives (the content) and observe how clients present this information (the process). Questions should be asked to further both the nurse's and the client's understanding of the client's experience. For example, a client may be describing the death of a parent and the subsequent breakup of the family (this is the content, i.e., *what* is said). Yet the client may relate all of this information in a matter-of-fact way (this is the process, *how* it is said). The nurse's response should be one that will broaden the client's knowledge of the experience. For example, the nurse could comment, "Please tell me more about what this was like for you." Or the nurse may simply reflect back an important key statement.* Rather than interpreting, nurses

---

Box 22-1   Nursing Skills to Establish a Therapeutic Relationship Within a Limited Time Frame

During the client's short-term hospitalization, the nurse will:

Make rounds on clients immediately after the shift report, and introduce self. Meet family/significant others as appropriate.

Explain the roles and responsibilities of the client, the nurse, and other disciplines as appropriate.

Discuss the time frame of the therapeutic relationship and client goals to be achieved within that time.

Help the client to prioritize achievable goals and list resources for long-term goals that may be met postdischarge.

Inform the client of his or her rights and of the expectations of the nurse and other caregivers.

Provide the client with a schedule of groups, activities, medications, and other treatments appropriate for the estimated length of stay and plan of care.

Educate the client/family/significant others about medications and other treatments and provide written literature approved by the treatment team to help the client meet discharge and aftercare needs.

Discuss discharge plans (with the client/family/significant others) in collaboration with the treatment team.

A key statement is one that is continually brought up by the client in conversation; one that the client stresses or emphasizes; or one that is not said or is deliberately omitted even though the topic is a known problem or conflict, given the client's history.

should encourage clients to recognize their own feelings (Peplau, 1952). These responses help clients to focus and expand their experiences. Questions are focused on clients' experiences and are open ended to allow clients to expand and clarify their thoughts.

Responses in Orientation

Very often, psychiatric clients have not been able to "tell their story." Families may develop their own version around specific issues, and the "family myth" is difficult to challenge. Friends may tire of the story or respond in a socially conventional way. As a result, clients have no one to tell their story to, and thus the story gets "stopped" at a certain point and is never allowed to reach a conclusion. Consequently, many of the emotions are also "blocked" and never worked through to resolution. The nurse's work in orientation is to help the client continue the story.

Although some clients are open to continuing their story, others do not welcome this opportunity or even know how to use it. There is a great deal of anxiety whenever one ventures beyond the known social conventions. When the client begins to challenge "the family myth" or the socially acceptable ways of dealing with aspects of the story, anxiety may be manifested in several ways. The client may test the nurse in some way, such as being late for meetings, ending them early, or questioning their usefulness. The client may focus on the nurse personally by questioning the nurse's competence, showing sexual interest, or attempting to shock the nurse through profanity, confrontation, or sharing bizarre experiences or behavior (Fortinash and Holoday-Worret, 1999).

The nurse needs to observe this behavior sensitively and objectively and consider it as both the client's interactive style and as a level of the client's anxiety. The nurse responds by focusing the client on the therapeutic work. For instance, to a client who demonstrates withdrawal, unusual behavior, or silence after being asked a question, the nurse might say, "That seems to be a difficult question for you right now. We don't have to talk about it now if you'd rather not." Or, to a client who continually focuses on the nurse rather than on self, the nurse could say, "It seems difficult for you to talk about yourself." In both cases the nurse acknowledges the client's situation and refocuses on the therapeutic relationship.

Assessment

In addition to establishing the relationship, the orientation phase gives the nurse an opportunity to assess the client.

Themes.   The nurse listens for themes that run throughout the client's stories. **Themes** are recurring patterns of interactions that the client experiences. The following are examples of themes: every close relationship ending in anger; clients doubting their abilities in every instance; clients blaming others for life situations and taking no responsibility themselves; clients portraying themselves as

victims. Themes are the underlying dynamics of many encounters. It is important to discern these patterns, and it takes time. The patterns become more evident as the work progresses; the client may or may not be aware of them.

Themes are often linked to the client's problem areas. Clients are usually aware of their problem areas and can assist in identifying them. Generally, clients can give the nurse some idea of what would make the situation "right" for them (i.e., their thoughts about what is unhealthy for them and what would "fix" it). For instance, the agitated borderline client may say, "I just want everything to be all right." The housewife in crisis may say, "I just can't do it all any more." The psychotic client may speak of voices tormenting him and of his desire for relief; the suicidal client may want to die. Only catatonic clients will be unable to verbalize any goal at all; other clients will give some clue to their understanding of their situation. The function of the psychiatric mental health nurse is to accept this understanding and work to safely create opportunities for the client to learn healthy ways of assessing and achieving appropriate parts of the goal. Together, the client and the nurse can prioritize the identified problem areas.

Observations.   The human mind can process language much faster than the mouth can speak it. As a result, the brain is not fully occupied when simply listening to another. Psychiatric mental health nurses can enhance their effectiveness by using this "extra brain power" to make observations about clients and the relationship between them. The nurse could make note of the client's affect and demeanor, noticing whether either changes when certain topics are discussed and in what way. The nurse also listens for what is *not* said—in terms of the major players in the client's life who are not part of the story and the omission of feelings, reactions, or thoughts. Nurses need to listen and identify their own feelings evoked in the relationship with the client. These feelings provide valuable information about the client's interactive style. The nurse must assess the client's mood, cognitive functioning, and potential for suicide or homicide.

Strengths.   One of the most important aspects of the orientation period is to assess the strengths and positive aspects of the client's personality. These healthy parts of the individual can be used to heal the more problematic areas. If the work of psychiatric mental health nursing is to move the client toward health, then it is critical to know "the allies." Much of the work of psychiatric mental health nursing is to expand and enlarge the healthy aspects of a person's personality while minimizing the dysfunctional aspects.

There is a story of the work of the great hypnotherapist, Milton Ericson, which emphasizes this point. Ericson was working at a Veterans Administration hospital for clients with chronic mental illness. One of the clients was convinced he was Jesus and acted as such for years. Ericson approached the client and said, "I hear you've had some experience as a carpenter." When the client acknowledged this was so, Ericson asked for some assistance with a minor woodworking project. The client agreed to assist. Over time, Ericson increased the complexity, functionality, and time frame of the woodworking projects, thus expanding the boundaries of the functional aspect of the personality. The client became less delusional and more reality oriented as time passed. Ericson found the functional part in all of the client's dysfunctional behavior and worked to expand it.

It is a skill to assist clients in using their own strengths in ways that benefit them. Together, the nurse and the client identify these strengths. It is helpful for clients to view themselves as more than the sum of their problems. Such an expanded self-view may be the first step toward altering clients' self-perception and increasing their objectivity; it will assist them as they begin to engage in problem solving.

Nursing care plan.   Once the assessment is completed, the nurse identifies the client's problems, nursing diagnoses, and outcome criteria; formulates the nursing care plan; implements the plan with nursing interventions; and evaluates the efficacy of the care plan, modifying it as needed (Fortinash and Holoday-Worret, 1999).

In summary, the work of the *orientation phase* is to (1) define the boundaries of the therapeutic relationship (i.e., identification of the work to be completed, the relationship between client and nurse, and the time frame; in effect, the "contract" between the nurse and the client); (2) begin the development of safety and trust by acting congruently within the defined boundaries; (3) complete the nursing assessment of the client; and (4) formulate the nursing care plan.

WORKING PHASE

There is no clear ending to the orientation phase or beginning to the next phase, known as the *working phase*. The phases of the relationship overlap. As the working phase begins, the boundaries of the relationship have been established and the client acts within these boundaries. Safety and trust have also developed to the point that the client is willing to risk further exploration of issues. The nurse and the client have come to know each other well enough to be able to cooperate in dealing with a problem.

There are two parts to the working phase:

Understanding the problem
Assisting clients in translating this understanding to actions that work to their benefit

Understanding the Problem

Understanding the problem includes facilitating both the nurse's understanding of the client's position and the client's own understanding. Sometimes this is called *problem*

formulating. To do this, nurses ask open-ended questions designed to promote clients' recognition and integration of their own experiences and perhaps gain a new perspective on them. In this part of the work the nurse functions very much in the counselor roles as described by Peplau. Counseling acknowledges that self-renewal, repair, and awareness come from within the individual. The function of the nurse counselor is to assist the individual's self-directed learning in ways that promote health and integration of experience (Peplau, 1952). The formulation of a daily goal can streamline this process. The nurse can interact throughout the day about the goal accomplishment and how it is influenced by varying events.

Necessary skills for this phase of work are careful listening and open-ended, nonjudgmental responses. The nursing response to a client's statement must not obstruct the possibility of identifying feelings or thoughts that assist clients in learning about themselves (Peplau, 1952). For example, consider the homemaker in crisis mentioned earlier. She had stated, "I just can't do it all anymore." The nurse's goal is to further the client's understanding of her own situation. Evaluate the following conversations to see which statement accomplishes this task.

Conversation 1

Client: It's overwhelming. I can't do it all anymore.
Nurse: We all have bad days.
Client: I've had a string of them.
Nurse: Then they must be almost over. Hang in there.
Client: Thanks. I will.

Conversation 2

Client: It's overwhelming. I can't do it anymore.
Nurse: I'm not sure I understand. What's "it"?
Client: My life.
Nurse: Your whole life is overwhelming?
Client: No, well, yes. There's so much to be done.
Nurse: You have a lot to do?
Client: I'll say. I take care of the kids and the house, and my husband is never around to help out.
Nurse: You're taking care of the kids and the house without much help?
Client: Much help? *No* help! He's never there for me, always out doing something while I'm stuck at home with his kids from his first marriage.
Nurse: What's that like for you?
Client: It makes me mad! I'm not his slave.
Nurse: So, you're angry about this?
Client: Sometimes. Sometimes I think it's more than I deserve. My first marriage was pretty bad.
Nurse: It sounds like you have more than one feeling about this.

In the first example, the nurse closed any chance for exploration by injecting her own viewpoint as a reassurance. The client could justifiably assume herself to be a self-pitying whiner. Most likely, the client will keep further "failings" from this nurse. In the second example, however, the nurse was simply open to exploring the client's reality with her. Her questions provided focus for this work of exploring but did not limit the client's responses, thereby allowing the client to begin to gain perspective on her situation.

To further demonstrate nursing responses that promote the client's understanding of the situation, consider the following example of a suicidal client.

Client:	I just want to die.
Nurse:	You're thinking about death very seriously.
Client:	Yes. It would take care of everything.
Nurse:	You're seeing death as a solution.
Client:	Yes.
Nurse:	I'm not sure I understand. Tell me more.
Client:	About what?
Nurse:	About death as a solution.
Client:	Well, the insurance money would pay off my debts, and my wife would have money to live on.
Nurse:	You're thinking it would be a financial benefit to your wife.
Client:	Yes. She'd probably be happier, too . . . without me. I'm not worth much these days.
Nurse:	You think your wife would be happier if you were to die.
Client:	Yes . . . well, not right away, of course. She'd be sad . . . but she'd get over it . . . find somebody worthy of her.
Nurse:	It sounds as if you think highly of her.
Client:	Oh, yes! I don't know why she puts up with me, though. I've been terrible to be around.
Nurse:	You sound puzzled that she could love you even during this difficult time.

In this case the nurse did not argue against the client's solution of suicide but explored the dynamics behind it. The questions/statements also helped to introduce different perspectives to the client (the fact that he is worthy of love even during his depression and the possibility that the depression is time limited).

Further exploration with both these clients would serve to clarify the patterns of thinking and acting that contribute to their dysphoria. This is crucial information. It is the meaning of the behavior, mood, or thoughts perceived by the client that offers the nurse clues to determine which needs must be met. The nurse obtains this information as purely as possible without contaminating it. To do this, the nurse acts as a neutral sounding board so that clients can voice their views in a relationship that is safely defined and nonjudgmental (Peplau, 1952).

Safety Development
It is during the working phase of the relationship that the concepts of safety and boundaries become important

again. As noted earlier, safety comes in knowing what the expectations are in a given situation, as well as one's responsibilities in meeting those expectations. Clients sense in some way that they are expected to tell their story; this may cause them a good deal of anxiety. The nurse assists the client by setting the pace to prevent the client from becoming overwhelmed (Peplau, 1952). By evaluating the client's anxiety level, the nurse ensures that the client does not become overly anxious in the process but instead moves at a pace with which the client feels safe.

Another part of understanding the problem involves the client and nurse determining what sorts of things trigger the maladaptive response. The nurse can help clients determine whether their reactions are a global response to any stressor or whether certain situations set them off or make them worse. This is important to know because it helps the nurse to assist the client in developing effective responses. To learn to deal in effective and healthy ways, the client needs to be aware of those situations that produce unhealthy responses. For example, suicidal clients noted earlier may experience what Beck calls *overgeneralization* (see Chapter 3) and tend to generalize their worthlessness to all situations. A homemaker may find that she manages the normal routine without undue distress but becomes overwhelmed when "extra" tasks are added (e.g., the car breaks down, a child gets sick, an organization requests volunteer time).

Both of the situations in the preceding examples could require different strategies. The nurse could elect to do cognitive work with the client with depression, and stress reduction and assertiveness work with the homemaker.

The nurse's teaching must be appropriate to each client's plan of care; this teaching can consist of both instruction and experience. For instance, the nurse must educate the clients about their diagnosis or the effects of any medications they may be receiving. This is done by evaluating clients' current levels of knowledge and then using their experience with their symptoms or medications to expand their levels of understanding. In other instances the nurse may have to teach the client new skills, such as the relaxation response, stress reduction techniques, assertiveness training, and cognitive work.

Translating Understanding Into Action
The second part of the working phase is to assist clients in translating their expanded understanding of the situation into behavioral changes or actions that promote health. There are many ways to do this, depending on the client's situation and the nurse's theoretic perspective. One aspect common to all client situations is that the behavioral changes are practiced in the "here and now." The client actually attempts behavioral change in the clinical situation with nursing support. For example, perhaps the suicidal man has learned that his days are much worse when he does not get out of bed in the morning. Together with the nurse, he has identified a behavioral pattern in which he

stays in bed isolated from his wife, reflects on his worthlessness, and becomes more despondent as the day goes on. This pattern has been repeated on the unit. The client and the nurse have decided to evaluate whether a change in this pattern would effect a change in his self-perception; they decide to test this by having the client get out of bed promptly in the morning and interact with at least one person at breakfast. (This would be consistent with a cognitive therapy approach.)

The homemaker has discovered an inability to say "no" to requests or to ask for any assistance at all. On the unit she has been very helpful to other clients, caring for them and deferring her own needs. After learning some assertiveness skills, she and the nurse devise a plan in which she has to say "no" to three requests made of her and to ask for help once. In both cases the nurse continues to help the client to clarify feelings associated with the task and integrate the experience into the client's life (see Chapter 8 for further information on assertiveness).

Working in the "here and now" is always possible and is especially appropriate for short-term hospitalizations. Beginners will often focus on the situation outside of the therapy as if it is a separate entity. If nurses focus on the problem situation as one occurring outside the client, they can assist clients in dissociating from the situation (Peplau, 1952). However, the nurse's function is to assist clients in seeing that the locus of control is within themselves and that they have or can learn the skills to deal with that and other situations. Clients must experience this to learn it.

Roles

Much of this learning is done within the client's relationship with the nurse, and it requires a sensitivity to the different roles that clients assign nurses. As noted earlier, clients will often respond to nurses *as if* they were someone else from a previous relationship. This unconscious pattern occurs when the client's situation reactivates feelings that were generated in a prior relationship (transference) (Peplau, 1952). For example, the needy client may respond to a female nurse *as if* she were a mother; the borderline client may view the nurse as a tyrant when she defines rules and limits; the client with low self-esteem may respond to the nurse as an authority figure. In addition, the client will anticipate the nurse's behavior to correspond to that of the earlier role model. The nurse's functions are to assist clients in recognizing the likenesses and differences between the nurse and the earlier role model and to assist clients in getting to know the nurse as a person just by being natural (Peplau, 1952).

By stereotyping the nurse, clients limit their own actions and reactions to those in the original experiences. This repetitive pattern of interacting is limited and can serve to reinforce maladaptive behavior. As nurses gradually reveal their own individuality, they demonstrate the variety of human responses to their clients, who are then free to explore their own various responses.

For example, imagine the homemaker in a creative group setting where she accidentally spills the paint. She seems horrified by this and begins to clean it up frantically. The nurse approaches her.

Client: I'm so sorry! I'm so sorry. I can't believe how clumsy I've been! I can't do anything right.

Nurse: [Recognizing that the client seems to want the nurse to participate in this "critical parent" stance] Are you expecting me to criticize you?

Client: Well, you should. I've made a mess of things. Don't you see what I've done?

Nurse: What I see is that you had an accident and you're cleaning it up. That looks like being responsible to me. Can I help you at all?

Client: No, it's almost done. The spill wasn't that big.

Nurse: I appreciate your taking care of it.

By being genuine and sharing her viewpoint, the nurse provided the client with an important learning experience. The nurse did not respond in the anticipated critical way, but instead offered her own point of view and acknowledged the client's appropriate response.

From the nurse's viewpoint the client was acting responsibly. The client may have never considered this, since her self-perceptions were locked in a self-critical mode, a pattern she enacted in the here-and-now in the presence of the nurse. The nurse used the opportunity to reject the critical role the client attempted to assign her and to acknowledge the client's strength.

The psychiatric nurse recognizes that *every* interaction provides an opportunity to be therapeutic and promote health.

Trust Development

In the preceding scenario, the nurse promoted trust between herself and the client by congruent words and actions. As noted earlier in this chapter, trust develops when there is congruence between words and actions. The nurse had agreed to work with the client's concerns. By being aware of the roles the client cast on her, yet refusing to interact as her mother, sister, teacher, or wife, but only as herself, the nurse fulfills her part of the therapeutic relationship by focusing on the client's issue of assuming criticism.

As clients learn to trust the nurse's genuineness and experience the nurse's acceptance, they begin to trust their own genuineness. This is one of the remarkable healing features of an effective therapeutic relationship: as clients experience trust and safety in the relationship, they begin to incorporate these elements into their sense of self. The nurse often has to point out the areas of growth or change in the "here and now," because there may not be another opportunity. It is especially helpful if these comments are geared toward clients' daily goals so that they can see the work they have done and may not recognize.

Eventually the client will develop an understanding of

the situation, its causes, some skills for dealing with it, and some self-confidence to enact those skills. It is then time to terminate the therapeutic relationship.

TERMINATION PHASE

Terminating relationships is not generally done effectively in many Western cultures. There is a tendency to ignore, belittle, or hasten terminations in relationships, whether they are superficial or intimate. *Termination* is often a difficult phase in therapy as well. Because it represents an "ending" and is consciously or unconsciously associated with death, termination brings out many fears and anxieties in people. Termination forces one to come to terms with the limits of the relationship and therefore acknowledges the limits of life itself. In a more concrete sense, termination is the real loss of the nurse for the client. The relationship ends, and the client must face life without the external support of the nurse. However, at the same time that endings are being acknowledged, so are accomplishments, growth, and individuality. The *therapeutic work* of the nurse is to help the client accept the closure of the boundaries of the relationship and the transfer of safety and trust to the client.

Before Termination

As noted earlier, termination work begins during the introductory phase. The nurse defines the time frame for the therapeutic relationship. The inpatient nurse may state, "*While you are in the hospital,* we will be working together." The outpatient nurse may say, "During the 6 weeks of this program . . ." The nurse defines the time frame of the work during the initial meetings and begins to prepare the client for the eventual end of the relationship. In addition, the work of the relationship, including specific goals, has been clearly defined during the introductory period. Given the current short lengths of stay, it is imperative that the nurse be as clear as possible about client goals, the time frame, the therapeutic regimen, and termination issues (see Box 22-1).

The nurse must also continue to acknowledge the end of the relationship during the working phase. Comments such as "While we're still working together . . ." or "During the time we have remaining . . ." reinforce the given time boundaries and help the client get used to the idea of termination.

It is also effective to acknowledge the client's growth or accomplishments toward goal achievement or attainment as they occur during the working phase. By noting movement toward goal achievement, the nurse marks the client's progress and reinforces the concept that the relationship exists to accomplish certain things. Such comments also promote trust and safety in clients by encouraging them to trust themselves to be effective in specific areas of their lives and consequently feel safer.

As clients begin to do more for themselves, the nurse can transition to the termination phase by spacing con-

---

> **Box 22-2   Acknowledging Client Goals in the Working Phase**
>
> 1. The nurse should assist the client in acknowledging the work done on the daily goal and the issues remaining. A review of the day is helpful and reinforcing.
> 2. The nurse should offer his or her observations of the client's progress toward goal accomplishment.
> 3. Preliminary goal setting for the next shift or day is appropriate because it helps the client to recognize progress made toward goal achievement.

---

tacts further apart to allow clients more time to "stand on their own" according to their capabilities. This gives clients the opportunity to support themselves gradually, which the nurse acknowledges.

During the transition to the termination phase (and during termination itself), new or intense topics should not be introduced. This is a time of solidifying gains and acknowledging the work accomplished. If other issues exist, they may be acknowledged as areas for future work. It is unfair to the client to raise issues that cannot be resolved within the time that remains (Box 22-2).

Responses in Termination

As the reality of termination approaches, clients may respond in a variety of ways depending on their personality and coping skills. Some may deny the occurrence or imminence of separation. Clients involved in denial will try to make plans to visit the nurse after discharge or will ask about making arrangements to "drop by" the hospital some time. By guaranteeing future contact, they can deny the impact of the current separation. Other clients will minimize the importance of the relationship and may make comments comparing the nurse with other supportive people in their lives, as if discounting the work done and the importance of the nurse's role. They may even ignore or avoid the nurse. Another common reaction is anger. The client may express anger at the nurse, the institution, or other clients in an attempt to cover the pain of separation. The client may experience the termination as a rejection, which may activate old feelings of inferiority or a negative self-concept. Some clients may attempt to avoid the whole situation through premature discharge or noninvolvement in groups. Others may regress as if to demonstrate their continuing need for the nurse, stemming from their perceived inability to deal with life on their own. A few clients may actually attempt suicide in order to keep the nurse involved. Finally, some clients will accept the termination and demonstrate some perspective on their various reactions (Fortinash and Holoday-Worret, 1999). Careful review of these various reactions will remind the reader of the stages of grief (denial, anger, bar-

Box 22-3	Client's Typical Response to Termination of the Relationship

Denial
Minimizing the relationship
Rejection
Regression
Anger
Suicide attempt
Acceptance

gaining, and acceptance [see Chapter 29]). This is not surprising when termination is viewed as a loss (Box 22-3).

Nurse's Role in Termination

As noted earlier, the American culture does not deal with endings well. Consequently, few clients have a frame of reference for handling this crucial aspect of life. The nurse has the unique opportunity to assist the client in a successful separation and ending, allowing the client to transfer this knowledge to the next situation. To do this, the nurse must model effective parting for the client. The first step is for the nurse to clearly understand the goal of termination, which is to dissolve the therapeutic relationship while assuring the client of an improved ability to function independently (Fortinash and Holoday-Worret, 1999).

The second step is for the nurse to have a clear understanding of the dynamics of loss (see Chapter 29) and how these concepts affect the client and the nurse. For instance, it is important that the nurse not respond to the client's anger or regression in a personal manner but instead continue to work to help clarify the client's feelings and reactions.

Preparing to terminate the therapeutic relationship takes time. A general rule is that one third of the entire length of the therapeutic relationship should be spent on termination issues. Although this may not always be possible, given the current system of health care, it does emphasize the importance of this aspect of care.

Although termination is addressed initially and throughout the relationship, it begins formally when the client has accomplished the appropriately defined goals and has improved to a higher level of self-sufficiency.

The nurse acknowledges the upcoming ending of the relationship by engaging the client in open discussions of his or her feelings. The nurse continues to be accepting and nonjudgmental even if the client expresses anger, apathy, or denial. By accepting the client's response, the nurse acknowledges that such reactions to loss are normal. The nurse's acceptance allows clients to accept and experience their own reactions (instead of defending them) and to view them as part of the whole process.

The nurse helps the client acknowledge the gains made during their work together. It is often useful to review the progress made throughout the relationship, acknowledging the client's initial distress, the significant learning that took place, and the changes in behavior at the end. Although most of this is done by the client, nurses also share their perceptions of the work. This sharing is incredibly powerful, and nurses need to express themselves positively to continue to promote health. The nurse's emphasis is on summarizing the important learning and the aspects of the client's growth. The nurse also shares what he or she has learned while working with the client. Clients are often surprised that nurses "learn" something from being with them, and such knowledge reinforces their self-esteem and self-worth. (After all, the client must have done *something* if the nurse benefited from the relationship.) The nurse also models the positive influence people can have on each other.

A realistic and natural part of any discussion of termination is the disappointment about what was not achieved. This will be a major part of the work for some, whereas for others it will be a mere footnote. In either case, the topic of things not achieved should not be avoided, since it provides the opportunity to help the client recognize that growth continues throughout life. Frequently the clients and nurses who are most disappointed at termination are those who set goals that are unrealistic or inappropriate to the time frame. Examples are clients who expect to be functioning optimally in all areas of their lives at the time of discharge and nurses who wish to have all of their clients become self-actualized during the course of therapy.

Nurses, like clients, need to express their own mixed feelings about the separation. For example, "I also feel sad that this relationship is ending, and I am happy about the work we've accomplished" is a statement that helps clients perceive their own reactions to termination as normal.

Even with the best preparation, most clients are anxious at the time of discharge or termination because of fears about their ability to cope on their own. A list of available community resources will help clients know "the door has not been closed" and that help is available whenever needed.

Because the focus of short-term hospitalization is often on assessment, medication stabilization, and crisis intervention, follow-up care is essential for treatment. Arrangements for follow-up care are best discussed throughout the hospitalization. At discharge, the patient should have an established link to care in the community. It is also important to help the client make initial plans on ways to accomplish unmet goals at a future time, outside the relationship.

THERAPEUTIC MILIEU

The therapeutic milieu is the environment designed to promote health. Since its earliest days nursing has recognized the importance of the environment, or milieu, to healing. Indeed, Florence Nightingale defined her work as organizing the environment to allow the body to heal. The same principle holds true in psychiatric mental health nursing.

The psychiatric unit is a social system in its own right, with clients at various points of length of stay, each with their own agenda, interacting and meeting unique personal and social needs. As such, the milieu can be seen both as a large work group with the definitive task of healing and as a community with all the tasks of communal living. The psychiatric mental health nurse is a constant in this system, interacting with clients and staff in a variety of ways. These interactions are very significant and greatly assist in creating the atmosphere or culture of each particular psychiatric unit.

HISTORICAL DEVELOPMENT

Maxwell Jones developed the concept of the therapeutic community in the 1950s. His goal was to design an entire culture that would promote healthy personalities (Jones, 1953). Jones's goal for patients was one of improved behavior, and he was one of the first to act on the knowledge that the hospital environment affects the symptoms, behaviors, and progress of clients.

Since the 1950s this work has been expanded and revised, although the language has changed from *therapeutic community* to the French term *therapeutic milieu,* meaning environment or setting. Thus a **therapeutic milieu,** much like a *therapeutic relationship,* is an environment designed to promote health. It is also an environment designed to provide corrective or healing experiences that enhance the client's coping abilities. A milieu can be hierarchic or democratic, open to problem solving or rigid in its application of rules. The environment can foster individual responsibility or behavioral control. It is one of the challenges of psychiatric mental health nursing to use this environment in a conscious manner to promote the healthy functioning of individuals and the group as a whole. The nurse, who is involved in most of the activities on the unit, is key to effective milieu development.

PRINCIPLES OF MILIEU THERAPY

In order to be effective, the nurse must understand the underlying assumptions of milieu therapy and promote its principles. The basic underlying assumption of milieu therapy is that *clients are active, not passive, participants in their lives.* This implies that clients "own" their behavior and environment and consequently need to be involved in the management of both. In the milieu, human beings are seen as independent. Distortions, conflicts, and inappropriate behaviors are dealt with in the "here and now" and in the context of their impact on others. Peers are assumed to be necessary for the learning that comes from various interactions, as well as the potential healing effect of peer pressure. The principles of milieu therapy are the following:

To promote a fundamental respect for individuals (both clients and staff)

To use the opportunities for communication between client and staff for maximum therapeutic benefit

To encourage clients to act at a level equal to their ability and to enhance their self-esteem

To promote socialization

To provide opportunities for clients to be part of unit management (Herz, 1969; Jones, 1953).

The nurse's function is to act in ways that consistently promote these goals.

BOUNDARY, SAFETY, AND TRUST DEVELOPMENT IN A MILIEU

The concepts of boundary, safety, and trust assist in formulating this task just as they help formulate the therapeutic relationship discussed earlier. At this level, however, they are expanded to meet the needs of a type of community, which is the psychiatric unit.

Boundary

As mentioned earlier, boundaries serve to define functions and consequently imply responsibility. The nurse must clarify boundaries for clients. It is not easy for anyone to walk into a new culture (such as a psychiatric unit) and make sense of it. It is considerably more difficult if that person is experiencing the cognitive or emotional stress of a psychiatric disorder. By defining functions and tasks of the various groups and activities offered on the unit, the nurse promotes the opportunity for each group or activity to be used efficiently. Appropriate task completion is essential for health.

For example, most units have some type of meeting for staff and client that is designed to orient clients to the staff, activities of the day, and any issues of communal living. This is frequently called the *community* or *contact meeting,* and it provides an excellent opportunity for boundary definition because one of its purposes is the orientation of clients. This roughly correlates with the orientation phase in the development of a therapeutic relationship. Introductions and explanation of purpose and role are needed, only now these introductions address the relationship of the client to the unit and staff, rather than to the individual therapist.

All too often, the community meeting is reduced to superficial introductions of the members (clients and staff) and a cursory schedule of activities. A rich opportunity to help clients structure their time and focus their work is wasted.

Consider the effects of these two examples of community meetings. In this first example, the nurse leader does little to define the structure, or purpose, of the work.

Example 1 (Nontherapeutic)

Leader defines function of the meeting as introductory.	**Leader:**	OK. This is community meeting, and we usually introduce ourselves. I'm Casey, the nurse. I'll be passing out meds today.
Clients follow defined function of introductions	**Client:**	I'm Sue.
	Client:	Carl.
	Client:	Mike.
	Client:	Peggy.
	Client:	Lynn.
	Client:	Carol.
	Staff:	I'm Judy. I'm the O.T. I'll see most of you at my group.
Leader offers minimal assistance in organizing.	**Leader:**	OK. The schedule of groups is posted on the board. Who are the contacts?
Leader does not define function of contacts	**Judy:**	I'll be working with Carl, Peggy, and Lynn today.
	Leader:	And I'll work with the rest.
Leader uses "stuff," a vague term that does not focus group to work.	**Leader:**	Any questions about unit stuff?
	Lynn:	I still don't have hot water in my room.
Leader does not allow for group problem solving.	**Leader:**	I know. Engineering's working on it. Anything else? [Pause] OK? Meeting adjourned.

On the surface, boundaries were addressed in a cursory way. The nurse defined one of her functions (giving medications) and informed the clients that groups would be formed. Clients picked up on this role modeling and responded with cursory information of their own. It is difficult to see how they could understand unit organization in order to function effectively within it. A rich opportunity was missed.

Now, consider the difference in tone and expectations when boundaries and tasks are more clearly defined as in the following example.

Example 2 (Therapeutic)

Leader defines purpose of meeting.	**Leader:**	Good morning. It's Tuesday, June 14, and this is our community meeting. This is the meeting where we get ourselves organized for the day and take care of any business that comes up just from so many people living together.
Leader provides structure for task.	**Leader:**	Let's do first things first and introduce ourselves and what we do here.
Leader defines tasks and explains how clients can use her in this role.	**Leader:**	I'm Casey, and I'm one of the nurses. I'll be passing out the medications today, so if any of you have questions about your medications, please see me. I'll also be leading the process group, and I'll tell you more about that later.
Leader provides structure.	**Leader:**	[To each client] Would you please introduce yourself to everybody and say something about yourself?
	Client:	Well, I think everybody knows me. I'm Sue. I've been here since Friday. I'll probably go home Wednesday or Thursday.
	Client:	I'm Carl. I don't know if I'll ever go home.
	Client:	I'm Mike. I'm Carl's roommate, and he snores! So loud!
Leader focuses on task.	**Leader:**	Please say something about yourself.
	Client:	I'm tired. I'm not sleeping well.
	Leader:	Thanks.
	Client:	I'm Peggy. I just came in yesterday, and I've met a few of you. This is a real nice place.
	Client:	I'm Lynn. I've got nothing to say.
	Client:	I'm Carol. Uh—I don't like to talk in front of people.
Leader models acceptance.	**Leader:**	I appreciate your effort.
	Staff:	I'm Judy. I'm the occupational therapist. I'll be leading the 9 AM and 2 PM groups today in the activity room. I also want to meet with you, Peggy, to get to know you and make some plans with you about how you can best use occupational therapy. Could you meet with me after the meeting to set up a time?

Example 2 (Therapeutic)—cont'd

	Peggy:	Sure.
	Leader:	Thanks for your introductions.
Leader defines role and how to use contact person to promote task accomplishment.	**Leader:**	Each one of the staff acts as a contact person for each of you. A contact is the person who is working with you for the day. You can talk to your contact about anything that concerns you. I'll be the contact person for Sue, Mike, and Carol. Judy will be the contact person for Carl, Mary, and Lynn. Any questions so far?
Leader promotes self-responsibility by telling clients how to meet their own needs.	**Leader:**	Let me introduce today's schedule to you. It's posted on the bulletin board if you forget the times. We mostly want to tell you about the activities.
	Judy:	From 9 AM to 10 AM is roles group. This group helps you look at the different parts you play in your various relationships. It's a good place to look for patterns that reoccur in your life. I will be the leader.
Leader defines purpose.	**Leader:**	You have free time until 10:30 AM. From 10:30 AM to 11:30 AM is process group. This is the group I'll be leading. This is the group where we pay attention to how we communicate with each other. It's a good place to look at any problems you may be having communicating with other people. Lunch is at 11:45 AM, and at 1 PM you have a choice of taking a walk (if you have privilege to do so) or playing a game like bingo here on the unit. From 2 PM to 3 PM is the activity group that Judy leads. This is where you can make something. It's a good opportunity to look at how you approach doing a task. At 3:30 PM we go home, and the evening staff will meet with you to go over the evening schedule and staffing. Any questions?
Client uses information and responds to cooperative style modeled by leaders.	**Carl:**	Do we have to play bingo? I hate that game.
	Leader:	No, that was just what came to mind. Actually, as a group you can choose any game you'd like at that time.
Leader supports client initiative, clarifies the situation, and models acceptance of question asking.	**Leader:**	Thanks for asking. It helps us to make ourselves clear and share understanding of what happens here on the unit.
Leader reiterates ways to be self-responsible.	**Leader:**	Any other questions about the schedule? [Pause] It's a lot to remember. If any questions come up during the day, check the schedule on the bulletin board or see your contact person.
Leader continues providing structure.	**Leader:**	I think we can move to the last piece of business for this meeting and that's to deal with any issues that come up whenever so many people live together. Anything you want to bring up?
	Lynn:	I still don't have any hot water.
Leader promotes interaction.	**Leader:**	I heard about that from night staff again. It's been a while, hasn't it?
	Lynn:	Three days, and nothing is happening.
Leader clarifies information.	**Leader:**	Well, actually, something is happening. Engineering found that the valve is broken and they're waiting for a replacement.
Group follows up on problem solving (probably based on leader's earlier modeled acceptance and encouragement to be self-responsible).	**Lynn:**	[Sarcastically] Great! They're waiting, and I don't have any hot water.
	Sue:	No hot water at all?
	Lynn:	Well, my shower works, but I don't have any hot water in my sink to wash up. I don't want to take a whole shower just to wash my face.
	Mike:	Why don't you just wet your washcloth in the shower?
	Lynn:	That's what I've been doing, but I get soaked and my clothes get soaked.
	Sue:	Well, I don't mind if you want to use my sink for washing up, as long as you ask first.
Clients have clarified their action appropriate to their role.	**Lynn:**	Really? Thanks. I'll do that.
Leader clarifies her action appropriate to her role as staff member.	**Leader:**	That worked out . . . I'll see what engineering can do today, Lynn.
	Lynn:	Thanks.
	Leader:	Any other issues?
	Mike:	The radio is broken.
	Carl:	No, it's not broken, just out of batteries.
Leader shares information not available to clients and offers solution.	**Leader:**	We keep batteries at the desk. Mike, would you bring the radio to the desk after this meeting and we'll see what new batteries can do.
	Mike:	Sure.
Leader acknowledges contribution.	**Leader:**	Thanks. What else?
	Peggy:	I just don't know what to do about my son. He never listens to me anymore. He used to be such a good kid and now I just worry all the time.

Example 2 (Therapeutic)—cont'd

Leader acknowledges issue and ways to work on it while keeping group focused to accomplish task of this meeting.

Leader: Peggy, this sounds very important to you and something I know you'll want to work on while you're here. Process group or role play, or even a talk with your contact would be good places to talk about that; that's their purpose. In this meeting we try to handle the nuts and bolts of living on this unit.

Peggy: I'm sorry.

Supportive and accepting approach.

Leader: It's OK. It takes a bit of time to learn how to use this place and what all the meetings are for. It sounds like you have a good idea of some of the issues you want to work on.

Peggy: Oh, yes!

Leader continues to focus client on task of meeting to promote goal accomplishment.

Leader: That's how it starts. Any questions about living here?

Peggy: You mentioned that you would be passing out medications? I know I'm on some. Where do I go?

Leader models self-acceptance of faults.

Leader: Thank you. That's an important point, and I forgot to mention it.

Leader provides further clarification on unit structure.

Leader: Medications are passed out at the medication cart at 9 AM, right after this meeting, and again at 1 PM. The evening shift will pass them out at 5 PM and 9 PM. Not everyone gets medications at all these times. If you'd like, I can meet with you after this meeting to see when you get your medicine.

Peggy: Thanks. I'd like to do that. There's so much.

Supportive comment from peer.

Sue: Don't worry. You'll get used to it.

Peggy: [Smiles at Sue]

Leader: Anything else?

Mike: I don't know if I should bring this up.

Leader continues to focus on task appropriateness.

Leader: Does it have to do with the business of living together?

Mike: Yes.

Leader: Then this is the place.

Mike: OK then—well, I like Carl, don't get me wrong, but I can't sleep with his snoring and I don't think that's healthy for me.

Carl: I do snore. I've heard that all my life.

Leader makes supportive and educational comment.

Leader: Sleep is important to being able to function. Any solutions?

Mike: Well, I'd like a new room.

Leader: That would be a great solution, but we don't have another room, and with our current mix of males and females we can't do any swaps.

Lynn: Well, it's not fair! He should be able to sleep, for God's sake. This is a hospital.

Leader models reality orientation and acceptance of limits.

Leader: I couldn't agree with you more. But a hospital has its limits, too. Apparently right now there is limited bed space. So we have to figure out a solution with what we've got.

Lynn: Isn't this ridiculous! What can we do? Sleep in shifts?

Leader keeps group focused on task of problem solving and does not allow group to degenerate into gripe session.

Leader: There's one idea on the table. Any others?

Peggy: Maybe he could get a bed on another unit?

Mike: Well, I actually have an idea that might work.

Leader: What is it?

Mike: Well, I was wondering if I could sleep in the quiet room, as long as it wasn't in use.

Leader: What do you all think?

Group: [Murmurs assent]

Leader supports client initiative and provides link to other shifts as appropriate for staff member role.

Leader: That's a very workable solution, Mike. I'll tell the evening and night staff, and you can start tonight.

Leader promotes functional communication by assisting in message completion.

Mike: Thanks! [To Carl] No hard feelings? [No response]

Leader: Any hard feelings, Carl? Mike wants to know.

Carl: No hard feelings. Like I say, this is an old problem.

Leader: OK, anything else? [Pause] It seems like we've taken care of a lot of business. Thanks for your contributions here. If there are no objections, this meeting is adjourned.

What a different meeting and tone! The first meeting had a rather superficial feeling, whereas this second meeting actually facilitated movement toward the stated goals of introductions, orientation, and organization. In addition, the nurse has had the opportunity to assess the general tone of the milieu—for example, Peggy seemed somewhat bewildered and Lynn appeared angry. This information will be extremely useful to the rest of the staff as they interact with the clients throughout the course of the day. In effect, the clearly defined boundaries greatly assist the nurse in becoming oriented to the tone of the unit and the status of the clients. This information will help the nurse to organize the day while considering the clients' needs.

Boundaries continue to be addressed throughout the day: groups are introduced, duties of staff and clients are defined, and responsibility for various actions is acknowledged. Just as boundaries provide structure for individual work by defining the work, its limits, and time frame, so do boundaries in the milieu.

Safety

Safety and trust are developed in a similar manner as well. As noted earlier, safety is developed by knowing what one's responsibilities are in a given situation, and trust develops through actions that are consistent with an individual's or group's stated intent. It is important that these issues be addressed in terms of the milieu. To feel safe, clients need to know what is expected of them in their role as clients. Do they make their own beds or not? Are they called to group or expected to arrive at the stated location on time? Do they go to a certain spot to get medications, or are medications delivered? How do they contact a staff member if they want to talk?

The psychiatric staff may not inform clients of their responsibilities, thinking that these expectations are obvious. By addressing these issues in a timely manner, however, the staff is able to ensure that safety is promoted, and work may proceed more quickly.

Development of safety is addressed consistently throughout a client's stay through this clarification of expectations and responsibilities. This clarification of responsibilities is often necessary as it relates to other clients. Often, psychiatric clients will attempt to "help" other clients in certain ways. One client may "help" another by doing a task for him; another may "help" by stating the other's case in a difficult interpersonal interaction. Such "help" is usually "unhelpful" because it violates the boundaries of each individual's responsibilities (completing a task, speaking for oneself). Safety is promoted by clarifying what each member's tasks are and are not and assisting all clients in meeting their appropriate responsibilities.

As an example of this, consider the following scenario that occurs on the same day as the community meeting just outlined.

Peggy:	I need to find a blanket.
Nurse:	We keep them on the linen cart.
Peggy:	Along with the pillowcases and sheets?
Nurse:	Yes. It sounds like you're making a bed. I thought you had already done that.
Peggy:	Oh, I have done mine. I just wanted to help Mike out and make up the quiet room for him.
Nurse:	How did you decide to do that?
Peggy:	Oh, it's just my way. I'm always doing things like that for people.
Nurse:	How does that work for you?
Peggy:	Pretty well; people always ask me for help, so I know I'm needed.
Nurse:	So, you're always needed.
Peggy:	Yes, and always tired.
Nurse:	It gets tiring doing things for other people.
Peggy:	Yeah, I don't know any other way, though.
Nurse:	So, you're doing the same thing here that you do outside?
Peggy:	Yes.
Nurse:	I wonder what would happen if you just took care of yourself and your needs here, and let others do the same for themselves. Do you think Mike can make his own bed?
Peggy:	He's grown, I don't see why not.
Nurse:	Do you think you can let him make his own bed and do his own work?
Peggy:	I suppose I could, but it would be so different.
Nurse:	It is a different way for you, to let each person do his or her own work. Are you willing to try it?
Peggy:	OK.
Nurse:	Let me know later on what it's been like for you.

In this scenario, the nurse was able to turn a casual question into a therapeutic conversation, using this interaction to reinforce the boundaries of personal responsibility (each does own task), focus Peggy on her work (exploring self-defeating patterns), and promote safety by clarifying the expectations of each person's work. The nurse functioned within the role of a nurse in the milieu by (1) performing within the role to use communication for therapeutic benefit, (2) helping the client to function within the limits of self-responsibility, (3) promoting the appropriate self-functioning of each client, and (4) demonstrating respect for both the client and the process.

Trust

Trust in a milieu is nurtured in a similar manner: the promotion of consistency between words and actions. Again, the nurse acts in a consistent manner to achieve defined purposes. For instance, nurses who say that they are medication nurses work to achieve the stated objectives: they pass out the medications on schedule and are available to answer questions about the medications. Nurses who say they will orient a new client to the unit follow up by actually doing so.

More subtle, however, is the accomplishment of the overall goal of promoting a functional milieu that fosters self-responsibility, growth, and clear communication patterns. Nurses are involved in creating this type of milieu each time they interact with clients and staff. In the preceding conversation between Peggy and the nurse, the nurse used a client's casual question to more clearly define areas of responsibility for both Peggy (the client) and her peers. Psychiatric mental health nurses must be aware of the various goals of the therapeutic milieu and their own role in facilitating trust; they must then work in a consistent manner to promote trust as a major goal of milieu work.

Working effectively in a milieu is some of the most challenging work for the psychiatric mental health nurse. Each nursing interaction affects the milieu in some way. The challenge, then, is to make every interaction a therapeutic one. This is accomplished by acting in a manner that promotes the achievement of identified therapeutic goals within the milieu.

GROUP THERAPY

Humans spend much of their time in some form of group interaction. We are raised in family groups, participate in work groups at all ages, and socialize in formal or informal group settings. Much of our "humanness" is defined in our interactions with others. Before looking specifically at the use of groups as a form of therapy, it would be helpful to examine some universal characteristics of all groups.

THE GROUP AS A MICROCOSM

Groups offer individuals the opportunity to interact with other individuals in a meaningful way. Groups provide the opportunity for self-definition through human interaction and task accomplishment. All groups have a task or purpose; family groups are for mutual nurturance and support (especially in caring for offspring); work groups are designed to accomplish or produce certain defined tasks; social groups of various types exist to foster interactions. Each group functions as a microcosm, or miniature universe, reflecting its own specific group culture and set of values. People interact within this microcosm to meet their own needs.

ROLES

For the group to do its work, specific duties need to be accomplished. These duties are formulated into roles. Individuals enact roles based on their own personal dynamics and group needs. Roles are described as either *ascribed* or *achieved*. Ascribed roles are based on certain intrinsic characteristics that are beyond a person's control, such as age or sex; *achieved* roles are based on a person's achievements through interests, education, and talents (Sampson and Marthas, 1990). Examples of achieved roles are teacher, nurse, musician, and athlete. Achieved roles are played out in relation to other roles; thus to fulfill the role, a parent

needs a child, a teacher needs a student, a nurse needs a client, and so on.

Roles exist in all groups and are related to the group's main issues of (1) accomplishing its defined task and (2) maintaining member relations (Sampson and Marthas, 1990). Special roles develop in the group to deal with these issues. A *task specialist* is someone within a group who works toward accomplishing the group's defined task. A *social specialist* is someone who maintains relative harmony in member relationships throughout the group process (Sampson and Marthas, 1990). Members enact these roles and others based on personal preference and group need. Roles that serve the individual's personal needs rather than the group's are referred to as *individual functions*; Box 22-4 summarizes these roles.

NORMS

Norms are the group's standards of behavior, attitudes, and perceptions of its members. They represent the shared expectations of appropriateness in behavior (Sampson and Marthas, 1990). Norms serve certain purposes for groups. One major function of norms is to allow a group to act in a fairly coordinated manner to accomplish its goals and tasks. In this way norms fulfill a *task function*. Norms also fulfill a maintenance function by regulating maintenance issues around attendance, conflict resolution, and personal relations. Finally, norms serve a *social reality function*. Much of what we "know" to be true has been socially determined. Overall, group norms provide a framework for the interpretation of data (Sampson and Marthas, 1990).

Norms vary in content, extent, and explicitness. Norm *content* refers to the extent to which the norm covers aspects of the member's life. For instance, it is the norm among some Roman Catholics not to eat meat on Friday; it is the norm for some Buddhists to never eat meat (the latter is a more extensive norm).

Explicitness refers to how obvious or clear the norms are. *Overt* norms are the usually stated expectations for behavior known to all members, such as groups always beginning and ending at a specific time (Northouse and Northouse, 1992). *Covert* norms are often practiced but not defined; they are a shared understanding about appropriate behavior rather than being verbally acknowledged, such as members sitting in the same place at every group session (Northouse and Northouse, 1992). Frequently a new member will conform with the explicit (overt) norms of a group quickly, but take more time to discover and understand implicit (covert) norms (Sampson and Marthas, 1990).

Norms can be *enabling* (assist the group in accomplishing its work) or *restrictive* (hinder movement toward goal accomplishment).

UNIVERSAL TASKS

Finally, all groups must deal with the issues of group life: forming, working, and ending. Often this work is un-

---

Box 22-4   Individual Functions Within a Group

Roles Involving Task Functions

Initiator: Proposes new ideas, directions, tasks, methods.
Elaborator: Expands on existing suggestions and develops the group's plans further.
Evaluator: Critically evaluates ideas, proposals, and plans, examining the practicality of proposals and the effectiveness of procedures.
Coordinator: Helps to pull together ideas and themes, to clarify suggestions that have been made, and to help various subgroups work more effectively together toward their common goals.

Roles Involving Group Maintenance Functions

Encourager: Offers praise to and agrees with other members; communicates acceptance of others and their ideas and an openness to differences within the group.
Harmonizer: Mediates conflicts and disagreements that crop up, trying to relieve or reduce tension within the group.

Compromiser: Seeks a position between contending sides; seeks a compromise that all parties can accept.

Roles Involving Primarily Personal, Individualistic Functions

Aggressor: Acts negatively, with hostility toward other members; criticizes others' contributions; attacks the group and its members.
Recognition-seeker: Calls attention to own activities; boasts; redirects things toward self.
Help-seeker or confessor: Uses the group as a vehicle either to gain sympathy or to achieve personal insight and self-satisfaction without consideration for others or the group as a whole.
Dominator: Asserts authority and seeks to manipulate others so as to be in control of everything that happens.

---

known to the group, but work in human relations theory implies that it is always being addressed. During the *forming phase*, group members deal with issues of joining a group. They wrestle with questions of how to join a group and issues of pairing with other group members. Acceptance/rejection by group members, issues of sexual attractions, and position within the group are also addressed at some level. During the group's working phase, task accomplishment is emphasized. The group deals with issues of leadership, completion, competence, and trust. At the final or termination phase, the group deals with issues that apply to endings, such as death, loss of the group, grief, separation, loneliness, and limitations.

These issues underlie all group processes and are always being addressed by the group, even if only at an unconscious level.

TYPES OF GROUPS

Groups in the health care setting vary according to whether they are *content oriented* or *process oriented*. Content refers to the discussion of goals and tasks. Process refers to the discussion of interpersonal relations. Although all groups contain both elements, they vary with the degree of emphasis given (Northouse and Northouse, 1992).

Task groups focus on content issues: defining the tasks and what work is needed to accomplish them. It is rare, however, to find a group that is totally task oriented. There is generally some processing going on among members. Examples of task groups are committees formed to develop clinical or critical pathways or to monitor quality improvement.

Process groups focus on relations among members and their communication styles or patterns. Therapy groups

designed to discuss client issues on an inpatient psychiatric unit fall into this category.

Finally, there are the *mid-range* groups that combine both functions of task and process. Many support groups with an emphasis on education and adjustment fall into this category (Figure 22-2).

ASPECTS OF GROUP THERAPY

Groups, like milieus, function as social communities, and individuals tend to function in groups as they do in other parts of their lives. Likewise, individuals' behavior in group therapy will imitate their behavior in other group settings. A key assumption of group therapy is that psychopathology has its source in disordered relationships (Yalom, 1985). The goal of the therapy group is to help individuals develop more functional and satisfying relationships. Because the individual dysfunction is demonstrated in the group, the task of the group is to assist members in understanding their patterns of interacting within the group so as to be able to generalize to the larger arena of life outside the group. To do this, members must (1) get information on how they present themselves to others, (2) assess whether their fixed patterns are realistic to continue in the current situation, (3) discover previously unknown parts of themselves (strengths, skills, abilities, desires), (4) gradually try new behaviors within the safety of the group, and (5) accept ultimate responsibility for the way they live (Yalom, 1985).

Cohesiveness

The extent to which group members work together to accomplish these stated goals is called *cohesion or cohesiveness:* the sense of "we-ness" that a group experiences that

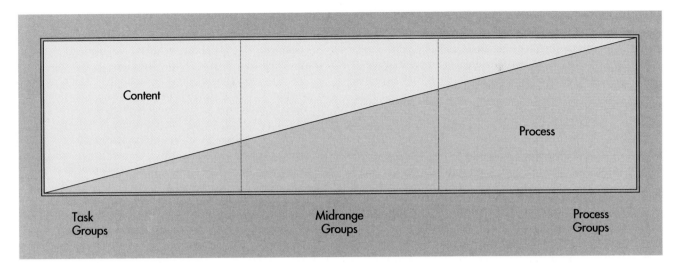

Figure 22-2   The emphasis on content and process in different types of groups. Psychiatric mental health nurses are most involved with process group therapy. (Modified from Loomis M: *Group process for nurses,* St. Louis, 1979, Mosby.)

Table 22-1	**Factors That Influence Group Cohesiveness**
Group goals	Clear goals, based on similar member values and interests, motivate members to seek or maintain group membership.
Similarity among members	Members are frequently attracted to other members who share similar values and beliefs. There are some instances, however, in which people are attracted to those who are dissimilar in values and attitudes.
Type of interdependence among members	Groups that function in a cooperative versus competitive manner tend to have higher cohesion among members.
Leader behavior	For the most part, democratic styles of leadership are associated with higher group cohesiveness than are other styles of leadership (e.g., autocratic).
Communication structures	Decentralized communication structures, characterized by increased member interaction, are associated with higher morale and increased satisfaction among members.
Group activities	Members who are asked to perform group activities they believe are beyond their capabilities will feel less attraction toward the group, whereas members who believe group activities are within their capabilities will feel more attracted toward the group.
Group atmosphere	Members are frequently attracted to groups that help them feel valued and accepted.
Group size	Group size should match the number of members needed to complete the task. Larger groups, in which the group size interferes with group goals, can decrease cohesiveness.

From Cartwright D: The nature of group cohesiveness. In Cartwright D, Zander A, editors: *Group dynamics: research and theory,* ed 3, New York, 1968, Harper & Row.

acts as a bond between group members. Cohesion has been associated with positive group outcomes: increased interactions, norm conformity and goal-directed behaviors, and member satisfaction (Northouse and Northouse, 1992). Factors that influence group cohesiveness are summarized in Table 22-1.

Therapeutic Factors

Researchers have attempted to define the factors of a group process that have a positive effect on its members. To be effective as a group leader, the nurse must have an appreciation of these therapeutic factors of group therapy

and be able to promote them. Yalom identified 11 curative factors, which are listed in Box 22-5.

INPATIENT GROUPS

To effectively lead an inpatient group, the nurse must be aware of the various factors influencing the group so as to develop a style that is responsive to the unpredictable conditions of inpatient group therapy.

The turnover of clients in today's psychiatric hospitals is rapid. This means it is probable that group membership will not be constant from one meeting to the next. It is likely that one or more members will be new to the group,

Box 22-5   Yalom's Curative Factors of Group Therapy

1. *Instill hope:* Group members are at various points of the health continuum. Those who are not coping well can gain hope from those who have benefited from the group experience.
2. *Universality:* Members come to learn they are not unique or alone in their discomfort. They learn that others have reactions and thoughts similar to their own.
3. *Imparting information:* Both formal and informal learning occurs in groups. Some groups such as AA and medication-education or symptom recognition groups are designed specifically to impart information. Through groups designed to assist with interpersonal dynamics, members learn about the effects of their interactions on group dynamics.
4. *Altruism:* By and large, members of groups give credit to the other group members for their support and insight. Members view their improvement as related to the work done by all group members. By learning they can be useful, members experience an improved sense of self-value.
5. *Corrective recapitulation of the family group:* As noted earlier, people act as they were taught to act in their families. As is often the case with psychiatric clients, these patterns are dysfunctional and the client continues to repeat these dysfunctional patterns in all interactions. Group therapy provides the opportunity for these patterns to be identified, evaluated, and changed.
6. *Development of social techniques:* By interacting with others, members can improve their social skills. Members will often give each other feedback on their reactions to each other's interpersonal style. This enriches member recognition of the various effects of their style on others and gives them opportunities to choose and practice styles that are more in keeping with their goals.
7. *Imitative behavior:* Very often group members are "caught" or trapped in ways of interacting because they

cannot conceive of another way. In a group situation members are able to see how others interact and can choose to model their behaviors on those of other group members or the therapist. By looking at options, group members get the help they need to dissolve their rigid behavioral styles and become more flexible in their interactions.

8. *Catharsis:* Catharsis is the release of intense emotions. Psychiatric clients are often hesitant to express these emotions for fear that they will be too overwhelming for anyone to handle and that the consequence of expressing them would be grievous. In group therapy, members learn how to express these emotions and experience the immediate relief catharsis can bring. In addition, members learn that they and the group have survived the expression of emotions without calamity.
9. *Existential factors:* All human beings must deal with one basic issue of existence: that we are ultimately alone despite the presence of others. Psychiatric clients (and others) may tend to be unrealistic in their expectations of human relationships, thinking that with the perfect mate, friend, or family all feelings of "aloneness" would vanish. In group therapy, members learn that feelings of loneliness can be decreased by human companionship but not completely eliminated. By not reaching for what is unattainable, members may be able to enjoy what is attainable.
10. *Cohesiveness:* This is one of the most powerful benefits of an effective group. Many members experience extreme isolation from others in their daily lives and consequently experience a feeling of disconnectedness from others. By being part of a group that is achieving its stated goals, members experience a sense of "belonging," a feeling of being part of a "whole" that is greater than each individual self.
11. *Interpersonal learning:* In groups designed to examine interpersonal relationships, the members learn to identify, clarify, and modify maladaptive behaviors.

From Yalom ID: *The theory and practice of group psychotherapy*, ed 3 New York, 1985, Basic Books.

whereas others will be ready to leave. Thus some members may be in totally different phases of the group process (e.g., orientation, working, termination). This has critical implications for how group routines and dynamics are played out and carried over from one group to the next. Rapid turnover may compromise group cohesion. This greatly affects safety development within the group. Because it is rare for all group members to share a single specific diagnosis, the variety of disorders also affects group safety and cohesiveness. Generally, all the clients on a unit will attend all of the groups. Therefore different levels of functioning and presentation will be represented, which may be frightening to some group members and may affect cohesion and safety development.

The clients are inpatients and, by definition, fragile.

They are often frightened, confused, and disorganized. Again, the creation of safety and structure becomes important. Many clients are unmotivated. They attend group sessions because they "have to" by unit rules, but it would not be their choice. The nurse leader must find ways to make the group relevant for them and their needs. There is often too little time to prepare the clients for the group experience. Staff may frequently be too busy to effectively orient the clients to the group. This implies that all too often the orientation must happen within the group.

Another issue affecting inpatient group therapy is varying leadership. Not only does the membership vary, so does the leadership based on staff scheduling. This affects the continuity of routine, as well as safety development.

Another consideration related to staffing is that the cli-

Table 22-2   Summary of Inpatient Group Considerations

Considerations of Inpatient Group Work	Clients' Requirements	Nurse's Technique/ Functions of Nurse	Nurse's Style to Promote Function	Promote Function
High severity of distress in group members caused by: Personal distress Secondary anxiety of hospitalization Rapid turnover Little preparation Many roles of therapist Brief duration of therapy Provide opportunity to explore (not necessarily resolve) questions of interpersonal relationship	Defined structure to work within	Lessen the ambiguity of therapy situation through clarification of details	Provide boundaries: Room Time frame Orientation Expectations for behavior (therapist's and client's) Sequence of group Norm clarification	Firm, explicit, and active Explain actions Model contradictory feelings and solicit feedback
	Goals that can be achieved: How am I seen by others? How does my behavior affect others Finding a safe arena to try new behaviors	Enhance client strengths by: Discouraging self-defeating behavior Acknowledging contributions	Support client by: Modeling feedback Providing positive interpretation Showing relevance of interactions to life outside hospital	Model respect as shown by: Being supportive, constructive, and accepting feedback Using data as learning opportunity Acknowledging client's contributions during summary statement
Group exists as part of a larger whole: Client is member of unit milieu Group session is only one of many groups	Facilitating client-to-client relations	Problem identification	Promote direct communication Client to client Abstract to specific Questions support furthering of relationships: What aspect of behavior gets in way of ideal relationship?	Modeling of openness, selective self-disclosure, risk taking
Fragility of patients	Avoiding and managing stress	Conflict management	Immediate intervention Promoting resolution, objectivity, and learning	

ents see the group leader in a variety of roles throughout the day. The nurse may be their contact person, their medication nurse, and part of the treatment team, in addition to leading the group. It would be easy for clients to confuse these various roles. Consequently, leaders have the responsibility to clarify their roles and functions in the group.

Finally, there is little time for the more subtle aspects of psychiatric treatment. Clients are generally preoccupied with seeking relief from their despair and are not interested in subtle nuances. This implies that the work must be direct, effective, and limited in scope to accomplish goals. In summary, the membership of an inpatient group requires leadership that provides orientation and continuity of group norms, defines the structure and limits of the group, promotes safety development, clarifies the relevant group task, and assists in the group's accomplishment of that task.

The careful leader will recognize the need for boundary definition, safety, and trust development as just noted. These concepts must be expanded to create a therapeutic relationship at the group level. Instead of applying these concepts to individuals, the nurse leader must now apply them so that they are useful to the unique requirements of group functioning. This is accomplished in some specific ways, as are summarized in Table 22-2.

GROUP BOUNDARIES

Boundaries refer to the definition of structure surrounding tasks, group norms, roles, and time. In working with groups, boundaries between people also must be defined clearly. Not only must members' responsibilities to self and others be clarified, but their obligation to task accomplishment must also be defined. In other words, guidance ought to be given to help group members understand how to work together to accomplish a specific task.

In expanding the concept of boundary to group work, location must be added. Previously the concept of spatial boundaries was identified as the inpatient unit. In group work, an area must be defined as the specific location for the group to do its work. As noted by Yalom (1985), an externally imposed structure is the first step to the internal structure needed by the frightened, confused, and disorganized inpatient. Therefore the group leader needs to

provide clear spatial boundaries for the group. The ideal space is a comfortable room with a door that can be closed when the group session begins and opened when the session ends. This not only provides privacy for the group, but also serves as a visual reminder of structure. Everyone in the group should be able to see each other (a further expansion of the therapeutic relationship); chairs should be arranged in a circle. This structure will serve to promote the task of interaction in the group. If the clients cannot see each other, they will tend to speak only to the nurse (Yalom, 1985). The space should be consistent from session to session. Group size is also a consideration. The ideal number for an inpatient process group is 6 to 10 clients (Yalom, 1985). This number allows for enough interactional material for processing yet is small enough for all members to interact.

Linked to the concept of spatial boundary is the temporal or time boundary. The group needs a definite time to begin and to end its work. The best way for this to occur is for the leader to model promptness. The leader should be in the room, ready to begin work at the appointed time. It is also the leader's responsibility to ensure that the group meets its tasks within the appointed time frame and ends on time. The leader must recognize that the effective life span of the group is one group session long. Because of the rapidly changing membership, it is unlikely that the same group members will ever meet twice; therefore the leader must provide a beginning, middle, and ending structure to every group session.

Perhaps the greatest opportunity for the leader to define group structure and boundaries is in the introductory comments to the group. As in developing a therapeutic relationship with an individual, the introduction serves to clarify:

The role of the nurse
The role of the client
The tasks of the group
The ways to accomplish these tasks
The time frame for accomplishing these tasks

An example of such an introduction follows (Yalom, 1985).

Orientation to names	"Hello, I'm Mary Webster, and this is the daily therapy group. We meet in this room every
Defining spatial and time boundaries	day for 1 hour, from 10 AM to 11 AM. I'll keep track of the time and make sure we end on
Defining a leadership function	time."
Task definition	"The purpose of this group is to help members understand their problems better and to
Limits of work defined	learn more about the way they communicate with others. I know there are many different
	reasons why people come into the hospital, and you may not want to talk about some of
	these reasons in a group."
Restating task	"But one thing almost all of the people here have in common is some unhappiness in their
	relationships with people who are important to them. What groups do better than any
	other form of therapy is help people understand more about their relationships with
	others."

Tasks definition (and method to accomplish)	"One of the ways we'll work on this task is to look at relationships that may go on between people in this room. We're not very different inside the hospital than we are outside of it, so the better we can understand relationships that happen here, the better we'll understand the important relationships outside the hospital."
Information boundary addressed Confidentiality issue to promote safety	"You'll be learning a lot about yourself and other people while you're in the group. It's very natural to want to share what you learn with your family and friends, but confidentiality is of utmost importance. We ask you to pass on the valuable information but to keep the names of the people or other identifying information confidential. This information is only for group members and staff."
Consistent explicit sequence (provides for method to accomplish task)	"As I mentioned before, the group lasts 1 hour. We start by going around the group and asking each member to say something about the kinds of problems he or she is having and would like to work on in group. Then we talk about as many of those as possible. We save the last 10 minutes or so, to check in on everybody again, about how everybody feels and what kind of work we saw happening, and to finish up any leftover business."

This type of structured and consistent introduction serves many purposes:

It provides an orientation to new members as to the purpose and sequence of the group, thus relieving some anxiety.

It facilitates the transfer of norms from one meeting to the next, even in the absence of returning members

It defines the work of the group (i.e., relating to others) in relevant terms.

It sets limits (i.e., not every problem is appropriate for group discussion).

It defines the role of the nurse implicitly as the one with the sense of group tasks and appropriateness, and explicitly, as timekeeper and organizer.

The introduction alone, however, will not meet all of the boundary issues. The group leader must actively continue to work to shore up the boundaries and structures of the group, throughout the meeting, by using an active, focused style of leadership that promotes task accomplishment. Yalom (1985) has suggested that clients are reassured by a leader who is firm, explicit, and decisive, and who also shares the reasons for his or her actions.

Thus the leader of an inpatient group will actively identify group themes, focus discussion on learning from relationships within the group, share his or her ambivalence and thinking about difficult decisions he or she makes within the group, and maintain a consistent order to the group. His or her choice of actions, directions, and words are consistent with the goal of furthering learning about relationships.

Safety and Trust

Safety has been defined in terms of knowing what is expected of oneself in a given situation. As has been mentioned earlier, in group situations this concept must be expanded to knowing what is expected in relationship to others. In this example, it is expected that group members explore their relationships with each other to understand their outside relationships better. Recognizing that psychiatric clients may have tumultuous relationships with others, the group leader strives to maintain a safe and supportive environment in which to do the work. In group work, as in other forms of the therapeutic relationship, safety is developed when the nurse demonstrates a personal acceptance or valuing of each member, treats each member with respect, and empathizes with each one's situation as much as possible within the boundary context. The nurse works to reinforce the client's strengths and encourages higher-level behavior (Yalom, 1985). The nurse models these safety-promoting behaviors by acknowledging each client's contributions openly to the group and by taking each client seriously. These tasks are often accomplished by providing a framework for the group to understand the client's behavior, discouraging self-defeating behavior before anger builds in the group, and acknowledging at some point each client's contribution to the group. The nurse must actively intervene if a client is being verbally attacked by another and use the opportunity to promote reflection on relationships appropriate to the group's goal. The leader consistently works to help the members meet their responsibilities to each other in a safe and nonthreatening manner.

FAMILY THERAPY
DEFINITION

Family therapy is a unique form of group therapy in that it deals with the most intimate of all groups, the family. Families are given the tasks of raising children within the expectations of the culture and of providing support and nurturance for its members. A well-functioning family is reflected in a collaborative power structure, an acceptance of the individuality of its members, mutual affection, and an ability to adapt to social change. Generally, families present for therapy when they are experiencing some difficulty in accomplishing these tasks. These difficulties frequently arise at times of transition for the family: births, deaths, marriage, changes in finances, illness, divorce, and the major growth transitions from childhood to adulthood.

The identified difficulty is generally expressed by one

member of the family experiencing symptoms. Most often, a child develops certain symptoms such as school failures, drug abuse, acting-out behavior, withdrawn or passive behavior, or sexual promiscuity. This behavior is usually of great concern to the parents, who initiate therapy. At times, however, the parents may be coerced into treatment by the various social systems with which the child interacts, such as schools, judicial organizations, and social welfare agencies. Often, these bodies will define the behavior as a problem and recommend therapy, even against parental wishes. Thus not everyone comes to family therapy willingly.

The child's behavior is usually seen as the child's problem by the parents, who assume that the family will become functional again once the child's problem is "fixed." Thus the child is seen as the **identified client** (i.e., the one whose behavior is causing the problem). Occasionally, an adult is the identified client. For example, the problem may be seen as the mother's drinking or the father's absenteeism, and the family belief is that once this behavior (or person) is "fixed," the family will be fine.

THEORETIC PERSPECTIVE

Family therapists view the behavior of the identified client as merely relaying a message about the overall functioning of the family in general. Instead of seeing the "identified client" as the cause of the family's distress, the family therapist sees that person more as the "symptom carrier" for the family. The process of family therapy is geared toward the family as a whole rather than toward any individual member.

Family therapy is based on systems theory. A family is seen as a system that will strive to maintain homeostasis or balance. Consequently, even if the identified client's behavior were to change, systems theory predicts that another symptom would develop in another member in an attempt to maintain the previous balance of a dysfunctional system. A dysfunctional system cannot tolerate health in one member; the entire system must be made functional in order to restore health.

GOALS

The goal of family therapy is to relieve the family's pain and to promote functional nurturing of its members. Satir (1972) has identified four areas that cause a family to be troubled. These areas are the following:

> Self-worth or the feelings and ideas one has about oneself
> Communication styles in the family, which can be indirect, vague, and dishonest
> The rules the family uses to define behavior, as well as the way the rules are negotiated
> The links to society (the way the family relates to institutions outside the family)

The goals of family therapy, therefore, are the following (Satir, 1972):

> To foster higher self-worth in family members
> To promote communication that is direct, clear, specific, and honest
> To create rules that are flexible, humane, and responsive to varying needs
> To link with society in a way that is open and hopeful

SETTINGS

Family therapy can be conducted in a variety of settings. It most often occurs in a nurse's office in a structured, formal outpatient setting. Families can be seen in the hospital as well, when the "identified client" is admitted. It is difficult to complete the work of family therapy on an inpatient basis, however, and arrangements must be made for follow-up family therapy after discharge.

One of the most valuable settings from the nurse's point of view is the home. The home provides the nurse with much information about the family's unique interactive style. For example, the use of space, the objects valued, and the interaction within the home (as opposed to the office) may reveal a great deal about the family dynamics. A family can be seen as a single unit, or groups of families can be seen together, which is called *multiple family therapy*, in which four or five families meet weekly with a nurse to discuss common issues. This form of therapy works well with families dealing with isolation and lack of familial or community support. Several couples can also be seen at a time in couples therapy to work on ways to strengthen the marital relationship.

BASIC CONCEPTS OF FAMILY THERAPY

As noted earlier, the family is a special kind of group. It has defined tasks, roles for its members, norms, and communication patterns. As with other groups, difficulties arise when any one of these aspects is jeopardized in some way. Nurses working as family therapists assess several areas of family functioning.

Role Confusion

According to the traditional concept of family roles, the parents form the primal unit. They are the authority figures in the family, making rules for behavior and decisions for family survival. The parents are seen as a unit. Children are seen as dependents and are given less authority in decision making. As the children grow in age, judgment, and decision-making ability, they are granted more independence and participation in the decision-making process. At times, family members may not be able to fulfill their roles properly, and dysfunctional patterns occur. Examples of role confusion follow:

• A parent dies, and the oldest same-sex child takes over the role functions of the deceased parent.

- A child becomes ill, and in an attempt to support the child, the family revolves around the desires of the ill child—in effect making the child the central authority figure.
- A couple is unhappy with their relationship, and each forms a strong alliance with one of the children, thus negating the spousal unit as the primary unit of the family.

Nurses working with a family evaluate how the family enacts their various roles and the effects this enactment has on the members.

Task Confusion

The family's tasks are to raise children and provide support and nurturance for its members. This is not always easy to accomplish. As noted earlier, families experience stress at times of transition because of a family's uncertainty about how to perform its tasks during transition points. Examples of this are the following:

- The birth of a new child. The family struggles to adjust to meeting the needs of the baby while continuing to meet the needs of other family members.
- The transition of a child to a teenager. The family must allow increasing separation and individuation and support the growing person in his or her new tasks.
- The geographic move of a family. The family task is to link to the resources of the community, but the family finds it difficult to locate these resources in a new community.

The nurse will assess the family's ability to meet its tasks and identify areas of difficulty.

Communication

Communication, both verbal and nonverbal, is the way family members develop trust and love and nurture one another. To do this, both verbal and nonverbal messages must match (see Chapter 8). Family members develop unique ways of communicating with each other as a way of establishing family norms, accomplishing tasks, and enforcing roles. These patterns generally become firmly established, and grown children often continue to use patterns learned in their family of origin.

Nurses examine the communication patterns of the family in several ways. A basic question to answer is: "Who has the right to say what to whom and in what situation?" This question addresses the issues of authority, family position, and content (i.e., what is talked about and what is not). For instance, can the child question a rule laid out by the parent? Can the husband and wife voice their differing opinions? Can they do so in front of the children? Is there a "family secret" that no one discusses?

Nurses also analyze the family's "double messages" or messages that conflict on the verbal and nonverbal levels. The nurse may ask: Does the family express one value verbally but act in ways that discourage the purported value? For example, does the family say that it wants to hear what a member has to say, but then go on to interrupt, become angry, or pay no attention when that member is speaking? Do the parents say they are open to negotiating family rules but then discount every option suggested? The nurse thus seeks to discern patterns in communication that make it difficult for the family to accomplish its tasks.

THERAPEUTIC PROCESS

Although the family is usually seen in therapy as a unit, occasionally the nurse may wish to work with one member on a particular issue, or perhaps meet with the couple to strengthen their bond. This is consistent with the systems theory viewpoint that a change in one part of the system will precipitate other changes. The overall goal, however, is to decrease the family's pain and increase its abilities to perform its tasks. Because communication is the link between all family members and the family's ability to perform its tasks, attention is always paid to the communication pattern of the family with the goal of changing the family system of interaction (Yalom, 1985).

In general, the process begins when the family makes contact with the nurse. It is important to note which family member makes the actual contact, since this may be the most motivated member. The family usually presents in disarray, its members frequently demoralized, frustrated, and angry. They have tried every solution they can think of but continue to have problems, so they must seek assistance either by their own choice or as prompted by the school or the judicial systems.

Initial meetings are often chaotic as the family demonstrates their way of "being" to the nurse. They frequently demonstrate their mixed messages and confusion; feelings of helplessness and loss of control are common.

The nurse seeks to focus the family's disorganized energy and information toward manageable tasks. Goals for therapy are set by family members. The nurse listens to all of the family members in addition to watching their interactions in order to determine the structure and dynamics of the family situation. Nurses consider the family's presenting problems when making assessments to help the family clarify issues. Problems related to roles, tasks, and norms are discussed, with the nurse providing a perspective that the family may lack. Frequently the nurse will educate the family on functional communication patterns. The nurse will assist the family with communication within the session and may assign "homework" for them to further their practice. Patterns of communication are identified and evaluated as to their usefulness.

The family is frequently encouraged to make changes in its routine. For example, if a family is always together, they may be encouraged to interact with the community more. Such an expansion of their social network would serve to decrease their overdependence on each other and provide other outlets for their individuation. On the other hand, if a family is rarely together, its members may be encouraged to spend an evening together for the sake of learning how to support each other and to communicate needed information.

As in other therapeutic relationships, the nurse must be seen as caring and responsive to the needs of the client. In this case the client is a family, and consequently the nurse must be careful to be responsive to each family member and not fall into an alliance or conspiracy with one member over another.

Summary of Key Concepts

1. The nurse in the therapeutic relationship acts as a resource person, counselor, surrogate, and technical expert for the client.
2. To be an effective counselor, a nurse must continually assess his or her own personal values and attitudes.
3. The basic concepts a nurse must develop in each therapeutic relationship are boundary development and maintenance, safety development, and trust development.
4. The orientation phase of the relationship serves to define the client's issue or conflict, the goal of the work, and the relationship between the client and the nurse.
5. In the working phase, the nurse demonstrates understanding of the client's problem and assists the client in finding beneficial coping actions.
6. The termination phase involves helping the client to acknowledge gains already made and progress yet to be made.
7. The basic purpose of milieu therapy is to facilitate clients to become active, not passive, participants in their lives.
8. Group therapy allows clients to define themselves through human interaction and task accomplishment.
9. Family therapy promotes the health and functionality of the whole family system.

REFERENCES

Brammer LM: *The helping relationship: process and skills,* Boston, 1993, Allyn & Bacon.

Cartwright D: The nature of group cohesiveness. In Cartwright D, Zander A, editors: *Group dynamics: research and theory,* ed 3, New York, 1968, Harper & Row.

Corey G: *Becoming a helper,* Pacific Grove, Calif, 1989, Brooks/Cole Publishing.

Corey G: *Case approach to counseling and psychotherapy,* ed 3, Pacific Grove, Calif, 1991, Brooks/Cole.

Corey G: *Theory and practice of group counseling,* ed 3, Pacific Grove, Calif, 1990, Brooks/Cole.

Cosgray E et al: A day in the life of an inpatient: an experiential game to promote empathy for individuals in a psychiatric hospital, *Arch Psychiatr Nurs* 6:6, 1990.

Denton PL: *Psychiatric occupations therapy: a workbook of practical skills,* New York, 1987, Little, Brown.

Fortinash KM, Holoday-Worret PA: *Psychiatric nursing care plans,* ed 3, St. Louis, 1999, Mosby.

Herz MI: The therapeutic milieu: a necessity, *Int J Psychiatry* 7:209, 1969.

Hogarth C: Families and family therapy. In Johnson B, editor: *Psychiatric mental health nursing: adaptation and growth,* ed 3, Philadelphia, 1993,

Jones M: *The therapeutic community,* New York, 1953, Basic Books.

Kennedy E: *On becoming a counselor,* New York, 1977, Seabury Press.

Northouse P, Northouse L: *Health communication: strategies for health professionals,* Norwalk, Conn., 1992, Appleton & Lange.

Peplau HE: *Interpersonal relations in nursing,* New York, 1952, GP Putnam's Sons.

Sadock BJ: Group psychotherapy, combined psychotherapy and psychodrama. In Kaplan HL, Sadock BJ, editors: *Comprehensive textbook of psychiatry,* ed 6, Baltimore, 1995, Williams & Wilkins.

Sampson E, Marthas M: *Group process for the health professions,* New York, 1990, Delmar.

Satir V: *Peoplemaking,* Palo Alto, Calif. 1972, Science & Behavior Books.

Sayre J: Common errors in communication made by students in psychiatric nursing, *Perspect Psychiatr Care* 5:175, 1978.

Yalom ID: *The theory and practice of group psychotherapy,* ed 3 New York, 1985, Basic Books.

INTERNET SOURCES

Internet Mental Health, *http://www.mentalhealth.com/copy/html*

Mental Health InfoSource, *http://www.mhsource.com/edu/index.html*

PsychPro Online, *http://www.onlinepsych.com*

Notes

CHAPTER 23

Psychopharmacology and Other Biologic Therapies

Jay Sherr

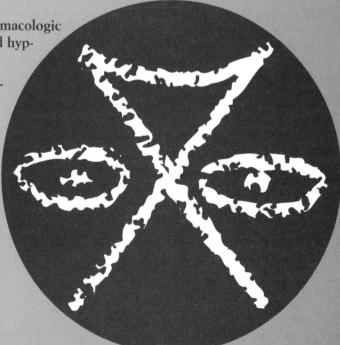

OBJECTIVES

- Describe and discuss the pharmacologic issues related to antipsychotic medication therapy.

- Describe and discuss the pharmacologic issues related to antidepressant medication therapy.

- Describe and discuss the pharmacologic issues related to mood stabilization therapy.

- Describe and discuss the pharmacologic issues related to anxiolytic and hypnotic medication therapy.

- Describe and discuss the pharmacologic issues related to stimulant medication therapy.

- Explain nonpharmacologic modalities related to the treatment of individuals with mood disorders.

- Explain the nursing issues related to psychopharmacology and nonpharmacologic treatment modalities.

Earliest historical records tell of major mental illnesses that disrupted lives and often went untreated. In fact, truly effective treatments have been available only since the mid-twentieth century. The impact of effective pharmacologic treatment has been striking.

Before the advent of chlorpromazine and thioridazine in the 1950s, the permanent inpatient population in mental institutions in the United States was approximately 500,000. These individuals had thought disorders so severe that they could not reside outside of a structured institutional setting. With the advent of pharmacologic interventions, the number of hospitalized clients was dramatically reduced to about 200,000 within 10 years. This decrease demonstrated the effectiveness of antipsychotic medications. Sadly, it also demonstrated that efficacy varied greatly from client to client. Millions continued to suffer from mental disorders that included psychotic symptoms, mood, anxiety, and other related disorders.

PSYCHOPHARMA-COLOGY
MODE AND MECHANISM

Even when most effective, medications for major mental disorders primarily treat symptoms but have little or no effect on the underlying pathophysiology. All drugs have both a *mode* and a *mechanism of action*. The mode of action describes what the drug does to the body, whereas the mechanism of action is defined specifically by how the drug works to affect symptoms, cure disease, or cause **side effects,** the undesired, nontherapeutic, and often predictable consequences of medication that frequently diminish with time. Often, much is understood about the mode of action for psychoactive drugs, but the mechanism of action is frequently unclear. For example, it is known that lithium affects nor-

Agranulocytosis A drop in the production of leukocytes, specifically the neutrophil cell line, leaving the body defenseless against bacterial infection.

Akathisia Literally, "not sitting." A syndrome caused by dopamine-blocking drugs, characterized by both motor restlessness and a subjective feeling of inner restlessness.

Anticholinergic delirium Toxic effects of anticholinergic drugs characterized by confusion, perceptive disturbances, sleep disturbance, increased or decreased psychomotor activity, and change in level of consciousness. Also called atropine psychosis, this syndrome may present as a psychotic state.

Extrapyramidal symptom (EPS) The collective term used to describe the motor side effect of dopamine-blocking medications. EPS includes acute dystonia, akathisia, parkinsonism, and tardive dyskinesia.

Metabolite The result of biotransformation of a drug.

Neuroleptic Literally, "to clasp the neuron," the term used to describe what are now called the typical antipsychotic medications.

Neuroleptic malignant syndrome (NMS) A rare but potentially lethal toxic reaction to dopamine-blocking drugs that presents with a constellation of symptoms, including fever, autonomic instability, increased muscular rigidity, and altered mental status.

Novel Term used interchangeably with *atypical* when referring to antipsychotic medications.

Psychotropic Literally, "mind nutrition," the term used to describe drugs that affect the central nervous system.

Refractory Failure to favorably respond to two antipsychotic medications of different classes.

Serum level monitoring The process of obtaining blood samples to determine drug concentration.

Side effect An undesired nontherapeutic and often predictable consequence of medication. Frequently diminishes with time. Contrast with *adverse drug reaction.*

Sustained release Medications designed to provide slow, controlled dissolution that allows longer dosing intervals.

Tardive dyskinesia (TD) A syndrome of abnormal involuntary movements occurring after months or years of treatment with drugs that block dopamine type 2 receptors. Often described as oral, buccal, and lingual masticatory movements, they can occur throughout the body.

Titration Incremental adjustment of dose to allow for tolerance of side effects.

Traditional Term used interchangeably with *typical,* when referring to antipsychotic medications.

adrenergic, serotonergic, and dopaminergic neuronal systems, but this knowledge does not specifically define how lithium helps control manic behavior.

The mode and mechanism of actions on multiple systems contribute to a wide variety of side effects that can be substantial and, in some cases, life threatening. The ideal drug would be specific and curative, convenient and economical, and have minimal side effects. Since the ideal drug does not yet exist, the process of pharmacologic treatment is always one of compromise. A goal of psychopharmacologic treatment is to provide maximum efficacy (efficiency) and minimum toxicity in a form that the client is willing and able to take and can afford.

PSYCHOTROPIC PHARMACOTHERAPY ASSESSMENT

Psychotropic literally means "mind nutrition." It is used to describe drugs that affect the central nervous system. The safe and effective use of psychotropic pharmacotherapy (use of drugs that affect the central nervous system) depends on an accurate assessment of the client's condition. In addition to taking into account both psychiatric and somatic diagnoses, a continually updated problem assessment before administration of medication includes answering these questions:

> What is the etiology of current symptoms?
> How severe is the problem?
> Why now?

Etiology is important because identification of the origins of a problem can lead to focused treatment of potentially correctable causes. For example, electrolyte imbalances or hyperthyroidism may underlie psychotic behavior. Also, understanding symptom severity guides one to decisions regarding rapidity of treatment. For example, nurses may need to decide the route of administration based on how imminent of a risk a client's current behavior presents.

A client's symptoms must always be assessed in the context of "why now?" For example, a client who has been treated for several days with an antipsychotic medication may develop increasing psychomotor agitation. The clinician needs to assess if this is due to worsening psychosis, perhaps implying additional medication, or if the client is developing akathisia. Optimal use of medications carefully considers not only the diagnosis, presenting signs and symptoms, and the specific drug used but also the context of administration.

When assessing clients before or during pharmacotherapy, it is necessary to incorporate information from both drug-related and client-related variables before initiating interventions. Common drug- and client-related variables are described in Box 23-1. Drug-related variables include pharmacologic characteristics of available dosage forms. Client-related variables include those factors about

---

Box 23-1   **Variables Affecting Drug Therapy**

Drug-Related Variables
Mode/mechanism of action
Available dosage forms—oral (solid, liquid, sublingual), parenteral
Bioavailability of various formulations
Onset, peak, and duration of action
Serum half-life
Method of elimination from the body (hepatic or renal)
Side effects/toxicities (both predictable and idiosyncratic)
Cost (drug price, administration, and monitoring costs)

Client-Related Variables
Diagnosis
Other disease states (cardiovascular, liver, renal disease)
Age
Weight
Anticholinergic susceptibility
History of side effects
Previous response
Family history of response
Willingness to comply/insight into illness
Financial and/or health insurance
Support systems

---

the individual that may facilitate, hinder, or interact with medication therapy. Correlation of drug- and client-related variables promotes optimization of therapy for an individual client. The success of psychopharmacologic therapy depends on (1) the optimal integration of the anticipated medication effects with the client's personal, physical, and psychosocial dimensions and (2) the nurse's assessment of the client's response to psychopharmacologic therapy and the communication of these data to the prescriber.

ANTIPSYCHOTICS

Major advances in science are often perceived as the result of coincidence or chance. What really occurs is that an individual with a prepared mind and a willingness for hard work observes something new and unusual. Rather than discarding what does not quite fit the norm, the well-trained observer wonders about the nature of such phenomena and investigates further. Chlorpromazine was discovered in this manner, when Henri Laborit, a French neurosurgeon, was searching for medications to decrease anxiety in preoperative clients. He noted that chlorpromazine caused a "beatific quietude" and recommended it to his psychiatric colleagues for use with agitated clients. In 1951 Delay and Deniker began to use chlorpromazine and observed that their psychiatric clients became more manageable (Deniker, 1990). They also quickly noted side ef-

Table 23-1	Antipsychotic Medications*			
Generic Name	**Trade Name**	**Potency†**	**Usual Dose (mg)**	**Comments**
Traditional (Typical) Agents				
Phenothiazines				
Aliphatic				
Chlorpromazine	Thorazine	100	60-2000	IM is painful
Piperazines				
Acetophenazine	Tindal	25	60-300	Tablets only
Fluphenazine	Prolixin	2	2-40	Available as immediate-release injectable and as 25 mg/ml decanoate
Perphenazine	Trilafon	10	8-64	
Prochlorperazine	Compazine	15	15-150	
Trifluoperazine	Stelazine	5	2-80	
Piperidines				
Mesoridazine	Serentil	50	50-500	
Thioridazine	Mellaril	100	50-800	No injectable form
Thioxanthenes				
Chlorprothixene	Taractan	100	100-1600	
Thiothixene	Navane	4	5-60	
Butyrophenone				
Haloperidol	Haldol	2	1-100	Available as immediate-release injectable and as 50 mg/ml and 100 mg/ml decanoate
Dibenzoxapine				
Loxapine	Loxitane	10	20-250	
Dihydroindolone				
Molindone	Moban	10	15-225	No injectable form
Novel (Atypical) Antipsychotics				
Dibenzodiazepines				
Clozapine	Clozaril	100	50-900	Tablets only
Quetiapine	Seroquel	100	100-800	Tablets only
Thienobenzodiazepine				
Olanzapine	Zyprexa	4	5-30	Tablets only
Benzisoxazole				
Risperidone	Risperdal	1	4-8	Tablets and concentrate
Imidazolidinone				
Sertindole	Serlect	3	12-24	

*All are available as tablet or capsule, liquid, and parenteral except as noted.
†Expressed as chlorpromazine equivalents for traditional and relative dosage potency for novel agents.

fects that reminded them of Parkinson's disease, a motor disorder known to affect motor neurons. Thus they coined the term **neuroleptic,** from the Greek, meaning "to clasp the neuron." In 1954 chlorpromazine (Thorazine) became the first effective antipsychotic available in the United States. Current antipsychotic medications available in the United States are listed in Table 23-1.

Antipsychotics can be divided into two basic types: typical, or **traditional,** and atypical, or **novel.** Since the introduction of chlorpromazine, no antipsychotic was demonstrated to be more effective than any other until the introduction of clozapine (Clozaril) in 1989. Until then, it was the side effect profile that distinguished differences among what are now called typical or traditional antipsychotics (e.g., haloperidol [Haldol]. Atypical antipsychotics (e.g., clozapine and risperidone [Risperdal]) are characterized by an improved response of negative symptoms, less deleterious effects on cognition, and a reduced propensity toward extrapyramidal side effects.

INDICATIONS

Antipsychotics (once called major tranquilizers) are effective in treating the symptoms of psychosis. Clients with schizophrenia, schizophreniform disorder, schizoaffective disorder, and delusional disorder may benefit from antipsychotic medications. Exacerbations of psychosis and hospitalizations may be prevented with continued medication use. Psychosis from secondary causes, such as electrolyte or hormonal imbalances, drug abuse, brain tumors, mania, or depression with psychotic features, may also benefit from short-term antipsychotic treatment while the underlying disorder is being treated.

The symptoms of psychosis are varied but have been organized into three domains: positive, negative, and cognitive (see Chapter 14). Positive symptoms are associated with increased mental and physical activity. Negative symptoms are related to decreased mental and physical activity. Cognitive symptoms result in difficulties in organizing thoughts, in learning, and in executive functions.

GOALS OF THERAPY

Antipsychotic medications are used to decrease psychotic signs and symptoms, including hallucinations, delusions, and feelings of paranoia. In assessing clients' symptoms at baseline and throughout treatment, it is important to document specific behaviors that demonstrate psychotic symptoms.

The overall goal in treatment of a psychotic client is to return control to the individual. Since these are powerful drugs, it is important to remain sensitive to the potential for their use in controlling the client. Overmedication places control of the individual in the hands of the clinician. Thus the goal of returning control to the individual is achieved through monitoring specific psychotic symptoms and improvement in the client's ability to provide self-care.

MODE OF ACTION

All known antipsychotics are dopamine receptor blockers. The drug occupies the dopamine receptor on the postsynaptic neuron and blocks endogenous dopamine from having its effect. Traditional antipsychotic potency has been related to its dopamine$_2$ receptor affinity. The dopamine$_2$ receptors are confined primarily to four major areas of the brain: the mesolimbic cortical, nigrostriatal, and tuberoinfundibular pathways. Dopamine receptor blockade in these different areas has very different effects. The mesolimbic pathway projecting from the mesencephalon to the anterior limbic brain is believed to play a major role in positive psychotic signs and symptoms. Dopamine recep-

tor blockade in this area, which may contain excess dopamine during psychosis, would relieve positive symptoms. A reduced level of dopamine in mesocortical pathways is thought to contribute to negative signs and symptoms of schizophrenic disorders. Blockade of dopamine receptors in this area would then potentially make negative symptoms worse (Davis et al, 1991).

Dopamine$_2$ receptor blockade is also responsible for many of the side effects of antipsychotics. The nigrostriatal pathway begins in the substantia nigra and ascends to the caudate nucleus and putamen in the extrapyramidal system. Blockade in the nigrostriatal tracts causes neuroleptic-induced pseudoparkinsonism (bradykinesia, stiffness, and tremor) and dystonic reactions (muscle spasms of the tongue, jaw, eyes, and neck). Akathisia and tardive dyskinesia appear to be related to dopamine$_2$ receptor blockade. These phenomena, collectively known as extrapyramidal symptom (EPS) are discussed in detail later in the chapter. The tuberoinfundibular pathway extends from the arcuate nucleus and terminates on the median eminence. These tracts mediate hypothalamic control of endocrine function. Dopamine blockade in this area causes increases in prolactin, resulting in gynecomastia and galactorrhea (breast development and milk expression, respectively).

Novel (atypical) antipsychotics also block dopamine receptors. In addition, currently available novel antipsychotics block serotonin to a greater degree than dopamine. The improved response of negative symptoms, improved cognitive functioning, and reduced EPS seen with the novel drugs may be related to this serotonin blockade.

Antipsychotic drugs vary greatly in their affinity for other receptors, resulting in additional side effects secondary to receptor blockade. Histamine (H$_1$) blockade causes sedation, cholinergic blockade causes anticholinergic side effects, and α-blockade causes hypotension and reflex tachycardia. Side effects caused by receptor blockade and the antipsychotic medications are listed in Table 23-2.

Thus it is important to understand the receptor-specific characteristics of the different medications, because these characteristics can help predict both the efficacy and side effects likely to be observed.

CLINICAL USE AND EFFICACY

Although they are important and effective medications, antipsychotics are also the most toxic drugs used in psychiatry. The lowest possible effective dose should be used for the shortest amount of time.

Target symptom response varies with time. Positive symptoms are the most responsive. Symptoms such as combativeness, hostility, psychomotor agitation, and irritability are often relieved within hours. Affective symptoms, anxiety, tension, depression, inappropriate affect, reduced attention span, and social withdrawal may take 2 to 4 weeks to respond. Cognitive and perceptive symptoms such as hallucinations, delusions, and thought broadcast-

Table 23-2	Side Effects Associated With Receptor Blockade			
Dopamine$_2$	Histamine$_1$	Cholinergic	Alpha$_1$	Serotonin$_2$
Extrapyramidal symptoms (EPS) Prolactin	Sedation Weight gain	Dry mouth Blurred vision Sinus tachycardia Constipation Impaired memory/cognition	Orthostatic hypotension Reflex tachycardia	Weight gain GI upset Sexual dysfunction

ing may take 2 to 8 weeks to respond. The most negative symptoms—poor social skills, unrealistic planning, poor judgment and insight—respond the slowest and the least. Many clients have fixed hallucinations and delusions that respond minimally to medications. Given the varied time course of different symptoms, it should be kept in mind that increases in medication dose will not hasten the relief of slow-responding symptoms.

Antipsychotic therapy may be started using divided doses, three or four times a day. This is a useful approach in determining a client's ability to tolerate a medication and to minimize the initial impact of side effects. Once an effective total daily dose has been established and the client has had time to develop tolerance to side effects, the medication is often reduced to once or twice a day. Reduced frequency of administration increases the likelihood of compliance with the regimen.

In general, antipsychotics are well absorbed from the gastrointestinal (GI) tract. They are extensively metabolized in the liver. The half-life varies highly among individuals but is usually between 20 and 40 hours in adults, with steady state being reached in 4 to 7 days. **Serum level monitoring,** obtaining blood samples to determine drug concentration, is not routinely useful. Serum level monitoring may be revealing in specific situations, including lack of response to normal doses after 6 weeks, severe or unusual adverse reactions, clients taking multiple medications, the physically ill, and as a check for compliance.

MEDICATION FORMS
Liquid
Most antipsychotic medications are available in liquid form. One of the most troubling symptoms of psychotic disorders is lack of insight. A client who believes that he or she is not sick will have little motivation to take medication and may be resistive to drug treatment. Such clients may "cheek" tablets or capsules in efforts to avoid medication. Liquid concentrates may be given at the initiation of therapy to help ensure compliance.

Injectable
Acute situations.   Immediate-release injectable forms of antipsychotic medications are available for psychiatric emergencies. Single intramuscular (IM) injections can of-

ten be rapidly effective for clients who present an imminent danger to self or others but refuse oral (PO) medication. Rarely, repeated injection every hour until the client is calm, a technique called rapid tranquilization, is used. This technique is associated with increased risk of acute dystonic reactions and neuroleptic malignant syndrome (NMS) (a potentially lethal toxic reaction to dopamine-blocking drugs) and therefore must be used judiciously. The simultaneous use of a benzodiazepine may help clients regain control more quickly. Haloperidol and lorazepam (Ativan), in combination, have been used for this purpose (Battaglia et al, 1992).

Chronic situations.   In the United States two antipsychotic drugs are available as long-acting injections. These sustained-release drugs may increase overall compliance and are useful in clients who are reluctant to take medications every day (Glazer and Kane, 1992). Haloperidol decanoate (Haldol Decanoate 50 and Haldol Decanoate 100) and fluphenazine decanoate (Prolixin Decanoate) are commonly given as monthly or biweekly injections, respectively. By linking the active drug molecule to a decanoate chain and dissolving it in sesame oil, a slow release of medication is achieved when given a deep IM injection. The half-lives of haloperidol decanoate and fluphenazine decanoate are approximately 21 days and 14 days, respectively.

An important consideration in the use of the decanoate injections is monitoring these medications in an outpatient setting. Conversions from oral to injectable doses are always approximations, since the exact degree of bioavailability varies substantially among clients. The long half-life of these drugs results in steady-state serum levels not being obtained until 2 to 3 months after injections are initiated. Thus loss of efficacy or increases in side effects can develop over time as serum levels fall or rise toward steady state. Clients need to be educated about this and encouraged to report any problems to their physicians. Clients also need to be examined for local irritation and sterile abscess at the injection sites, which can result from repeated injections.

TOXICITY OF TYPICAL ANTIPSYCHOTICS
The side effect profile differentiates typical antipsychotic drugs. The low-potency drugs are more likely to cause se-

dation and hypotension, whereas the high-potency drugs tend to cause more EPS. These drugs vary greatly in the amount of anticholinergic side effects they cause. The severity of these effects—dry mouth, blurred vision, tachycardia, urinary retention, constipation, and disorientation/delirium—vary greatly among individuals. Note that the drugs more likely to cause EPS have less anticholinergic side effects; those drugs with the most anticholinergic effects have relatively less EPS. EPS is often treated with adjunctive anticholinergic drugs. Therefore it is likely that the relatively reduced EPS caused by the low-potency drugs is due to the anticholinergic profile of the low-potency drugs.

EXTRAPYRAMIDAL SIDE EFFECTS

The dopamine blockade of antipsychotics can cause a variety of movement-related side effects collectively known as **extrapyramidal symptom (EPS)**. These side effects are troublesome to clients and are a major cause of noncompliance. EPS presents as acute dystonia, neuroleptic-induced pseudoparkinsonism, akathisia, and tardive dyskinesia. The unifying factor in the presentation of these side effects is disruption of normal motor activity.

Acute Dystonia

Acute dystonia is muscular spasm that may occur in up to 10% of clients. Taking the client by surprise, this painful and often frightening reaction may affect different muscle groups. Symptoms may present as blepharospasm (eye closing), torticollis (neck muscle contraction pulling the head to the side), oculogyric crisis (severe upward deviation of the eyeballs), and/or opisthotonos (severe dorsal arching of the neck and back). Severe presentations involving the tongue and/or laryngospasm can result in dysphagia (difficult swallowing) and jeopardize the airway.

Fortunately, anticholinergic drugs are rapidly effective. Mild presentations may be treated with oral anticholinergic drugs. Severe, painful presentations will benefit from the rapid onset of IM treatment. Benztropine (Cogentin) 2 mg IM and diphenhydramine (Benadryl) 50 mg IM are commonly used and may be repeated in 30 minutes if the symptoms have not resolved.

Neuroleptic-Induced Pseudoparkinsonism

Dopamine and acetylcholine exist in balance in the brain. Dopamine blockade in nigrostriatal pathways results in relative cholinergic predominance that produces clinical symptoms. Neuroleptic-induced pseudoparkinsonism presents with tremors, bradykinesia/akinesia (slowness, absence of movement), cogwheel rigidity (slow, regular muscular jerks), postural instability, hunched posturing, shuffling gait, loss of associated movements, masked facies (loss of mobility in the facial muscles), hypersalivation, and drooling. Pseudoparkinsonism affects as many as 15% of clients. Symptoms generally start 5 to 30 days after initiation of therapy.

Anticholinergic drugs or dopamine agonists are usual treatments for pseudoparkinsonism. Some of the same medications used to treat idiopathic parkinson's disease (degradation of dopamine neurons in the substantia nigra) are useful for relieving symptoms of neuroleptic-induced parkinsonism. Table 23-3 lists drugs ordinarily used as adjunctive treatments to counteract EPS. Anticholinergic medications are generally used initially, unless contraindicated. Acute-closure (sometimes called narrow-angle) glaucoma is an absolute contraindication.

Relative contraindications include dehydration, cardiac arrhythmias, and benign prostatic hypertrophy (BPH). Signs and symptoms of dehydration may be exacerbated by anticholinergic medications. Anticholinergics frequently increase the pulse rate. Clients with existing cardiac arrhythmias may be at increased risk as the heart rate increases. Clients with existing BPH may have increased difficulty initiating urine flow when treated with anticholinergics. Older clients and clients taking additional medications with anticholinergic effects must be monitored with particular diligence. Excess anticholinergic medication can result in urinary retention requiring catheterization; paralytic ileus; and memory problems with confusion, disorientation, and delirium

Table 23-3	Adjunctive Medications Used to Treat Extrapyramidal Side Effects			
Generic Name	Trade Name	Equivalent Dose (mg)	Dose Range (mg)	Dosage Forms (All Available as Tablets Unless Noted)
Anticholinergic				
Benztropine	Cogentin	1	1-8	Injectable
Trihexyphenidyl	Artane	2	2-15	Capsule-extended release, elixir
Antihistamine				
Diphenhydramine	Benadryl	50	50-400	Capsules, liquid, injectable
Dopamine Agonist				
Amantadine	Symmetrel	N/A	100-400	Capsule and liquid only

(that can resemble psychosis). The latter, sometimes called **anticholinergic delirium,** may present with a full spectrum of anticholinergic effects, including blurred vision, mydriasis, tachycardia, tachypnea, diminished bowel sounds, and mental status impairment. This syndrome remits with anticholinergic medication discontinuation but can be treated with a cholinergic agonist. When anticholinergics are contraindicated or not tolerated, dopamine agonists can be helpful. Amantadine (Symmetrel) is frequently used. Amantadine facilitates the release of dopamine and thus aids in the restoration of dopamine/acetylcholine balance. The risk in using dopamine agonists is that an excess of the medication can worsen the psychosis. This is seldom seen when amantadine doses are 200 mg/day or less. Amantadine is eliminated by the kidneys; therefore clients with renal dysfunction are at increased risk of accumulating amantadine and worsening their psychosis.

Clients should be counseled that in most cases anticholinergic side effects, whether from primary medications (e.g., high-dose, low-potency antipsychotics) or adjunctive medications (e.g., benztropine [Cogentin], trihexyphenadyl [Artane]) will diminish over several weeks. This gradual reduction of effect is called tolerance. Most clients develop substantial tolerance to the parkinsonian side effects of antipsychotic medications within 3 months. Thus trial reductions of adjunctive medications will simplify medication regimens, reduce the potential for drug interactions, and improve compliance.

Akathisia

Akathisia literally means "not sitting" and presents with subjective and objective components. The objective symptoms of akathisia, namely motor restlessness, pacing, rocking, and foot tapping, are common. Most clients with akathisia complain of inner restlessness described as tension, irritability, and the inability to sit still or lie down. However, clients with akathisia may not have or cannot verbalize these feelings of inner disquiet. Although some clinicians believe that virtually all clients receiving typical antipsychotics experience some form of akathisia, it clearly occurs in approximately 25% of those treated.

Differentiating between akathisia and the psychomotor agitation/irritability of worsening psychosis can be difficult. This differentiation is important because akathisia responds best to dose reduction. Misinterpretation of akathisia as psychomotor agitation or anxiety (secondary to psychosis) could result in increasing the dose of antipsychotic. This would result in worsening the akathisia. Conversely, worsening psychosis interpreted as akathisia could result in the inappropriate reduction of needed antipsychotic medication, resulting in continued or worsened symptoms, prolonged hospital stays, increased risks to clients and staff, and needless adjunctive medications. The nurse must assess the client thoroughly and report observations to the prescriber.

Akathisia may respond to a reduction of the antipsychotic medication. When this is not clinically practical—for instance, when psychotic symptoms are responding well—β-blockers and benzodiazepines are the most common adjunctive treatments (Adler et al, 1993; Dumon et al, 1992). β-Blockers may be the most effective adjunctive treatment; up to 160 mg daily of propranolol (Inderal) or 80 mg daily of nadolol (Corgard) has been found useful. The benzodiazepines are an alternative adjunct. Lorazepam (Ativan) 1 to 4 mg daily or clonazepam (Klonopin) 0.5 to 2 mg daily has shown benefit. Occasionally benztropine (Cogentin) may be beneficial at relatively high doses of up to 6 mg daily, but many clients cannot tolerate the high dose.

Tardive Dyskinesia

Tardive dyskinesia (TD) literally means late-occurring, abnormal movements. Although classically described as oral, buccal, lingual, and masticatory movements (tongue thrusting and writhing, lip pursing and smacking, facial grimaces and chewing movements), these choreoathetoid (rapid, jerky, and slow, writhing) movements may first occur anywhere in the body. Arm, finger, leg, feet, and truncal movements are often noted. Less commonly, involvement of muscles in the swallowing reflex or the diaphragm can lead to choking or respiratory compromise. The client is frequently unaware of the potentially irreversible movements.

The movements wax and wane over time. Thus family members and providers who spend a lot of time with clients are frequently the first to report abnormal movements. Although these abnormal involuntary movements are generally not seen before at least 6 months of antipsychotic treatment, they may be seen substantially earlier or after years of treatment. The overall incidence of TD appears in approximately 4% of clients taking antipsychotics.

Clients on a stable antipsychotic regimen who develop abnormal involuntary movements and then have their antipsychotic discontinued have about a 50% probability of having permanent abnormal movements. Clients who must remain on drug therapy are even more likely to have permanent abnormal movements.

Prevention of TD is important because there are no truly effective treatments for TD. Formal monitoring procedures should be performed at least every 6 months while the client is taking antipsychotics.

The pathophysiology of TD is only partially understood and involves complex interactions of multiple neurotransmitter systems. When these antipsychotic drugs block dopamine receptors, over time, the neurons manufacture more dopamine receptors, a process called upregulation or supersensitivity. If the drug is suddenly removed, increased numbers of dopamine receptors are exposed to endogenous dopamine, resulting in increased abnormal movements. Dose reduction can cause a temporary increase in severity of movements that gradually subside as neurons readjust to the absence of dopamine-blocking drugs.

Withdrawal dyskinesia presents as TD-like movements that occur with antipsychotic dose reduction. Typically these movements fully resolve in 2 weeks to 2 months. Withdrawal dyskinesia is most common and most severe in children. Conversely, increasing the dose of antipsychotic, and covering more dopamine receptors, will usually cause a reduction in abnormal involuntary movements. This strategy furthers the toxic process that originally brought about the movements and will eventually result in a return of the movements. Thus increasing the dose merely "masks" TD and is not an acceptable treatment. Benzodiazepines may be a useful treatment in TD, but response is usually temporary, lasting only several months. Some clients with severe TD have been treated with clozapine (Clozaril) with benefit (Tamminga et al, 1994).

Vitamin E has been used as a TD treatment at 800 to 1200 IU daily, but reductions in movements are inconsistent and modest at best. TD and novel antipsychotics are discussed later.

◆ *CLINICAL ALERT*

Nurses who administer antipsychotic medications must continually observe clients for potential adverse effects of these medications. Neuroleptic malignant syndrome (NMS) may occur during any stage of treatment but usually occurs early. It is an emergency. Symptoms include high fever and muscle rigidity. NMS can be fatal, so early symptom recognition is essential.

NEUROLEPTIC MALIGNANT SYNDROME

Neuroleptic malignant syndrome (NMS) is a medical emergency. It is a potentially fatal reaction to antipsychotic medication and is characterized by muscular rigidity, hyperthermia, altered consciousness, and autonomic dysfunction. Kinross-Wright first described the syndrome in 1958, and Delay and Deniker named it neuroleptic malignant syndrome in 1968. Researchers have suggested that cases of NMS were for years underreported or misdiagnosed (Caroff et al, 1991; Gurrera et al, 1992). The reported incidence of NMS is approximately 0.5% to 1.4% of the population who receive antipsychotic medications (Pope et al, 1986). Laboratory findings can include leucocytosis (15,000 to 30,000 cells/mm^3), elevated creatine phosphokinase (may be >3000 IU/ml), and myoglobinuria. NMS may occur any time during treatment but is more frequent shortly after initiation of antipsychotics or dose increases. There are other factors that may predispose the client to development of NMS. Rapid administration of a high-potency antipsychotic (rapid tranquilization) and an increased number of IM injections increase the risk of NMS.

The underlying pathophysiology associated with NMS remains unclear. A relationship exists between NMS and the blockage or depletion of dopamine in the basal ganglia (which also causes extrapyramidal symptoms). This blockade is also associated with the generation of heat through muscle contraction and through effects in the hypothalamus, which controls central thermoregulation (heat dissipation).

NMS may develop within hours after taking antipsychotic medications or after years of exposure. It may present as mild and self-limiting or fulminate progressively over 48 to 72 hours. Early recognition and treatment may minimize potentially fatal complications that include myocardial infarct, hepatic failure, disseminated intravascular coagulation (DIC), and pulmonary edema. Rapid destruction of muscle tissues (rhabdomyolysis) releases large amounts of myoglobin that can be seen in the urine as myoglobinuria. In extreme cases myoglobin can saturate the serum, which results in crystallization in the kidney and causes renal failure or permanent renal impairment.

Treatment

The first and most important step in the treatment of NMS is discontinuation of the antipsychotic. Hydration and cooling are also of paramount importance. Intravenous (IV) administration of a muscle relaxant has been used to reduce the sustained muscle rigidity and thereby reduce fever and the results of muscle tissue breakdown. The dopaminergic drugs (e.g., bromocriptine [Parlodel]), amantadine (Symmetryl), and anticholinergics have also been used.

Clients who require continued antipsychotic treatment are usually changed to an antipsychotic with a different chemical structure using low starting doses and slow **titration** (incremental adjustment of dose to allow for tolerance to side effects). Whenever possible, reinitiation is delayed until 2 weeks after symptoms have subsided. The resolution of NMS is related to clearing the antipsychotic from the body. Therefore the long half-life depot antipsychotics (haloperidol decanoate, fluphenazine decanoate) are avoided in clients with a history of NMS.

OTHER SIDE EFFECTS

Antipsychotic medications are associated with a wide variety of additional side effects. Some of these effects are an extension of the known pharmacology of the agents, whereas other effects are idiosyncratic and unpredictable. Dopamine blockade can lead to gynecomastia and galactorrhea. Small breast pads may be useful for those suffering from galactorrhea. Amenorrhea occasionally occurs in women soon after antipsychotics are first started. Most commonly, one or two cycles are missed before normal cycles resume. Weight gain from unclear mechanisms is common, although molindone (Moban) may be associated with weight loss. Incontinence is more common in older clients. Impaired temperature regulation can put clients at risk for hypothermia in winter and hyperthermia in the summer. Seizures caused by these agents in clients without any seizure history are well documented. Clients with a seizure history or current seizure disorder must be monitored closely when started on these drugs. All of these agents can reduce the seizure threshold, but this is more common with the low-potency agents (e.g., chlorpromazine [Thorazine] and thioridazine [Mellaril]).

The low-potency agents are more commonly associated with a variety of problems. Electrocardiographic changes (conduction delays) are more common with thioridazine and chlorpromazine. Sudden death via unknown mechanisms, while extremely rare, is more common with low-potency agents. Rare cholestatic jaundice presenting 2 to 4 weeks after the client has begun therapy is more commonly associated with a phenothiazine. Photosensitivity, dramatically increased predisposition to sunburn, may last a month after drugs are stopped. Liberal use of hats and sunscreens is advised before sun exposure. High doses of thioridazine can lead to pigmentary retinopathy and permanent blindness. Sexual dysfunction is vastly underreported but likely affects approximately 25% of treated clients. Up to one third of men taking thioridazine may experience retrograde ejaculation. Complaints of impaired erection are also common. Both men and women may complain of inhibition of orgasm. When side effects persist, dose reduction, switching to another drug, and adding an adjunctive agent need to be considered in context. The severity of the problem, the current benefit the client is receiving, other drugs the client is taking, and any other psychiatric and somatic conditions affecting the client must all be evaluated to determine the best intervention.

ATYPICAL (NOVEL) ANTIPSYCHOTICS

Agents that avoid the major problems associated with traditional antipsychotics have long been sought. A number of such medications are now available. Nomenclature to describe these agents is still evolving. The term *atypical antipsychotic* was initially applied to drugs that have an improved negative symptom response and minimal EPS. Because of negative connotations of the term *atypical*, *novel antipsychotic* is often used. Traditional (typical) antipsychotic efficacy has been related to dopamine$_2$ antagonism. The most discriminating pharmacologic feature of novel agents is that they block serotonin more than dopamine, making them serotonin-dopamine antagonists (SDAs). Although the nondescriptive terms, *traditional* and *novel*, suffice for now, newer agents with different modes of action will soon make these terms obsolete. As psychopharmacology matures, terminology that relates to pharmacology (e.g., SDA) will be most meaningful for the clinician.

CLOZAPINE

The arrival of clozapine created a great deal of excitement in the psychiatric community. It is the first antipsychotic to demonstrate a significantly greater improvement of negative symptoms compared with typical antipsychotics. Clozapine brought substantial improvement in symptoms and the quality of life to many individuals who failed to adequately respond to typical antipsychotics. Numerous side effects, including potentially fatal agranulocytosis, and its extremely high cost have tempered the enthusiasm of many. Regardless, clozapine is the first major advance in the pharmacotherapy for major psychosis in almost 40 years.

Indications

Clozapine is indicated for use in treatment of refractory schizophrenia. Being treatment **refractory** is defined as failing to respond to two antipsychotics of different chemical classes given at doses of 800 chlorpromazine equivalents a day for at least 6 weeks. Clozapine is the only drug that has demonstrated an improved response in treatment of refractory clients (Hagger et al, 1993; Kane et al, 1988; Meltzer et al, 1993). Clozapine has restricted indication because of side effects. Although not indicated by the Food and Drug Administration (FDA), clozapine is sometimes useful in schizoaffective disorder (McElroy et al, 1991), bipolar disorder, and severe tardive dyskinesia (Tamminga, 1994) when standard treatments have failed.

Mode of Action

The pharmacologic reasons for clozapine's unique effects are unclear. Clozapine, like typical antipsychotics, blocks dopamine receptors. Clozapine also has considerable serotonin (5-hydroxytryptamine [5-HT]) blockade. Still, the specific reasons for the unique clinical response to clozapine remain elusive. Current investigations are centering on the ratio of serotonin to dopamine blockade as well (Lichter, 1993; Pickar et al, 1992). Clozapine has less penetration into the striatum where EPS is caused, as compared with the typical antipsychotics. Thus there is minimal EPS. Blockade of other receptors, including histamine, alpha, and cholinergic receptors, causes substantial side effects.

Clinical Use and Efficacy

The recommended starting dose of clozapine is 12.5 mg. This dose reduces the risk of orthostatic hypotension and syncopal episodes, an unusual first-dose effect. This effect may be more common in clients who have had benzodiazepines in the previous 7 days. Most clients respond to the drug given in the 300 to 600 mg/day (usually bid or hs) range. Very gradual titration is necessary because of hypotension, tachycardia, and sedation. The slow development of tolerance to these side effects can result in full evaluation of clinical response to clozapine taking up to 6 months. Because of the risk of agranulocytosis, clients taking clozapine must have blood drawn for a white blood cell (WBC) count periodically. Typically, responding clients gradually demonstrate improvements in socialization and thought organization. Although positive symptoms respond to clozapine, the improved response in negative symptoms and improvement in disorganization are what most distinguish clozapine. In robust responders the psychologic effects of recovering from chronic schizophrenia can be dramatic, and many of these clients can demonstrate continuous improvement over many months. However, clients who gain insight into their illness and organization in their thoughts may be rapidly confronted with the seriousness of their previous mental state and an awareness of the consequences of their illness. These clients can then suffer from serious depression and dysphoria.

Side Effects

Agranulocytosis.   Life-threatening **agranulocytosis** develops in approximately 0.5% of monitored clozapine-treated clients. The risk peaks at approximately 3 months and is greatest during the first 6 months of treatment (Alvir and Lieberman, 1994). Subsequent agranulocytosis is rare. Recovery is usually complete if the drug is stopped before clinical symptoms of infection appear. Thus weekly monitoring of the WBC count is required for the first 6 months and biweekly thereafter as long as treatment continues. Clients receive a 7- or 14-day supply of clozapine only after an adequate WBC count (>3000 cells/mm^3) has been obtained.

Agranulocytosis is not dose related. Reductions in the WBC count serious enough to endanger clients require discontinuation of the drug. WBC counts should include a WBC differential each week for at least the first 18 weeks to 6 months of treatment. The differential will determine the percentage of different types of leukocytes in the blood. Clients with WBC counts below 2000 cells/mm^3 must discontinue clozapine immediately, and these clients can *never* receive clozapine again. Clients with WBC counts between 2000 and 3500 should be monitored closely. Often, additional WBC counts are drawn during the week in clients who have intermediate values or have had a sudden decrease from their normal values.

Seizures.   Seizures are a dose-related side effect and the main reason clozapine's maximum daily dose is 900 mg. Overall seizure incidence is approximately 3%. These generalized seizures may respond to dose reduction. The antiseizure medication valproate, most commonly administered as Depakote, may be added if needed. Carbamazepine (Tegretol), also an antiseizure medication, is avoided because of its propensity to reduce WBC counts. Myoclonic jerking may precede seizures and may indicate the need to hold or reduce the total daily dose.

Miscellaneous.   Other common side effects caused by clozapine include sedation, tachycardia, hypotension, GI upset, benign hyperthermia, anticholinergic effects, and sialorrhea (hypersalivation). Although most side effects diminish substantially with time, fatigue and sedation can be quite persistent. Fatigue can be overwhelming during the titration phase for some clients. Tachycardia with increases of 25 beats per minute or greater may also persist and is sometimes treated with β-blockers. Some clients may complain of a vague burning in the stomach, which is relieved by food, and resultant weight gain can be significant. During the first 3 weeks of therapy, some clients develop a mild fever for a few days. This benign hyperthermia remits on its own and has no clinical consequence. Acetaminophen can be used to provide comfort.

Clozapine has moderate anticholinergic effects, but, paradoxically, there is approximately a 30% incidence of sialorrhea. When sialorrhea is persistent and problematic, dose reduction or the addition of anticholinergics may help. Anticholinergics should be added with caution because of the risk of anticholinergic delirium, particularly in the elderly and in individuals with a bowel impaction.

Clozapine is a drug with great potential benefits and risks. Rapid changes in clozapine dosage can be serious. Sudden discontinuation of clozapine can result in serious rebound psychosis and anticholinergic rebound (e.g., nausea, vomiting, diarrhea). Noncompliance for more than a few days and abrupt reinstitution of the previous dosage (commonly 300 to 600 mg/day) could result in syncopal episodes, orthostatic hypotension, or seizures. Thus while clozapine is indicated for treatment of refractory clients, an individual's ability to comply is important. This overall response results not only in medication compliance, but also in clients remaining in treatment. It is important to note that slow, gradual improvement, particularly in negative symptoms, occurs over at least several months. Clients may continue to improve throughout the first year.

The difference between the novel antipsychotic clozapine and the traditional antipsychotic haloperidol can be dramatically demonstrated using positron emission tomography (PET) scan techniques as illustrated in Figure 23-1.

OTHER NOVEL ANTIPSYCHOTICS
Mode of Action

Although clozapine remains unique in the robustness of its efficacy, particularly in treatment refractory clients, other novel antipsychotic drugs with more benign side effect profiles are available. These include risperidone (Risperdal), olanzapine (Zyprexa) and quetiapine (Seroquel). By definition, these atypical (novel) antipsychotic drugs differ from typical drugs by reduced EPS and improved negative symptom response. Many clients also show improvements in cognitive functioning.

Just as with the traditional drugs, novel antipsychotics differ in their side effect profile (Table 23-4). Unlike traditional agents, the pharmacology of antipsychotic efficacy

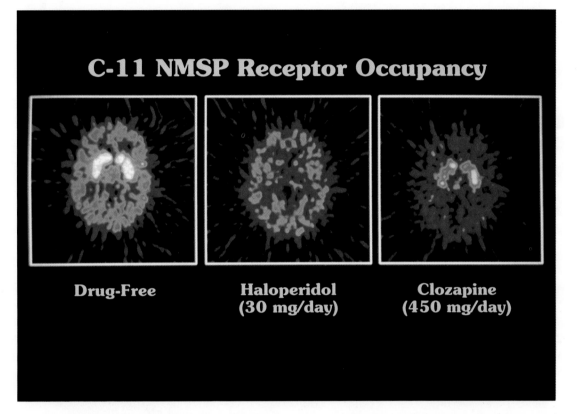

Figure 23-1   A transaxial PET scan image at the level of the basal ganglia. Carbon-11 *N*-methylspiperone (NMSP) is a radioactive tag that binds, and thus highlights dopamine type 2 (D$_2$) receptors. The three panels are from the same 36-year-old man with schizophrenia. In the first panel the man is drug free, and the D$_2$-rich basal ganglia are highlighted by the NMSP. Note the absence of NMSP in the next panel, 6 weeks later, with the man taking haloperidol 30 mg/day, with 85% of his basal ganglia D$_2$ receptors occupied with haloperidol. Finally, with the man taking clozapine 450 mg/day, only 37% of the D$_2$ receptors are occupied by drug. Although his psychosis was responsive to both medications, motor side effects were considerable with haloperidol and absent with clozapine. (Data from Tamminga CA et al, Maryland Psychiatric Research Center, University of Maryland at Baltimore, unpublished research.)

Table 23-4   Common Side Effects of Novel Antipsychotics

	Clozapine	Risperidone	Olanzapine	Quetiapine
EPS	0	+	+	0
Cardiac	+++	++	+	+
Sedation	++++	++	+	+
Anticholinergic	++++	+	++	0
Weight gain	+++	++	++++	+

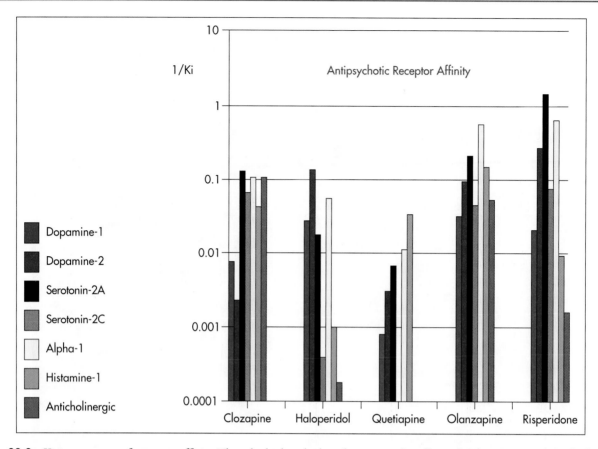

Figure 23-2   Ki is a measure of receptor affinity. Thus the higher the bar, the greater the affinity for the receptor. Note the log scale indicating a tenfold increase in affinity whenever a bar crosses a line. (Courtesy Jay Sherr, University of Maryland at Baltimore, Schools of Pharmacy and Medicine.)

appears to vary among novel drugs. This is illustrated in Figure 23-2. Observe that haloperidol has 10 times more dopamine$_2$ receptor affinity than it does for other receptors. Thus at usual prescribed clinical doses, haloperidol has negligible effects on blood pressure (α_1-receptor), sedation (H$_1$ receptor), weight gain (serotonin$_{2c}$ and H$_1$ receptors), or anticholinergic receptors. Next, note that all of the novel antipsychotics have more than 10 times more serotonin$_{2A}$ blockade than dopamine$_2$ blockade. It has been proposed that this is the reason why these drugs are different from the typical agents. Observe that risperidone has even more dopamine$_2$ blockade than haloperidol, whereas clinically it has much less EPS. Thus it appears that relationships of receptor pharmacology are just as important in overall effects as the binding to a specific receptor.

The relationship of receptor-binding effects does not always correlate directly with clinical effects. Even so, these relationships are useful in thinking about potential effects in clients. For example, even with the proposed protective benefit on EPS of serotonin$_{2A}$ blockade, clients taking higher doses of risperidone and olanzapine are more likely to need anticholinergic medication for EPS than clients taking clozapine or quetiapine. This is consistent with the high dopamine$_2$ blockade of risperidone and olanzapine compared with that of clozapine and quetiapine.

Clinical Use and Efficacy

The novel antipsychotics are first-line therapy for psychotic disorders. While offering an improved response in negative symptoms compared with traditional agents, optimal drug use will consider multiple causes of negative symptoms. Figure 23-3 graphically represents multiple etiologies of negative symptoms. The availability of the novel drugs actually allows the clinician the opportunity to do a more in-depth assessment of secondary negative symptoms than was possible with traditional antipsychotics, which sometimes make negative symptoms worse.

All novel agents have a reduced incidence of EPS and appear to have a reduced risk of causing tardive dyskinesia. The lack of EPS may be a major reason for improved compliance with novel agents. The improved compliance has resulted in reductions in rehospitalization rates compared with typical agents (Conley et al, 1998).

Risperidone (Risperdal) is a high-potency drug. Like other antipsychotics, risperidone is well absorbed and may be taken with or without food. The starting dose in adults is 1 mg bid. Unless there are limiting side effects, the dose may be increased by 1 mg bid each day to an initial daily dose of 4 to 6 mg/day. In geriatric clients, who metabolize medications more slowly, dosing should be halved, starting at 0.5 mg bid and titrating to 1.5 mg bid. Some studies

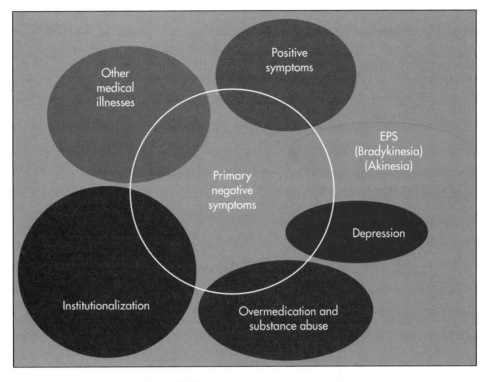

Figure 23-3 Primary negative symptoms.

suggest that clients are more likely to be discharged on doses <6 mg/day (Love, Conley, and Kelly, 1998). Risperidone has dose-related EPS usually seen at doses >6 mg/day. Other common side effects include anxiety, rhinitis, somnolence, tachycardia, and mild weight gain.

Olanzapine (Zyprexa) is a medium potency antipsychotic. The starting dose in adults is 5 to 10 mg/day (2.5 mg/day in geriatric clients). The effective dose range is 5 mg/day to 40 mg/day. Mild EPS, particularly akathisia, can be seen at doses >10 mg/day. Other side effects include postural hypotension, dizziness, constipation, and substantial weight gain.

Quetiapine (Seroquel) is a low-potency antipsychotic. The starting dose is 25 mg bid in adults, with dose increases of 25 to 50 mg bid to reach an initial target dose of 300 mg/day. Twice-daily dosing is usually maintained because of a mean serum half-life of 7 hours. The maximum dose is 800 mg/day. There is virtually no EPS with quetiapine, nor does it increase serum prolactin. Common side effects include postural hypotension, tachycardia, dizziness, and somnolence. Cataract formation discussed in the package insert has not been observed as a significant clinical problem.

Novel antipsychotics are better tolerated and may offer improved response to many clients. Unfortunately, 20% to 30% of clients may have inadequate response and require traditional therapy. Definitive, well-designed, comparative studies of these atypical agents are lacking.

SUMMARY

Since the 1950s when the first truly effective medications for the treatment of major psychotic disorders became available, antipsychotic drugs have remained a double-edged sword. The great benefits have been counterbalanced by serious toxicities such as neuroleptic malignant syndrome and tardive dyskinesia. Also, a significant portion of the schizophrenic population has remained refractory to treatment. Atypical antipsychotic medications in development herald a new era in treatment, with improved efficacy and reduced or absent extrapyramidal side effects. However, as tardive dyskinesia and NMS were not predicted when chlorpromazine and thioridazine were introduced, these new medications may contain unanticipated side effects and adverse reactions. The astute physician may observe a new level of efficacy but must remain alert for unanticipated toxicities.

ANTIDEPRESSANTS

The first modern antidepressant medication, marketed in 1958, was imipramine. This tricyclic compound is a modification of the structure of the antipsychotic chlorpromazine. The reason imipramine and similar drugs are called *tricyclics* can be readily seen by the three-ring chemical structure of the compounds (Figure 23-4). Dr. Roland Kuhn, a Swiss psychiatrist, originally administered imipramine to clients with schizophrenia and found no clinical efficacy. Astute observation and the persistence of Dr. Kuhn, who proceeded to study imipramine in clients with depression, quickly led to proving imipramine's efficacy in the treatment of depression. This success served as the catalyst for the search for additional antidepressant medications exhibiting improved efficacy and reduced side effects. At the same time, advances in the understanding of

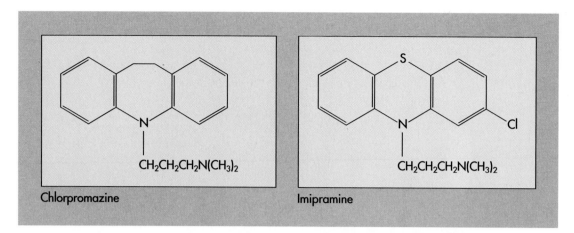

Figure 23-4   Chlorpromazine and imipramine are referred to as tricyclics because of their three-ring chemical structure.

the role of serotonin in depression pointed toward a new class of antidepressants, the serotonin selective reuptake inhibitors (SSRIs).

INDICATIONS

As their name implies, antidepressants are indicated in the treatment of major depressive disorders. However, research has indicated the use of antidepressants in a wide variety of disorders, such as enuresis, eating disorders, and anxiety disorders.

MODE OF ACTION

The biogenic amine hypothesis of depression proposes that depression is caused by a reduced quantity or function of the catecholamine neurotransmitters norepinephrine and/or serotonin.

Antidepressant drugs affect the fate of the neurotransmitters norepinephrine and/or serotonin. Presynaptic neurons synthesize norepinephrine and serotonin, which are incorporated into vesicles. Action potentials cause the vesicles to release their contents into the synapse. Normally, once released from the vesicles, the neurotransmitter crosses the synapse to impact receptors on the postsynaptic neuron. Most of the released neurotransmitter is taken back up into the presynaptic neuron in an effort to conserve this valuable resource. There, it reenters the synthesis process and is incorporated into vesicles for future use. The cyclic antidepressants partially block the reuptake of norepinephrine and serontin. Initially, this reuptake blockade results in increased amounts of neurotransmitter in the synapse. The increased amount of neurotransmitter in the synapse is associated with a reduction in the number of receptors on the postsynaptic membrane. This change in receptor density, called downregulation, can take several weeks to occur and is temporally associated with antidepressant response (Figure 23-5). In clients who have failed to respond to an an-

tidepressant more specific for one neurotransmitter, it is rational to switch to a drug more specific for the other neurotransmitter.

The pathophysiology of depression remains elusive. It is unlikely that a single theory will explain the etiology of depression. The efficacy of medications and the ability to measure interneuronal effects give important clues toward understanding the causes of depression. It is likely that there are multiple causes of depression. A single, underlying process has not been identified, and the cause of depression remains unclear.

CYCLIC ANTIDEPRESSANTS
Clinical Use and Efficacy

Approximately 70% of clients with major depression will respond to antidepressant therapy (Andrews, 1994). One individual may respond better to one drug rather than another. The likelihood of response is not predictable on the basis of the presenting symptoms of depression. Thus the initial selection of an antidepressant is based on the client's history and how the anticipated side effects of the drug interact with the client's specific physical and psychiatric status. (See Box 23-1 for common client-related variables.)

Antidepressant drugs are well absorbed, and there is extensive first-pass metabolism. Initial doses and dosage ranges are listed in Table 23-5. Cyclic antidepressant dosing begins with low doses to allow the client time to tolerate the side effects. The most common reason for failure to respond to cyclic antidepressant treatment is inadequate dose or duration of therapy. This can result from a prescriber's reluctance to prescribe enough, in an effort to avoid serious toxicity, or from client noncompliance secondary to side effects. Serum levels may be most useful when monitoring imipramine (Tofranil), desipramine (Norpramin), and nortriptyline (Pamelor). Target symp-

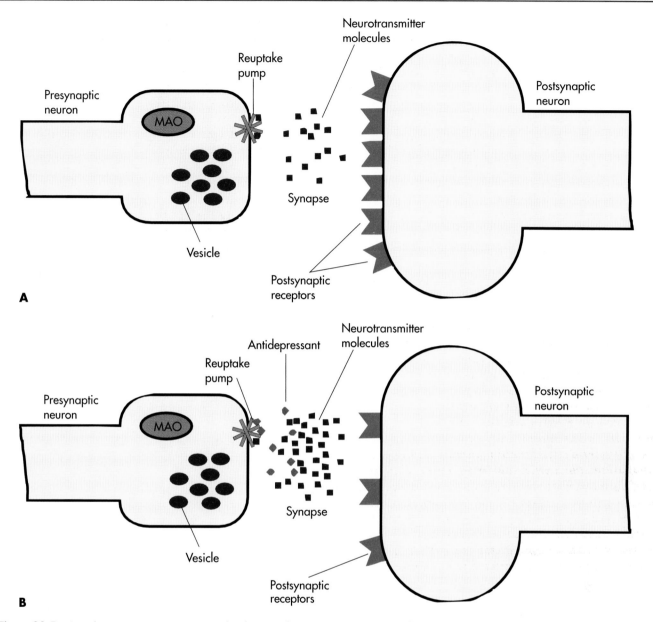

Figure 23-5   Antidepressant response. **A,** In the depressed state, sparse amounts of neurotransmitter are available in the synapse of a depressed person. **B,** With treatment, the reuptake of neurotransmitter is blocked by the antidepressant drug *(in red)*. The result is increased amounts of neurotransmitter in the synapse, and, finally, after several weeks the postsynaptic receptors have decreased (i.e., down-regulated), which is associated with resolving depression. For the sake of clarity, this drawing omits numerous receptors and postsynaptic intracellular mechanisms that may ultimately prove to be important components of the pathophysiologic substrate of depression and antidepressant response.

tom response in depression is gradual, usually occurring over several weeks. The time course of response to antidepressant therapy is summarized in Box 23-2.

Clients should be advised early of potential side effects and that therapeutic response will take some time (Pollack and Rosenbaum, 1987). Clients and families often become impatient when suffering from the side effects of medication while the original symptoms remain. Compliance is often facilitated when there is a discussion with cli-

ents and families about expectations regarding medications. There are times when the depression has resolved and the side effects remain. It is therefore important to communicate that compliance with medication after the depression has cleared is vital. Letting clients know that side effects will diminish with time or that there are management alternatives also helps ensure compliance for the total duration of therapy.

When clients have been receiving therapeutic doses

Table 23-5	Antidepressant Dosing		
Generic (Trade Name)*	Starting Dose (mg/day)	Maintenance Dose (mg/day)	
Cyclic Antidepressants			
Tricyclics			
Amitriptyline (Elavil, Endep)	25-50	100-300	
Clomipramine (Anafranil)	25	100-250	
Desipramine (Norpramin)	25-50	100-300	
Doxepin (Sinequan)	25-50	100-300	
Imipramine (Tofranil)	25-50	100-300	
Nortriptyline (Aventyl)	25-50	100-300	
Maprotiline (Ludiomil)	50	100-225	
Protriptyline (Vivactil)	10	15-60	
Trimipramine (Surmontil)	25-50	100-300	
Tricyclic Dibenzoxazepine			
Amoxapine (Asendin)	50	100-400	
Triazolopyridines			
Nefazodone (Serzone)	200	300-600	
Trazodone (Desyrel)	50	150-500	
Piperazinoazepine			
Mirtazapine (Remeron)	15	15-45	
Monoamine Oxidase Inhibitors			
Phenelzine (Nardil)	15	15-90	
Tranylcypromine (Parnate)	10	10-40	
Serotonin-Selective Reuptake Inhibitors†			FDA Indications
Citalopram (Celexa)	20	20-40	Depression only
Fluvoxamine (Luvox)	50	100-300	Obsessive-compulsive disorder only
Fluoxetine (Prozac)	5-20	20-80	Obsessive-compulsive disorder, bulimia nervosa
Paroxetine (Paxil)	10-20	20-50	Obsessive-compulsive disorder, panic
Sertraline (Zoloft)	50-100	50-200	Obsessive-compulsive disorder, panic
Indolamine			
Bupropion (Wellbutrin)	200	300-450	
Phenylethlyamine			
Venlafaxine (Effexor)	75	150-350	

*Use about half the dose for the elderly.
†Note FDA indications in addition to depression.

for 3 or 4 weeks and are not demonstrating clinical improvement, changing medications may be indicated. Adjunctive medications in partial and nonresponding clients are sometimes useful.

"First break" (meaning the first episode of major depression) treatment should continue for 6 to 12 months. Many clinicians treat recurrence of major depression for at least 5 years, and lifelong treatment may be indicated for some clients (American Psychiatric Association [APA], 1993). Decisions regarding duration of treatment need to consider the severity of the depression and the history and risk of suicidal gestures. Major depression with psychotic features is often treated by adding an antipsychotic. As the depression resolves, the psychotic symptoms will also clear, and the antipsychotic can be discontinued.

Side Effects

These drugs are routinely associated with increased sedation and anticholinergic effects. These effects are directly related to the degree of histamine and cholinergic receptor blockade of each drug. The secondary amine drugs (nortriptyline, protriptyline, and desipramine) are less sedating and less anticholinergic than the tertiary amines (amitriptyline, imipramine, trimipramine, and doxepin). Clients often complain about these side effects, and they are a significant cause of noncompliance. These sedating and drying effects, so-called nuisance side effects, generally diminish with time. Over time, cyclic antidepressants are associated with substantial weight gain.

A wide variety of side effects may be caused by central nervous system (CNS) receptor activity, allergy, or unclear mechanisms. Whenever possible, the best way to treat problematic side effects is to remove the offending agent. Of course, this is not always possible. Allergies excluded, most side effects will substantially diminish with time. When they do not diminish, a variety of interventions can be offered to help clients who are demonstrating adequate efficacy and are continuing to suffer from bothersome side effects. Interventions for helping clients with both initial and persistent side effects are listed in Table 23-6. The significance of "minor" side effects should not be underestimated. Constipation, particularly in the elderly, can lead to paralytic ileus, bowel obstruction, and the need for hospitalization. Noncompliance due to "minor" side effects can lead to relapse and increased suicide risk.

One of the most serious side effects of antidepressants is directly related to their efficacy. During the gradual response of depressive symptoms, clients may demonstrate increased energy and physical activity while suicidal ideation remains. It is in this intermediate stage of response, often the second week of therapy, that clients may be at the highest risk to act on self-destructive thoughts. Careful monitoring is essential as clients begin to emerge from depression (APA, 1993).

Tricyclic antidepressants are associated with significant cardiac toxicity. All tricyclics cause a dose-related widening of electrocardiographic (ECG) intervals. It is unfortunate that medications effective in the treatment of depression can also be fatal in overdose.

While helping clients rise from depression, antidepressants can sometimes elevate mood beyond the desired effect. In clients with bipolar disorder, it is not uncommon for antidepressants to "push" clients into mania. A first episode of mania sometimes occurs during antidepressant therapy (Pickar et al, 1984).

MONOAMINE OXIDASE INHIBITORS

Iproniazid, an antitubercular drug in the 1950s, was a monoamine oxidase inhibitor (MAOI). Some patients receiving iproniazid were noted to become euphoric. This observation ultimately led to the use of MAOIs as antidepressant agents. The use of MAOIs has been limited as a result of the side affects and dietary modifications. Thus investigation for antidepressant agents continued.

Mode of Action

The neurotransmitters norepinephrine, serotonin, and dopamine are chemically described as monoamines. In the CNS these molecules are synthesized inside the presynaptic neuron. Maintenance of cellular homeostasis requires a mechanism to degrade monoamines. Monoamine oxidase (MAO) is an enzyme found in the mitochondria of cells that participates in the normal process of degradation of these amines. MAOIs are drugs that inhibit this enzyme. This inhibition initially results in increased availability of these neurotransmitters. As with other antidepressants, these initial neurotransmitter increases result in postsynaptic receptor down-regulation that is temporally related to antidepressant response.

Clinical Use and Efficacy

MAOIs are indicated in the treatment of atypical (novel) depression, major depression without melancholia, or depressive disorders resistant to tricyclic antidepressants. Atypical depression is characterized by hypersomnia, hyperphagia, anxiety, and the absence of vegetative symptoms. In addition, MAOIs have been used with variable success in the treatment of other disorders such as certain anxiety disorders, eating disorders, and some pain syndromes (e.g., migraines).

The MAOIs are rapidly absorbed, liver metabolized, and have average half-lives of approximately 24 hours. A majority of individuals metabolize MAOIs relatively slowly. This metabolic difference among individuals results in wide variation with respect to required doses for efficacy and sensitivity to side effects at a given dose (Johnstone and Marsh, 1973). There is no clinically available test for this metabolic rate. Thus many clinicians begin MAOI therapy with a 10- or 15-mg test dose and monitor vital signs and complaints of side effects closely before beginning titration.

Contraindications to the use of MAOIs include cere-

Table 23-6 · Side Effects of Antidepressants With Nursing Interventions

Side Effect	Nursing Interventions
Anticholinergic Effects	
Dry mouth	Offer sugarless gum and candy, artificial saliva. For persistent problems treat with pilocarpine 1% rinse and spit (4 drops of 4% pilocarpine and 12 drops water) or bethanechol (Duvoid, Urecholine) 5 mg sublingual or 10-30 mg qd-bid.
Blurred vision: disturbance of presbyopia (near vision), far vision usually preserved	Ask if vision prescription is current; try pilocarpine 1% eye drops or bethanecol 10-30 mg tid.
Urinary retention	When not caused by benign prostatic hypertrophy (BPH) may be treated with bethanecol 10-30 mg tid.
Constipation	Prevention: encourage fluids (medication givers may offer), fruits and vegetables, mild physical exercise (walks). Treat with bulk-forming laxatives (e.g., Metamucil 1-2 tablespoons qAM or docusate 100 mg qd-bid). Avoid stimulant laxatives when possible; if needed, limit duration to avoid laxative dependence. Or treat with bethanecol 10-30 mg qd-bid.
Anticholinergic delirium (also known as atropine psychosis)	Monitor for agitation restlessness, psychotic signs and symptoms, myoclonic jerking. May occur with or without peripheral anticholinergic signs. Hold anticholinergic drugs. Physostigmine 5 mg IV can rapidly reverse but requires life-support backup and cardiac monitoring.
α-Blockade	
Orthostatic hypotension	Consider other contributing factors such as low-salt diets, restricted fluid intake, dehydration. Antihypertensive medications may exacerbate. Advise client to change positions slowly, dangle feet 1 minute in sitting position when rising from prone; sit immediately when lightheaded. Offer support hose, exercise to strengthen calf muscles to improve venous return.
Sexual Dysfunction	Obtain a clear history that the complaint does not predate the depression or medication use.
Decreased libido	Neostigmine 7.5-15 mg 30 minutes before anticipated intercourse.
Impaired erection	Often an anticholinergic problem; change to less anticholinergic drug or try bethanecol.
Priapism	Rare disorder associated with trazodone. Prolonged painful, nonsexual erection. Medical urgency treated with epinephrine injections to the corpus cavernosa. May require surgical intervention leading to permanent impotence.
Impaired ejaculation	May require switching drug. Try Neostigmine 7.5-15 mg 30 minutes before anticipated intercourse.
Inhibition of orgasm	Less serotonergic drug. Try cyproheptadine 4 mg qd. Note that cyproheptadine, a serotonin antagonist, has caused loss of antidepressant efficacy in some clients. The addition of buproprion has been used successfully.
Hematologic	
Agranulocytosis	Exceedingly rare allergic reaction usually occurring in the first 3 months of treatment. Monitor for fever, sore throat, mucosal ulceration, weakness. Discontinue drug, change to a different chemical class.
Petechia, ecchymosis, easy bruising, bleeding	Associated with SSRI effect on platelet. May occur with normal or decreased platelet counts. Discontinue drug. Monitor CBC, dizziness, lightheadedness.
Other	
Weight gain	Associated with cyclic antidepressants and MAOIs. Recommend diet and exercise. Treat with diuretics (e.g., hydrochlorothiazide for edema).
Weight loss	Associated with SSRI; rarely clinically significant.
Tremor	Advise caffeine may exacerbate. Determine degree of interference with daily activities. Propranolol 10-20 mg tid-qid may be useful.
Antidepressant withdrawal	Anticholinergic rebound can result in GI upset, cramps, diarrhea. Educate client on potential withdrawal symptoms. When discontinuing, taper slowly over several weeks. SSRI withdrawal symptoms include nausea, lightheadedness, dizziness, faintness, fatigue, parasthesias, flulike syndrome. Taper slowly.

From Andrews JM, Nemeroff CB: Contemporary management of depression, *Am J Med* 97(6A):24S, 1994; modified from Pollack MH, Rosenbaum JF: Management of antidepressant-induced side effects: a practical guide for the clinician, *J Clin Psychiatry* 48(1):3, 1987.

| Box 23-3 | Dietary Restrictions for Clients Taking Monoamine Oxidase Inhibitors |

Prohibited

Aged cheeses
Ripe avocados
Ripe figs
Anchovies
Bean curd/fermented beans
Broad beans (fava/Italian)
Yeast extracts and yeast-derived vitamin supplements
Liver
Delicatessen meats (especially sausage)
Pickled herring
Meat extracts (Marmite, Borvil)
Fermented foods
Chianti and sherry

Allowed with Moderation

Beer and ale *(tyramine content varies with brand and can be especially high in imported beers and some nonalcoholic beers)*
White wine/distilled spirits
Cottage cheese, cream cheese
Coffee (<2 cups/day)
Chocolate
Soy sauce (tyramine content varies with brand)
Yogurt and sour cream
Spinach, raisins, tomatoes, eggplant, plums

brovascular defects, major cardiovascular disease, and pheochromocytoma (tumor of the adrenal medulla). The elderly do not tolerate MAOIs well, so use is uncommon in individuals over age 65. MAOIs have been known to worsen symptoms of Parkinson's disease, induce manic states in bipolar clients, and exacerbate psychotic symptoms in clients with schizophrenia. Clients with diabetes may require adjustment of their hypoglycemic medication. MAOIs are contraindicated in pregnancy.

The use of MAOIs requires additional considerations. As with cyclic antidepressants, initial dosing must be titrated to give clients time to tolerate side effects. Table 23-5 lists initial and maintenance dosing ranges. Clients taking MAOIs must comply with a tyramine-restricted diet (Box 23-3) and must studiously avoid stimulant medications to avoid the risk of a potentially fatal hypertensive crisis. Thus the client's ability to comply with dietary and medication restrictions is an important consideration before initiating therapy. Response to therapy may take 3 to 6 weeks. Except in emergencies, discontinuations should be tapered.

Side Effects

Orthostatic hypotension is a common initial and sometimes persistent side effect of MAOIs. Dangling feet on rising, changing positions slowly, support stockings, and increased fluid and salt intake can be effective treatments. A caffeinated drink in the morning may be useful as long as vital signs are monitored initially. Edema, sexual dysfunction, and weight gain are also common and can lead to drug discontinuation. Complaints of insomnia occur with all MAOIs. Moving the last dose of the day to an earlier time may be helpful. Complaints of confusion or feeling drunk may indicate an excessive dosage. Although these drugs do not have direct effects on cholinergic receptors, anticholinergic-type side effects (e.g., dry mouth, urinary hesitancy, constipation) are seen. Parasthesias (numbness, prickling, tingling feelings) may be caused by MAOI-induced pyridoxine (vitamin B_6) deficiency and is treated with oral pyridoxine (Goodhart et al, 1991).

Avoiding certain foods is essential when clients are taking MAOIs. Dietary tyramine is a precursor in the synthesis of norepinephrine. In the presence of an MAOI, foods high in tyramine (an amino acid by-product formed by the bacterial breakdown of tyrosine in fermented foods) can lead to a sharp increase in available norepinephrine and potentially fatal hypertensive crisis. Box 23-3 lists some foods that may interact with MAOIs. Tyramine is not the only factor in food that can interact with MAOIs. For instance, fava beans contain dopamine, which can affect blood pressure in the presence of MAOIs. Previously, dietary restrictions for MAOIs were extensive and made compliance unlikely. Estimates of compliance with an MAOI diet have been as low as 40%. Yet, for several reasons, there are not an overwhelming number of MAOI hypertensive reactions. Foods, different brands of prepared foods, and a client's susceptibility to this interaction all vary widely. For instance, although a cup of coffee may elevate blood pressure and cause headaches in some clients, others taking MAOIs benefit from a cup of coffee as an adjunct to treat hypotension on awakening. Thus client education should consist of simple, clear, written and verbal instructions to absolutely avoid certain foods. Warnings of other foods that may cause problems in some clients or when taken in large quantity should be reviewed. Dietary restrictions should be maintained for 2 weeks after MAOIs are discontinued. All clients need to know the warning signs of hypertensive crisis, which include headache, stiff neck, sweating, nausea, and vomiting. Clients with such symptoms should seek medical attention immediately.

> ⚠ **CLINICAL ALERT**
>
> Clients receiving MAOI antidepressants must be cautioned about ingesting foods containing tyramine or drugs that may interact with the MAOIs. Potential results are hypertensive crisis or extreme hypotension. Symptoms include headache, stiff neck, nausea/vomiting, and diaphoresis. Client teaching is essential with these medications.

| Box 23-4 | Drugs to Avoid When Taking Monoamine Oxidase Inhibitors |

Antiasthmatics
  Theophylline and inhalers containing epinephrine or
    β-agonists (e.g., albuterol [Proventil, Ventolin])
Antihypertensives
  Methyldopa (Aldomet), guanethidine (Ismelin), reser-
    pine
Anesthetics with epinephrine
Allergy, hayfever, cough and cold products, deconges-
    tants, diet pills
  (Many combination over-the-counter products. Look
    for inclusion of phenylpropanolamine, ephedrine,
    phenylephrine, dextromethorphan.)
Buspirone (Buspar)
Meperidine (Demerol)
Serotonin selective reuptake inhibitors
  Fluoxetine (Prozac), sertraline (Zoloft), paroxetine
    (Paxil), fluvoxamine (Luvox), nefazodone (Serzone)
Yohimbine (Yocon)

Understanding & Applying Research

The role of serotonin in depression was demonstrated by this important study by Delgado et al. They examined a group of 21 hospitalized clients with depression who were medicated with a variety of antidepressants and whose depression had remitted. These clients were placed on tyrosine-free diets. Tyrosine, an essential amino acid, is required in the diet. In the brain, the synthesis of 5-HT is limited by the availability of tyrosine. When deprived of all tyrosine for 24 hours, two thirds (14/21) of the clients in the study rapidly became depressed. Some became suicidal. Depression quickly remitted when tyrosine was restored to the diet. This is the first study to demonstrate that for some depressed clients, a functional serotonin system is required for antidepressant efficacy.

It is not yet possible to predict which depressed clients are more likely to respond to an SSRI versus a more adrenergic cyclic antidepressant. However, similar studies are beginning to elucidate more precisely how the depressed brain responds to medication, and are bringing us closer to understanding the underlying etiology of depression, as well as more effective ways to treat it.

Delgado PL et al: Serotonin function and the mechanism of antidepressant action, *Arch Gen Psychiatry* 47:411, 1990.

Many drugs can also interact with MAOIs and can lead to a hypertensive crisis or dangerous hypotension. These drugs are listed in Box 23-4. Many over-the-counter medications may be dangerous when taken with MAOIs, including diet pills, nasal decongestants, asthma medications (including inhalers), and cough suppressants (dextromethorphan). Literally hundreds of over-the-counter and prescription combination products under many different brand names contain sympathomimetics that are unsafe to use with MAOIs. Therefore every client taking an MAOI must be educated to consult a physician, dentist, nurse, or pharmacist before taking any additional medication. Although hypertensive events are generally more dangerous and more common, the response to a sympathomimetic medication or dietary indiscretion can be hypotension rather than hypertension. Whether a hypotensive or hypertensive reaction ensues is a function of the overall adrenergic tone of the client and is not predictable.

Treatment for hypertensive crisis may be started with nifedipine (Procardia, Adalat) 10 mg. Absorption from oral administration is extremely rapid, and reductions of blood pressure may be seen in a matter of minutes. Vital signs should be monitored every 10 to 15 minutes until the client is stable. Other therapies that have been used include the α-adrenergic blockers phentolamine (Regitine) 5 mg IV and chlorpromazine 50 mg PO.

Clients who fail to respond to a non-MAOI antidepressant should usually wait at least 2 weeks before starting an MAOI. An important exception to this is fluoxetine (Prozac). Because of the long half-life of fluoxetine and its active metabolite norfluoxetine (approximately 7 to 10

days), clients discontinuing fluoxetine should wait at least 5 weeks before starting an MAOI.

SEROTONIN SELECTIVE REUPTAKE INHIBITORS

There has been an explosion of research and interest in the role of serotonin in depression in recent years, such as the study in the Understanding & Applying Research box. Important findings include:

In some depressed clients, reduced serotonin and its major metabolite 5-hydroxy indole acetic acid (5-HIAA) are found in the cerebrospinal fluid.

Reduced serotonin has been noted in the brains of individuals who were depressed and committed suicide.

Blood platelet serotonin receptors are altered in some clients with depression.

All known SSRIs are clinically effective antidepressants (Risch and Nemeroff, 1992).

Mode of Action

As their name implies, SSRIs act primarily to block the reuptake of serotonin. These drugs, listed in Table 23-5, have minimal direct effects on other receptors, including the cholinergic, adrenergic, and histamine systems (Cole, 1992; Dechant and Clissold, 1991; De Wilde et al, 1993; Wilde et al, 1993).

Clinical Use and Efficacy

In addition to the treatment of major depression, and although FDA indications vary between the drugs, all of the

SSRI antidepressants have also been found to be useful in the treatment of obsessive-compulsive disorder, panic disorder, and bulimia nervosa.

Serotonin-specific (selective) reuptake inhibitors now comprise more than half of all antidepressant use. The huge success of the SSRI antidepressants, starting with the release of fluoxetine in 1988, is due to several factors. The side effect profile is relatively mild compared with that of other antidepressants (Richelson, 1991). There is minimal cardiac toxicity, eliminating the need for ECGs. Serum levels are not clinically useful to determine dose or monitor for toxicity. Dose titration is minimal, and in the treatment of major depression the starting dose is also the maintenance dose for the majority of clients. Finally, all SSRIs currently on the market are comparatively safe in overdose. When taken as a single agent, SSRI overdoses are serious and can cause seizures, but complete recovery is common.

SSRIs are absorbed from the GI tract relatively slowly, and peak serum concentrations are obtained in 4 to 10 hours. All marketed SSRIs have serum half-lives averaging 15 to 24 hours, except fluoxetine (Prozac). Fluoxetine's half-life in adults averages 2 to 3 days, and its active metabolite norfluoxetine has a half-life of 7 to 10 days. This means that frequent dosage adjustments of fluoxetine are not generally warranted. Elimination can be substantially longer in older clients and those with hepatic disease where norfluoxetine half-lives of 14 to 21 days are well documented. Also, it is not possible to abruptly discontinue fluoxetine. This has important implications for drug interactions. A minimum 5-week washout is required before MAOI use. Clients switched to a cyclic antidepressant must be started on low doses and titrated slowly, because remaining fluoxetine can inhibit metabolism of the cyclic antidepressant and yield toxic serum levels (Vaughn, 1988).

Side Effects

Common initial side effects of SSRIs include nausea, drowsiness, dizziness, headache, sweating, anxiety, insomnia, anorexia, and nervousness. These are generally milder and more tolerable to the client than the sedation and anticholinergic effects of cyclic antidepressants. Often these are substantially more tolerable within a few weeks. Although all SSRIs share these side effects, the susceptibility of an individual to a particular agent varies. Paroxetine (Paxil) may be slightly anticholinergic and more sedating than other SSRIs (Tulloch and Johnson, 1992). These medications, particularly fluoxetine, have been associated with insomnia. This also diminishes significantly with time but can be persistent in some clients. Dose reduction should be considered before adding an adjunctive agent for sleep. Trazodone (Desyrel) 50 mg is sometimes used.

Fluoxetine may cause more agitation and anxiety, but this may be a dosing issue, since the commonly used 20-mg starting dose is too much for many clients. Some-times SSRIs, and most commonly fluoxetine, can cause substantial anxiety and restlessness that appears to be a form of akathisia. These symptoms warrant close scrutiny because akathisia is associated with increased aggression and suicide. All SSRIs have been linked to occasional EPS.

A great deal of publicity has surrounded fluoxetine (Prozac) and the risk of increased suicidal ideation when taking fluoxetine. This reaction was first described in a case report of six clients during fluoxetine's premarketing studies (Teicher, 1990). Paradoxic increased suicidal ideation has been reported for virtually all antidepressants (Damluji and Ferguson, 1988; Fava and Rosenbaum, 1991). Unfortunately, popular media sensationalism has blown this risk way out of proportion. This jaded perception continues to persist in the minds of many individuals despite considerable scientific evidence to the contrary. Fluoxetine has become a cultural icon, and stories of benefits and risks have reached mythic proportions. Clients should be allowed to express feelings about this medication regimen. Noncompliance can result from unaddressed concerns.

An often overlooked side effect of SSRIs is sexual dysfunction. As many as 20% to 40% of clients may suffer from loss of libido, erectile dysfunction, ejaculatory dysfunction, or anorgasmia. Clients are often reluctant to discuss these issues. Therefore sensitive inquiry can reveal side effects that could lead to noncompliance and a relapse of depression. Side effects and considerations in treating antidepressant sexual dysfunction are found in Table 23-6.

OTHER ANTIDEPRESSANT AGENTS

In recent years, antidepressant medications with a variety of chemical structures and varied modes of action have appeared on the market. These agents are not easily characterized into groups and thus are discussed individually below.

Clomipramine (Anafranil) was the first drug indicated for the treatment of obsessive-compulsive disorder (OCD) in the United States. Clomipramine has been used in Europe to treat depression for more than a decade. It is structurally a tricyclic and shares the anticholinergic, sedative profile of these agents. The most serotonergic of the cyclic agents, clomipramine can cause GI upset, sweating, insomnia, and nervousness typical of these agents. It must be titrated to effective doses like the tricyclics. The starting dose is 25 mg/day, and the maximum daily dose is 250 mg. This drug does have an increased risk of causing seizures by lowering the seizure threshold. Fluoxetine (Prozac) and fluvoxamine (Luvox) are also FDA-indicated drugs for the treatment of OCD (Pigot et al, 1990; Wilde et al, 1993). However, the use of fluvoxamine in depression is still under investigation.

Bupropion (Wellbutrin) has a somewhat different mechanism of action in that it blocks the reuptake of dopamine while having only minimal reuptake effects on norepinephrine (Ferris and Cooper, 1993). Yet, bupropion has demonstrated efficacy against depression. It has a mild side effect profile, causing less sedation, anticholinergic, and cardiac conduction side effects than tricyclic antidepressants. The most common side effects are agitation and insomnia. The starting dose is no greater than 75 mg tid. Bupropion can cause dose-related seizures. Therefore it must never be dosed greater than 150 mg at one time; when the maximum dose is required, the recommended regimen is 150 mg tid. Depressed individuals with a history of bipolar disorder taking bupropion need to be assessed for symptoms of mania.

Venlafaxine (Effexor) is the first of a new class of antidepressants that significantly block the reuptake of both serotonin and norepinephrine (Montgomery, 1993). Venlafaxine has mild dopamine reuptake blockade effects. It is rapidly absorbed and has a short half-life of approximately 5 hours. Its active metabolite has a half-life of 11 hours. Because of the short half-life, venlafaxine is dosed two or three times a day, starting at 75 mg, either 37.5 mg bid or 25 mg tid. Preliminary data suggest that outpatient clients have responded to doses between 75 and 225 mg/day while hospitalized; presumably more severely depressed clients may require the maximum dose of 375 mg/day.

Venlafaxine has side effects similar to those of SSRIs and may have mild anticholinergic-like effects. Nervousness and anxiety sometimes seen at lower doses may resolve at higher doses. Hypertension, increased diastolic blood pressure to greater than 90 mm Hg and greater than 10 mm Hg over baseline, is a dose-related side effect and an indication to reduce the dose or discontinue the medication.

Mirtazapine (Remeron) has a unique mechanism of action. By blocking presynaptic α_2-receptors, it causes an increased release in both norepinepherine and serotonin. It effectively blocks serotonin$_2$ and serotonin$_3$ receptors. This serotonin$_2$ blockade likely results in an antidepressant with minimal sexual side effects. With a half-life of 20 to 40 hours, it can be given once a day. Mirtazapine dosing starts at 15 mg/day, and the effective dose range is 15 to 45 mg/day. Common side effects include somnolence, increased appetite, weight gain, and dizziness. The serotonin$_2$ blockade appears to be the reason this is a serotonergic antidepressant with minimal sexual side effects. Liver enzymes should be monitored periodically. Rare WBC suppression is a serious potential adverse reaction. Nurses should educate clients to report any signs or symptoms of infection.

SUMMARY

Depression is a common and potentially deadly illness. Pharmacotherapy for depression, although effective, has many liabilities. Tricyclics are deadly in overdose. MAOIs require dietary discipline and particular vigilance for drug interactions. SSRIs are effective antidepressants that have fewer side effects than other agents. SSRIs cause sexual side effects that many clients may be reluctant to discuss and that may lead to noncompliance. Nurses should know the efficacy and toxicity of these agents. Moreover, teaching clients what to expect is a crucial component in helping to maintain safety, compliance, and optimal therapeutic response.

ANTIMANIC AGENTS
LITHIUM

For decades lithium was the treatment of choice for mania. Lithium is the simplest possible drug, a single ion. This single ion has had purported medical uses for more than 100 years. In the late nineteenth century, lithium was used as a treatment for gout, for seizures, and as a sedative. Around this time, Trousseau in France and Carl and Fritz Lange in Denmark reported efficacy of lithium in mania and depression, respectively. In the early 1900s, fashionable spas touted lithium waters as healing and rejuvenating. Actually, these "lithia" waters contained only rare traces of lithium with inconceivable medical benefit. Unfortunately, in the United States in 1949 lithium was given to some cardiac clients as a salt substitute. The subsequent toxicity resulted in some deaths and cast a pall on the use of lithium. Interestingly, that same year in Australia, John Cade, in noting that guinea pigs given lithium became sluggish, wondered if lithium would help his agitated and manic clients. His astute observation resulted in the rediscovery of Trousseau's observation, that lithium had a specific effect in his clients with mania.

Indications

Since Cade first used lithium in the treatment of bipolar disorder in 1949, it has remained one of the most effective psychotropic medications. Approximately 70% to 80% of clients with bipolar disorder respond to lithium in the treatment of both acute manic episodes and maintenance treatment (Baastrup et al, 1970; Prien, 1992). Lithium is also commonly used in the treatment of schizoaffective disorder and as an adjunct to antidepressant therapy in depression. It has also been used in treating impulse-control disorders, self-injurious behaviors in conduct disorder, pervasive developmental disorder, and mental retardation.

Mode of Action

Lithium affects the neurotransmitters of multiple systems, including dopamine, norepinephrine, serotonin, acetylcholine, and γ-aminobutyric acid (GABA). These effects are modest; none of them has been directly linked to lithium's efficacy in bipolar disorder. Promising research suggests that lithium may work inside the neuron by interfering with guanine nucleotide (G-protein) binding (Manji et al, 1995). G proteins may be thought of as signal transducers or chemical messengers inside the cell. The effects of many endogenous substances and drugs that impact receptors are subsequently manifest through the intracellular actions of G proteins. Thus the effects of neurotransmitters may be altered by lithium's effects on this signal transduction system. Future research in clarifying lithium's effects on G proteins holds great promise in leading to a better understanding of the pathophysiologic nature of bipolar disorder.

Clinical Use and Efficacy

Lithium's most important clinical feature is its narrow therapeutic index. Because serious toxic effects can occur with small increases in lithium plasma concentrations, conscientious monitoring is required. Lithium is rapidly absorbed from the GI tract and is widely distributed throughout the body. Lithium is not metabolized and is excreted primarily by the kidney. Its clearance is directly proportional to the glomerular filtration rate. The average half-life is 24 hours in adults and 36 hours in geriatric clients. Because of the potential for toxicity, rigorous baseline laboratory monitoring is common. Conventional pre-lithium baseline monitoring is shown in Box 23-5. Baseline values are vital in the assessment of both acute and chronic lithium toxicity.

Starting doses for clients with normal renal function are generally 900 to 1200 mg/day in divided doses. Available lithium products are shown in Table 23-7. **Sustained-release** lithium may be useful in clients who persistently suffer GI upset. The slow absorption of sustained-release lithium preparation results in 12-hour postdose serum lithium levels that are approximately 30% higher than those obtained with immediate-release products. Subsequent dose adjustments are based on lithium plasma concentrations. Clients with normal renal function will reach steady state in 4 to 5 days, which is when first serum levels should be obtained. It is common to obtain levels earlier in clients with impaired renal function or in those prone to lithium toxicity. Routinely monitored serum lithium levels should be obtained 12 hours after the previous dose.

The therapeutic range for lithium is customarily defined as 0.5 to 1.2 mEq/L measured 12 hours after the last dose. Acute mania may require plasma levels as high as 1.2 to 1.5 mEq/L. Maintenance treatment serum levels are

lower. Recent studies suggest that relapse and hospitalization are reduced by plasma levels of 0.8 to 1.0 mEq/L in adults (Gelenberg et al, 1989). Geriatric clients may respond well to lower levels (0.4 to 0.6 mEq/L). Older clients are generally more sensitive to the neurotoxic effects of higher doses.

During maintenance, lithium is usually dosed two or three times a day. It has been suggested that once-a-day dosing at bedtime can reduce side effects, such as polyuria. Once-a-day-at-bedtime dosing is practical when the total daily dose is 1500 mg/day or less. Larger single doses often result in significant GI upset.

In the treatment of mania, initial response to lithium may take a week or longer. Therefore, concomitant antipsychotic therapy is often added temporarily to assist with the acute treatment of psychotic arousal symptoms (e.g., agitation, irritability, insomnia). Manic symptoms such as euphoria, grandiosity, pressured speech, flight of ideas, and hypersexuality may take somewhat longer to respond. Lithium alone may be effective to treat depression in individuals who are, in reality, bipolar but have not had their first manic episode. Low-dose lithium therapy (e.g., 300 mg bid) can be effective in treating major depression as an augmenting agent to antidepressant therapy.

Side Effects

Continuous monitoring for signs and symptoms of toxicity is a requirement for the safe use of lithium. Lithium side effects can be divided into those occurring early in therapy and those that tend to persist. Box 23-6 delineates these side effects. Most early-onset symptoms resolve or diminish considerably but persist to a lesser extent in many clients.

A variety of problems caused by lithium may yield to

Box 23-5   Lithium Baseline Monitoring

Vital signs
Weight
Blood urea nitrogen/creatinine
Electrolytes
Thyroid function tests
Complete blood count with differential
Urinalysis
Electrocardiogram*
Pregnancy test

*For those older than age 40 or with a history of cardiovascular disease.

Table 23-7	Lithium Products
Generic	**Trade Name**
Capsules	
150 mg lithium carbonate	
300 mg lithium carbonate	Eskalith, Lithonate
600 mg lithium carbonate	
Tablets (Scored)	
300 mg lithium carbonate	Eskalith, Lithane
Extended-Release Tablets	
300 mg lithium carbonate	Lithobid
450 mg lithium carbonate	Eskalith CR
Syrup	
Lithium citrate syrup	Cibalith-S syrup
8 mEq/5 ml*	

*300 mg of lithium carbonate = 8.12 mEq of lithium.

simple interventions. Lithium-induced hypothyroidism is treatable with thyroid supplementation and is reversible if lithium is discontinued. Weight gain with lithium may be greater than 10 kg but will respond to diet adjustments. Mild leukocytosis is benign and does not require treatment. Acne may be treated with benzoyl peroxide or erythromycin topical solutions. Exacerbation of psoriasis can be serious and may require discontinuation of lithium treatment.

Lithium's effects on cardiac function are generally mild and of little consequence. Lithium may substitute for potassium in ion channels in the heart. ECG changes resemble those seen in hypokalemia, but usually these are benign. Despite this, idiosyncratic cardiotoxicity is rarely observed, and the astute clinician must remain alert. Baseline and yearly ECGs are advisable in clients over age 40 or those with cardiac disease. Lithium can cause sinus node depression and should be avoided in clients with sick sinus syndrome.

Lithium is generally avoided in pregnancy, especially in the first trimester, because of a possible low-incidence association with Ebstein's anomaly, a cardiac malformation (Jacobson et al, 1992; Schou et al, 1973). Often, low doses of a high-potency antipsychotic agent is substituted if drug treatment is required during pregnancy. When the behavioral toxicity and/or physical health risks of being manic while pregnant clearly outweigh the risks of lithium use, extra monitoring must be performed because of changes in renal function during pregnancy. Lithium should be discontinued several days before delivery. Nursing mothers should not use lithium.

The polyuria caused by lithium is a mild nephrogenic diabetes insipidus. When it is persistent and problematic, this polyuria can be treated with amiloride, a potassium-sparing diuretic, 5 to 10 mg/day. Contrary to popular belief, even with long-term treatment, lithium is rarely toxic to the kidney unless plasma levels rise (Schou, 1988). Permanent damage to nephrons and subsequent loss of renal function can occur with substantially elevated lithium levels.

Many side effects of lithium toxicity are dose-related (see Box 23-6). If a client receiving stable lithium therapy experiences a return of some of his or her original transient side effects, this may be an indication of impending lithium toxicity. GI complaints and coarsening of the fine lithium tremor should result in examination of plasma lithium levels. If these dose-related warning signs were reliable, there would be little need to monitor serum levels. Unfortunately, sometimes seizures or cardiovascular collapse are the first signs of lithium toxicity. For this reason, particular attention should be paid to factors that expose clients to the risk of lithium toxicity.

Because lithium is excreted primarily by the kidney, factors that affect sodium and water metabolism are intimately linked to lithium elimination. Stable diets, whether high or low in sodium, are not problematic. It is

Box 23-6   Serum Lithium Levels and Side Effects

Transient effects and mild toxicity:
  Fine tremor
  GI upset
  Mild polyuria, polydipsia
  Muscle weakness, lethargy
Persistent effects:
  Fine tremor
  Mild polyuria, polydipsia
  Increased WBC count
  Nontoxic goiter, hypothyroidism
  Exacerbation of psoriasis
  Acne
  Alopecia
  Weight gain
Effective acute treatment and prophylaxis—0.5-1.2 mEq/L
Moderate toxicity—lithium level >1.5 mEq/L:
  Coarsening of tremor
  Reappearance of GI symptoms
  Confusion
  Sedation, lethargy
As levels increase:
  Ataxia
  Dysarthria
  Mental status deterioration
Severe toxicity—lithium level >2.5 mEq/L:
  Seizures
  Coma
  Death
  Cardiovascular collapse

the change in dietary salt intake that will affect lithium levels. Addition of salt to the diet will result in lower lithium levels and possible loss of efficacy. Less salt in the diet or conditions that cause sodium loss, such as fever or dehydration, will increase lithium levels. For example, clients leaving the hospital and returning to a substantially different diet at home may be at increased risk for lithium toxicity.

As lithium levels rise, CNS toxicity becomes more pronounced. Clients who become ataxic, dysarthric, or have any change in mental status should be evaluated immediately for lithium toxicity.

Summary

For more than 40 years, lithium has been the most effective psychopharmacologic agent in the treatment of bipolar disorder. Although extensively studied, the exact mechanism of action remains a mystery. Because of a narrow therapeutic range and side effects, the search for alternative treatments continues.

Anticonvulsants are also important in the treatment of mood disorders. The anticonvulsant valproic acid is the other first-line agent indicated in bipolar disorder. This is addressed in detail in the following section. At present, lithium remains a cornerstone in the treatment of bipolar disorder.

ANTICONVULSANTS IN PSYCHIATRY

The use of terminology to group medications by the description of a drug's initial indication, while useful, can at times be misleading. Such drugs may have vastly different chemical structures, pharmacokinetics, modes of action, side effects, and, in the case of anticonvulsants, a variety of uses. Two anticonvulsants originally used in the control of seizure disorders, carbamazepine (Tegretol) and valproate (Depakene and Depakote), are being used with increasing frequency in the treatment of psychiatric disorders.

INDICATIONS

Carbamazepine has long been used in the treatment of simple partial, complex partial, and tonic-clonic seizures, whereas valproate has been indicated for only the latter and in absence of seizures. Recently, valproate received FDA approval for the initial control of acute mania (Bowden et al, 1994). All other uses of these agents for psychiatric indications are based on the scientific literature and medical standards of care. Bipolar disorder, in which, both valproate and carbamazepine have been used effectively, is the best-studied indication. The broad scope of research into potential uses for these agents in psychiatry is summarized in Table 23-8. Studies have examined these two drugs in various mood and anxiety disorders. Carbamazepine does not appear to have a role in panic disorder, and valproate has had little effect on unipolar depression.

MODE OF ACTION

The mode of action of these agents on psychiatric neurobiology is uncertain at this time, although several issues

are clear. The effects of these agents in psychiatric disorders appear to be separate from their antiseizure mechanisms. Valproate and carbamazepine work via different mechanisms. For example, valproate has mild effects on CNS GABA receptors, whereas carbamazepine does not. It appears likely that these drugs have substantial effects on the inner chemistry of neurons via pathways known as second-messenger systems (Post et al, 1992). The term *second messenger* refers to a broad variety of intracellular chemical reactions that influence both the metabolism and action potential transmission of neurons. Stimulation or inhibition of receptors on the cell membrane is one way of affecting second-messenger systems. Some drugs (e.g., carbamazepine, valproate, and lithium) appear to affect second-messenger systems directly. The study of these systems in health and disease and the effects of drugs on the systems are leading toward greater understanding of the pathophysiology of psychiatric disease.

GOALS OF THERAPY

The goals of therapy for mood and anxiety disorders have been described previously. However, the role of anticonvulsants in the pharmacotherapy of chronic aggression has not been addressed. Anticonvulsants were first used to treat aggression after the relationship between seizure disorders and aggression was noticed (Monroe, 1970). One important step in titrating the medication is to objectively note the type of aggression (e.g., verbal and/or physical, against self, inanimate objects, or others) and the frequency of the occurrences over time both before and after medication changes.

CLINICAL USE AND EFFICACY

It is a mistake to think of both of these agents as similar in efficacy because they are both anticonvulsants. Bipolar clients who have failed to respond to lithium and subsequent treatment with one of these anticonvulsants may eventually respond to the other anticonvulsant. Usually, these drugs are titrated gradually to allow for tolerance to side effects. Baseline monitoring after a medical history and physical examination includes electrolytes, liver function tests, complete blood counts (CBCs), ECGs, and pregnancy testing. Valproate is teratogenic and is associated with neural tube defects—most commonly spina bifida—and should be avoided in pregnancy.

Valproate

Valproate is available in several dosage forms as different salts of valproate. Valproate is the common compound that is measured in the plasma. Depakene is the trade name for both an immediate-release tablet and a liquid concentrate. Depakote is an enteric-coated capsule with a slower release. Depakote sprinkles are capsules that contain coated particles that can be taken intact or pulled apart and sprinkled on food. The half-life averages 6 to 16 hours. Serum levels should be monitored and dosing ad-

Table 23-8	Anticonvulsants in Psychiatry	
Potential Use	**Carbamazepine**	**Valproate**
Bipolar disorder	XX	XX
Unipolar depression	X	—
Aggression/dyscontrol syndromes	XX	X
Panic disorder	—	X
Posttraumatic stress disorder	X	X
Substance withdrawal	XX	X

XX, Documented efficacy for some clients; X, some potential usefulness but more study is needed; —, usefulness not demonstrated.

justed accordingly. There may be a response threshold because response to valproate is rarely seen with serum levels less than 50 μg/ml (McElroy et al, 1992). Efficacy is generally found with levels of 50 to 120 μg/ml, although levels up to 150 μg/ml may be useful in the treatment of acute mania. An exception to the initial titration of these agents is the use of a so-called loading regimen of valproate in the treatment of acute mania. Given as Depakote 500 mg tid, clients with acute mania can frequently tolerate this aggressive dosing without the GI upset and sedation often seen. With this regimen some clients with acute mania may respond within 3 days, more than twice as fast as with standard lithium therapy (Keck et al, 1993).

Carbamazepine

Carbamazepine has a unique pharmacokinetic profile. Initially it has a half-life of approximately 36 hours. However, carbamazepine induces its own metabolism. That is, in the presence of the drug, the liver gradually manufactures more of the enzymes that metabolize carbamazepine, which results in faster metabolism. After 4 to 6 weeks, the approximate half-life is 24 hours. For this reason, clients taking carbamazepine are not at steady state for at least 1 month after a dosage change. When carbamazepine is used to treat the signs and symptoms of substance withdrawal, dosing is low (200 to 400 mg/day) and the duration of therapy is brief. For other indications the starting dose is usually 200 mg bid and may be taken with meals to reduce GI upset. The average dose is titrated to about 1000 mg/day in divided doses, but dosage requirements vary widely and should be guided by serum levels. Efficacy for psychiatric indications is associated with serum levels of 7 to 12 μg/ml, although some clients become overly sedated or ataxic at serum levels greater than 7 μg/ml.

SIDE EFFECTS
Valproate

GI complaints—nausea and vomiting, anorexia, dyspepsia, and diarrhea—are the most common side effects of valproate. GI complaints usually occur early and usually subside with continued treatment. Persistent complaints can be treated with dose reduction, a switch to sprinkles, or H_2 blockers (e.g., ranitidine [Zantac]). Initial somnolence is common. Minor liver enzyme elevations (less than three times normal) may occur. Regardless, in the presence of substantial therapeutic benefits, valproate is usually continued in the face of minor liver enzyme elevations (McElroy et al, 1992). Tremor is common. If tremor persists and is a problem, propranolol (Inderal) has been used effectively. Weight gain with and without increased appetite may occur. Hair loss, usually transient, affects approximately 10% of clients. More serious but less common side effects include thrombocytopenia, coagulopathies, pancreatitis, edema, and hepatic failure. Hepatic failure is a greater risk in children under the age of 10 and in clients

taking other anticonvulsant drugs. Liver enzymes should be monitored closely.

Carbamazepine

During the initiation of carbamazepine therapy, clients may complain of sedation, lethargy, GI upset, and blurred vision. These side effects tend to diminish with time and are the primary reason for dose titration. Mild fluid retention and edema may occur. Liver enzyme elevations similar to those with valproate occur, and periodic liver enzyme monitoring is the standard of care for both drugs.

Carbamazepine causes a predictable suppression of the WBC count. In most cases this reduction is benign and will stabilize at 10% to 15% below baseline levels. Thus the WBC count is monitored at baseline and periodically after treatment is initiated. Agranulocytosis, a life-threatening absence of WBCs, is associated with carbamazepine but is extremely rare and should not be confused with the mild neutropenia. Similarly, a mild reduction in platelets (thrombocytopenia) is usually not clinically significant.

Ataxia is a sign of carbamazepine toxicity usually associated with increased serum levels. Nurses should consider holding the dose of carbamazepine in a client with ataxia. Urticaria and pruritic and erythematous rashes occur occasionally. These rashes may be mild and self-limiting but must be evaluated closely and monitored continuously.

SUMMARY

Although the use of anticonvulsants in psychiatry is rapidly increasing, with the exception of valproate in the treatment of acute mania, unequivocal evidence of efficacy is not always available. Side effects and toxicity can be substantial. Thus clear expectations of response and well-defined target symptoms must be specified before pharmacotherapy is begun. Several newer anticonvulsants may have some utility in bipolar disorder. These medications include gabapentin (Neurontin), lamotrigine (Lamictal), and topiramate (Topamax). Open-use series and case reports, mostly in clients who are refractory to more standard treatments, suggest that some clients may benefit. However, randomized, controlled, double-blind studies will be required before the usefulness and ultimate role of these medications in psychiatry is determined. Nurses should be aware that lamotrigine has been associated with serious drug rash requiring hospitalization.

ANXIOLYTICS AND HYPNOTICS

The sensation of extreme anxiety triggers the "fight or flight" reaction. This reaction elicits a series of observable physical changes or responses. The client's emotionally charged response may include dramatic physical symptoms, such as chest pain or pressure with radiation to the shoulder and arm, rapid heartbeat or palpitations, and shortness of breath. This syndrome is not a new malady of the twentieth century, and documented reports of it are found from the Civil War in the 1860s.

Today, symptoms such as these often motivate people to seek medical treatment. Once underlying somatic medical causes are ruled out, a variety of treatment alternatives is available. Commonly, comprehensive treatment involves a combination of psychotherapy and adjunctive pharmacotherapy.

Sleep is commonly reported to be disrupted in anxiety. In the treatment of anxiety disorders, the appropriate initiation and maintenance of sleep are intrinsically related to the use of a variety of compounds with sedative properties. Whether the medication is being used as an anxiolytic (antianxiety) or a hypnotic, the effect of sedative agents on sleep requires consideration.

BARBITURATES

Indications

Historically, barbiturates were the primary agents used to treat anxiety and insomnia. Their use in anxiety predates the advent of benzodiazepines. However, almost all barbiturate use has been replaced by benzodiazepines, which are safer and more effective anxiolytics and hypnotics.

Barbiturates have several disadvantages. First, they are not good anxiolytics and provide mostly sedation. As hypnotics, tolerance develops rapidly in many clients. Thus therapeutic and toxic doses converge with continued use. In acute overdose, barbiturates can be fatal when taken as a single agent. Death occurs secondary to respiratory depression, which is exceedingly rare for benzodiazepines.

All barbiturates have the potential to be habit forming. Barbiturates induce hepatic enzymes and can thus result in increased metabolism, decreased serum levels, and reduced efficacy of other hepatically cleared drugs, including cyclic antidepressants, anticonvulsants, anticoagulants, and some cardiac medications. Barbiturates can also interfere with oral contraceptives, and alternative methods of birth control should be used if barbiturates are added to the regimen.

Mechanism of Action

The mechanism of action of barbiturates is unknown. Researchers have found that the mesencephalic reticular activating system is remarkably sensitive to barbiturates. It is likely that barbiturates diminish neuronal responsiveness. Unlike benzodiazepines, as doses increase, barbiturates reduce the respiratory drive and mechanisms responsible for the rhythmic character of respiration. Barbiturates are differentiated primarily by their pharmacokinetic half-lives. Amobarbital has the shortest-acting half-life, and phenobarbital has the longest. Half-lives and usual dosages are listed in Table 23-9.

Despite their liabilities, barbiturates still retain some legitimate uses. Barbiturates may be used as hypnotics in clients in whom benzodiazepine therapy has failed. Phe-

nobarbital is still used occasionally in the treatment of seizure disorders. IV amobarbital is used in narcoanalysis, a technique of medication-induced mental relaxation/hypnosis, that may help properly prepared clients address suppressed memories and emotions.

BENZODIAZEPINES

Indications

Benzodiazepines are one of the most widely used classes of medications in all of medicine and have a variety of indications. In general medicine they are used for preoperative relief of anxiety and for sedation, for light anesthesia, and to induce anterograde amnesia (an inability to remember events that occurred after ingesting the medication) for perioperative events (King, 1992). They are used in higher doses as skeletal muscle relaxants. Diazepam (Valium) is used intravenously to treat status epilepticus, and oral clonazepam (Klonopin) is indicated for the treatment of Lennox-Gastaut seizures. Benzodiazepines are frequently used as hypnotics to treat insomnia and in the management of anxiety disorders.

Although indicated as hypnotic and antianxiety agents, benzodiazepines are commonly used in a broad array of settings. There is limited evidence that benzodiazepines may be useful in the treatment of some clients with mood disorders. Clonazepam (Klonopin) has been used with some success in the treatment of bipolar disorder and as an adjunct to lithium in partially responsive clients (Sachs, 1990). Akathisia may be treated with benzodiazepines. Chlordiazepoxide (Librium) has long been used to treat the acute signs and symptoms of alcohol withdrawal. Catatonic clients are sometimes aroused by benzodiazepines. Finally, lorazepam (Ativan), along with antipsychotics, has become a standard in the treatment of psychotic agitation in emergency situations.

Mechanism of Action

GABA is the primary inhibitory neurotransmitter in the brain. Receptors, dubbed benzodiazepine receptors, serve as chloride ion gates. GABA interacts with these chloride ion channels to allow chloride ion into neurons, thus hyperpolarizing the neuron and reducing the firing rate. In the presence of a benzodiazepine, the activity of GABA is enhanced, resulting in further opening of the chloride ion channel and a further inhibition of neuronal activity.

Goals of Therapy

In the treatment of anxiety, medications are best viewed as an adjunct to therapy. During drug treatment, clients may find relief from their symptoms, which allows them to benefit from a variety of psychotherapies. Some clients may require maintenance treatment with antianxiety agents. Target symptoms of anxiety and panic should be clearly identified.

The goal of therapy in the treatment of sleep disorders

Table 23-9	Hypnotic and Anxiolytic Agents					
Generic Name	**Trade Name**	**Approved Indication**	**Approx. Benzodiazepine Equivalency (mg)**	**Active Metabolite**	**Usual Dosage Range (mg/day)**	**Half-Life Hours**
Barbiturates						
Amobarbital	Amytal	Hypnotic	NA	—	100-200	8-42
Butabarbital	Butisol	Hypnotic	NA	—	50-100	34-42
Pentobarbital	Nembutal	Hypnotic	NA	—	100-200	15-48
Phenobarbital	Luminal	Hypnotic	NA	—	100-200	80-120
Secobarbital	Seconal	Hypnotic	NA	—	100-300	15-40
Benzodiazepines						
Alprazolam	Xanax	A, AD, P	0.5	No	0.75-4 (A) 4-10 (P)	12-15
Clonazepam	Klonopin	LGS	2.5	No	1-6*	20-50
Clorazepate	Tranxene	A	7.5	Yes	7.5-90	20-80
Chlordiazepoxide	Librium	A, AW, PS	10	Yes	25-200	5-30
Diazepam	Valium	A, PS, SE	5	Yes	2-40	20-80
Estazolam	ProSom	Hypnotic	2	No	1-2	10-15
Flurazepam	Dalmane	Hypnotic	15	Yes	15-30	8-40
Halazepam	Paxipam	A	20	Yes	20-160	10-20
Lorazepam	Lorazepam	A, PS	1	No	0.5-10	10-20
Oxazepam	Serax	A, AD, AW	15	No	30-120	5-20
Prazepam	Centrax	A	10	Yes	20-60	20-80
Quazepam	Doral	Hypnotic	2	Yes	30-50	30-50
Temazepam	Restoril	Hypnotic	15	No	15-30	10-20
Triazolam	Halcion	Hypnotic	0.25	No	0.125-0.25	1.5-5
Nonbarbiturate, Nonbenzodiazepine						
Buspirone	Buspar	A	NA		10-60	2-4
Chloral hydrate	Noetec	Hypnotic	NA		500-2000	8-11
Ethchlorvynol	Placydyl	Hypnotic	NA		500-1000	18-20
Diphenhydramine	Benadryl	Hypnotic	NA		25-100	3-9
Doxylamine	Unisom	Hypnotic	NA		25-100	8-12
Zolpidem	Ambien	Hypnotic	NA		5-10	1.5-4

A, Anxiety; *AD*, anxiety associated with depression; *AW*, alcohol withdrawal; *LGS*, Lennox-Gastaut syndrome (seizures); *P*, panic disorders; *PS*, psychotic disorders; *SE*, status epilepticus.
*Dosed up to 20 mg/day for seizure.

is the (re)establishment of normal sleep patterns. Again, short-term intervention is the standard of care.

Clinical Use and Efficacy

The benzodiazepines are the drugs of choice for the treatment of anxiety and sleep disturbances. All benzodiazepines have anxiolytic effects. A particular benzodiazepine may be sedative at low doses, provide improved relief from anxiety at higher doses, and be a hypnotic at even higher doses. The available benzodiazepines are listed in Table 23-9. This table points out the speed of oral absorption, the elimination half-lives, active **metabolites,** and the relative potency of the agents.

The main difference between benzodiazepines is in their pharmacokinetic profiles and potency. Thus the rational use of benzodiazepines is derived from applying ef-

fects of their pharmacokinetic differences to the clinical setting. When used for the treatment of acute anxiety or agitation, rapid oral absorption is desirable, whereas in the chronic treatment of an anxiety disorder, rapid oral absorption is less important. Parenteral and concentrate forms of some benzodiazepines are sensitive to light and temperature, and significant degradation may occur if they are left at room temperature for more than a few hours. For example, liquid lorazepam should be refrigerated until immediately before use to prevent degradation.

There is an additional absorption issue that is important with benzodiazepines. Once the drug is in the bloodstream, it must be absorbed into the brain. The two benzodiazepines absorbed the fastest from the blood are diazepam (Valium) and alprazolam (Xanax). This rapid penetration into the brain is the likely reason for the "buzz" effect commonly reported for these two drugs. People who do not abuse drugs may find this "buzz" unpleasant and may report feeling spacey, out of it, or disconnected.

Benzodiazepine should be started at low doses and gradually increased as needed to achieve clinical response. There is a rapid onset of clinical efficacy once an appropriate dose is achieved. In anxiety disorders some reduction of anxiety may be apparent almost immediately. The antianxiety effect, with initial dosing, may not last as long as the serum half-life would suggest. This is probably due to the drug redistributing out of the brain. With continued dosing, steady-state brain levels and sustained efficacy are achieved. For the treatment of anxiety, benzodiazepines are usually dosed at bedtime or bid. Only occasionally is tid dosing required.

Ideally, hypnotics should be rapidly absorbed and thus have a short onset of action and a short elimination half-life so that next-day carry-over effects such as sedation and impaired cognition are minimized. Realistically, individuals may experience a sedation "hangover effect" the next day.

As with antianxiety treatment, hypnotic pharmacotherapy should be for as short a time as possible. Medication should be an adjunct to help clients (re)establish a regular sleep pattern. Along with improved sleep hygiene techniques taught to the client, benzodiazepines should be used for 7 to 10 days and discontinued. Clients who require longer pharmacotherapy are at greater risk to develop rebound insomnia and anxiety on drug discontinuation.

Side Effects

Unwanted sedation is the most common side effect of benzodiazepines and affects at least 10% of clients. Sedation may diminish with time or a decrease in dose. Clients should always be counseled not to drive or use dangerous machinery when initiating these drugs. This is important even in clients taking hypnotic medications at bedtime only. Next-day, or carry-over, sedation can affect driving, as well as result in cognitive dysfunction that can affect work or school performance. Dizziness and ataxia occur less frequently and are more common in the elderly and physically debilitated. A paradoxic excitability, hyperarousal, or increase in aggression may be seen. However, these side effects are rare and may be more common in children and in the elderly with organic brain disease. Clients with chronic obstructive pulmonary disease or sleep apnea may develop clinically significant respiratory impairment.

Benzodiazepines may be teratogenic and should not be used during pregnancy. If used during the third trimester and immediately before delivery, newborns may develop withdrawal reactions. Benzodiazepines are secreted in breast milk in sufficient concentrations to cause symptoms such as dyspnea, bradycardia, and drowsiness in nursing infants.

When used for more than brief periods, the accumulation of active metabolites can be clinically significant. During this time clients may gradually develop increasing sedation, decreased cognitive functioning, and even ataxia. This is especially true in the elderly population and clients with hepatic dysfunction. Even for drugs without active metabolites, clients on these potent drugs should be monitored closely for ataxia and risk for falls.

ABUSE AND WITHDRAWAL OF BENZODIAZEPINES AND BARBITURATES

Before any use of either benzodiazepines or barbiturates, the clinician must consider their abuse potential. Use of these agents in clients with a history of substance abuse, particularly in the outpatient setting, must be carefully considered. Barbiturate intoxication presents with confusion, drowsiness, irritability, hyporeflexia, ataxia, and nystagmus. More serious overdoses can result in coma. Intoxication with benzodiazepines does not generally present with nystagmus (Roy-Byrne and Hommer, 1988). Barbiturate overdose can easily result in death from respiratory depression and is especially dangerous in the presence of alcohol and/or other CNS depressant drugs. Benzodiazepines as single-agent overdoses are not usually life threatening. However, a possible benzodiazepine overdose must always be taken seriously because it is often unclear in the clinical situation if other medications are present. As with barbiturates, benzodiazepine overdose is potentially fatal when combined with alcohol or other CNS-depressant agents.

Physical withdrawal symptoms can occur any time these drugs are taken continuously for more than 2 weeks and occur in almost half of clients who have taken these drugs for more than 4 weeks. Accordingly, drug discontinuation should be gradual. The most severe withdrawal symptoms are experienced by clients who have been taking high doses for long periods of time and suddenly stop taking the drug. Long half-life drugs tend to have milder withdrawal phenomena, whereas short half-life drugs are associated with more severe withdrawal. Barbiturate withdrawal symptoms occur more often and are generally more severe than with benzodiazepines. Withdrawal presents as a hyperarousal state, including anxiety, irritability, insomnia, fatigue, muscle aches, tremors, sweating, and difficulty in concentrating. These signs and symptoms closely resemble the original sleep or anxiety complaints. The nurse communicates the client's response to the detoxification protocol with the treatment team.

NONBENZODIAZEPINES

The first nonbenzodiazepine anxiolytic is buspirone (Buspar). Buspirone is indicated for the treatment of anxiety disorders—specifically, generalized anxiety disorder. It is notable for its mild side effect profile. Common side effects include dizziness, headache, drowsiness, and lightheadedness. The CNS sedation and cognitive impairment occur much less frequently than with other anxiolytics.

Clients whose anxiety responds to buspirone may report that they do not feel like they are taking a drug. That is, they now feel normal, their symptoms are relieved, and they are without side effects. It is important to note that the antianxiety effects of buspirone begin to occur gradually over the first 2 weeks of therapy, and full efficacy may not be apparent for 3 to 6 weeks. For this reason, some individuals can become impatient waiting for the drug to work, particularly if they are under a great deal of stress. Furthermore, many clients have previously been treated with a benzodiazepine whose antianxiety effects begin almost immediately. Thus clients who hold the same expectations for buspirone may require education about the gradual onset of efficacy to remain motivated and compliant with treatment.

Buspirone's mechanism of action is unknown. It is a partial agonist at the serotonin receptor (Eison et al, 1986). This means that it stimulates the receptor but not as much as serotonin. Overstimulation of serotonin receptors has been hypothesized to cause anxiety. Thus buspirone's partial agonist activity may restore more "normal" serotonergic tone in anxiety disorders. At high doses, buspirone can block the dopamine receptor. It is unknown at this time if prolonged use at high doses may result in the development of abnormal involuntary movements.

Safer and commonly used hypnotics for the treatment of short-term insomnia include chloral hydrate (Noctec) and the antihistamines diphenhydramine (Benadryl) and doxylamine (Unisom, Nitetime Sleep-Aid, and Sleep 2-Nite).

The first of a new class of hypnotics is zolpidem (Ambien). Zolpidem is indicated for the short-term treatment of insomnia and is a schedule IV controlled substance.

Zolpidem's mechanism of action is different from that of benzodiazepines. The GABA chloride ion channel has several different binding sites. Although zolpidem interacts with the benzodiazepine receptor, this selectivity for only part of the benzodiazepine receptor results in quite a different effect profile. Zolpidem, unlike benzodiazepines, does not have anticonvulsant or myorelaxant effects (Sanger et al, 1987). Sleep studies have revealed that zolpidem does not suppress REM sleep. Furthermore, abrupt discontinuation in clients taking zolpidem for up to 30 days has resulted in little rebound insomnia (Lader, 1992; Scharf et al, 1991).

The most common side effects are drowsiness and dizziness. At doses greater than 10 mg (the maximum recommended dose), the incidence of nausea and dizziness increases dramatically (Merlotti et al, 1989). This suggests that although zolpidem is potentially habit forming, it will not be popular with substance abusers.

SUMMARY

Hypnotics and anxiolytics, although effective agents, can produce their own set of clinical problems. First, the appropriate duration of therapy is often unclear. Also, even gradual discontinuation can result in a recurrence of the original signs and symptoms. Finally, an addictive potential must often be considered.

STIMULANTS
INDICATIONS

The use of stimulants in psychiatry has a checkered history. Before the advent of antidepressant medications, stimulants were used to treat depression with little efficacy. In the 1950s these drugs were widely prescribed to reduce appetite in the treatment of obesity. Failure to achieve lasting weight loss and the high abuse liability of these drugs have substantially curtailed this practice. Today stimulants are used in psychiatry primarily to treat attention-deficit/hyperactivity disorder (ADHD). Drugs used to treat ADHD include methylphenidate (Ritalin), dextroamphetamine (Dexedrine), pemoline (Cylert), and a combination product consisting of a mixture of amphetamine and dextroamphetamine salts (Adderall). These stimulants are controlled substances. Amphetamine, dextroamphetamine, and methylphenidate are schedule II agents, and pemoline is a schedule IV agent. Stimulants are also used in the treatment of narcolepsy and, less commonly, to treat withdrawn and apathetic states in the elderly.

MODE OF ACTION

Stimulants are widely used in the treatment of ADHD. The exact pathophysiology of ADHD is not known, but it clearly involves both dopamine and norepinephrine. All stimulants block the reuptake of dopamine and norepinephrine. Dextroamphetamine also blocks serotonin reuptake and blocks the enzyme MAO. In higher doses dextroamphetamine also facilitates release of dopamine and norepinephrine. Methylphenidate affects dopamine and norepinephrine reuptake more than dextroamphetamine and affects release less than dextroamphetamine. Pemoline's reuptake effect appears to be greater for dopamine than for norepinephrine. The ascending reticular activating system is particularly affected by the psychostimulants.

GOALS OF THERAPY

Clients with ADHD suffer from increased motor activity, impulsiveness, and inattention. The goal of pharmacotherapeutic treatment is to decrease motor activity and impulsivity. However, optimal treatment integrates medication use and behavioral interventions.

CLINICAL USE AND EFFICACY

Although both methylphenidate and dextroamphetamine are effective in the treatment of ADHD, methylphenidate is used more often. Many clinicians suggest that optimal therapy should involve sequential trials of both methylphenidate and dextroamphetamine to determine which offers better effect in a particular individual (Calis et al, 1990). Both drugs are rapidly absorbed, and some

Table 23-10	Stimulants			
Drug Name	Dosage Forms	Starting Dose (mg/day)	Average (Maximum) Daily Dose)	Half-Life (hr)
Amphetamine and dextroamphetamine (Adderall)	5-, 10-, 20-, 30-mg tablets	5-10	15-40	8-10
Dextroamphetamine (Dexadrine)	5-, 10-mg tablets 5 mg/5 ml elixir 5-, 10-, 15-mg sustained-release tablets	2.5-10	10-20	8-12
Methylphenidate (Ritalin)	5-, 10-, 20-mg tablets 20-mg sustained-release tablets	5-10	20-30	1-2
Pemoline (Cylert)	18.75-, 37.5-, 75-mg tablets 37.5-mg chewable tablets	18.75-37.5	56.25-75	9-14

therapeutic efficacy may be initially noted almost immediately. Full effects are often seen in 2 or 3 days. Dosage forms, half-lives, and starting and maintenance doses are listed in Table 23-10. The short half-lives of methylphenidate and dextroamphetamine can result in a return of symptoms in the afternoon or evenings. Thus dosing is often with breakfast, again at midday, and in the afternoon when symptoms begin to break through. Dosing later in the day may increase the potential for insomnia. (Adderall is given once or twice a day.) Pemoline's longer half-life allows for once-a-day dosing.

SIDE EFFECTS

These three medications cause many similar side effects. GI upset, nausea, cramps, and anorexia are common. Initial GI symptoms often diminish with time. Lack of appetite for several hours after dosing may persist. Weight loss and growth suppression have been reported for all three stimulants. Dosing strategies that include drug holidays (e.g., school days only or periods off medication in the summer) allow for a correction of the growth suppression and result in children remaining within normal physical growth and development guidelines. All of these medications are occasionally associated with headache, dizziness, nervousness, irritability, and, rarely, emotional lability and psychosis. When these side effects are persistent, dose reduction or changing medication is a useful tactic.

Emergence of tics may be observed. Tics may diminish with dose reduction. However, these medications are often initiated in children during ages when the tic disorder Tourette's syndrome may first emerge. Whether tics are a part of Tourette's syndrome or not, their presence may make it difficult to use stimulants at any dose, and alternative ADHD treatments (e.g., antidepressants) may need to be tried.

There are differences in side effects between methyl-

phenidate, dextroamphetamine, and pemoline. Both of the former can cause palpitations, tachycardia, and increases in blood pressure, although these are seldom clinically significant. Nonetheless, these medications are sympathomimetics, and cardiac status, particularly hypertension and tachyarrhythmias, should be monitored at baseline and with dose titration. Pemoline has been occasionally associated with liver toxicity, usually during the first 3 months of therapy (Pratt and Dubois, 1990). Thus baseline and periodic monitoring of liver function tests are warranted.

SUMMARY

There is a great deal of public misunderstanding about the use of stimulant medication. An urban myth, that stimulants cause brain damage, is unsubstantiated but persists in some areas. Families must be provided with accurate information about anticipated efficacy and side effects. Optimal therapy involves the client, family, teachers, and clinicians working together.

OTHER BIOLOGIC THERAPIES
ELECTROCONVULSIVE THERAPY
Historical Perspective

Electroconvulsive therapy (ECT), sometimes referred to as electroshock therapy (EST), was first used as a treatment modality in 1934 to "cure" psychotic disorders by inducing convulsions. Throughout the years, ECT has been a topic of much controversy, some of which can be linked to the criticism of consumer groups. As a result of this criticism, ECT fell into disfavor and was rarely used. Used appropriately, ECT can be an effective therapy for many clients who have not responded to other treatment modalities.

ECT is not a new innovation. Paracelsus, a sixteenth-century Swiss physician, gave camphor to induce convulsions as a method of treating lunacy. This intervention also was used by von Auenbrugger in 1764. However, Auenbrugger's treatment was to ameliorate symptoms of mania. The "modern era" of convulsive therapy dates back to von Meduna's original work with a client who had been in a catatonic stupor for 4 years. In 1934 Meduna administered the injection of camphor oil to a client with schizophrenia, which resulted in a remarkable recovery after a series of treatments. Inspired by that success, Meduna administered the convulsive treatment to an additional 26 clients, of which 13 demonstrated considerable improvement.

Reports of the success of the new therapy spread and served as an impetus to explore additional methods to induce convulsions. This investigation led to the examination of an electrical stimulus as a seizure induction agent. By 1938 Cerletti and Bini achieved worldwide notoriety after administering 11 separate transcerebral treatments to a client with schizophrenia who demonstrated a full recovery from his illness (Abrams, 1988). It is unlikely that this client would be diagnosed with schizophrenia by today's standards, but the relative safety and potential efficacy of the procedure opened an entirely new treatment technique in psychiatry.

Even though modern ECT bears little resemblance to early ECT, there remains a stigma attached to its use. Confusion regarding the current practice of ECT is due to the lack of accurate information. Media versions of ECT portray barbaric methods of psychiatric treatment regimens.

Nurses play an integral role in the use of ECT by providing accurate education to the client and family to ameliorate fear and prevent distortions regarding the use of ECT. Nurses must fully understand the indications, contraindications, procedures, and side effects of ECT to educate, monitor, and support the client recommended for ECT and his or her family.

Modern ECT

ECT is a safe and effective treatment for major depression. The most appropriate candidates are clients experiencing a major mood disorder. Melancholic, delusional, and psychotic depression tend to respond well to ECT. Other indications for ECT include previous positive results from ECT, clients who cannot tolerate side effects of antidepressants, acute suicidal ruminations and behavior, and clients in danger of fluid and electrolyte imbalances secondary to inability to eat or drink as a result of severe depression. ECT has also been used in the treatment of mania, severe catatonia, and schizophrenia unresponsive to antipsychotic medications. ECT is also considered in the first trimester of pregnancy when pharmacotherapy is contraindicated.

Absolute contraindications include clients with space-occupying lesions with increased intracranial pressure. Risk factors to be considered are clients with recent myocardial infarction, aneurysms, acute respiratory infection, cardiac arrhythmias, organic syndromes, thrombophlebi-

tis, and narrow-angle glaucoma. ECT is not indicated for clients with a diagnosis of drug dependence, personality disorder, reactive depression, and paranoid schizophrenia.

Before and after the procedure, the client and family require education. Informed consent, which nurses frequently witness, can be obtained only after the client is thoroughly educated. Consent is given before treatment and authorizes the physician to perform it. The consent discusses the purpose of the treatment, the proposed number of treatments, and risk factors associated with ECT. Preliminary baseline tests (CBC, SMA, urinalysis, ECG, and physical examination) are obtained.

Today, the client may receive ECT on either an inpatient or outpatient basis. Clients scheduled for the procedure are fasted overnight (NPO) and are routinely prepared for an operative procedure (i.e., clients are asked to empty their bladder and remove jewelry, dental work, and nail polish). Approximately 30 minutes before the procedure, the client receives an IM atropine injection, typically 0.5 mg. This will reduce secretions and protect against vagal bradycardia, which can occur after application of the stimulus. In the ECT suite, blood pressure, cardiac, and electroencephalographic (EEG) monitors are placed to assess vital functions. Wherever ECT is given, emergency equipment, including oxygen, suction, and a cardiac arrest cart, must also be available. Staff attendance includes at minimum a psychiatrist, anesthetist, and nurse. A short-acting anesthetic and a muscle relaxant are given intravenously. Muscle paralysis prevents increased movement to decrease the risk of fracture or injury. A mouthguard and 100% oxygen is administered. Once anesthesia and paralysis are obtained, the ECT electrodes are placed. For bilateral ECT, electrodes are placed on the anterior portion of the client's temples; in unilateral ECT, the electrode is placed on the anterior portion of the client's nondominant temple (i.e., right handed—right temple). Once the electrodes are placed, a brief electrical stimulus (usually less than 2 seconds' total duration) is applied. The body does not move, and the seizure is confirmed by EEG monitoring. The client wakes in a few minutes, and oxygen is discontinued. The client is monitored closely for any respiratory distress and excess secretions that may need to be suctioned. The client remains in a recovery room, usually 1 to 3 hours, until vital signs are stable and the client is alert, oriented, and able to walk without assistance. The client may now eat and resume normal activity. Some clients may feel sleepy and return to bed.

Side effects most associated with ECT are headache and memory loss. Clients who experience headache may be given mild analgesia and instructed to rest. Memory impairment tends to be more pronounced with bilateral treatment. It can be quite severe during the course of treatment but generally improves significantly after completion of a series of treatments. The nurse will reorient clients and offer support and reassurance to those who are distraught regarding the memory loss. It is important to remember, especially with clients suffering memory loss, that client teaching will require repetition throughout the course of treatment. Nurses will allow clients to ventilate fears while offering support and education to assist in decreasing anxiety expressed in relation to ECT.

SEASONAL AFFECTIVE DISORDER AND PHOTOTHERAPY

Alterations in mood have been related to seasonal changes in some individuals. Research indicates that attacks of mania are more frequent in the summer (Rosenthal et al, 1983). Conversely, statistics indicate that the incidence of depression is more common in late fall. In 1981 Aschoff made an environmental observation that seasonal variation in mood disorders was greater in the least industrialized countries than in industrialized nations. He hypothesized that factors such as artificial light, central heating, and adherence to a work day based on clock hours as opposed to available natural light may reduce risk for affective episodes. Seasonal variation was increased in temperate climates and not in the north, as one might expect. Environmentally, this pattern correlated with clear sunshine and not with the length of the day, thus implicating brightness and duration of light in affecting mood.

Seasonal changes in time and duration of daylight trigger many changes seen in the behavior of various organisms. Artificial light has been used in industry to bring plants into bloom out of season, to increase productivity in egg-laying chickens, and to breed animals out of season. Bright, full-spectrum light may improve the productivity and irritability of shift workers whose work schedules force a discordance between "normal" sleep patterns and natural sunlight. Thus multiple observations suggest that phototherapy is potential treatment for seasonal affective disorder (SAD) (Lewy et al, 1986; Rosenthal et al, 1985; Terman et al, 1986).

Researchers have investigated seasonal depression. The depression usually begins in November and is characterized by hypersomnia, anergia, carbohydrate craving resulting in weight gain, decreased libido, social withdrawal, and suicidal thoughts. This depression lifts in March and may be followed by hypomania in spring (Kukopulos and Reginaldi, 1973).

Investigators of SAD have noted that some biologic markers may be more common in clients with this disorder. Altered sleep architecture has been observed on sleep EEGs (Rosenthal et al, 1983). Prolactin and melatonin, two hormones that have seasonal rhythms, are often abnormally high in clients with SAD.

Clinical trials have yielded several generalizations regarding the effectiveness of phototherapy. Often up to 80% of clients have been rated as much improved with phototherapy (Lewy et al, 1986; Rosenthal et al, 1985). The light used must be several times brighter than that which is usually encountered during indoor activities. Typically, clients are exposed to eight 4-foot fluorescent bulbs at a distance of 3 feet. Light administration in the middle of the day is as effective as light in the early morning or late at night. Effective treatment regimens require at least 2 hours of light exposure; greater effectiveness may be seen with 4 hours of exposure. The therapeutic effect appears to be mediated by the quantity of light that strikes the eyes and not the skin.

Response to phototherapy can be quite rapid. Some clients report improvement with 1 to 2 treatments, and maximum benefit may be seen in 4 to 7 days. Conversely, relapse with the withdrawal of light is reported to be just as rapid.

The mechanism of action of phototherapy, like the mechanism underlying SAD, is not clearly understood. Investigations into these issues, as well as practical devices and procedures to provide light therapy to clients, are active areas of investigation.

Summary of Key Concepts

1. Both typical (traditional) and atypical (novel) antipsychotics block dopamine receptors, but atypical antipsychotics have an improved efficacy against negative symptoms. Despite the high toxicity of antipsychotics, for many clients their benefits outweigh their risks.

2. Symptom response to antipsychotics varies. The order of response time from quickest to slowest follows: positive symptoms, affective symptoms, cognitive and perceptive symptoms, and negative symptoms.

3. Neuroleptic malignant syndrome (NMS) is a potentially fatal reaction to typical antipsychotics and must be recognized early to minimize fatal complications. However, NMS is often misdiagnosed as heat stroke, pneumonia, or lethal catatonia.

4. Seventy percent of clients with major depression will respond to antidepressants. The 30% failure rate is generally due to inadequate dosage or duration of therapy.

5. Antidepressants may cause increased energy and physical activity. Suicidal ideations may persist, so clients are at the highest risk to act on harmful impulses during the second week of therapy.

6. Pharmacotherapy for depression has many liabilities. Thus knowledge of toxicity and efficacy is essential to achieve optimal therapeutic response.

7. Because response to lithium may take a week or longer, concomitant antipsychotic therapy is often used to decrease acute psychotic symptoms.
8. Anxiolytics and hypnotics such as benzodiazepines are an adjunct to therapy. Short-term (7- to 10-day) intervention is the standard treatment.
9. Withdrawal symptoms from barbiturates closely resemble the original sleep or anxiety complaints.
10. Although barbiturates and benzodiazepines are commonly used, they have a highly addictive potential that must be considered.
11. Use of anticonvulsants should occur only with clear response expectations and well-defined target symptoms.
12. ECT, despite common consumer beliefs, is a safe and effective treatment for major depression.
13. Phototherapy has been found to be effective for clients with seasonal affective disorder (SAD).

REFERENCES

Abrams R: *Electroconvulsive therapy,* New York, 1988, Oxford University Press.

Adler LA et al: A controlled comparison of the effects of propranolol, benztropine and placebo on akathisia: an interim analysis, *Psychopharmacol Bull* 29(2):283, 1993.

Alvir JM, Lieberman JA: A reevaluation of the clinical characteristics of clozapine-induced agranulocytosis in light of the United States experience, *J Clin Psychopharmacol* 14(2):87, 1994.

American Psychiatric Association: Practice guidelines for major depressive disorder in adults, *Am J Psychiatry* 150(suppl):1, 1993.

Andrews JM, Nemeroff CB: Contemporary management of depression, *Am J Med* 97(6A):24S, 1994.

Aschoff J: Annual rhythms in man. In *Handbook of behavioral neurobiology,* New York, 1981, Plenum Press.

Baastrup PC et al: Prophylactic lithium: double-blind discontinuation in manic-depressive and recurrent depressive disorders, *Lancet* 2:326, 1970.

Baldessarini RJ: Drugs and the treatment of psychiatric disorders. In Gilman AG et al, editors: *Goodman and Gilman's the pharmacologic basis of therapeutics,* ed 8, New York, 1990, Pergamon.

Battaglia J et al: *Rapid tranquilization of agitated psychotic patients in the emergency room.* Presented at New Clinical Drug Evaluation Unit, Boca Raton, Fla., May 1992.

Borison RL et al: Risperidone: clinical safety and efficacy in schizophrenia, *Psychopharmacol Bull* 28(2):213, 1992.

Bowden C et al: Efficacy of divalproex vs lithium and placebo in the treatment of mania, *JAMA* 271:918, 1994.

Calis KA et al: Attention-deficit hyperactivity disorder, *Clin Pharmacy* 9:632, 1990.

Caroff SN et al: Neuroleptic malignant syndrome: diagnostic issues, *Psychiatr Ann* 21(2):130, 1991.

Cole J: New directions in antidepressant therapy: a review of sertraline, a unique serotonin reuptake inhibitor, *J Clin Psychiatry* 53(9):335, 1992.

Conley RR et al: Rehospitalization rates of recently discharged patients on risperidone and clozapine. Presented at the New Clinical Drug Evaluation Unit Annual Meeting, Boca Raton, Fla., June 10-13, 1998.

Damluji NF, Ferguson JM: Paradoxical worsening of depressive symptomatology caused by antidepressants, *J Clin Psychopharmacol* 8(5):347, 1988.

Davis KL et al: Dopamine in schizophrenia: a review and reconceptualization, *Am J Psychiatry* 148:1474, 1991.

De Wilde J et al: A double-blind, comparative, multi-center study comparing paroxetine with fluoxetine in depressed patients, *Acta Psychiatr Scand* 87:141, 1993.

Dechant KL, Clissold SP: Paroxetine—a review of its pharmacodynamic and pharmacokinetic properties and therapeutic potential in depressive illness, *Drugs* 41(2):225, 1991.

Delgado PL et al: Serotonin function and the mechanism of antidepressant action, *Arch Gen Psychiatry* 47:411, 1990.

Deniker P: The neuroleptics: an historical survey, *Acta Psychiatr Scand* 82 (suppl 358):83, 1990.

Dumon JP et al: Randomized, double-blind, crossover, placebo-controlled comparison of propranolol and betaxolol in the treatment of neuroleptic-induced akathisia, *Am J Psychiatry* 149:647, 1992.

Eison AS et al: Review of its pharmacology and current perspectives on its mechanism of action, *Am J Med* 80 (suppl 3B):1, 1986.

Fava M, Rosenbaum JF: Suicidality and fluoxetine: is there a relationship, *J Clin Psychiatry* 52:108, 1991.

Ferris RM, Cooper BR: Mechanism of antidepressant activity of bupropion, *J Clin Psychiatry* 11(1):2, 1993.

Gelenberg AJ et al: Comparison of standard and low serum levels of lithium for maintenance treatment of bipolar disorder, *N Engl J Med* 321(22):1489, 1989.

Glazer WM, Kane JM: Depot neuroleptic therapy: an underutilized treatment option, *J Clin Psychiatry* 53:426, 1992.

Goodhart RS et al: Phenelzine-associated peripheral neuropathy, clinical and electrophysiologic findings, *Aust NZ J Med* 21:339, 1991.

Gurrera RJ et al: A comparison of diagnostic criteria for neuroleptic malignant syndrome, *J Clin Psychiatry* 53:56, 1992.

Hagger C et al: Improvement in cognitive functions and psychiatric symptoms in treatment-refractory schizophrenic patients receiving clozapine, *Biol Psychiatry* 34:702, 1993.

Jacobson SJ et al: Prospective multi-center study of pregnancy outcome after lithium exposure during the first trimester, *Lancet* 339:530, 1992.

Johnstone EC, Marsh W: The relationship between response to phenelzine and acetylation status in depressed patients, *Proc R Soc Lond Biol Sci* 66:947, 1973.

Kane JM, Marder SR: Psychopharmacologic treatment of schizophrenia, *Special Report: schizophrenia,* 19(2):113, 1993.

Kane J et al: Clozapine for the treatment of schizophrenia, *Arch Gen Psychiatry* 45:789, 1988.

Keck PE et al: Valproate oral loading in the treatment of acute mania, *J Clin Psychiatry* 54:305, 1993.

King DJ: Benzodiazepines, amnesia and sedation: theoretical and clinical issues and controversies, *Human Pharmacol* 7:75, 1992.

Kukopulos A, Reginaldi D: Does lithium prevent depression by suppressing manias? *Int J Pharmacopsychiatry* 8:152, 1973.

Lader M: Rebound insomnia and newer hypnotics, *Psychopharmacology* 108(3):649, 1992.

Lewy AJ et al: Treatment of winter depression with light. In Shagass C et al, editors: *Biological psychiatry*, vol 6, New York, 1986, Elsevier.

Lichter JB et al: A hypervariable segment in the human dopamine receptor D_4 (DRD4) gene, *Hum Mol Genet* 2(6):767, 1993.

Love RC, Conley RR, Kelly DL: A Dose-outcome analysis of risperidone use in the Maryland State Mental Health System, XXIst CINP Congress, Glasgow, Scotland, July 12-16, 1998.

Manji HK et al: Signal transduction pathways, molecular targets for lithium's actions, *Arch Gen Psychiatry* 52:531, 1995.

McElroy SL et al: Clozapine in the treatment of psychotic mood disorders, schizoaffective disorder and schizophrenia, *J Clin Psychiatry* 51:411, 1991.

McElroy SL et al: Valproate in the treatment of bipolar disorder: literature review and clinical guidelines, *J Clin Psychiatry* 12:42S, 1992.

Meltzer HY et al: Cost effectiveness of clozapine in neuroleptic-resistant patients, *Am J Psychiatry* 150:1630, 1993.

Merlotti L et al: The dose effects of zolpidem on the sleep of healthy normals, *J Clin Psychiatry* 9(1):9, 1989.

Monroe RR: *Episodic behavioral disorders*, Cambridge, Mass, 1970, Harvard University Press.

Montgomery S: Venlafaxine: a new dimension in antidepressant pharmacotherapy, *J Clin Psychiatry* 54:3:119, 1993.

Pickar D et al: Mania and hypomania during antidepressant pharmacotherapy: clinical and research implications. In Post RM, Ballenger JC, editors: *Neurobiology of mood disorders*, Baltimore, 1984, Williams & Wilkins.

Pickar D et al: Clinical and biologic response to clozapine in patients with schizophrenia, crossover comparison with fluphenazine, *Arch Gen Psychiatry* 49:345, 1992.

Pigot TA et al: Controlled comparison of clomipramine and fluoxetine in the treatment of obsessive-compulsive disorder, *Arch Gen Psychiatry* 47(10):926, 1990.

Pollack MH, Rosenbaum JF: Management of antidepressant-induced side effects: a practical guide for the clinician, *J Clin Psychiatry* 48(1):3, 1987.

Pope H et al: Frequency and presentation of neuroleptic malignant syndrome in a large psychiatric hospital, *Am J Psychiatry* 143(10):1227, 1986.

Post RM et al: Mechanism of action of anticonvulsants in affective disorders: comparisons with lithium, *J Clin Psychopharmacol* 12:23S, 1992.

Pratt DS, Dubois RS: Hepatotoxicity due to pemoline: a report of two cases, *J Pediatr Gastroenterol Nutr* 10:239, 1990.

Prien RF: Maintenance therapy. In Paykel E, editor: *Handbook of affective disorders*, London, 1992, Churchill Livingston.

Quitkin FM et al: Response to phenelzine and imipramine in placebo nonresponders with atypical depression, *Arch Gen Psychiatry* 48:319, 1991.

Richelson R: Side effects of old and new generation antidepressants: a pharmacologic framework, *J Clin Psychiatry* 9(1):13, 1991.

Risch SC, Nemeroff CB: Neurochemical alterations of serotonergic neuronal systems in depression, *J Clin Psychiatry* 53(10, suppl):3, 1992.

Rosenthal NE et al: Seasonal variation in affective disorders. In Wehr TA, Goodwin FK, editors: *Biological rhythms and psychiatry*, Pacific Grove, Calif, 1983, Boxwood Press.

Rosenthal NE et al: Antidepressant effects of light in seasonal affective disorder, *Am J Psychiatry* 142:163, 1985.

Roy-Byrne PP, Hommer D: Benzodiazepine withdrawal: overview and implications for the treatment of anxiety, *Am J Med* 84(6):1041, 1988.

Sachs GS: Use of clonazepam for bipolar affective disorder, *J Clin Psychiatry* 51(5, suppl):31, 1990.

Sanger DJ et al: The behavioral profile of zolpidem, a novel hypnotic drug of imidazopyridins structure. *Physiol Behav* 4:(2):39, 1987.

Scharf MB et al: Dose response effects of zolpidem in normal geriatric subjects. *J Clin Psychiatry* 52:77, 1991.

Schou M: Effects of long-term lithium treatment on kidney function: an overview, *J Psychiatr Res* 22:287, 1988.

Schou M et al: Lithium and pregnancy. I. Report from the register of lithium babies, *BMJ* 2:135, 1973.

Stimmel et al

Tamminga CA et al: Clozapine in tardive dyskinesia: observations from human and animal model studies. *J Clin Psychiatry* 55(9, suppl B):102, 1994.

Teicher MH et al: Emergence of intense suicidal preoccupation during fluoxetine treatment, *Am J Psychiatry* 247(2):207, 1990.

Terman M et al: Bright light treatment of seasonal affective disorder, *New Research Abstracts*, 139th annual meeting of the American Psychiatric Association, 1986.

Thomas H et al: Droperidol versus haloperidol for chemical restraint of agitated and combative patients, *Ann Emerg Med* 21(4):407, 1992.

Tulloch IF, Johnson AM: The pharmacologic profile of paroxetine, a new selective serotonin reuptake inhibitor, *J Clin Psychiatry* 53(suppl 2):7, 1992.

Vaughn DA: Interaction of fluoxetine and tricyclic antidepressants, *Am J Psychiatry* 145:1478, 1988.

Wilde MI et al: Fluvoxamine: an updated review of its pharmacology and therapeutic use in depressive illness, *Drugs* 46(5):895, 1993.

Wysowski DK, Barash D: Adverse behavioral reactions attributed to triazolam in the food and drug administration's spontaneous reporting system, *Arch Intern Med* 151:2003, 1991.

CHAPTER 24

Alternative Therapies

Ruth N. Grendell

OBJECTIVES

- Describe the philosophic differences between alternative and traditional (conventional) therapies.

- Discuss the influence of mind-body inter-relationships on wellness and health promotion.

- Identify the current alternative therapies used in treatment of physiologic and psychologic health problems, particularly chronic disease management.

- Discuss the nurse's role in providing holistic nursing care.

- Discuss the impact of alternative therapies on the nurse's role in applying therapeutic interventions.

- Describe incorporation of alternative therapies in the plan of care.

- Discuss client education concerning concurrent use of alternative therapies and traditional (Western) therapies.

- Discuss the impact of alternative therapies on nursing practice, education, and research.

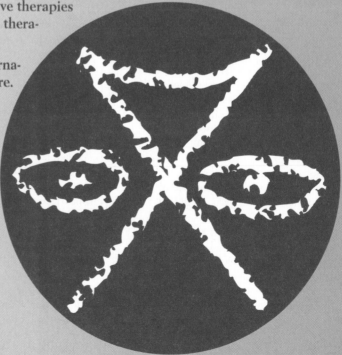

The biomedical model is based primarily on identifying external causes of **disease** and implementing external treatment methods of cure, whereas the focus of the holistic or alternative care model is on strengthening one's inner resistance to disease and "healing from within," or enhancing the body's innate healing powers. Although **nursing** has been strongly influenced by biomedical practices, it also has deep roots in the holistic perspective that considers the impact of all intrapersonal, interpersonal, and environmental interactions as contributing factors to a person's well-being or **illness.**

Some alternative medical practices have been accepted into conventional medicine, particularly in pain management and treatment of chronic illness, anxiety, depression, and the prevention of disease. The following discussion centers around the contrast in philosophies and treatment modalities of the biomedical and holistic models of care, descriptions of selected alternative therapies, and their significance to the practice of nursing.

ALTERNATIVE THERAPY FIELDS

"Complementary and **alternative medicine** covers a broad range of healing philosophies, approaches, and therapies. It generally is defined as those treatments and health care practices not taught widely in medical schools, not generally used in hospitals, and not usually reimbursed by medical insurance companies" (National Institutes of Health [NIH], 1998). Some therapies are based on physiologic principles of traditional medicine, whereas others arise from concepts that are in contrast to the accepted medical practices. Alternative therapies can be arranged into seven fields of practice (Dossey, 1998; Reed et al, 1994). These are (1) mind/body biobehavioral inter-

Alternative medicine Alternative (complementary) medicine covers a broad range of healing philosophies, approaches, and therapies. It generally is defined as those treatments and health care practices not taught widely in medical schools, not generally used in hospitals, and not usually reimbursed by medical insurance companies.

Disease A term used to describe altered body functions and a condition that places limitations on daily activities with the presence of recognizable disease symptoms. It is a result of the inability to adapt to certain stressors. Formerly it was believed that a specific disease had one particular cause. Today, multiple stimuli are known to be involved, as well as the individual's response to those factors and prescribed remedies.

Health The absence of disease and a state of total well-being. The various definitions imply that health is dynamic, with its focus on living rather than on disease categories. Health has been referred to as a condition of adjustment, or adaptation, to physical, psychologic, and social environmental changes. A person's *health status* refers to that status at a given point in time. For some individuals, health is defined in terms related to the ability to work.

Illness A feeling of disease, or discomfort. Illness is a subjective experience and must be interpreted by the individual. Illness may or may not be associated with disease. Illness has been labeled as an unexpected stressful event in individuals' lives that can interrupt them from fulfilling their usual tasks or roles. Illness is often perceived to be a crisis event. The terms *illness* and *disease* are often used synonymously; however, the disease process may be present without the person feeling ill, such as a lump in the breast that has not yet been detected. A number of factors are now being considered as causes of illness and determinants of an individual's response. *Chronic illness* is a health

problem with symptoms or disabilities requiring long-term management that affect persons across the life span. The incidence of chronic illnesses increases with aging, and many elderly persons develop multiple chronic health problems. This includes learning to live with any identity changes, and the common associated symptoms of pain and fatigue. Maintaining a regimen to keep symptoms under control, thus preventing complications, becomes a part of the person's lifestyle; however, some chronic illnesses permit people to function independently with little disruption to their lives, whereas others must rely on frequent assisted care or placement in long-term care facilities.

Nursing The science that occupies all of the relative processes of care of the health of the individual, family, and community in order to promote, maintain, or bring them to a state of wellness. It is dynamic and evolutionary, humanistic, and a discipline that is fundamentally based on scientific and technical knowledge and founded on moral, ethical, and spiritual values. It uses the nursing process with a holistic approach and promotes an essential environment for the health care of the human being (definition provided by the Universidad Politecnia de Nicaragua School of Nursing [Lockhart, 1998]).

Stress (1) A term that refers to both a stimulus and a response. It can denote a nonspecific response of the body to any demand placed on it whether the causal event is negative (a painful experience) or positive (a happy occasion). (2) A state produced by a change in the environment that is perceived as challenging, threatening, or damaging to the person's dynamic equilibrium. (3) The wear and tear on the body over time. (4) Psychologic stress has been defined as all processes, whether originating in the external environment or within the person, that demand a mental appraisal of the event before the involvement or activation of any other system.

ventions; (2) bioelectromagnetics; (3) alternative systems of medical practice (e.g., oriental medicine); homeopathy and environmental medicine; (4) manual techniques, which are sometimes included under the alternative systems category; (5) medications that are not accepted by traditional practitioners; (6) herbal medications; and (7) diet, nutrition and supplements, and lifestyle changes. Selected alternative therapies are listed in Box 24-1.

HISTORICAL OVERVIEW
ANCIENT CULTURAL BELIEFS

In ancient times illness was often believed to be punishment for sin or at the whim of the gods—a matter of fate; healing came through purification of the body by incantations and the use of herbs. Evil spirits were believed to cause illnesses and adverse events; good spirits intervened on the behalf of an individual or group. Animal sacrifices were made to appease the gods, and spirits became part of healing rituals. In some countries, however, laws were also passed to regulate the practices of hygiene, sanitation, and preservation of food to protect people from disease.

Hippocrates, born in 400 BC and known as the father of modern medicine, introduced beliefs that health was not controlled by the gods but was dependent on the harmony, or balance, between the body, the mind, and the environment. He employed a patient-centered approach to treat the whole person. The dominant beliefs in most Asian countries considered that this balance between humans and nature could be attained through finding inner peace and spiritual contentment and by understanding and practicing the interactive powers of the mind and body. In many cultures healers were priest-physicians referred to as holy men, or shamans, and the care they provided was referred to as shamanistic medicine (Ellis and Hartley, 1998).

BIOMEDICINE MODEL CONCEPTS

During the seventeenth century the interconnections of body, mind, and spirit were considered of minor importance within the biomedical model. Medical practitioners treated the ailments of the body while matters of the mind and spirit were delegated to the church. This separation permitted dramatic advances in understanding of the biologic processes and in the discoveries of treatments of disease. This practice has continued up to modern times as physicians treat physical illness, psychiatrists deal with mental disorders, and the clergy attend to spiritual needs. Today there is still a strong tendency to consider a human as a complex system composed of many interconnecting subsystems. The total person is, then, a sum of the individual parts (Achterberg, et al, 1994; Bellamy and Pfister, 1992).

Conventional medical practice primarily uses standardized treatments such as drugs and/or surgical intervention, and the care regimen is tailored to the client's

---

Box 24-1   Alternative Therapy Fields and Selected Examples

Mind-Body Interventions
Meditation
Prayer
Yoga
The arts: music, dance, drama, art, literature, humor
Psychotherapy
Hypnosis

Alternative Systems of Medical Practice
Traditional Oriental medicine
    Acupuncture
Ayurvedic medicine
Homeopathic medicine
Naturopathy
Environmental medicine
Culture-based community medicine

Pharmacologic and Biologic Treatments
Vaccines and medicines not yet approved by mainstream
    medicine
    Animal cartilage
    Ethylene diamine tetraacetic acid (EDTA) as chelating
    chemical

Diet, Nutrition, Supplements, and Lifestyle Changes
Vitamins, minerals, and supplements
Designer diets—macrobiotic, cancer, weight reduction
Food elimination diets—allergy detection
Vegetarian
Ethnic-based diets

Bioelectromagnetics
Light therapy
Bone growth stimulation
Magnet therapy

Manual Healing Methods
Osteopathy
Chiropractic
Massage
Acupressure
Foot reflexology
Therapeutic touch

Herbal Medications
Chinese herbals
European
American

---

match with a disease category of defined signs and symptoms. Dr. Andrew Weil (1995), physician, professor, and author of several books on mind/body healing, commented that medical students are mainly exposed to the world of hospital medicine, where very sick clients represent only a small portion of the general population. "Curing rather than healing has dominated the Western mode of health care with emphasis on technology, power, analysis, and the repair of damaged parts" (Kozier, Erb, and Blais, 1997). Medical education is also *physician centered*, granting the caregiver authority for making decisions and placing the client in a passive, somewhat powerless, position that limits the client's responsibility in the recovery process.

HOLISTIC MODEL CONCEPTS

In contrast, the holistic perspective is more concerned with healing of the total person rather than the cure of a specific disease. Each person is viewed as uniquely separate from another human being and is *more* than the sum of the individual parts—what affects one aspect affects all (Bellamy and Pfister, 1992; Dossey and Dossey, 1998; Keegan, 1998). In addition to examining physical symptoms, the clinician considers the influence of cultural and genetic factors, past and current experiences, family structure, and role functions on the person's perception of **health** and illness and the use of coping mechanisms. Individuals are encouraged to take active responsibility for their own health and participate in the recovery process when illnesses do occur. A change in attitude and lifestyle, a sense of control, peace, and loss of anxiety can indicate healing even though the particular disease is not cured. Multiple methods may be incorporated into the individualized plan of care. Many of the therapies are based on Oriental and Far Eastern beliefs and practices. Although there is a wide variety of alternative therapies, there are some unifying themes, including a person's inherent recuperative ability, the importance of self-esteem, and the influence of spiritual and emotional beliefs on health. Treatment methods are based on maintaining or restoring a balance within all aspects of the individual. A detailed listing of themes is provided in Box 24-2.

Box 24-2   Common Themes of Alternative Therapies

Humans have innate recuperative powers.

There is importance in religious and spiritual values to the state of health.

Self-esteem and purpose of life are a positive influence in the healing process.

Thoughts, feelings, emotions, values, and perceived meanings affect physical function.

Most therapies rely on diet, exercise, relaxation techniques, lifestyle, and attitude changes.

Focus is on the total person—physical, emotional, mental, and psychosocial health.

Illness is viewed as an imbalance; interventions are directed toward restoring balance.

Energy is the force needed to achieve balance and harmony.

RISE IN DOMINANCE OF THE BIOMEDICAL MODEL

Before the 1800s, biomedicine and alternative medicine coexisted and competed on a somewhat equal basis. However, during the latter part of that century, the biomedical model was validated as being superior because of the scientific discovery of microbes as the cause of many infectious diseases and the development of methods to eradicate those causes. Disease cure rates rose, and favorable surgical outcomes soon followed through the use of proper aseptic techniques and new anesthesia discoveries. Another significant event that legitimized biomedicine was the research report by Abraham Flexner in 1910 that indicated the need for standards in education and licensing of physicians. Philanthropic funding of medical education institutions quickly halted any financial assistance to the schools with the nonmedical, nonscientific curricula.

As a result of the medical model acceptance, credibility of alternative therapy practitioners and their methods became questionable, and these practices were soon relegated to the fringes of health care and often referred to as "quackery." Although chiropractic and osteopathic practices continued, others such as homeopathy and naturopathy were almost forgotten (Dossey and Swyers, 1994; Kozier, Erb, and Blais, 1997). Currently, health care professionals often ignore the fact that people use many alternative methods in managing their illnesses (Ellis and Hartley, 1998).

MERGING TRENDS OF PHILOSOPHIES

Orthodox medicine however, could not explain either function or disease of the mind; nor did it interpret the interactions between mind, spirit, and body. (The brain was considered a part of the body.) The discovery that some people exposed to pathogens did not become ill led researchers to challenge the existing biologic theory and to explore other possible influencing causes. Subsequent epidemiologic studies revealed that diet, smoking, and environmental pollution were strongly associated with increased incidences of lung cancer; widowed persons had higher death rates than married persons in the same age-group; socioeconomic factors had impact on disease; and certain religious groups had fewer reports of illness and death from specific diseases. The strong possibility of a cause-effect relationship between the mind, spirit, and body in health and illness encouraged further investigation. These findings indicated that many chronic conditions are not amenable to the one-dimensional solutions prescribed by conventional medicine (Berman and Larson, 1994).

Scientists, then, explored the age-old mind-body healing modalities of other societies, particularly Oriental medicine. As a result, acupuncture, meditation, relaxation techniques, massage, and other related interventions have been integrated into mainstream health care. Some medical schools have included courses in alternative therapies in the curriculum; additional research has been undertaken; and several articles have been published (Bassick, 1996; Dossey and Swyers, 1994; Reed et al, 1994; Weil, 1995). However, progress in using these modalities as alternative and complementary techniques may be slowed because of regulatory and reimbursement measures, values and misconceptions still held by many traditional practitioners, and the lack of large-scale clinical trials to demonstrate their effectiveness.

CURRENT ISSUES
THE CHANGING COMPLEXION OF HEALTH CARE

Modern medicine has become so expensive that it is straining the economy of the United States and of many developed nations, putting itself beyond the reach of much of the world's population, particularly for long-term regimens. Nearly 70% of the nation's health care budget is spent on treatment of persons with chronic diseases, and costs will escalate as the "baby boomer" generation grows older. Approximately 160 million people in the United States are covered by managed care, and almost $1 trillion is spent annually on treatment of disease, illness, and injury. People often need assistance in negotiating the complexities of the maze of the modern health care system.

Unfortunately, biomedical treatments and advanced technology can also have adverse consequences. Microbes have become resistant to medications; some chronic diseases that still defy scientific interventions have replaced infectious diseases as the major cripplers and killers. Side effects of many of the new "wonder" drugs can have devastating psychologic and physiologic effects.

Consumer confidence in conventional treatment methods has deteriorated, and citizens are turning to legislators to bring about change in the health care system. Reasons given for the growing dissatisfaction include the spiraling costs and restrictions imposed by managed care and health maintenance organizations and the desire to have more control in health care decisions. Health care reform requires a focus on disease prevention and health promotion rather than on disease treatment (Dossey and Swyers, 1994; Ellis and Hartley, 1998; Moran, 1995; Weil, 1995). A large portion of the population now depend on nontraditional therapies to manage their own health care.

Exposure to the various alternative therapies through the merger of cultures and abundant information provided by the media have a strong influence on the public's acceptance and use of alternative therapies. Information on health care is covered almost daily by newspapers, radio, and television and is easily accessible on the Internet. Articles frequently appear in popular magazines, and many book stores have substantial space allocated to self-help books that have become "best sellers." Convenience and fewer side effects from "natural" substances, less-invasive techniques, the possibility of an overall decrease in cost, and the ability to choose are appealing alternatives to traditional medicine.

According to a 1993 national survey of 1539 respondents over 18 years of age, approximately 70% to 90% used at least one alternative therapy during the previous year. People frequently tried home remedies first, often in consultation with friends and family members, and then turned to cultural or spiritual "healers" before seeking care from traditional medical professionals for acute illnesses. The participants also reported using both traditional and alternative therapies for chronic conditions with or without informing their medical care providers. Approximately one third of the respondents took over-the-counter (OTC) drugs, and 50% took vitamins and nutritional supplements.

The study revealed that $14 billion was spent in out-of-pocket expense by these respondents using alternative remedies for treatment of chronic diseases, with the average number of visits to alternative care clinicians exceeding the average number of visits to traditional care providers. The investigation was limited to the 16 most commonly used alternative therapies, which included acupuncture and chiropractic manipulation. The largest group represented were in the 25- to 49-year age range, had college educations, and were in a higher-than-average income bracket. Among the chronic conditions reported were back problems, digestive disturbances, headaches, allergies, asthma, hypertension and cardiovascular problems, diabetes mellitus, cancer, arthritis, and substance abuse, particularly alcohol (Eisenberg et al, 1993).

Similar findings were found in a national study conducted in 1997 with 1752 respondents over the age of 18 years. In addition to findings in the previous study, anxiety was reported by 18% of the respondents, and 14% reported episodes of depression. Feeling stressed was reported by 43%, with half of these individuals stating they realized that stress can be a contributing factor to physical illnesses. They commented that mental stress produced more fatigue than physical stress (Clements and Hales, 1997).

Common alternative therapies chosen by the respondents in both studies were chiropractic manipulation, exercise, nutrition and supplements, stress reduction techniques, biofeedback, meditation, yoga, spiritual counsel and prayer, herbal and folk remedies, and energy healing strategies (Clements and Hales, 1997; Eisenberg et al, 1993). A summary of findings of these studies is given in Box 24-3.

Another recent study revealed that the major health concerns for the elderly were related to quality-of-life issues and the availability of resources for coping with age-related psychologic, social, and physiologic changes. Many of these individuals experienced social isolation and anxiety, had multiple chronic health problems accompanied by pain, had poor nutritional intake, and had limited activity. Financial concerns and access to health care were also primary concerns (Dossey, 1997).

Box 24-3   Data Collected in Two Independent National Telephone Surveys

Studies were conducted in 1993 (Eisenberg et al) with 1539 subjects over 18 years of age and in 1997 (Clements and Hales) with 1752 subjects over 18 years of age. The largest group represented in the Eisenberg et al study were in the 25- to 49-year age range, had college educations, and were in a higher-than-average income bracket.

Seventy percent used at least one alternative therapy during the previous year.

Several used traditional and alternative therapies concurrently.

Alternative therapies were used for chronic illnesses with or without informing the health care provider.

One third took OTC drugs.

Fifty percent took vitamins and nutritional supplements.

Home remedies used were usually associated with consultation with family/friends or cultural/spiritual counsel.

Several believed that most illnesses are self-limiting and preferred to try their own remedies before trying conventional practices.

Primary reasons cited for these practices were the high costs of medical care and persons accepting responsibility for their own health.

Chronic conditions reported included back problems, digestive disturbances, headaches, allergies, asthma, hypertension and cardiovascular problems, diabetes mellitus, cancer, arthritis, and substance abuse, particularly alcohol. (Anxiety and depression were included in the Clements and Hales study.)

Alternative therapies chosen included chiropractic manipulation, exercise, nutrition and supplements, stress reduction techniques, biofeedback, meditation, yoga, spiritual counsel and prayer, herbal and folk remedies, and energy healing strategies.

Alternative therapies frequently used by the elderly include folk remedies passed down through family or cultural generations. Some remedies include drinking a mixture of honey, safflower oil, and cider vinegar; wearing copper bracelets; and, more recently, using magnets in the treatment of arthritis and muscle pain.

BARRIERS TO ACCEPTANCE OF ALTERNATIVE THERAPIES

Although alternative practices have been in vogue for centuries in Europe, Asia, and Far Eastern countries, therapeutic results have primarily been reported via anecdotal reports, so the rigor of the research methods has been questioned. The traditional medical world continues to call for clinical studies conducted within strict, controlled parameters. The Food and Drug Administration (FDA) has also expressed great concern over the lack of guide-

lines to ensure purity and dosage accuracy of herbal remedies and supplements (Dossey and Swyers, 1994). Currently these substances are exempt from FDA approval. There is also a concern over claims that one substance can be a "cure-all" for many health problems. The FDA continues to argue for the right to regulate these products. Another great concern is the validity of media reports and the credentials of the report writers. "The public has been bombarded with information that is difficult to sort out," therefore encouraging the possibility of misuse and overdependence on these products (Keegan, 1998).

The tremendous costs for investigation are prohibitive for many advocates of alternative therapies; thus many methods will not be tested. Additional barriers are the heavy reliance on high-technology treatments by society, the dependence on pharmaceuticals, and state laws that limit the practice of medicine or the healing arts to those with professional medical licensure. The political lobbying and advertising influence of drug manufacturers is another major barrier, although most companies produce OTC compounds that are attractive substitutes to costly prescriptive medications.

Many of the barriers are the typical ones encountered by innovative proposals that challenge any current traditional practices (Dossey and Swyers, 1994; Jessup, 1995). Additional concerns focus on the dangers of self-diagnosis, potential and critical delay in seeking appropriate medical care, the potential interactions during the concurrent use of herbal and other drugs with prescribed medications, and the detrimental effects of not informing health care providers about the use of alternative products.

IMPACT OF THE *HEALTHY PEOPLE 2000 REPORT*

As early as the 1970s, the rising costs of medical care directed several physicians and educators to see the need for integrating technical sophistication with humanistic values. The debate over quality-of-life issues required a focus on changes in education of the public and the profession. Alternative strategies evolved, such as permitting family members to assist in patient care in intensive care units, creating a homelike atmosphere during labor and delivery, presenting health education programs, and establishing self-help support groups. Health appraisal questionnaires were made available in physicians' offices and hospital rooms, and illnesses were used as "creative opportunities" for instruction on self-care. A limited number of alternative therapies, including acupuncture and stress reduction measures, were introduced into the system (Berman and Larson, 1994; Weil, 1995).

Health care reform became a major issue in the 1980s, and as a result, several nationwide studies were conducted. The *Healthy People 2000 Report* published under the auspices of the U.S. Public Health Department in 1990 contained three major goals: (1) to increase the healthy life span for all Americans, (2) to reduce the discrepancies in care provided among Americans, and (3) to provide access to preventive services for all. Primary, secondary, and tertiary levels of illness/disease prevention were referred to as healthy lifestyle practices, early screening and treatment, and rehabilitation measures to inhibit complications. These protective and preventive measures required active participation by both the people and health care providers. The report also targeted specific needs of several high-risk groups, including infants, children, ethnic and low-income groups, and the elderly.

EXPLORING EFFECTIVENESS OF ALTERNATIVE THERAPIES

In 1992 Congress established the Office of Alternative Medicine (OAM) under the direction of the National Institutes of Health (NIH). Its major purposes are to investigate the efficacy of alternative therapies for several serious health problems in the United States, to establish a clearinghouse for information exchange, and to support research education in alternative therapies that are not ordinarily included in mainstream medical care curricula. Ten regional centers have been established nationwide for the evaluation of alternative therapies that have the *potential* for improving the health of a large number of people. (An eleventh center was established recently to specifically examine chiropractic medicine.) To date, government funding has been increased each year ($20 million in fiscal 1998), and several studies are in various stages of progress. In actuality, the distinction between some areas of conventional and alternative medicine is not clear-cut because of the movement of some "fringe" therapies into mainstream practices. Therefore there is a great need for testing to take place (Clark, 1998; Dossy, 1997; Dossey and Swyers, 1994; Keegan, 1998; NIH, 1998).

Examples of OAM-funded research include a study in progress at Bastyr University in Seattle, which is investigating the use of alternative therapies on survival rates, the quality of life, and evidence of infections for people with AIDS. So far, the use of 70 alternative therapies has been mentioned. Following the initial analysis, the research design will be refined for use with participants from a wider geographic distribution. Data collection will continue with 1500 participants every 6 months. Preliminary findings from another study at Bastyr University produced promising results on the effects of acupuncture used on 327 identified substance abusers of alcohol and cocaine. Alcohol users experienced less craving, and there were fewer readmissions for detoxification for cocaine users (Villaire, 1995). Newly OAM-funded studies are listed in Box 24-4.

THE INFORMED CLIENT

Physician control over disease information may be ebbing as consumers become more active in decisions about their methods of treatment. The Internet is commonly used by self-help and discussion groups for the exchange of infor-

---

Box 24-4   Ongoing Research Funded by the Office of Alternative Medicine

NOTE: Many of the studies are longitudinal and will require several months or years to produce results. Preliminary findings have been reported on some of the studies. The following list is a sample of the many ongoing and proposed research works. Much of the funding is for new research that will be conducted over the next 5 years or more. Some studies receive grant funds from other agencies as well. $20 million was pledged for 1998.

Current Research

Funded in 1993—herbal treatment for Parkinson's disease to study the effects of plants used in Ayurvedic medicine (Southern Illinois University); currently—a multicenter clinical trial being conducted in India

Alternative therapies in treatment of persons with AIDS and substance addiction (Bastyr University)

New Research Grants

Pilot trials using acupuncture for a variety of clinical situations (sites to be announced)

Dietary supplements—glucosamine sulfate and chondroitin sulfate in treatment of osteoarthritis—safety and effectiveness (Georgetown University—3-year study)

Randomized clinical trial on effectiveness of St. John's wort (Hypericum perforatum) for moderate to severe depression (Duke University Medical Center, 1998)

The eleventh center for the study of chiropractic medicine effects

Future Considerations

Trials on effects of *Ginkgo biloba* for dementia and traumatic brain injury following cerebrovascular accident

Herbal treatments for benign prostatic hypertrophy

Use of garlic for cardiovascular disease (cholesterol reduction)

Use of acupuncture and herbs in treatment of alcoholism and abuse

Dietary supplements, such as dehydroepiandrosterone (DHEA)

Alternative methods and pain relief (acute and chronic)

---

mation and has provided a pooling of current expertise about a variety of health problems that often goes beyond current information known by the practicing health care provider. Families and clients faced with life-threatening situations have located information about the particular problem, and by sharing it with their physicians, they have often been effective in changing the course of medical protocol (Bassick, 1996; Jessup, 1995).

Public awareness of developments in health care and alternative therapies has also been enhanced by the broadcasting of documentary films. Health care providers depicted in the humanities and sciences film produced by

Alternative Therapies

Mental health nurses working in the community may be amazed at how many alternative treatments are being used by clients with mental health problems. Although these therapies are not free of side effects and interactions with other medications, they are widely regarded as "safer" by clients than conventional medicine because they are "natural." Individuals may be self-medicating with a variety of vitamins, minerals, and herbal preparations for mental health difficulties. Many of them are trying St. John's wort for depression or melatonin for insomnia. Adult children are giving their aging parents *Ginkgo biloba* tablets and vitamin E, and they are encouraging them to participate in energizing experiences such as tai chi and yoga.

Many physicians are also aware of recent studies for treating dementia and prescribing vitamin E megadose therapy, as well as conventional medications. They may also order *Ginkgo biloba* for memory loss and St. John's wort for depression when their clients refuse more conventional treatments. For some clients, treatments such as acupuncture, meditation, biofeedback, and massage are being prescribed with some success, especially for stress reduction and to reduce symptoms of drug withdrawal. Some types of hypnotherapy are being used for addictive behaviors and for traumatic stress disorders.

Because of the widespread use of these therapies, both initial and ongoing nursing evaluations should include questions about alternative treatments, since some may interact with allopathic medicines and produce serious effects such as reduced clotting time because of antioxidant agents. Participation in alternative therapies is more pervasive in some areas of the country than in others, but assessing a client for utilization is an important part of a comprehensive mental health evaluation.

The community mental health nurse must also be aware of another form of self-medication—illicit drug use. Some clients believe that the herb marijuana is more effective in controlling their symptoms than medications prescribed by their physicians. They may use other street drugs or mind-altering substances for the same reasons. It is extremely important that the community mental health nurse both recognize signs of psychoactive drug use and gain the client's trust, so that a meaningful dialogue about the dangers of these substances may develop.

Bassick (1996) commented on the need for more physicians to be educated in multidisciplinary methods. Recognizing that 1 in 3 Americans use alternative therapies is a wake-up call for the field of medicine. A gynecologist stated that she had been educated about the effectiveness of alternative therapies for menopausal symptoms by her clients, who initially did not inform her that they were using them. She subsequently introduced these methods to other clients with similar problems. Another physician established a center in New England for women where acupuncture, massage, and counseling are routine treatments of menopausal symptoms. Others commented on their use of Ayurvedic concepts of meditation, relaxation techniques, and massage as adjuncts to their standard practices. One pediatric physician used **naturopathic** dietary and **homeopathic** methods and vitamins in the treatment of allergies to increase children's immune responses to repeated infections. One segment of the film describes the benefits of herbal remedies from the Far East and Europe and of herbs first introduced by the American Indians to the early colonists. Advocates of alternative therapies stated that there is unlimited potential for discovering additional natural remedies.

THE NURSE'S ROLE

"Nurses have a primary responsibility in health promotion, health maintenance, and prevention activities; in fact, these are the essence of professional nursing practice" (Nunnery, 1997). The health of individuals, families, and communities is a major focus of nursing, with consideration for the effect of the individual's health status, health beliefs, and interactions with self, others, and the environment. Several practice models have been developed to guide the nurse in carrying out these practices. All of the models are designed around a holistic view of the client giving consideration to the ability for adapting and coping with life events, the impact of social and cultural values on health/illness beliefs, and personal responsibility for healthy outcomes (Kozier et al, 1997; Nunnery, 1997).

The American Holistic Nurses' Association has published standards for holistic practice, and several resources are available through the National League for Nursing (Keegan, 1998). Wayne B. Jonas, MD, Director of OAM, commented on the significant role that nurses fulfill in implementing alternative and complementary practices along with mainstream medicine. "They have often provided interventions that address some of the biopsychosocial aspects that get overlooked in an environment that is increasingly driven by technology and health care management pressures. Nursing care can provide the gap between alternative and conventional worlds" (Keegan, 1998).

APPLICATION OF SELECTED ALTERNATIVE THERAPIES: AN OVERVIEW

Although alternative therapies have been used in a variety of acute illness situations, their greatest benefit has been in promoting healthy lifestyles and in the management of chronic illnesses and diseases. The greater incidence of chronic illnesses today has been linked to environmental and emotional stresses. Anxiety, depression, anger, frustration, low self-esteem, despair, hopelessness, and isolation are common emotions experienced by persons with chronic diseases. Chronic illness and pain permeate the person's total existence. They feel victimized and powerless. The world is seen through eyes accustomed to chronic sorrow over their ongoing losses (Eakes, Burke, and Hainsworth, 1998; Thorne and Paterson, 1998). During the past 30 years there has been a major effort to identify strategies to assist individuals with acute diagnoses and chronic health problems (e.g., heart disease, hypertension, cancer, arthritis, and depression) in coping with and managing sudden and long-term life changes.

This search process led scientists to examine meditation, yoga, and tai chi practices, used primarily in Far Eastern cultures, to aid in quieting the mind and to identify and control internal and external sources of **stress**. Newer techniques of biofeedback and visual imagery, which are based on these principles, have been designed to interpret links between mental processes, the autonomic nervous system, and functions of the immune system, and to aid in modifying detrimental effects. In fact, psychoneuroimmunology is a new discipline that grew out of these endeavors (Achterberg, et al, 1994). These methods can be used both as preventive and as healing measures.

MIND-BODY INTERVENTIONS
Meditation
The relaxation response to meditation consists of a wide range of beneficial physiologic and psychologic effects, including lowered heart and blood pressure rates, decreased serum levels of adrenal corticosteroids, increased immunity to disease, a sense of calmness and peace, and mental alertness. Meditation, joined with biofeedback, visual imagery, and other stress reduction measures, including yoga and progressive relaxation techniques, has been used for a variety of situations (e.g., pain relief, decrease in anxiety levels, alleviation of depression, increased healing rates, and lessening of substance abuse). Originally, meditation was considered a religious practice; saying prayers, reciting scripture, or saying the rosary can be considered forms of meditation. Meditative techniques can be taught, and a number of audiotapes have been designed to facilitate mastery of concentration. Guidelines for meditating include a routine of selecting a special time and place, assuming a comfortable position, using deep breathing and progressive relaxation exercises, and focusing attention on a chosen mental image (Achterberg et al, 1994; Keegan, 1998; Kozier, Erb, and Blais, 1997; Taylor, 1994).

Prayer
Prayer differs from meditation in that it involves communication with God or a superior being, who is believed to answer the prayer. Prayer can be an individual or group action, or an "intercessory prayer" conducted by other people without the knowledge of the individual for whom the prayers are said (Kozier et al, 1997). The "laying on of hands" and anointing the ill person with oil while praying for healing is an ancient form of intercessory prayer. Prayer can be silent or spoken, conversational or formal, or a recitation of a favorite psalm. Illness can interfere with an individual's ability to pray because of feelings of isolation, guilt, grief, or anxiety. Prayer is one of the therapeutic tools nurses use when providing spiritual care to allay a client's distraught feelings (Carson, 1989; Dossey and Dossey, 1998).

Yoga
Living a balanced life is central to yoga principles. The use of specific body postures, breath control, minimizing stimulation of the senses, leading a simple life, and directed meditation are achieved through daily practices. Concentration on purity of body and mind, self-restraint and contentment with life, studying relevant literature, and daily dedication to God are the means to attain that balance. Originally practiced in India, it has become a popular practice as a part of health enhancement and as a therapy for people with chronic diseases (Achterberg et al, 1994; Kozier, Erb, and Blais, 1997; Taylor, 1994; Wanning, 1993).

Biofeedback
Biofeedback is a technique that uses electrical equipment to assist persons in gaining conscious control over body processes that normally are thought to be beyond voluntary command (Kozier, Erb, and Blais, 1997). It is often combined with controlled breathing techniques and/or meditation to provide individuals with information about their bodies, of which they are unaware. Electrodes that are attached to the affected area send information into the monitoring device, which emits a signal to alert the person to changes in a particular body function (e.g., an increase or decrease in muscle tension).

By watching the device, clients can learn to use mental processes to control that particular body action. A therapist instructs the client in the mental exercises during a series of sessions. Eventually the client is able to practice the exercises without the aid of the machine. Biofeedback has been used in the treatment of multiple physical, cognitive, and behavioral symptoms. Among these are hypertension, temperature control, gastrointestinal activity, substance abuse, stress, sleep disorders, migraine headaches, and other vascular disorders (Achterberg et al, 1994; Kozier, Erb, and Blais, 1997).

Use of the Arts
The use of music, dance, drama, literature, humor, and art are part of environmental therapy. Quiet background music provides a soothing atmosphere and can be a distract-

ing medium during times of stress and pain. Music is often used in intensive care units, in birthing rooms, during dental procedures, and even as a stimulus for people with lowered levels of consciousness. "Mood" music allows the listener to express emotions and feelings through dancing, singing, and creative thinking (Pope, 1995).

The dance is an expression of joy and celebration throughout the world. It has been used as a means to increase self-esteem and body image; lessen depression, fear, and isolation; and express emotions—even anger (Achterberg et al, 1994). Collaborative nursing research has been undertaken in Canada and Korea on the positive effects of music and dance on wellness. Joining a therapy group in ethnic folk dance has been shown to reduce social isolation for elderly Korean women and as a therapeutic intervention with mentally ill clients (Choe and Heber, 1997). Music and art were major components of a nurse-managed community rehabilitation care model in Seoul, Korea, for mentally ill persons, which produced remarkable results. Findings from the 2-year-old study, sponsored by the United Nations, revealed that a majority of the participants were able to live normal, independent lives; family relationships were improved; and recurrence of illness episodes and rehospitalization decreased (Kim, 1998) (see Understanding & Applying Research box).

Art has often been used with children and adults for expression of their feelings about stressful situations and unconscious concerns about their illnesses. As with music and dance, art can produce a calming or exciting effect. Art expression has been a psychotherapy tool in geriatric centers, with children and adolescents, in hospices, in alcohol treatment programs, and in prisons (Achterberg et al, 1994; Samules, 1995).

Books, poetry, and religious writings can be inspirational and can cause a person to become immersed for long periods in the reading situations. Journals and diaries are also forms of expressing one's emotions and have been referred to as "process meditation" and a conversation with the self (Carson, 1989).

Humor

Humor and laughter are also used for expressing emotions, for relieving tensions and anxiety, and for coping with painful or unpleasant situations. Laughter can have positive effects on respiratory and heart rates, blood pressure, and muscle tension. "Humor" rooms supplied with videocassettes and audiotapes, books, cartoons, and artwork have been created for clients, families, and agency staff (Kozier, Erb, and Blais, 1997). Gibson (1994) encouraged the use of humorous artwork on bulletin boards in patient rooms and staff work areas. Sharing a chuckle with a client by wearing a humorous button, or by telling a funny story, an anecdote, or a riddle can be an effective tool. In his article *Anatomy of an Illness* (1979), Norman Cousins, a famous journalist, wrote about the value of hu-

Understanding & Applying Research

This study, which was conducted in several stages, evaluated the effectiveness of a new nursing model developed by Dr. Susie Kim in Seoul, Korea. Eight interpersonal therapeutic concepts included the following: noticing, participating, sharing, active listening, companioning, complimenting, comforting, and hoping.

Background
Government statistics (1995) place the number of psychiatric clients at 1,000,020, or 2.2% of the Korean population. Approximately 9% need to be hospitalized; however, many cannot be accommodated, and much of the institutionalized care consists of custodial and medical-based care beyond the reach of many. Korean culture places a social stigma on the mentally ill, especially people with schizophrenia.

Program Design
The emphasis of Kim's rehabilitation program was on self-care and rehabilitation of the person back into the family and community. The program was funded by the United Nations Development Project and resulted in 15 replications. Major interventions were designed to prevent revolving-door hospitalizations and to increase the psychosocial functioning. These included (1) home visits for aiding the client in developing skills such as stress reduction and coping strategies, and informing family of their role; (2) day care in which the client can practice social skills; and (3) weekend seminars for family members for instruction on helping the person in the rehabilitation process.

Participant Data
Participants (314) in the treatment and control groups were 54% male; 64.6% had never married; and the average age was 39 years; 55.8% were college educated or college dropouts; 86% had never been employed. The average duration of the illness was 14.9 years. The leading diagnosis was schizophrenia (80.5%).

Findings
Members in the treatment group reported more social support, adhered to the medication regimen, and believed they could recover. Family members reported having a better relationship with their relative and could identify significant improvements. Members in the control group received the typical care and were transferred to the rehabilitation program.

Qualitative data related how a man's piano talent was nourished by a professional pianist and he was able to perform Beethoven's "Moonlight" sonata in concert at the Ewha Woman's University. A man with manic depression made a public debut in a gospel singing contest and cut a record, which went on sale. An elderly woman used her expertise in making beautiful thimbles to ease her chronic depression.

Kim S: Out of darkness, *Reflections* 24(3):8, 1998.

mor in relieving the severe pain he experienced from ankylosing spondylitis by stating that a "good belly laugh" allowed him to be pain free for at least 2 hours at a time. Cousins wrote that humor healed him.

Exercise

The benefits of physical exercise are well known. It can bring a general sense of well-being and vitality, increase respiratory and cardiovascular efficiency, and promote a longer life. People who exercise often sleep better and have improved appetites; exercise is now considered a major factor in self-care. Even simple exercises can be performed by people with disabilities. Special Olympics for wheelchair athletes is an excellent example of using exercise to enhance the self-image and general health.

Animals

This discussion of mind-body interventions would not be complete without the mention of using companion animals to enhance emotional and physiologic well being. Studies have shown a reduction in hypertension, heart rate, and social isolation when pets are introduced as a treatment modality. Studies have also shown the benefits to the morale of staff and caregivers. Companion animals have been used by individuals who are blind, deaf, or paralyzed to assist in accomplishing activities of daily living (Jorgenson, 1997). A recent report described the use of trained dogs to assist persons with Parkinson's disease to remain independent for longer periods. While walking, these individuals often "freeze" in place and have a loss of balance. The dogs are taught to recognize freezing and to tap on the person's foot, which breaks the cycle and subsequently prevents possible falls. The dogs are also trained to assist with everyday tasks such as opening doors, flipping light switches, and picking up dropped objects (Huff, 1998). Acute and long-term health care agency policies have been altered to allow pets into intensive care units, pediatric wards, hospices, rehabilitation units, and geriatric and other areas. Nurses have been active supporters of animal-assisted therapy.

Psychotherapy and Hypnosis

Psychotherapy is the medium and basis of all care (Achterberg et al, 1994). A variety of social support and self-help groups have implemented many of the psychologic methods such as multiple therapy approaches and cognitive, behavior, and body-oriented therapies to bring about beneficial effects for the participants. Groups are commonly used as adjunct therapy for substance abuse control, weight loss, cancer, grief counseling, and caregiver support.

Hypnosis has been in use since the eighteenth century as a deep relaxation technique and has become a useful tool in the treatment of substance addiction, pain control, fears, and phobias. It has also been used successfully before anesthesia induction, as a means in reducing hypertension, and for dietary management. Hypnosis involves the use of mental images, concentration, use of repetitive words or sounds, and total relaxation. Hypnosis produces an altered state of consciousness that permits the person to focus concentration with minimal distraction. Education in self-hypnosis through the aid of guided audiotapes tailored to meet the individual's specific problem has been used for therapy at home (Actherberg et al, 1994; Kozier, Erb, and Blais, 1997).

BIOELECTROMAGNETICS

Concepts of magnetic field therapy relate to the electrical currents that exist within and external to the body, the influence of external currents on the body, and the result of physical and behavioral changes. Examples are the electromagnetic energies produced by x-rays, television, microwaves, and light rays. Prolonged exposure to such fields can produce hazardous effects. However, scientists have also discovered that lower-level energy frequencies can be beneficial in designing diagnostic and treatment tools.

Recent bioelectromagnetic (BEM) research has also discovered a visible low-level light that is emitted by most living organisms. There is some indication that this extremely low-level light, or biophoton emission, may be valuable in bioregulation, membrane transport, and gene expression. Nonthermal electromagnetic fields, which do not cause heating of tissues, have been used for bone repair, nerve stimulation, and wound healing; as electrostimulation via acupuncture needles for stimulation of the immune system; and for neuroendocrine modulations (Rubik et al, 1994). Unipolor magnets have been used for pain relief, particularly of arthritis. Magnets can be taped to various areas of the body, inserted inside shoes, and placed in mattress covers. Anecdotal accounts have yielded very favorable responses (Keegan, 1998; Lawrence, 1996).

ALTERNATIVE SYSTEMS OF MEDICAL PRACTICE

Alternative systems include traditional Oriental medicine; acupuncture; Ayurvedic, homeopathic, naturopathic, and environmental medicines; and anthroposophically extended medicine (which builds on naturopathy, homeopathy, and modern scientific medicine).

Traditional Oriental Medicine

A variety of therapies are practiced within traditional Oriental medicine, including acupuncture and acupressure, massage, herbal medicine, qigong, and tai chi (a slow-motion dancelike martial art). Variations of traditional Oriental medicine are practiced in Japan, Korea, and Vietnam. The core principles of Oriental medicine center on the diagnosis of disturbances of qi, or the vital energy and the balance between yin and yang (female and male, cold and hot, dark and light) forces.

Diagnostic procedures consist of observing facial expressions and body movements, careful listening and questioning, and palpating body pulses. The relationship of physical and emotional behaviors is used to plan a range of traditional therapies. The most frequent methods used in the United States are acupuncture and Oriental massage.

Acupuncture.   Acupuncture is a process in which small needles are inserted at selected energy points of the body that correspond to energy pathways, or meridians, that traverse from the body surface to inner organs. Its purpose is to activate the qi, or life energy, and achieve a balance when imbalance exists. The needles can be heated and attached to mild electrical current or be twirled by hand to cause vibrations. Numerous studies have revealed the positive effects of acupuncture on a wide range of disorders, including gynecologic, mental, and neural problems and substance addiction. Its effectiveness in pain control and anesthesia is attributed to the release of endogenous opioids (endorphins) that are produced within the central nervous system (Achterberg et al, 1994; Kozier, Erb, and Blais, 1997). Acupuncture is one of the most thoroughly researched and documented alternative medical practices (Reed et al, 1994).

Ayurveda/Ayurvedic Medicine

Ayurvedic (science of life) medicine originated in India and dates back thousands of years. This method may use a combination of therapies, employing meditation, yoga, massage, herbs, aromatherapy, and biofeedback. The body is viewed as a pharmacy that can make its own natural drugs to heal the self (Carson, 1989; Kozier, Erb, and Blais, 1997; Reed et al, 1994).

The human body is also considered a microcosm of the universe, endowed with principles, or doshas, that interact in maintaining balance. The basic nature (prakriti), or genetic code, and the relationship among the doshas remain unaltered throughout a person's life. Each dosha has a principal location in the body. Emphasis is placed on the interdependence of health and the quality of the person's sociocultural life. When any imbalance occurs, a restoration of balance of the internal environment is achieved through proper diet and lifestyle. A recent study funded by the NIH Alternative Medicine Branch demonstrated the positive effects of Ayurvedic practices with healthy adults (see Understanding & Applying Research Box).

Homeopathic Medicine

Homeopathic medicine is based on the belief that a drug that will produce certain disease symptoms in a healthy person can provide a cure for a sick person experiencing the same symptoms. Diluted substances are used to elicit a cure (e.g., a very dilute solution containing poison ivy compound may be prescribed for a skin rash). The medication must be shaken vigorously or "potentized" for the

Understanding & Applying Research

The purpose of this study was to evaluate the effects of a health education program on the use of Ayurvedic or Western health promotion techniques with healthy adults. The hypothesis was that one or both interventions would be beneficial in decreasing health risks and improving the health-related quality of life (HQRL) in this group over that of a control group 1 year later. The study was funded by a grant from the NIH Alternative Medicine Branch.

A random sample was taken from a Southern California preferred provider organization (PPO).

Selection criteria included ages 20-56, free of serious disease (e.g., cancer), and English speaking.

Participants were randomly assigned to treatment groups: Ayurvedic (n = 41), Western (n = 38), or control group (n = 45).

Educational interventions consisted of philosophically varied content on relaxation, activity, and diet over a weekend followed by reinforcement phone calls and refresher sessions at 3-month intervals.

The Ayurveda group received primordial sound meditation, yoga, and an Ayurvedic diet. The Western group received aerobic exercise, progressive muscle relaxation, and a high-fiber diet.

Measurements consisted of body mass index and blood pressure at baseline and every 3 months. Lipids, a health risk appraisal, and the SF-36 and supplementary items were measured at 0, 6, and 12 months.

There were 124 participants, with 88 (71%) completing the year-long study. The typical person was female (78%), Caucasian (82%), with an average age of 42, and a college graduate (31%). Results indicated that individuals in both treatment groups reported overall improved general perceptions of health, resistance to illness, more energy, fewer illness symptoms, lower blood pressure readings, and better adherence to diet than the control group. Use of prescription medications also decreased.

When adherence to treatment was correlated with outcome, the Ayurveda group reported more significant outcomes than might occur by chance in health perceptions, less depression, and better adherence to therapy practices than the Western Group.

The study was presented at the Joint Southern California Sigma Theta Tau Chapters Nursing Research Conference (October 10-12, 1996) by Barbara Riegel, DNSc, RN, CS, FAAN, and David Simon, MD.

greatest effectiveness as the solution picks up energy from the dissolved substance. These products are used for acute and chronic health problems, as well as for health promotion.

The homeopathic drug market has become a multimillion-dollar industry today. The remedies are currently regulated by the FDA, and drugs manufactured by reputable pharmaceutical companies are listed in the

Homeopathic Pharmacopoeia of the United States. Some are sold as OTC drugs; products used for serious conditions require dispensing by a licensed practitioner (Kozier, Erb, and Blais, 1997; Reed et al, 1994).

Naturopathy.   Naturopathy is a method primarily used by a small group of physicians who have been educated in the sciences and receive specialized training in the disciplines of alternative medicine. They use an eclectic selection of herbs, homeopathy, nutrition, traditional Oriental medicine, hydrotherapy, and manipulative therapy in conjunction with modern scientific medical diagnostic methods and standards. Naturopathy focuses on self-healing, and health care is tailored to the individual's needs. The basic principles include use of therapies that do no harm, the physician's primary role as teacher, establishing and maintaining an optimal health and balance, treatment of the whole person, prevention of disease through a healthy lifestyle, and therapeutic use of nutrition (Reed et al, 1994).

Environmental medicine.   Allergy treatment was the original drive for the development of environmental medicine in the 1940s. Scientists noted that the sensitivity and allergy symptoms of some individuals were improved when certain foods or chemicals, molds, dust, pollens, etc., were eliminated. Emotional stress was also identified as a source of immune system dysfunction. The person's environmental history became an important component in the diagnostic process by providing a chronologic account of etiologic circumstances leading to the health problem. The elimination of health hazards from the environment has become a major health issue. Examples include the removal of asbestos building insulation materials; instillation of devices for recapture of gasoline fumes and smog emissions on automobiles; removal of certain pesticides from the market; and elimination of preservatives and color additives from foods, medicines, and nutrition supplements (Reed et al, 1994).

Culture-based community medicines.   The many culture-based practices follow naturalistic methods, and religious rituals, which are a major component, are usually provided by a spiritual healer or shaman. Symbols such as prayer wheels, sand paintings, meditation, group singing, chanting, and dancing ceremonies are part of the healing rituals. On the Navajo reservation, modern hospitals and the shaman's healing room are under the same roof. Some people believe that spells cast by the witch doctor, at times, have proved to be more powerful than Western medicines.

MANUAL HEALING METHODS
Included in manual healing methods are osteopathic and chiropractic medicines, massage, reflexology, and the techniques of pressure point and other various touch therapies.

Osteopathy and Chiropractic Medicines
These practices involve manipulation of soft tissues and joints. Both require specialized education and licensure to practice. Osteopathic practices are considered to be mainstream medicine by much of the public, and the practitioner often is the primary health care provider. Chiropractic practitioners study the relationship between pressure, strain, or tension on the spinal cord and the ability of the neuromusculoskeletal system to act efficiently. Manual adjustments of the spine to correct alignment is a mainstay of treatment. Chiropractic medicine has now been approved by some insurance carriers, and the most recent center has been established by OAM to study its effects (NIH, 1998).

Massage
More than 80 different forms of massage therapy have been identified. These forms vary from gentle stroking to deep kneading, rubbing, and percussion. Most massage is done with the hands; however, the forearms, elbows, or feet are sometimes used. The primary purposes of massage therapy are to result in muscle and total-body relaxation and increased circulation. Massage techniques, at one time, were included in the fundamental nursing courses. Touch, which is the basic medium of massage therapy, is a form of communication and caring (Wanning, 1993).

Acupressure
The same meridian points used in acupuncture are manipulated in pressure point therapies. The fingertips are used to apply pressure to over 600 designated points in soft tissues. Acupressure can be used both as a diagnostic tool and as treatment. The sessions can last up to an hour, with the recipient spending equal time lying in the prone and dorsal positions for a total body treatment. The therapist also places a strong emphasis on mind-spirit-body balance in counseling the client. Shiatsu is similar to acupressure, with pressure being applied by the palm of the hand, as well as the fingers (Kozier, Erb, and Blais, 1997; Rubik et al, 1994).

Foot Reflexology
Reflexology, which originated in Egypt, is also referred to as zone therapy. This technique is based on the premise that the feet (and hands) are mirrors of the body, with reflex points that correspond to glands, organs, and other structures in the body. (The feet are considered to be more responsive to massage than the hands.) Massage of a reflex point stimulates the corresponding organ in that zone. The main goal is to provide relaxation by removing tension in a zone area (Kozier, Erb, and Blais, 1997; Slagle, 1996).

Therapeutic Touch
Healing through touch can be traced back to early civilizations. Various forms of therapeutic touch have been

practiced by nurses for many years. Benefits of contact touch such as massage have recently been identified as providing a sense of spiritual balance, relieving mental and emotional tension and anxiety, improving blood flow, easing pain, and stimulating the immune system.

Therapeutic touch (TT) also refers to a noncontact technique derived from the "laying on of hands" associated with Far Eastern, European, and religious philosophies. This method is based on a theory that the release of excess energy from the healer assists the ill person in the healing process. The basic principles can be learned, and workshops have been offered throughout the country. Healing touch is a similar technique and became a certificate program of the American Holistic Nurses' Association in 1993 (Kozier, Erb, and Blais, 1997; Mackey, 1995).

PHARMACOLOGIC AND BIOLOGIC TREATMENTS

Pharmacologic and biologic alternative therapies consist of a variety of drugs and vaccines that have not yet been included in mainstream medicine. Some are designed to stimulate the immune system to ward off diseases and may consist of older herbal remedies. All are considered to be nontoxic. Two examples are shark and other animal cartilage used as treatment for AIDS, cancer, and arthritis, and ethylene diamine tetraacetic acid (EDTA) chelation therapy, a popular treatment for cardiovascular problems. Cartilage is believed to inhibit tumor growth by cutting off the blood supply to the tumor, to suppress autoimmune reactions, and to promote wound healing. EDTA is a chemical that binds with metallic ions and is used as a treatment for lead poisoning and other toxic metals. It is now being proposed as treatment for ridding the body of free radicals and thus removing fat deposits from artery walls and improving cardiovascular circulation (Moss et al, 1994).

Herbal Medicine

The use of herbal and plant medicine is an ancient practice worldwide. Tree barks, plant roots, berries, leaves, resins, seeds, and flowers have all been ground into powders, mixed with solutions, brewed in teas, and used singly or in combination as the treatment of ailments. Herbal remedies are used by an estimated 4 billion people, or 80% of the world population (McIntyre, 1996). (Approximately one fourth of prescription medications contain at least one active ingredient derived from a natural plant.) Scientists believe that only 1% of the world's plants have been analyzed, leaving many potential medicinals to be found. The rain forests, where many of today's medicines have their origins, are quickly disappearing, and urgent international efforts in the search for new drugs are being funded before these sources are lost. The popularity of herbal remedies has also caused some of the wild plants to be harvested indiscriminately. Botanists have warned that overharvesting

of slow-growing plants could eliminate the crop within a few years (Associated Press, 1998).

Records of herbal medicines appeared in Egypt extending back to 2000 BC, in Greece and Rome at the time of Aristotle, in the Muslim world, in India, and in the Orient. Each culture compiled a *materia medica*—a listing of drugs and their uses. The American Indians contributed a vast array of herbals to the Colonial American medicine formulary, and herbals continued to be a mainstay of medical practices for many years. Today, herbal products can only be marketed as food supplements and are considered to be worthless, or even potentially dangerous, by the FDA and other regulatory agencies. No safety guidelines have been established. Nevertheless, the public is purchasing alternative medicines at a greater rate than ever before and adopting many of the remedies from other cultures.

The formulas of Chinese medicine are based on the correct ratio or balance of a variety of "food herbs" that are harvested and prepared at an appropriate time to enhance their effects. The various herbal ingredients are mixed according to the diseases caused by imbalance of yin and yang rather than the chemistry makeup of the herb. Yin and yang characteristics and their related properties of cold and heat are used to categorize diseases and medicines (Bellamy and Pfister, 1992; Carson, 1989; Kozier, Erb, and Blais, 1997). These mixtures are used as supplements to a well-balanced diet and are often prescribed in conjunction with daily exercise and positive thinking, in the belief that a balanced body is a result of a balanced life. Many Chinese herbal stores have captured a large share of the U.S. alternative medicine market.

Aromatherapy was initially used in Egypt to relieve pain. More recently, it is being used for relaxation or as an adjunct to stress reduction measures. More than 300 essential plant oils are currently in use as inhalants, for massage and compresses, or as additions to bathwater, and candles. The burning of aromatic woods was used in ancient times to purify the air; incense is still used today as part of healing ceremonies, and room deodorants aid in masking unpleasant odors. Other examples include birch oil as an antiinflammatory agent, lavender for headache relief, rosemary added to vaporizers, and peppermint for nausea relief and as an antipyretic and respiratory stimulant (Kozier, Erb, and Blais, 1997). Aromatherapy is included in Ayurvedic therapy.

Examples of commonly used herbs are *Ginkgo biloba*, echinacea, saw palmetto, *Prunus africanum*, ginseng, and St. John's wort. Both European and Oriental varieties of *Ginkgo biloba* are used to increase circulation, particularly to bring oxygen to the brain, and to retard the effects of aging. European studies have shown its effectiveness for improvement in mental alertness, increased circulation to the extremities, lowered cholesterol, and improved blood flow to the retina. Echinacea, or purple coneflower, is prized for its antiseptic properties and ability to stimulate the immune system, particularly against infections such as flu, colds, and wound healing. Saw palmetto berries and *Prunus africanum* have become popular treatments for benign prostatic hypertrophy. Ginseng root has been used in China for more than 3000 years as a tonic. It has also been used as an antistress agent and to alter circadian rhythms and amounts of circulating corticosterone. *Hypericum*, the principal ingredient of St. John's wort, has been termed "Nature's Prozac" because of its very popular use as an antidepressant (Huff, 1998; McIntyre, 1996). Additional herbal remedies are given in Box 24-5.

DIET AND NUTRITION

Diet and nutritional needs are integral to both traditional and alternative therapies. Today's "affluent" diet, which is high in animal fats, refined carbohydrates, and partially hydrogenated vegetable oils, contributes to many of the current health problems in the United States. Alternative healthy diets and a change in lifestyle have been included

in educational information to prevent or correct obesity, cardiovascular disease, and diabetes and other chronic health problems. Vitamins and other food supplements are frequently added to the health maintenance plan. Recent studies include research on the value of the antioxidant vitamins C, E, and β-carotene in the prevention of cataracts and cancer, and on the effects of vitamin C and nicotinic acid as replacement therapy for psychiatric clients receiving electroconvulsive and tranquilizer therapy. Megadoses of niacin have been shown to aid in reducing serum cholesterol. Nutritional supplements are given to offset the effects of medicines prescribed for people with AIDS.

Several diets have been developed as specific treatments for cancer. Among these is the Gerson diet, which is low in sodium, fat, and protein and high in vegetable juices, and includes potassium and thyroid supplements. Macrobiotic cancer diets are based on Oriental beliefs regarding creating the balance of yin and yang. The Pritikin diet, designed as a cardiac diet, also has a high content of

---

Box 24-5   Examples of Herbs and Food Herbals Used as Alternative Therapies and as the Basis for Allopathic Traditional Medicines

Most of the herbs come from tropical rain forests; others are derived from the sea, and still others come from countries around the world. Flowers, seeds, leaves, woods and barks, vines, tubers, roots, and even grasses have been the basis of alternative and traditional allopathic medicine therapy. (Over one fourth of traditional medicines are based on plant properties.) Different portions of a plant or tree may have different properties and different concentrations and also can be used for different purposes. These products can be used as inhalants, taken internally, added to bathwater, or applied externally. The following is a small list of examples.

Analgesics: Meadowsweet, poplar (balm of Gilead) tree, willow tree (aspirin), wintergreen, oil of clove (used in dentistry), feverfew, nutmeg (for migraine), marijuana (nausea and pain for cancer patients and people with AIDS)

Narcotics: Belladonna, celandine, nightshade, opium poppy

Aromatics: Allspice, angelica, anise, avicena, camomile, ginger, juniper, lavender, mint, nutmeg, pennyroyal, rosemary, wormwood, pine and balsam woods, cinnamon (as incense); used as relaxants, for bronchodilator effects, etc.

Stimulants: Marijuana, nutmeg, peyote, Scotch broom for euphorics and hallucinogens; ginseng (American and Asian) for mental and physical energizer—also considered a panacea for its variety of healing properties; belladonna for atropine effects on the central nervous system

Sedatives: Celery, feverweed, hops, Indian pipe, lavender, monkshood, wild black cherry, mountain laurel, passion flower, peachtree, peony, periwinkle, heliotrope (valerian)

Antidepressant/antianxiety agents: Borage, St. John's wort, lobelia (in correct dosage), rosemary, pasqueflower, aromatics

Antiaging agents: Ginkgo biloba (increases circulation)

Antiseptics: Garlic (also used to reduce cholesterol), onion, wintergreen, camphor

Diaphoretics: Seneca snakeroot

Antioxidants: Ginger, spices (Indian)

Cardiotonics: Foxglove (digitalis), lily of the valley, *Strophantus* (ouabain)

Ophthalmic agents: Calabar bean (physiostigmine) used for glaucoma

Antihypertensives: Parsley, skullcap, garlic, hawthorn, wild black cherry, seneca snakeroot (rauwolfia)

Contraceptive agents: Mexican yam—diosegenin that can be converted to progesterone (Syntex)

Muscle paralyzing agents: *Strychnos toxifera* produces a powerful poison—curare (used to create intercostal muscle paralysis during surgery)

Antineoplastic agents: Yew tree bark (paclitaxel), rosy periwinkle (vincristine, vinblastine); used for childhood leukemias and Hodgkin's disease

Gastrointestinal agents: Papaya for dyspepsia, liquorice flower (carbenoxolone) as treatment for peptic ulcer

Antidiarrheal agents: Opium poppy (paregoric)

Cathartics: Ricinus communis (castor oil)

Dermatologic agents: Aloe vera, wintergreen (ointment)

Antibiotic agents: Fungi (penicillin), iris versicolor (antisyphilitic), lobelia (antisyphilitic)

Antimalarials: Chinchona bark or Peruvian bark (quinine)—also used as antiarrhythmic

Antiviral agents: May apple—venereal warts and AIDS

vegetables, is low in fat, and is high in fiber and complex carbohydrates. It requires a 45-minute daily exercise program as well. Vegetarian diets are common today in the United States as a means of weight control, for religious reasons, and for ethical reasons by people who dislike the killing and eating of animals. Research by environmental medicine scientists has helped to identify potential food antigens such as chemical additives and natural food substances. Food elimination diets have been used to reduce sensitivity to certain substances and hasten recovery from

allergic responses. These diets have also been used in the treatment of children with attention-deficit/hyperactivity disorder (Baer et al, 1994). Health care providers must be sensitive to ethnic and cultural diets when planning health care activities. Some of these diets may pose health risks because of a lack of essential ingredients or interaction with prescribed medications. Incorporating familiar foods into the diet may also facilitate a person's recovery, and substances in the diet may actually facilitate healing.

Summary of Key Concepts

1. There still seems to be a stigma attached to alternative methods, with the scientific community labeling alternative methods as a hoax, witchcraft, or magicoreligious practices, and attributing results to placebo effects. However, nurses must become knowledgeable about the many methods that clients use to manage their lives and be nonjudgmental about these practices. Taking a comprehensive history, documenting the findings, and sharing them with others on the health care team are important steps in the plan of care.

2. Education of the public regarding the potential harmful effects of concurrent use of alternative and prescription medicines and the need to inform their health care providers is also essential. People must also understand the consequences of self-diagnosis and delay in seeking help. The informed client must be a well-informed client.

3. Dossey (1997) suggested that alternative and traditional therapies can complement each other in providing holistic care and urged nurses to become familiar with the alternative methods and to incorporate them into the plan of care whenever possible.

4. The concepts of caring and healing, and commitment to global health are integral components of nursing. Some nursing leaders predict that nursing care of the future will be administered in holistic centers that provide many of today's so-called alternative therapies (Keegan, 1998).

5. According to the definition provided by the Universidad Politecnia de Nicaragua School of Nursing (Lockhart, 1998), nursing is the science that occupies all of the relative processes of care of the health of the individual, family, and community in order to promote, maintain, or bring them to a state of wellness. The nursing profession is qualified to perform independent and interdependent actions that are largely technical, such as teaching, administration, and research. It is dynamic and evolutionary, humanistic, and a discipline that is fundamentally based on scientific and technical knowledge and founded on moral, ethical, and spiritual values. It uses the nursing process with a holistic approach and promotes an essential environment for the health care of the human being.

REFERENCES

Achterberg J et al: Mind-body interventions. In *Alternative medicine: expanding medical horizons*, Torrance, Calif, 1994, Homestead Schools.

Associated Press: Echinacea roots prized by diggers, *San Diego Union-Tribune*, p, A7, August 10, 1998.

Baer R et al: Diet and nutrition in the prevention and treatment of chronic disease. In *Alternative medicine: expanding medical horizons*, Torrance, Calif, 1994, Homestead Schools.

Bassick J, producer: *The doctor is in: alternative medicine*, Princeton, NJ, 1996, Films for the Humanities and Sciences.

Bellamy D, Pfister A: *World medicine: plants, patients and people*, Mass, 1992, Blackwell.

Berman B, Larson D: Preface. In *Alternative medicine: expanding medical horizons*, Torrance, Calif, 1994, Homestead Schools.

Carson V: *Spiritual dimensions of nursing practice*, Philadelphia, 1989, WB Saunders.

Choe M, Heber L: Listen to the music, *Reflections* 23(2):17, 1997.

Clark C: Cancer specialists hear spiritual guru, *San Diego Union-Tribune*, p B-7, March 28, 1998.

Clements M, Hales D: How healthy are we? *Parade Magazine*, September 7, 1997 (national survey).

Cousins N: *Anatomy of an illness as perceived by the patient*, New York, 1979, WW Norton.

Dossey B: Using imagery to help your patient heal, *Am J Nurs* 95(6):41, 1995.

Dossey B: Complementary and alternative therapies for our aging society, *J Gerontol Nurs* 23(9):45, 1997.

Dossey B: Holistic modalities and healing moments, *Am J Nurs* 98(6):44, 1998.

Dossey B, Dossey L: Body-mind-spirit: attending to holistic care, *Am J Nurs* 98(8):35, 1998.

Dossey L, Swyers J: Introduction. In *Alternative medicine: expanding medical horizons*, Torrance, Calif, 1994, Homestead Schools.

Eakes G, Burke M, Hainsworth M: Middle-range theory of chronic sorrow, *Image J Nurs Sch* 30(2):179, 1998.

Eisenberg D et al: Unconventional medicine in U.S.: prevalence, costs, and patterns of use, *N Engl J Med* 328(4):245, 1993.

Ellis J, Hartley C: *Nursing in today's world: challenges, issues and trends*, Philadelphia, 1998, JB Lippincott.

Gibson L: Healing and humor, *Nursing* 94(9):56-57, 1994.

Huff C: Nature's Prozac, *Remedy*, p 8, March/April 1998.

Jessup A: The democratization of expertise: information-sharing on the Internet, *Alternative Ther Health Med* 1(4):22, 1995.

Jorgenson J: Therapeutic use of companion animals in health care, *Image J Nurs Sch* 29(3):249, 1997.

Keegan L: Getting comfortable with alternative and complementary therapies, *Nursing* 98(4):50, 1998.

Kim S: Out of darkness, *Reflections* 24(3):8, 1998.

Kozier B, Erb G, Blais K: *Professional nursing practice*, Menlo Park, Calif, 1997, Addison-Wesley.

Lawrence R: Magnets stop pain . . . ease arthritis, help heal broken bones and more, *Health Confidential*, p 7, January 1996.

Lockhart J: Hallowed ground: Managua, Nicaragua, *Reflections* 24(3):24, 1998.

Mackey R: Discovering the healing power of therapeutic touch, *Am J Nurs* 95(4):27, 1995.

Malik, T: The safety of herbal medicine, *Alternative Ther* 1(4):27, 1995.

McIntyre A: Healing with flowers. In *Flower power*, New York, 1996, Henry Holt.

Moran J: Making alternative therapies everyone's issue, *Alternative Ther Health Med* 1(4):79, 1995.

Moss R et al: Pharmacological and biological treatments. In *Alternative medicine: expanding medical horizons*, Torrance, Calif, 1994, Homestead Schools.

National Institutes of Health, Office of Alternative Medicine: *Complementary and alternative medicine at the NIH* (online), Springfield, Md, Spring 1998.

Nunnery R: *Advancing your career: concepts of professional nursing*, Philadelphia, 1997, FA Davis.

Pope D: Music, noise, and the human voice in the nurse-patient environment, *Image J Nurs Sch* 27(4):291, 1995.

Reed J et al: Alternative systems of medical practice. In *Alternative medicine: expanding medical horizons*, Torrance, Calif, 1994, Homestead Schools.

Riegel B, Simon D: *Effectiveness of Ayurvedic or Western health promotion strategies in healthy adults*. Presentation at Sigma Theta Tau research conference, San Diego, Calif, October 10, 1996.

Rubik B et al: Bioelectromagnetics applications in medicine. In *Alternative therapies: expanding medical horizons*, Torrance, Calif, 1994, Homestead Schools.

Samules M: Art as a healing force, *Alternative Ther Health Med* 1(4):38, 1995.

Slagle N: Issues of alternative therapies, Nurs Pract 21(2):16, 1996.

Taylor E: Yoga and meditation, *Alternative Ther Health Med* 1(4):77, 1994.

Thorne S, Paterson B: Shifting images of chronic illness, *Image: J Nurs Sch* 30(2):173, 1998.

Villaire M: OAM funded programs at Bastyr University provide updates, *Alternative Ther Health Med* 1(4):14, 1995.

Wanning T: Massage, acupuncture, yoga, t'ai chi and Feldenkrais, *J Occup Health Nurses* 41(7):349, 1993.

Weil A: *Spontaneous healing*, New York, 1995, Fawcett Columbine.

Notes

CHAPTER 25

Crisis Intervention

Donna C. Aguilera

OBJECTIVES

- Describe the historical development of crisis intervention.

- Identify and define the phases of crisis.

- Discuss the balancing factors that affect emotional equilibrium.

- Compare and contrast maturational crises, situational crises, and adventitious crises.

- Compare and contrast the generic and individual approaches of crisis intervention.

- Define and describe the steps of crisis intervention and apply them to the problem-solving process.

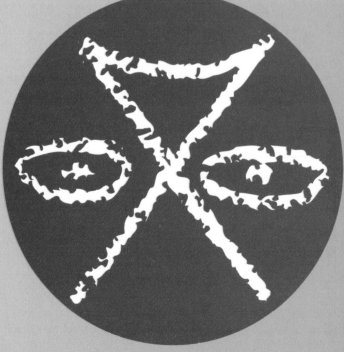

A psychologic crisis results from an individual's inability to solve a problem. People strive to exist in a state of emotional **equilibrium,** a state of balance, or homeostasis. When something occurs that is different (either positive or negative), such as a change, threat, or loss, it creates a state of disequilibrium. The individual attempts to regain and maintain the previous level of equilibrium and is at a turning point. The individual faces a problem that he or she cannot readily solve by using previously successful coping mechanisms or skills. This results in an increase in tension and anxiety, and the person becomes less able to find a solution to the problem. In a situation like this, the individual feels helpless. He or she is in a state of great emotional upheaval and feels unable to take action on his or her own to solve the problem.

Crisis intervention can offer immediate help for a person in crisis to reestablish equilibrium. It is an inexpensive, short-term therapy that focuses on solving the **immediate problem.**

HISTORICAL DEVELOPMENT

The crisis approach to therapeutic intervention has been developed only within the past few decades. It is based on a broad range of theories of human behavior, including those of Freud, Hartmann, Rado, Erickson, Lindemann, and Caplan.

Eric Lindemann (1944) and his colleagues observed the psychologic symptoms of the survivors following the Coconut Grove fire in Boston on November 28, 1942. It was the worst single-building fire in the country's history (at that time); 493 people perished from the flames that swept through the crowded nightclub. Lindemann and others from Massachusetts General Hospital played an active role in helping survivors who had lost loved ones in the disaster.

Lindemann's report on the psychologic symptoms became the cornerstone for subsequent theorizing on the grief process, a series of stages through which a mourner progresses toward accepting and resolving loss. Lindemann came to believe that the clergy and other community caregivers could play a critical role in helping bereaved people through the mourning process and thereby head off later psychologic difficulties. This concept was further developed with the establishment of the Wellesley Human Resources Services in Boston in 1948, one of the first community mental health services noted for its focus on short-term therapy in the context of preventive psychiatry.

From his experience working with grief reactions, Lindemann concluded that a conceptual framework built around the concept of an emotional crisis as shown by bereavement reactions would be worthy of investigation and useful for the development of preventive efforts. Certain inevitable events in life can be described as "hazardous" situations (e.g., bereavement, the birth of a child, and marriage). He proposed that in each of these situations emotional strain is generated, stress is experienced, and a series of adaptive mechanisms occur that can lead to mastery of the new situation or to failure with more or less lasting impairment of function. Although such situations create stress for all people exposed to them, they become crises for those who are especially vulnerable to this stress and who do not have the emotional resources to adapt.

Lindemann's theoretic frame of reference led to the development of crisis intervention techniques. In 1948 he and Gerald Caplan established the Wellesley Project, a community-wide mental health program in Boston.

According to Caplan (1961), the most important aspects of mental health are the state of the ego, the stage of its maturity, and the quality of its structure. Assessment of the ego's state is based on three main areas: (1) the capacity of the person to withstand stress and anxiety and to maintain ego equilibrium, (2) the degree of reality recognized and faced in solving problems, and (3) the repertoire of effective coping mechanisms the individual can employ in maintaining a balance in the biopsychosocial field.

Caplan believes that all of the elements that compose a person's total emotional milieu or environment must be assessed in an approach to preventive mental health. The material, physical, and social demands of reality, as well as the individual's needs, instincts, and impulses, must all be considered important behavioral determinants.

CRISIS
DEFINITION AND DESCRIPTION

Caplan (1961) defines crisis as occurring "when a person faces an obstacle to an important life goal that is, for a time, insurmountable through the utilization of customary methods of problem solving. A period of disequilibrium ensues, a period of upset, during which many abortive attempts at solution are made." In essence, the individual is viewed as living in a state of emotional equilibrium—with the goal always to return to or maintain that state. The individual must either solve the problem or adapt to nonsolution. In either case, a new state of equilibrium develops, sometimes better and sometimes worse in terms of positive mental health. There is a rise in inner tension, there are signs of anxiety, and there is disorganization of function, resulting in a prolonged period of emotional upset. This Caplan refers to as "crisis." The outcome is governed by the kind of interaction that takes place during the crisis period between the individual and the key figures in his or her emotional milieu.

Crisis is characteristically self-limiting and lasts from 4 to 6 weeks. This transitional period represents both the danger of increased psychologic vulnerability and an opportunity for personality growth. In any particular situation the outcome may depend to a significant degree on the availability of appropriate help. On this basis the length of time for intervention is from 4 to 6 weeks, with the average time being 4 weeks (Jacobson, 1965). Because time is so important, the therapeutic intervention commands the concentrated attention of both therapist and client. A goal-oriented sense of commitment develops, in sharp contrast to the more modest pace of traditional treatment modes.

PHASES

According to Caplan (1974), a crisis has four developmental phases:

1. There is an initial rise in tension as the stimulus continues and more discomfort is felt.
2. A lack of success in coping occurs as the stimulus continues and more discomfort is felt.
3. A further increase in tension acts as a powerful internal stimulus that mobilizes internal and external resources. In this stage, emergency problem-solving mechanisms are tried. The problem may be redefined, or there may be resignation and the giving up of certain aspects of the goal as unattainable.
4. If the problem continues and can be neither solved nor avoided, tension increases and a major disorganization occurs.

A stressful event is seldom so clearly defined that its source can be determined immediately. Internalized changes occur at the same time as the externally provoked stress. As a result, some events may cause a strong emotional response in one person, yet leave another person apparently unaffected. Much is determined by the presence or absence of factors that can effect a return to equilibrium.

Whenever a stressful event occurs, certain recognized balancing factors can bring about a return to equilibrium; these factors are the person's perception of the event, available situational supports, and coping mechanisms, as shown in the paradigm in Figure 25-1. A **paradigm** is a side-by-side example to show a clear pattern. The upper portion of the paradigm illustrates the "normal" initial reaction of an individual to a stressful event.

In the left column of Figure 25-1, the balancing factors are operating and crisis is avoided. However, in the right column the absence of one or more of these balancing factors may block resolution of the problem and thus increase disequilibrium and precipitate crisis.

BALANCING FACTORS AFFECTING EQUILIBRIUM

Between the perceived effects of a stressful situation and the resolution of the problem are three recognized balancing factors that may determine the state of equilibrium: **perception of the event**, situational supports, and coping mechanisms. Strengths or weaknesses in any one of the factors can be directly related to the onset of crisis or to its resolution.

Perception of the Event

Cognition, or the awareness and subjective meaning of a stressful event, plays a major role in determining both the nature and the degree of coping behaviors. Differences in cognition, in terms of the event's threat to an important life goal or value, account for large differences in coping behaviors. The concept of *cognitive style* (Cropley and Field, 1969) suggests uniqueness in the way people take in, process, and use information from the environment.

Cognitive styles, or the characteristic modes for orga-

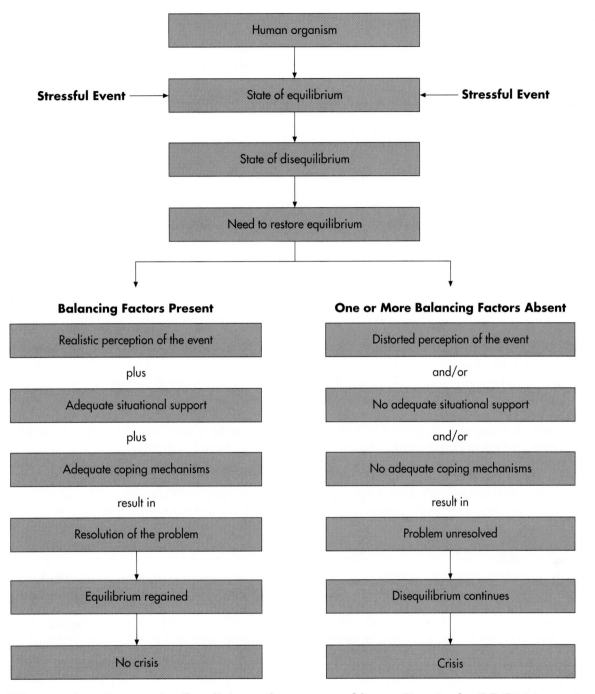

Figure 25-1   A paradigm illustrating the effect of balancing factors in a stressful event. (From Aguilera DC: *Crisis intervention: theory and methodology,* ed 8, St. Louis, 1998, Mosby.)

nizing perceptual and intellectual activities, play an important role in determining an individual's coping responses to daily life stresses. According to Inkeles (1966), cognitive style helps to set limits on information seeking in stress situations. It also strongly influences perceptions of others, interpersonal relationships, and responses to various types of psychiatric treatment.

For example, in stressful situations a person whose cognitive style is identified as "field dependent" is very dependent on external objects in the environment for orientation to reality. This type of individual tends to use such coping mechanisms as repression and denial. In contrast, the person who is "field independent" tends to prefer intellectualization as a defense mode.

If the event is perceived realistically, the relationship between the event and feelings of stress is recognized.

Problem solving can be appropriately oriented toward reduction of tension, and a successful solution of the stressful situation is more probable.

Lazarus (1966) and colleagues (1974) focused on the importance of the mediating cognitive process, appraisal, to determine the various coping methods individuals use. **Appraisal,** in this context, is an ongoing perceptual process by which a potentially harmful event is distinguished from a potentially beneficial or irrelevant event. It has been found that an individual's sense of coherence (SOC) significantly affects cognitive appraisal, specifically secondary appraisal (McSherry and Holm, 1994). SOC is a global orientation that expresses the extent to which one has a pervasive, enduring though dynamic feeling of confidence to comprehend, manage, and learn from a crisis (Antonovsky, 1987).

When a threatening situation exists, a *primary* appraisal is made to judge the perceived outcome of the event in relation to one's future goals and values. This is followed by a *secondary* appraisal whereby one perceives the range of coping alternatives available either to master the threat or to achieve a beneficial outcome. As coping activities are selected and initiated, feedback cues from changing internal and external environments lead to ongoing *reappraisals* or to changes in the original perception.

As a result of the appraisal process, coping behaviors are never static. They change constantly in both quality and degree as new information and cues are received during reappraisal activities. New coping responses may occur whenever new significance is attached to a situation. One's SOC level appears to be associated with the way in which one appraises and copes with stressful situations (McSherry and Holm, 1994).

If, in the appraisal process, the outcome is judged to be too overwhelming or too difficult to be dealt with by using available coping skills, an individual is more likely to use defense mechanisms to repress or distort the reality of the situation. An appraisal of a potentially successful outcome, however, more likely leads to the use of direct action modes of coping, such as attack, flight, or compromise. It has been recognized that high SOC persons report significantly higher levels of perceived coping resources than low SOC persons (McSherry and Holm, 1994).

If the perception of the event is distorted, a relationship between the event and feelings of stress may not be recognized. Thus attempts to solve the problem are ineffective, and tension is not reduced. In other words, what does the event mean to the individual? How is it going to affect his or her future? Can the person look at it realistically, or does the person distort its meaning?

Situational Supports

Situational supports are those persons who are available in the environment and who can be depended on to help solve the problem. By nature, human beings are dependent on others to supply them with reflected appraisals of their own intrinsic and extrinsic values. In establishing life patterns, certain appraisals are more significant to the individual than others because they tend to reinforce the individual's self-perception. Dependency relationships may be more readily established with those whose appraisals tend to support the individual against feelings of insecurity and with those who reinforce feelings of ego integrity.

These meaningful relationships with others provide a person with nurturance and support, resources vital for coping with stressors. Social isolation denies a person availability of social interactions and opportunities to develop meaningful relationships. Sudden or unexpected social isolation results in the loss of usual resource supports. Lacking these, a person is much more vulnerable to daily living stressors.

Loss, threatened loss, or feelings of inadequacy in a supportive relationship may also leave a person in a vulnerable position. Confrontation with a stressful situation, combined with a lack of situational support, may lead to a state of disequilibrium and possible crisis.

Appraisal of self varies across ages, sexes, and roles. The belief system that forms the basis of the self-concept and self-esteem develops out of experiences with significant others in a person's life. Although self-esteem is fairly stable within a certain range, it does fluctuate according to internal and external environmental variables. To achieve and maintain a sense of value and self-worth, a person must feel loved by others and capable of achieving an ideal self, one that is strong, capable, good, and loving of others.

When self-esteem is low or when a situation is perceived as particularly threatening, the person is strongly in need of and seeks out others from whom positive reflective appraisals of self-worth and ability to achieve can be obtained. The lower the self-esteem or the greater the threat, the greater the need to seek situational supports. Conversely, a person avoids or withdraws from contacts with those perceived as threatening to the person's self-esteem, whether the threat is real or imagined. Any potentially stressful situation can set off questions of self-doubt about how one is perceived by others, the kind of impression being made, and the real or imagined inadequacies that might be disclosed (Mechanic, 1974). However, not everyone who faces a threat to self-image will suffer a decrease in self-esteem (Jalajas, 1994). Whether self-esteem decreases will depend on whether the threat to the self-image can be reaffirmed (Jalajas, 1994).

Success or failure of a coping behavior is always strongly influenced by the social context in which it occurs. The environmental variable most centrally identified is the person's significant others. From them, a person learns to seek advice and support in solving daily problems in living. Confidence in being liked and respected by these peers is based on past testing and reaffirmation of the expected supportive responses.

Self-esteem has an important influence on how threats to the self-concept result in a loss of well-being (Jalajas,

1994). Any perceived failure to obtain adequate support to meet psychosocial needs may provoke, or compound, a stressful situation. The receipt of negative support could be equally detrimental to a person's self-esteem.

Coping Mechanisms

People use many methods to cope with anxiety and reduce tension. Lifestyles are developed around patterns of response that, in turn, are established to cope with stressful situations. These lifestyles are highly individual and quite necessary to protect and maintain equilibrium.

Over the years, it has been common to find the term *coping* used interchangeably with such similar concepts as adaptation, defense, mastery, and adjustive reactions. Coping activities take a wide variety of forms, including all of the diverse behaviors that people engage in to meet actual or anticipated challenges. In psychologic stress theory, the term **coping** emphasizes various strategies used, consciously or unconsciously, to deal with stress and tensions arising from perceived threats to psychologic integrity. It is not synonymous with mastery over life problems. Rather, it is the *process* of attempting to solve them (Lazarus, 1966).

Coleman (1950) defined coping as an adjustive reaction made in response to actual or imagined stress in order to maintain psychologic integrity. Within this concept, human beings are perceived as responding to stress by attack, flight, or compromise reactions. These reactions become complicated by various ego-defense mechanisms whenever the stress becomes ego involved.

Attack reactions usually attempt to remove or overcome the obstacles seen as causing stress in life situations. They may be primarily constructive or destructive in nature. Flight, withdrawal, or fear reactions may be as simple as physically removing the threat from the environment (such as putting out a fire) or removing oneself from the threatening situation (such as running away from the fire area). They might also involve much more complex psychologic maneuvering, depending on the perceived extent of the threat and the possibilities for escape.

Compromise or substitution reactions occur when attack or flight from the threatening situation is thought to be impossible. This method is most commonly used to deal with problem solving and includes accepting substitute goals or changing internalized values and standards.

Masserman (1946) demonstrated that in situations of extended frustration individuals find it increasingly possible to compromise with substitute goals. This often involves use of *rationalization*, a defense mechanism whereby "half a loaf" does indeed soon appear to be "better than none."

Tension-reducing mechanisms can be overt or covert and can be consciously or unconsciously activated. They have been generally classified into such behavioral responses as aggression, regression, withdrawal, and repression. The selection of a response is based on tension-reducing actions that successfully relieved anxiety and reduced tension in similar situations in the past. Through repetition, the response may pass from conscious awareness during its learning phase to a habitual level of reaction as a learned behavior. In many instances the individual may not be aware of *how*, let alone *why*, he or she reacts to stress in given situations. Except for having vague feelings of discomfort, the individual may not notice the rise and consequent reduction in tension. When a new stress-producing event arises and learned coping mechanisms are ineffectual, discomfort is felt on a conscious level. The need to "do something" becomes the focus of activity, narrowing perception of all other life activities.

Normally, defense mechanisms are used constructively in the process of coping. This is particularly evident whenever there is danger of becoming psychologically overwhelmed. Almost all defense mechanisms are seen as important for survival. None is equated with a pathologic condition unless it interferes with the process of coping, such as being used to deny, to falsify, or to distort perceptions of reality.

According to Bandura et al (1977), the strength of the individual's conviction in his or her own effectiveness in overcoming or mastering a problematic situation determines whether coping behavior is even attempted in the first place. People fear and avoid stressful, threatening situations they believe exceed their ability to cope. They behave with assurance in those situations in which they judge themselves able to manage and in which they expect eventual success. It is the perceived ability to master that can influence the choice of coping behaviors, as well as the persistence used once a coping behavior is chosen.

Available coping mechanisms are what people *usually* do when they have a problem. They may sit down and try to think it out or talk it out with a friend. Some cry it out or try to get rid of their feelings of anger and hostility by swearing, kicking a chair, or slamming doors. Others may get into verbal battles with friends. Some may react by temporarily withdrawing from the situation in order to reassess the problem. These are just a few of the many coping methods people use to relieve their tension and anxiety when faced with a problem. Each coping mechanism has been used at some time in the developmental past of the individual, has been found to be effective in maintaining emotional stability, and has become part of the lifestyle in meeting and dealing with the stresses of daily living.

TYPES

Maturational Crises

A maturational crisis involves the normal life transition that creates changes with individuals and how they perceive themselves, their role, and their status. Transitional periods throughout the life cycle are key times for maturational growth to occur. Examples of these crucial times are adolescence, parenthood, midlife, and retirement. How an individual has accomplished developmental tasks throughout the life span significantly determines whether the new transitional period will be viewed as a crisis or an opportunity for maturation.

A young adult who has had difficulty with the task of middle childhood (i.e., industry versus inferiority) and learning the necessary socialization skills for that age-group is also likely to experience difficulty leaving the parental home, establishing a new family, and obtaining employment and social competence. A transitional crisis can be an out-of-sequence life transition, such as a normal occurrence happening unexpectedly (e.g., premature death of a parent). Out-of-sequence events tend to be more difficult to experience because the individual is unprepared for such traumatic occurrences; thus they can have negative maturational effects.

Situational Crises

A situational crisis occurs when a specific, external event disturbs an individual's psychologic equilibrium. This can be an event that affects the person individually or within that person's peer group. Situational crises usually center around losses that impact the individual and result in **ego dissonance** (inconsistency between attitudes and behaviors). Examples of situational crises are loss of employ-ment, loss of a loved one or valued object, loss of health, and loss of status.

The loss of an important person in one's life may result in confusion and ambivalent, unresolved feelings surrounding the loss. The loss may be compounded by a change in one's status, finances, and support systems. The loss of employment can result in financial stress, resulting in a deeper sense of loss of one's role and a possible sense of failure, as well as decreased self-worth and self-esteem.

It is normal to mourn the loss of a loved one and to experience grief, but it is also common to mourn the loss of an idea, an idealized object, or changes within oneself. The changes that occur in one's body over time and in loved ones help define and redefine the self. In periods of stability, one defines one's life by attempting to understand its meaning and finiteness. Each transition from one developmental stage to another leads to termination of a previous life structure; each transition is an ending, a process involving separation or loss. Levinson described transition as an opportunity to review and evaluate one's past, to take what was best from one's life and separate it from the difficult and traumatic events. A transition is a time of bridging the past with the hopes and promises of the future. During transitions, changes can be attempted in both the self and the individual's world. It involves a letting go of unfinished or painful experiences and incor-

---

Nursing Care in the Community

Crisis Intervention

Crisis intervention acts as a lifeline to the public. A skilled crisis nurse acts as the gatekeeper for the entire mental health system, as well as activating the law enforcement network in emergency situations. The nurse must often make decisions that have a direct impact on the life or death of clients in the community when assessing an individual's danger to self or to others. The entire community could be considered, as well as the client.

Psychiatric mental health nurses working in the community are especially warranted in catastrophic situations such as fires, floods, or earthquakes, both for those who have been traumatized by the event itself and for those who have lost significant others in the tragedy. Victims of the event may have a psychiatric diagnosis that is intensified by the event. They may experience delusions in which they believe they are responsible for the disaster and may not be amenable to rational reassurance. Immediate psychiatric assessment and intervention are necessary to help these individuals manage the effects of the trauma through personal comfort and medication. Hospitalization may also be necessary.

Friends and relatives of trauma victims may also be adversely affected by an overwhelming emotional response that requires psychiatric intervention. They should be given brief reassurances, referred to a community contact, and provided with information about the possible duration of their symptoms.

The nurse must be able to triage the needs of the individual, as well as the community, and may also offer support to individual clients who are expressing fear, loneliness, and other stress-related problems. Some callers may need to check in daily with familiar workers and become well known to crisis service personnel. Strategies focus on identifying an immediate precipitant, evaluating the client's personal safety, and working with him or her to reestablish emotional equilibrium.

Interventions range from giving referrals to programs such as Alcoholics Anonymous and suggesting private therapists, to commonsense advice about daily crises. It is routine to counsel a heartbroken lover, a recently discharged patient with adjustment difficulties, or a parent whose child has become estranged through behaviors such as drug abuse. Some people call crisis centers as proxies for friends or family members who are too upset or disorganized to be coherent.

Although a psychiatrist is always on call for consultation and orders, the crisis nurse must be familiar with the most recent diagnostic manual and be capable of making assessments based on sparse information. He or she must be aware of personal limitations yet be able to take responsibility for rapid independent actions, which may include calling EMTs (emergency medical technicians, or paramedics) or the police. As in other community situations, it is safer to err on the side of caution than to hesitate because of fear of intruding on individual clients.

porating the best of one's development and experience (Levinson et al, 1978).

Adventitious Crises

Adventitious crises are precipitated by providence, or fate. They are the unpredictable tragedies that occur without warning. Examples are earthquakes, tidal waves, floods, famine, and other natural disasters. Civil uprising, riots, and war are also included in this category. Often, it is the unpredictability of such disasters that leaves such fear, confusion, and ego dissonance in their victims. Only a minority of those who experience a natural disaster develop psychologic disorders, suggesting that there are individual differences in responses to such stressors (Phifer, 1990).

METHODS OF CRISIS INTERVENTION

According to Jacobson et al (1968), crisis intervention may be divided into two major complementary categories: generic and individual.

Generic Approach

The **generic approach** proposes that there are certain recognized patterns of behavior in most crises. Many studies have substantiated this (e.g., Lindemann's [1944] studies of bereavement of a relative). He referred to these sequential phases as "grief work" and found that failure of a person to grieve appropriately or to complete the process of bereavement could potentially lead to future emotional illness. Kaplan and Mason (1960) and Caplan (1974) studied the effect on the mother of the birth of a premature baby and identified four phases or tasks that she must work through to ensure healthy adaptation to the experience. Janis (1958) has suggested several hypotheses concerning the psychologic stress of impending surgery and the patterns of emotional responses that follow a diagnosis of chronic illness. Rappoport (1963) had defined three subphases of marriage during which unusual stress could precipitate crises.

The generic approach focuses on the characteristic course of the *particular kind of crisis* rather than on the psychodynamics of each individual in crisis. A treatment plan is directed toward an adaptive resolution of the crisis. Specific intervention measures are designed to be effective for all members of a given group rather than for the unique differences of one individual. Recognition of these behavioral patterns is an important aspect of preventive mental health.

Jacobson et al (1968) state that generic approaches to crisis intervention include:

direct encouragement of adaptive behavior, general support, environmental manipulation and anticipatory guidance. . . . In brief, the generic approach emphasizes (1) specific situational and maturational events occurring to significant population groups, (2) intervention oriented to crisis related to these specific events, and (3) intervention carried out by non–mental health professionals.

This approach has been found to be feasible as a mode of intervention that can be learned and implemented by nonpsychiatric physicians, nurses, social workers, and others. It does not require a mastery of knowledge of the intrapsychic and interpersonal processes of an individual in crisis.

Individual Approach

The **individual approach** differs from the generic approach in its emphasis on assessment by a professional of the interpersonal and intrapsychic processes of the person in crisis. It is used in selected cases, usually with those who are not responding to the generic approach. Intervention is planned to meet the unique needs of the individual in crisis and to reach a solution for the particular situation and circumstances that precipitated the crisis. It differs from the generic approach, which focuses on the characteristic course of a particular kind of crisis.

Unlike extended psychotherapy, the individual approach deals relatively little with the developmental past of the individual. Information from this source is seen as relevant only for the clues that may result in a better understanding of the present crisis situation. Emphasis is placed on the immediate causes for disturbed equilibrium and on the processes necessary for regaining a **precrisis,** or higher, **level of functioning.**

Jacobson (1968) cites the inclusion of family members or other important persons in the process of the individual's crisis resolution as another area of differentiation from most individual psychotherapy. In comparison with the generic approach, the individual approach is viewed by Jacobson as emphasizing the need for greater depth of understanding of the biopsychosocial process, intervention oriented to the individual's unique situation, and intervention carried out only by mental health professionals.

PROBLEM SOLVING IN CRISIS INTERVENTION: APPLICATION OF CRISIS THEORY

John Dewey (1910) proposed the classical steps of problem solving:

1. A difficulty is perceived.
2. The difficulty is located and defined.
3. Possible solutions are suggested.
4. Consequences are considered.
5. A solution is accepted.

With minor changes, this approach to the steps in problem solving has persisted over the years. Johnson (1955) simplified problem solving by reducing the number of steps to three: preparation, production, and judgment.

According to Guilford (1967), the general problem-solving model involves the following processes:

Input (from environment and soma)
Filtering (attention aroused and directed)

Cognition (problem sensed and structured)
Production (answers generated)
Cognition (new information obtained)
Production (new answers generated)
Evaluation (input and cognition tested, answers tested; new tests of problem structure, new answers tested)

When professional help is sought because a person is in crisis, the nurse must use logic and background knowledge to define the problem and plan the intervention. The *crisis approach to problem solving* involves an assessment of the individual and the problem, planning of therapeutic intervention, intervention, and resolution of the crisis and anticipatory planning (Morley, Messick, and Aguilera, 1967).

STEPS IN CRISIS INTERVENTION

Specific steps are involved in crisis invention and were first outlined for nursing by Morley, Messick, and Aguilera (1967).

ASSESSMENT

When help is needed because an individual is in a crisis, the nurse must use logic and background knowledge to define the problem and plan interventions. Nurses are familiar with the problem-solving approach that is used in crisis intervention. Assessment requires the nurse to use active focusing techniques to obtain an accurate appraisal of the precipitating event and the crisis that caused the individual to seek professional help. The nurse must decide if the individual presents a high suicidal or homicidal risk. If the lethality is high (e.g., the client has a loaded gun and a specific plan), then hospitalization is necessary to protect the client or others in the community. Assessment questions are very direct and specific. If the lethality is low (no method or specific plan), then hospitalization is not considered necessary.

In this phase, determination is made of the length of time since the onset of the crisis. It is important to know how much the crisis has disrupted the individual's life and the effects of this disruption on others. Information is also sought to determine the individual's strengths, what coping skills have been successful in the past, what coping skills are being used presently, and what people might be engaged as situational supports. Search is made for alternative methods of coping that for some reason are not presently being used.

The first therapy session is directed toward finding out the crisis-precipitating event and the factors affecting the individual's inability to solve his or her problem. It is vital that both the nurse and the client define the situation clearly before taking any action to change it. Questions to ask are: "What do I need to know?" and "What must be done?" The more specifically the problem can be defined, the more likely the "correct" answer will be found. One of the nurse's first questions is *always* "Why did you come for

help today?" The word *today* should always be emphasized. Sometimes the individual will try to avoid stating the reason by saying, "I've been planning to come for some time." The usual reply is "Yes, but what happened that made you come in *today?*" Other questions to ask are "What happened in your life that is *different?*" and "*When* did it happen?"

It is important to remember that the nurse's task is to focus only on the immediate problem. There is not enough time and *no need* to go into the client's past history in depth or to discuss unrelated issues or problems. The nurse politely indicates that any unrelated issues the client discusses may be important but that the focus will remain on the immediate problem.

The next area to focus on is the *individual's perception* of the event. What does it mean to the person? How does it affect the future? Is the event perceived realistically, or is the meaning distorted?

The client is then questioned about available *situational supports*. Who in the environment can the nurse find to support the person? With whom does the client talk about problems? Who is the client's best friend? Who does the client trust? Is there a member of the family to whom the client feels particularly close? Crisis intervention is so sharply time limited that the more people involved in helping the person, the better. Also, if others are involved and familiar with the problem, they can continue to give support when therapy is terminated. Supports may also be organizations or agencies (church, formal self-help groups, social services).

The next area of focus concerns what the person usually does with a problem that is difficult to solve. What are the client's usual *coping skills*? Has anything like this ever happened before? How does the individual usually reduce tension, anxiety, or depression? Has the client tried using this method to relieve this problem? If not, why not, if it usually works? What does the person think would reduce symptoms of stress? Methods of coping with anxiety that have not been used for years may be remembered. The client usually can think of something. Coping skills are very individual.

PLANNING THERAPEUTIC INTERVENTION

The plan for the client is aimed at resolution of the individual's immediate crisis and restoring the client to *at least* the precrisis level of functioning. The plan considers the length of time since the onset of the crisis, how much the crisis has disrupted the person's life, and the effects of this disruption on others. Also incorporated are the individual's strengths, coping skills that have been successfully used in the past, and coping skills that are being presently. Alternative methods of coping are considered. Situational supports are included in each client's plan of care.

INTERVENTION

The nature of intervention techniques is highly dependent on preexisting skills, creativity, and flexibility of the nurse.

The following suggestions by Morley, Messick, and Aguilera have been found to be useful:

- *Assist the individual in gaining an intellectual understanding of the crisis.* Often the individual sees no relationship between a hazardous situation occurring in life and the extreme discomfort of disequilibrium it causes. The nurse may use the direct approach, describing to the client the relationship between the crisis and the event, if the client is unable to gain insight on his or her own.
- *Assist the individual in bringing into the open present feelings that were not previously accessible.* Frequently the person may have suppressed some very real feelings such as anger or other inadmissible emotions toward someone that "should be loved or honored." It may also be denial of grief, feelings of guilt, or failure to complete the mourning process following bereavement. An immediate goal of intervention is the reduction of tension by providing a means for the individual to recognize these feelings and bring them into the open. It is sometimes necessary to produce an emotional catharsis and reduce immobilizing tension. This is usually done by a nurse who is skilled in managing the client's strong emotional reaction.
- *Explore coping mechanisms.* This requires helping the individual to examine alternate ways of coping. If behaviors used in the past for successfully reducing anxiety have not been tried, the possibility of their use in the present situation is also explored. New coping methods are sought, and frequently the person devises some highly original methods that have not been tried. This phase of intervention provides the opportunity for learning new skills, and for growth.
- *Reopen the social world.* If the crisis has been precipitated by the loss of someone significant to the person's life, the possibility of introducing new people to fill the void can be highly effective. It is particularly effective if supports and gratifications provided by the "lost" person in the past can be achieved to a similar degree through new relationships.

RESOLUTION OF THE CRISIS
During this phase the nurse reinforces those adaptive coping mechanisms that the individual has used successfully to reduce tension and anxiety. As coping abilities increase and positive changes occur, they may be summarized to allow the person to reexperience and reconfirm the progress that was made. Assistance is given as needed in making realistic plans for the future (Box 25-1). There is discussion of ways in which the present experience may help in coping with future crises.

VIOLENCE IN OUR SOCIETY
The twentieth century has not been very tranquil or serene. Seldom does a week go by that we are not confronted by the news of apparently random acts of violence, including killing, rape, and kidnapping; spousal abuse; abuse of the elderly; child abuse and neglect; and murder. There have been a multitude of traumatic events. Violence is escalating in our society and in the lives of those we love. Perhaps the violence we encounter in our lives does not always appear in banner headlines. Sometimes it appears as a headline for a brief period, but it neither affects as many people nor receives the same notoriety over a lengthy period. All violence perpetuates crisis.

Some of the events that occur daily may not affect us directly, but they still affect us. How can we as individuals *not* care when we read about children being neglected, sexually abused, or murdered by their family members or caregivers? Do some of us identify with the wife or husband when we read that a husband has killed his wife and three children because she has been unable to contend with his verbal and physical abuse and leaves him, seeking a divorce? Are we not concerned about our children's exposure to drugs and violence in schools and with their peers? We are, of course, very concerned when we read about "gangs" who shoot and kill innocent young boys and girls because they were *thought* to be members of a "rival" gang. The police in most metropolitan cities are understaffed, overworked, and underpaid. They try to do the best they can, but they can only do so much.

VIOLENCE IN THE SCHOOLS
The problem of violence in schools, which is a part of the overall problem of violence in society, has become one of the most pressing issues in the United States. In many school districts concerns about violence have even surpassed academic achievement—traditionally the most persistent theme on the nation's educational agenda—as having the highest priority for reform and intervention (Noguera, 1995). Public clamoring over the need to do something about violence in schools has brought the issue to a critical juncture; if schools fail to respond decisively to this problem, popular support for public education may be endangered. The escalation of violent incidents and the apparent inadequacy of traditional methods to curtail them has led to a search for new strategies to ensure the safety and security of children and teachers in schools (Toby, 1993/1994).

Accepting the fact that it may not be realistic to expect

Box 25-1   Crisis Intervention Method

Assist and encourage insight and understanding of the present situation/crisis.
Encourage expression of feelings to assist client in finding release of tension and anxiety.
Foster problem solving while exploring thoughts.
Explore new coping techniques.
Assist expansion of social supports.
Summarize the progress client has made and methods that were used.
Guide anticipatory planning for future challenges.

that schools can ever be completely immune from the violence that plagues society, we seek to understand why schools may be especially vulnerable to its occurrence. Current efforts aimed at combating violence may in fact have the opposite effect, particularly given the weakening of the moral authority schools once enjoyed.

The goal of maintaining social control through the use of force and discipline has persisted too long. Although past generations could be made to accept the passivity and constraint that such practices engender, present generations will not. Most urban youth today are neither passive nor compliant. The rewards that are dangled before them, such as a decent job and material wealth for those who do

well in school, are perceived by too many as either overvalued or unattainable. New strategies must be devised and supported to help our young people see education as meaningful, relevant, and attainable, and as a viable means of achieving greater personal fulfillment. Anything short of this will leave us mired in a situation that grows increasingly depressing and dangerous every day.

The urban schools perceived as safe by those who spend their time there do not have metal detectors or armed security guards, and their principals do not carry baseball bats. What these "safe" schools do have is a strong sense of community and collective responsibility. Such schools are seen by students as sacred territory, too special

---

CASE STUDY

Ricardo was assigned to a particular therapist at the crisis center because the volunteer assumed (incorrectly) that the therapist also was Latino. The therapist met Ricardo and introduced herself and asked him to come to her office. When they reached her office, she asked him to have a seat while she looked briefly at the form that he had completed. He had stated that his problems were "problems at school."

The therapist asked Ricardo what school he was attending. He answered with the name of an inner-city school that was notorious for being the "hub" of two well-known rival gangs. The therapist asked Ricardo if he was an active member of one of the gangs. Ricardo was quiet for a few minutes and then asked the therapist, "You aren't Latino, are you?" The therapist answered, "No, but my husband is from Spain—that is why everyone assumes that I am a Latino. Why do you ask, Ricardo?" He answered, "Maybe you won't be able to understand my problem." Smiling, the therapist replied, "Well we won't know until you tell me what the problem is, will we?"

Ricardo returned her smile and said, "I haven't talked to anyone about this. I just don't know what to do." She replied, "Ricardo, please tell me what you are so concerned about. Maybe I can help, and maybe I can't." He looked at the therapist intently and said, "Okay, I've got to trust someone."

Ricardo began by asking the therapist if she knew anything about the two rival gangs at his school. The therapist told him that almost everyone had heard about them. She knew that one gang was Latino and the other was African-American. The rivalry frequently erupted into violence, with fights between the two with guns and knives. Not only some of the members, but also some innocent bystanders, had been killed. Some had been shot and killed or severely injured by cars when one of the gangs assumed, wrongly, that those in the car were members of the rival gang. She related this to Ricardo.

The therapist asked Ricardo if he was a member of the Latino gang. He answered, "No, and that is the problem!" He continued, saying that he had a friend in the gang and had overheard him talking about one of the members of the other gang. He heard him say that this member was on a "hit" list and that "it" was planned for the next evening, and even where they were planning to do the "hit." He said that he had refused to be-

come a member of the Latino gang because he did not believe that violence achieved anything. He continued by saying that he didn't want to get his friend in trouble. So he couldn't say anything to anyone at school. There were too many "snitches," so if he went to the police, someone would find out that he was the one who had leaked the information of the "hit."

The therapist asked Ricardo if he had told anyone that he was coming to the crisis center. He answered in the negative, saying, "God, no! No one must know that I've been here."

The therapist asked him if he *wanted* to let the police know about the "hit." He looked at the therapist and said, "Yes, I just don't know how I can without someone finding out." The therapist said, "Ricardo, What if I just accidentally, of course, left the telephone number of a hot line on my desk that would not ask you anything about yourself but that handles problems like the one you are faced with? I, of course, will not be in my office with you." She paused, "I am going to get some coffee. Would you like me to bring you a soft drink?" In almost a whisper she added, "In case you want to make a telephone call while I am gone, just dial 9 for an outside line." Ricardo hesitated, "Can they trace this number?" "No," the therapist replied, "they never have in the past." He looked at her knowingly and said, "You have done this before, haven't you?" "Done what?" she replied. They exchanged glances. "Did you decide if you wanted a soft drink?" Ricardo followed her lead, "I would like a Coke, if you have one." The therapist put a card from her Rolodex in the center of her desk and placed the telephone next to it. "I'll be back with my coffee and your Coke in about 10 minutes, okay?" Ricardo smiled and said, "Thanks." She returned his smile, walked out of her office, and closed the door firmly behind her.

When the therapist returned, the card had been replaced in the Rolodex and Ricardo had left her a note, "Thanks, friend. Your pal, R." He had left "no clues."

Ricardo was not her first experience with gangs, and she doubted it would be her last.

Critical Thinking Exercise

1. Complete the paradigm for this case study (Figure 25-2). Refer to the paradigm in Figure 25-1.

to be spoiled by crime and violence and too important to risk being excluded. Such schools are few, but their existence serves as tangible proof that there are alternatives to chaotic schools plagued by violence and controlled institutions that aim to produce docile bodies (Noguera, 1995).

The Case Study box illustrates how a psychotherapist of one culture can work effectively with a client of a different culture. Not only do they have different cultures, but they also have different backgrounds, values, and ideals.

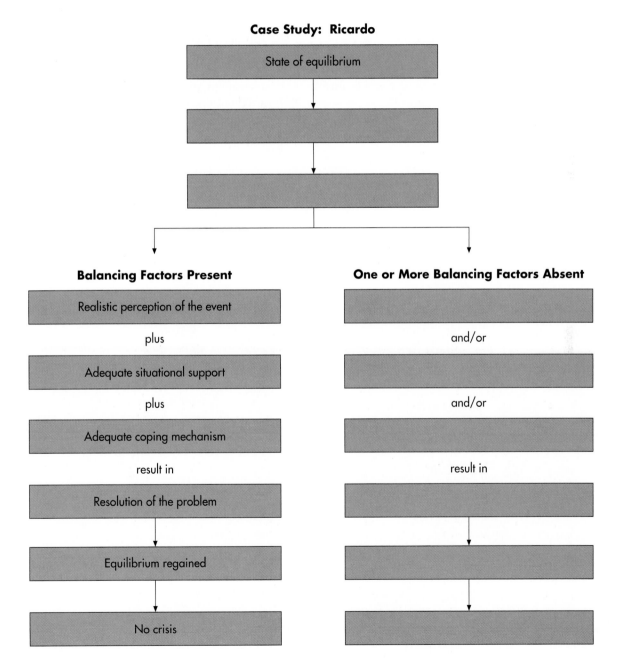

Figure 25-2   Case study: Ricardo. (From Aguilera DC: *Crisis intervention: theory and methodology,* ed 8, St. Louis, 1998, Mosby.)

Summary of Key Concepts

1. The most important aspects of mental health are the state of the ego, the stage of its maturity, and the quality of its structure.

2. Caplan refers to a crisis as showing a rise in inner tension, signs of anxiety, and disorganization of function, all of which result in a prolonged period of emotional upset.

3. If adaptive mechanisms are used and a state of equilibrium is regained, a crisis can result in personal growth.

4. Differences in coping mechanisms are influenced by the way each individual perceives the threat.

5. The more realistically an individual views the stressful event, the more success the individual has in solving the problem quickly.

6. Because appraisal of the event is an ongoing process, coping behaviors are never static, as new significance is attached to the event.

7. Lack of situational support may compound a stressful situation into a crisis.

8. Coping is the process of attempting to solve problems—not the mastery over life problems.

9. There are three basic reactions to stress: attack, flight, or compromise.

10. Tension-reducing responses—aggression, regression, withdrawal, and repression—are based on past successful responses.

11. Success in handling maturational, or transitional crises depends on how the individual accomplished developmental tasks.

12. There are two approaches to crisis intervention. The generic approach focuses on the characteristic course of a particular kind of crisis. The individual approach focuses on meeting the unique needs of an individual.

13. There are four typical phases in crisis intervention: assessment, planning therapeutic interventions, intervention, and resolution of the crisis and anticipatory planning.

REFERENCES

Aguilera DC: *Crisis intervention: theory and methodology*, ed 8, St Louis, 1998, Mosby.

Antonovsky A: *Unraveling the mystery of health: how people manage stress and stay well*, San Francisco, 1987, Jossey-Bass.

Bandura A et al: Cognitive processes mediating behavioral change, *J Pers Soc Psychol* 35:125, 1977.

Canatsey K, Roper JM: Removal from stimuli for crisis intervention: using least restrictive methods to improve the quality of patient care, *Issues Ment Health Nurs* 18(1):35, 1997.

Caplan C: *An approach to community mental health*, New York, 1961, Grune & Stratton.

Caplan C: *Support systems and community mental health: lectures in concept development*, New York, 1974, Behavioral Publications.

Coleman JC: *Abnormal psychology and modern life*, Chicago, 1950, Scott, Foresman.

Cropley A, Field T: Achievement in science and intellectual style, *J Appl Psychol* 53:132, 1969.

Dewey J: *How we think*, Boston, 1910, DC Heath.

Dyehouse JM, Sommers MS: Brief intervention after alcohol-related injuries, *Nurs Clin North Am* 33(1):93, 1998.

D'Zurilla TJ, Maydeu-Olivares A: Conceptual and methodological issues in social problem–solving assessment, *Behav Ther* 26(3):409, 1995.

Guilford JP: *The nature of human intelligence*, New York, 1967, McGraw-Hill.

Hales A et al: Role of the psychiatric clinical nurse specialist in the emergency department, *Nurse Spec* 11(6):264, 1997.

Helms S: Experiences of stress in accident and emergency nurses, Belgrave Department of Child Psychiatry, King's College Hospital, London, UK, *Br J Hosp Med* 33:152, 1996.

Inkeles A: Social structure and the socialization of confidence, *Harvard Educ Rev* 36:265, 1966.

Jackson G: Crisis theory, *New Dir Ment Health Serv* 6:1, 1980.

Jacobson G: Crisis theory and treatment strategy: some sociocultural and psychodynamic considerations, *J Nerv Ment Dis* 141:209, 1965.

Jacobson G et al: Generic and individual approaches to crisis intervention, *Am J Public Health* 58:339, 1968.

Jalajas DS: The role of self-esteem in the stress process: empirical results from job hunting, *J Appl Soc Psychol* 24(22):1984, 1994.

Janis IL: *Psychological stress, psychoanalytical and behavioral studies of surgical patients*, New York, 1958, John Wiley & Sons.

Johnson DM: *The psychology of thought and judgment*, New York, 1955, Harper & Row.

Kaplan DM, Mason EA: Maternal reactions to premature birth viewed as an acute emotional disorder, *Am J Orthopsychiatry* 30:539, 1960.

Lazarus RS: *Psychological stress and the coping process*, New York, 1966, McGraw-Hill.

Lazarus RS et al: The psychology of coping: issues in research and assessment. In Coehlo GV et al, editors: *Coping and adaptation*, New York, 1974, Basic Books.

Levinson DJ et al: *The seasons of a man's life*, New York, 1978, Alfred A Knopf.

Liefland L et al: A crisis intervention program: staff go the extra mile for client improvement, *J Psychosoc Nurs Ment Health Serv* 35(2):32, 1997.

Lindemann E: Symptomatology and management of acute grief, *Am J Psychiatry* 101:101, 1944.

Littlepage GE et al: An input-process-output analysis of influence and performance in problem-solving groups, *J Pers Soc Psychol* 69(5):877, 1995.

Masserman JH: *Principles of dynamic psychology*, Philadelphia, 1946, WB Saunders.

McSherry WC, Holm JE: Sense of coherence: its effects on psychological and physiological processes prior to, during, and after a stressful situation, *J Clin Psychol* 50(4):476, 1994.

Mechanic D: Social structure and personal adaptation: some neglected dimensions. In Coelho GV et al, editors: *Coping and adaptation*, New York, 1974, Basic Books.

Morley WE, Messick JM, Aguilera DC: Crisis: paradigms of intervention, *J Psychiatr Nurs* 5:538, 1967.

Neely KW, Spitzer WJ: A model for a statewide critical incident stress (CIS) debriefing program for emergency services personnel, *Prehosp Disaster Med* 12(2):43, 1997.

Noguera P: Preventing and producing violence: a critical analysis of response to school violence, *Harvard Educ Rev* 63:2, 1995.

Phifer JF: Psychological distress and somatic symptoms after natural disaster: differential vulnerability among older adults, *Psychol Aging* 5(3):412, 1990.

Rappoport R: Normal crises, family structure and mental health, *Fam Process* 2:68, 1963.

Riley B: *Application of Aguilera's crisis model to caregivers of elders relocating to nursing homes*, doctoral dissertation, Birmingham, 1993, University of Alabama at Birmingham, unpublished.

Thomas, SP: Assessing and intervening with anger disorders, *Nurs Clin North Am* 33(1):121, 1998.

Toby J: Everyday school violence: how disorder fuels it, *Am Educator*, p 4, Winter 1993/1994.

Tomic W: Training in inductive reasoning and problem solving, *Contemp Educ Psychol* 20(4):483, 1995.

CHAPTER 26

Activity Therapies

Theresa Williams-Hessling

OBJECTIVES

- Distinguish between occupational, recreational, art, music, psychodrama, and movement/dance therapies.

- Describe common settings in which activity therapies are found and give examples of therapeutic modalities for each.

- Identify the goals and objectives of activity therapies when used for specific DSM-IV diagnoses.

- Compare and contrast activity therapies with traditional verbal therapies.

- Describe effective nursing roles for each of the activity therapies.

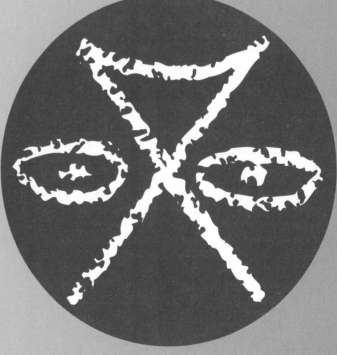

Activity therapies, also known as expressive, experiential, or adjunct therapies, include occupational, recreational, art, music, movement/dance, and psychodrama therapies. Activity therapists provide services to children, adolescents, adults, and elderly of all functional levels and diagnostic categories. They can be found in a broad range of therapeutic settings, including medical and psychiatric hospitals, nursing homes, psychosocial and physical rehabilitation centers, homeless shelters, clinics, public and private schools, group homes, correctional centers, home health agencies, community mental health centers, day care centers, and private practices.

The techniques involved in these modalities become therapeutic when the primary intention is to increase the client's awareness of feelings, behavior, perceptions, cognitions, and sensations to minimize pathology and promote health. The "action" in activity therapies can be physical and/or imagined. Activity therapies are not limited by the same constraints of verbal therapies, such as the clients' censorship of thoughts and feelings. Instead, these therapeutic modalities allow clients to be expressive on multiple levels at once, including physical, emotional, and symbolic levels. They also allow clients to demonstrate conflicts, strengths, and limitations, both developmentally and psychologically, and to resolve these issues in the present. The creative process is recognized as curative because it involves problem solving, experiencing hope, and connecting with the inside (the psyche) and the outside world. These expressive experiences are important, especially for in-patient settings, because they allow clients to be viewed as whole people, rather than being identified by pathology and subsequently depersonalized.

Activity therapy
Action-oriented process with the primary intention to increase awareness of feelings, behaviors, perceptions, and cognitions to minimize pathology and promote health.

Art medium Materials or technical means used for artistic expression.

Art therapy The use of the creative art process for psychotherapy and rehabilitation.

Closure Also called sharing; the last stage in psychodrama or movement/dance therapy in which the experience is verbally processed to promote insight and provide a sense of completion.

Double
The individuals in psychodrama who operate as the "inner voice" of the protagonist to express repressed thoughts, feelings, and conflicts.

Enactment The action portion in psychodrama in which a scene or sequence of scenes is portrayed.

Mirroring
A technique in psychodrama and movement/dance therapy in which one individual imitates the behavior patterns of another to demonstrate how others perceive and react to him or her.

Movement
Kinesthetic behavior in which individuals communicate by the use of body motions.

Movement/dance therapy The psychotherapeutic use of movement as a process that furthers the emotional, cognitive, and physical integration of the individual.

Music The science or art of assembling or performing intelligible combinations of tones in an organized, structured form.

Music therapy The use of music in the accomplishment of therapeutic aims: the restoration, maintenance, and improvement of mental and physical health.

Occupation The goal-directed use of time, energy, interest, and attention to foster adaption and productivity, to minimize pathology, and to promote the maintenance of health.

Occupational therapy The application of goal-directed, purposeful activity in the assessment and treatment of individuals with psychologic, physical, or developmental disabilities.

Protagonist The individual in psychodrama who presents and acts out his or her emotional problem or issue.

Psychodrama The use of guided dramatic action to examine problems or issues raised by an individual to clarify issues, increase physical and emotional well-being, enhance learning, and develop new skills.

Recreation To create again by some form of play, amusement, or relaxation.

Recreational therapy To restore, remediate, or rehabilitate through play to improve functioning and independence and reduce or eliminate the effects of illness or disability.

Theme development The part of movement/dance therapy in which a specific issue or feeling is actively being explored.

HISTORICAL PERSPECTIVES

Activity therapies date back to early Greek, Roman, and Egyptian times when, as early as 2000 BC, exercise and the arts were found to be healing, especially for melancholia, known today as *depression*. It was not until the increased moral treatment of people with mental illness in the eighteenth and nineteenth centuries that these activities became widely recognized and used in therapeutic settings. For many of the activity therapies, it was nurses who first recognized their therapeutic value. Florence Nightingale and Susan E. Tracy, for example, were major contributors to the birth of recreational therapy (RT) and occupational therapy (OT). As the activity therapies evolved, they became more complex in their theory and practice. It was with this evolution that each activity therapy became recognized as a specialty with its own professional, ethical, and educational standards. These standards were developed to ensure that facilitators are knowledgeable about the dynamics, limitations, and risks in their applications. Activity therapists generally specialize in a specific field, namely occupational, recreational, art, music, dance, or psychodrama therapy. Their formal training usually includes a master's degree with a pregraduate and postgraduate internship.

Through the 1980s, activity therapy departments were commonly found in psychiatric settings. It was not unusual for these settings to employ several recreational and occupational therapists, an art therapist, a music therapist, a dance therapist, and/or a psychodramatist. With the presence of managed care, many activity therapy departments have been reduced to one or two recreational or occupational therapists or they have been eliminated entirely. Often, activity therapists are limited to consultant roles, and these therapies are discounted as "diversionary extras." This downsizing has left other disciplines, usually nursing, to incorporate these important modalities into the therapeutic milieu. Without the commitment of nursing to continue the use of these therapies, they would become unavailable to clients in some instances. It is, therefore, a collaborative effort between activity therapists and nurses that allows clients to continue to benefit from a multidisciplinary approach that can significantly increase the successfulness of treatment outcome (Folsom, Hildreth, and Blair, 1992). This chapter presents activity therapies in their strict theoretic framework as they are used in an optimal collaboration between activity therapists and nurses.

THE ROLE OF NURSING IN ACTIVITY THERAPY

Special considerations must be made by nurses before they decide to direct experiential therapy sessions. In deciding to use these methods, nurses must assess whether they have sufficient skills, or the interest and ability to obtain the skills, necessary to facilitate a particular experiential therapy. Nurses may vary in their degree of comfort with specific techniques (e.g., being physically active or directive with clients). Even if one is uncomfortable with directing or participating in an activity therapy, it is still beneficial for the nurse to become familiar with the specific therapies to recommend them to the primary physician and to support the contributions of all treatment team members. When there is a comfort level but not enough expertise to direct a particular activity therapy experience, the nurse's participation is still extremely valuable and adds an additional trained observer to the group, as well as decreasing many of the clients' inhibitions.

As the reader becomes familiar with each modality and its objectives, it will become obvious that there is an overlapping of treatment goals. A team approach using as many combined therapies as possible has proven to be the most effective and efficient approach for many of the acute diagnoses. This variety allows clients to explore the same problem or symptom from many different perspectives. It also increases the opportunity for clients to use therapeutic strategies that are comfortable, familiar, and safe to resolve conflicts and experience success.

OCCUPATIONAL THERAPY

Occupational therapy was developed in the twentieth century by Adolf Meyer, a neuropathologist who realized the importance of viewing the individual holistically and creating balance in productivity, self-care, and leisure. In 1905 Susan E. Tracy, a nurse and the first practicing occupational therapist, noted the benefits of OT in relieving nervous tension and making bed rest more tolerable. She also observed that these benefits carried over to discharge. Despite this awareness, the use of OT services was limited primarily to the physically disabled through World War I and World War II. Dr. William Rush Dunton, Jr., a psychiatrist who is credited with being the "Father of Occupational Therapy," stated that the goal was "to divert the patient's attention from unpleasant subjects, to keep the patient's train of thought in more healthy channels, to control attention, to secure rest, to train in mental processes by educating hand, eyes, muscles, etc., to serve as a safety valve, and to provide a new vocation" (Dunton, 1915).

It was not until the 1950s that intrapsychic issues were incorporated into OT services, when it was recognized that medical treatment alone was not sufficient for a client with an illness that also impaired social skills. At that time the emphasis was placed on the integration of the client into social settings and the appreciation for activities as therapy. At present, OT focuses on the assessment of task performance, cognitive functioning, and psychosocial development. Treatment is directed toward recognizing strengths, minimizing weaknesses, and adapting to change.

The American Occupational Therapy Association (1994) defines **occupational therapy** as "the use of purposeful activity or interventions designed to achieve functional outcomes which promote health, prevent injury or disability, and which develop, improve, sustain or restore the highest level of independence of any individual who has an injury, illness, cognitive impairment, psychosocial dysfunction, mental illness, developmental or learning disability, physical disability, or other disorder or condition. The word **occupation** means "the goal-directed use of time, energy, interest, and attention to foster adaptation and productivity, to minimize pathology, and to promote the maintenance of health" (Kaplan and Sadock, 1995).

Like nurses, occupational therapists treat physical dysfunction and psychosocial impairment. The treatment goals of OT in mental health are as follows:

1. Provide task-oriented activities, such as crafts, to assess levels of concentration, impulsivity, frustration tolerance, and problem solving.
2. Assist with living skills involving self-care and maintenance to teach or reestablish good habits of personal grooming and health.
3. Promote independent living skills, such as communication and stress management, through psychoeducational groups using didactic materials, discussion, or creative media.
4. Improve sensorimotor skills through sensory-integrative activities and exercise.
5. Assist with discharge planning and community reentry through outings and information about community resources.
6. Provide a prevocational assessment, which may include a practice job interview, an occupational interest inventory, and exposure to work-related tasks.

RECREATIONAL THERAPY

As far back as 2000 BC, Egyptians used games, songs, and dances as therapy, specifically noting their benefits with melancholia *(depression)*. In 1854 Florence Nightingale introduced recreational services to hospitalized soldiers and became known as the "Mother of Hospital Recreation." She came to appreciate the significant therapeutic value of such services as she observed that clients who were involved in the care and feeding of pets experienced increased feelings of self-worth and self-esteem. In 1892 Dr. Adolf Meyer, a neuropathologist, observed that the proper use of time in some helpful and gratifying activity appeared to be a fundamental issue in the treatment of the neuropsychiatric patient. During World War I the American Red Cross used recreational services in hospital settings. In the 1920s and 1930s, recreational programs began appearing in state mental hospitals and schools for individuals with mental retardation. It wasn't until World War II, however, that recreational services began to be recognized as legitimate, curative therapy that could be used to meet specific medical goals and objectives.

CLINICAL APPLICATION
Occupational Therapy

A 35-year-old, divorced, unemployed female is hospitalized for depression on a psychiatric unit. Her hospitalization was prompted by an overdose of prescription medication. She has two adolescent children. She held jobs for a short time in food service but has not worked for 10 years. She overdosed on prescription medication because of self-derogatory hallucinations. She has a DSM-IV, Axis I diagnosis of schizoaffective disorder, depressive type.

Nursing Diagnosis

Social interaction, impaired; self-esteem disturbance; cognitive impairment, related to poor concentration, limited problem-solving abilities, and limited frustration tolerance; coping, ineffective individual, related to difficulty completing daily tasks; role performance, altered; parenting, altered; self-care deficits related to bathing/hygiene, dressing/grooming; violence, risk for: self-directed.

Activity and Objectives

- Self-care and maintenance tasks are divided into small, manageable steps specific to hygiene, dress, makeup, and laundry. The occupational therapist or nurse will follow up with daily contact with the client to review these tasks and provide encouragement.
- A task-oriented craft group is provided to evaluate concentration, planning, and sequencing of tasks, self-confidence, and problem-solving skills. Additionally, these groups allow for reality testing and increasing tolerance for socialization.
- Educational groups, such as assertiveness and stress management, are provided to help the client recognize and use more effective coping techniques. The nurse also provides similar teaching on an individual basis and reinforces positive changes in behavior.
- As acute symptoms decrease, the client's progress is assessed and he or she is assisted in setting goals for the current occupational role. Possible options are suggested, including a parenting class and a gradual return to the work process.

During that time, mental health professionals began to realize the disadvantages and limitations of the sterile hospital environment. Psychiatric hospitals limited their services to physical examinations, balanced meals, pharmacology, and a "safe place to rest." Not only did this stress-free environment prevent an accurate observation of the client's coping skills and adaptive skills, but it also promoted the depersonalization of the client. "The hospitalized patient tended almost inescapably to be depersonalized—to be regarded as an instance of pathology rather than an afflicted and suffering being with all of the sensitivities, needs, hopes and discouragements" (Haun, 1965).

Recreation can be thought of as "creating again," or "refreshing oneself," by some form of play, amusement, or relaxation. Play can also be a powerful tool for venting aggression, achieving motor mastery in children, and recalling childhood successes as adults. Within the regressive elements of play, there are also limits and structures set by the rules of the game.

Recreational therapy is defined by the American Therapeutic Recreation Association (1991) as "treatment services which: restore, remediate or rehabilitate in order to improve functioning and independence as well as reduce or eliminate the effects of illness or disability." The recreational therapist "plans, organizes and directs such activities as adapted sports, dramatics, social activities, and arts and crafts" (Dictionary of Occupational Titles, 1991). In addition, the recreational therapist may organize events such as audiovisual activities; dances; hobbies and special interest programs; musical activities; cooking sessions; and special outings, such as ball games, sightseeing, or picnics. Recreational therapy incorporates the active process of demonstrating and applying observable skills within the curative elements of play (Figure 26-1). The recreational therapist selects an activity based on the treatment goals, taking into account the client's functional abilities, physical requirements, degree of coordination, tolerance for social involvement and interaction, and the level of difficulty of the activity. The four primary goals of recreational therapy are as follows:

1. Provide clients with structured, "normal" activities of daily living.
2. Assist clients in developing leisure skills and interests suitable to their lifestyles.
3. Augment verbal psychotherapy and other activity therapies.
4. Assist clients in bridging the gap between the hospital and the community.
5. Observe clients' reactions and evidence of progression or regression.

ART THERAPY

Throughout history, art has been an important means of expression. In prehistoric times, symbols and images were the primary forms of communication. In 2500 BC, the Greeks used stone carvings to represent their gods. The early Christian church used paintings and sculpture to educate and stimulate intense emotion in people who were predominantly illiterate.

It was not until 1922, when Hans Prinzhorn put to-

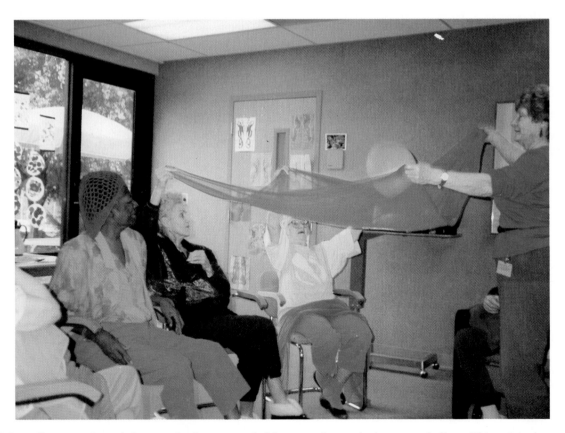

Figure 26-1   Balloon toss. Several clients and a therapist are holding a scarf as a vehicle to toss a balloon. This activity has several purposed: it provides an opportunity for cooperative effort to keep the balloon afloat; it stimulates the senses with colors; and it provides physical existence.

gether a collection of artwork from asylum clients in Europe, that art was additionally appreciated for representing inner psychologic processes. It was then that an established connection was made between illness and its expression through art. Art was also recognized as a bridge between the client's inside and outside world when, in 1933, Sigmund Freud described the unconscious and its expression in imagery, especially in dreams. Freud often provided his clients with paints to re-create their dreams because they had difficulty describing dream images in words alone. As Freud wrote: "Part of the difficulty of giving an account of dreams is due to our having to translate these images into words. 'I could draw it,' a dreamer often says to us, 'but I don't know how to say it.' " (Freud, 1963). In 1964, Carl Jung took the symbolism in artwork a step further when he realized that art gave form to the con-scious and the unconscious (Jung, 1998). Jung observed that many symbols crossed over cultures and generations, which suggested that a "universal unconscious" was being communicated in art.

Art therapy was formalized in the United States as a therapy in its own right in the 1940s. Margaret Naumburg and Edith Kramer were two leaders of this movement. Naumburg, influenced by Sigmund Freud, viewed art therapy from a psychoanalytic perspective. She recognized the art experience as a release of unconscious material and encouraged her clients to engage in free associations about their artwork (Naumburg, 1966). Edith Kramer, on the other hand, concentrated on the creative process itself as curative. She believed that art paralleled life, and in art, life could be "practiced," "changed," and "repeated" without negative consequences (Kramer, 1971).

Elinor Ulman expanded the scope of art therapy for psychotic clients by increasing directiveness and focusing more on building defenses against unconscious material. Ulman saw art therapy as "a way to bring order out of chaos—chaotic feelings and impulses within, the bewildering mass of impressions from without. It is a means to discover both the self and the world, and to establish a relation between the two" (Ulman and Dachinger, 1975).

Art therapy is defined by the American Art Therapy Association as follows:

Art therapy is a human service profession that utilizes art media, images, the creative art process and patient/client responses to the created products as reflections of an individual's development, abilities, personality, interests, concerns and conflicts. Art therapy practice is based on knowledge of human developmental and psychological theories which are implemented in the full spectrum of models of assessment and treatment including educational, psychodynamic, cognitive, transpersonal, and other therapeutic means of reconciling conflicts, fostering self-awareness, developing social skills, managing behavior, solving problems, reducing anxiety, aiding reality orientation, and increasing self-esteem.

Art therapy can be viewed from many of the same schools of thought as can verbal therapies. The most common theories applied are psychoanalytic, gestalt, developmental, and behavioral. Despite the range of theories, it is generally agreed by art therapists that art allows for diverse elements of experience to be communicated simultaneously in a single expressive way.

The **art medium,** or art materials generally used, require little or no technical knowledge, and artistic training is not necessary. In fact, as developmental theorists have observed, healthy people physically and intellectually progress naturally through stages of artistic development up to the age of 12, without any artistic training or talent. For example, children scribble until they are age 1, and children between the ages of 9 and 12 deal in "schemas," or repeated symbols. Viktor Lowenfield (Lowenfield and Brittain, 1970) observed and documented these stages, adding further insight and validity to the interpre-

---

CLINICAL APPLICATION
Recreational Therapy

The recreational therapist is presented with a mixed adult population in an inpatient psychiatric setting with a variety of DSM-IV, Axis I diagnoses, including major depressive disorder, schizophrenia, and bipolar disorder.

Nursing Diagnosis
Verbal communication, impaired; social interaction, ineffective; social isolation; self-esteem disturbance; coping, ineffective individual, related to poor problem-solving skills and difficulty accepting responsibility.

Activity and Objectives
- A unit dance is planned with the highest-functioning clients, and they are assigned specific preparation tasks to foster independence, responsibility, and problem-solving skills. These tasks include decorating the craft room, preparing snacks, selecting music, and designing a flyer to announce the dance to the staff and other clients on the unit. The recreational therapist and nurse demonstrate enthusiasm, encouragement, and support and assist clients with problem solving these tasks through role modeling.
- A safe, "normal" environment is provided for clients to decrease isolation and increase the opportunity to practice appropriate social skills. The recreational therapist and nurse engage the clients in a discussion regarding the upcoming dance, thus promoting anticipation and modeling social interaction.
- Participation in dancing styles that clients are familiar with or can easily learn is encouraged. This increases self-confidence and social contact and provides an outlet for emotions through movement, spontaneity, and play. The recreational therapist and nurse encourage clients to participate in the dancing and involve the more timid clients by dancing with them. They also engage lower-functioning clients who are on the periphery by sitting with them and conversing whenever possible.
- The clients are provided with a safe, enjoyable activity that will promote fun and mental health.

CLINICAL APPLICATION
Art Therapy

A group of ten adolescent boys and girls, ages 14 to 17, who are being treated in an adolescent residential treatment facility, present with a range of DSM-IV, Axis I diagnoses that include major depressive disorder and conduct disorders. These adolescents have family histories that include physical and mental abuse, alcohol and drug use, and school histories of failed grades and suspensions. Two of the adolescents have expressed suicidal ideation.

Nursing Diagnosis

Verbal communication, impaired; social interaction, impaired; self-esteem disturbance; coping, ineffective individual; violence, risk for: self-directed; related to poor problem-solving abilities, poor impulse control, and low frustration levels; and acting-out behavior.

Activity and Objectives

- A variety of art materials are provided, such as liquid tempera paints, pastels, self-hardening clay, watercolors, colored marking pens, pencils, erasers, and white drawing paper of varying sizes. The variety of materials for this group allows for a wide range of expression and an opportunity for the therapist to observe the level of defenses used. The art therapist and nurse observe the clients as they interact with the materials, noting which materials they select and whether they are using these materials appropriately.

- The art therapist suggests a theme for the clients to draw by saying: "Draw a picture of yourself in a box and show how you would get out of the box. The box can be any size or shape and made out of any material you choose. You can get out of the box any way you choose." This theme addresses problem-solving skills, both in dealing with the blank piece of paper and with the theme of getting out of the box. Also, working individually with the art promotes individuation and, as with all art production, a healthy outlet for expression of thoughts and feelings. The art therapist and nurse participate in the art production, creating their own drawings. This is beneficial because it reduces the level of anxiety within the group and serves as another means for connecting with the clients.

- The group is told at the outset that anything they put down on paper is acceptable. For example, at the beginning of each session, the therapist may state: "There is no right or wrong, good or bad, or censorship here." This establishes a safe, judgment-free environment that allows for increased self-expression. This unconditional acceptance also enhances self-esteem by providing a successful experience. It is important that participants do not comment on the artistic value of the art productions or influence its content by suggesting additions or deletions. The most important contribution of the art therapist and nurse is to model that all art productions have merit and value, even a blank piece of paper presented as a finished product.

- Clients are encouraged to verbally share their finished products with the group. The art therapist leads a discussion exploring the metaphor of the box as a problem and the act of getting out of the box as representation of how the clients solve their problems. This promotes further awareness and appreciation of the content of the artwork. Members are encouraged to share any honest observations or feelings elicited by the artwork, without judgment, and to value all expression (e.g., "When I look at your picture, I see/feel . . ." or "I wonder if . . .").

- As the group begins to draw, one client appears anxious about the theme and selects controlled materials including pencil and pastel crayons. He scribbles out his first attempt, further demonstrating his anxiety. He then draws a box with a house, labeled "dynomite," and displays himself blowing up the box (Figure 26-2). During the discussion, the client is encouraged to talk about how he "blows up" to solve problems and how these problems seem to center around a home that has its own potential for "exploding" (as evidenced by the label "dynomite"). The group addresses the consequences of "blowing up" the box and explores alternative choices for getting out of the box. This provides the client with a safe and constructive outlet and a vehicle for problem solving that does not include "exploding."

- After the art therapy session, the art therapist assesses the artwork for additional information regarding intellectual capacity, level of depression, elements of suicidal ideation, impulse control, and defenses used. The art therapist and nurse also exchange observations about the medium that was used, the clients' verbal responses to the artwork, and how the content relates specifically to clients' individual issues.

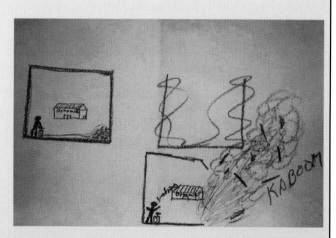

Figure 26-2 Draw a picture of yourself in a box, and show how you would get out of the box. (Courtesy Theresa Williams-Hessling.)

tation of art. In fact, the level at which a client draws can be extremely valuable information in determining his or her intellectual capacity, as well as the age of emotional or cognitive injury. For example, a verbally articulate and high-functioning adult may appear comfortable working with the art materials until a theme about relationships is introduced, at which time the art style regresses to age 5. This would suggest issues regarding relationships that began at the age of 5.

It is critical that clients' diagnosis and level of functioning be taken into consideration when selecting the art materials and the theme to be used. The choice of art medium is important for protecting clients' ego defenses and preventing decompensation. For example, finger paints and clay promote regression, whereas pencils and marking pens promote defenses against regression. In other words, clients with obsessive-compulsive disorder might be encouraged to progress from pencils to paints and to a larger piece of paper, and clients with schizophrenia would be given more structured materials, such as colored pencils and marking pens and a defined space within which to draw. A theme, or topic, is often suggested by art therapists to provide clients with direction and structure. Themes can be as specific as "Draw a picture of yourself and your family doing something together" or as vague as "Use the art materials to say something about yourself."

The primary goals of art therapy are as follows:

1. Provide a safe environment free of judgment and censorship for the expression of feelings, cognitions, and unconscious material.
2. Select a medium that will promote the therapeutic balance between regression and the use of healthy defenses.
3. Encourage clients to verbally share their artwork with the therapist, individually or with a group, to increase insight and promote a connection with others.
4. Provide a creative experience as an outlet for emotions, cognitions, and perceptions.
5. Expose clients to art materials so that they may benefit from the curative effects of color and design.

MUSIC THERAPY

Music can be found in every culture throughout history. Although originally used in rituals and ceremonies for religious and curative purposes, music has come to be recognized as both a science and an art. In our contemporary society, music is used to achieve ambiance in the home, in restaurants, in places of business, and in shopping malls. It creates mood in movies and is an accompaniment for dance. It is also an entertainment medium in its own right. Since the eighteenth century, music has been documented as effecting healing; it was used during both World War I and World War II as therapy with wounded soldiers.

Music is defined as "the science or art of assembling or performing intelligible combinations of tones in organized structured form, with infinitive varieties of expression possible, depending on the relation of its several component factors of rhythm, melody, volume and tonal quality" (Gaston, 1957).

Music becomes **music therapy** when it is used to bring about a specific change in the person who listens to it or performs it. "The responses will be neurophysiological, endocrinological, psychological, and sociological. . . We react through our own interpretations, integrated through our own experiences, augmented by our own emotional feedback system, which makes it even more forceful and meaningful" (Gaston, 1968). The National Association of Music Therapy (1997) defines music therapy as "the use of music in the accomplishment of therapeutic aims: the restoration, maintenance and improvement of mental and physical health. It is the systemic application of music, as directed by the music therapist in a therapeutic environment, to bring about desirable changes in behavior. Such changes enable the individual undergoing therapy to experience a greater understanding of himself and the world around him, thereby achieving a more appropriate adjustment of society."

CLINICAL APPLICATION
Music Therapy

Six adult clients attending a day treatment program are admitted with the DSM-IV, Axis I diagnosis of major depression.

Nursing Diagnosis
Verbal communication, impaired; social interaction, impaired; self-esteem disturbance; social isolation; knowledge deficit related to low attention span and difficulties with concentration; coping, ineffective individual, related to avoidance of conflict.

Activity and Objectives
- Each member of the group is directed to select a song that describes how he or she feels and another song that describes how he or she would like to feel. This allows each person to individually explore his or her own feelings in a nonverbal, nonthreatening way.
- Each member's songs are played for the group and discussion is encouraged. This provides further awareness and identification of feelings, catharsis of feelings, increased spontaneous verbalization, decreased isolation, and increased attention span. The music therapist and nurse provide nonjudgmental validation of feelings and modeling of interpersonal social skills.
- After the music therapy experience, the music therapist and nurse share observations, including verbal and nonverbal feelings expressed by the clients. They also note which clients were active and which were passive and discuss how these observations relate to the clients' individual issues.

Music therapy allows for an immediate experience within a defined structure, promoting both self-organization and social connection. The music medium is selected based on the age of the clients, their level of cognitive functioning, and their ego strengths. The therapeutic process may incorporate recorded music, songwriting, movement and music, or the use of instruments that allow clients to create music easily, with little or no formal training. For music to be universally accepted by a diverse group of people, it must contain neutral sounds instead of recognizable tunes embraced only by a specific age group. "Technically, the musical qualities should be characterized by a slow tempo; a slow, irregular, and unpredictable rhythm; and a certain homogenous monotony throughout" (Goddaer and Abraham, 1994). The long-term goals of music therapy are as follows:

1. Improve self-esteem and body awareness.
2. Increase communication skills.
3. Increase the ability to use energy purposefully.
4. Reduce maladaptive (stereotypic, compulsive, self-abusive, assaultive, disruptive, perserverative, impulsive) behaviors.
5. Increase interaction with peers and others.
6. Increase independence and self-direction.
7. Stimulate creativity and imagination.
8. Enhance emotional expression and adjustment.
9. Increase attending behavior.
10. Improve fine and gross motor skills.
11. Improve auditory perception.

MOVEMENT/DANCE THERAPY

Dance has been used throughout history for celebration, worship, mourning, and healing. Movement/dance therapy is often described as the oldest of the expressive therapies, with many of its concepts taken from the classical Greeks and the religious and healing application of dance from the Orient.

In the early twentieth century, Isadora Duncan developed a framework by which modern dance and movement/dance therapy are defined. Duncan's basic concept was that "physical movement is the natural, biological reaction of man to inner emotion or the soul" (Rosen, 1974). Movement/dance therapy was formally described in the United States in 1942 by Marion Chase (Charklin, 1975). Chase recognized **movement** as a direct expression of the self through the body, promoting increased awareness of the body and changes in feeling states, cognitions, and behavior. She also noted that this increased awareness of the body in space allowed distorted body image perceptions to be confronted and corrected.

Movement/dance therapy is defined as "the psychotherapeutic use of movement as a process which furthers the emotional, cognitive and physical integration of the individual" (American Dance Therapy Association).

CLINICAL APPLICATION
Movement/Dance Therapy

Six female clients in a partial hospitalization eating disorders program, with DSM-IV, Axis I diagnoses of anorexia nervosa or bulimia nervosa, are prescribed a weekly movement/dance therapy group.

Nursing Diagnosis

Self-esteem disturbance; body image disturbance; sensory/perceptual alterations, kinesthetic, related to the experience of feeling detached from the body; verbal communication, impaired; social interaction, impaired; social isolation; knowledge deficit, related to self-deprecating thoughts, low tolerance for error, and difficulty identifying feelings; coping, ineffective individual, related to poor physical, sexual, and internal boundaries.

Activity and Objectives

- A warm-up exercise is presented with relaxation techniques that include lying on mats and using diaphragmatic breathing to relax. The clients are encouraged to note any specific tension in their bodies and to observe any emotions. This experience decreases anxiety and promotes body awareness and attention to feelings.
- The clients are presented with a theme regarding boundaries and are instructed to select one partner to explore the issues of defining and defending boundaries. A towel is given to one member in each pair and told that the towel "belongs" to him or her alone. The partner is instructed to attempt to take the towel away and claim it as his or her own. This experience allows the emotional and kinesthetic (movement) experiences of defending that which belongs exclusively to the individual, whether the towel represents physical, sexual, or internal boundaries. Self-esteem is also increased as clients are presented the opportunity to successfully "take a stand" in their own defense. Also, it allows for an increased awareness of the body and its strength and promotes spontaneity and creative problem solving. The movement/dance therapist and nurse observe and encourage those clients who display passivity, ambivalence, or difficulty maintaining boundaries. They note the various attempts, effective or ineffective, by clients to defend their boundaries. They are prepared to participate if modeling or an additional partner is needed.
- The theme is followed by closure in the form of an open discussion in which clients are encouraged to talk about the experience and problem solve alternative ways to deal with the situation. The movement/dance therapist and nurse share observations honestly, draw quiet or withdrawn clients into the discussion whenever possible, and acknowledge when clients have taken a risk and validate their efforts.

Movement/dance therapists observe clients' movements as they reflect psychologic difficulties. The therapist then presents themes to alter the movements, thereby affecting the emotions and cognition. The flow of the session is established as the movement therapist facilitates a client's spontaneous movements and connects them to the movements of others with such methods as **mirroring** the action, extending it, changing it, or moving in opposition to it. This linking of movements is based on the movement therapist's assessment of the process as it unfolds. There are three parts to this process:

1. The warm-up heightens clients' awareness of their physical and emotional states and increases comfort with movement. The warm-up focuses on introducing group members, increasing their comfort level, and determining the theme or issues to be addressed.
2. The **theme-development** stage explores specific issues or feelings.
3. In **closure,** the experience is processed verbally and nonverbally to promote insight and a sense of completion.

As Marian Chase observed about movement/dance therapy: "Those who have been helped are the ones who know what happened" (Charklin, 1975).

PSYCHODRAMA

Psychodrama was developed in the early 1900s by Jacob L. Moreno, a Romanian psychiatrist, and grew out of the principle that play is therapeutic. In 1934 he founded the Psychodrama Institute in Beacon, New York. Moreno viewed people as "natural role players" and believed that health was promoted from the spontaneous expression of many diverse roles. He observed that when this spontaneity is curtailed, the self cannot emerge and growth and change are not permitted to take place. Through psychodrama, Moreno focused on developing spontaneity, increasing a repertoire for responding to new situations, and resolving repressed emotions from the past (Moreno, 1964).

Psychodrama is the use of "guided dramatic action to examine problems or issues raised by an individual. Using experiential methods, sociometry, role theory, and group dynamics, psychodrama facilitates insight, personal growth, and integration on cognitive, affective, and behavioral levels. It clarifies issues, increases physical and emotional well-being, enhances learning, and develops new skills" (American Society of Group Psychotherapy and Psychodrama, 1998).

Psychodrama uses dramatic techniques to "act out" the emotional problem. The drama includes six operational aspects, which are listed in Box 26-1.

Clients may use this modality to reenact past situations, address present dilemmas, or explore future expectations and fantasies. Addressing these problems in the "here and now" allows for increased awareness of the problems and an opportunity to actively work through them. The primary goal of psychodrama is to provide an experience that allows behavior to become "visible and

CLINICAL APPLICATION
Psychodrama

Eight men and women, ranging from ages 20 to 35, are participating in an outpatient group for unresolved grief. All of the group members have lost a significant family member. A 20-year-old woman is identified during the warm-up as the protagonist. She is a single college student with a DSM-IV, Axis I diagnosis of major depressive disorder. Her grief manifests itself by isolation from friends and family, alternating binge eating and fasting, and uncontrollable crying episodes. These symptoms were precipitated by the untimely death of her older sister, who was killed in a car accident when the client was 17 years of age. The woman describes her grief and her regret that she arrived too late to the hospital to say goodbye to her sister before she died.

Nursing Diagnosis

Grieving, dysfunctional, related to guilt and repressed anger; denial, ineffective; adjustment, impaired; hopelessness; social isolation; social interaction, impaired.

Activity and Objectives

• The protagonist is selected by observing who speaks first in the group or appears most tense or anxious. This client is then invited into the preliminary warm-up discussion.

• During the warm-up, the protagonist is encouraged to choose someone to act as her auxiliary ego (her sister) and other group members to act as doubles (inner thoughts) to help her verbalize her repressed thoughts, feelings, and conflicts. A hospital stage is set, and the other group members position themselves where they can observe unintrusively. The client describes how her sister would have been expected to respond (e.g., nurturing, withdrawn, hostile, responsive). As the protagonist talks about her loss and sets the scene for the enactment, she is addressing denial, obtaining closure, and increasing contact with others.

• The enactment allows the protagonist to have the dialogue with her sister that she was unable to have before her sister died. The client is encouraged to tell her sister anything she wishes, especially those things that have felt unfinished. This is an opportunity for guilt and anger to be resolved and the grieving process to finally be initiated. The nurse is prepared, if asked, to participate in the enactment, either as the auxiliary ego or as a double.

• The closure involves discussion with the protagonist, auxiliary ego, doubles, and group members regarding feelings and thoughts resulting from the enactment. Feedback and observations are also made at this time. This is an opportunity for the therapist and nurse to assess the degree of movement in initiating the grieving process for the protagonist and other group members. The therapist and nurse also use this time to help the group move out of the intense feeling state and reinstate a healthy distance from the experience. They observe if any clients appear anxious or withdrawn or markedly upset and encourage them to process their reactions within the group. These reactions are "normalized" whenever possible by relating them to the stages of grief, using reflective and empathic listening skills.

Box 26-1	Elements of a Psychodrama

The **protagonist,** usually the client, who presents and acts out his or her emotional problems and interpersonal relationships

The **auxiliary ego,** or alter ego, who is chosen from the group by the protagonist to portray significant others in the life of the client

The **director,** or psychodramatist, who facilitates the psychodrama and the client's development of new perceptions, behaviors, and connection with others

Doubles, who operate as the "inner voices" of the protagonist to express repressed thoughts, feelings, and conflicts

The **group,** which provides observation and support and benefits from its own catharsis and identification

The **space,** which can symbolize any environment or time that the protagonist has experienced or imagined

measurable, then reintegrate the behavior into the client's unconscious" (Landy, 1986).

There are three phases of a psychodrama:

1. The warm-up prepares the group by introducing the members to each other and deciding on the protagonist and enactment.
2. The **enactment,** or action portion, is a scene or sequence of scenes that are acted out to portray the problem and explore new methods of resolving it.
3. The sharing promotes discussion among the group members about the enactment, as well as the individual experiences and reactions to the process (Fleshman and Fryrear, 1981).

Psychodrama is a powerful form of therapy. Therefore the techniques must be applied carefully with specific attention given to the level of functioning and ego strengths of the clients in the group. For example, fantasy and emotionally charged expression can be used for high-functioning, nonpsychotic groups, whereas reality-based role-play is best used when working with clients with schizophrenia or even clients with borderline personality disorder.

Summary of Key Concepts

1. Activity therapies, also known as expressive, experimental, or adjunct therapies, include occupational, recreational, art, music, movement/dance, and psychodrama therapies.
2. The primary intention of activity therapies is to increase the client's awareness of feelings, behaviors, perceptions, cognitions, and sensations.
3. Activity therapies are used in a variety of therapeutic settings.
4. It is important for the nurse to become familiar with specific activity therapies to recommend them to the primary physician and to collaborate with activity therapists in providing these therapeutic experiences to clients.
5. Occupational therapy focuses on assessment of task performance, cognitive functioning, psychosocial development, recognizing strengths, improving weaknesses, and adapting to change.
6. The nurse's role in occupational therapy includes daily contact with clients to provide encouragement, support, role modeling, teaching, discussion, and reality testing of prescribed tasks.
7. Recreational therapy incorporates the active process of demonstrating and applying observable skills within the curative elements of play to assist clients

in developing leisure skills and interests that are suitable to their lifestyles.

8. The nurse's role in recreational therapy includes promoting activities and interactions that foster independence, responsibility, and problem-solving skills.
9. Art therapy utilizes art media as a nonverbal means of communication for the purpose of reconciling conflicts and fostering self-awareness.
10. The nurse's role in art therapy includes observing clients' use of the art media, encouraging their verbal responses to the artwork, and noting the specific content of the artwork as it relates to clients' individual issues.
11. Music therapy involves the use of music in a defined structure to bring about specific change and promote self-organization, social connection, and expression.
12. The nurse's role in music therapy includes observing which clients are active or passive during the music experience and noting any verbal and nonverbal feelings expressed by the clients.
13. Movement/dance therapy encourages the expression of emotions to work off tensions, develop improved body image, and achieve body awareness

and social interaction through rhythmic exercises and responses to music.

14. The nurse's role in movement/dance therapy includes participation in the activity, observing and encouraging all clients with honest observations, and promoting discussion when possible.

15. Psychodrama uses spontaneous expression and dramatic techniques to act out emotional problems to promote health through the development of new perceptions, behaviors, and connections with others.

16. The nurse's role in psychodrama includes observing clients' reactions and encouraging clients to relate these reactions to their own issues. It may also involve participation in the psychodrama as an auxiliary ego or a double.

REFERENCES

Boxill EH: *Music therapy for the developmentally disabled*, 1985, Pro-Ed.

Charklin H: *Marion Chase, her papers*, Columbia, Md, 1975, American Dance Therapy Association.

Dictionary of Occupational Titles, ed 4, Washington, DC, 1991.

Dunton WR: *Occupational therapy: a manual for nurses*, 1915.

Fleshman B, Fryrear JL: *The arts in therapy*, Chicago, 1981, Nelson-Hall.

Folsum JC, Hildreth NH, Blair DT: Behavioral interventions in the dementias by a multi-therapist team. In *Memory function and age-related disorders*, New York, 1992, Springer.

Freud S: *Dreams, new introductory lectures on psychoanalysis*, vol xv, London, 1963, Hogath Press.

Gaston E: Factors contributing to responses in music. In *Book of proceedings*, Kansas City, Kansas, 1957, National Association for Music Therapy.

Gaston F: *Music in therapy*, New York, 1968, Macmillan.

Goddaer J, Abraham IL: Effects of relaxing music on agitation during meals among nursing home residents with severe cognitive impairment, *Arch Psychiatr Nurs* 8(3)150, 1994.

Goldenson RM, editor: *Longman dictionary of psychology and psychiatry*, New York, 1984, Longman.

Haun P: *Recreation: a medical viewpoint*, New York, 1965, Teachers College.

Jung CG: *Man and his symbols*, New York, 1998, Doubleday.

Kaplan HI, Sadock BJ: *Comprehensive textbook of psychiatry*, ed 6, Baltimore, 1995, Williams & Wilkins.

Kramer E: *Art as therapy with children*, New York, 1971, Schocken Books.

Landy RJ: *Drama therapy: concepts and practices*, Springfield, Ill, 1986, Charles C. Thomas.

Lepola I, Vanhanen L: The patient's daily activities in acute psychiatric care, *J Psychiatr Ment Health Nurs* 4:29, 1997.

Lowenfield V, Brittain WC: *Creative and mental growth*, ed 5, New York, 1970, Macmillan.

McCaffrey G: The use of leisure activities in a therapeutic community, *J Psychiatr Ment Health Nurs* 5:53, 1998.

Moreno J: *Psychodrama*, vol 1, New York, 1964, Beacon House.

Naumburg M: *Dynamically oriented art therapy: its principles and practice*, New York, 1966, Grune & Stratton.

Rosen F: *Dance in psychotherapy*, New York, 1974, a Dance Horizons Republication.

Sadock BJ: Group psychotherapy, combined psychotherapy and psychodrama. In Kaplan HL, Sadock BJ, editors: *Comprehensive textbook of psychiatry*, ed 6, Baltimore, 1995, Williams & Wilkins.

Ulman E, Dachinger P, editors: *Art therapy in theory and practice*, New York, 1975, Schocken Books.

PROFESSIONAL ASSOCIATIONS

American Art Therapy Association, Baltimore, Md.

American Dance Therapy Association, Columbia, Md.

American Music Therapy Association, Silver Springs, Md.

American Occupational Therapy Association, Bethesda, Md.

American Society of Group Psychotherapy and Psychodrama, Princeton, NJ.

American Therapeutic Recreation Association, Hattiesburg, Miss.

PART•SIX

Contemporary Issues

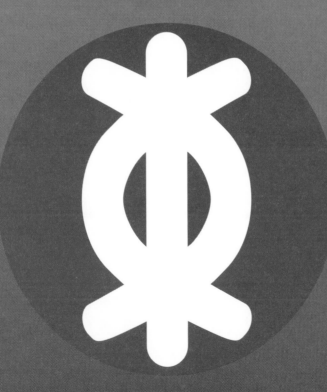

Wawa Aba
Ashanti, West Africa

The seeds of the owawa tree that are represented by this symbol are extremely hard. The symbol infers that hardiness and a sense of purpose can assist individuals to overcome difficult events, situations, and circumstances. The chapters in Part Six discuss significant contemporary issues that can have psychiatric implications.

CHAPTER 27

Survivors of Family Violence

Joan C. Urbancic

OBJECTIVES

- Analyze various theories of family violence for application to nursing practice.

- Discuss conditions that discourage a battered woman from leaving her violent situation.

- Discuss the role of "control" in the etiology of domestic violence.

- Compare the child physical offender with the child sexual offender.

- Describe the common characteristics of victims of family violence.

- Apply the nursing process in the care of victims of family violence.

- Construct examples of how women who are raped are revictimized by society.

FAMILY VIOLENCE

The United States is the most violent of all industrialized nations; this violence is one of the most urgent social problems of contemporary American society. In 1994 the United States Bureau of Census reported an increased rate of 9 murders per 100,000 from the 1985 rate of 7.9 per 100,000. One million residents of the United States die each year as a result of intentional homicide or suicide. The primary cause of death for both black and white male teenagers in the United States is gunshot wounds; suicide is the third leading cause of death among children and adolescents.

Criminal justice experts claim that the family is the birthplace of violence and that interpersonal violence is usually perpetrated by a close friend or family member of the abused. The belief that people are safe in their own homes and that family violence is rare are myths that are difficult to dispel. A woman is much more likely to be beaten, raped, and/or murdered by a partner or ex-partner than by a stranger. Approximately 3 to 4 million women are battered by their partners each year (American Medical Association Council on Scientific Affairs [AMACSA], 1992). Stark and Flitcraft refer to this pattern of violence as **woman battering** (1996). Experts estimate that 10 million children are exposed to marital/woman battering each year (Holden, Geffner, and Jouriles, 1998).

Violence against women affects their family members, as well as society. Research indicates that 28% to 70% of children who are exposed to woman battering are also physically and sexually abused and suffer multiple consequences, both short- and long-term, which include posttraumatic stress, social, cognitive, emotional, and behavioral problems. Rarely do the children receive assis-

Child neglect Harm or threatened harm to a child's health or welfare by a parent, legal guardian, or any other person responsible for the child's health or welfare either through failure to provide adequate food, clothing, shelter, or medical care or by placing the child's health or welfare at unreasonable risk.

Child physical abuse Inflicted injury to a child that can range from minor bruises and lacerations to severe neurologic trauma and death. Psychologic abuse is also included.

Child psychologic abuse Rejection, degradation/devaluation, terrorization, isolation, corruption, exploitation, denying essential stimulation to a child, or unreliable and inconsistent parenting.

Childhood incest Any type of exploitative sexual experience between relatives or surrogate relatives before the victim reaches the age of 18.

Elder abuse Includes psychologic or emotional neglect, psychologic or emotional abuse, violation of personal rights, financial abuse, physical neglect, or direct physical abuse to persons over 65 years of age.

Enmeshed Lacking clear relationship boundaries or role definition; excessively involved.

Machismo
Compulsive masculinity characterized by a male's excessive need to control and dominate his wife at all costs.

Rape The act of physically forcing sexual intercourse.

Social learning theory Bandura's theory that aggression is not instinctual but a learned behavior.

Transgenerational violence
When violence within the family is an accepted, everyday occurrence and a natural, normal component of family living.

Woman battering Physical and/or mental abuse of women by their intimate partners or those with whom they have been intimate.

tance or support to deal with their trauma (Edelson and Eisikovits, 1996; Graham-Bermann and Levendosky, 1998; Holden, Geffner, and Jouriles, 1998).

Battered women also report that their male partners often harm or even kill the family pets. Children may model the batterer by abusing pets as well. Many experts view the exposure of children to the torture and/or killing of a family pet as a form of psychologic abuse. Because shelters for battered women do not typically accept pets, some women hesitate to leave because of concern for their pets (Ascione, 1998).

All family members are at much greater risk of being abused by another family member than they are by a stranger. Family violence is known to occur in multiple generations in the same family, which is termed **transgenerational violence.** "In 1997 over 3 million (3,195,000) children were reported for child abuse and neglect to child protective service agencies in the United States" (Wang and Daro, 1998). Children are much more likely to be sexually abused by a family member than someone who is unknown to them. Abuse occurs in all age groups. Each year 2 million older persons are typically abused by their own children or spouses (Wolf, 1995).

Family violence is multicausal and highly complex. Usually it is insidious in onset and occurs in tandem with a variety of interrelated factors. Despite the many contributing factors, it is the sociocultural attitudes toward women, children, and older persons and the value placed on violence to solve problems that underlie and support family violence. Significantly, societal attitudes toward family violence seem to be changing. Society is beginning to recognize family violence as a social issue and social problem rather than as a private family problem (Gelles, 1997).

Nevertheless, because of beliefs about the privacy and sanctity of the family, violence within the family generally remains hidden. Often, nurses, doctors, and other health care professionals maintain the dark secret of family violence by their conspiracy of silence despite the heavy media attention given to family violence in recent years and efforts to educate health care professionals.

The most dramatic examples of failure by health care professionals to address family violence are reflected in studies that examine battered women's experiences when seeking health care services. In general, these studies (AMACSA, 1992; Stark and Flitcraft, 1996; Warshaw, 1989) report a lack of assessment, intervention, and responsiveness by doctors and nurses in the treatment of battered women.

The Joint Commission on Accreditation on Healthcare Organizations (JCAHO) has mandated policies and procedures for the assessment, treatment, and referral of victims of violence. After the JCAHO mandate, in 1992 the American Medical Association took steps to recognize and intervene in domestic violence by developing guidelines for practice. The result is a developing awareness that the growing problem of family violence must be addressed on multiple levels. Because nurses interact with families and individuals in a wide variety of settings, they are frequently the first to identify and therapeutically intervene with those experiencing family violence. A question remains as to why nurses often do not intervene therapeutically in family violence. Some explanations include lack of knowledge, stereotypes, prejudices, and poor role models as factors. According to a study by Limandri and Tilden (1996), nurses often feel frustrated because of the ineffectiveness of the system of protective services. King and Ryan (1989) find that 18% of nurses in their study report being victims of physical and emotional abuse, and another 28% report abuse among family members. Certainly, nurses are not exempt from violence in their own lives; to confront violence in the lives of others may be too painful a reminder of what is or has occurred in their own lives. It may be less painful to deny the existence of family violence than to confront it.

This chapter discusses the various types of family violence: woman battering, child physical and sexual abuse, and elder abuse. Although it is recognized that domestic violence may at times be mutual, it is the woman who is typically injured. More important, repeated studies indicate that women usually do not initiate the violence, and when they are violent toward their partners, it is usually in self-defense (Gelles, 1997; Kurz, 1993; Stark and Flitcraft, 1996). Because of their lack of power and authority in many families, women are much more vulnerable to battering and abuse. The authors cited above claim that the type of violent abuse that is repetitive, extensive, and escalates over time, with minimal or no provocation, and is characterized by coercive control is limited to male abuse of females.

Reports are now available on violence in gay and lesbian relationships. These researchers claim that the incidence of violence among gays and lesbians is comparable with that of heterosexuals, if not higher (Bourg and Stock, 1994; Gelles, 1997; Renzetti, 1992).

DEFINITIONS OF VIOLENCE AND ABUSE

A major problem in the field of family violence has been the difficulty of developing useful and clear definitions of violence and abuse. Some researchers define violence on the basis of physical injury only, whereas others insist that mental injury must also be included in the definition. Often, severe psychologic abuse can occur without visible physical symptoms. Therefore it is critical to use a broad, holistic approach in the assessment of family violence.

Disagreement exists on whether spanking constitutes violent and abusive behavior. Because many parents use spanking at least occasionally, there is major resistance to include spanking as violent and abusive behavior. Gelles and Cornell (1990) suggest making a distinction between so-called "normal" acts of force such as spanking versus harmful acts of violence. However, the question is: What is harmful? Such determinations may be significantly different from one cultural group to another.

THEORIES OF FAMILY VIOLENCE

The following discussion will focus on a number of models that attempt to explain family violence (Box 27-1). Although some models have greater explanatory power than do others, no single model is able to fully explain the phenomenon of family violence. Various statistics on family violence are listed in Box 27-2.

THE PSYCHIATRIC MENTAL ILLNESS MODEL

This model focuses on the individual characteristics of the abuser or survivor to explain the phenomenon at hand. In the past, a person who severely injured a child was considered to be psychotic or mentally disturbed; however, when the victim was a woman, she (rather than the abuser) was the focus of attention and was judged to be mentally defective (masochistic) for remaining with the

Box 27-1   **Etiologic Theories Related to Family Violence**

Psychiatric/mental illness model
Social learning theory
   Aggression as a learned behavior, not instinctual
   Family role modeling
   Desensitization to violence through repeated exposure
     via the media
Sociologic theory
   Unemployment
   Poverty
   Crime
   Teenage pregnancy
   Isolation
Anthropologic theory
   Sexual inequalities
   Social organization
   Cultural patterning
Feminist theory
   Explanatory utility of constructs of gender and power
   Analysis of the family as a historically situated institution
   Importance of understanding and validating women's experiences
   Employing scholarship for women

abuser. Only recently has the spotlight turned to examining the characteristics of the abuser instead of placing blame on the victim. Some psychiatrists continue to maintain that battered women are masochistic and choose to remain in an abusive relationship to satisfy their unconscious need for punishment. Within the psychiatric model, the causative factors in family violence are defects in the abuser such as mental illness, alcohol and drug abuse, and personality disorders. Interventions focus on changing the mental disorder or personality characteristics of the abuser. External factors are not the focus of this model. The psychiatric model is very popular and is commonly used because it is comforting for society to believe that it is the "abnormal or deranged" person who abuses others or chooses to remain in an abusive relationship (Gelles and Cornell, 1990). Because most people do not consider themselves mentally ill, they neither question their potential for abuse nor do they examine their behavior if they are abusive.

Abusers and the abused are not significantly different from the rest of the population in terms of mental disorders (Ammerman and Hersen, 1992; Campbell and Humphreys, 1993; Gelles and Cornell, 1990). In addition, no evidence supports the theory that women remain in abusive relationships because they are masochistic (Gelles, 1997; Walker, 1994). Pagelow (1993) maintains that although some batterers have been found to exhibit men-

---

Box 27-2   Epidemiology for Violence

Battered Women

1.8 million wives in the United States are abused every year by their husbands.
25% to 50% of all women are abused by their intimate partners at least once.
20% to 25% of women who seek treatment in emergency rooms are there because of battering injuries.
2% to 8% of these women identified abuse as the cause of their injuries.
7% to 17% of pregnant women experience physical abuse by their partners.

Physically Abused Children

2 million children are seriously abused each year by their parents and caregivers.
Of these, 1000 die from results of these injuries.
25% of the 2 million abused children are physically abused; 20% are sexually abused; 55% are neglected.
25% of the 2 million abused children are under age 5; 60% are between ages 5 and 14.
Children under age 3 are at a greater risk for fatal abuse than are older children.

Abused and neglected children are at greater risk for later delinquency, adult criminality, and violent crimes than are nonabused or nonneglected children.

Sexually Abused Children

50% of psychiatric clients have histories of physical and sexual abuse.
The average age at which child incest begins is age 6, with an average duration of 7 years.

Rape

Only one in 10% to 20% of rapes are reported to the police.
Over 90% of rape victims are women.
20% of female college students are raped at some time during their college education.
The most common age group for rape victims is 16 to 25 years.
In 84% of rape cases, the victim is acquainted with the perpetrator.
Only 5% of rapists were psychotic when they raped their victims.
In 90% of rape cases, victims and perpetrators are of the same race.

tal disturbances, the majority are not mentally disordered. Stronger evidence seems to exist for psychopathology in sexual abusers. Some studies find that some sexual abusers exhibit more antisocial behaviors and personality disorders than do nonabusers (Chaffin, 1994; Quinsey, Rice, and Harris, 1995; Quinsey and Walker, 1992). Clearly, more research on abuser psychopathology is needed.

SOCIAL LEARNING THEORY

Psychologist Albert Bandura's **social learning theory** model (1973) is based on research on aggression. This model combines components of behavioral and sociologic theories. Contrary to earlier writings by a variety of people, Bandura's model of social learning theory states that aggression is a learned behavior rather than instinctual. Although Bandura recognizes that neurophysiology can produce aggressive behavior, he maintains that the biologic mechanisms depend on appropriate stimulation for activation and that even when activated, aggressive behavior is still under cognitive control.

Bandura's research demonstrates that children learn how to behave by observing the role models in their own families. Values, attitudes, and behaviors are shaped and developed by significant others in a child's life. The way parents cope with stress, anger, and frustration becomes a powerful lesson for the impressionable, unlearned child.

Because family role models are usually the ones to which children are exposed, children assume that family behavior is normal and acceptable even though it may be highly violent and abusive. Physical discipline by parents gives children the message that punishment is necessary to enforce rules and gain compliance. In this sense, the use of violence or physical force is reinforced because of the power derived from its use. In addition to role modeling in the family, children learn aggressive behavior through direct experience, practice, and observation of other mediums of violence.

Support for the social learning theory is seen in repeated generational patterns of family violence. Although exposure to family violence does not guarantee that the pattern of violence will be repeated in subsequent generations, it does increase the child's risk of using violent behavior in adulthood.

Much has been written about the influence of television, films, music, and other media to promote violence. Campbell and Humphreys (1993) describe multiple studies that support the contention that violence in the media (1) encourages aggressive behavior through modeling, (2) disinhibits aggressive acting-out behaviors by repeated exposure, and (3) desensitizes people to violence around them. The desensitization to violence results in people becoming apathetic or unimpressed with the impact of violence on others. Research studies also suggest that repeated exposure to media violence increases feelings of insecurity, distrust, and suspicion of others. In classic studies, Bandura (1973), and other researchers who replicated

his work, acknowledged that the vast majority of people do not act out the violence that they observe in the media; however, for the majority of people who are heavy television viewers of violence, their perception of the world is that of a dangerous, unsafe place. Believing that the world is unsafe may predispose some people to misinterpret social cues and respond as though they are under attack when they are not.

SOCIOLOGIC THEORY

Sociologic models recognize the influence of neurophysiologic and psychologic factors, but their focus is on environmental and socioeconomic forces that underlie violence. Like social learning theory, sociologists reject the notion that aggression is instinctual. According to these theories, conditions such as unemployment, crime, poverty, isolation, teenage pregnancy, and stress are of major concern in addressing violence in families. Many sociologists view violence in families as gender neutral, that is, both sexes play out a role in the problem. This stance is criticized by feminists because it minimizes the impact of male domination and power.

A wide variety of sociologic theories abounds. Gelles and Cornell (1990) maintain that violence occurs in families because it "can" occur. The challenge is to provide social controls by increasing the cost of violence (e.g., imprisonment, fines, loss of status in the community, loss of family) and decreasing the rewards (e.g., power and control over family members).

ANTHROPOLOGIC THEORY

Cultural attitudes and definitions of abuse and violence vary significantly from one society to another. Some societies may view particular behaviors by its members as violent, whereas other societies may not. This lack of agreement on the perception of violence and abuse makes it difficult to establish a universal definition of family violence that will be culturally acceptable to various societies.

FEMINIST THEORY

Multiple studies report that batterers are characterized by patriarchal attitudes that include an excessive need to control and dominate their wives. Feminist researchers claim that these patriarchal values are the underlying basis for violence against women (Avni, 1991; Campbell and Humphreys, 1993; Stark and Flitcraft, 1996).

Campbell and Fishwick (1993) use the concept of machismo, or compulsive masculinity, to explain wife abuse and violence against women. Although machismo is not the direct cause of family violence and wife abuse, it is helpful in understanding some of the complex factors that contribute to violence. According to these two researchers, violence is a central component of male social standing in Western culture. Male heroes are "Rambo" and "James Bond" types who are able to achieve success, admiration, and acceptance through machismo. Their relationships with women are characterized by disdain, control, dominance, and treatment of women as commodities and sexual objects. Typically the male with strong needs to dominate and control believes it is his right and responsibility to control and beat his wife and children because they are his property to do with as he pleases. Campbell and Fishwick (1993) define **machismo** as "male attitudes and behavior arising from and supported by the patriarchal social structure that express sexism and male ownership of women, glorify violence, emphasize virility, and despise gentleness and the expression of any emotions except anger and rage."

Barbee (1992) describes how men use culture, custom, and tradition as excuses for the continuation of violence against women. In particular, she describes the combined impact of racism, sexism, and patriarchy on the black woman. The patriarchal cultural argument seems to be that if beating your wife has been the tradition in a particular cultural group, then the male is not responsible, because he is merely carrying on traditions of his cultural group.

Feminists strongly believe that woman abuse must not be subsumed under terms such as family violence or spouse abuse because such language obscures the reality that in the great majority of domestic violence cases, it is the woman who is battered. With generic terms, the issues of power and control are not given the focus they need to fully understand the dynamics of woman battering (Bograd, 1988).

THE BATTERED WOMAN

Battering is the most common cause of injury to women in the United States. Although some women escape from their abusive partners, many remain in a violent relationship that gradually escalates in frequency and severity.

Sampselle (1992) cautions nurses to be aware that one out of every 10 women in any health care setting is abused by her male intimate partner. Emergency department presentation of domestic violence is even higher. In one study that examines emergency room (ER) records retrospectively, only 2.8% of the women who were treated in the ER were identified by physicians as abused on their medical records, even though 25% were actually there because of battering injuries (Stark and Flitcraft, 1996).

Among pregnant women, 7% to 21% experience physical abuse by their partners. Effects of physical abuse on the pregnant woman are usually direct or indirect. Direct effects include low birth weight, preterm labor, preterm infants, and infant injury and death (Stark and Flitcraft, 1996). These researchers report that indirect effects of physical abuse have a more profound effect on womens' health than do direct effects. Indirect effects include chronic pain, depression, high anxiety, use of drugs and alcohol, or suicide attempts by these women to escape their violent situations.

A number of studies have been done on battered women and their experiences with the health care system (Brendtro and Bowker, 1989; Kurz, 1993; Stark and Flitcraft, 1996) that document (1) the failure of doctors and nurses to make direct inquiries as to how the women received their injuries, even when women wanted to provide this information; (2) subtle blaming and pejorative labeling of the women; and (3) unnecessary or inappropriate dispensing of medication such as tranquilizers. In an extensive survey of battered women who had sought support from various health care and helping professions, Brendtro and Bowker (1989) report that "battered wives find health care services to be less effective than any other formal source of help, including the clergy, lawyers, police, district attorneys, social services and counseling agencies, women's groups and battered women's shelters."

DEFINITION OF THE BATTERED WOMAN

The term *battered woman* is used in this chapter to mean a woman who is battered by her intimate partner, including a lesbian partner. A woman is in greatest danger when she attempts to leave the controlling mate. Although it is recognized that violence exists between homosexual couples, this discussion is focused on the most common type of domestic violence, that of the male abuser and the abused female.

When describing the battered woman, violence is not limited to physical abuse. One survivor lived under the constant threat of a loaded gun frequently pressed to her temple by her abuser, but she never received a bruise on her body. Such psychologic abuse is devastating. Other battered women report that over time the physical abuse actually ends but profound psychologic abuse continues. This happens because the threat of violence is so terrorizing to the woman that this threat alone becomes the controlling force. For this reason, advocates for battered women define *domestic violence* as physical, psychologic,

---

Box 27-3   Behaviors of the Abuser

Economic abuse—strict control of money (even when the woman earns it), food, clothing, transportation, and other resources.

Sexual abuse—includes marital rape and forcing the woman to participate in sexual activities against her will.

Threats and intimidation, including threats of taking the children from the woman or hurting them or other family members.

Threatening to injure or kill family pets.

Isolating the woman from any support system, including her family, friends, and health care professionals.

Constantly demeaning and insulting the woman.

Intentionally breaking material objects to terrorize the woman.

and sexual abuse that is primarily directed at women by men for the purpose of maintaining power and control over the women (Box 27-3).

Battered women represent all ethnic, religious, and socioeconomic groups. However, middle and upper socioeconomic women can more easily hide their abuse. Material resources allow middle class and upperclass women to be seen by a private physician who is more likely to keep their secret and frequently ask no questions. Other resources that may be available are extended family members who may agree to provide temporary shelter, summer homes where women may retreat, or the financial assets to leave their battering spouses and go to a hotel for a few days. Women without financial resources often have extended families who are already overburdened and unable to help them. They may not have the finances that allow them to stay in a hotel for a few days. Consequently, most women who are seen in shelters for battered women are those without other options (Figure 27-1).

THE BATTERER

Too often the batterers are portrayed as males who have temporarily lost control, usually under provocation. This loss of control is frequently blamed on alcohol or drugs. Actually, batterers abuse their partner whether batterers are drunk or sober; however, they typically use drunkeness as an excuse. Despite numerous studies on the characteristics of batterers, no evidence supports the belief that the typical batterer is an alcoholic or mentally ill. Usually batterers are described by fellow workers as average, normal males who give no hint of the abusive behavior they demonstrate in the privacy of their own homes. Few batterers have criminal records or have physical altercations with others outside of their homes. Such physical abuse against a stranger would result in arrest and incarceration, but the privacy of their homes protects batterers and continues to do so as society turns a blind eye. Batterers learn that there are few if any consequences to their abusive behaviors. The privacy and secrecy in which abuse toward women occurs are the main reasons that abuse is perpetuated.

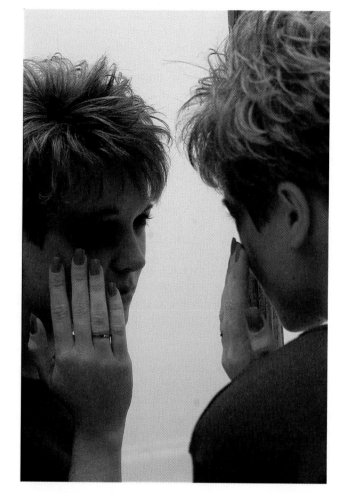

Figure 27-1   Physical abuse is the most common cause of injury to women in the United States. Battering occurs in all ethnic, religious, and socioeconomic groups. Although the batterer is unprovoked, the woman is made to feel it is her fault. (Copyright Cathy Lander-Goldberg, Lander Photographics.)

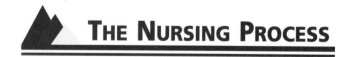

THE NURSING PROCESS

ASSESSMENT

Assessment of the battered woman begins with the nurse critically examining her own beliefs and biases about battered women. For example, if the nurse believes that the woman has brought the problem on herself for not leaving the abusive relationship, then this attitude, consciously or unconsciously, will most likely be communicated to the battered woman. The nurse's attitude and resulting interactions may revictimize the woman.

Because holistic assessments are the foundation of the nursing process, culture is an important consideration in that assessment. Culture often defines how the battered woman will interpret and respond to the violence that has been perpetrated against her. Understanding the battered woman's culture is also critical for developing a treatment plan for her.

Culture is also an important determinant of whether the battered woman seeks assistance from community resources such as the police and shelters. Some ethnic women are very isolated and unaware of community resources for abuse, are suspicious of caregivers outside of their own cultural group, and fear being ostracized by their cultural group if they reach out to the broader community. Most battered women's shelters make a concerted effort to reach out to women of all colors and ethnic groups. When caring for a client from a minority culture, it is the nurse's responsibility to learn about the client's culture to provide culturally sensitive care. Questions about the woman's culture are appropriate but must be presented in a sensitive, respectful manner so that the woman understands that the nurse is concerned and is intent on learning more about the woman's values and customs to provide effective holistic nursing care.

An understanding of culture is as important when working with the male batterer as it is when working with the battered woman. Before treatment strategies can be planned for the abuser, his cultural attitudes, values, and beliefs must be acknowledged and respected. No cultural beliefs and traditions, however, can be accepted or tolerated at the expense of another person's health and well-being. Barbee (1992) suggests that the defense of abusive behaviors as being culture bound serves to maintain the status quo of patriarchy.

Because physical abuse (that includes **rape**) of women by the partners is common, it is critical to ask about physical, sexual, and emotional abuse in the histories of all women. The nurse must also ask if the abuser hits the children. Protective services must be notified if the children have been abused.

A complete physical examination must be given to any woman who is suspected of being battered. This includes a neurologic examination and x-rays if necessary to determine the existence of previous injuries. Because battering during pregnancy (Bohn and Parker, 1993) is one of the major causes of complications during pregnancy, nurses need to assess for it. Even older widows may have serious unresolved issues relating to abusive relationships with their deceased husbands. Many battered women report a myriad of physical problems without disclosing the source of violence. Because they have been programmed to believe that somehow they provoked the violence, they feel guilty and ashamed. Nevertheless, if asked directly and under appropriate conditions, most women will disclose the nature of their injuries. These conditions include being respectful and sensitive to the woman's disclosures and informing her that she is not at fault and that no human being has the right to abuse another. In addition, the nurse must provide a safe environment that is conducive to disclosure. The first step is to separate the woman from her abuser. On many occasions it will be obvious that the woman's partner is determined not to be separated from her. Nevertheless, separation must occur, even if it means calling security for assistance.

During assessment and when taking the woman's history, it is recommended that the nurse begin with the least sensitive questions and gradually progress to the more sensitive ones. Questions should be simple and direct and reflect the language and terms that the woman herself uses. The Nursing Research Consortium on Violence and Abuse has developed a simple four-item questionnaire, which was adapted by Campbell and Humphreys (1993) for taking general case history (Box 27-4).

When women do present with current physical trauma, a delay in seeking treatment and/or an illogical explanation for the injury are cues that may indicate abuse. Often, abused women seek treatment for indirect effects of their violent relationships. Complaints may reflect the stress of these violent relationships and/or residual pain from past injuries. Often, the woman appears depressed, anxious, and fatigued. The battered woman typically has more chronic, pain-related, vague complaints than her nonbattered counterpart. Health history may indicate frequent accidents and other traumatic injuries such as lacerations, bruises, and fractures. Spontaneous abortions, suicide attempts, and substance abuse also may be reported.

Other potential indicators of abuse may be identified in the family history. Potential indicators that relate to the woman's partner include the following:

Very strict disciplinarian
Believes in physical punishment
Abuses children
Abuses alcohol and drugs
Extremely possessive and jealous
History of violence in his family of origin
Unemployed
Seeks to isolate family members

Box 27-5 presents the most important physical examination indicators of wife/woman abuse.

The nurse must accurately document all statements the woman makes. Open-ended questions that reflect what the woman is disclosing should be used so that she feels in charge of the interview. Documented information must include the name of the abuser and when and how

---

Box 27-4   **General Case History Questions for the Abused**

1. Have you ever been emotionally or physically abused by your partner or someone important to you?
2. Within the last year, have you been hit, slapped, kicked, or otherwise physically hurt by someone? If yes, by whom and how many times?
3. Within the last year, has anyone forced you to have sexual activities? If yes, who and how many times?
4. Are you afraid of your partner or anyone else listed above?

Off, Pause

Box 27-5   Physical Indicators of Possible Wife/Woman Abuse

General Appearance

Anxious and frightened, depressed and passive, ashamed and embarrassed, poor eye contact, weight problems, looks to partner for answers, partner does all of the talking, partner exhibits smothering and extremely possessive behavior

Skin

Contusions; abrasions and minor lacerations; scars; burns, particularly on breasts, arms, abdomen, chest, neck, face, and genitals

Musculoskeletal

Fractures and sprains, especially of distal versus proximal bones (e.g., skull, facial bones, extremities), dislocated shoulder, and evidence of old fractures

Genital/Rectal

Evidence of vaginal/anal rape such as bruising, edema, and bleeding; also evidence of direct kicks or punches

Abdominal

Internal bleeding or other injuries; chronic pelvic pain

Neurologic

Acute stress disorder, hyperactive reflexes, chronic headaches and backaches, paresthesias from old injuries

---

the abuse occurred. When possible, the nurse should record the exact words of the woman because such documentation is very powerful legally. The nurse must also ask if the abuser hits the children. Protective services must be notified if the children have been abused.

A complete physical examination must be performed on any woman who is suspected of being battered. This includes a neurologic examination and x-rays, if necessary, to determine the existence of previous injuries. A detailed description of the woman's injuries must be documented in the narrative, and a body chart diagram should be used to indicate the location and type of injury. The nurse should ask the woman if she was forced into sexual acts against her will and then examine her for anal and vaginal tears. If there is a possibility of marital rape, the nurse should follow the rape protocol and use the evidence collection kit. The nurse should also assess the woman for sexually transmitted diseases (STDs) and document all laboratory and x-ray results. The American Medical Association Guidelines on Treatment of Domestic Violence (Flitcraft, 1992) assert that at least two photographs should be taken of each trauma area. The woman must sign a consent form first. The nurse should place one set of photographs in the woman's record with identifying data on the back that includes the date, woman's name, hospital number, and the name of photographer. Because of the possibility of future legal proceedings, the nurse should re-

---

Survivors of Violence

Survivors of trauma may be of any age, gender, or nationality. They share a bond in that their ability to enjoy fully functional lives has been altered by a disruptive event, be it experiencing molestation as a child, rape as an adult, or armed conflict in war. The event may involve family members or strangers and be life threatening or totally demeaning. The responses of family, friends, or society may be problematic.

The nurse in the community setting, who works with such a disparate group of clients, must be extremely flexible and accepting. As in other emotional disturbances, the presence of a strong supportive network is critical. Debriefing a traumatic incident requires a team effort in which the nurse may play a role as the individual counselor, hearing every detail, or the group facilitator, helping the victims begin to repattern their lives and social interactions. The relationship will be more ongoing than a crisis intervention in the controlled hospital environment.

Assessing the truth in such a situation is often difficult because a molester, rapist, or batterer is usually involved, who may still be threatening to the survivor and perhaps to anyone assisting. Nurses may feel angry at or fearful of the perpetrator and must carefully monitor personal reactions to the situation. Other professions, including child protective services (CPS) or the police, may become involved, and communication channels must be clear and overt. There is no margin for error when dealing with such a potentially volatile

situation as a parent molesting a child or a husband battering his wife.

Survivors of combat are often diagnosed with posttraumatic stress disorder (PTSD). These persons often lead lives that are estranged from mainstream society and complicated by drug/alcohol abuse. They may respond to questions with anger toward any type of proffered help and require prolonged, specialized counseling before they are willing to participate in group therapy. The community psychiatric mental health nurse may encounter these persons in homeless shelters or living on the street. The nurse must be able to tolerate frequent rebuffs before any sort of therapeutic relationship is established. Patience and a sense of humor in a tension-filled situation may often be the keys to effective interaction.

The nurse working in the community may encounter victims with a strong sense of entitlement, who will emphasize their victimization to get special treatment. These individuals will quickly exhaust even the most patient mental health professional. The nurse must know the system of entitlements well and must circumscribe the client's expectations. Such clients must be offered what is available and told that no more will be forthcoming, despite their distress or anger. Such a situation often requires a concerted effort from other mental health disciplines, so that one person does not have to bear the brunt of the clients' irritation.

quest a safe address from the woman where the second set of photographs can be mailed.

It is crucial to reassure the woman that the documentation is confidential and that her partner will not be allowed access to it without her permission (unless it goes to court; then the documentation becomes public record). Retaliation by the batterer is always a major concern for the abused woman. However, the woman should understand that she has the right to access her records and that they will be valuable to her in child custody cases or if she chooses to file charges against the abuser.

Campbell and Fishwick (1993) caution against the use of such terms as *abuse* and *battering* because many abused women do not have this image of themselves. Direct questions are more helpful, such as "Did someone hit you?" It is also important to understand that the woman may love her partner and desperately wants to believe him when he promises that it will never happen again.

It is imperative to assess the woman's potential danger in cases of domestic violence. Information about the pattern of abuse and if it has increased in severity and frequency is vital. Other critical signs that indicate increased danger are that the abuser has a weapon, has been violent outside the house, is a substance abuser, has been stalking the woman, and has threatened suicide/homicide. At times the woman may contemplate suicide. It is well documented that the battered woman is at greatest risk of harm when she tries to leave her abuser (Campbell and Humphreys, 1993; Gelles, 1997). Therefore the woman must become aware of this risk, and the nurse must assist her to develop a safety plan. Such a plan typically involves providing the woman with phone numbers of nearby shelters, crisis lines, and community resources. The woman should also be referred to the local crime victims compensation board.

NURSING DIAGNOSIS

The following nursing diagnoses are examples of those that are relevant to the case study on Nina. They are based on information identified in the case study. However, all nursing diagnoses are formulated from information obtained during the assessment phase of the nursing process. The accuracy of the diagnoses depends on a careful, in-depth assessment. Based on the information that was provided, can you identify additional nursing diagnoses?

CASE STUDY

Nina was brought to the emergency room by her husband to whom she has been married for 10 years. Her husband was very attentive to her, spoke reassuringly, and appeared very concerned about Nina's condition. According to her husband, a day ago Nina slipped as she was getting out of the bathtub. When she slipped, she bumped her head on the faucet and then fell on her arm. As her husband spoke, Nina sat quietly with her head down. She cradled her right arm and appeared to be in severe pain. Her right eye was red and swollen shut, and she seemed to have some difficulty breathing. Despite protests from her husband, the nurse interviewed Nina separately from her husband in a private consultation room. Although the nurse inquired directly whether Nina's husband had beaten her, Nina denied the abuse. A complete physical and neurologic examination was performed by the physician and a series of x-rays were taken. When Nina returned from the radiology department, she was told by the physician that she had fractures of the wrist, facial bones, and several ribs. Nina was also informed that the x-rays indicated multiple old, healed fractures of the ribs and pelvic girdle. The nurse spent time explaining to Nina how unlikely it was for her injuries to result from a fall in the bathtub. The nurse also reassured Nina that nothing she could have done would deserve such abuse by another person. Nina finally acknowledged that her husband had abused her but insisted she had no intention of leaving him because he was a good husband. According to Nina, the only time her husband is abusive is when she fails to fulfill her domestic responsibilities and therefore provokes him into losing his temper and beating her. Nina has no children and no family nearby, except for a younger sister who is currently overwhelmed with her own family problems. Nina is psychologically and economically dependent on her husband and has no means of financial or psychologic support.

Critical Thinking—Assessment
1. What is the first priority for the nurse who suspects abuse when assessing a woman?
2. How should the nurse respond to the shame, guilt, and self-blame of the battered woman.
3. What should a nurse do if he or she becomes angry and rejecting with a battered woman who is in denial about being battered?
4. If you suspected that your neighbor was in an abusive situation, what signs would you look for in the relationship?

NURSING ASSESSMENT QUESTIONS

For the Battered Woman

1. We often see women who have been hurt by their partners. Is your partner responsible for your injuries?
2. Has your partner ever hurt you?
3. Have you noticed any pattern to this behavior such as an increase in frequency and severity?
4. Does he threaten to use or has he ever used a weapon to hurt you?

Pain related to injuries sustained by battering as evidenced by difficulty breathing deeply and sleeping (multiple fractures)

Injury, risk for, related to present and past abuse by husband

Anxiety and fear related to threat of further battering

Family coping, ineffective, related to abuse by husband and denial by wife

DSM DIAGNOSES

The DSM-IV has not assigned a diagnosis for the battered woman. Stark and Flitcraft (1996) recommend the DSM-IV designation of "physical abuse of adult" because although it is a psychiatric diagnosis, it is nonstigmatizing and will allow the woman access to resources. Some researchers and clinicians maintain that posttraumatic stress disorder is an appropriate diagnosis for many battered women who are repeatedly and severely abused (Briere, 1996; van der Kolk, McFarlane, and Weisaeth, 1996). The battered-woman syndrome is a description of what happens over time to the battered woman. This syndrome, as described by Walker (1994), has been allowed in courtrooms in all states as a defense in cases in which battered women have murdered their abusers.

OUTCOME IDENTIFICATION

The following outcome criteria are derived from the nursing diagnoses identified in the case study on Nina. These outcomes are the expected behaviors that Nina will demonstrate as a result of her plan of care. Stabilizing Nina's physical condition and securing her safety are the immediate short-term goals.

Client will:

1. Report a decrease in her pain resulting from injuries sustained during her abuse.
2. Demonstrate no difficulty breathing and verbalize feeling more relaxed.
3. Demonstrate less fear and anxiety by being able to discuss her abuse and explore possible options for resolving it with the nurse.
4. Verbalize an awareness of her increasingly dangerous situation because her abuse has intensified over time.
5. Discuss with the nurse the implications for herself, her spouse, and other family members if she remains in the present abusive situation and explore alternative means of family coping.
6. Demonstrate an awareness of the need for safety by taking steps to protect herself in the future.
7. Explore the possibility of pursuing litigation against her husband and requesting a restraining order if her husband is not jailed.
8. Devise plans to secure her safety in case of future threats of abuse.

9. Take advantage of community resources that increase her self-esteem and independence and become involved with an outreach group for battered women.

PLANNING

The plan of care for any survivor of violence should focus on addressing critical physical problems, securing the immediate safety of the victim, examining the implications of the abuse on the woman and other family members, and discussing future plans for safety. In the case of a battered woman such as Nina who acknowledges the abuse only when confronted by the nurse, all possible options must be explored because she may need to use them in the future. The nurse should develop the care plan with the client and recognize that any effort to impose personal beliefs on the battered woman is fated for failure. Instead, the battered woman needs reassurance that she is capable of making appropriate decisions for herself—even if her decision is to return to her abuser. It is only through empowerment, not threats and intimidation, that the woman is most likely to develop the strength to make growth-producing decisions independently.

IMPLEMENTATION

Once the battered woman's physical condition has been stabilized, it is critical to assess her future safety and collaboratively explore her fears, anxieties, and concerns. Despite the need to leave the abusive situation, the woman may strongly believe that she has no other option except to return. If the woman chooses to return to the batterer, it is important to respect this decision. Making a decision to leave the batterer is usually a gradual process. However, it is critical that the woman realize that she has options. The nurse may serve as the key factor in a beginning awareness that other options do exist.

At present, all states have laws that provide some level of protection for survivors of domestic violence, and there is a definite trend across the country to pass further legislation to ensure this protection. However, the reality is that there is a large gap between the actual laws and their implementation by the police and criminal justice system. In some localities police are mandated to arrest the abuser if there is evidence of probable violence. In many states the police must provide the battered woman with information on local shelters, domestic violence crisis lines, and her legal rights. However, the police may not always respond appropriately, so it is important that the nurse be able to inform the battered woman of her legal rights.

In recent years, some women's rights advocates and criminal justice experts have been debating mandatory reporting laws on domestic violence (Reel, 1997). Women's rights advocates claim that mandatory domestic violence reporting laws discourage battered women from seeking treatment for their injuries because the women fear that their situation will be reported to the police. Because some women will not be ready to deal with the police, being forced to do so could be nontherapeutic and disempowering and even increase their danger of abuse. If no mandatory reporting laws exist, then the police should not be notified unless the woman consents (Gelles, 1997; McFarlane and Parker, 1994). Although some professionals choose to maintain confidentiality if the battered woman requests it, the deciding factor on reporting is the degree of danger that the woman faces.

NURSING INTERVENTIONS

Primary prevention for woman abuse begins with identifying families at risk and changing societal views toward wife abuse. Nurses must become politically active to promote social, economic, and psychologic independence for all women. Societal acceptance of violence against women as portrayed in films, television, magazines, and music must not be tolerated. Nurses must become more knowledgeable about factors such as poverty, drugs, gun control, and unemployment, which increase the risk of domestic violence, and must work with other members of the community to establish public policy and programs to address these issues.

Secondary prevention of woman battering involves early case finding and decisive intervention. Specific nursing interventions will depend on the stage that the battered woman is in, because a woman in denial about the abuse will require a different strategy than one who is determined not to return to the relationship. In relationships where the abuse is just beginning and is mild, it may be possible to work with the marital dyad when both partners choose to do so. In these cases, the male accepts all responsibility for the abuse and the counseling focuses on preventing any further abuse. In many situations the advanced practice nurse will be the appropriate professional to work with the battered woman.

Tertiary prevention is required when the woman has been repeatedly abused, as with Nina. In such cases the focus is on assisting the abused woman to overcome the physical and psychologic effects of the abuse and to prevent future abuse. Because the abuser frequently threatens and harasses the woman when she attempts to leave, it may be very difficult for her to follow through. Frequently, these women will seek assistance from local shelters that can provide safety and counseling. Nurses are often in the position to provide support and counseling to battered women in shelters. The nursing interventions identified in Table 27-1 relate to the case study describing Nina, who requires tertiary prevention measures in an emergency department setting.

Table 27-1	Nursing Interventions for Battered Women
Interventions	**Rationales**
Report abuse to police.	Provide for safety.
Provide medications to relieve pain and anxiety.	Relieve her pain and reduce anxiety.
Discuss validity of the woman's anxiety.	
Encourage the woman to discuss events leading to past and present abuse.	Reduce her guilt and shame.
Point out the increasingly violent nature of the relationship and concern for her safety.	
Insist that no person has the right to abuse another.	
Explore effectiveness of her current coping skills and suggest additional skills.	Increase her independence and effective coping skills.
Focus on strengths, endurance, and abilities.	Increase her self-esteem.
Discuss destructive societal expectations of women.	
Discuss frequency of woman abuse among women like her.	
Explore family and/or friends as support possibilities.	Increase her awareness of potential support.
Discuss potential for using community resources (e.g., shelters and/or hotlines and police).	
Describe current laws on domestic violence.	Increase her awareness of abuse implications.
Explore implications of pressing charges against the batterer.	
Explore meaning of potential relationship loss.	
Explore various options for the future.	Identify long-term goals.
Provide fact sheet on domestic violence.	
Provide referrals.	
Develop a safety plan with critical papers, money, clothing, and other essentials to be set aside for emergency exits.	
Offer to be available for further questions.	Provide continuity of care.

EVALUATION

Evaluation is a critical component of the nursing process. With the battered woman it is especially critical because inadequate or inappropriate nursing interventions may result in more serious abuse or even death for the woman. Nurses who work in settings where battered women seek treatment must be knowledgeable about the many different responses that may occur in the battered woman. Correct evaluation of outcomes and interventions depends on this recognition. Once a complete nursing care plan is developed, the evaluation is based on achievement of the patient goals.

CHILD ABUSE

Based on data collected from each state, the National Center on Child Abuse and Neglect has conducted three surveys (1980, 1988, 1996) on child maltreatment in the United States (Gelles, 1997). The latest survey indicates that agencies identified 2.9 million maltreated children in the year that the survey was last taken (1993). Based on this total of maltreated children, 620,000 were physically abused, 302,000 were sexually abused, 536,400 were emotionally abused, and the largest number of 2,481,800 children were neglected.

Researchers have only recently begun to document the effects of domestic violence on children. Barnett and colleagues (1997) identify four general areas of adverse effects: (1) immediate trauma, (2) adverse effects on development, (3) living under high stress, and (4) exposure to violent role models. Overall, children exposed to domestic violence demonstrate more behavioral and emotional problems, cognitive deficits, and health problems than nonexposed children; as adults, the exposed children experience a wide variety of long-term psychologic effects as well. Finally, children who are exposed to marital violence are themselves at high risk for battering by the abuser (Gelles, 1997).

In the 1940s the introduction of x-ray technology dramatically facilitated the identification of abused children. During this time, some physicians began to notice patterns of healed fractures in small children. However, it was not until 1962 when the classic article, "The Battered Child Syndrome" (Kempe et al, 1962), was published that child abuse was thrust into the public consciousness. In 1974 the U.S. government established the National Center on Child Abuse and Neglect. By that time, mandatory reporting requirements for child abuse and neglect were instituted by all 50 states.

Humphreys and Ramsey (1993) report that most child physical abuse is classified as moderate in severity and includes injuries such as bruises, depressions, and emotional distress, which are not severe enough to warrant medical attention. Therefore most children who are physically abused do not come to the attention of emergency room doctors and nurses; instead they will likely be identified at clinics, schools, and through the efforts of community health nurses.

Social science research indicates that the majority of parents use physical punishment to discipline their children. Gelles and Cornell (1990) claim that spanking is the most common form of family violence in the United States. Parents tend to discipline their children the way in which they were disciplined as children, and they often insist that the only language a child understands is physical punishment. It is difficult to change repeated generational patterns of family discipline, even though social science research finds no potential benefit from physical punishment as discipline and much to condemn it.

Straus, an eminent sociologist who researches family violence, has been condemning physical punishment of children for many years. His latest study (Straus, Sugarman, and Giles-Sims, 1997) finds that physical punishment remains a strong predictor of antisocial behavior for as long as 2 years after the punishment. Although Straus admits that not everyone who is physically disciplined will become antisocial, he cautions that because there are multiple, complex relationships that influence the development of antisocial behavior, society can only benefit by eliminating one of the strongest contributing factors, physical punishment.

DEFINITIONS OF CHILD ABUSE AND NEGLECT

Definitions of child abuse and **child neglect** vary from state to state and among clinicians and researchers. The American Medical Association (Berkowitz et al, 1992) defines **child physical abuse** as "inflicted injury to a child and can range from minor bruises and lacerations to severe neurologic trauma and death." In many states child abuse is defined as actual or threatened physical violence.

Ammerman and Hersen (1992) reflect on the difficulties of operationalizing child abuse and state that "arriving at a universally accepted operational definition of maltreatment has proven to be a dilemma that is virtually insurmountable." This is due primarily to the fact that definitions have such a wide application that many parents and institutions would be viewed as abusive in the United States. Nevertheless, it is clear that nurses and other health care professionals must conduct holistic assessments and search for psychologic trauma, as well as physical, because abuse that leaves no physical scars can disrupt normal growth and development of children in profound ways.

Inherent in all physical abuse is a psychologic component. Briere (1992) describes eight parent/caretaker behaviors that make up his definition of **child psychologic abuse.** These behaviors are rejecting, degrading/devaluing, terrorizing, isolating, corrupting, exploiting, denying essential stimulation or availability, and unreliable and in-consistent parenting.

THEORETIC FRAMEWORKS OF CHILD ABUSE

There is no single theory that explains the causation of child abuse. It is generally recognized that many complex interacting factors are involved that place children at risk for abuse. Box 27-6 summarizes the various theories of child abuse and neglect.

THE ABUSED CHILD

Younger children, especially those under 3 years old, are at greater risk for fatal abuse than are older children. Because younger children are more fragile than older ones, the fatality risk is easy to understand. Earlier studies report that premature infants, handicapped, and developmentally disabled children are also at higher risk. However, recent studies do not find this association (Gelles, 1997).

Data from a national study by the National Center for Child Abuse and Neglect (Gelles, 1997) indicate that child abuse actually increases as a child gets older and plateaus by age 14. Although the researchers do not find any gender differences in child neglect in this study, they do report significant differences between abused males and females; females are more likely to experience physical, emotional, and sexual abuse than are males.

In a discussion of the long-term consequences of childhood abuse, Gelles (1997) reports that abused and neglected children are at greater risk for later delinquency, adult criminality, and violent crimes than are children in the control group. Abused and neglected children also have more intellectual deficits, learning disabilities, drug and alcohol abuse, and psychiatric problems.

THE CHILD PHYSICAL ABUSER

Research on the characteristics of child physical abusers describes them as immature; lacking in self-esteem; and having unrealistic expectations of children, poor impulse control, and minimal or no external support systems. Males and females are equally likely to be abusers. However, in fatal child abuse cases the mother's boyfriend is most commonly identified as the abuser; the natural mother and the natural father are next (Humphreys and Ramsey, 1993).

When analyzing the likelihood of males versus females as child abusers, it must be considered that mothers are frequently the only adults in the household. When data are adjusted for situations in which no male caregiver is present, mothers account for only one third of the abuse (Humphreys and Ramsey, 1993).

THE NURSE'S ATTITUDE IN CHILD ABUSE

When nurses work in settings in which they may encounter abusive families, it is critical that they take time to assess their own attitudes and feelings before interacting with such families. Humphreys and Ramsey (1993) describe three typical reactions by the nurse: (1) horror that parents could perpetrate abuse on their children, (2) denial of the abuse, and (3) fantasies of saving or rescuing the child. None of these responses are helpful to the child, family, or nurse because each will interfere with meeting the therapeutic needs of the child and the family, as well as preventing the nurse from providing effective nursing care.

If the nurse has a history of abuse in his or her own family, to acknowledge the present abuse may initiate some powerful reexperiencing of his or her own abuse. Sometimes the realization of child abuse is so repugnant that nurses may use avoidance to protect themselves. If nurses believe that they are the only ones who are capable of helping the child, they deny the parents the opportunity to understand how their behavior has affected the child and how they must change if the family is to survive and become functional. It is critical that nurses accept that most families, given the necessary conditions, have the potential for abusing and neglecting their children

---

Box 27-6   Etiologic Theories Related to Child Abuse

Biologic Theory
Parents who were abused as children are at risk for abusing their own children.

Social Learning Theory
Family teaches and accepts violent behavior.
Violence is glorified in the media.
Violence is accepted in families, schools, and churches.

Environmental Theory
Socioeconomic class
Unemployment
Stressful life events

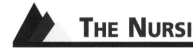

THE NURSING PROCESS

ASSESSMENT

The following discussion focuses on the nurse's responsibilities in making a holistic assessment of the abused child. The areas of assessment cover physical and emotional abuse and neglect of the child. Assessment of the sexually abused child is covered in the next section.

HISTORY

It is the nurse's responsibility to identify abuse and neglect and to intervene in a nonjudgemental and nonthreatening manner. An open and honest attitude with parents is much more likely to gain cooperation and trust than a hostile, blaming one. Direct, honest questions are necessary. All states require nurses and other health care professionals to report any suspicions of child abuse to protective service. Failure to report may constitute a misdemeanor.

Typically, the history format will first focus on parental concerns, then on general family history, and finally on the present concern. This progression moves from the least to the most threatening issue and affords the nurse the opportunity to establish rapport with the parents before requesting information about the most sensitive issue—the possibility of abuse.

When taking the history, the nurse must be alert for discrepancies between the parental explanation of the child's injuries and the physical findings. An example of a discrepancy could be the parents' claim that they have no knowledge of how the child broke his or her femur. The nurse should suspect child abuse when fractures of the femur are diagnosed without some history of significant trauma, such as a car accident. Other clues include parental delay in seeking treatment for the child's injuries, failure to use hospitals closer to home, the child's history of multiple injuries, reluctance by parents to give a history, or discrepancies in the histories that each parent gives. To identify inconsistencies in the history, each parent should be interviewed separately. Whenever possible, children should also be interviewed separately from parents, although children may often deny abuse in an effort to protect parents out of feelings of loyalty or fear of retaliation.

It is often extremely helpful to observe the parent-child relationship while taking the history. Taking the history also allows the nurse to role model appropriate child-

---

Box 27-7   Child Abuse and Neglect—Possible/Actual Physical Indicators

General Appearance
Excessive fearfulness and watchfulness
Disheveled and malnourished
Failure to thrive

Multiple Injuries
No history of significant trauma

Skin
Unexplained bruises, welts, and scratches in various stages of healing (different colors)
Regular patterns of bruises and welts such as bite marks or marks from electrical cords
Untreated infected wounds
Lacerations from rope burns; especially on the neck, wrists, ankles, and torso
Bruises on buttocks, genitalia, thighs, side of the face, trunk, and upper arms

Burns
Small round cigarette burns (infected insect bites resemble cigarette burns)
Immersion burns (even boundaries that are glovelike, sock-like, or symmetric; accidental burns are asymmetric with splash marks)
Patterned burn marks (e.g., from an iron or grill)

Fractures
Fractures in infants younger than age 1
Fractures of femur, humerus, posterior ribs, skull, and long bones and any uncommon fractures

Head Injuries
Skull fractures and subdural hematomas (leading cause of death among abused children)
Brain hemorrhages or contusions without external signs of injury (e.g., shaken baby syndrome)
Alopecia caused by hair pulling

Abdominal Injuries
Ruptured liver or spleen
Ruptured blood vessels
Kidney, bladder, or pancreatic injuries
Injuries to jejunum or duodenum

Injuries to Eyes, Ears, Nose, and Mouth
A wide variety of injuries including missing teeth, bruising, perforation of tympanic membrane, epistaxis and nasal fractures, retinal hemorrhage or detachment corneal abrasions, and periorbital hematomas

Other Types of Abuse/Neglect
Munchausen's syndrome by proxy
Deprivational syndromes

NURSING ASSESSMENT QUESTIONS

For Parents Who Are Suspected of Child Abuse

1. Is there anything in particular that you would like to share about your child or your family as we begin this history?
2. Does your child have any particular health or behavior problems?

3. Have any of your other children ever had similar injuries?
4. How did your child receive these injuries?

---

rearing skills and allows the parents to express their fears, concerns, and problems.

All physical findings should be documented on the child diagram on the history form and direct quotations of the parents should be included whenever possible (Box 27-7). At present, photographs are being used more extensively, although they are not a substitute for a detailed history and physical examination. State laws vary regarding authorization for taking photographs without parental consent. Therefore nurses who work in settings that provide care for children should familiarize themselves with state laws in this regard.

NURSING DIAGNOSIS

Nursing diagnoses in a situation like the case study on Marilee must include the parents because the identified patient is an infant who depends on her parents for care and nurturance. Therefore the following diagnoses relate to both parents and child. Multiple nursing diagnoses may be identified; the following diagnoses are examples. Nursing diagnoses are formulated from information obtained during the assessment phase of the nursing process. The accuracy of the diagnoses depends on a careful, in-depth assessment.

Family-Related Diagnosis

Parenting, altered, related to inexperience with care giving, unrealistic expectations, marginal family adaptation, social isolation, lack of resources, and poverty.

Child-Related Diagnoses

Sensory/perceptual alterations, related to cerebral trauma (subdural hemorrhage)
Fear, related to physical and emotional abuse
Anxiety, related to physical and emotional abuse

OUTCOME IDENTIFICATION

The nurse derived outcome criteria for Marilee from the diagnoses that were formulated for her in collaboration with her parents. These outcomes are the expected behav-

CASE STUDY

Eighteen-month-old Marilee was brought into Southside Hospital emergency room by her parents, Betty and Jim Brown. Although the Browns live on the north side of town, they chose to bring their daughter to the Southside Hospital. Marilee was unconscious when she arrived at 7:00 AM. The physical examination revealed no external signs of trauma on the body except for bruises on the child's upper arms, which resemble grip marks. The Browns reported that Marilee was put to bed the night before in the usual manner but that this morning they were unable to arouse her. The Browns were unaware of any trauma or significant event that could account for their daughter's unconscious state. Both parents were teenagers and clearly agitated about their infant daughter's condition. Mr. Brown refused to have his wife interviewed without him. During the interview and history taking, Betty sat across the room crying softly while Jim answered the nurse's questions. The young couple stated that they are estranged from their own parents and rarely see them. Mr. Brown is currently unemployed.

Critical Thinking—Assessment
1. What is the first priority for the nurse and health care team in this scenario?
2. What criteria make this young couple at risk for child abuse?
3. How would you establish trust with this young couple?
4. If you suspect child abuse, how would you protect the future safety of this child?
5. Why is an understanding of child developmental stages a critical component of effective parenting?

iors that Marilee and her parents will demonstrate as a result of the implementation of the plan of care and the nursing interventions.

For Marilee the first priority is the short-term nursing goal of stabilizing her critical physical condition, the subdural hemorrhage, that resulted from the vigorous shaking by her father. This outcome will be demonstrated by Marilee's renewed ability to respond to stimuli, that is, Marilee will be able to respond to sounds, sights, touch, motion, and smell at the same developmental level she had before her injury. She will recognize her parents, be able to ambulate, and tolerate a light diet.

The nursing diagnoses of fear and anxiety related to Marilee's abuse will involve the long-term nursing goal of helping her reestablish the trust of her father and mother.

OUTCOME IDENTIFICATION FOR AN ABUSED CHILD
Client will:

1. Demonstrate trust by being receptive to her father and not exhibiting any fear of him. This outcome depends on her father's outcome.

OUTCOME IDENTIFICATION FOR AN ABUSING PARENT
Client will:

1. Attend parenting classes to improve his knowledge and understanding of normal growth and development in children.
2. Learn positive parenting skills and use them consistently with his daughter.
3. Cooperate with protective services when they investigate him for the alleged abuse.

PLAN OF CARE WITH OUTCOME CRITERIA
In all child abuse cases the primary concern is the health and safety of the child. Because Marilee is experiencing a medical crisis, the first priority is to stabilize her physical condition. Next, steps must be taken to secure her short- and long-term safety and to support the family in meeting these goals. Because the child's future health and safety depends on her family, it is critical that the nurse establish a trusting relationship with the family and collaborate on developing goals that are mutually acceptable. At times mutually agreed-on goals in child abuse cases may be difficult to achieve because many parents firmly believe that "sparing the rod spoils the child." However, children are sometimes punished because parents are ignorant of normal child development and interpret the child's inability to achieve parental demands as obstinacy or disobedience. Therefore classes in basic child growth and development are a critical component in addressing the needs of families who abuse or neglect their children. Child discipline and anger-control classes are also important in preventing future child abuse.

IMPLEMENTATION
All too frequently in child abuse cases, the child's physical trauma is addressed without addressing the underlying problem of the abuse. Hospitals and agencies that provide primary care are mandated by the Joint Commission on Accreditation of Healthcare Organizations to identify patients who are abused and to provide treatment and referrals for them and their families. This mandate usually requires a concerted and collaborative effort by the health care team. The nurse is usually in an optimal position to coordinate this effort. In particular, the nurse must secure the physical and psychologic safety and health of the child, assist the parents to understand the consequences of their abusive behavior, and develop strategies with the parents that will prevent any reoccurrence of abuse.

When nurses plan interventions for abusive families, they must go beyond the focused family and think in terms of primary prevention for all families, that is, from families that appear normal through high risk. Potential settings for educating and identifying parents are hospital obstetric and pediatric units, substance abuse programs, health clinics, schools, churches, and the community at large. Because of their access to families in their own homes, community health nurses are in an excellent position to assess, teach, and model parenting skills and intervene on the primary prevention level before child maltreatment occurs.

NURSING INTERVENTIONS
Primary prevention is focused on identifying families at risk and implementing interventions directed at preventing abuse. For Marilee, the nursing interventions will be on the secondary prevention level because abuse has already occurred; the present focus is on addressing this current crisis and preventing future occurrences of abuse. In tertiary prevention the child is removed from the home because the safety of the child cannot be secured there. The goal is to maximize the future potential of the child within the constraints of the existing damage. The nursing interventions listed in Table 27-2 focus on secondary prevention for Marilee.

EVALUATION
Because the nursing care of this family will be necessary after hospital discharge, the nursing evaluation will continue throughout the nursing involvement with the family. Evaluation will focus on the family achievement of identified goals. The nurse will conduct a final evaluation when the public health nurse determines that the family has achieved their goals and that there is minimal risk for child abuse.

INTRAFAMILIAL SEXUAL ABUSE OF CHILDREN

OVERVIEW
The most commonly cited study of the incidence of childhood sexual abuse is derived from Diane Russell's work (1986), which includes a random sample of 953 women. Russell reports that approximately one third

Table 27-2	Nursing Interventions for the Physically Abused Child	
Nursing Interventions (Secondary Prevention)	**Rationales**
Develop a trusting relationship with parents. Be direct and open but supportive. Obtain a holistic history, including the stresses and problems the family is experiencing.	Provide environment for parents that facilitates their sharing the sequence of events leading to abuse.
Explore how events that led to abuse might be altered in the future. Explore alternative strategies for child care problems. Discuss basic child growth and development. Provide parents with basic materials on child growth and development. Have parents apply child development principles. Discuss need for parenting classes. Discuss strategies for anger control. Discuss reporting laws on child abuse.	Problem solve and educate on how to avoid similar scenarios in the future. Gain parental agreement to cooperate with protective services.
Explain child welfare function of protective services. Take steps to inform protective services. Observe parent-child interactions unobtrusively. Involve parents in child care during hospitalization when appropriate. Discuss physical impact of abuse with parents. Discuss short- and long-term psychologic effects of child abuse. Provide referral to postdischarge public health child nursing. Public health nurse will coordinate services and monitor parental progress. Public health nurse will role model and assist parents to apply principles learned in parenting classes in their own lives. Public health nurse will reinforce positive parenting skills. Have father discuss how he will maintain anger skills. Teach mother to intervene if father exhibits negative parenting. Assist parents to develop social support systems. Explore community resources with family.	Role model providing care and support for child. Have parents verbalize their understanding of abusive behavior on child. Support parents in the prevention of future abuse. Involve parents in child care classes. Demonstrate anger control skills. Prevent isolation of problem and expand support system.

of her sample were sexually abused as children; 16% of this sample were incestuously abused by a relative before the age of 18. Wyatt's (1985) study corroborates Russell's results with female subjects. Other studies report that sexual abuse to male children is 15% to 20% (Briere, 1992; Jacobson and Herald, 1990). The Gallup Poll (1995) validates these statistics with the report that 23% of surveyed adults claim that they were sexually abused during their childhood by an adult or an older child.

Throughout this discussion on childhood sexual abuse, the pronoun "she" will be used in reference to the child victim; however, it is recognized that male children are also victims of sexual abuse. Also, the term *sexual abuse* will be used interchangeably with *incest*, because most childhood sexual abuse is perpetrated by a relative or someone the child knows and trusts (Courtois, 1988). Therefore many researchers argue that most childhood sexual abuse is incestual.

Many studies (Eilenberg et al, 1996; Jacobson and Herald, 1990) indicate that at least 50% of psychiatric clients have histories of physical and sexual abuse. Although many studies indicate that childhood sexual abuse is a core issue in mental health disorders, the effects of sexual abuse are frequently compounded by concurrent severe physical and emotional abuse.

Many experts claim that sexual abuse is the worst kind of child abuse because it is hidden and, therefore, more difficult to detect and address. The vast majority of children who have been sexually abused will demonstrate no physical evidence of having been abused. Their trauma is primarily psychologic. Conversely, physical abuse of children is much easier to identify because it is more visible and easier to document.

DEFINITION OF INTRAFAMILIAL SEXUAL ABUSE

Traditionally, intrafamilial sexual abuse, or *incest*, has been defined as sexual intercourse between blood relatives who are too close to marry. However, incest is no longer defined in such restricted terms, because intercourse with small children is not typical and a multitude of other exploitative sexual activities do occur that can be equally traumatic for the child. In addition, many researchers and clinicians no longer restrict the offender to a blood relative. At present, many clinicians and researchers use the quality of the relationship between the perpetrator and the child to determine whether the abuse was incestual. If the perpetrator is in a caregiver or surrogate parent role to the child, many consider such abuse incestual. Examples of such relationships include stepfathers, mothers' boyfriends, grandmothers' boyfriends, close family friends, close neighbors who might baby-sit, ministers, and teachers. Because such people assume a position of trust, nurturance, and protection for the child, the potential for trauma is great because of the betrayal of trust. Because children do not have the cognitive, physical, and psychologic maturity to understand the implications of the sexual activity and the perpetrator is always in a powerful position, the children are unable to give true consent. Therefore children must be viewed as victims, and the adults must always be viewed as the responsible party in sexually abusive activity.

The definition of **childhood incest** is any type of exploitative sexual experience between relatives or surrogate relatives before the victim reaches 18 years of age (Urbancic, 1993). Exploitative actions involve behaviors that the perpetrator uses for his/her sexual gratification with the child. This includes disrobing; nudity; masturbation; voyeurism; fondling; digital or object penetration; and oral, anal, or vaginal penetration. In the typical incestual relationship, the abuse begins very gradually with gentle fondling and gradually escalates over time, often progressing to vaginal or oral penetration. Initially, some children may derive pleasure and gratification from the attention and the sexual activity and may actually seek the abuser out. It must be remembered that children are capable of experiencing sexual pleasure when stimulated sexually and that this is a natural physical and biochemical response to the stimulation. Sometimes children feel very special to be the object of such focused attention, particularly if their emotional needs have not been met by others and if the sexual activity provides them with feelings of pleasure, love, and attention. However, despite the pleasurable aspects of the abuse, children usually feel confused and ashamed and in adulthood may find that the pleasurable memories of the abuse become the basis for serious guilt and shame. Such feelings can be difficult to overcome because the adult survivor believes she or he gave consent and does not view the activity as abusive. It cannot be overemphasized that the adult is always the responsible person, regardless of how the child responds. It is the adult's task to nurture, set boundaries, and teach age-appropriate behaviors rather than to exploit children for their own sexual gratification.

HISTORICAL AND THEORETIC PERSPECTIVES ON INCEST

Herman (1992) states that it was not until the rise of the feminist movement in the late 1970s that it became clear that the most common posttraumatic stress disorders were not those of men in war but of women in everyday life. At this time, adult female survivors of childhood sexual abuse began to speak out, establish self-help groups, and document their abuse experiences. Clinicians began to publish anecdotal works on their experiences with survivors of childhood sexual abuse. However, as late as 1975, Henderson reported in the *Comprehensive Textbook of Psychiatry* that incest rarely occurred and was of little consequence.

Since the late 1970s and early 1980s, research on childhood sexual abuse has increased; currently there is an explosion of research on the topic. Many researchers attempt to explain the basis of the traumatic effects of childhood sexual abuse. Most incorporate the posttraumatic stress disorder or various aspects of psychologic trauma into their conceptual model. Some researchers use a cognitive model and maintain that if the traumatic events are not processed and neutralized, they cannot be stored in distant memory. Instead, these traumatic memories remain in active memory and the person has to make a constant effort to defend against them through a variety of cognitive defense mechanisms. Burgess et al (1987) term this effort to defend oneself from traumatic memories *trauma encapsulation.*

Carmen and Rieker (1989) and Briere (1992) propose models similar to the Burgess et al (1987) model that explain the traumatic effects as being efforts by a defenseless child to cope in the best way possible. The cognitive defense mechanisms include denial, repression, disassociation, splitting, and compartmentalization. There is no doubt that these defenses are helpful and adaptive in coping with the trauma of the abuse during childhood. However, as adults the same defenses become entrenched, counterproductive, and the basis for mental health problems.

CHARACTERISTICS OF THE INCESTUAL FAMILY

Research on intrafamilial sexual abuse indicates that these families are highly dysfunctional, although overtly they may appear quite normal. Studies do not find a correlation with incest and such characteristics as socioeconomic status, culture, race, and ethnicity. Rather, incest seems to cross all boundaries.

Within incestual families, multiple forms of abuse are likely to be present including physical and other forms of psychologic/emotional abuse. Most incestual families are described as **enmeshed,** which means that they are relatively isolated from those outside the family and tend to focus most of their energies on relationships within the family. Boundaries within the family are poorly defined and characterized by excessive dependency on each other for physical, social, and psychologic needs. Role reversals often occur with the abused child assuming a caregiver role for the parents and other family members. However, it must be emphasized that no single pattern can accurately describe the complexity of the incestual family.

OFFENDERS

Characteristics of offenders are primarily based on research of those cases that are examined within the criminal-justice system and, therefore, are more serious abuse cases. Most cases of sexual abuse are never reported, so these criminal cases are not representative of all offenders. More recently researchers have begun to focus on non-incarcerated offenders.

At present, experts recognize that child sexual offenders are a diverse population that are difficult to classify. They vary in age, occupation, income, marital status, and ethnic group (Becker, 1994). Some researchers are also beginning to study the female perpetrator, because they believe female perpetration is more common than studies indicate (Barnett, Miller-Perrin, and Perrin, 1997). Existing research on female perpetrators indicate that they are often accomplices to males or to a general pattern of abuse among all family members (Elliot, 1993; Urbancic, 1993). Sometimes a female perpetrator is attracted to an adolescent boy and will develop a sexual relationship and insist she is "in love" with the child.

Criminal justice experts have expressed great concern in recent years because of the descending age of offenders (Barnett, Miller-Perrin, and Perrin, 1997; Becker, 1994). More juveniles are being identified as offenders, and they demonstrate more violent behavior than do typical adult offenders. In addition, more of these juvenile offenders are prepubescent and include growing numbers of female offenders. These juvenile offenders range in age from 5 to 19 years and represent all ethnic, racial, and socioeconomic classes; 90% are males (Ryan and Lane, 1991). The majority of adult offenders reports beginning their deviant sexual behavior during adolescence.

There is a critical need for research that will identify typologies of sexual offenders and nursing interventions that are effective. Sexual offenders are appropriate for treatment only if they acknowledge their guilt, express remorse, and recognize their need for treatment (Becker, 1994).

CHARACTERISTICS OF THE NONOFFENDING PARENT

When the abuser is the father, the mother is typically blamed for failing to satisfy her husband's psychologic and sexual needs, of being rejecting and dominating, and of expecting her daughter to assume the lover role with the father and be caregiver to both parents. The literature has also blamed the mother for being absent when the incest occurred, even if she was working to support the family. In addition, when the child discloses the abuse to the mother, it has been claimed that the mother commonly denies that the abuse has occurred or blames the child for initiating or encouraging it.

Although these have been common themes in the literature, little or no research exists to support the contentions. In fact, recent research suggests that the majority of nonoffending mothers believe their children and take steps to protect them by notifying protective services. Deblinger et al (1993) report that mothers of children who are sexually abused by partners are more likely to be battered by the abusive partners than are mothers of children abused by other relatives or nonrelatives. Consequently, these researchers suggest that it is more appropriate to view these battered mothers as secondary victims of abuse rather than as colluders and deniers. In addition, they find that the vast majority of mothers believe their children's reports of being abused.

In Urbancic's clinical practice (1993), many nonoffending mothers are initially shocked and ambivalent about the disclosure of sexual abuse by their children. It is especially devastating to the woman if she loves and trusts her partner, because she must now cope with her partner's betrayal in addition to her child being violated and traumatized. It is much simpler and less painful to believe that it did not occur. Nevertheless, many mothers who are initially in shock experience a process involving a crisis of disbelief and/or ambivalence that is followed by gradual acceptance and eventual dedication to the healing of the child's trauma, as well as their own.

It is probably most accurate to recognize that a variety of scenarios exist with regard to the nonoffending mother and that it is inappropriate to try to categorize the complexity of the nonoffending mother according to any one particular pattern or description.

SEXUALLY ABUSED CHILDREN

Most of the research on child victims of sexual abuse has been directed toward female children. Much less is known about the male child victim. Typically, the incest victim is the oldest daughter in the family, and often when she is able to extricate herself from this role, the next daughter replaces her. Some research indicates that the average age at which the incestual relationship begins is 8 or 9. However, in Urbancic's study (1993) the average age of the child when the incest begins is 6 years, with an average duration of 7 years.

Often the secret is never revealed; however, at other times the child may disclose the incest to a close friend or trusted relative. Sometimes the child discloses the incest during a family argument in which her acting-out behavior is being criticized by her parents. Although acting-out behavior by the child is common, there is no unique pattern of behavior that might indicate the presence of abuse. Indeed, sometimes the victim is a model child in every way.

EFFECTS OF SEXUAL ABUSE ON CHILDREN

Briere (1992) and Herman (1992) emphasize that frequently physical, psychologic, and sexual abuse are combined and the resulting combined effects are extremely traumatic. However, Briere and Herman emphasize that even when the effects of other abuse are considered and analyzed in research studies, sexual abuse effects are still significant and usually a key issue. This is a crucial point because some writers discount the trauma of childhood sexual abuse and insist that it is the chaotic family, not the sexual abuse, that is the core problem. Nevertheless, it is important to use a holistic view in the assessment and treatment of abused clients and to address whatever abuse issues are salient to the client.

Recently, an extensive review of the literature was reported by Kendall-Tackett, Williams, and Finkelhor (1993). After reviewing 45 studies, these researchers conclude that no single core of symptoms exist as a common denominator among sexually abused children. Instead, a multitude of symptoms have been identified. Symptomatology seems to depend on a complex blend of factors including developmental age of the child when the abuse occurs; maternal support; individual coping skills; positive influences that may neutralize the abuse; severity, duration, and frequency of the abuse; relationship of the abuser; and degree of force.

The literature review by Kendall-Tackett and colleagues (1993) indicates that childhood sexual abuse has serious repercussions that are reflected in a wide variety of symptoms and pathologic behaviors. The most common symptoms are the sexual acting-out behavior and posttraumatic stress disorder. Other commonly experienced symptoms and behaviors in abused children include anxiety, fear, depression, somatic complaints, aggressive antisocial behavior, withdrawn behavior, school learning problems, and hyperactivity. Sexual acting-out behaviors are evidenced by the child's preoccupation with sexual play behavior with dolls and other children, inserting objects into anal and vaginal openings, compulsive masturbation, sexual knowledge beyond her age, and promiscuity. Many of the symptoms are developmentally specific, so the researchers caution about generalizing all symptoms across all age groups.

LONG-TERM EFFECTS OF CHILDHOOD SEXUAL ABUSE

Just as there is no specific profile for the sexually abused child, there is none for the adult survivor. Most survivors of childhood sexual abuse report being treated by multiple therapists before finding one who effectively identified and facilitated their recovery process (Urbancic,

1993). With the explosion of clinical literature, training workshops, and research, it is hoped that this scenario is rapidly changing. A growing awareness that people can heal from childhood sexual abuse is reflected in the use of the term "survivor" rather than victim by professionals and those who have been abused. A *survivor* is viewed as a person who has discarded the helpless victim mentality in favor of an empowerment attitude in which the person acts on the belief that she is capable of overcoming and recovering from the trauma.

Clinicians and researchers categorize the long-term effects of childhood sexual abuse in a variety of ways. Jehu (1992) identifies the most common psychosocial problems of survivors who seek treatment as posttraumatic stress disorder, self-damaging behavior, mood disturbances, interpersonal problems, and sexual difficulties. Sexual difficulties include rape, prostitution, compulsive sexuality, and confusion about sexual orientation.

For many survivors of childhood sexual abuse, posttraumatic stress disorder is a reality that is characterized by a reexperiencing of the trauma via flashbacks and recurrent dreams (van der Kolk, McFarlane, and Weisaeth, 1996). Other symptoms of posttraumatic stress disorder include numbing or constricted affect, memory problems, difficulty concentrating, irrational guilt and shame, constant vigilance, sleep problems, and anxiety attacks. The traumatic memories can be experienced through the senses of smell, touch, taste, sight or sound. Thus the survivor may experience an overwhelming sense of terror when some cue in the environment triggers such a sensory memory. For example, the survivor is exposed to someone who resembles her abuser and she experiences an overwhelming sense of fear, panic, and dread. Because she is unaware of the connection between her powerful reaction and this person as a trigger to her abusive childhood experience, she is unable to give a logical explanation for her reaction and may fear that she is "going crazy."

On many occasions the survivors will report recurring physical symptoms for which no organicity can be found. Recently clinicians, researchers, and survivors have begun to relate many of these symptoms to specifics of the abuse. These symptoms are referred to as *body memories*. In Urbancic's research (1993), approximately 35% of her sample of adult survivors report symptoms that can be categorized as body memories. Women who report being forced into oral sex tended to describe such symptoms as absent gag reflex, teeth clenching, difficulty swallowing, and severe biting of the inside of the mouth. Women who were penetrated vaginally or rectally often report pelvic or rectal pain or severe pain during intercourse. Other body memories are represented by symptoms such as heavy pressure on the chest and difficulty breathing (abuser lying on top of child) and periodic numbness of the hand (hand that masturbated the abuser).

Survivors with body memories typically consult many doctors to no avail because there is no organic explanation for these symptoms. It is also likely that many survivors have had multiple unsuccessful surgeries to treat these symptoms. Again, because the survivor and the health care professional are unaware of the relationship between these physical symptoms and the abuse, one can see how these conditions could contribute to the survivor's feelings of anxiety, confusion, helplessness, and depression.

Most survivors in the Urbancic study (1993) report having difficulty trusting others, feeling isolated, different, depressed, vulnerable, and helpless. Most also complain of low self-esteem and feeling deep shame and guilt. About 20% of the women report dissociative and depersonalization experiences, panic attacks, and agoraphobia. A wide variety of symptoms are reported by adult survivors of childhood sexual abuse, leaving no doubt that there can be and often are serious repercussions from such experiences.

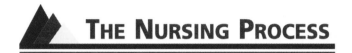

THE NURSING PROCESS

ASSESSMENT

As with the assessment of other victims of violence, the nurse should begin with an assessment of her own assumptions, beliefs, and attitudes about childhood sexual abuse. Nurses who believe that the child is responsible in any way for the sexual abuse will find it difficult to be supportive toward the child. The nurse must be comfortable when speaking with the child about the abuse so that an attitude of discomfort is not conveyed to the child. Children are very adept at picking up nonverbal cues, and the nurse's discomfort may be interpreted by the child as a sign that she is not to talk about the abuse or that she is disbelieved.

As with all nursing assessments, a holistic approach is essential. Because childhood sexual abuse trauma is highly complex and is affected by multiple interacting factors, it is important to gain as much information as possible without subjecting the child to unnecessary and repeated probing and questioning. Most often the nurse will encounter the sexually abused child in the emergency department or outpatient clinic. Often, the mother or other caregiver will bring the child to a medical facility to determine if the child has been sexually abused. Whenever there is a suspicion of childhood abuse, a complete physical examination must be given.

The primary focus is to establish a trusting relationship with the child so that she is as comfortable as possible in relating relevant events and cooperating with the physical examination. It is important to assess the relationship between the caregiver and the child to determine if the child is more comfortable with or without that person. Usually younger children will not want to be separated from this caregiver, whereas older children may be too inhibited to disclose in front of the caregiver for a variety of reasons, such as fear of being blamed by family members, disbelieved, or instrumental in the family break-up. Sometimes the child may retract her disclosure in an effort to protect the abuser with whom she may have a love/hate relationship. Finally, the developmental age of the child is an important factor in her ability to successfully provide data about the abuse; the younger the child, the less able she is to describe events and understand the interviewer's questions.

The majority of children who have been sexually abused will not display any physical signs of abuse because the most common type of abusive activity is fondling, and it seldom leaves physical manifestations. The occurrence of oral copulation or mock intercourse is also difficult to physically document unless the child is examined within a short time after the activity. Giardino et al (1992) report that even serious physical injuries from sexual abuse can heal without any significant residual signs. Evidence such as enlargement of the hymenal orifice alone is not conclusive for proving sexual abuse. Thus it is very difficult to demonstrate physical signs of sexual abuse.

In addition to the lack of physical evidence, the sexually abused child may not display any signs of emotional trauma and she may deny, retract, and be inconsistent in her description of the abuse. Caregivers often interpret this behavior to mean that the abuse did not occur and the child is lying. The significance of absent physical or emotional signs must be clearly explained to the child's caregivers. Conversely, multiple emotional/psychologic indicators may be present; however, because many of these signs can also reflect other problems, their presence alone is not a conclusive sign that sexual abuse has occurred. The diagnosis of sexual abuse is difficult and challenging because there is no single profile or set of symptoms that guarantee its presence. Many of the following signs and symptoms must be viewed as potential indicators of sexual abuse only, whereas others are highly probable indicators. Detailed psychosocial protocols and guidelines for health care professionals who interview and evaluate children for sexual abuse have been developed by the American Professional Society on Abused Children (APSAC) Task Force (1990). Guidelines for evaluation of physical signs of sexual abuse have been published by Giardino et al (1992). The following indicators are derived from these two sets of guidelines and from clinical observation.

Box 27-8   Possible/Probable Physical, Behavioral, and Psychosocial Indicators of Childhood Sexual Abuse

General Appearance

Varies from normal to anxious, fearful, and depressed

Probable Physical Examination Indicators

Bruises, lacerations, or bite marks on breasts, neck, buttocks, extremities, and oropharynx

Presence of sexually transmitted disease, including HIV

Presence of adult pubic hair and semen

Edema, abrasions, petechiae, and erythema of genital area

Lacerations to vagina or anus

Alterations and/or enlargement of hymenal orifice

Dysuria due to periurethral trauma

Rectal fissures, chafing and erythema, bruising, lacerations, and perianal scarring

Semen in the oropharynx and/or nasopharynx

Scar tissue of labia minora, hymenal membrane, and anus

High-Risk Family History Indicators

Substance abuse in caregivers

History of abuse in parents

Domestic violence

Inadequate impulse control/mental illness in caregivers

Alleged offender with sexual dysfunction and/or poor coping skills, poor social skills

Socially isolated family

Sexual abuse of sibling

Behavioral Indicators

Disclosure and spontaneous discussion of the abuse

Preoccupation with drawing genitals or anxious avoidance of anything to do with genitals/sex

Inappropriate sexual play behavior with dolls or other children, compulsive masturbation, inserting objects into vagina and/or anus, sexualized kissing, fondling genitals of others, and imitating intercourse

Dissociation

Avoidance of particular people, school/learning problems

Possible Psychosocial Indicators

Increased anxiety, fears, depression, low self-esteem

Multiple somatic complaints

Signs of posttraumatic stress disorder

Antisocial behavior, promiscuity, substance abuse

Running away, self-destructive behavior

As noted earlier, there is no single profile or set of signs and symptoms that indicate the presence of sexual abuse, and in some cases there is an absence of obvious indicators. However, when caregivers look back at the child's behavior after the disclosure of the abuse, they are often able to identify signs and symptoms that seemed to have no significance at the time.

Clearly, the meaning of any child's acting-out behavior needs to be explored. Such behavior in abused children usually reflects the anger, confusion, and sense of betrayal that the child is experiencing and is unable to discuss. Although many abused children are able to act out their feelings through rebellious and delinquent behavior, others withdraw, blame themselves, become guilt ridden, and continuously try to be a "better" or "good" child. Such children may function at a high level in school and even be praised and admired for what appears to be mature behavior because they often assume major responsibility for adult caregiver roles in their homes. Finally, some children with abusive histories do not exhibit signs of trauma during childhood but do exhibit them later in life, whereas others seem to escape trauma from abuse throughout their life. As previously discussed, the presence of sexual abuse trauma depends on a wide variety of complex factors; in particular, the degree to which the child receives validation, protection, and support after disclosure is crucial to the resolution of the trauma.

The assessment of child sexual abuse should include a physical examination, interviews with the child and family members, outside information from sources such as teachers and baby-sitters, and psychologic tests if needed.

In general, the interview with the child should take place in an environment in which the child can feel safe and comfortable. As with all sensitive topics, questions should begin with the least sensitive and most positive topics and progress to the most sensitive and direct ones. Initial questions are meant to gain the trust of the child and assist her to relax and become more spontaneous. The developmental age of the child is a critical factor in the type and level of question that is used; therefore all techniques must be modified according to the child's needs. Small children may have difficulty with nondirective, open-ended questions. Interviewers must be extremely cautious *not* to use leading questions. An example would be, "Daddy likes to tickle your bottom, doesn't he?"

The nurse's role is to provide comfort and safety for the child. Thus the immediate physical and psychologic needs of the child must be determined and addressed. Once these needs have been addressed, it is always critical for the nurse and other health care professionals to make a determination as to whether the child will be safe if returned to her home.

Some sexual abuse may constitute an emergency situation because of severe physical trauma to the child. In this case the physical condition must be stabilized as soon as possible, keeping in mind that the child will be in great pain and very frightened. Most often the abuse will involve fondling rather than physical injury.

NURSING ASSESSMENT QUESTIONS
For the Sexually Abused Child

1. Who do you like to play with best of all?
2. What kind of fun things do you and (name) do together?
3. What kinds of games do you and (name) play when mom isn't around?
4. Are there any games that you and (name) play that you don't like?

Eventually, the child must be asked directly about the possibility of sexual abuse. In a nonemergency situation, questions such as those in the Nursing Assessment Questions box could be used with a small child whose father, stepfather, or other male caregiver is suspected of the abuse.

NURSING DIAGNOSIS

The following nursing diagnoses are based on data identified in the case study on Suzy. Nursing diagnoses are formulated from the information obtained during the assessment phase of the nursing process. The accuracy of the diagnoses depends on a careful, in-depth assessment.

CASE STUDY

Suzy is a 5-year-old female who was brought to the emergency room by her mother and stepfather, Mr. and Mrs. Jones, because she was bleeding from the vagina. Mrs. Jones reported that while she was bathing Suzy in the tub, the phone rang, so she left Suzy for a few minutes to answer it. Mr. Jones claims that he went in to check on Suzy when he heard her crying and found her standing in the tub crying and bleeding from the vagina. Mr. and Mrs. Jones maintained that Suzy tried to get out of the tub but slipped and injured herself on the tub faucet. No other persons were in the home at the time of the accident. Suzy was obviously distressed and unable to give a history. She clung to her mother and would not allow anyone, including her stepfather, to touch her. On physical examination Suzy was found to have lacerations of the hymenal membrane and vaginal wall, trauma to surrounding perineal area, and old scarring.

Critical Thinking—Assessment

1. What are the possible mechanisms for the injury that Suzy received?
2. How would you best prepare Suzy for her physical examination?
3. What kind of questions and comments would be appropriate and helpful to Suzy?
4. How can the nurse structure the environment so that Suzy will feel more safe?

Pain related to injuries sustained from sexual abuse

Anxiety and fear related to further abuse

Injury, risk for, related to sexual abuse by stepfather (increased chances of recurrence and possible prior incidents of sexual abuse by stepfather)

Coping, ineffective family related to sexual abuse by stepfather and mother's possible denial as evidenced by the mother's inability to protect her daughter

OUTCOME IDENTIFICATION

Outcome criteria for Suzy are derived from the nursing diagnoses that were identified earlier. These outcomes are the expected behaviors that Suzy and her mother will demonstrate as a result of the plan of care.

For Suzy, the first priority is addressing the physical trauma of the sexual abuse, which is the hymenal and vaginal laceration and localized trauma to the perineal area. Presence of scar tissue indicates prior abuse. Depending on the extent of damage and bleeding, Suzy may require surgical repair of her injuries. Based on her plan of care, the first outcome will be focused on stabilizing her physical condition. The second priority will be to ensure that the abuse will not recur and the child will be protected in the future.

OUTCOME IDENTIFICATION FOR CHILD SEXUAL ABUSE

Child will:

1. Report a decrease in pain and anxiety.
2. Verbalize an awareness that she will be protected in the future and that no one will be allowed to injure her again.
3. Discuss her present perceptions, distortions, and fears with the nurse.

Child and parent will:

1. Follow through on referral sources for herself and her family. Because Suzy's abuse was ongoing and severe, she will require an individual therapist.
2. Participate in individual or group therapy. Many organizations exist that conduct groups for survivors, non-offending parents, offenders, and siblings in families in

which sexual abuse has occurred. All family members need to be assessed for the level of their therapy needs.

3. Mother will attend parenting classes because she will require assistance in learning how to nurture, support, and protect her daughter in the future.

No specific diagnosis exists in the DSM-IV for childhood sexual abuse. Many adult survivors have been identified as experiencing posttraumatic stress disorder, but symptoms for both children and adult survivors of abuse vary greatly and no single profile has been identified that would clearly describe sexual abuse survivors. However, sexual abuse can be reported under the DSM-IV Axis IV, which focuses on psychosocial and environmental problems.

PLANNING

The plan of care for the abused child begins with stabilizing the child's physical needs, securing the child's safety, and addressing the child's psychologic needs (Table 27-3). Because the child depends on the parents for the continuation of these goals outside of the hospital, the family system must also be assessed. In the case study on Suzy, the stepfather is the suspected abuser; therefore it must be clearly established that the stepfather will not have access to his stepdaughter and that the mother is capable of nurturing and protecting her child in the future. Police and protective services reports must be completed by the attending staff.

IMPLEMENTATION

Nurses need to be educated about the signs and symptoms of childhood sexual abuse so that they are able to recognize them and take swift action in all potential cases. Because the child's safety is critical, nurses should be knowledgeable about the laws in their state and the policies and procedures of their institution for caring for all survivors of abuse, especially children who are the most vulnerable. In severe cases such as Suzy's, the stepfather will be removed from the home. Nurses are often the coordinators who ensure that protective services and law enforcement agencies are notified and that treatment referrals are made and are followed through. Usually treatment will be mandated by the court after investigations by protective services and the criminal justice system are made.

Types of long-term treatment will depend on the child's developmental level and the mother's potential for supporting and protecting the child in the future. With a younger child, play therapy is often used because the child will often have difficulty verbally expressing feelings about her abuse. Group therapy with other young children is also very useful because common fears and misperceptions can be addressed. As the child becomes able to repeatedly address these fears and misperceptions, they will gradually be resolved. Group therapy with other children is also a powerful modality for teaching them self-assertive behavior and how to protect themselves in the future.

EVALUATION

Ongoing evaluation of the client and family outcomes reveals the efficiency of the nursing interventions and is critical to ensure that the child is protected and supported to recover from the trauma of the abuse. In addition, an ongoing evaluation of the caregiver is needed to determine if this person is following through with the plan of care and to address any problems that may arise. A reliable

Table 27-3	Nursing Interventions for the Sexually Abused Child	
Nursing Interventions	**Rationales**
Call police and protective services.	Provide for safety needs.
Provide medication prn; reassure child that she is safe and that no one will hurt her again.	Relieve the child's pain and anxiety.
Encourage her to talk about her fears and concerns.	Allow expression of feelings.
Reassure her that she is not to blame and that her abuser did a bad thing to hurt her.	Reduce guilt.
Verify that the appropriate agencies have been notified and will follow through.	Coordinate contact of appropriate agencies.
Document the mother's responses in terms of supporting her child and being committed to protecting her child in the future.	Assess and strengthen the mother's coping abilities.
Provide support and educate about potential resources (e.g., treatment centers, role of social services and criminal justice system).	
Educate the mother about the signs and symptoms of abuse that the child may exhibit and how to support her.	
Assess the mother for her ability to cope with possible feelings of grief and betrayal.	

evaluation of the mother's motivation and ability to support and protect her child requires both short- and long-term assessment. Sometimes the mother may become involved with another partner who is at high risk for child abuse. Thus the mother must be able to confront her own behavior and the decisions she makes with regard to the safety of her children.

ELDER ABUSE

Elder abuse is the last area of family violence to break through public awareness and consciousness. Because it is the most recent family violence phenomenon to gain public attention, it is also the least researched and the least understood. In the past 10 years a growing body of knowledge has developed on the issue of elder abuse that has dispelled some of the earlier beliefs about this type of family violence. The first medical publication about elder abuse appeared in the British Medical Journal in 1975. The phenomenon of "granny battering" was described. The emerging belief was that elder abuse was the result of stressed caregivers who occasionally became overwhelmed and beat their unruly parents. Victim blaming was implicit in this explanation. Just as abused children and battered women are blamed for provoking or somehow initiating the abuse, so too the elderly "asked for it."

Because of demographic changes in the United States, an ever-increasing number of elderly are living much longer and accounting for a greater proportion of the population. This large block of elderly citizens has caused a heightened interest by the public in the concerns of the aged. Elderly citizens have also become more political, with organizations such as the Association for Retired Persons and the Grey Panthers. However, because so many elderly are isolated and depend on the people who abuse them, it has been difficult to accurately describe and explain the parameters of this hidden problem. Wolf (1995) estimates that approximately 5% of people who are 65 years of age or older are victims of some type of abuse or neglect each year. This figure translates into a yearly figure of 2 million abused elders.

Even when abuse is clearly documented, the elderly frequently refuse to acknowledge it. Reporting of abuse by the elderly accounts for only 5% of elder abuse (Tatara (1993). As with other victims of abuse, the elderly feel too ashamed and guilty to disclose the abuse and frequently believe that somehow they provoked or deserved the abuse. Because their abusers are frequently family members, the elderly may hesitate to report abusive incidents for fear of possible institutionalization or loss of the only home they know. Furthermore, as with the battered women and the abused children, the elderly may have strong feelings of affection and loyalty to their abusers.

DEFINITION

Six major categories of **elder abuse** are commonly identified (Sengstock and Barrett, 1993) as follows:

1. Psychologic or emotional neglect
2. Psychologic or emotional abuse
3. Violation of personal rights
4. Financial abuse
5. Physical neglect
6. Direct physical abuse

Psychologic neglect involves ignoring or consistently failing to address the concerns of the elderly. *Psychologic abuse* includes isolating the elderly, threatening their safety in some way, inducing fear, and being verbally assaultive. Elderly persons' rights are violated when they are forced to act against their will. An example of such a violation would be forcing the elderly to move into a nursing home against their will. *Financial abuse* is characterized by theft or misuse of the elder's money, property, or other possessions. *Physical neglect* involves the failure to provide the basic necessities of daily living for the elderly. Sengstock and Barrett (1993) claim that the major difference between direct abuse and neglect is that in neglect there is no intent to injure. Finally, *direct physical abuse* is described as deliberate actions to injure the elderly. These may include such actions as beatings, punches, sexual assaults, and threats with an actual weapon.

THE ABUSED ELDER

The abused elder has been defined as over 65 years of age. There are no other specific characteristics because the abused elder can be male or female, healthy or unhealthy, and competent or incompetent. In terms of severity, abuse of wives by husbands was found to be more severe than that inflicted by wives on husbands.

THE ABUSER

The earlier image of elder abuse was that of an elderly white female who is abused by her middle-age, overwhelmed caregiver daughter. However, recent research indicates that the most likely person to abuse the elderly is the person who lives with them—a son, daughter, or spouse. This contention is supported by the research of Pillemer and Finkelhor (1988), who find that spouses are the most frequent abusers and that elderly people who live alone are abused only 25% as often as those who live with others. Although the abuse typically occurs in the elder's home, it is not uncommon for relatives to visit and abuse elderly relatives in nursing homes. As with other types of abuse, the typical pattern in elder abuse is one of gradually increasing violence and frequency.

With child-to-parent abuse, sons and daughters are equally likely to abuse. Sons are more likely to inflict physical abuse, whereas psychologic abuse or neglect is more common with daughters.

THEORIES ON ELDER ABUSE

Although there are many theories that seek to explain elder abuse, no single theory is completely adequate (Box 27-9). Sengstock and Barrett (1993) identify three main foci for theories on elder abuse: abuser characteristics, situational stress, and family relationships. Pillemer (1986) identifies five risk factors for elder abuse, and these five factors can be articulated within the three theoretic foci of Sengstock and Barrett. These factors are (1) psychopathology of the abuser, (2) external stress, (3) dependency, (4) social isolation, and (5) transgenerational violence.

Elder abuse is frequently compared with child abuse because in both cases neglect is common. However, with elder abuse, the elderly continue to have the rights of adults unless they are declared incompetent by a judge. Therefore decisions cannot legally be forced on the elderly as they can with children. Elders have the right to choose to remain in a particular environment, even when it is obvious that they are being abused or neglected.

Box 27-9	**Etiologic Factors Related to Elder Abuse**

Biologic
Psychopathology of the abuser

Social Learning
Dependency (financial and relational)
Social isolation
Transgenerational violence

Environmental
External stress

THE NURSING PROCESS

ASSESSMENT

As with other types of family abuse, it is critical to interview the elder apart from the caregiver. In the hospital it is quite easy to simply assert that hospital policy mandates that clients be seen alone. If the nurse is conducting the interview at home, it may be much more difficult to gain access to the elder; nurses may even jeopardize their own safety by insisting on privacy. In these cases, suspected abusers must be assessed for their potential to harm non-family members. This assessment must determine whether the abuser is a substance abuser or has a history of mental illness and/or violence because these factors may further compromise the nurse's safety. Sometimes it is possible to identify a family member who is trusted and is able to provide the nurse with an opportunity to visit the elder, as well as security. Having another nurse present during a home visit is always an option, but at no time should the nurses intentionally place themselves in dangerous home-visit situations.

It is not uncommon for both the abuser and the abused to maintain secrecy about the abuse. As with other types of family violence, abusers frequently threaten their victims with harm if they disclose the abuse. However, even without threats of retaliation, a great deal of time often lapses before the abused elderly are comfortable disclosing their mistreatment. Their reluctance is usually due to shame; self-blame; or fear of abandonment, institutionalization, and serious consequences for the abuser. Sengstock and Barrett (1993) state that some elderly victims are unable to report their abuse because it is too devastating to accept the reality of being abused by their loved ones.

Box 25-10 identifies physical indicators of actual or potential elder abuse. Many of these symptoms are present with normal aging. Therefore, as with other types of family violence, the nurse must do a comprehensive assessment and consider the physical symptoms within the broader context of the client's life history.

In addition to the signs and symptoms in Box 27-10, the elderly may experience abuse by being overmedicated, socially isolated, and threatened with physical punishment if their behavior is not deemed appropriate.

Besides possible physical signs and symptoms of elder abuse and neglect, it is also necessary to assess the elderly for signs of exploitation and/or abandonment. Signs of *exploitation* include complaints by the elderly or evidence of misuse of their money, loss of control over their finances, material goods taken without consent or approval, and unmet financial needs that are inconsistent with their actual financial status. Signs of *abandonment* include reports by the elderly or evidence of being left alone and helpless for extended periods without adequate assistance.

NURSING DIAGNOSIS

The following nursing diagnoses are based on the assessment data gathered by the nurse who interviewed and ex-

NURSING ASSESSMENT QUESTIONS
For the Abused Elderly

1. Are you happy living with your ----?
2. Can you tell me about your financial assets and how they are managed?
3. Whom do you turn to when you are feeling down?
4. How are family disagreements handled in your household?
5. Has anyone ever hurt you or touched you when you didn't want to be touched?

---

amined Marjorie. These diagnoses represent a few of the possibilities that might be relevant for similar cases. Nursing diagnoses are formulated from the information obtained during the assessment phase of the nursing process. The accuracy of the diagnoses depends on a careful, in-depth assessment.

Cardiac output, decreased and activity intolerance related to change in health status (congestive heart failure).

Depression related to physical illness, loss of role functioning, and lack of social support.

Anxiety, moderate to severe, related to change in health status and role functioning.

Family coping, ineffective related to alcohol abuse by caregivers and caregiver role strain.

Personal identity disturbance related to changes in health status and role functioning.

No diagnosis in the DSM-IV is currently appropriate for the abused elderly person.

OUTCOME IDENTIFICATION

Outcome criteria for this section are based on the nursing diagnoses derived from the case study on Marjorie. These outcomes are the expected behaviors that someone like Marjorie will demonstrate or achieve as a result of the implementation of the plan of care and the interventions. Because Marjorie came to the emergency department with severe cardiac distress, the first priority is stabilizing her congestive heart failure so that she can regain normal cardiac output as evidenced by normal vital signs, freedom from chest pain and dyspnea, and decreased anxiety and fear. The remainder of Marjorie's nursing diagnoses relate to her psychosocial needs, including her depression. Because of her change in health status and her dependency on caregivers who are exploitative and neglectful, Marjorie is feeling helpless, frightened, and depressed.

OUTCOME IDENTIFICATION FOR ELDER ABUSE
Client will:

1. Explore options that may exist in relation to her home situation. Because Marjorie is an adult, she cannot be forced to leave her children's home or press charges

---

Box 27-10   **Physical Indicators of Actual or Potential Elder Abuse/Neglect**

General Appearance
Anxious, fearful, and passive
Poor eye contact
Looks to caregiver for answers
Poor hygiene and inappropriate dress
Underweight or malnourished
Physically handicapped
No glasses, false teeth, or hearing aid despite need

Skin
Contusions, abrasions, burns, and scars in various stages of healing
Decubitus ulcers, urine burns
Rope marks

Abdominal/Rectal
Distended
Internal bleeding
Fecal impactions

Musculoskeletal Fractures
Evidence of old, healed fractures
Current fractures and sprains
Limited range of motion
Contractures

Genital/Urinary
Vaginal lacerations, bruises, and infections
Urinary tract infections

Neurologic
Slurred speech
Confusion

---

against them. If there are mandatory reporting laws in Marjorie's state, her children's abusive behavior will have to be reported.
2. Verbalize feelings about her change in health care status, her dependency on her children, the treatment she has received from her children, and available options for dealing with these concerns.

CASE STUDY

Eighty-year-old Marjorie Jones is brought to the emergency room by her daughter and son-in-law and is anxiously holding her chest and gasping for breath. Marjorie is currently on medication for congestive heart failure. She is underweight, dehydrated, without dentures, and has poor hygiene. When asked about her missing dentures, she states that they have been lost for several months and that no one has been able to find them. After receiving medical treatment to stabilize her heart condition, Marjorie begins to feel much better and is able to give a brief history to the nurse in the privacy of her hospital room.

Marjorie appears depressed, withdrawn, and had difficulty making eye contact. She states that because of her inability to maintain her own apartment any longer, she had moved in with her daughter and son-in-law 18 months ago. Until that time Marjorie had a full life with her widowed friends and had participated in social activities. She had had a part-time housekeeper since her husband died 5 years ago, and she had been able to maintain her independence quite well until she developed congestive heart failure.

Marjorie reports that life is quite different for her now that she is no longer independent. She states that she is having a difficult time adjusting to being "so dependent" and that she "misses her friends." She denies ever being hurt by anyone. After gentle questioning, Marjorie gradually admits having difficulty living with her daughter and son-in-law because of their alcohol abuse. Although neither have harmed her physically, they have discouraged her friends from visiting her and have continually demanded exorbitant room and board payments. Recently, she has noticed that some of her jewelry has disappeared. Marjorie is left alone for long periods, sometimes for an entire weekend, which is frightening to her because she is physically unable to provide for her own needs and has no access to the telephone. In addition, she becomes dyspneic periodically and experiences chest pressure.

Critical Thinking—Assessment

1. What is the first priority for the nurse in the care of an elderly person who may be a victim of abuse, neglect, or exploitation?
2. What is the best way to assist an elderly patient like Marjorie to disclose feelings, concerns, and fears?
3. What type of mistreatment has Marjorie been experiencing from her daughter and son-in-law?
4. What characteristics require assessment in Marjorie's daughter and son-in-law?

PLANNING

As with other victims of family violence, securing safety is a major aspect in the plan of care for the abused elderly. In the case of Marjorie, stabilizing her congestive heart failure had to be achieved before her abusive home situation could be assessed and before a plan of care for this aspect of her life could be established. Because most states have mandatory elder abuse reporting laws, it is critical that nurses and other health care professionals remain open to the possibility of elder abuse whenever there are potential indicators for it. As noted earlier, many times the elderly will deny the existence of the abuse; therefore it is necessary to establish a trusting relationship with elderly clients to facilitate disclosure. Sengstock and Barrett (1993) suggest that the establishment of trust is the most critical component in planning the care of the abused client. In particular, they warn about being critical of the abuser because the elderly are most likely to strongly defend their loved ones, despite the abuse they have experienced. Because nurses have time constraints in such settings as emergency rooms and clinics, it can be difficult to establish the trust necessary to facilitate disclosure by elderly abused clients. Nevertheless, often it will be the nurse who is in the best position to assess and identify abused clients. Thus the plan of care should include the nurse's taking time to communicate concern, compassion, and a desire to explore options and resources, which can determine whether clients disclose critical information or continue to suffer in silence.

IMPLEMENTATION

As with other cases of family violence, the nurse will often be called on to function as the coordinator of care. In Marjorie's case, the nurse may need to work closely with the social worker to develop and implement the plan of care. Because the nurse has frequent opportunities to discuss Marjorie's problems with her, she will be a key person in assisting Marjorie to identify her feelings, recognize her strengths, realistically assess the situation, and explore all possible options before making decisions. Thus the nurse is in a position to address the total biopsychosocial, spiritual, and cultural needs of the client.

NURSING INTERVENTIONS

As previously mentioned, nursing interventions will focus on meeting the biopsychosocial, spiritual, and cultural needs of the client. Thus the nurse can assist Marjorie to accept the limitations of her congestive heart failure and encourage her to optimize her self-care abilities. It is also very important to assist Marjorie to learn about the community resources that are available to her in terms of maximizing her mental and physical health. Marjorie will require assistance dealing with the guilt and shame she feels about being a burden to her daughter and son-in-law and the abuse they mete out. A plan must be made with the family if Marjorie insists on remaining with them. This plan must clearly explain the family's obligations, Marjorie's rights, and the consequences of abusive or neglectful behavior in the future. As Marjorie's care requirements increase, the potential for greater abuse increases proportionately. Ongoing monitoring and evaluation are necessary, a role that is becoming more important for nurses as they provide ever increasing amounts of care for elderly clients in their homes.

The home health care nurse must be prepared to provide counseling, referrals, support, and education to elderly clients and their families (Table 27-4). Sometimes the caregiver may be in desperate need of stress management techniques, general information on the aging process, basic nursing care principles, and community agencies that provide assistance for the elderly. Providing such support may dramatically ease the burden of caring for the elderly relative and prevent the occurrence of abuse and neglect.

EVALUATION

Evaluating the effectiveness of the outcomes and nursing care plan for elderly who have been abused is important because the abuse may continue and even escalate if elderly clients choose to return to the abusive environment. In a situation like Marjorie's, the potential for escalating abuse is significant because she will probably require increasing assistance from dysfunctional caregivers who are at high risk for continuing the abuse as a result of their substance abuse. However, nurses often are not in a position to follow up with clients once they leave the hospital.

Sengstock and Barrett (1993) claim that certain clues can be helpful in determining whether the nursing inter-

ventions will be successful. These include the willingness of the elderly client to acknowledge the abuse and the willingness of the elderly client and the abusive family members to accept outside interventions and/or removal of the elder from the abusive environment. Although many resources for the elderly exist in most communities, the family cannot be assisted if they deny the existence of the abuse. Like battered women, elderly clients may experience multiple occasions of abuse before they gradually make the decision to leave their abusive environment.

RAPE

In recent years much energy and attention have been devoted to the public discussion of rape. Rape cases involving high profile males are especially prominent in the media. Recently, the U.S. Congress held hearings on sexual assault in the Naval Tailgate event and sexual assault incidents in the U.S. Air Force. As a result of the growing public concern about female sexual assault and feminists' demands for action to prevent this violence, many states have passed laws to protect rape victims and more aggressively prosecute rapists.

The National Institute of Mental Health has also responded to the call for action by increasing funding for

Table 27-4	**Nursing Interventions for the Abused Elderly**
Nursing Interventions	**Rationales**
Monitor the client's response to decreased cardiac output.	Support return of normal cardiac output.
Monitor the client's response to medications.	
Provide reassurance and support.	
Educate the client about medications and limitations.	
Monitor the client for increased depression and suicide potential.	Reduce the client's sense of helplessness and grief; increase feelings of control.
Explore with the client the reasons for feelings of helplessness and grief.	
Discuss the client's capabilities and strengths.	
Explore options that provide the client with increased control.	
Explore ways for the client to increase self-care.	
Explore the client's feelings related to family abuse.	Increase the client's awareness of feelings related to abuse by family.
Explore the client's options for remaining with family versus alternate living arrangements.	Increase the client's awareness of options relating to living arrangements.
Coordinate referrals.	
Show respect for the client's decisions.	
Evaluate the caregiver's motivation for seeking and using assistance.	Evaluate the caregiver's motivation and ability to provide care in the future.
Evaluate family's coping skills.	
Evaluate possible substance abuse by caregiver.	
Evaluate the caregiver's willingness to acknowledge and work on family problems.	

rape research. In addition, stronger federal policies for prosecuting perpetrators of sexual harassment and assault have forced corporations and universities to develop policies and procedures for addressing sexual harassment and sexual assault.

Despite the positive steps that have been taken in recent years to support rape victims, prosecute offenders, and prevent sexual assault, victim blaming persists. Instead of placing blame on the rapist where it belongs, victims are blamed and revictimized in a myriad of ways. The following scenarios are common examples of victim blaming and revictimization.

If a woman cannot provide evidence of resisting a rapist, she is often accused of consenting to the sexual activity.

If the woman was drinking, she is often viewed as causing her own rape.

If the woman was dressed "sensually" or was out late at night, she was "looking for it."

If the woman acted friendly to the rapist, she "led him on or seduced him."

If the rapist spent money on the woman, she "owed" it to him.

No one has the right to verbally or physically force another into sexual activity against his or her will. If a person says "no," that means "no," even if he or she said "yes" first, then changed his or her mind later. Research indicates that programs on rape education can be effective in changing attitudes and myths about rape in college students (Lonsway, 1998).

DEFINITION

The traditional legal definition of **rape** is forced penile-vaginal penetration against the will of the woman. In the last few years, this traditional definition has been expanded by most states and the federal government to include cunnilingus, fellatio, anal intercourse, or any intrusion of any part of a person's body (Koss, 1993). Nonconsent involves physical force, the threat of physical force, or the inability of the victim to consent for reasons such as age, developmental disability, or intoxication.

Estimating the prevalence of rape is difficult because most rapes are not reported and because research studies that attempt to report accurate figures are based on a variety of definitions, screening questions, and samples that are not always representative of the population. Koss (1993) emphasizes that failure to report rape is a much greater problem than false reports of rape. False reports of rape are projected at 2% of reports, the same rate as with other crimes. Conversely, only 10% to 20% of rapes are reported (Botash, Braen, and Gilchrist, 1994).

Studies demonstrate that a range of 20% to 25% of attempted rapes are completed (Koss, 1993; Russell, 1984).

Koss reports that women who are incarcerated and those with a history of psychiatric inpatient treatment have a much higher prevalence of reported rape. Koss concludes that the United States has a major rape problem.

Twenty percent of college women are raped at some time during their college careers. This is consistent with the statistic that the most common age group for rape victims is women between the ages of 16 and 25. In 84% of rape cases the victim is acquainted with the offender. Thus rape by a stranger is the exception rather than the rule (Warshaw, 1988). Furthermore, the physical violence perpetrated by husbands and boyfriends on their intimate female partners is similar to violence perpetrated by strangers (Stermac, DuMont, and Dunn, 1998).

Rather than the dark alley, rapes most commonly occur on dates, at parties, and at other social functions. Although society may believe that rapists are "sick or psychopathic," research has failed to find support for such general personality patterns. A growing body of research indicates that many males are sexually aggressive and force their partners into sex. A common male attitude is that women exist to satisfy males, therefore consent is unnecessary. Scully and Marolla (1993) discuss several decades of research on male sexual aggression and conclude that such behavior is viewed as "normal." By not addressing the sexually aggressive behavior of many males and by maintaining the myth that all rapists are psychotic, society avoids its responsibility to examine most rapes within the context of learned and socially sanctioned male behavior.

CHARACTERISTICS OF A RAPIST

A common myth about rapists is that most are males of color. Botash, Braen, and Gilchrist (1994) report that most perpetrators and victims are white; in 90% of cases victims and perpetrators are of the same race.

Although research has focused on individual characteristics of rapists rather than group behavior, in recent years more attention has been focused on fraternities on college campuses as a rape-prone social context. Martin and Hummer (1993), in their study on fraternities and rape on campus, conclude that fraternities provide a physical and sociocultural context that encourages the sexual coercion of women. These researchers acknowledge that not all fraternity men are rapists. Nevertheless, they insist that because of the type of men that are recruited, the social expectations of these organizations, and the lack of university or community supervision, the incidence of rape increases in fraternities. Martin and Hummer dismiss the notion of peer pressure as an excuse and suggest "that fraternities create a sociocultural context in which the use of coercion in sexual relations with women is normative and in which the mechanisms to keep this pattern of behavior in check are minimal at best and absent at worst." They also report that fraternity men acknowledge using alcohol as a weapon to gain sexual mastery over reluctant women and the very proper sorority girl is particularly prized as a sexual trophy.

EFFECTS OF RAPE ON THE VICTIM

Many rape victims experience devastating effects from their rape. In the past, rape was frequently viewed as unwanted sex with few if any negative consequences. At present, society is much more aware of the serious short- and long-term effects of rape.

In a literature review of the psychologic consequences of rape, Resick (1993) reports that 1 month after the rape a majority of women continued to experience significant fear, depression, sexual dysfunction, and social adjustment problems. Most women report a decrease of symptoms after 2 to 3 months. One year after the rape, however, many victims continued to experience these symptoms when compared with a control group of women who had not been raped. About one third of women continued to experience distress 3 to 6 years after the rape. Resick reports that the symptoms in this third of the women became chronic and generally involved posttraumatic stress disorder, depression, anxiety, sexual dysfunctions, and social adjustment problems. In addition, rape victims reported feeling more anger, hostility, and confusion than nonvictims and were more likely to use alcohol and drugs.

Not all women experience long-term serious effects from being raped. Many factors can account for these differences among rape victims, but much more research is needed before the interrelationships among these factors can be understood (Resick, 1993). Currently, research evidence is unclear as to whether demographic factors such as age, socioeconomic status, and race have significant effect on rape trauma. However, prior psychologic functioning and life stressors are reported to be important in the development of long-term effects from rape. Women with mental health problems, revictimization, and multiple-incident revictimization seem to have more difficulty overcoming long-term effects of rape. Resick reports that preassault, assault, and postassault factors may all influence the psychologic functioning of the rape victim.

Although a variety of victim responses to rape occur, rape is a traumatic experience and its victims require immediate attention and support from health care professionals. Evidence of the rape must be gathered and documented, laboratory tests for pregnancy and sexually transmitted diseases must be performed, and the victim must be referred to an experienced counselor or rape crisis center.

As with victims of family violence, nurses are often in a position to assist victims of rape. It is incumbent on the professional nurse to accept responsibility for becoming knowledgeable and skillful in assisting rape victims. This assistance may take a variety of forms including identification and support for disclosure, as well as therapeutic interventions to facilitate recovery of this often neglected population.

Summary of Key Concepts

1. Violence and abusive behaviors are major public health concerns.
2. Because nurses assume many roles in such a variety of settings, they are in prime positions to advocate and intervene for those who are victims of family violence.
3. Interpersonal violence is more likely to be done by someone the victim knows.
4. Battering is the most common cause of injury to women in the United States.
5. Domestic violence is generally defined as physical, psychologic, and sexual abuse primarily directed at women by men for the purpose of maintaining control and power.
6. Emotional and psychologic abuse can be just as devastating as direct physical abuse.
7. Most child physical and sexual abuse is perpetrated by an adult the child knows.
8. Actions that ensure protection and safety for the victim are the most important nursing interventions in abusive situations.
9. Elder abuse is becoming a greater public concern because the number of elderly persons in the population is growing.

REFERENCES

Ammerman RT, Hersen M: *Assessment of family violence: a clinical and legal sourcebook*, New York, 1992, John Wiley & Sons.

American Medical Association Council on Scientific Affairs: Violence against women: relevance for medical practitioners, *JAMA* 267:3184, 1992.

American Professional Society on Abused Children Task Force: *Guidelines for psychosocial evaluation of suspected sexual abuse in young children*, Chicago, 1990, The Task Force.

Ascione FR: Battered women's reports of their partners' and their children's cruelty to animals, *J Emotional Abuse* 1:119, 1998.

Avni N: Battered wives: characteristics of their courtship days, *J Interpers Violence* 6:232, 1991.

Bandura A: *Aggression: a social learning analysis*, Morristown, NJ, 1973, Prentice Hall.

Barbee EL: Ethnicity and woman abuse in the United States. In Sampselle C, editor: *Violence against women*, New York, 1992, Hemisphere.

Barnett OL, Miller-Perrin CL, Perrin R: *Family violence across the lifespan: an introduction*, Thousand Oaks, Calif, 1997, Sage.

Becker JV: Offenders: characteristics and treatment. In Behrman RE, editor: *The future of children: sexual abuse of children*, Los Altos, Calif, 1994, The Center for the Future of Children, The David and Lucille Packard Foundation.

Berkowitz CD et al: American Medical Association diagnostic and treatment guidelines on child physical abuse and neglect, *Arch Fam Med* 1:187, 1992.

Bograd M: Feminist perspectives on wife abuse: an introduction. In Yllo K, Bograd M, editors: *Feminist perspectives on wife abuse*, Newbury Park, Calif, 1988, Sage.

Bohn D, Parker B: Domestic violence and pregnancy. In Campbell J, Humphreys J, editors: *Nursing care of survivors of family violence*, St. Louis, 1993, Mosby.

Botash AS, Braen GR, Gilchrist VJ: Acute care for sexual assault victims, *Patient Care* 28:112, 1994.

Bourg S, Stock HV: A review of domestic violence arrest statistics in a police department using pro-arrest police, *J Fam Violence* 9:177, 1994.

Brendtro M, Bowker LH: Battered women: how can nurses help? *Issues Ment Health Nurs* 10:169, 1989.

Briere J: *Child abuse trauma*, Newbury Park, Calif, 1992, Sage.

Briere J: *Therapy for adults molested as children: beyond survival*, New York, 1996, Springer.

Burgess A et al: Child molestation: assessing impact in multiple victims (part 1), *Arch Psychiatr Nurs* 1:33, 1987.

Campbell JC, Fishwick N: Abuse of female partners. In Campbell JC, Humphreys J, editors: *Nursing care of survivors of family violence*, St. Louis, 1993, Mosby.

Campbell JC, Humphreys J: *Nursing care of survivors of family violence*, St. Louis, 1993, Mosby.

Carmen E, Rieker PP: A psychosocial model of the victim-to-patient process, *Psychiatr Clin North Am* 12:431, 1989.

Chaffin M: Research in action: assessment and treatment of child sexual abusers, *J Interpersonal Violence* 9:224, 1994.

Cohen MA, Miller T: The cost of mental health care for victims of crime, *J Interpersonal Violence* 13:93, 1998.

Courtois C: *Healing the incest wound*, New York, 1988, Norton.

Deblinger E et al: Psychosocial characteristics and correlate of symptom distress in nonoffending mothers of sexually abused children, *J Interpersonal Violence* 8:155, 1993.

Edleson JL, Eisikovits ZC: *Future interventions with battered women and their families*, Thousand Oaks, Calif, 1996, Sage.

Eilenberg J et al: Quality and use of trauma histories obtained from psychiatric outpatients through mandated inquiries, *Psychiatr Serv* 47:165, 1996.

Elliot M: *Female abuse of children*, New York, 1993, Guilford.

Flitcraft AH: American Medical Association diagnostic and treatment guidelines on domestic violence, *Arch Fam Med* 1:39, 1992.

Gelles RJ: *Intimate violence in families*, Thousand Oaks, Calif, 1997, Sage.

Gelles RJ, Cornell CP: *Intimate violence in families*, Newbury Park, Calif, 1990, Sage.

Giardino A et al: *A practical guide to the evaluation of sexual abuse in the prepubertal child*, Newbury Park, Calif, 1992, Sage.

Graham-Bermann SA, Levendosky AA: Traumatic stress symptoms in children of battered women, *J Interpersonal Violence* 13:111, 1998.

Henderson J: Incest. In Freedman AM, Kaplan HI, Sadock BS, editors: *Comprehensive textbook of psychiatry*, Baltimore, 1975, Williams & Wilkins.

Herman J: *Trauma and recovery*, 1992, New York, Basic Books.

Holden GW, Geffner R, Jouriles EN: *Children exposed to marital violence: theory, research and applied issues*, Washington, DC, 1998, American Psychological Association.

Humphreys J, Ramsey AM: Child abuse. In Campbell J, Humphreys J, editors: *Nursing care of survivors of family violence* St. Louis, 1993, Mosby.

Jacobson A, Herald C: The relevance of childhood sexual abuse to adult psychiatric inpatient care, *Hosp Community Psychiatry* 41:154, 1990.

Jehu D: Adult survivors of sexual abuse. In Ammerman R, Hersen M, editors: *The assessment of family violence*, New York, 1992, John Wiley & Sons.

Kempe CH et al: The battered child syndrome, *JAMA* 181:17, 1962.

Kendall-Tackett K, Williams LM, Finkelhor D: Impact of sexual abuse on children: a review and synthesis of recent empirical studies, *Psychol Bull* 113:164, 1993.

King MC, Ryan J: Abused women: dispelling myths and encouraging intervention, *Nurse Pract* 14:47, 1989.

Koss MP: Detecting the scope of rape, *J Interpersonal Violence* 8:198, 1993.

Kurz D: 18 Social science perspectives on wife abuse: current debates and future directions. In Bart PB, Moran EG, editors: *Violence against women*. Newbury Park, Calif, 1993, Sage.

Limandri BJ, Tilden VP: Nurses' reasoning in the assessment of family violence, *Image J Nurs Sch* 28:247, 1996.

Lonsway KA: Beyond "No means no": outcomes of an intensive program to train peer facilitators for campus acquaintance rape education, *J Interpersonal Violence* 13:73, 1998.

Martin PY, Hummer RA: Fraternities and rape on campus. In Bart PB, Moran EG, editors: *Violence against women*, Newbury Park, Calif, 1993, Sage.

McFarlane J, Parker B: *Abuse during pregnancy*, White Plains, NY, 1994, March of Dimes Birth Defects Foundation.

Pagelow MD: Response to Hamberger's comments, *J Interpersonal Violence* 8:137, 1993.

Pillemer KA: Risk factors in elder abuse: results from a case-control study. In Pillimer KA, Wolf R, editors: *Elder abuse: conflict in the family*, Dover, England, 1986, Auburn House.

Pillemer KA, Finkelhor D: The prevalence of elder abuse: a random sample survey, *Gerontologist* 28:51, 1988.

Quinsey VL, Rice ME, Harris GT: Actuarial prediction of sexual recidivism, *J Interpersonal Violence* 10:85, 1995.

Quinsey VL, Walker WD: Dealing with dangerousness: community risk management strategies with violent offenders. In Peters RD, editor: *Aggression and violence throughout the life span*, Newbury Park, Calif, 1992, Sage.

Reel SJ: Violence during pregnancy, *Crit Care Nurs Clin North Am* 9:149, 1997.

Renzetti CM: *Violent betrayal: partner abuse in lesbian relationships*, Newbury Park, Calif, 1992, Sage.

Resick P: The psychological impact of rape, *J Interpersonal Violence* 8:223, 1993.

Russell D: *Sexual exploitation*, Beverly Hills, Calif, 1984, Sage.

Russell D: *The secret trauma*, New York, 1986, Basic Books.

Ryan G, Lane S, editors: Juvenile offenders: defining the population. In Ryan G, Lane S, editors: *Juvenile sexual offending*, Lexington, Mass, 1991, Lexington Books.

Sampselle CM: *Violence against women*, New York, 1992, Hemisphere.

Scully D, Marolla J: Riding the bull at Gilley's: convicted rapists describe the rewards of rape. In Bart EP, Moran G, editors: *Violence against women*, Newbury Park, Calif, 1993, Sage.

Sengstock MC, Barrett S: Abuse and neglect of the elderly in family settings. In Campbell JC, Humphreys J, editors: *Nursing care of survivors of family violence*, St. Louis, 1993, Mosby.

Stark E, Flitcraft A: *Women at risk: domestic violence and womens' health*, Thousand Oaks, Calif, 1996, Sage.

Stermac L, DuMont J, Dunn S: Violence in known-assailant sexual assaults, *J Interpersonal Violence* 13:398, 1998.

Straus MA, Sugarman DB, Giles-Sims: Spanking by parents and subsequent antisocial behavior of children, *Arch Pediatr Adolesc Med* 151:761, 1997.

Tatara T: Understanding the nature and scope of domestic elder abuse with the use of state aggregate data: summaries of the key findings of a national survey of state APS and aging agencies, *J Elder Abuse Neglect* 5:35, 1993.

Urbancic J: Intrafamilial sexual abuse. In Campbell J, Humphries J, editors: *Nursing care of survivors of family violence*, St. Louis, 1993, Mosby.

U.S. Bureau of Census: *Statistical abstract of the U.S. 1994 census*, ed 114, Washington, DC, 1994, The Bureau.

U.S. Department of Labor, Women's Bureau: Domestic violence: a workplace issue. In *Facts on working women*, No. 96.3, Washington, DC, 1996, The Bureau.

van der Kolk BA, McFarlane AC, Weisaeth L: Traumatic stress: the effects of overwhelming experience on mind, body, and society, New York, 1996, Guilford.

Walker LE: *Abused women and survivor therapy*, Washington, DC, 1994, American Psychological Association.

Wang CT, Daro D: *Current trends in child abuse reporting and fatalities: the results of the 1997 annual fifty state survey*, Chicago, 1998, Prevent Child Abuse America.

Warshaw C: Limitations of the medical model in the care of battered women, *Gender Sociology* 3:506, 1989.

Warshaw R: *I never called it rape*, San Francisco, 1988, Harper Row.

Wolf R: Abuse of the elderly. In Gelles R, editor: *Visions 2010: families & violence, abuse and neglect*, Minneapolis, 1995, National Council on Family Relations.

Wyatt GE: The sexual abuse of Afro-American and White-American women in childhood, *Child Abuse Negl* 9:507, 1985.

CHAPTER 28

Suicide

Pamela E. Marcus

OBJECTIVES

- Discuss the scope of suicide by age, gender, ethnicity, socioeconomic status, and familial factors.

- Compare and contrast biologic, psychologic, and sociologic theories regarding the etiology of suicide.

- Distinguish between suicidal ideation, gesture, threat, attempt, and successful suicide.

- Discuss key elements in the assessment of suicide risk.

- Apply the nursing process for suicidal clients and their families.

- Construct a nursing care plan for a client admitted to the psychiatric care unit with depression and suicidality.

- Describe the responsibility of mental health professionals in protecting patients from self-harm.

- Debate the role of parents and significant adults in observing self-destructive clues in youth and in offering guidance and assistance.

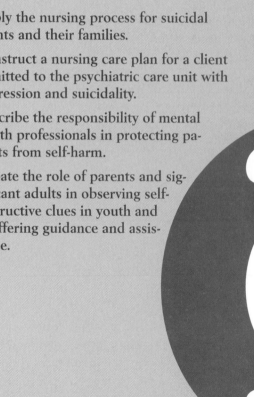

SUICIDE

Suicide, the act of taking one's own life, is a major public health and mental health problem in the United States. It is among the leading causes of death for youth between the ages of 15 and 24. The suicide rate for the elderly population is growing faster than the rate for any other age-group. In 1992 McIntosh noted that the completed suicide rate for older adults was 21 per 100,000 in the United States. It is anticipated that this rate will increase as more individuals enter their older years.

Suicidal thoughts, threats, and attempts often precede clients' search for mental health treatment in a variety of settings. Imminent risk for suicide is one of the leading criteria for medical care of clients admitted to psychiatric hospitals. Health professionals in all disciplines increasingly are being called on to assist with assessing suicide risk and ensuring that clients receive prompt intervention to provide physical and psychologic safety. Nurses are positioned strategically to contribute to these efforts by the nature of the broad scope of their practice in multiple health care settings.

HISTORICAL AND THEORETIC PERSPECTIVES

World history includes many references to suicide as a religious, psychologic, or social phenomenon. Suicide was considered both a spiritual offense and a legal offense against the king in Europe, dating back to 673 AD. Those who commited suicide were not allowed a Christian burial, and all of their possessions were forfeited to the king unless it was determined that the suicide was a result of madness or physical illness (Celo-Cruz, 1992). Shakespeare wrote of suicide in *Romeo and Juliet* and in *Macbeth*. Suicides increased

Cognitive rigidity The inability to adequately identify problems and corresponding solutions.

Comorbidity The occurrence of two or more disorders in the same individual at the same time.

Conscious suicidal intention A state of awareness characterized by a desire to bring about one's own death.

Imminence The likelihood that an event will occur within a specific time period.

Lethality The potential for causing death related to the level of danger associated with the suicidal plan, along a continuum from low to high probability (e.g., aspirin overdose versus a gunshot wound to the head).

Parasuicidal behavior Suicidal gestures and attempts that are unsuccessful and of low lethality (e.g., superficial cutting of the wrists).

Perturbation A determination of an individual's level of distress, developed by Shneidman and rated on a scale of 1 to 9. Refers to how upset, disturbed, or perturbed the individual is.

Suicide The act of taking one's own life.

Suicidal ideation Thoughts of suicide; including a plan and thoughts about how it would be to end one's life.

Suicidology The scientific and humane study of human self-destruction.

Unconscious suicidal intention A state outside of awareness during which persons engage in risk-taking behaviors that have a high likelihood of causing their deaths.

following the stock market crash in 1929 and during the Great Depression as people took their own lives rather than face financial ruin and humiliation. Japan's kamikaze pilots of World War II elevated suicide to a high cultural level as they sacrificed their lives for their country and their religious principles.

Throughout history, suicide has served as a solution to the disappointments and obstacles that people have faced. It was not until the late 1800s that pioneers such as Durkheim, a sociologist, and Freud, a psychoanalyst, began to study the phenomenon from theoretic viewpoints.

SOCIOLOGIC THEORY

Durkheim, in his classic work of 1897, classified the social and cultural aspects of suicide into four subtypes: anomic, egoistic, altruistic, and fatalistic (Durkheim, 1951). He defined anomic suicides as acts of self-destruction by individuals who have become estranged from important relationships in their groups, especially as this estrangement relates to their standard of living (e.g., the suicides after the 1929 stock market crash). Durkheim characterized egoistic suicides as self-inflicted deaths of individuals who are influenced to turn against their own conscience (e.g., the suicide of a devout Catholic adolescent after she has had an abortion forbidden by her religion). Durkheim described altruistic suicides as self-inflicted deaths based on obedience to a group's goals that override the person's own best interests (e.g., the kamikaze pilot incidents). Finally, he defined fatalistic suicides as self-inflicted deaths resulting from excessive regulation (e.g., the suicides of felons who hang themselves in prison to escape oppression).

PSYCHOANALYTIC THEORY

Freud viewed suicide from a psychoanalytic viewpoint. At the 1910 psychoanalytic meeting on suicide in Vienna, he and Stekel described self-destruction as hostility directed inward toward the internalized love object (Freud, 1920; Stekel, 1967). These early formulations ignored other critical feeling states, such as shame, hopelessness, helplessness, worthlessness, and fear. Later, Freud incorporated many accompanying psychologic and sociologic clinical features, such as guilt, into his views about suicide (Litman, 1967). Freud identified three features that he believed made each individual somewhat vulnerable to suicide (Litman, 1967):

1. The death instinct
2. The splitting of the ego when the individual is unable to assume mastery over his or her instincts and has to conform to others' wishes or die
3. The influence of group institutions, such as family and society, that require compliance from each member of the group through guilt

Psychoanalytic theorists following Freud have added their own perspectives to the notion of suicide (Weiss, 1966). Menninger described several sources of suicidal impulses: the wish to kill, the wish to be killed, and the wish to die. According to Jung, the suicidal person holds an unconscious wish for spiritual rebirth after feeling that life has lost its meaning. Adler identified the importance of inferiority, narcissism, and low self-esteem in suicidal acts. Horney believed suicide to be a solution for someone experiencing extreme alienation of self as a result of great disparity between the idealized self and the perceived psychosocial self (Weiss, 1966).

INTERPERSONAL THEORY

Sullivan broadened the theoretic knowledge base of suicide by emphasizing the importance of interpersonal relationship factors. According to him, persons can never be isolated from the interactions of significant people in their lives (Sullivan, 1931). Therefore, Sullivan believed, the suicidal act should be understood within the context of the perceptions of the suicidal person by his or her significant others. He viewed suicide as evidence of failure to resolve interpersonal conflicts (Sullivan, 1956).

These classic sociologic, psychodynamic, and interpersonal theories formed the foundation for the major contemporary etiologies that followed in the 1960s.

ETIOLOGY

The contemporary, scientific, and humane study of suicide, called **suicidology**, began in the early 1960s when several important events occurred (Shneidman, 1969):

1. The Center for Studies of Suicide Prevention was established at the National Institute of Mental Health in 1966.
2. The American Association of Suicidology was founded in 1967.
3. The *Bulletin of Suicidology*, the first professional journal devoted to the study of self-destruction phenomena, began publication in 1967.
4. There was an increase in the number of suicide prevention centers, from 3 in 1958 to more than 100 in 1968.
5. The 1910 Viennese psychoanalytic meetings on suicide were reconvened at the first annual conference of the American Association of Suicidology in Chicago in 1968. Shneidman and his colleagues led the discussion of innovations in the prevention of suicide.

BIOLOGIC FACTORS

The structure and chemistry of the brain have been studied most thoroughly in relation to affective or mood disorders (see Chapter 13). Neurotransmitters, or certain chemicals in the brain that regulate mood, have been identified (e.g., serotonin, dopamine, norepinephrine, and γ-aminobutyric acid [GABA]). Recently, research with adults has suggested that irregularities in the serotonin system are found in suicidal clients. In a 1994 study by Nielson and colleagues, the major metabolite of serotonin, 5-hydroxyindoleacetic acid (5-HIAA), which is found in cerebrospinal fluid, was studied in conjunction with the genotype, tryptophan hydroxylase (TPH). This was the first report to implicate a specific gene in the predisposition to certain antisocial and suicidal behavior that were postulated to be regulated by serotonin (Nielson et al, 1994) (See Understanding & Applying Research box).

Currently there are no medications that specifically affect suicidal behavior. However, medications that regulate serotonin levels are effective in the treatment of mood disorders that often accompany suicidal ideation (see Chapters 13 and 23).

Another psychologic factor is the neurobiologic correlation of depression and suicide. Suicide is most often correlated with depression, and as depression resolves, suicide risk diminishes. According to Cummings (1993), the dimensions of depression can be correlated with alterations in specific areas of the brain (see Chapters 4 and 13).

Mood: Sadness and dysphoria are associated with limbic lesions that can be moderated with dopamine.

Affect: Separate motor systems of the limbic and brain stem regions of the brain influence control of the face and facial expressions and the muscular responses associated with emotional affect (e.g., crying).

Motivation: Changes in the pleasure response, which is moderated by dopamine and dopamine antagonists, are correlated with motivational levels.

Understanding & Applying Research

Family and twin studies have suggested a genetic component to certain antisocial and suicidal behaviors. This study found that the genotype tryptophan hydroxylase (THP) was a factor influencing the neurotransmitter serotonin and its principal metabolite, 5-hydroxyindoleacetic acid (5-HIAA), found in the cerebrospinal fluid.

The THP genotype was found in 56 impulsive and 14 nonimpulsive Finnish alcoholic violent offenders and in 20 healthy volunteers with no mental disorders. All subjects were evaluated for documented histories of severe suicide attempts. THP analysis and 5-HIAA concentration levels in the cerebrospinal fluid were obtained by investigators who were unaware of whether they were studying the subjects or the volunteers. A significant association of the THP genotype with violent offenders who had histories of severe suicide attempts was found. If replicated, the findings of this study could lead to an improved ability to identify individuals at risk for suicide and to suggest pharmocologic or genetic interventions. This information could assist nurses in improving their assessment of clients for suicide risk and in determining the most appropriate interventions.

Nielsen D et al: Suicidality and 5-hydroxyindoleacetic acid, concentration associated with tryptophan hydroxylase polymorphism, *Arch Gen Psychiatry* 51:34, 1994.

Cognitive content: Frontal lobe dysfunction is thought to be related to feelings of hopelessness and worthlessness, both of which are precursors to suicidal thoughts.

The explosion of knowledge in psychobiology requires that nurses integrate the psychophysiologic aspects of illness with the behavioral sciences in their own nursing practice. Trygstad (1994), in a descriptive study of the perceived psychobiologic learning needs of psychiatric mental health nurses, identified five areas of focus, which are listed in Box 28-1.

PSYCHOLOGIC FACTORS

Intrapsychic and interpersonal theories continue to dominate the psychologic view of suicidal behavior. Contemporary etiologies include (Linehan, 1993; Masterson, 1976):

Self-directed aggression or self-destruction as an act of murder directed at the love object toward whom the person feels ambivalent, leading to states of isolation and loneliness

Death as an atonement for wrongdoings

Death as a way to recapture the lost love object

Suicidal death as a secondary result of the major depressive processes

Suicidal ideation and parasuicidal behavior due to abandonment anxiety

Box 28-1   Focus Areas for Psychiatric Mental Health Nurses

1. Knowledge of medications
2. Recognition of medications and physical conditions interacting with other substances (e.g., illicit drugs and over-the-counter drugs)
3. Skills to manage the therapeutic milieu as it is influenced by both chronic and acute medical problems
4. Maintenance of client safety and the management of sensory and environmental factors influencing safety
5. Self-care skills for the caregiver

Most psychodynamic theorists following Freud have theorized that depression follows the loss of a significant love object and leads to feelings of helplessness, hopelessness, guilt, and diminished self-esteem. Suicide can serve as a way to end those painful feeling states (Toolan, 1974). This model emphasizes the functioning of the psyche and the reporting of subjective experiences. Case studies of individuals and a small series of similar cases were examined to identify the mental mechanisms that led to suicide attempts or completions (Andreasen, 1984).

Cognitive theory adds to the understanding of suicidal episodes by emphasizing the role of particular thought patterns: negativism, self-worthlessness, and a bleak view of the future. **Cognitive rigidity**, the inability to identify problems and solutions, has been hypothesized as a factor in suicide when accompanied by stress (Rudd et al, 1994).

Shneidman (1985) developed the term **perturbation**, defined as a determination of an individual's level of distress and rated on a scale of 1 to 9. Perturbation refers to how upset, disturbed, or perturbed the individual is. Shneidman (1985), building on his 35 years of work as a suicidologist, lectured about the common psychologic features of suicide. He defined suicide as a "response to an inner decision that the pain is unendurable, intolerable, and unacceptable. It is an unwillingness to endure that pain rather than the pain itself." He outlined the 10 psychologic commonalities of suicide from his studies (Box 28-2).

Feelings of abandonment and abandonment anxiety are important to understand in order to prevent a suicidal gesture in clients with interpersonal disturbances, especially in individuals with borderline personality disorder (Linehan, 1993; Masterson, 1976) (see Chapter 15).

In addition, the development of behavioral approaches based on learning theory contributed to the understanding and treatment of mental health problems. Interventions for suicidal ideation based on learning theory are directed toward decreasing unpleasant events and increasing pleasant events. Tension-reducing relaxation techniques, stress management skills, and rehearsal of problem-solving techniques are valuable adjuncts to reducing depression and suicidal behavior (Lewinsohn and Mischel, 1980).

**Box 28-2   Psychologic Commonalities
                             of Suicide**

1. The common *purpose* of suicide is to solve a
   problem. The health care professional must assist
   the suicidal person in identifying the life problem
   that needs to be solved or changed.
2. The common *goal* of suicide is the cessation of consciousness (i.e., death).
3. The common *stimulus* of suicide is intolerable psychologic pain, along with the decision not to experience that pain.
4. The common *stressor* in suicide is frustrated psychologic needs, such as achievement, affiliation, aggression, autonomy, dominance, harm avoidance, shame
   avoidance, nurturance, order, or play.
5. The common *emotions* of suicide are helplessness
   and hopelessness.
6. The common *cognitive state* is ambivalence.
7. The common *perceptual state* is constriction with
   pain, frustration of needs, and helplessness.
8. The common *action* of suicide is aggression or
   exiting the scene.
9. The common *interpersonal act* is the communication
   of intention.
10. The common *consistency* in suicide is lifelong pat-
    terns of failure, stress, duress, and threats to self-
    esteem.

**Box 28-3   Etiologic Factors Related
                             to Suicide**

Biologic Factors

The neurotransmitters—principally serotonin, dopamine,
   norepinephrine, and γ-aminobutyric acid (GABA)—
   have been linked through extensive research to emotional responses.
Serotonin plays a major role in regulating mood and influences the occurrence of depression and suicidality.
Genetic influences are being found; a specific gene has
   been implicated in the predisposition to suicide.
Others have found that dimensions of depression, such
   as mood, affect, motivation, and cognitive content, are
   correlated to alterations in specific brain structure.

Psychologic Factors

Self-directed aggression
Unresolved interpersonal conflicts
Negativistic thinking patterns
A reduction in positive reinforcement

Sociologic Factors

Isolation and alienation from social groups
Biopsychosocial influences

SOCIOLOGIC FACTORS

Contemporary sociologists have reinforced Durkheim's
earlier work on suicide. Contemporary social scientists
have supported the idea that alienation from social groups
after disruption of family, community, or social relationships leads some individuals to attempt or commit suicide
(Maris, 1985; Richman, 1986). In a prospective study of
almost 100,000 women from 1970 to 1975 in Norway, sociologists Hoyer and Lund (1993) found empiric support
for Durkheim's notion that marriage and parenthood lead
to a lower suicide rate for women.

Thus the findings of sociologic studies have provided
added dimensions to the biologic and psychologic explanations of suicidal behavior. A more holistic approach is to
consider a biopsychosocial model that integrates all of
these schools of thought in explaining such complex human concepts as suicide (Box 28-3).

EPIDEMIOLOGY
PREVALENCE

Suicide and suicidal behavior are found among persons of
all ages (including young children), among both sexes, and
among all ethnic groups and socioeconomic levels. Wilson
(1994) reported that suicide accounts for nearly 1% of all
deaths in the world. The Hungarians and Finns have suicide rates two to three times those of the United States

and most of Europe. Interestingly, that figure holds true
even when persons of those nationalities emigrate to other
countries, suggesting some biologic influence. Currently in
the United States, there are slightly more than 30,000 suicides annually, or a suicide every 17 minutes, with 12 of
every 100,000 Americans killing themselves. Suicide is
the eighth leading cause of death in the United States
(*Facts About Suicide in the USA*, 1993).

Age

The two most vulnerable age-groups for suicide are the elderly and youth ages 15 to 24 years.

The elderly.   Rates of suicide are highest among the older
population, age 65 years and above. Older adults have suicide rates 50% higher than those of the nation as a whole.
In 1987, older Caucasian men had a suicide rate of 46
deaths per 100,000 population. The prevalence rate for
older Caucasian men is substantially higher than that for
African-American men, Caucasian women, and African-
American women (U.S. Senate Special Committee on Aging, Federal Council on Aging, and U.S. Department of
Health and Human Services, 1991). Figure 28-1 shows
that Caucasian men age 85 years and older are most at
risk, with a suicide rate of 72 deaths per 100,000.

Shneidman (1985) has suggested that the high suicide
rates among the elderly represent failure to adapt to significant losses, the inability to endure emotional pain, and
pessimistic attitudes toward the aging process that are related to loneliness, illness, rejection by family and society,

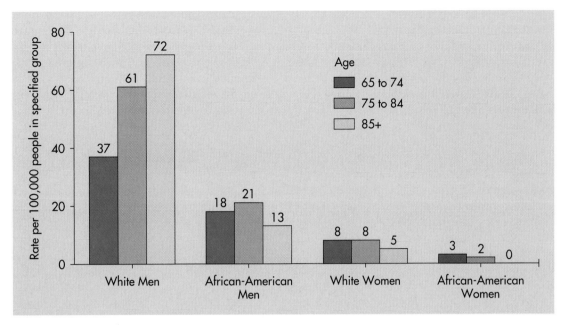

Figure 28-1   Suicide rates of people 65 and older by age and race, 1987. (From National Center for Health Statistics: *Health, United States, 1989*, DHHS Pub No. [PHS]90-1232, Washington, DC, 1990, U.S. Department of Health and Human Services.)

sudden termination of meaningful work, disruption of long-standing relationships, and feelings of emptiness. As the population ages and seniors become the dominant subgroup, suicide may increasingly become a major public health problem. A study relating to suicidal thought and self-transcendence found that elderly clients who experienced a loss of meaning in their lives were at greater risk for suicide completion, especially if they had lost the will to live (Buchanan, Farran, and Clark, 1995).

Youth.   Young people ages 15 to 24 have a suicide rate approximately 200% higher than that in the 1950s. The rates have stabilized since the 1970s. However, suicide now ranks as the third leading cause of death for youth, after accidents and homicides (*Facts*, 1993). Currently the rate is about 6000 suicides a year, with 400,000 teenagers attempting suicide a year. As many as 11% of all high school students have made at least one suicide attempt.

Although there are few studies related to suicide rates for children under the age of 15, some statistical and anecdotal studies have chronicled successful suicide attempts in this age-group. Children as young as 2½ years of age have attempted suicide. In 1985 there were 278 suicide deaths of children 5 to 14 years of age in the United States (Valente, 1989). Wolk and Weissman (1996) studied data from 226 individuals who had been depressed as children to determine the rate of suicidal behavior. They concluded that 4% of these individuals had completed suicide and that 37% of the individuals who had depression as chil-

dren had reported suicide attempts. The authors found that 16% of the group who had anxiety disorders as children had attempted suicide and that 6% of the individuals in the normal control group had attempted suicide. This study emphasizes the importance of childhood depression as a risk factor to assess in order to decrease the potential for suicide attempts in individuals, especially during adolescence.

Gender and Ethnicity

National suicide rates tend to obscure the importance of gender and ethnicity in defining the scope of suicidal behavior. Caucasian suicide rates are approximately twice those of non-Caucasian rates as a whole. Although the high suicide rates of older Caucasian men have been highlighted, it is important to note that suicide rates for African-American men have tripled during the past 25 years among the 85+ age-group. This increased rate of suicide among the oldest African-American men rivals the increased rate among young men ages 15 to 24 for both races (Monk, 1987).

After older Caucasian men, African-American young adult men have the next highest rate of suicide. Males commit suicide at rates three to four times those of females. Although Figure 28-1 indicates that Caucasian and African-American women have comparatively low completed suicide rates, females have the highest rate of suicide attempts (Valente, 1989). Females have been found generally to make three to four times as many attempts, and the female Hispanic suicide attempt rate is higher than that of any other ethnic minority group in the United States (Heacock, 1990).

African-Americans and Hispanics rank below the midrange when compared with the suicide rates of other reporting nations of the world. In the United States, Hispanic and Asian rates of suicide are similar to those of Caucasians. However, there are very few publications detailing the incidence of suicide among Hispanic youth. One article points out that the Hispanic population is not homogeneous and that what may be characteristic of one subgroup may not be of another. For example, rates vary among Puerto Ricans, Dominicans, Cubans, and Mexican-Americans (Smith et al, 1985). Zayas (1978), in an early study, noted that several cultural factors have a bearing on suicide attempts among Hispanic adolescent females, including socioeconomic disadvantages, traditional gender roles, socialization, acculturation, cultural identity, and intergenerational conflict.

Another infrequently studied ethnic group is Native Americans. This oversight is particularly alarming in that Native Americans are often noted to be the ethnic group with the highest suicide rates in the United States, according to the American Association of Suicidology. As with Hispanics, there are great tribal group differences, and Shore demonstrated that suicide rates for certain tribes varied from higher to lower than that of the general population (Shore, 1975). May and Dizmang (1974) stressed that suicide in Native Americans was largely a problem within the male adolescent subgroup. Epidemiologic research focusing on Native American suicide factors warrants a higher profile.

Socioeconomic Status

Suicide crosses all socioeconomic levels. In fact, studies show that poverty and unemployment contribute to high suicide rates and, conversely, that a high gross national product per capita and a high quality of life with associated stresses also contribute to suicidal behavior. Yang et al (1992) studied the sociologic and economic theories of suicide and found high unemployment rates to be positively related to suicide rates. They argued that people's expectations of decreased future income because of unemployment lead to an increased probability of suicide. Marshall (1978) found a correlation between increased suicide rates and decreased income status among older Social Security recipients.

Zayas (1978) found that socioeconomic disadvantages such as poverty, substandard housing, unemployment, crime, victimization, poor health care, and poor education contributed to the high rate of suicidal behavior among Hispanics. By contrast, Lester (1984) demonstrated that nations with a higher quality of life and income also had higher suicide rates but for different reasons. A high quality of life leaves fewer external events on which to blame one's misfortune and failures, and thus inner-directed ag-

gression may occur. Yang et al (1992) have postulated that economic prosperity produces a social environment that is conducive to suicidal behavior: urbanization, often a by-product of prosperity, leads to a decline in social cohesion or an increase in social isolation, and a quickened pace of life increases stress for individuals. Thus both economic well-being and poverty can create circumstances leading to the choice of suicide as a solution to stressful events.

Familial Influences

Suicidal behavior is frequently a symptom of prolonged and progressive family disruption and dysfunction. In addition, significant changes in the family, such as divorce; death of a spouse, parent, or child; and social isolation contribute to high suicide rates (Blazer, 1989).

The family is most influential in the lives of children and adolescents and contributes to the incidence of suicidal behavior in those age-groups. A suicidal adolescent may feel estranged from family members and may experience rejection and a loss of love. Actual physical or psychologic loss, as in death, separation, or emotional distancing from the family, is thought to be one of the most significant factors in the high incidence of adolescent suicides (Husain, 1990).

There is a familial predisposition to suicide in that many suicidal adolescents often have histories of suicidal behavior among their immediate and extended families. Those adolescents who completed suicide more often lost their mothers by suicide before their own deaths than did those who attempted suicide. According to Tishler et al (1981), suicidal behavior among many family members serves as a means of communication or as a language that is understood when other forms of communication fail. Suicidal behavior becomes a learned familial adaptation to problems and stressors.

Familial cultural values also are strong factors in suicidal behavior. For example, in Hispanic families, family honor and family centeredness and cohesiveness are variables that buffer against suicidal behavior or contribute to it. Hispanic youth may experience conflict between traditional Hispanic values and the values of the dominant culture. Intergenerational tension, language barriers, and role conflicts may contribute to mental health problems. Adolescents who can relate positively to the main culture and still have positive relationships with their family members who have more traditional values are often sheltered from such problems.

CO-OCCURRENCE WITH RELATED HEALTH ISSUES

Suicidal behavior is strongly associated with the occurrence of psychiatric disorders and other health-related problems. Psychiatric illness, alcohol and other drug use and abuse, and medical illnesses are important adjuncts to suicidal events. Tanskanen et al (1998) studied smoking and suicidal behavior. They found that individuals who smoked cigarettes had a 43% higher risk of having mild to severe suicidal ideation, as compared with a nonsmoking sample of individuals.

Psychiatric Disorders

The presence of a diagnosable mental disorder increases the risk for suicide, regardless of age. Miles (1977) reviewed more than 100 longitudinal studies of psychiatric clients and concluded that nearly all suicides committed in the United States are committed by persons with a mental disorder. Others concur that the **comorbidity** of mood disorder and substance abuse with suicide is very high. Most investigators report that suicide risk secondary to a mental disorder is higher in men than in women (Monk, 1987). Beautrais et al (1996) found that 90.1% of their research population had an emotional illness at the time of their suicide attempt. The most commonly identified emotional illnesses in this study were mood disorder, substance abuse, conduct disorder or antisocial disorder, and nonaffective psychosis.

Depression.   The single best predictor of suicidal thinking is the presence of a mood disorder. Research indicates that 30% to 70% of all completed suicides are related to depression. Other studies indicate that 10% to 15% of completed suicides are committed by persons specifically diagnosed with major depressive disorder. Depression is a major factor for persons attempting suicide as well (Arato et al, 1988).

Schizophrenia.   Another diagnostic category linked with suicide is schizophrenia. Suicide is the leading cause of premature death in that population, with an estimated 10% incidence of suicide in the first 10 years of the illness and a 15% lifetime incidence (Nyman and Jonsson, 1986). One study reported that clients with schizophrenia expressed high levels of subjective stress and feelings of hopelessness, loneliness, and dissatisfaction with social relationships (Cohen et al, 1990). Since schizophrenia most often has its onset in late adolescence or early young adulthood, the high-risk period for suicide is in the 20- to 30-year age-group. Other risk factors that are associated with suicide completion in this population are active psychotic symptoms, depression, and a history of prior suicide attempts. Other factors include women having a higher completion rate after an acute exacerbation of the illness, as well as depressive symptoms and the use of alcohol (Heilä et al, 1997). This population must be carefully evaluated and reevaluated for suicide risk, particularly during the first 10 years of the illness.

Panic disorder.   There is controversy among views of a co-occurrence factor with panic disorder and suicide attempts. Some studies indicate that there is a high comorbidity of suicidal behavior with panic disorder, major depression, and substance abuse (Lepine et al, 1993). Others

---

> ### ⚠ CLINICAL ALERT
>
> Conflicting findings among researchers may lead nurses and other clinicians to overlook the possible lethality of clients with panic disorder, obsessive-compulsive disorder, and phobias. A careful suicide assessment is required to ensure that this possibility is considered because clients with anxiety disorders may develop depression that could result in suicidality (see Chapter 12).

report that panic disorder is an independent risk factor for suicide or suicidal behavior (Weissman et al, 1989). Others assert that there is evidence to support panic disorder, in conjunction with phobias and obsessive-compulsive disorders, as a risk factor for suicide and suicide attempts (Sakinofsky et al, 1991).

Some researchers have concluded that clients with panic disorder have an increased risk for suicide attempts comparable to that of clients with major depression and are at greater risk than persons without a psychiatric disorder (Johnson, 1990).

Borderline personality disorder.   DSM-IV criteria for borderline personality disorder include "recurrent suicidal behavior, gestures, or threats of self-mutilating behavior" (American Psychiatric Association, 1994). Often the individual with this disorder experiences suicidal behavior when there is a loss or a perceived loss (Gunderson, 1984; Masterson, 1976). Brodsky et al (1997) studied the relationship between the characteristics of individuals with borderline personality disorder and their suicidal behavior. These authors found the trait of impulsivity to be an important risk factor for suicide attempts. It is therefore imperative that the nurse assess the client for impulsive behavioral patterns. This study also found individuals with a history of childhood abuse to have a higher possibility for self-destructive behaviors (Brodsky et al, 1997).

Alcohol and Other Drugs

Of special clinical relevance is the high incidence of concurrence of the use of alcohol and other drugs with suicidal behavior. In a clinical review of eight clients who committed suicide less than 60 days after discharge from one of two psychiatric hospitals from 1988 to 1993, all had been drinking or using other drugs at the time of the completed suicides (Barbee, 1993).

One study of 93 outpatient clients who completed suicide found that the majority of them were young, were male, had a history of drug and alcohol abuse, and had a primary diagnosis of depression. Of the outpatient clients who completed suicide, 62% used drugs, as compared with 18% of all outpatient clients (Earle et al, 1994). In another study of 44 youths who completed suicide, 25% had used alcohol weekly, 11% had used marijuana weekly,

---

Box 28-4   Epidemiology of Suicide

Age, Gender, and Ethnicity

Of the 30,000 completed suicides in the United States annually, the majority are Caucasian males of all ages.

The two groups most at risk are youth ages 15 to 24 years (with suicides increasing at the fastest rate in African-American men ages 19 to 24 years) and Caucasian men over age 65 (with suicides increasing at the fastest rate in men in the 85+ age-group).

Native American adolescent males and Hispanic females are high-risk groups among ethnic minority populations.

Females in general attempt more suicides than males.

Socioeconomic and Familial Factors

Suicide crosses all socioeconomic levels.

Affluent, educated overachievers are as vulnerable to suicide as people at the poverty level who are unemployed, undereducated, living in substandard housing, and often the victims of crime.

Prolonged family disruption and familial predisposition to depression and suicide, biologically or as a learned behavior from other family members, contribute to the incidence rates.

Family turmoil, disturbed parent-child relationships, physical and sexual abuse by family members, and hostile and rejecting parental attitudes have been found to promote suicidal behavior.

Co-occurrence With Related Health Issues

Suicidal behavior is strongly associated with psychiatric disorders.

Mood disorders, substance abuse, schizophrenia, borderline personality disorder, and panic disorders have a co-occurrence with high-risk suicidal behavior.

Depression remains as the single best predictor of suicide risk in all ages.

Suicide is the leading cause of death during the first 10 years of the course of schizophrenic illness.

The research is mixed on the correlation of suicide with panic disorders, but it is thought by most to be associated with suicide risk, especially when panic disorder co-occurs with obsessive-compulsive disorder or phobias.

Independent of another specific psychiatric diagnosis, alcohol use and abuse are highly correlated with most suicidal acts, especially among youth. It is underdiagnosed and underreported among the elderly.

Similarly, chronic physical illness contributes to suicidal behavior. Physical health problems, such as heart disease, hypertension, obesity, and diabetes were found in more than half of the outpatient clients who committed suicide in several studies. The elderly are particularly prone.

---

and 14% had used marijuana daily (Litman and Farberow, 1986). Drugs contribute to poor, impulsive decisions that can lead to high-risk, self-injurious behaviors. A high percentage of alcohol- and drug-related automobile accidents among teens may be suicide attempts (Barbee, 1993).

Research related to the role that alcohol and drugs play in suicidal behavior is somewhat conflicting. Mellick et al (1992) conducted a study focusing on completed suicides of 84 elderly white men in Iowa. The men were found not to have been addicted to drugs and did not have a strong reliance on drugs. These findings contradict the 1976 study by Miller that Mellick and colleagues were replicating. In contrast, Miller's original findings indicated a statistically significant difference between completed suicides and controls in that the former group was addicted to or had a strong reliance on drugs (Miller, 1979). Conflicting results from these studies may result from the the underreporting and underdiagnosing of alcohol and drug problems among the depressed elderly.

Medical Illnesses

Physical health problems have been identified as a component of the profile for persons at risk for suicidal behaviors because of their co-occurrence with depression. The Medical Outcomes Study, one of the first major national studies to link medical illnesses and depression (Wells et al, 1989), found the physical and social dysfunctions associated with depression to be greater than with most chronic medical conditions. Depression is thought to cause as much physical and social impairment as chronic heart disease. In the study, depressed persons perceived their current health as being poor and experienced greater body pain. In comparison with chronic illness, the physical functions of depressed clients were found to be worse than those of clients with hypertension, diabetes, arthritis, and gastrointestinal and back problems. When depression and a medical condition such as advanced coronary artery disease coexisted, the client was noted to suffer nearly twice the loss of social functions that occurred when either condition existed by itself. Suicide risk also was noted to increase in such coexisting conditions (Gonzales et al, 1985).

A complicating factor is that these clients often seek medical care for their health problems, and the coexistence of a depressive disorder is overlooked or missed. A study of 93 completed outpatient suicides found that physical health problems were reported for more than half of the clients who committed suicide. The mean age of the sample was 42 years. The most common problem identified was obesity (14%), followed by heart disease and hypertension (10%), diabetes (8%), asthma (8%), loss of hearing or sight (8%), severe acne or abscess (6%), arthritis (5%), ulcer or stomach problems (4%), epilepsy (4%), and HIV seropositivity (3%) (Earle et al, 1994) (Box 28-4).

Physical health problems often enhance the emotional

```
╔═══════════════════════════════════════════════╗
║ ◆ CLINICAL ALERT                              ║
╠═══════════════════════════════════════════════╣
║ A sudden change in affect for the better or a ║
║ dramatic lifting of depression may be an      ║
║ indication that the person may have resolved  ║
║ ambivalence about living or dying and has     ║
║ made the decision to commit suicide. Increased║
║ energy and the ability to concentrate and plan║
║ the suicidal act facilitate the suicidal      ║
║ actions. Be alert.                            ║
╚═══════════════════════════════════════════════╝
```

CLINICAL DESCRIPTION

The assessment of suicide risk is an important skill for the professional nurse practicing in all clinical settings. Merely voicing a concern about a patient's possible suicidality to other members of the health care team is no longer an adequate or safe response. The nurse needs to use interviewing skills to talk directly with the client and family about suicide during the initial nursing assessment and at points of reassessment in the treatment process. Being alert to the client's past medical history and psychiatric history of suicidal behavior gives the nurse clues for identifying areas for further inquiry.

This section highlights the background information needed to complement the assessment phase of the nursing process. Definitions of the five levels of suicidal behavior are given in Box 28-5, and risk factors are discussed.

Often the five levels of suicidal thought or action are described collectively as "suicidal behaviors," yet it is very important to be specific in naming the types of thoughts and/or actions in the nursing assessment with clear descriptions or examples so that others may judge the level of intent themselves.

pain experienced by suicidal persons and may contribute to their decision to end their life. Nurses play a critical role in assessing clients for depression and suicide risk in medical-surgical health care settings. Alerting the health care team to these findings may help to avert suicide attempts and deaths.

ERRONEOUS BELIEFS ABOUT SUICIDE

Despite the numerous studies done on suicide, the massive efforts to educate people about suicide risk, and the efforts of mental health advocacy groups to break the stigmatized silence about suicidal behavior, erroneous beliefs and myths still exist. It is important to highlight several long-standing erroneous beliefs that can contribute to errors in judgment when assessing for suicidal intent. These beliefs are summarized in Table 28-1.

RISK FACTORS FOR SUICIDE

Nurses should use a knowledge of risk factors to assist in assessing intent and lethality. Risk factors based in part on key points from the epidemiologic findings discussed earlier in the chapter are presented in Box 28-6.

Understanding & Applying Research

An important risk factor to consider when assessing a client for suicide potential is any aborted suicide attempts. This study of a random sample of 135 adult individuals on an inpatient unit dealt with the effect that aborted suicide attempts had on actual suicidal behavior. The authors defined an aborted suicide attempt as occurring when an individual had thoughts about committing suicide and had a lethal plan (e.g., jumping off a high bridge) but aborted the attempt immediately before the planned action. The authors set up the following criteria for an aborted suicide attempt:

The intent to kill oneself
A change of mind immediately before the actual attempt
The absence of injury

The authors interviewed the 135 study participants using a structured interview to collect information about the client's past aborted suicide attempts, the client's actual suicide attempts, the degree of self-destructive intent, and the seriousness of the injuries sustained from the past and present actual suicide attempts. The authors developed a questionnaire called the Aborted Attempts Inventory that collected information about past aborted suicide attempts. For each occurrence of an aborted suicide attempt, the researchers administered the Beck Suicidal Intent Scale.

The information collected from the clients showed that of the 135 subjects, 71 (52.6%) had a lifetime history of having made at least one aborted suicide attempt. Thirty-three (24.4%) had made one aborted attempt, and 38 (28.1%) had made many aborted attempts. Therefore half of the study participants with histories of actual suicide attempts had made at least one aborted suicide attempt; the other half had made several aborted suicide attempts. Individuals who had made aborted suicide attempts actually attempted suicide twice as often as those individuals without aborted suicide attempts. The most common method of an aborted attempt was jumping from a height; the most common method of an actual suicide attempt was an overdose. The authors had no information on aborted attempts and actual suicide completion. This information would be important to gather at a future study.

This research points out the importance of assessing an individual for aborted suicide attempts in the assessment for the individual's level of potential dangerousness to self. This information would allow the nurse to plan and carry out early suicide prevention.

Barber ME et al: Aborted suicide attempts: a new classification of suicidal behavior, *Am J Psychiatry* 155(3):385, 1998.

Table 28-1	Erroneous Beliefs and Facts About Suicide
Erroneous Belief	**Fact**
People who talk about suicide will not commit suicide.	Most people communicate directly about their suicidal intent verbally, in writing, through artwork, and behaviorally through previous suicide attempts. These are all high-risk indicators of suicidal intent. Manipulation is not usually a factor. All messages of intent should be treated seriously.
People who are serious about committing suicide do not give clues.	Most suicidal people give warnings of their intent by giving away possessions; wrapping up business affairs; isolating from friends; demonstrating an increased incidence of accidents; being preoccupied about death in writing, music, and art; and making self-deprecating comments related to worthlessness and hopelessness.
Young children do not commit suicide.	There were 278 suicide deaths of children between the ages of 5 and 14 in 1985 in the United States. All threats from young children should be considered seriously. Suicidal behavior is the leading precipitating event for the psychiatric hospitalization of young children.
An improved mood means the suicide crisis is over.	Persons who completed suicide often showed improved mood and energy before their deaths. It is thought that the improved mood and energy level mean that the person's ambivalence has ended and he or she has made the decision to commit suicide.
Only people with the diagnosis of depression kill themselves.	While depression is the single best indicator of suicial risk, some people who commit suicide are not diagnosed as depressed, although they may experience depressed feelings. At risk are those with schizophrenia, substance-related disorders, panic disorder, posttraumatic stress disorder, obsessive-compulsive disorder, and the manic phase of bipolar disorder. Some people do not exhibit a specific mental disorder at all (e.g., an elderly man who commits suicide after learning that he has terminal cancer or after his beloved wife of 60 years dies suddenly).

Box 28-5   Five Levels of Suicidal Behavior

The following terms are used often in clinical settings to describe the five levels of suicidal thought or action.

1. *Suicidal ideation.* Direct or indirect thoughts or fantasies of suicide or self-injurious acts expressed verbally or through writing or artwork without definite intent or action expressed. May be veiled or expressed symbolically.
2. *Suicide threats.* Direct verbal or written expressions of intent to commit suicide but without action.
3. *Suicide gestures.* Self-directed actions that result in no injury or minor injury by persons who neither intended to end their lives nor expected to die as a result, but were done in such a way that others would interpret the act as suicidal in purpose (e.g., minor scratches on the wrist with a plastic knife).
4. *Suicide attempts.* Serious self-directed actions that may result in minor or major injury by persons who intend to end their lives or cause serious harm to themselves. Gestures and attempts that are unsuccessful and of low lethality are sometimes called **parasuicidal behavior.**
5. *Completed or successful suicides.* Deaths of persons who ended their lives by their own means with conscious intent to die. However, it is important to note that some suicides may occur based on unconscious intent to die (e.g., engaging in high-risk activities).

CLINICAL ALERT

Adolescents who completed suicides experienced the loss of their mothers by suicide before their own deaths more often than those who attempted suicide. A careful family history and a record of previous attempts are critical to the thoroughness of the nursing assessment and the determination of suicide risk.

Of special note is that young children and older adults are less likely to have an explicit plan, thus making the assessment of risk more difficult.

LETHALITY ASSESSMENT FACTORS

In addition to the suicide risk factors, the assessment of **lethality** (the potential for causing death related to the level of danger associated with the suicide plan) must be considered. **Imminence** (the likelihood that an event will occur within a specific time period), intent, and the method chosen and its accessibility are often the three determinants that indicate the level of lethality and the extent of interventions required for safety.

Box 28-6   Risk Factors for Suicide

- *Age.* Persons most at risk for suicide are youth ages 15 to 24 and older adults age 65 and older, with those 85 years and older being the most vulnerable.
- *Sex.* Men by far have a greater incidence of completed suicides. Women have a higher rate of suicide attempts and gestures.
- *Race/ethnicity.* Suicide rates for Caucasians are twice those of non-Caucasians. However, rates for African-American men over age 85 are increasing faster than those for any other group. Second most at risk are young African-American and Native American males.
- *Physical and emotional symptoms.* High-risk indicators are serious depression, significant changes in weight, serious sleep disturbances, extreme fatigue and loss of energy, self-deprecation, anger, feelings of hopelessness, and pre-occupation with themes of death and dying. Serious depression is often the precursor to suicidal behavior.
- *Suicide plan.* The presence and the nature of the suicide plan is one of the most critical factors in assigning suicide risk. A plan clearly signals forethought and intent and often helps determine the level of lethality. Plans that are more precise, detailed, and explicit about the method to be used in the suicide act indicate high risk. If the method described is highly lethal (e.g., a gunshot to the head versus an overdose of pills), and if the method is readily available, the risk is elevated even more. Add alcohol and other drugs, poor impulse control, and limited time for rescue attempts, and the risk reaches a critical level. Plans often include instructions regarding the distribution of possessions and may mention the intent to join a deceased loved one in afterlife, especially if the loved one had committed suicide.
- *History of previous attempts.* The majority of persons who complete suicides have made previous suicide attempts.
- *Social supports and resources.* The availability of a support system for a suicidal person often determines the outcome of an emotional crisis. This "life line" of caring, support, confrontation, and limit setting, as appropriate from family, friends, and community resources, assists suicidal persons in choosing other alternatives in solving their problems. Real or perceived lack of support systems or failure to use the support system that is available increases the risk for suicide significantly.
- *Recent losses.* One of the major emotional determinants of suicidal behavior is real or perceived losses, separations, or abandonments. Unresolved grief reactions can lead to depression and suicidal behavior.
- *Medical problems.* Persons who suffer painful, debilitating, acute or chronic conditions, or terminal illness are of special concern for suicide risk.
- *Alcohol and other drugs.* These substances are often lethal companions to suicidal acts. Drugs may lower inhibition, heighten depression, and quicken impulsivity. It is generally thought that at least 50% of adolescents are legally drunk at the time of their death by suicide and that an even higher percentage have a history of recent alcohol or other drug abuse.
- *Cognition and problem-solving ability.* The inability to identify problems and corresponding solutions adequately greatly contributes to the choice of suicide as a solution to problems.

Imminence Versus Nonimminence

The determination of imminence is critical. If persons are imminently in danger of killing themselves, rapid action must be taken. Determination of imminence, however, is subjective and at best is a clinical judgment based on the professional's experience, knowledge base, and intuition. The specifics of the suicide plan often offer clues as to when the individual will be ready to act.

Some mental health professionals arbitrarily define imminence as the likelihood that the person will engage in suicidal behavior within the next 24 hours. A specific plan, access to lethal measures, behaviors that signal a decision to die, and admission of wanting to die suggest imminent risk for the client. Those who refuse treatment and are at high risk (judged to be imminently dangerous to themselves) can be placed on an involuntary hold-and-treat status by a qualified person, usually for 72 hours, depending on specific state statutes. This allows clinicians to hospitalize these individuals for an evaluation of risk and to determine appropriate treatment recommendations. These clients' rights are protected in order to prevent exploitation and punishment. Those judged not to be imminently in danger of hurting or killing themselves may choose less restrictive treatment options such as partial hospitalization programs or outpatient programs. *Any suicidal thoughts or behaviors, whether ideation, threat, gesture, or attempt, indicate an emergency situation and require prompt assessment* (Bongar, 1991). Suicide risk and imminence usually decrease after support systems are established for those at risk and the cry for help has been answered.

Ideation Versus Intent

Suicidal ideation, or thinking about suicide without clear intent, places a person at lower risk than a person who intends or proposes to die through a suicidal act. There are two categories of intention: conscious and unconscious. **Conscious suicidal intention** is usually characterized by various aspects of awareness (Farberow, 1980):

Awareness of the outcomes or anticipated results of the suicidal behavior

Awareness of others' responses to suicide threats or attempts

Awareness of the lethality index of the chosen method

Awareness of rescue possibilities (i.e., part of the plan includes various avenues of rescue, or the plan is designed so that rescue is difficult or remote; the latter is a more lethal attribute than the former)

Unconscious suicidal intention is often more difficult to assess because it requires a higher level of skill and knowledge of psychodynamic theory. Often, there is a cluster of symptoms characteristic of the dynamics of self-destruction: depression, anxiety, guilt, hostility, and dependency, along with fantasies symbolic of death, hurting others, killing oneself, failure, and hopelessness. The motivation to hurt or kill oneself is outside of awareness yet is often expressed by extreme risk-taking behaviors. For example, some platform parachutists who jump from low heights off stationary objects such as buildings, towers, or cliffs may have unconscious wishes to hurt themselves or end their lives under the guise of an "extreme sport." Others may seek dangerous occupations such as skyscraper workers, bridge builders, and high-wire artists without nets as metaphors for suicidal wishes. Some persons may place themselves in dangerous, vulnerable situations that result in their deaths at the hands of others (e.g., victim-precipitated homicides). Some psychiatric clients unconsciously manipulate others through suicide threats or attempts and unconsciously arrange to be found or rescued. Unfortunately, the rescue plans may fail, resulting in completed suicides.

Fawcett et al (1969) wrote about the importance of the communication of intent among suicidal persons. These authors found that 50% to 70% of higher-risk persons who completed suicides communicated their intent in advance, often only to their significant other. The group that was at moderate risk of suicide communicated by threatening suicide to family members or health care providers.

Nurses should carefully observe and listen for direct and indirect communication regarding clients' suicidal intent. They should listen not only for the words, but also for the underlying themes that the words refer to or symbolize. *Suicidal intent accompanied by imminence represents a high level of lethality.*

Chosen Method and Accessibility

The third determinant of lethality is perhaps the most critical. The method and its availability determine the outcome of the suicidal behavior. One is more likely to seriously injure or kill oneself if there is an easily accessible means or method.

Persons who complete suicide tend to engage in only one high-lethality act through violent methods: using firearms (the most prevalent high-lethality method used in the United States), piercing of vital organs, hanging, jumping from high places, or using carbon monoxide poisoning. Men who complete suicides are more likely to select more violent means and use guns or knives or hang themselves; women are more likely to jump from high places or over-

dose. Nonfatal attempters tend to engage in multiple, low-lethality acts and use self-poisoning by pill ingestion (the most common method for suicide attempts), followed by wrist cutting. These methods allow time for rescue because of the slowness of their physiologic actions. Most who attempt suicide will use the same method for repeated suicide attempts.

Boyd and Moscicki (1986) noted that *accessibility to dangerous weapons raises the suicide risk*. They observed the increase in youth suicide rates to be in proportion to the increased use of firearms. The most rapid increase in firearm suicides has been in the 15- to 24-year age range. Because of the increasing availability of firearms and other weapons, it is important for parents to be aware of the activities and peers of their children. Any clues or signs of self-destructive behavior or any verbalizations regarding violence toward self and or others should be investigated by parents and significant adults so that help and guidance can be offered, which may prevent a possible tragedy.

> ⚠ **CLINICAL ALERT**
>
> Asking suicidal clients and their family members about their access to dangerous weapons must be a part of the nursing assessment. Many will verify that there are guns and other dangerous weapons in the home that are easily accessible. If the clients are experienced in firearms use (e.g., policemen, military personnel, or hunters), the risk for suicide rises sharply. Provisions must be made at the end of the assessment to secure the weapons and have family and friends remove them from the home or from automobiles and trucks. Usually, a physician's order is required before dangerous weapons are returned to the at-risk client.

Suicidal clients in psychiatric hospitals or on psychiatric units in general hospitals are high suicide risks. Hospitals report a wide range of 20 to 90 completed suicides per 100,000 client years. The most vulnerable periods for attempts are within the first 24 hours after admission and as discharge approaches. Close observation is required as clients move from one suicide precaution level to another. Remember that *a sudden brightening of affect or lifting of depression may signal that the client has resolved his or her ambivalence about living or dying, has made the decision to commit suicide, and is awaiting the opportunity.* Some clients have attempted or completed suicide while they were not on suicide precautions at all. Observation of all clients at least every 30 minutes, whether or not they are suicidal, is vital in detecting early clues to self-destructive behavior.

Hanging is the most prevalent suicide method used in hospital settings and is a lethal one. Sharp objects are usually not available to clients, as part of the safety program of the unit. However, sheets, towels, belts, cords, plastic garbage bags, shoe strings, and articles of clothing have been used to create nooses. Other clients may "cheek" their psychotropic medications and use them later in overdose attempts. Some chronically suicidal clients who sneak sharp objects into the hospital are prone to cutting attempts, usually of the wrists or antecubital areas of the arms. Clients diagnosed with borderline personality disorders or dissociative disorders are prone to these attempts. Searching the client on admission and when returning from off-ground passes is an important safety intervention to detect contraband such as razors, knives, pieces of glass, and aluminum cans.

It is not possible to prevent all suicides, even in the most secure facilities such as psychiatric hospitals and jails, but *close observation and continued reassessment of suicide risk minimize the chances of completed suicides.* Mental health professionals have an obligation to protect clients from harming themselves, just as parents and significant adults must be responsible for youth who demonstrate signs of self-destructive behavior requiring prompt intervention.

PROGNOSIS

Suicidal behavior is a treatable mental health problem. The prognosis for many suicidal clients is related to the severity of their accompanying mental disorder. Since most suicidal behavior is correlated closely with major depressive disorders, effective treatment of depression results in a rapid reduction in suicide risk. The majority of patients with depression who are treated with antidepressant medications demonstrate increased improvement or complete remission of their depressive symptoms according to the Clinical Practice Guidelines (Cummings, 1993). Patients with schizophrenia and panic disorder who main-

tain therapeutic blood levels of the prescribed psychotropic medications also have a favorable response and a positive outcome related to reduction in suicide risk (see Chapter 23 for further information about medication).

DISCHARGE CRITERIA

Discharge criteria are necessary guidelines for both the client and the nursing staff and lead toward a completion of treatment goals. The admission assessment establishes the groundwork for discharge criteria. Without an accurate, thorough, and knowledgeable assessment and appropriate treatment plan, effective interventions and timely discharge activities can be delayed. Discharge criteria help to establish time frames in which goals are achieved, designate areas of responsibility and accountability by way of documentation, and meet specific institutional, professional, certifying, legal, or funding requirements.

Discharge criteria for the suicidal client must include:

Indications that the client is no longer imminently suicidal

Determination that the client's living environment is safe for his or her return

A consistent, available support system for the client to access if he or she is feeling self-destructive

A commitment from the client to use psychotherapy to understand the crises that precipitated the suicidal ideation and/or attempt

An agreement by the client to use a suicide hot line or call a supportive friend or family member if suicidal ideation is experienced again in the future

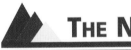

THE NURSING PROCESS

ASSESSMENT

The nursing assessment is a critical step toward ensuring the client's safety. Accurate assessment, continuing throughout the course of hospitalization, helps the nurse provide appropriate intervention and discharge planning. Determining an individual's risk for self-harm requires a thorough evaluation of factors that contribute to suicidality (e.g., a mental status examination and an evaluation of the client's support resources).

The initial assessment helps determine the presence of specific risk factors. Noting the presence of symptoms does not necessarily mean that a client is suicidal. However, recognizing a cluster of certain symptoms within a given time frame is necessary to accurately assess suicidal intent (see Nursing Care in the Community box).

When assessing the client's potential for suicide, the nurse will observe for the following:

1. *The observable behavior of the client.* A calm client may be highly suicidal, whereas an agitated client may not be dangerous. Although appearances can be deceiving, increased perturbation (Shneidman, 1985, 1996) often signals an imminent suicide attempt and is characterized by impulsivity, restlessness, excessive motor agitation, and a brightening of affect. With some clients, however, withdrawal, apathy, irritability, and immobility may intensify with suicidality.

Suicides do occur in hospitals. It is important that nurses consistently monitor a suicidal client's behavior, affect, and interactions with others. Lethality levels can

Suicide

Everyone working in mental health recognizes that it is standard procedure to assess all individuals experiencing depression for suicidality and the ability to agree to a no-harm contract with his or her mental health professional. Evaluation is based on the lethality of the suicide plan and the availability of the means to carry it out. The community mental health nurse's personal knowledge of the client's family and lifestyle and the ability to offer access to the mental health system are distinct advantages. The nurse's availability on an extended basis may help to establish credibility with clients so that agreements are based on relationships and trust.

It is important to consider the individual in the context of daily life, which is also an advantage of being in the community. The elderly individual, living alone, may be at high risk for suicidal acts, as are young persons newly diagnosed with a major psychiatric illness. Assessment can be made, not only on the basis of the client's demographics, but also on the basis of interviews with the persons in the client's support system. The interview should be focused on the appearance of the vegetative signs of depression, as well as religious orientation, personal habits, and medication compliance. The capability of the person, especially his or her ability to organize, is significant. Those who seem to be improving are often at increased risk, since they are better able to plan and implement a lethal attempt. Other elements that must be considered as risk factors are the disinhibiting effects of certain medications and the mind-altering effects of substance abuse.

Assessment of suicidality remains a difficult issue in the community, because many clients desire the security of the hospital psychiatric unit and have found that expressing suicidal intent will lead to admission. They have become adept at manipulating the system to get what they feel they need without making an effort to change themselves.

Although the community mental health nurse may recognize system abuse, by certain clients, preserving life remains a central duty no matter how frequently the client has used suicidality as a ploy to enter the hospital. Each situation must be individually evaluated, and all options must be explored regardless of a client's past behavior. The nurse's paramount role is as an advocate for the client. Sometimes the human contact and focused attention, along with a personalized no-harm contract, will make a difference in the client's feeling of despair, isolation, and subsequent suicidal behavior. A partial hospitalization or day treatment program may offer enough individual support. At other times, only the constraints imposed by hospitalization will prevent suicide.

increase during hospitalization, particularly as depression lifts and discharge becomes imminent.

2. *The history from the client.* Careful scrutiny will sometimes reveal precipitating events that contribute to current self-destructive thoughts. It is important to determine why the client is feeling suicidal at this time. In gathering the client's history, the nurse may identify self-defeating coping patterns and past experiences that have negatively affected the client's self-esteem. Making note of significant anniversary dates may help to predict a future suicide attempt.

3. *Information from friends or relatives.* Useful information regarding the client's history can be obtained from friends or relatives. Often it is helpful to interview the client and family together and separately (in case the friend or relative is hesitant to speak openly in front of the client). The nurse should assess how family members and friends feel about the client's suicidal behavior. Family members who are angry, disgusted, or frustrated with the self-destructive client may actually provoke the client to complete a plan of suicide.

4. *History of suicidal gestures or attempts.* The suicide attempt is often used as a way of coping with painful feelings. People who have used this coping style in the past are at greater risk for using it again.

5. *The mental status examination.* Disturbance in concentration, orientation, and memory suggest possible organic brain syndrome, which may reduce the client's impulse control and increase the potential for self-harm. Disturbance in thought processing, evidenced in command hallucinations, places the client at greater risk to act destructively.

6. *The physical examination.* A physical examination should always be conducted when there are obvious signs and symptoms of substance abuse (e.g., impaired attention, irritability, euphoria, slurred speech, unsteady gait, flushed face, psychomotor agitation, needle tracks), previous suicide attempts (e.g., scars on wrists), or debilitating medical conditions.

7. *The nurse's intuition.* The nurse's own feelings of uneasiness, anxiety, or unexplained sadness may be the only clues that a seemingly calm client is barely able to refrain from acting on suicidal impulses. Although these feelings may be described as intuition, research suggests that "intuitive feelings" tend to be based on previous experiences in similar client care situations (Aguilera, 1998). Nevertheless, if the nurse does not "feel right" about a client, this important source of information should not be ignored.

Nurses can use the assessment questions in Figure 28-2 to determine the client's risk for suicide.

The following discussion refers to the Case Study box on p. 668. The nurse knew the first task of assessment was to make psychologic contact with the client. She planned to listen to how John viewed his situation and then communicate her understanding of his thoughts and feelings. The nurse realized that it was important to establish rap-

NURSING SUICIDE RISK SCREENING SCALE

Name _____ Age _____ Sex _____ Date _____

Evaluator _____ Screening Score _____

Lethality Level	Low 1	2	Moderate 3	4	High 5	Score
AGE	0–4	5–14	15–25	25–49	50+	
SEX		Male	Male	Female/Male	Male	
RACE		Hispanic, Asian African-American Women	African-American	Urban African-American, Caucasian	Native American, Caucasian over 65	
EMOTIONAL SIGNS AND SYMPTOMS	Stress-related, transient emotional problems		Presence of psychiatric illness physical, emotional exhaustion	Symptoms of major depression, panic attacks, schizophrenia	Apathy, despondency, hopelessness, preoccupation with death	
SUICIDE PLAN	Ideation without plan	Ideation, vague plan, no means to carry out, rescue plan	Plan, previous low-level attempt, rescue plan	Explicit plan, previous high-level attempt, less immediacy	Lethal plan, means, intent to die, previous high-level attempt, no rescue plan	
SOCIAL SUPPORT, RESOURCES	Friends, family	Friends, family	Family, history of suicide in nuclear or extended family	Withdrawal from family or friends	Isolated, lives alone	
RECENT LOSS OR CHANGES		Success, promotion, increased obligations	Health, job problems, loss of self-esteem	Divorce, separation	Death of loved one, anniversary date of significant loss	
MEDICAL PROBLEMS				Debilitating illness	Terminal illness	
ALCOHOL, OTHER DRUGS				Prescription medication availability	Alcohol or other drug use/abuse	
COGNITION, PROBLEM SOLVING ABILITY		Ineffective coping skills	Problem solving impaired	Cognitive rigidity	Limited divergent thinking, hopelessness	
METHOD		Limited knowledge or access to pills or wrist-cutting	Availability of lethal prescriptions	Guns, knives, jumps, hangings, CO poisoning	Weapons in home, knowledge of use	

SCORING
    High Risk Level - 25–40
    Moderate Risk Level - 15–24
    Low Risk Level - 0–14

Total Score _____

Figure 28-2 Nursing Suicide Risk Screening Scale. (Developed and copyrighted by P. Bricker and M. Barbee.)

CASE STUDY

John, age 24, had been hospitalized at age 18 after overdosing on tricyclic antidepressants. At the time, John's suicide attempt seemed to be linked to the end of a 2-year relationship with his girlfriend. Since the initial episode of major depression, John successfully graduated from college and, following the sudden death of his father, returned home to live with his mother. Soon, however, he began to feel frustrated and inadequate when unable to find employment commensurate with his educational background and intellectual capabilities. John was forced to accept a part-time position that paid minimum wage and lacked benefits. When his steady girlfriend suddenly relocated to another state, he felt rejected and abandoned.

John's mother, who noticed that he had become more withdrawn and isolative, was concerned that John might be self-destructive. After finding a loaded pistol lying on a table alongside John's bed, John's mother phoned the local mental health crisis intervention center to discuss her concerns about her son's behavior. While talking with the intake nurse, she added that John had recently instructed her to donate his body organs to medical science if "anything should happen" to him.

The nurse requested that John come to the center for an immediate assessment to determine his risk for suicide.

Critical Thinking—Assessment

1. What information did the nurse gather during the phone conversation with John's mother that alerted her to his need for an immediate suicide assessment? Why is this information pertinent to suicidal ideation?
2. What other factors will the nurse consider when assessing John's risk for suicide during the face-to-face evaluation?
3. Identify one factor noted in the assessment that may help reduce John's risk for self-harm.

---

port and trust with John. She believed that the client-centered approach, developed by Rogers (1961), would facilitate open communication and in turn assist her in more accurately assessing John's risk for suicide (see Chapter 3 for further information about Carl Rogers).

The nurse used empathic listening techniques by listening for both facts and feelings (i.e., what happened and how the client felt about it). The nurse demonstrated caring and interest by using reflective statements so that John knew the nurse had heard what he had been saying.

When feelings were obviously present but not yet expressed, the nurse would gently comment, "I sense how upset you are by the way you are speaking. It seems like you are also angry and frustrated about what has happened."

Psychologic contact is not always made solely through verbal communication. Sometimes, nonverbal, physical contact is quite effective. A gentle touch on the forearm or placing an arm around a shoulder can have an important calming effect and signify human concern as well.

The nurse demonstrated concern for John by offering him a tissue when his eyes filled with tears. The nurse not only recognized and acknowledged his feelings, but also responded in a calm, controlled manner, resisting the tendency to become anxious, angry, or depressed because of the intensity of the client's feelings. During the assessment of John, the nurse included the questions in the Nursing Assessment Questions box.

Following a suicide attempt, an individual may continue to be at high risk for attempting suicide again. When clients are admitted to the hospital following a suicide attempt, ongoing assessments are necessary to determine whether the person continues to be at high risk.

NURSING DIAGNOSIS

Suicidal clients are frequently admitted to psychiatric units, emergency departments, and intensive care units of general medical hospitals. Suicide attempts can occur before or during hospitalization. Hangings, medication overdoses, and jumps from high places are frequent methods of suicide in hospitals. An accurate nursing diagnosis based on a thorough, ongoing assessment is necessary when identifying and prioritizing the client's needs for nursing interventions.

A complete nursing diagnosis is individualized and related to the client's behaviors and nursing needs. Validation of the nursing diagnosis with the client is required. However, the client may deny suicidal intent or the need for extra precautions. In the case of the diagnosis of violence, risk for: self-directed, caution is recommended in determining the level of risk. *It is best to err on the side of caution when diagnosing suicidality than to allow serious injury or death to occur.*

NURSING DIAGNOSES RELATED TO SUICIDE

Primary diagnosis:

Violence, risk for: self-directed

Secondary diagnoses may include:

Coping, defensive
Coping, ineffective individual
Hopelessness
Powerlessness
Self-esteem, chronic low
Social isolation
Thought processes, altered

COLLABORATIVE DIAGNOSES

Clients with chronic mental illness are at higher risk for suicide. Several medical diagnoses include a group of symptoms that relate to the nursing diagnosis of violence, risk for: self-directed.

Major depression and bipolar disorder are affective

NURSING ASSESSMENT QUESTIONS

Suicide

1. What does the client understand about why his mother suggested he come to the center for a mental health assessment?
   (To determine if the client will validate his mother's concerns or deny that a problem exists.)
2. What was John's intention in having a loaded gun lying next to his bed? Did he intend to kill himself or someone else?
   (Asking directly about a client's intentions can decrease anxiety and feelings of humiliation and shame.)
3. Has John taken antidepressants or mood-stabilizing medications in the past? Currently?
   (Have medications used in the past been effective in improving John's mood and lowering his lethality level? Does he have access to other lethal means of suicide?)
4. When was the last time John used alcohol or other drugs? When was he last intoxicated?
   (Clients who use alcohol and other drugs are at higher risk to complete a suicide attempt. Increased impulsivity, disorientation, and confusion, which often accompany drug and alcohol use, place people at higher risk for suicide.)
5. With whom does John share his feelings?
   (To determine if John has a trusted and reliable support system. If so, the lethality level could be lower.)
6. What were the circumstances surrounding his father's death? Is there a history of depression or suicide on either side of John's family?
   (To determine the nature of John's father's death, family history of depression, or family style of coping, all of which increase the risk of suicide.)
7. The nurse asked John's mother: "How do you feel about John's thoughts of suicide?"
   (To determine if John's mother is a support resource for him.)

---

disorders that may include the symptoms of suicidal ideation, plans, gestures, and recurring suicide attempts.

Schizophrenia, with associated psychotic features such as delusions and command hallucinations, can also manifest as life-threatening behaviors. Hostile voices may direct the client to kill himself or herself.

Mental disorders due to a medical condition (such as substance abuse) may involve increased suicide risk if the client is repeating negative or self-defeating patterns. The client may be subject to an increased potential for self-directed violence when attempting to deal with stress by using alcohol or other drugs, demonstrating impulsive behavior, or having limited adaptive responses, mood swings, or confusion.

Indirect, self-destructive behaviors, sometimes identified as passive forms of suicide, are exhibited in the medical diagnoses of anorexia nervosa, bulimia nervosa, and noncompliance with medical treatment.

Clients with personality disorders such as borderline personality disorder, antisocial personality disorder, or schizotypal personality disorder may have a potential for suicide completion, especially if there is another Axis I diagnosis or if substance abuse is involved (see Collaborative Diagnoses box).

OUTCOME IDENTIFICATION

Outcomes are derived from the nursing diagnoses and are defined as anticipated, expected client behaviors or responses that are achieved as a result of nursing interventions. Outcomes must be stated in clear behavioral or measurable terms.

COLLABORATIVE DIAGNOSES

DSM-IV Diagnoses*‡	NANDA Diagnoses†
Major depression, single episode	Violence, risk for: self directed‡
Major depression, recurrent	Coping, ineffective individual
Major depression with psychotic features	Self-esteem, chronic low
	Hopelessness
	Powerlessness
Bipolar disorder	Thought processes, altered
	Coping, defensive
	Social interactions, impaired
	Communication, impaired verbal
Schizophrenia	Sensory/perceptual alterations
	Thought processes, altered
	Social isolation
Mental disorders caused by a general medical condition	Coping, ineffective individual
	Self-care deficit

*From American Psychiatric Association: *Diagnostic and statistical manual of mental disorders,* ed 4, Washington, DC, 1994, The Association.
†From North American Nursing Diagnosis Association: *NANDA nursing diagnoses: definitions and classifications, 1999-2000,* Philadelphia, 1999, The Association.
‡Risk for violence may be present in all DSM-IV diagnoses listed above.

▲ NURSING CARE PLAN

Tiffany, a 15-year-old, was admitted to the adolescent psychiatric unit of a local community hospital after her nurse therapist assessed that she was imminently suicidal. Over the past year Tiffany had become preoccupied with wanting to die. She reported that she had overdosed on analgesics and antibiotics three times in the past 6 months but never told anyone and did not seek medical attention. She reported that she made her first suicide attempt when she was 10 by self-inflicting lacerations to her wrists with a razor blade. Within the past year she had cut her wrists five or six times. Tiffany complained that she felt helpless to change her relationship with her mother, who she felt misunderstood her and from whom she felt alienated. She reported poor school performance, increased irritability, morbid thoughts, decreased appetite, periods of insomnia, low self-esteem, and a history of sexual abuse by a babysitter's boyfriend when she was 8.

During her weekly therapy session, Tiffany announced to her therapist: "I am no longer willing to honor our contract not to harm myself. Nothing is changing at home. My mother hates me and doesn't want me in her life. My stepdad is the only person Mom really cares about outside of herself. I hate how I look, and I hate how I am. I saved most of the pain pills

my doctor gave me when I injured my leg." Laughing, she added, "I think there's enough to really put me out of my pain this time."

When questioned further, Tiffany admitted she was planning to kill herself. She indicated that she didn't know exactly when she would attempt to do so but promised, "I am not going to wait much longer."

To provide for her immediate safety, the nurse therapist ordered Tiffany's admission to the hospital.

DSM-IV Diagnoses

Axis I	Major depression, recurrent
	Adjustment disorder
Axis II	Developmental reading disorder
	Borderline personality traits
Axis III	Fractured left tibia; healing
Axis IV	Severe: two overdoses, self-inflicted wrist lacerations, persistent morbid thinking, severe depression, dysfunctional family relationships
Axis V	GAF = 10 (current)
	GAF = 35 (past year)

Nursing Diagnosis: Violence, risk for: self-directed. Risk factors: dysfunctional family relationships, ineffective coping style, low self-esteem, effects of sexual abuse, verbalized intent to die, history of several previous suicide attempts, lethal suicide plan, severely depressed mood.

Client Outcomes	Nursing Interventions	Evaluation
• Tiffany will verbalize an absence of suicidal ideation, intent, plan.	• Check the client and room for potentially dangerous items and observe for any secretive behavior. *Protecting the client from self-destructive behavior promotes safety and gives a message of caring and concern.*	• On the third day of hospitalization, Tiffany told her primary nurse that she wanted to live. She reported that suicidal ideation had ceased by the fifth day of hospitalization.
• Tiffany will express a desire to live and will list several reasons for wanting to live.	• Support Tiffany in developing a hopeful attitude. Reinforce her efforts at positive self-evaluation, self-control, and goal-setting *to promote self-esteem and provide hope for change.*	• The client reported looking forward to summer vacation. She accepted a job as a veterinarian's assistant. She identified her appearance and intelligence as positive attributes.
• Tiffany will make plans for the future that include identification of a viable support system and a daily plan for structured activities with friends and family, routine exercise, weekly therapy sessions, and medication compliance.	• Encourage Tiffany to list people she will contact for support and help her develop a daily plan of structured activities that include a health care regimen. *Additional support and success-oriented activities will increase the client's sense of self-worth, decrease feelings of alienation, and lessen the suicide risk.*	• Tiffany developed a weekly plan of activities that included a health care regimen and a part-time job. She listed her mother, stepfather, and two friends as people she would talk with.

▲ NURSING CARE PLAN —cont'd

Nursing Diagnosis: Coping, ineffective individual, related to negative thinking patterns, self-defeating behaviors, disturbance in self-concept, multiple stressors, and ineffective support system, as evidenced by self-destructive behaviors, lack of assertive communication, impaired judgment and insight, misdirected anger, and social isolation.

Client Outcomes	Nursing Interventions	Evaluation

• Tiffany will demonstrate improved coping skills by:
  • Discussing feelings and needs assertively.
  • Taking responsibility for feelings and not blaming others
  • Making a written list of healthy coping skills to use in times of increased stress
  • Keeping a daily journal of thoughts and feelings related to her relationships
  • Engaging in efforts to socialize with peers and reestablish communication with family
	• Teach cognitive and behavioral techniques to assist Tiffany in limiting negative thought patterns and self-defeating behaviors and using more realistic self-evaluations. Encourage attendance at all psychoeducation groups. Review journal daily. Point out any self-defeating thoughts. Role-model assertive communication. *Therapeutic modalities can help the client to identify and replace self-defeating thoughts and behaviors with an improved, healthy coping style.*	• Tiffany directly confronted her feelings with others in group, individual, and family therapy.
		• Tiffany labeled and challenged her "thinking errors" in journal work, owned responsibility for her feelings/actions, and progressively stopped accusing or blaming others.

Nursing Diagnosis: Coping, ineffective family, related to highly conflicted family relationships, enmeshed relationship with mother, hostile relationship with stepfather, and ineffective communication and parenting skills, as evidenced by distancing behaviors toward client, inability to set consistent limits, and inappropriate parent-child boundaries.

Client Family Outcomes	Nursing Interventions	Evaluation
• Family will attend all scheduled family therapies and parents' support group, where they will discuss their feelings of fear, guilt, and frustration related to Tiffany's suicide attempts.	• Encourage parents to actively participate in Tiffany's treatment. Routinely update parents on any changes in Tiffany's behaviors. Encourage Tiffany and parents to directly confront their feelings. Role-model effective listening skills and assertive communication. *Demonstrating involvement in Tiffany's treatment will convey a message of caring and concern and parents' willingness to make needed changes.*	• Parents attended all family groups. Mother planned one afternoon each week for special time with Tiffany. Parents openly discussed feelings with the client and each other. They asked for referral to a parenting skills workshop.
• Parents will demonstrate willingness to listen to daughter's concerns and self-doubts. Parents will praise Tiffany when she engages in healthy coping behaviors.	• Apprise parents of any changes in Tiffany's behavior. Provide support and reassurance when Tiffany's mood and/or behavior fluctuate. Discuss warning signs of impending decompensation such as increased irritability, isolation, failure to maintain medication regimen, and depressed mood. Inform parents of risk factors following hospitalization (e.g., significant losses or disappointments that forewarn decompensation). Reinforce attempts at improved communication and parenting skills. *Maintaining supportive communication with families enhances the client's support resources, decreases family members' anxiety, and promotes healthy coping.*	• Parents reassured Tiffany when she voiced self-doubts. Parents requested involvement in parents' aftercare group following Tiffany's discharge.

Client will:

1. Remain safe and free from self-harm.
2. Verbalize an absence of suicidal ideation/plan/intent.
3. Verbalize a desire to live and list several reasons for wanting to live.
4. Agree to maintain a signed "no self-harm contract" with the nursing staff, attending psychiatrist, or individual therapist for a specified length of time. Agree to inform staff immediately if suicidal feelings/thoughts recur.
5. Display brightened affect with broad range of expression and spontaneity and cheerful content of speech that reflects a hopeful, optimistic attitude.
6. Initiate social interactions with peers and staff (individually and in groups).
7. Use effective coping methods to counteract feelings of hopelessness.
8. Express a sense of self-worth.
9. Meet own needs through clear, direct methods of communication.
10. Verbalize realistic role expectations and goals for meeting them.
11. Demonstrate absence of psychotic thinking (e.g., delusions, command hallucinations directing self-harm).
12. Make plans for the future that include follow-up psychotherapy and prescribed medication compliance.
13. List several friends or supportive individuals (such as a clergy member) or use a suicide hot line to prevent a possible suicide attempt when experiencing increased suicidal thoughts.

PLANNING

The nurse's awareness of a client's risk for suicide and the recurrent nature of suicide attempts warrant a plan of care aimed at saving lives and restoring biopsychosocial stability. The plan of care for the suicidal client emphasizes a reduction in the risk of self-destructive behaviors by monitoring client behaviors and providing a safe environment, promoting the client's feelings of self-worth and hope, improving coping skills, limiting social isolation, and building self-esteem.

IMPLEMENTATION

Primary nursing responsibilities involve the prevention of suicide. The nurse must recognize and effectively intervene in the potentially lethal behaviors of clients at risk. This process involves a continuing assessment of lethality factors to determine the client's risk level while working with the client to restore hope, connect with support resources, and develop positive alternatives to assist in improved coping.

NURSING INTERVENTIONS

The following interventions must be consistently implemented with all hospitalized suicidal clients.

To provide safety and prevent violence:

1. All unit precautions for preventing suicide should be strictly enforced. This includes vigilantly maintaining a safe environment by:
   a. Routinely counting silverware and all other sharp objects before and after the client's use
   b. Having awareness of the client's whereabouts at all times
   c. Providing one-to-one supervision for the client as warranted, based on assessment of the client's current lethality level
   d. Planning so that the unit is always covered by experienced staff, especially at staff mealtimes, breaks, vacations, change of shift, or unit staff meetings (times during which most suicides occur in hospitals)
   e. Providing a roommate for the suicidal client
   f. Requesting that visitors clear all gifts with staff
   g. Searching the suicidal individual for drugs, sharp objects, cords, shoelaces, and other potential weapons following a return from a pass
   h. Thoroughly assessing the client before any passes to determine the client's current risk level.
   i. Encouraging the client to sign a "no suicide" contract* for a specified length of time, which is reviewed during hospitalization and before discharge and renegotiated before its expiration, *to indicate to the client the nurse's caring, concern, and consistent follow-through*
2. Being mindful that most suicides occur within 90 days following hospitalization, the nurse must reinforce with families, guardians, social services, or legal authorities the necessity of removing any possible weapons (e.g., guns or drugs) in the person's home environment to a safe location before the client's return home.
3. Because working with suicidal clients is emotionally draining and anxiety producing, the nurse must help create a supportive environment for self and other staff, which includes daily supervision and informal discussions regarding feelings about suicide, death, hostility, anger, depression, and other painful feelings. Developing an ongoing relationship with a suicidal client is an intense experience in which the client and nurse both examine their feelings about the meaning of life and death. It is an opportunity for the nurse to share a commitment to life, hope, and caring for another person. *Receiving support and supervision will enable the nurse to develop this kind of intense, caring relationship so that both the nurse and the client will experience less anxiety and have increased energy to work toward hope and health.*

---

*"No-suicide" contracts do not preclude the need for constant observation/supervision.

To assist in development of improved coping skills:

1. Nurses use specific techniques that include nonjudgmental, empathic listening, encouragement, tolerance of expressions of pain, flexible responses to client needs, and consistent limit setting.

2. The nurse encourages the client to focus on strengths rather than weaknesses so that the client becomes aware of positive qualities and capabilities that have helped with coping in the past. Nurses provide learning opportunities for improved coping by introducing the client to therapeutic modalities that assist in more positive thinking. *By replacing or substituting irrational, self-deprecating thoughts, beliefs, and images, the client can become more capable of viewing life realistically and rationally.*

3. Nurses help reduce the overwhelming effects of problems by helping clients prioritize their concerns. This is done by breaking them down into more manageable parts. The nurse can assist in this process by:
   a. Encouraging the client to prioritize problems from most to least urgent
   b. Supporting the client in finding immediate solutions for the most urgent problems
   c. Postponing finding solutions to those problems that do not require immediate remedy
   d. Encouraging the client to delegate problem solving to others when appropriate
   e. Helping the individual to acknowledge problems that are beyond his or her control
   f. Identifying, defining, and promoting healthy adaptive behaviors in clients
   g. Encouraging continuance of healthy behaviors when improved coping strategies are demonstrated (positive reinforcement)
   h. Encouraging the individual to discuss the feelings generated by ineffective coping (e.g., frustration, anger, inadequacy)
   i. Affirming the patient's rational decisions that have been based on accurate judgment
   j. Reinforcing the client's attempts to make independent decisions
   k. Acknowledging the client's demonstrated willingness to implement improved coping behaviors such as assertive communication
   l. Responding to delusional statements by stating the reality of the situation without arguing with the client's reality

To enhance family and social support systems:

1. Enlist the family as allies in the client's treatment. *Family attendance at psychoeducation groups and family therapy are crucial components in helping the client work through and understand complex and toxic family struc-* tures, systems, and dynamics that may contribute to the individual's suicidal feelings.

2. Determine the degree of available family support that contributes to overall risk management. Inform family members about critical signs that the client may exhibit as depression lifts and discharge occurs. Encourage the removal of any lethal weapons from the client's home environment.

3. Provide understanding and encouragement when family members express feelings (e.g., frustration, helplessness, or guilt) and intense affect.

4. Contact social services to assist with any needed vocational and financial support.

5. Refer the client to aftercare groups, support groups, and 12-step groups as needed.

6. Refer the client to a suicide hotline that can be used when the client is feeling overwhelmed and suicidal in the future

ADDITIONAL TREATMENT MODALITIES

Depending on the client's diagnosis, pharmacologic intervention is often a primary consideration in the treatment of the suicidal client. Antidepressants, anxiolytics, and antipsychotic medications are frequently used, depending on the individual's need, history, and previous response to medication intervention.

Psychotherapeutic interventions may vary and can include insight-oriented techniques, cognitive reframing, and brief, solution-focused crisis interventions.

Electroconvulsive therapy (ECT) may be used with adults whose response patterns reflect a lack of positive response to medication (i.e., "intractible" or "refractory" depression). These adults concurrently present with long-standing histories of severe depression while expressing imminent intent to die. ECT is discussed in detail in Chapter 23.

EVALUATION

An evaluation of the client's response to the plan of care is crucial in working with suicidal individuals. An ongoing, all-encompassing evaluation considers the accuracy of the nursing diagnosis, the appropriateness of the intervention based on the client's response, and the timeliness with which the intervention occurred. Evaluation helps the nurse target areas of outcome that are critical to the client's continued survival. A client's lack of positive response to nursing interventions may indicate a need to alter the interventions, implement other treatment modalities, or reexamine target dates for completion of outcomes.

Deliberate, conscientious evaluation of a suicidal client's response to nursing interventions that are directed toward promoting safety and biopsychosocial stabilization help ensure the client's continued safety and readiness for discharge.

Summary of Key Concepts

1. Suicide is a major public health and mental health problem in the United States.
2. Durkheim classified four subtypes of suicide relating to social and cultural aspects: anomic, egoistic, altruistic, and fatalistic.
3. Etiologies of suicide include biologic factors, which deal with chemical imbalances; psychologic factors, which dominate the understanding of suicide and define the dynamics of intrapsychic, interpersonal, cognitive and behavioral approaches in explaining suicidal behavior; and sociologic factors, relating to influences of social groups that contribute to suicide.
4. Around the world, suicide accounts for nearly 1% of all deaths. The United States reports 30,000 suicides annually.
5. The most vulnerable groups for suicide are the elderly and youth ages 15 to 24. Caucasians and men are more likely to be at risk for suicide. Suicide crosses all socioeconomic levels.
6. Suicidal behavior is strongly associated with the oc-currence of psychiatric disorders and other health-related problems such as depression, schizophrenia, panic disorders, substance abuse, some personality disorders (such as borderline personality disorder) and medical disorders.
7. Imminence, intent, and the method chosen and its accessibility are the three determinants that indicate the level of lethality and the levels of interventions necessary for safety.
8. Suicidal behavior is treatable.
9. Discharge criteria for the suicidal client must include indications that the client is no longer imminently suicidal, that the client's environment is safe to return to, and that a support system is in place for the client to access.
10. The plan of care emphasizes a reduction in the risk of self-destructive behaviors by monitoring the client's behaviors and providing a safe environment, promoting feelings of self-worth and hope, improving coping skills, limiting social isolation, and building self-esteem.

REFERENCES

Aguilera DC: Suicide: theoretical concepts. In Aguilera DC: *Crisis intervention: theory and methodology*, ed 8, St. Louis, 1998, Mosby.

American Psychiatric Association: *Diagnostic and statistical manual of mental disorders*, ed 4, 1994, Washington, DC, The Association.

Andreasen N: *The broken brain*, New York, 1984, Harper & Row.

Arato M et al: Retrospective psychiatric assessment of 200 suicides, *Acta Psychiatr Scand* 77:454, 1988.

Barbee M: Professionally speaking: what are the warning signs for suicidal adolescents? *J Psychosoc Nurs Ment Health Serv* 31:37, 1993.

Barber ME et al: Aborted suicide attempts: a new classification of suicidal behavior, *Am J Psychiatry* 155(3):385, 1998.

Beautrais AL et al: Prevalence and co-morbidity of mental disorders in persons making serious suicide attempts: a case-control study, *Am J Psychiatry* 153:1009, August 1996

Blazer D: *Suicide risk factors in the elderly: an epidemiological study.* Paper presented at the conference, Suicide Risk in the Elderly, Boston, 1989, Boston Society for Gerontologic Psychiatry.

Bongar B: *The suicidal patient, clinical and legal standards of care*, Washington, DC, 1991, American Psychological Association.

Boyd J, Moscicki E: Firearms and youth suicide, *Am J Public Health* 76:1240, 1986.

Brodsky BS et al: Characteristics of borderline personality disorder associated with suicidal behavior, *Am J Psychiatry* 154(12):1715, 1997.

Buchanan D, Farran C, Clark D: Suicidal thought and self-transcendence in older adults, *J Psychosoc Nurs Ment Health Serv* 33(10):31, 1995.

Celo-Cruz M: Aid-in-dying: should we decriminalize physician-assisted suicide and physician-committed euthanasia? *Am J Law Med* 4:369, 1992.

Cohen L et al: Suicide and schizophrenia: data from a prospective community treatment study, *Am J Psychiatry* 147:602, 1990.

Cummings J: The neuroanatomy of depression, *J Clin Psychiatry* 54:14, 1993.

Depression in primary care: detection, diagnosis, and treatment: a quick reference guide for clinicians based on Clinical Practice Guidelines, U.S. Department of Health and Human Services, vols 1 and 2, *J Psychosoc Nurs Ment Health Serv* 31:19, 1993.

Durkheim E: *Suicide*, Glencol, 1951, The Free Press (originally published as *Le Suicide* in 1897).

Earle K et al: Characteristics of outpatient suicides, *Hosp Community Psychiatry* 45:123, 1994.

Egan MP et al: The "no suicide contract": helpful or harmful? *J Psychosoc Nurs Ment Health Serv* 35(3):31, 1997.

Facts about suicide in the USA, Denver, 1993, American Association of Suicidology.

Farberow N, editor: *The many faces of suicide: indirect self-destructive behavior*, New York, 1980, McGraw-Hill.

Fawcett J et al: Suicide: clues from interpersonal communication, *Arch Gen Psychiatry* 21:129, 1969.

Fortinash KM, Holoday-Worret PA: *Psychiatric nursing care plans*, ed 3, St. Louis, 1999, Mosby.

Freud S: *Mourning and melancholia,* Collected papers, London, 1920, Hogarth Press (originally published in Germany in 1917).

Gonzales L et al: Longitudinal follow-up of unipolar depressives: an investigation of predictors of relapse, *J Consult Clin Psychol* 53:461, 1985.

Green E, Katz J, Marcus P: Practice guideline for suicide/self-harm prevention. In Green E, Katz J, editors: *Clinical practice guidelines for the adult patient,* St Louis, 1994, Mosby.

Gunderson JG: *Borderline personality disorder,* Washington, DC, 1984, American Psychiatric Press.

Heacock D: Suicidal behavior in black and Hispanic youth, *Psychiatr Ann* 20:134, 1990.

Heilä H et al: Suicide and schizophrenia: a nationwide psychological autopsy study on age- and sex-specific clinical characteristics of 92 suicide victims with schizophrenia, *Am J Psychiatry* 154:1235, September 1997.

Hoyer G, Lund E: Suicide among women related to number of children in marriage, *Arch Gen Psychiatry* 50(2):134, 1993.

Husain S: Current perspectives on the role of psychosocial factors in adolescent suicide, *Psychiatr Ann* 20:122, 1990.

Johnson J: Panic disorder, comorbidity, and suicide attempts, *Arch Gen Psychiatry* 47:805, 1990.

Lepine J et al: Suicide attempts in patients with panic disorder, *Arch Gen Psychiatry* 50:144, 1993.

Lester D: The association between quality of life and suicide and homicide rates, *J Soc Psychol* 124:247, 1984.

Lewinsohn P, Mischel W: Social competence and depression: the role of illusory self-perceptions, *J Abnorm Psychol* 89:203, 1980.

Linehan MM: *Cognitive-behavioral treatment of borderline personality disorder,* New York, 1993, Guildford Press.

Litman R, Farberow N: *Youth suicide in California,* Sacramento, 1986, California Department of Mental Health CMV 85-2482.

Litman R: Sigmund Freud on suicide, *Bull Suicidology,* p 11, July 1967.

Maris R: The adolescent suicide problem, *Suicide Life Threat Behav* 15:91, 1985.

Marshall J: Changes in aged white male suicide: 1948-1972, *J Gerontol* 33:763, 1978.

Masterson JF: *Psychotherapy of the borderline adult: a developmental approach,* New York, 1976, Brunner/Mazel.

May P, Dizmang L: Suicide and the American Indian, *Psychiatr Ann* 4(9):22, 1974.

McIntosh J: Older adults: the next suicide epidemic? *Suicide Life Threat Behav* 22: 322, 1992.

Mellick E et al: Suicide among elderly white men: development of a profile, *J Psychosoc Nurs Ment Health Serv* 30:29, 1992.

Miles C: Conditions predisposing to suicide: a review, *J Nerv Ment Dis* 164:231, 1977.

Miller M: *Suicide after sixty: the final alternative,* New York, 1979, Springer.

Monk M: Epidemiology of suicide, *Epidemiol Rev* 9:51, 1987.

Monk M, Warshaur E: Completed and attempted suicide in three ethnic groups, *Am J Epidemiol* 100:333, 1974.

Nielson D et al: Suicidality and 5-hydroxyindoleacetic acid concentration associated with tryptophan-hydroxylase polymorphism, *Arch Gen Psychiatry* 51:34, 1994.

North American Nursing Diagnosis Association: *NANDA nursing diagnoses: definitions and classifications, 1999-2000,* Philadelphia, 1999, The Association.

National Center for Health Statistics: *Health, United States, 1989,* DHHS Pub No. (PHS)90-1232, Washington, DC, 1990, U.S. Department of Health and Human Services.

Nyman A, Jonsson H: Patterns of self-destructive behavior in schizophrenia, *Acta Psychiatr Scand* 73:252, 1986.

Richman J: *Family therapy for suicidal people,* New York, 1986, Springer.

Rogers C, editor: *On becoming a person,* Boston, 1961, Houghton Mifflin.

Rudd D et al: Problem-solving appraisal in suicide ideators and attempters, *Am J Orthopsychiatry* 64(1):136, 1994.

Sakinofsky I et al: Problem resolution and repetition of parasuicide: a prospective study, *Br J Psychiatry* 156:395, 1991.

Shneidman E: *Definition of suicide,* New York, 1985, John Wiley & Sons.

Shneidman E: Fifty-eight years. In Shneidman E, editor: *On the nature of suicide,* San Francisco, 1969, Jossey-Bass.

Shneidman ES: *The suicidal mind,* New York, 1996, Oxford University Press.

Shore J: American Indian suicide—fact and fantasy, *Psychiatry* 38:86, 1975.

Smith J et al: Comparison of suicide among Anglos and Hispanics in five Southwestern states, *Suicide Life Threat Behav* 15:14, 1985.

Stekel W: Suicide and will. In Freidman P, editor: *On suicide,* New York, 1967, International Universities Press.

Sullivan H: Socio-psychiatric research: its implications for the schizophrenia problem and mental hygiene, *Am J Psychiatry* 10:977, 1931.

Sullivan H: The manic-depressive psychosis. In Perry H et al, editors: *Clinical studies in psychiatry,* New York, 1956, WW Norton.

Tanskanen A et al: Smoking and suicidality among psychiatric patients, *Am J Psychiatry* 155:129, January 1998.

Tishler C et al: Adolescent suicide attempts: some significant factors, *Suicide Life Threat Behav* 11:86, 1981.

Toolan J: Depression and suicide. In Caplan G, editor: *Child and adolescent psychiatry, sociocultural and community psychiatry,* New York, 1974, Basic Books.

Trygstad L: The need to know: biological learning needs identified by practicing psychiatric nurses, *J Psychosoc Nurs Ment Health Serv* 32(2):13, 1994.

U.S. Senate Special Committee on Aging, Federal Council on Aging, U.S. Department of Health and Human Services: *Aging America: trends and projections,* Washington, DC, 1991, U.S. Government Printing Office.

Valente S: Adolescent suicide: assessment and intervention, *J Child Adolesc Psychiatr Nurs* 2(1):34, 1989.

Weiss J: The suicidal patient. In Arieti S, editor: *American handbook of psychiatry*, New York, 1966, Basic Books.

Weissman M et al: Suicidal ideation and suicide attempts in panic disorder and attacks, *N Engl J Med* 321:1209, 1989.

Wells K et al: The functioning and well-being of depressed patients, *JAMA* 262:914, 1989.

Wilson D: *New York Times*, April 9, 1994.

Wolk SI, Weissman MM: Suicidal behavior in depressed children grown up: preliminary results of a longitudinal study, *Psychiatr Ann* 26:331, June 1996.

Wright J, Beck A: Cognitive therapy of depression: theory and practice, *Hosp Community Psychiatry* 34:1119, 1983.

Yang B et al: Sociological and economic theories of suicide: a comparison of the USA and Taiwan, *Soc Sci Med* 34:333, 1992.

Zayas L: Towards an understanding of suicide risks in young Hispanic females, *J Adolesc Res* 2:1, 1978.

Notes

CHAPTER 29

Grief and Loss

Charles Kemp

OBJECTIVES

- Discuss four major categories for symptoms of grief.

- Describe three components of the normal grief process.

- Distinguish between symptoms/behaviors of grief and those of depression.

- Analyze the risk for complicated grief reactions in selected high-risk clients.

- Discuss the major goals for intervention in acute grief.

- Evaluate the "points of intervention" with respect to intervention efficacy.

- Compare and contrast chronic sorrow with other types of grief, and list persons at risk for chronic sorrow.

- Explain how posttraumatic stress disorder can be a feature of complicated grief.

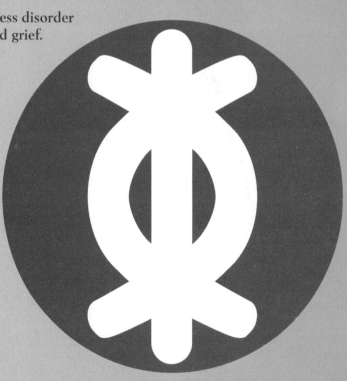

GRIEF AND LOSS

Grief is the painful psychologic and physiologic response to loss. Although it is most commonly associated with the death of a loved one, grief occurs when there is any significant loss, including loss of self-esteem, identity, dignity, or sense of worth. Grief descends on the client newly admitted to a psychiatric hospital, the client who undergoes mutilating surgery, the parents of an infant with birth defects, the child who changes schools, the victim of violence, the nurse who works with victims of violence, the betrayed lover, and the person who loses a job or retires. Grief comes to everyone. Most nurses are in daily contact with grief—other people's and their own.

This chapter describes grief in the following terms: definitions, responses or manifestations, stages or process, and types of grief, including anticipatory, acute, complicated, and chronic sorrow. Assessment information, diagnoses, interventions, and case studies are included.

The terms **grief, bereavement,** and **mourning** are often used interchangeably and there is sometimes disagreement about their exact meanings (see Key Terms) (Parkes, 1998b).

In some cases a grieving person may benefit from psychosocial or pharmacologic intervention, and in other cases, grief may become pathologic (see later discussion on complicated grief). However, although it is terribly painful, it is important to understand that grief is a normal (and, indeed, an inevitable) aspect of life (American Psychiatric Association [APA], 1994; Freud, 1917; Lev and McCorkle, 1998).

RESPONSES

Responses to bereavement (loss) may be examined as a range of physical, cognitive, relating, and affective manifestations of pain—the intensity

Acute grief The initial response to loss. Although it diminishes over time, acute grief may last for as long as several years, depending primarily on the meaning of the lost person or object for the survivor.

Anticipatory grief Grief experienced before death or loss occurs (e.g., when a loved one has a terminal illness).

Bereavement The situation of a person who has lost a person or object to whom or which he or she was attached; the state of grieving.

Chronic sorrow Grief in response to an *ongoing* loss such as long chronic illness in a loved one.

Complicated grief Grief that is expressed to a significantly greater or lesser intensity over a significantly longer or shorter time than is culturally expected. It may manifest itself in serious physical and/or emotional disabilities.

Delayed grief Grief that is not expressed or experienced until well after a loss, often as a result of circumstances such as being focused on survival (as among refugees).

Grief The dynamic natural response to loss. Grief affects physical, cognitive, behavioral, emotional, social, and spiritual aspects of the individual.

Grief work The intense psychologic effort to (1) fully express the feelings associated with grief, (2) understand the relationship with the deceased, and, paradoxically, (3) carry on with essential activities of daily living.

Mourning The social expression of grief.

Postvention Grief therapy after the death occurs but before a pathologic condition develops.

Social support The presence of other individuals who are able to give understanding, encouragement, and other assistance in life, especially during difficult times.

Tasks in grief Tasks or activities common in the psychosocial experience of grieving. Accomplishing these tasks helps resolve grief.

of which are often a surprise to the mourner. Lindemann's seminal study of grief (1944) identified many of the manifestations of grief, including physical distress, preoccupation with the image of the deceased, guilt, hostile reactions, and disruptions in patterns of conduct. These and other physical and psychologic manifestations can be summarized as follows.

PHYSICAL MANIFESTATIONS

Physical manifestations of grief include weakness, anorexia, feelings of choking, shortness of breath, tightness in the chest, dry mouth, and gastrointestinal disturbances. Fatigue, exhaustion, and insomnia are common. Bereaved persons frequently seek medical assistance for vague symptoms, such as chest discomfort or gastrointestinal problems, some of which seem to have no physiologic basis (Steen, 1998). In addition, although grief is seldom a direct cause of illness or death, grief does often result in decreased immune responses (Lev and McCorkle, 1998), and there is a clear link between grief and increased vulnerability to physical and mental illness, especially myocardial infarction, hypertension, rheumatoid arthritis, depression, alcohol and other drug abuse, and malnutrition (Carman, 1997).

COGNITIVE MANIFESTATIONS

Cognitive manifestations center on preoccupation with the image and thoughts of the deceased. The involuntary nature and intensity of the preoccupation are surprising and distressing to some. It is common for the preoccupation to take the form of conversations with the deceased. Especially in the elderly, these conversations may continue for the rest of the survivor's life. Over time, preoccupation usually diminishes, although links with the deceased may be maintained for many years and, in some people, continue until death (Weiss and Richards, 1997). These links may be in the form of remembrances such as treasured things or renegotiated relationships with the deceased. Formerly thought by some to be a symptom that needed resolution, the drive to maintain links between the living and the dead is increasingly recognized as normative behavior (Silverman and Worden, 1992; Weiss and Richards, 1997). Indeed, in some cultures (e.g., Chinese and Vietnamese) the failure to maintain formal links with deceased ancestors is thought to be pathologic. Another common symptom is difficulty concentrating, such as complete lapses of focus or even orientation to time and place. Seeking and longing for the lost person or object are universally experienced. Hallucinations are experienced by some grieving persons. These are most often described as momentary glimpses of the person who died, or brief (two or three words) shortly sensed auditory messages perceived to be spoken by the deceased. In most cases hallucinations diminish within a month or two after the loss and thus may be considered as part of the normal grieving process. In a few cases hallucinations persist, increase in number or intensity, or become derogatory or threatening, such as beckoning the survivor to join the deceased. They are then considered negative hallucinations, and therapeutic interventions, including hospitalization and/or antipsychotic medications, may be indicated.

BEHAVIORAL AND RELATING MANIFESTATIONS

Behavioral and relating manifestations of grief include disruptions in patterns of conduct ranging from an inability to perform even basic activities of daily living; to dragging through daily activities; to a restless, disorganized behavior that includes "searching" for that which is lost and obsessive rumination and reminiscence (Lindemann, 1944; Weiss and Richards, 1997). The old life and patterns lose meaning and satisfaction without the lost object or person, and there does not seem to be a new life or patterns to which the bereaved individual can turn. This loss of relating and meaning is a major etiology of despair or hopelessness.

AFFECTIVE MANIFESTATIONS

Affective manifestations of grief are often overwhelming, with sadness, guilt, and anger being the most common. Sadness, loneliness, and hopelessness tend to predominate and may, along with other symptoms, meet the criteria for diagnosis of an affective disorder (e.g., major depression or dysthymic disorder). The most common differences between symptoms of bereavement versus major depression or dysthymic disorder are that psychomotor retardation, morbid guilt, and suicidal ideation are less common in bereavement and that affective disorders are of longer duration than bereavement (APA, 1994; Nuss and Zubenko, 1992). However, dysfunctional or unresolved grief may result in major depression.

Guilt is a pervasive theme in grief, even in children as young as 2 years (Gibbons, 1992; Jacob, 1996). Many survivors search for their failures or omissions in the relationship, and when significant mistakes are not found, they proceed to magnify whatever small transgressions might exist (Lindemann, 1944). Guilt may be especially troublesome for those whose relationships with the deceased were ambivalent and characterized by unresolved or unexpressed feelings. "Survivor guilt" is common among people who go through an intense experience (e.g., war) and survive when others do not. A similar guilt is experienced when survivors believe that they should have died instead of the loved one. Grief accompanied by "guilt about things other than actions taken or not taken by the survivor at the time of death," sustained loss of self-esteem, and ambivalence about living is an indication that suicide risk is increased and help is needed (APA, 1994). Anger is common and may be directed toward the person who died, to family members, to the health care staff, or to God, or it may be turned inward to self.

Anger is generally a response to the anxiety derived from the powerlessness and vulnerability resulting from the death of a loved one and other losses. Anger toward the deceased is common: "How could she do this to me? It's not fair!" Many survivors feel it is "wrong" to feel anger toward a deceased loved one and thus turn the anger inward. Anger turned inward may also reflect a survivor's inability to release the lost person or object. To those who have spent a lifetime suppressing anger, these overwhelming and "wrong" or ego-dystonic feelings are very distressing and indicate to some individuals that they are "going crazy." Some need permission to express anger. If the death itself is not enough to engender anger, tending to the business, such as funeral preparations, surrounding the death may result in anger. Death, usually the greatest and most painful loss in life, is seen by some morticians, lawyers, and others only as a point of vulnerability through which survivors can be exploited for profit.

The impulse to use drugs, including prescription drugs and alcohol, may occur or, if the survivor already uses, increase. Bereaved persons with a history of any sort of drug misuse or mental illness are at risk for recurrence or exacerbation of these problems.

STAGES AND PROCESS OF GRIEF
STAGES
Grief is often described in terms of stages. Although there exists variation among the different conceptions, many stage-oriented theories can be summarized as having three basic stages: avoidance (numbing and blunting), confrontation (disorganization and despair), and reestablishment (reorganization and recovery) (Kemp, 1999; Parkes, 1998b). Avoidance includes both the initial denial and subsequent brief periods of time when the survivor "forgets," then "remembers" with shock and pain, the losses and grief. Confrontation is the often lengthy period of active mourning and includes the previously discussed most acute physical, cognitive, behavioral and relating, and affective manifestations of grief. Reestablishment occurs, not as a distinct stage but as the *gradual* decrease of symptoms and adjustment to life without that which was lost. The problem with stages is that they tend to be neater in theory than they are in reality and thus may mislead some individuals into thinking that grief is a matter of progressing in an orderly manner through stages and then being finished with grief.

PROCESS
Characteristics
Rather than well-defined stages, it is more helpful to think in terms of a process of common and dynamic responses to grief. Thus a person might initially respond to the death of a loved one with shock and disbelief, then protest and despair; go through a period of emotionless cognitive activity (planning the funeral, etc.) interspersed with waves of despair; then experience yearning, despair, and disorganization (sobbing, confusion, wandering); and gradually begin the long, painful, and varied process of rebuilding a life without the person who died. An essential feature of this process is its dynamic, changing nature (Cowles and Rodgers, 1991; Parkes, 1998b). Periods of apparently normal functioning, for example, may be interspersed with periods of psychologic distress or symptoms (almost indistin-

---

| **Box 29-1** | **Summary of Grief Theories** |

Lindemann
Grief is manifested by predictable psychologic and somatic symptomatology. Acute mourning is characterized by somatic distress, preoccupation with the deceased person's image, guilt, hostile reactions, and loss of patterns of conduct. Dysfunctional or "morbid" grief reactions are defined as distortions of some aspect of "normal grief." The duration of grief and development of dysfunctional grief are largely dependent on the success with which the mourner *works* through the grief.

Kübler-Ross
Elisabeth Kübler-Ross' stages of dying (denial, anger, bargaining, depression, acceptance) are often applied to grief. The initial response to loss may include denial, anger, and bargaining. Denial is characterized by refusal to accept the loss. Anger may initially be directed at the health care staff and then, later in the process, at the person who died. Bargaining and denial are often mixed in a futile attempt to "reverse reality." Depression tends to be the lengthiest phase, and in dysfunctional grief it may become chronic and meet DSM-IV criteria for major depression. Acceptance of the loss is a gradual process that includes aspects of previous stages. As the grief work progresses, acceptance increases.

Bowlby
Grief and loss are characterized first by numbness in which the loss is recognized but not necessarily felt as real. Numbness is followed by yearning and searching, in which the loss is still not fully realized. In the third phase, disorganization and despair, the loss is real, and intense emotional pain and cognitive disorganization occur. Reorganization is the final phase and is characterized by a gradual adjustment to life without the deceased.

Engel
The initial response to loss is shock and disbelief. Awareness of the loss and the meaning of the loss develop during the first year of mourning. Eventually, the relationship is resolved and put into perspective.

Shneidman
Conceptualizing less structure or stages than other theorists in regard to grief, Shneidman views the expression of grief as being dependent primarily on an individual's personality or style of living. An individual who goes through life feeling depressed and guilty is likely to grieve similarly. One who avoids emotional investments with others will also tend to try to avoid grief as well.

Theory Synthesis
Grief tends to occur in several phases. The initial response to loss may be shock, numbness, denial, or other attempts to defend against the reality and pain of loss. This initial phase is followed by painful psychologic and physical disequilibrium—which, in the case of chronic grief, may last indefinitely. The third phase of resolution or recovery is a gradual process in which "the good days begin to outnumber the bad." Ultimately, although not forgotten, the relationship with the deceased is resolved and placed into perspective.

guishable from those of major depression). Countless people say, "It seems like I'm doing fine, and then, for no reason at all, I start crying." (As if some external or practical reason were needed!)

The grief process might include all of the aforementioned responses, phases, or symptoms, or only several of them. There might be no "stage of avoidance" or no period of organized cognitive activity, or very little in the way of resolution, reorganization, or adjustment to the environment in the absence of the deceased. Moreover, when death is expected, the grief process begins before the person dies. Grief occurring before the death or other loss is called anticipatory grief and is discussed later.

A summary of grief theories is provided in Box 29-1.

Grief Work

Stages and process are associated with another common characteristic of grief, which is work. Named first by Lindemann (1944), **grief work** is the means by which people move through the stages or process of grief. Grief work is both a struggle to not give in to despair and a willingness to confront the reality of despair. Thus within the grief process, the bereaved person must continue to some extent to move forward with the business of life, which includes paying the bills, making decisions, and at the same time, being able to express the deep, painful emotions of grieving.

Tasks in Grief

There are certain **tasks in grief,** the accomplishment of which helps in the resolution of grief (Kemp, 1999). These tasks are:

> Telling the "death story" or describing (in detail) events surrounding the death (or loss)
> Expressing and accepting the sadness of grief
> Expressing and accepting guilt, anger, and other feelings perceived as negative
> Reviewing the relationship with the deceased
> Exploring possibilities in life after the loss (e.g., new relationships, activities, sources of support, and so on)
> Understanding common processes and problems in grief
> Being understood or accepted by others

Complicating Factors

Grief work is complicated by several factors. First, it is extremely painful. Many people are surprised at the intensity and depth of the pain experienced in grieving and often make an attempt, consciously or unconsciously, to avoid the distress, often by throwing themselves back into a busy schedule or taking a vacation. Second, the work is inherently contradictory. The pain demands expression, but there is often the fear that if the pain is expressed, the control over feelings will be lost. "I know that if I start cry-

ing, I will never stop." Third, both emotion-based coping (such as expressing deep, powerful feelings) and problem-solving coping (such as developing strategies for going on with life) are needed to most successfully complete the work. Finally, in most of the Western world cultural values exist that support avoiding the expression of grief. For example, self-control is highly valued, especially by men. There is a tendency to try to rush through grief and get back to work or get on with one's life (or as TV newscasters say, *ad nauseum*, "let the healing begin"). Rituals that formerly helped in individual and community expression of grief are now often brief "celebrations" of the deceased's life or other upbeat and usually brief events. The expression of grief, therefore, is limited to what is "appropriate" in public and then what occurs when the bereaved individual is alone—with the pain.

TYPES OF GRIEF

Types of grief include anticipatory, acute, and complicated, as well as chronic sorrow. There is disagreement about definitions, especially in terms of the time required for resolution of a particular form of grief.

ANTICIPATORY GRIEF

Anticipatory grief, or premourning, is defined as grief associated with anticipation of a predicted death or loss (Shneidman, 1980). Anticipatory grief may begin with a catastrophic diagnosis when the patient and family enter a new dimension of being characterized by a sharp sense of vulnerability. The old and comfortable illusory dimension of being, in which death, suffering, or loss does not exist, then dies—and grief for that life ensues. Here, as in other situations, the grief may be complex. For example, in a family in which a loved one develops dementia, grief may be acute (related to the current condition), ongoing (as the family continuously loses aspects of the loved one), and anticipatory (as the long-term reality of the disorder is clarified).

Early in the development of the anticipatory grief model, anticipatory grief was viewed as an adaptive process that could help resolve relationships and prepare survivors, to some extent, for the anticipated loss. Ideally, the realization that loss was approaching would afford the people involved an opportunity to work on interpersonal and spiritual reconciliation and provide support for one another (Parkes, 1998a; Rando, 1988). More recently, anticipatory grief has been seen by some clinicians and researchers as being associated with a high incidence of depression (Levy, 1991) or with family withdrawal from the patient (McCabe, 1997). There is general agreement that (1) grief begins when a serious physical or mental illness occurs (Walker and Pomeroy, 1997); (2) this grief may be termed anticipatory and involves pain, as do other forms of grief (Chapman and Pepler, 1998); and (3) a lack of emotional response to serious illness or other loss is an indication that complicated or dysfunctional grief is likely (Sheldon, 1998) (see Understanding & Applying Research box below). Thus anticipatory grief may be viewed as normative, and persons experiencing it may benefit from intervention.

ACUTE GRIEF

Acute grief, usually referred to simply as grief, is the prototypic painful experience after a loss. Its symptoms and process are described earlier in the chapter. Although there is agreement that acute grief is time limited, an issue that has never been satisfactorily resolved is the question of how long acute (or normal) grief lasts. An early theory is that acute grief lasts approximately 1 year (Shneidman, 1980). More recently, the time span for acute grief has been interfaced with the severity of symptoms, severity of trauma or loss, nature of the relationship, and cultural values (APA, 1994; Kemp, 1998, 1999). Acute grief does not have a clear ending; gradually the sadness lessens, the pain diminishes, and eventually the mourner moves forward with his or her life—even though complete recovery may never occur (Weiss and Richards, 1997). In some traditional cultures (e.g., East Indian) and among some individuals in certain religions (e.g., Jewish and Hindu), grief may be ongoing and not limited by time (Goodman et al, 1991).

Within the process of healing and moving on, there are times of acute exacerbation; times when some situation or event brings back the pain and the mourner again feels overwhelmed with grief. Holidays, birthdays, and other significant milestones are obvious events with the potential to rekindle the grief. Other precipitants are less obvious, and thus the mourner is unable to prepare for them: For example, a song, an image, or a smell may occur in an unguarded moment and the sadness returns as powerful as it was in the beginning. These moments of exacerbation also decrease over time.

COMPLICATED GRIEF

Complicated grief has been described in multiple ways. Lindemann (1944) and a host of contemporary writers and researchers (e.g., Bowlby, 1980; Cowles and Rodgers, 1991; Parkes, 1998a) have emphasized normative and dysfunctional aspects of grief. In other words, up to some point, grief is "normal," and beyond that point, grief is variously considered "dysfunctional," "pathologic," or, more recently, "complicated" (Horowitz et al, 1997). Posttraumatic stress disorder (PTSD) is sometimes a feature of complicated grief (Kemp, 1998). If depression is the predominant feature of bereavement and is incapacitating 2 months after the loss, the client may be diagnosed as having a major depressive disorder (APA, 1994) (see Understanding & Applying Research box below).

All sources refer to essentially the same phenomenon when describing complicated grief: grief that lasts longer and is characterized by greater disability or other dysfunctional patterns than usual as defined by cultural values. Types of complicated grief (Hospice and Palliative Nurses

Understanding & Applying Research

ANTICIPATORY GRIEF

The purpose of this exploratory, cross-sectional, correlational study was to examine the relationships among general coping style, hope, and anticipatory grief in a convenience sample of family members of people with terminal cancer. Data were collected using tools such as a coping scale, hope index, grief inventory, and background information. Anticipatory grief patterns were found to be individualized, and anxiety regarding death was found to be an important component of anticipatory grief. Common dimensions of anticipatory grief were anxiety regarding death, despair, anger/hostility, and somatic distress. Emotive coping was the only coping style that accounted for variance in anticipatory grief. Women used more emotive coping strategies than men, including expressing more anger than men, but there was no relationship between gender and somatic distress. Hope was negatively associated with anticipatory grief. Based on study findings and other research, it may be predicted that some anticipatory grief is likely to contribute to resolution of postdeath grief and decreased incidence of complicated grief. Study findings were consistent with hospice and palliative care practices encouraging confronting feelings and working toward resolution of relationships in terminal illness.

Chapman KJ, Pepler C: Coping, hope, and anticipatory grief in family members in palliative home care, *Cancer Nurs* 21:226, 1998.

Understanding & Applying Research

COMPLICATED GRIEF DISORDER

The purpose of this clinical investigational study was to establish criteria for the diagnosis of complicated grief disorder separate from major depressive disorder (with the latter being a common diagnosis for persons experiencing unresolved or complicated grief). Using a structured diagnostic interview that included questions on 30 symptoms previously noted as being related to complicated grief, researchers interviewed subjects whose spouses had died. Interviews took place 6 and 14 months after the death to avoid the common increased distress of the death anniversary. Seven grief symptoms were extracted that could serve as potential diagnostic criteria for complicated grief disorder. These symptoms (at 14 months) included intense intrusive thoughts, pangs of severe emotion, distressing yearnings, feeling excessively alone and empty, excessively avoiding tasks reminiscent of the deceased, unusual sleep disturbances, and maladaptive levels of loss of interest in personal activities. These symptoms offer both assessment parameters to use and a rich opportunity for further research into more exact definitions of complicated grief.

Horowitz MJ et al: Diagnostic criteria for complicated grief disorder, *Am J Psychiatry* 154:904, 1997.

Association [HPNA]; Kemp, 1999; Parkes, 1998a) include:

- *Traumatic grief* occurs when there is traumatic loss such as a spouse murdered, a child dying suddenly and unexpectedly, rape, or multiple deaths. Posttraumatic stress disorder (PTSD) is often a concurrent or complicating factor, and the grief/PTSD may be characterized by psychic numbing, intrusive thoughts, avoidance of stimuli, increased arousal, and other aspects of PTSD (APA, 1994). There may also be distortion, usually exaggeration, of one or more normative components of grief, with anger and guilt being most common.
- *Absent or inhibited grief* is characterized by minimal emotional expression of grief and is sometimes related to trauma as noted above. Absent grief may convert to **delayed grief** and thus be experienced years after the loss. Precipitating factors for conversion to delayed grief often are powerful experiences such as psychotherapy or religious conversion.
- *Conflicted grief* may occur when the relationship with the deceased or lost object is characterized by ambivalence or conflict. Initial responses to the loss may be minimal and then intensify rather than diminish over time, and the survivor may feel "haunted" by the deceased. An adult survivor of childhood sexual abuse whose abusing parent dies is an example of a person at risk for conflicted grief.
- *Chronic grief* is unending grief after a loss. Chronic grief may be related to the survivor and the deceased having a highly dependent relationship. In other cases chronic grief is a result of (1) severe loss and (2) lack of resources or support to deal with the loss. Chronic grief may be especially common in some cultural groups such as Cambodian refugees or Native Americans.

In general, complicated grief is associated with unresolved issues in the relationship with the person who died; inhibited expression of grief; lack of social support; the "deritualization" of Western culture (e.g., mourning periods of 1 or 2 days); uncertain loss (e.g., prisoners of war);

⚠ CLINICAL ALERT

The following increase a client's potential for developing dysfunctional grief:
Premorbid psychiatric history
Social isolation
Relationship with the deceased that was characterized by unresolved conflict, ambivalence (e.g., "love-hate")
Relationship with the deceased that was characterized by enmeshment and a high level of introjection, hence difficulty "letting go"
Person who suppresses grief
Young age

---

traumatic loss (e.g., by murder); multiple losses; loss that is seldom discussed (e.g., rape); undervalued loss such as that felt by some who have an abortion, miscarriage, or other losses that may not be recognized by others as a significant loss; and by the accumulated effects of current grief on past unresolved grief.

CHRONIC SORROW

Only sparsely described in the literature, **chronic sorrow** is a form of grief that may include characteristics of other forms of grief but differs in several essential aspects. First, chronic sorrow is a response to *ongoing* loss such as the chronic illness of a loved one. Second, persons experiencing chronic sorrow seldom experience disability such as major depression but typically function at a higher level in activities of daily living than those experiencing other forms of grief (Burke et al, 1992). Persons at risk for chronic sorrow include parents with children who have mental retardation, schizophrenia, or other chronic illness; spouses of persons with long-term chronic illnesses such as multiple sclerosis, alcoholism, or Alzheimer's disease; and persons with similar disorders (Hainsworth, 1996; Lindgren, 1996). It is still undocumented what effects on the grief process result when the etiology of chronic sorrow is removed (i.e., when the disabled person dies).

GRIEF AND DEPRESSION

Grief and depression are often compared with one another. Grief, especially dysfunctional or complicated grief, also shares characteristics with PTSD, particularly in that both invariably involve loss (Table 29-1).

BEREAVEMENT CARE ACROSS THE LIFE SPAN
PREVENTION
Before Loss

Grief is a universal experience that may come with or without warning and occurs many times and with varying intensity throughout life. The major psychosocial determinants of pathology in grief are a psychiatric history before the loss and inadequate social support (Nuss and Zubenko, 1992). It follows, then, that grief is best addressed by the primary promotion of mental health, such as family involvement in community and faith activities, improved parenting, and other such efforts to promote mental and spiritual health.

When Loss Is Impending

A second point at which health promotion or disability prevention should be considered in relation to grief work is in the case of terminal illness or other anticipated loss. Interventions in these situations include assisting individuals and families in working toward personal, interpersonal, and spiritual reconciliation—and not necessarily anticipa-

Table 29-1	Comparison of Grief, Depression, and Posttraumatic Stress Disorder	
Grief	**Depression**	**Posttraumatic Stress Disorder**
Process related to loss.	Relatively static or cyclic affective disorder not necessarily related to loss.	Relatively static anxiety disorder related to trauma. Precipitating event is outside the range of usual human experience.
Symptoms usually appear shortly after the loss.	Symptoms may or may not be associated with an identified loss.	Symptoms often appear years after the trauma.
Depressive symptoms include dysphoric mood of sadness, hopelessness, and despair; anger is common, as are periods of agitation.	Depressive symptoms are similar to but more intense than grief, except that anger is seldom expressed and psychomotor retardation, morbid guilt, and suicidal ideation are more common.	Depressive symptoms are common. Other symptoms include persistent reexperiencing of the trauma (versus preoccupation with the image of the deceased, as in grief). Increased arousal is common.
Physical symptoms cover a wide spectrum. Physical sequelae may include heart disease and other chronic illness.	Physical symptoms are primarily neurovegetative.	Sleep disturbances may resemble those of grief or depression; hypervigilance is common.
Spiritual beliefs may provide meaning or context.	Spiritual beliefs seldom provide context or meaning.	Seldom any relation to spiritual beliefs.

tory grief. Even in the best of relationships, there may be unresolved issues or areas in which growth is possible, and whether interpersonal issues are addressed or not, promoting health in this stage of life includes promoting participation of the *client and family* in care. Clearly, effective participation in care has a positive effect on the grief process after death (although long-term effects are not known for caregivers in Alzheimer's disease, schizophrenia, and other similar chronic illnesses). A variety of means exist for intervention at this point, including individual informal or formal counseling in acute care settings, family support groups, hospice care, and church support. Nurses and other health care professionals should address the health needs of family members, as well as those of clients.

Preventive grief therapy is offered as a matter of course to survivors in several circumstances. Hospice and palliative care programs, for example, typically offer bereavement calls or visits at specified intervals to survivors. Many hospice programs also periodically hold picnics or other activities for bereaved adults or children. Churches and synagogues hold "grief workshops" for members and others in the community. These are generally weekend or time-limited groups similar to self-help groups such as I Can Cope, and others. Religiously oriented grief activities are also held in some cases in association with significant religious holidays related to death or remembrance.

After the Loss

The third intervention point is after the loss occurs. This was called **postvention** by Shneidman (1973) and simply called grief therapy by others. Intervention at this point may be preventive and directed toward addressing existing problems that are interpersonal in nature or related to normative or dysfunctional grief. The tasks in grief (see earlier discussion) provide a framework for intervention after loss.

PROBLEM-ORIENTED GRIEF THERAPY

Grief therapy is offered when a problem—not necessarily dysfunctional grief—exists or is anticipated. Like other of life's unavoidable processes, the difficult and painful transitions in normative grief usually respond to understanding and support. Grief therapy often focuses on emotional responses to the loss and problem solving related to moving forward in life (i.e., undoing bonds of attachment [Worden, 1982]). Emotional issues center around the telling and retelling of the details of the story (of the death and surrounding issues) and the history of the relationship, with emphasis on the experience and expression of the feelings, particularly sadness, anger, guilt, or other troubling feelings. In earlier phases of the process, the bereaved person may only recall the positive qualities of the deceased. As the mourner progresses through the grief work, both positive and negative qualities of the deceased and the relationship emerge. Problem-focused strategies may address questions of developing support, relationships, and other issues inherent in "the new life" or life after a loved one dies. Family-oriented therapy focuses on improving communications, increasing cohesiveness, and enhancing problem solving (Kissane et al, 1998).

In response to frequent overuse of medications to mask grief, some practitioners discourage the use of anxiolytic or antidepressant medications for bereaved persons. However, even in cases of "normal" grief, mourners may require short-term use of these drugs at certain stages of the grief process.

Reassurance is an essential component in grief therapy. The absence of cultural norms for expressing or otherwise dealing with grief results in some people feeling as if their grief is the beginning of insanity. Although some will not initially believe it, they need to hear from the nurse that their experience is grief and is normal and not mental illness. The tasks in grief, described earlier, provide a framework for therapy.

INTERVENTIONS IN COMPLICATED OR DYSFUNCTIONAL GRIEF

In complicated grief there is often unresolved grief from the past and/or a preexisting psychologic condition that must be addressed as part of the grief therapy. Thus therapy includes the issues noted above and other interpersonal issues. Often, a central issue in complicated grief is the promotion of the client's ability to express the pain of the grief rather than only the anger or guilt. It is common for bereaved persons to have ill-defined fantasies of catastrophe if their pain is expressed: "If I ever start crying, I will never stop." Clients with complicated grief are at increased risk for suicide or, to a lesser extent, for hurting others. They may also experience physical and mental disorders as previously discussed.

The client's primary physician, nurse practitioner, or other source of primary health care should be involved or at least kept aware of treatment for several specific reasons. First, it is common for such clients to frequently seek medical care, often for vague or difficult-to-evaluate complaints that are actually somatic expressions of grief. Awareness of complicated grief and ongoing therapy may help health care providers avoid unnecessary tests and treatment. Second, there is significant risk of suicide in complicated grief, and an informed health care provider can be alert to suicidal hints, gestures, and attempts to obtain lethal amounts of medications. All health professionals involved in the care of a person with complicated grief should be alert to the possibility of the client's seeking help from multiple sources and the potential for lethal medication admixture.

SPIRITUALITY AND GRIEF

All basic spiritual needs or issues may be threatened by the grief experience: meaning, hope, relatedness, forgiveness, and transcendence may fall away and leave the mourner in a spiritual vacuum. The nature of God and previously held beliefs, including any easy answers to life's problems (e.g., that faith protects one from pain), are called into question and may not support the reality of the current feelings. Grief may then be experienced as a test of faith, and the awareness or acknowledgment of anger may be interpreted as a personal spiritual failure (a source of more guilt). Although dreams and visions are seen as significant spiritual events in some cultures, in the context of Western cultures they may be discounted as either immaterial or pathologic. There may be reluctance by the grieving individual to discuss these experiences and feelings with family, friends, or clergy. As mourners struggle to find a context for the doubt and confusion that may accompany these experiences, it is important for the nurse to listen with openness, determining how these experiences either confirm or challenge the mourner's spiritual and religious beliefs. Some individuals are confirmed in their traditional beliefs; others see the dissolution of their faith; some find or rediscover a deeper faith (see Chapter 34).

• • •

Grief has the potential to transform those who experience it, for better or worse. Grief can be an "invitation to a new life" in which the discontinuity of death/loss and grief can be taken to a "higher continuity" (Carse, 1980), or grief can be a context for retreat into an impoverished life. Interventions in grief are most efficacious when used to promote health and prevent dysfunction. Interventions are less efficacious in the postvention period and least efficacious in treating complicated grief.

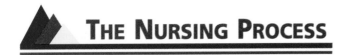

THE NURSING PROCESS

ASSESSMENT

Nursing assessment of a person who is bereaved is based on knowledge of normative and pathologic aspects of the grief process, influences on the grief process, and the person's resources. Assessment encompasses the following: (1) the grief experience of the mourner; (2) factors that inhibit or promote working through the grief process, including cultural and religious norms; and (3) the mourner's ability to mobilize cognitive, behavioral, and emotion-based coping strategies. The client's current level of functioning should be assessed, with the understanding that up to a point (about which there is disagreement), impaired functioning is to be expected.

PHYSICAL DISTURBANCES

Physical disturbances in acute grief include weakness, anorexia, shortness of breath, tightness of the chest, dry mouth, and gastrointestinal disturbances such as constipation or diarrhea, abdominal pain, gas, and nausea and vomiting. Cardiovascular and gastrointestinal problems predominate in chronic grief.

COGNITIVE DISTURBANCES

Cognitive disturbances are often focused on preoccupation with images and thoughts of the deceased. This preoccupation may be so pervasive that the bereaved person is unable to carry on with some activities of daily living. The inability to control thoughts is distressing to many mourners. In acute grief these obsessive thoughts are normal; they are simply part of the process. Preoccupation that results in significant disturbance of daily life (e.g., work) is widely considered pathologic after about 1 year past the date of death when the person who died was an adult and 2 or more years past the date of death when the deceased was a child.

BEHAVIORAL AND RELATING DISTURBANCES

Behavioral and relating disturbances may result from the depressive aspects of grief. People who are bereaved may describe themselves as "stopped" and thus unable to participate in relationships. There is a tendency in survivors to ruminate about the death and the relationship with the deceased. In at least the earlier phases of the process, talk of the deceased tends to focus only on his or her "good" qualities and ignore the multifaceted nature of the individual. Many people who are bereaved cry with little apparent provocation, which often results in discomfort for the mourner and others. In chronic grief the talk of the death and the relationship tends to be repetitive and superficial rather than progressive and insightful.

AFFECTIVE DISTURBANCES

Affective disturbances are primarily those of sadness or depression, anger, and guilt. Cultural norms of "carrying on" inhibit expression of these feelings. People who are bereaved soon learn that "nobody wants to hear your sad story." Sadness and even feelings of depression are not considered pathologic unless they persist a year or two past the death or include suicidal ideation.

NURSING DIAGNOSIS

Nursing diagnosis of grief or problems occurring in grief may be complicated by the more common approach of identifying problems of a physical or psychologic nature and seeking to alleviate the discomfort. The grief process by itself includes discomfort, and attempts to avoid or eliminate the discomfort, no matter how well intentioned, may impede the grieving process. On the other hand, extreme discomfort may require pharmacologic intervention. The point at which discomfort is classified as extreme or abnormal versus normal has not been defined. Thus an insightful diagnosis may focus on the *expression* of normal feelings (e.g., anger, guilt, sadness) as much as on what feelings exist.

NURSING DIAGNOSES FOR ACUTE GRIEF

Personal identity disturbance related to change in role and relationships, as evidenced by the inability to establish new patterns of relating to others and the environment after the death of a spouse or loved one

Self-esteem, situational low, related to pervasive feelings of guilt and cognitive distortions secondary to guilt, as evidenced by ruminating about inadequacies in the relationship with the deceased and blaming self for all problems in the relationship

Social interaction, impaired, related to altered role performance and disruptions in usual patterns of conduct/interactions, as evidenced by difficulty in adapting to life changes and developing relationships according to the current situation

---

NURSING ASSESSMENT QUESTIONS

Persons Experiencing Grief

1. Describe how it has been for you since your husband died.
2. How have you reacted to other major losses in your life?
3. Whom do you depend on when you are having a hard time, like now? Talk about how it is when you ask for help.
4. Let's go over all the prescription and other medicine and vitamins you are taking.

5. How often do you have alcoholic drinks (or other drugs)? When you drink (take drugs), how much do you take, and how does it make you feel?

A question not to ask is, "How are you doing?" Cultural norms are to respond to such questions with "pretty good," "OK," or "fine." These answers are essentially meaningless.

NURSING DIAGNOSES FOR COMPLICATED OR DYSFUNCTIONAL GRIEF

Grieving, dysfunctional, related to unresolved guilt, as evidenced by frequent references to personal failings in the relationship with the deceased

Grieving, dysfunctional (unexpressed), related to fear of catastrophe if grief is expressed, as evidenced by absence of expression of feelings related to the grief process

Violence, risk for: self-directed. Risk factors: feelings of hopelessness and anger and reports and observed incidents of rage over perceived inability to live without the deceased

NURSING DIAGNOSES FOR CHRONIC SORROW

Chronic sorrow is a concept being explored and developed. A nursing diagnosis for chronic sorrow has not yet been approved by NANDA, but one that might apply to chronic sorrow is:

Caregiver role strain related to chronic sorrow, as evidenced by caregiver withdrawal from community life to care for a loved one with chronic schizophrenia

OUTCOME IDENTIFICATION

Outcome criteria focus on enhancement of emotional coping skills or methods (e.g., greater expression of feelings of grief) and cognitive and behavioral coping abilities (e.g., strategies to develop more functional patterns of living, appropriate to changed life circumstances). Outcome criteria include that the client will:

1. Verbalize absence of suicidal ideations.
2. Express any guilty and/or angry feelings related to the death and grief versus suppression of grief.
3. Express both positive and negative feelings about the deceased versus idealizing the qualities of the deceased.
4. Explore the relationship with the deceased in a multifaceted way that includes both positive and negative aspects.
5. Formulate and implement reasonable plans for adapting life and the identified role to present circumstances.
6. Participate in at least one social or community activity each week.

PLANNING

The plan of care for a person with acute grief consists primarily of (1) supporting mobilization of the person's personal and community resources, (2) providing normative data about the grief process, and (3) supporting the person in her or his grief work. Each of these is discussed below.

Assistance may be needed in mobilizing resources

COLLABORATIVE DIAGNOSES

DSM-IV Diagnoses*	Nursing Diagnoses†
Adjustment disorder	Adjustment, impaired
Dysthymic disorder	Coping, ineffective family, disabling
Major depressive disorder	Coping, ineffective individual
	Denial, ineffective
	Family processes, altered
	Fatigue
	Grieving, anticipatory
	Grieving, dysfunctional
	Hopelessness
	Personal identity disturbance
	Posttrauma syndrome
	Powerlessness
	Role performance, altered
	Self-esteem, situational low
	Sexuality patterns, altered
	Sleep pattern disturbance
	Social interaction, impaired
	Social isolation
	Spiritual distress (distress of the human spirit)
	Thought processes, altered
	Violence, risk for: directed at others
	Violence, risk for: self-directed

*From American Psychiatric Association: *Diagnostic and statistical manual of mental disorders,* ed 4, Washington, DC, 1994, The Association.
†From North American Nursing Diagnosis Association: *NANDA nursing diagnoses: definitions and classifications, 1999-2000,* Philadelphia, 1999, The Association.

(e.g., family, friends, and spiritual supports), because individuals often are reluctant to ask for help and resources often do not know how to provide help. In addition, some of the symptoms of grief (e.g., fatigue, sadness, and anger) promote isolation rather than relating. Frequently, if either the bereaved person or his or her support systems can initiate contact, the other will respond appropriately. Too often, however, the mourner and resources exist in isolation, each wishing they knew how to make contact with the other.

Normative data on grief (i.e., explanation of physical, emotional, social, and spiritual difficulties inherent in the grief process) can be provided to both the bereaved and his or her support systems. In a culture in many ways lacking in ritual and tradition, grief may sometimes seem mysterious and/or pathologic even to those one might expect to be helpful (e.g., clergy). The nurse teaches survivors and others (such as family members) what they might experience in the grief process. Bereavement (survivor) groups are an excellent forum for such teaching.

Supporting the mourner in his or her grief work includes facilitating the telling of how the deceased died and related events and exploring both positive and negative aspects of the relationship with the deceased, positive and negative aspects of the deceased, and cognitive and behavioral coping strategies. Assistance with mobilizing

Grief and Loss

Grief and loss may be encountered anywhere in the community. The aging wife may be losing her husband after a year of declining health, the young person with schizophrenia may feel the loss of hope for the future, or the mature adult may experience unexpected unemployment. Each person perceives the world as changing dramatically without the prospect of immediate stabilization. The mental health nurse in the community responds to each of these crises with both compassion and practicality. The nurse must assess the client's need to voice emotional pain or to maintain silence. Expressing emotional empathy with the client and acknowledging the pain is not unprofessional as long as the nurse maintains emotional objectivity.

During the initial grief reaction the nurse should encourage expression of memory and emotion. The nurse may also assess the individual's ability to tolerate difficult emotions and use prescribed medication, if appropriate, while assisting the individual in adapting to change and loss. The nurse needs to be sensitive to both the client and the support network, to gauge how much intervention is necessary and can be tolerated.

The community is an ideal environment to support the grieving process. The community mental health nurse can ensure that referrals to appropriate support groups are accessed, as well as offer individual comfort and assistance. Rituals that are performed and expressed by cultural preferences should be respected and encouraged. Spiritual counselors such as clergy may be used to offer the client comfort, sustenance, and ceremony for grief.

The time of grieving varies widely among individuals, so the concept of well-delineated, consecutive stages may have to be individualized. Some individuals have difficulty focusing on grieving, and for them the process seems to take longer. A person may appear to have returned to a normal, pre-grief state, but still feel numb and anguished inside. The nurse assists by acknowledging the length of the process and educating the family and community to also respect the time necessary for the client's recovery.

The nurse should allow at least a year's follow-up with both the client and the support system to evaluate the client's level of function, food consumption, and sleep patterns. If the client appears extremely dysfunctional and depressed for more than 6 months, the grief may have become pathologic, and thoughts of suicide should be explored. If there are substantial concerns and the client appears to be clinically depressed, the client should be referred to a psychiatrist and may require hospitalization and medication. After a significant loss, client safety is always of major concern.

resources and providing normative data is also part of support.

The plan of care for a person with dysfunctional grieving focuses on the specific pathologic condition of the patient. Normative aspects of grief are also addressed.

Plans can also be directed toward the community. In community-focused planning the nurse helps churches, synagogues, community centers, hospitals, and other organizations develop self-help groups for bereaved persons. Nurses also serve as facilitators for such groups.

IMPLEMENTATION

The first priority in planning care for a person with dysfunctional grief is to assess the risk for violence toward self or others. The client's physical health may also be a major concern. The plan will include efforts to work toward resolving the grief through emotional, cognitive, and behavioral means. Chemical dependency presents a major barrier to the individual's goal attainment and must be addressed. Dependence on anxiolytic medications is common. In many cases the approach can be growth oriented rather than directed only to treatment of symptoms.

NURSING INTERVENTIONS

Bereavement care should ideally take place in the community before the client deteriorates to the extent that hospitalization is required.

1. The nurse assesses the client for intent to kill self or others *to ensure safety and prevent violence.*

CASE STUDY

Mrs. Jones is 70 years old and lives alone in the apartment she shared with her husband for the past 17 years since retirement. Her husband died last month, after a 2-year struggle with prostate cancer. Since her husband's death, Mrs. Jones has felt sad and depressed. She wants to spend time with others but says, "They are happy, and I'm sad, and it's no good for anyone." For the past week, except for "forcing" herself to take her daily walk around the block, Mrs. Jones has spent most of her time alone in her apartment. She has a poor appetite, difficulty sleeping, and feels guilty about "all the things I could have done to help my husband." Most of the other residents in the complex are similar in age to Mrs. Jones, and she is very close to several of them. Her only son lives in another state and has offered to let her move into a bedroom in his home.

Critical Thinking—Assessment
1. According to your assessment, what type of grief is Mrs. Jones experiencing?
2. From your knowledge of the grieving process, what are three important needs of Mrs. Jones?
3. What personal resources are likely to be most helpful to Mrs. Jones at the present time?

NURSING CARE PLAN

Mr. Smith and his wife had been married for 41 years when she died 18 months ago from bacterial endocarditis. Since his wife's death, Mr. Smith has become increasingly seclusive. He expresses extreme anger toward the physicians and nurses involved in his wife's care. Mr. Smith keeps his home exactly as it was when Mrs. Smith was alive. He has not disposed of any of her belongings and has renewed subscriptions to magazines that only Mrs. Smith read. Both Mr. and Mrs. Smith drank heavily but denied alcoholism. They had no children, and their relationship was characterized by frequent verbal and occasional physical abuse. Mr. Smith continues to drink daily. He complains of heart problems and is angry with his physician, who insists that Mr. Smith has only mild hypertension that should respond to dietary changes. Mr. Smith has begun keeping his curtains drawn and denies the need for interpersonal relationships.

DSM-IV Diagnoses

Axis I	Major depression; alcoholism
Axis II	None known
Axis III	Hypertension
Axis IV	Severity: Extreme-6 (death of spouse)
Axis V	GAF = 45 (current)
	GAF = 45 (past year)

Nursing Diagnosis: Grieving, dysfunctional (chronic distorted), related to inability to appropriately express the full spectrum of feelings associated with wife's death, as evidenced by social isolation, projected danger, daily alcohol use, and somatic complaints.

Client Outcomes	Nursing Interventions	Evaluation
• Mr. Smith will engage in a therapeutic alliance with the nurse.	• Visit Mr. Smith's home at a regular time on the same day once each week. *Constancy and dependability are essential in developing productive relationships.*	• Mr. Smith agrees to visits.
• Mr. Smith will cease intake of alcohol at least 4 hours before and during visits with nurse.	• Develop a contract with Mr. Smith in which he agrees to sobriety during visits. *Sobriety is essential to therapeutic relationships and personal growth.* • Institute chemical dependency care plan (see Chapter 16).	• Mr. Smith maintains sobriety during visits. • Mr. Smith enters and continues in a 12-step or other program intended to promote sobriety.
• Mr. Smith will express angry, sad, and other feelings concerning his wife's death.	• Gradually present Mr. Smith with aspects of his grief experience that will help him uncover his sadness and ambivalence. *Feelings of sadness and ambivalence are threatening to Mr. Smith and should not be introduced too rapidly.* • Recognize the legitimacy of Mr. Smith's anger. Demonstrate acceptance and understanding of the ambivalence and other feelings such as sadness and confusion. *Anger is the means by which Mr. Smith may be expressing other feelings not yet in his awareness. Facilitating other feelings helps to better manage anger and promote resolution of grief.*	• Mr. Smith is able to express sadness, confusion, ambivalence, and other feelings in addition to anger. • Mr. Smith begins to accept the validity of anger and feelings other than anger that may be hidden behind the expression of anger and rage.
• Mr. Smith will discuss his hopes (fulfilled and unfulfilled) and his disappointments about his relationship with his wife.	• Assist Mr. Smith in reviewing his relationship with his wife, and the hopes each one held, including those fulfilled and those that led to disappointments. *Although Mr. Smith's problems are attributed to his wife's death, they are also, to a great extent, attributable to his relationship with his wife and his difficulty coping with the loss of his wife.*	• Mr. Smith discusses his relationship with his wife in realistic terms (neither idealized nor all negative) and expresses both positive and negative feelings about their relationship.
• Mr. Smith will grieve in a functional manner for his wife, for their relationship, and for himself.	• Facilitate Mr. Smith's linking together all of his feelings and responses related to his relationship with his wife, to his life, and to his current dysfunctional behavior. *(This is the full expression of grief.)*	• Mr. Smith fully expresses his grief.

NURSING CARE PLAN —cont'd

Nursing Diagnosis: Social isolation related to seclusive behavior patterns secondary to unresolved grief, as evidenced by refusal to engage in interpersonal relationships.

Patient Outcomes	Nursing Interventions	Evaluation
• Mr. Smith will agree to regular visits in his home with the nurse.	• Adhere to 30-minute time limit for visits; be prompt according to schedule. *Structure in care increases order, understanding, and predictability and will help promote Mr. Smith's developing cognitive coping strategies, such as making realistic plans for the future.*	• Mr. Smith tolerates visits and eventually remarks that he looks forward to them.
• Mr. Smith participates in one social activity weekly. (Alcohol should not be served or available.)	• Give Mr. Smith choices of time-limited social activities that are likely to be enjoyable and convenient for him. *Activities that are enjoyable and sociable are more likely to be repeated; too many choices are likely to be overwhelming; time limits will reduce anxiety.*	• Mr. Smith follows through and attends activities, and expresses a favorable response.
• Mr. Smith participates in the termination phase of the relationship by increasing his social activities and continuing in his recovery from alcoholism.	• Include Mr. Smith in plans for termination by working *with* him to make plans for increased social activity as the relationship is terminated. Together, the nurse and Mr. Smith should write a schedule for termination that decreases the frequency of visits and ultimately ends the visits. *The therapeutic alliance progresses from collaboration between the nurse and client to the client's achieving independence.*	• Mr. Smith (1) participates in planning for termination, (2) initiates additional social activities, and (3) continues in his recovery.

2. Promote a therapeutic alliance between the client and the nurse. *Developing a working relationship may be difficult because of the client's suppressed feelings. Death and other major losses are often experienced as complete destruction of the certainty and order around which people structure their lives. It is therefore necessary for the nurse to be certain and orderly with respect to following through on all obligations, such as schedules and appointments.*

3. Facilitate the client's expression of feelings related to the loss, and validate the feelings already expressing by the client. Also, begin to introduce the possibility of other feelings related to the loss, such as ambivalence. Help the client take an increasingly active role in exploring and understanding the full response to the grief. *Ambivalent feelings are especially difficult for many clients to acknowledge. Many clients are prone to merely repeat feelings and thoughts rather than explore, expand, and understand them. Although some repetition of feelings, concerns, and experiences is unavoidable and somewhat helpful, it is important for the client to understand the full grief response to begin the healing process.*

4. Help the client understand the relationship between self and the lost person or object and to express and understand the grief and attendant feelings. Facilitate a review of the client's relationship with the deceased, and help the client to discuss and understand meanings

within the relationship, hopes fulfilled, disappointments, and strengths and weaknesses of the relationship. *It is essential that the client move beyond the grief that is related to the death or loss and begin to understand the full meaning of the relationship, both good and bad.*

5. Facilitate the full expression of grief by assisting the client in linking together the full spectrum of feelings, both positive and negative, regarding the loss and the relationship with the deceased. *It is necessary for the client to remember the deceased as a real human being with both positive and negative qualities, to "let go" of the idealistic image of the person, and begin to move forward without guilt and remorse. Some survivors are more successful at this than others.*

6. Promote interactions with others, and offer limited and specific options for the client to increase **social support,** both individually and in the community. Encourage the client to continue engaging in social relationships—even when, as some mourners say, it feels as if "it's just going through the motions." *It is important for the client to begin to move forward and "join the living," even if it means "going through the motions" at first. With encouragement from family and friends, the client should eventually develop a healthy social life while experiencing (in a healthy sense) both good and bad memories of the deceased.*

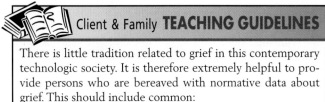

There is little tradition related to grief in this contemporary technologic society. It is therefore extremely helpful to provide persons who are bereaved with normative data about grief. This should include common:

Physical responses to grief
Cognitive responses to grief
Behavioral responses to grief
Affective responses to grief

It is helpful to write a list (in layperson's terms) and review the list with the person who is bereaved. The power or intensity of feelings in response to loss is especially important to discuss with the bereaved person.

COLLABORATIVE INTERVENTIONS

A multidisciplinary approach by a team consisting of nurse, psychiatrist, psychologist, social worker, occupational therapist, and other health care providers is not usually necessary, although community resources are an important part of care. Because of the frequency and vagueness of physical complaints, the most important discipline other than nursing is the client's general practitioner or other source of primary care.

EVALUATION

The nurse evaluates the client's increasing ability to express feelings and to develop effective coping strategies such as increasing social interactions. It is important for the client to express the full spectrum of feelings that are (1) associated with the loss and (2) related to the relationship with the deceased. Expressing feelings only about the loss itself is not sufficient for successful progress in grief work (see Client & Family Teaching Guidelines box). The nurse should remember that grief is a normal response to loss and that the feelings associated with grief are necessarily painful. The key to successful grief work depends on the individual's understanding of the relationship with the deceased. When that occurs, the client is able to continue the work of investing in new relationships.

CASE STUDY

Mr. and Mrs. Mason have a 26-year-old son, Jim, who has chronic undifferentiated schizophrenia. Jim lives at home most of the year, except when he is admitted to the state hospital (two or three times per year). Jim has never worked, has no friends, is withdrawn most of the time, has violent episodes about once a month, and is noncompliant with medications. The Masons have tried different hospitals (they no longer have any insurance coverage for Jim), a variety of antipsychotic medications, different therapists, prayer, and "alternative therapies," but nothing has changed the course of the illness. Mr. Mason works long hours at an auto parts store, and Mrs. Mason stays home with Jim. Mr. and Mrs. Mason have begun seeing the clinical nurse specialist from the state hospital community outreach program. Their chief complaints as a couple and individually are overwhelming feelings of hopelessness and physical and mental exhaustion. The clinical nurse specialist has diagnosed their problem as caregiver role strain related to chronic sorrow, as evidenced by the caregivers' withdrawal from community life in order to care for their son with chronic schizophrenia. The nurse has implemented a plan of care that includes (1) weekly couples' counseling, a (2) regular family support group in a community facility, and (3) biweekly home visits by an outreach staff member to assist Jim with medication compliance.

Critical Thinking—Planning

1. What is your opinion about whether Jim will experience significant improvement in his disorder?
2. Part of the care is directed to the parents. Why are they also receiving care instead of Jim alone, since he is the one who is mentally ill?
3. Discuss potential success in relation to this plan. Are the Masons likely to achieve happiness as a result of receiving care?
4. Discuss each of the following feelings that family members sometimes experience about relatives with chronic mental illness: anger, sorrow, love, disgust, and despair.

Summary of Key Concepts

1. Grief encompasses all spheres of being. Symptoms include physical, cognitive, behavioral, and affective reactions.
2. Although grief is commonly presented in stages, it is more effective to conceptualize grief in terms of a dynamic process in which certain tasks are usually accomplished.
3. Grief may be classified as acute, anticipatory, dysfunctional, or complicated, and as chronic sorrow. Types of dysfunctional grief include traumatic grief, absent or inhibited grief, conflicted grief, and chronic grief.
4. The potential for dysfunctional grief is decreased in situations where clients have a healthy family life,

provide care for the person who is dying, participate in community-oriented bereavement programs, and receive therapy if they are at risk. Therapy for persons experiencing dysfunctional grief includes facilitating expression of suppressed feelings, mobilizing cognitive and behavioral coping skills, dealing with unresolved aspects of the relationship, and encouraging reentry into socialization.

REFERENCES

American Psychiatric Association: *Diagnostic and statistical manual of mental disorders*, ed 4, Washington, DC, 1994, The Association.

Bowlby J: *Loss: sadness and depression*, vol 3, *Attachment and loss*, New York, 1980, Basic Books.

Burke ML et al: Current knowledge and research on chronic sorrow: a foundation for inquiry, *Death Studies* 16:231, 1992.

Carman MB: The psychology of normal aging, *Psychiatr Clin North Am* 20:15, 1997.

Carse JB: *Death and existence*, New York, 1980, John Wiley & Sons.

Chapman KJ, Pepler C: Coping, hope, and anticipatory grief in family members in palliative home care, *Cancer Nurs* 21:226, 1998.

Cowles KV, Rodgers BL: The concept of grief: a foundation for nursing research and practice, *Res Nurs Health* 14:119, 1991.

Engel G: Grief and grieving, *Am J Nurs* 64:93, 1964.

Freud S: Mourning and melancholia. In Strachey J, editor, *The standard edition of the complete psychological works of Sigmund Freud*, vol 14, London, 1917, Hogarth Press.

Gibbons MB: A child dies, a child survives: the impact of sibling loss, *J Pediatr Health Care* 6:65, 1992.

Goodman M et al: Cultural differences among elderly women in coping with the death of an adult child, *J Gerontol* 46:321, 1991.

Hainsworth MA: Helping spouses with chronic sorrow related to multiple sclerosis, *J Psychosoc Nurs Ment Health Serv* 34:36, 1996.

Horowitz MJ et al: Diagnostic criteria for complicated grief disorder, *Am J Psychiatry* 154:904, 1997.

Hospice and Palliative Nurses Association: *The hospice nurses study guide: a preparation for the CRNH candidate*, ed 2, Pittsburgh, 1997, The Association.

Jacob SR: The grief experience of older women whose husbands had hospice care, *J Adv Nurs* 24:280, 1996.

Kemp C: Refugee mental health issues, *Refugee health*, http://www.baylor.edu/~Charles_Kemp/refugee_health.htm, 1998.

Kemp C: *Terminal illness: a guide to nursing care*, ed 2, Philadelphia, 1999 Lippincott–Williams & Wilkins.

Kissane DW et al: Family grief therapy: a preliminary account of a new model to promote healthy family functioning during palliative care and bereavement, *Psycho-Oncology* 7:14, 1998.

Kubler-Ross E: *On death and dying*, New York, 1969, Macmillan.

Lev EL, McCorkle R: Loss, grief, and bereavement in family members of cancer patients, *Semin Oncol Nurs* 14:145, 1998.

Levy LH: Anticipatory grief: its measurement and proposed reconceptualization, *Hosp J* 7:1, 1991.

Lindemann E: Symptomatology and management of acute grief, *Am J Psychiatry* 101:141, 1944.

Lindgren CL: Chronic sorrow in persons with Parkinson's disease and their spouses, *Sch Inq Nurs Pract* 10:351, 1996.

McCabe MJ: Clinical responses to clinical issues. In Portenoy RK, Bruera E, editors: *Topics in palliative care*, vol 1, New York, 1997, Oxford University Press.

Nuss WS, Zubenko GS: Correlates of persistent depressive symptoms in widows, *Am J Psychiatry* 149:346, 1992.

Parkes CM: Bereavement in adult life, *BMJ* 316:856, 1998b.

Parkes CM: Bereavement. In Doyle D, Hanks GWC, MacDonald N, editors: *Oxford textbook of palliative medicine*, ed 2, Oxford, 1998a, Oxford University Press.

Rando TA: *Grieving*, Lexington, Mass, 1988, Lexington Books.

Sheldon F: ABC of palliative care: bereavement, *BMJ* 316:456, 1998.

Shneidman ES: *Deaths of man*, New York, 1973, Quadrangle/The New York Times Book Co.

Shneidman ES, *Voices of death*, New York, 1980, Harper & Row.

Silverman PR, Worden JW: Children's reactions in the early months after the death of a parent, *Am J Orthopsychiatry* 62:93, 1992.

Steen KF: A comprehensive approach to bereavement, *Nurse Pract* 23:54, 1998.

Walker RJ, Pomeroy EC: The impact of anticipatory grief on caregivers of persons with Alzheimer's disease, *Home Health Care Q* 16:55, 1997.

Weiss RS, Richards TA: A scale for predicting quality of recovery following the death of a partner, *J Pers Soc Psychol* 72:885, 1997.

Worden J: *Grief counseling and grief therapy: a handbook for the mental health practioner*, New York, 1982, Springer.

CHAPTER 30

Persons With HIV/AIDS

Gwen van Servellen

OBJECTIVES

- Discuss the prevalence of HIV/AIDS in vulnerable, hard-to-reach populations.
- Examine the risk of psychiatric and psychologic morbidity for those coping with HIV/AIDS.
- Distinguish between adjustment disorders and Axis I mood disorders in persons with HIV/AIDS, using the criteria of severity of symptoms, treatment, and prognosis.
- Examine behavioral characteristics of those persons placing themselves at high risk for the acquisition of HIV infection.
- Discuss why persons practicing high-risk behaviors may have difficulty changing these behaviors.
- Apply the nursing process for persons with HIV/AIDS.

HIV/AIDS

This chapter identifies and discusses the skills and knowledge needed to provide care to clients experiencing the neuropsychiatric and psychosocial aspects of **human immunodeficiency virus (HIV)** infection and **acquired immunodeficiency syndrome (AIDS)**. To understand the impact of HIV disease on the mental and emotional functioning of clients and their families, it is important to first define HIV disease.

HIV disease has been identified by the U.S. Department of Health and Human Services as a major public health problem in the nation. AIDS, the advanced stage of illness in HIV disease, is fatal. HIV disease is characterized by a defect in the natural immunity against disease, especially against certain opportunistic infections and AIDS-related cancers (e.g., Kaposi's sarcoma [KS] or non-Hodgkin's lymphoma). Although individuals in the symptomatic state are identifiable by a specific set of signs and symptoms, those who are infected but asymptomatic may go undiagnosed for long periods of time. Neither health care providers nor clients themselves may suspect HIV infection. Since the infected asymptomatic individuals are capable of transmitting the disease to others, even if they remain asymptomatic for a long time, HIV disease is unquestionably a serious public health threat.

Both clinical and research evidence indicate that HIV infects the brain and results in central nervous system impairment in some individuals. In addition to the troublesome neuropsychologic and neuropsychiatric consequences of HIV, many more, if not all, individuals with asymptomatic HIV infection, as well as those who perceive themselves to be at high risk for infection and their families and significant others, experience a wide range of psychosocial needs. All of them need

help in varying degrees in order to cope with psychologic symptoms that are a result of the AIDS epidemic. Although this includes care and counsel to those infected, it also includes information and counseling services to those who need to change high-risk behaviors or to regain or maintain low-risk activities. Since sexual transmission and infection through needle exchange in drug abuse are the primary modes of transmission, efforts to change behaviors effectively are exceedingly complex. They involve curbing behaviors that are not easily discussed or readily changed. Since African-Americans and Hispanics are disproportionately represented in the AIDS community, focus on culture-specific needs of these groups related to the prevention and treatment of HIV is needed.

Feelings of anxiety and depression in persons with HIV/AIDS are of concern to clinicians caring for these individuals for a variety of reasons. First, these conditions are negative-affective states reflective of subjective distress. In turn, this subjective distress can significantly alter clients' quality of life in the short and long term. Also, these conditions, when present as enduring clinical syndromes, present with behavioral, somatic, and cognitive features (in addition to affective symptoms) that affect clients' health status and ability to follow medical treatment protocol. These include negative affect, irritability, decreased energy and lethargy, altered performance, restlessness and/or interrupted sleep, feelings of helplessness, punitive and self-accusatory evaluations, and persistent fear and worry. These conditions further tax clients' resources and affect their quality of life. Although suicide in clients with HIV/AIDS may be understandable, it is preventable, and suicidal risk should always be included in assessments. Life-threatening illnesses increase the incidence of psychologic distress, particularly depression. Although some debate exists regarding exact figures, higher rates of depression and suicide risk have been associated with HIV infection (Marzuk et al, 1988). In light of available and appropriate pharmacologic therapy and concomitant counseling and/or social support, relief from depression is possible (Buck and Duffy, 1993; Rabkin et al, 1994) (see Understanding & Applying Research box below).

Understanding & Applying Research

HIV/AIDS is reported to impose significant psychosocial stressors, among which are stigmatization, lifestyle changes, illness-related uncertainty, and existential issues related to diagnosis with a life-threatening chronic illness. The purpose of this study was to measure the impact of a stress management training program on measures of psychologic distress and quality of life in men with HIV disease. The investigators used a 6-month pretest-posttest design to compare the effectiveness of a 6-week stress management program (progressive muscle relaxation training, yogaform stretching with integrative breathing, and mental techniques such as thematic imagery and beginning meditation) on several outcome measures: stress levels, coping patterns, quality of life, psychologic distress, illness-related uncertainty, and CD4 T lymphocyte levels. At 6 weeks those patients receiving the intervention (stress management training program) were reported to have increases in the emotional well-being dimension of the quality-of-life measure. Although changes in other measures were in the predicted directions, indicating improvement, only the emotional well-being subscale was found to be significantly higher immediately following the program. After 6 months, the intervention group had a relative decline in HIV-related intrusive thinking, a measure of illness-related psychologic distress. The investigators concluded that the stress management training program may have buffered illness-related stress over time, the exact mechanism by which is still incompletely understood. It may be that stress management may enhance quality of life and mitigate psychologic distress by virtue of its impact on the sense of personal control and/or optimism patients experience using stress management strategies. Future studies should include measures of personal control and/or optimism.

McCain NL et al: The influence of stress management training in HIV disease, *Nurs Res* 45:246, 1996.

In HIV/AIDS, as in other life-threatening illness (e.g., advanced cancer), somatic symptomatic health status carries both primary and secondary implications for quality of life and functional performance. Both physical and psychologic symptoms have a direct effect on quality of life but also an indirect effect through the process of secondary appraisal. These symptoms in and of themselves can be perceived as threatening. Likewise, their consequences (e.g., deficits in role performance, functional decline, and altered social activities) are also felt to be as threatening. Adaptation at this stage of HIV disease requires realignment of goal-related activities in order to achieve a positive emotional state. When viewed as being outside the individual's control, this decline leads to anxiety. Symptoms can also be perceived as stable (recurrent) and global (affecting many outcomes important to the individual). To the extent that one or more symptoms are perceived as uncontrollable, stable, and global, their presence may produce additional psychologic distress.

EPIDEMIOLOGY

The Centers for Disease Control and Prevention (CDC) publish a quarterly HIV/AIDS surveillance report. This publication typically identifies the numbers of full-blown cases of AIDS in the United States reported to the CDC. Since cases of HIV infection are not reportable in many states, the total number of persons in the United States infected with the virus at any one point in time is unknown and can only be estimated.

HIV surveillance data indicate that there have been 612,078 cases of AIDS reported to the CDC to date (CDC, 1997). With 379,258 reported deaths, the cumulative case-fatality rate to date is 62%. Treatment advances are extending the period between initial infection and the onset of AIDS-related conditions; thus it becomes increasingly important to rely on estimates of infection as health care policy makers attempt to address needs for HIV/AIDS services to U.S. residents. Estimates of the number of HIV infections in the United States range from 1 to 2 million, indicating that the threat of HIV/AIDS is much more serious than what can be gleamed from surveillance reports of either the current or cumulative number of AIDS cases.

In addition, it is important to understand that to derive meaningful predictions of the threat of HIV/AIDS, many different factors that seem to influence the rate of new infections and reportable cases of AIDS must be considered. These factors include a host of demographic characteristics, including regional differences, gender, age, ethnicity, and exposure category. HIV/AIDS does not discriminate; rural and urban, heterosexual men and women, children, adolescents, and elders are living with HIV/AIDS. Once a disease of gay white men in largely urban areas of the United States, HIV/AIDS has permeated most populations, creating a challenge not unlike that of major serious epidemics in history. Although men who have sex with men remain at highest risk for HIV infection, the number of cases of HIV/AIDS as a result of reported heterosexual transmission is rising at rates surpassing that of homosexual transmission. Although exposure continues to occur through homosexual encounters and injection drug use (blood exposure), the dramatic shift to those reporting heterosexual exposure (particularly among African-American women) have increased the need to think differently about those at risk for HIV/AIDS.

CULTURAL CONSIDERATIONS

Once primarily an affliction of gay white men in major urban epicenters, HIV/AIDS has spread with faster-than-average increases in populations difficult to reach from the perspective of both prevention and treatment. One such shift has been the rising number of cases of HIV/AIDS in rural areas of the United States. Recent reports have drawn attention to rural areas despite the fact that the number of reported AIDS cases is still lower in rural regions as compared with urban areas (U.S. Department of Health and Human Services [USDHHS], 1995), because the rate of increase in cases has risen faster than that in urban areas (Mainous et al, 1997). Some reasons postulated for the rise in reported AIDS cases in rural areas include the observation that individuals who migrated from rural to urban areas are moving back to rural communities once they have been diagnosed as having HIV infection. This backward migration has raised concern about the adequacy of health care and supportive services in regions where HIV/AIDS may be poorly understood and where specialists are typically not available. Rural communities have been challenged to design shared-care models in order to improve the care to this underserved population (Mainous et al, 1997).

A second population of concern that has also been difficult to reach is women and adolescent girls, a category accounting for almost 1 out of 5 new cases of AIDS diagnosed in 1996 in the United States (USDHHS, 1997). One of the groups with the greatest proportionate increases in incidence (12%) is non-Hispanic African-American women with heterosexual risk/exposures (USDHHS, 1997). Over 44,000 women with AIDS are faced with the day-to-day issues of dealing with this profoundly life-threatening illness in themselves and, for many, in their young children and spouses or partners. They are both the infected and affected, coping with their own disease course and the challenges of caring for children who are infected. Clearly, one of the most critical psychosocial concerns in this population (persons acquiring HIV infection through heterosexual activity) is the disbelief that they could be or are infected. Typically, those who do not perceive themselves to be at risk are less likely to suspect infection and are more likely to delay testing. Once tested, they may have significantly greater difficulty in coming to

terms with their infection, having never suspected that they could be infected. In some instances their heterosexual partners were also unaware of or hid their HIV serostatus. Thus these women and teens may experience greater distress, more denial, and poorer psychosocial adaptation, at least in the initial period of learning of their infection. Addressing the shock and disbelief surrounding their diagnosis and their perceived fantasies related to their prognosis has been identified as critical to the care of these women.

Clients with HIV/AIDS may not trust the traditional medically oriented health care system or have trouble accessing it. Many rely on alternative treatments (e.g., herbs) or adjunctive treatment (e.g., acupuncture) to manage their illness and their specific symptoms. To maintain rapport, it is critical that the nurse understands clients' beliefs and honors their alternative treatment choices. In some cases clients will not take their medications or miss appointments, suggesting problems with adherence. Nonadherent behaviors have been linked with higher levels of depression and anxiety and lower levels of optimism. Finally, in otherwise disenfranchised populations (e.g., incarcerated and undocumented residences), access to and adherence with treatment are of concern not only because of clients' potential mistrust of the system but also because of their fear of deportation (undocumented residents).

In summary, the specific cultural and regional differences displayed in clients with HIV/AIDS influence all aspects of health care, from prevention of infection to treatment of late-stage AIDS illness. Culturally sensitive interventions must take into account subtle, as well as more obvious, regional and ethnic characteristics of these populations.

ETIOLOGY OF EMOTIONAL DISTRESS IN HIV/AIDS

In establishing the basis for emotional distress in clients with HIV disease, it is important to understand various etiologic departures. Psychoneurologic and psychosocial theories are discussed only as they explain the etiology of emotional distress in persons (primarily adults) with HIV disease. Comorbid mental disorders such as schizophrenia, bipolar disorder, and borderline personality disorder are not addressed. The focus is on mood and/or cognitive disorders related to HIV/AIDS diagnoses. The primary DSM-IV diagnoses for review are adjustment disorders with anxiety, depression, and/or disturbance of conduct.

NEUROPSYCHIATRIC FACTORS

Soon after the discovery of AIDS, health care providers were puzzled not only by the frequency of cognitive impairment among hospitalized clients, but also by the severity of impairment.

The profound dementia noted in some clients with

AIDS seemed disproportionate to the clinical condition, laboratory values, and gross neuropathologic findings present in these clients (Perry and Markowitz, 1986). To confound this discovery even more, the histories of many of these clients revealed that psychologic and cognitive problems predated signs of immune deficiency. It is now known that HIV has a direct effect on the central nervous system and causes a subacute encephalopathy. Cortical atrophy and ventricular dilation have been shown on computed tomography (CT) scans, indicating possible permanent and significant damage to the central nervous system (Perry and Jacobsen, 1986).

With this knowledge of histopathology, accurate diagnosis of cognitive and affective changes in clients can be made. Changes in mood can be evidence of clinical depression or represent signs of AIDS-related dementia. Even with organically based changes, the signs and symptoms can be subtle, and laboratory findings may not immediately point to irregularities. The insidious emotional problems tend to mimic functional disorders. Also, initially, the neurologic examination, laboratory values, electroencephalogram, cerebrospinal fluid, and CT scan of the brain may appear normal. Additionally confusing is the fact that many of these high-risk and sometimes socially impaired individuals have psychosocial stresses that can explain the emotional distress they exhibit. Differential diagnosis is aided by seropositivity, the absence of a premorbid or family history of psychiatric illness (including substance abuse), positive signs on neuropsychologic testing, and signs of organicity (e.g., imbalance, tremor, avoidance of complex tasks, and sensitivity to drugs and alcohol). Although AIDS dementias vary, they can generally be categorized into two primary types: a dementia chiefly characterized by moderate signs of depression and a more acute psychotic presentation. The first of these is evidenced in apathy, withdrawal, fatigue, hypersomnia, weight loss, anorexia, psychomotor retardation, and subtle cognitive deficits. The acute psychotic presentation can include delusions, hallucinations, psychomotor agitation, mania with grandiosity, and profound cognitive impairment.

When clients' impairment is determined to be primarily organically based, the influence of psychosocial phenomena may be present but is not the initial target for intervention. Rather, clients with AIDS-related dementia are treated like clients with other organically based dementias.

In summary, AIDS clearly carries the potential for neuropsychiatric complications. AIDS-related moderate to severe cases of dementia occur in approximately 7% of clients newly diagnosed with HIV/AIDS and in up to 30% of those with more advanced HIV disease. Behavioral and cognitive symptoms of AIDS dementia complex are:

Organic psychosis
Apathy
Social withdrawal

Dysphoric mood
Regressed behavior
Forgetfulness
Loss of concentration
Confusion
Slowness of thought
Motor deficits that may include loss of balance, leg weakness, and deterioration of handwriting

It is confounding that many of these clients are also abusing alcohol and/or cocaine and other drugs and are frequently undergoing severe stress. There are multiple potential reasons for much of this symptomology. Cocaine psychosis may closely resemble and mask psychosis caused by HIV (Shaffer and Costikyan, 1988).

PSYCHOSOCIAL FACTORS

With HIV disease there is a spectrum of disorders in which psychosocial, particularly stress-related, disorders are important. Essentially, four categories of individuals may need intervention.

First, there are those who believe they are at risk for HIV infection but have not gone for testing. These individuals are "the worried well," some of whom experience ongoing stress, assuming they are indeed seropositive. They tend to exaggerate their risk rather than deny it. They may display low self-esteem, anxiety, uncertainty, and at times irrationality. They may appear somewhat histrionic and indecisive. They may offer clues to their concern, indicating a desire for help. Still, their fear of being seropositive may prevent them from taking care of themselves and confronting their irrationally based concerns.

The second category of individuals needing attention are *those who are asymptomatic but HIV positive.* Although one tends to think of HIV as an acute fatal illness, most clients are either asymptomatic or symptomatic but do not meet the criteria for full-blown AIDS. Even those who have been symptomatic may remain highly functional between symptomatic episodes. After a prolonged incubation period of months or years, most clients will go on to develop AIDS-related symptoms and AIDS. Of primary concern to the individuals is the uncertainty that is with them on a day-to-day basis.

The third category of individuals are *those who are symptomatic but have not yet developed an AIDS-defining condition.* Early in the epidemic these clients were diagnosed with AIDS-related complex (ARC). Symptomatic individuals are not acutely ill but tend to suffer from various AIDS-related conditions (e.g., fatigue, fever, night sweats, and nausea).

In studies of symptomatic versus asymptomatic HIV disease, persons with symptoms were reported to exhibit more distress. It is this group that seems to wait in dread of a drop in their **CD4 count,** or a diagnosable malignancy that would usher in fears of impending demise. The CD4 count (T4 cell count) is the most commonly used marker to determine HIV progression. HIV attacks CD4 cells, which help fight infection. The increased dependency in these individuals has been attributed to a "state" phenomenon (psychologic reaction to diagnosis and/or illness) and not a characterologic condition. Many of these clients exhibiting dependency, helplessness, and anxiety would not display these characteristics if not for their HIV disease.

The fourth and final category of individuals suffering directly from HIV disease is *clients with full-blown AIDS*. The clinical course of many AIDS-related conditions may be quite varied. Kaposi's sarcoma, a malignant neoplastic vascular proliferation in immunocompromised clients with AIDS, for example, may present as a slowly progressive disease over many years, or a rapidly fulminant progression over weeks to months. With the refinement of medications to combat opportunistic infections and the advent of new antiviral medications (protease inhibitors), the median survival rate has markedly increased. Available data on the client's disease course, immune status (current CD4 count and **viral loading**), and general health status can offer a clearer prognosis for clients. The depression these clients experience may not be simply a normal grief response about having a fatal illness. For some individuals, a pathologic process characterized by alienation, irrational guilt, diminished self-esteem, and pronounced suicidal ideation may be present.

The data about suicidal ideation and numbers of suicide attempts in clients with HIV/AIDS has been limited. Studies suggest that suicide is a common occurrence in these clients and that suicidal ideation is high (Brown and Rundell 1989; Frierson and Lippmann, 1988; Glass, 1988; Kieger et al, 1988; Marzuk et al, 1988; Plott et al, 1989). Increasing evidence suggests that declining physical health status may increase suicide risk, but with the advent of new therapies neither decline in physical health status nor overwhelming hopelessness may occur. Hopelessness is seen as an important risk factor for both suicidal ideation and suicide, and when it occurs, in the presence or absence of physical decline, it should be addressed aggressively.

CLINICAL DESCRIPTION

The primary DSM-IV diagnostic condition addressed here is adjustment disorder. Adjustment disorders are coded according to the subtype that best characterizes the predominant symptoms. Diagnoses include adjustment disorder:

> With depressed mood
> With anxiety
> With anxiety and depressed mood
> With disturbance of conduct
> With disturbance of emotions and conduct
> Unspecified, referring to maladaptive reactions to psychosocial stressors that are not classifiable as one of the specific subtypes

Note that although clients may also display other psychiatric disorders (e.g., a major depressive episode and/or psychoactive substance abuse), adjustment disorders with anxious and/or depressed mood are more commonly diagnosed in these clients, especially in outpatient clients. This diagnosis pertains to their reaction to having a fatal illness. Other disorders generally refer to conditions that predated seroconversion. Clients with HIV/AIDS have reported previous psychiatric histories. The exact rate of previous psychiatric illness and/or substance abuse in HIV-infected individuals is not known, but it is believed to be higher than for some community samples.

Two additional diagnostic categories are important in assessing these clients: bereavement reaction and organic manifestations related to HIV disease. Although diagnostic assessments may vary, substance abuse, bereavement reactions, and organicity are frequently seen as comorbid conditions in clients whose Axis I diagnosis is either major depressive episode or adjustment disorder with mixed emotional features. Specific HIV-related problems observed on psychiatric hospital admissions are anxiety and depression over deteriorating physical health status, social rejection related to HIV seropositive status, increased drug use as a response to HIV seropositivity, shame or guilt concerning stigmatized sexual practices, guilt or fear over having put others at risk (including fear of retribution), and homicidal ideation toward the presumed party who infected the client.

PROGNOSIS

The prognosis for resolution of anxiety and depression in clients with HIV/AIDS is not well documented. Scientists who study the emotional effects of this disease attempt to isolate crisis points where psychosocial stressors or other precipitants can lead to depression, anxiety, and other psychiatric problems.

Since HIV infection is a chronic stressful life event depicted by a series of physical, functional, and psychosocial losses, anxiety and depression are likely to occur intermittently and relate to the psychologic pain accompanying different phases of the disease process. Some experiences may be severe enough to precipitate a dysphoric mood and/or a crisis (Duffy, 1994). Although the concept of "crisis points" seems to be applicable to this population, several considerations are important.

The experience of HIV/AIDS as a crisis is highly individualized. Some clients struggle with the disease, and this struggle is evident. Other clients with HIV infection cope well and even seem to take a new lease on life. In addition, not everyone will experience a confirmed diagnosis of seropositive status as a crisis. Thus caution should be used in predicting psychologic distress, the crisis points that will occur, and any outcomes of the process of adapting to HIV disease.

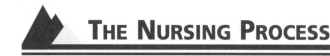

THE NURSING PROCESS

ASSESSMENT

The psychosocial assessment of a client with HIV/AIDS with a medical diagnosis of adjustment disorder, anxiety, and/or depression requires a thorough appraisal of primary and secondary nursing diagnoses. The emotional and behavioral symptoms that occur may develop in response to the stress of having, or being diagnosed with, a general medical condition.

The clinical assessment that enables nurses to derive pertinent nursing diagnoses must be all-inclusive. Identifying data, current symptoms, and history of the present problem (anxiety, depression, and/or conduct) must all be addressed. Specific data about sleep patterns, appetite, and change in weight are important in assessing the severity of the mood disturbance. Details about previous psychiatric contacts (both outpatient and hospitalizations), including precipitating events, will establish any preexisting psychiatric disorders that may place the client at risk for future episodes.

CASE STUDY

Rocio is a 29-year-old Hispanic woman married to José, who is reported to be behaviorally bisexual and HIV positive. Two months ago, Rocio was diagnosed as HIV positive with symptomatic HIV disease. She is positive for AIDS-related fatigue, fevers, nausea, diarrhea, dyspnea, and wasting syndrome. A thorough gynecologic examination reveals that Rocio is in the early stages of cervical dysplasia. The nurse practitioner in the women's clinic asked to have Rocio evaluated by the psychiatric team. She is 5 months' pregnant and has three additional children under age 5. Rocio and José are undocumented residents who have lived in the United States for 1½ years. Their primary language is Spanish. When questioned about her pregnancy and her personal health, Rocio sobbed uncontrollably. She explained that she is really worried about her children and what will happen to them. She cannot eat or sleep, and she has not told any friends or family that she is HIV positive, because she is ashamed and worried that they would not be kind to her children if they knew her diagnosis.

Critical Thinking—Assessment

1. What are the client's most immediate problems or needs related to her HIV diagnosis?
2. What assessment data reflect the client's sensitivity to her diagnosis?
3. Why might the client be reluctant to seek the social support she needs?
4. What stressors could contribute to fear, anxiety, a sense of helplessness, and depression?

Data about the client's family unit and current social network is particularly relevant. A description of the family unit of origin, including the family's history of traumatic events, migration, and cultural factors, will help to sensitize providers to the contextual nature of the client's responses to his or her illness. These same data about current relationships is also critical because they influence ways in which clients cope with HIV/AIDS and the availability of coping resources (see Case Study box).

Social history information is of general importance, but there are certain data that hold special significance. The nature of the client's social network and history of (and current) sexual practices are important. In many cases, clients are not only living with the personal threat of HIV, but they are also dealing with the possibility of placing others at risk. A diagnosis of HIV positivity brings with it an array of responsibilities to those with whom clients have been intimate. Finally, in assessing emotional distress, a thorough mental status examination should be conducted as part of the assessment process because of the prevalence of neuropsychiatric complications.

A final area of assessment is the client's previous and current suicidal or homicidal tendencies, as well as tendency for violent behavior. As previously noted, severe medical problems place people at risk for suicide. Anger and rage also may be manifested through violent behaviors, homicidal threats or gestures directed at those believed to be the source of infection, and occasionally toward society at large. Clients with disturbances of conduct may violate the rights of others, social norms, or even commit minor infractions of the law.

NURSING DIAGNOSIS

Nursing diagnoses are formulated from the data gathered by the nurse during the assessment phase of the nursing process. The accuracy of nursing diagnoses relies on the careful, comprehensive assessment of the client's history, presenting symptoms, behavior, and responses to actual and potential life stressors. The reliability of all informants, whether the sources are clients themselves, their significant others, and/or previous data from charts during this phase, is extremely important. Multiple sources of data can confirm information and ensure appropriate diagnoses.

NURSING DIAGNOSES FOR PERSONS WITH AIDS

Anxiety
Coping, defensive
Denial, ineffective
Fear

Hopelessness
Noncompliance
Powerlessness
Self-esteem disturbance
Social isolation
Violence, risk for: directed at others
Violence, risk for: self-directed

OUTCOME IDENTIFICATION

Outcome criteria are derived from the nursing diagnoses and are the expected client responses to be achieved.
　　Client will:

1. Verbalize absence of suicidal ideation and plans.
2. State reduced frequency/intensity of feelings of hopelessness and powerlessness.
3. Engage in a therapeutic alliance with staff to evaluate coping options.
4. Initiate social interactions with others with HIV/AIDS (both individually and in groups) to gain information and support about coping effectively with HIV/AIDS.

COLLABORATIVE DIAGNOSES

DSM-IV Diagnoses*	NANDA Diagnoses†
Adjustment disorder	Coping, ineffective individual
With depressed mood	Hopelessness
	Powerlessness
	Self-esteem disturbance
	Social isolation
	Violence, risk for: directed at others
	Violence, risk for: self-directed
With anxiety	Anxiety
	Coping, ineffective individual
	Fear
With mixed anxiety and depressed mood	Ineffective individual coping
With disturbance of conduct	Coping, defensive
	Coping, ineffective individual
	Denial, ineffective
	Noncompliance
	Violence, risk for: directed at others
	Violence, risk for: self-directed

DSM-IV diagnoses of adjustment disorder with mixed disturbance of emotions and conduct, and adjustment disorder, unspecified, are not addressed here, given the overlap with the previous diagnostic subtypes.

*From American Psychiatric Association: *Diagnostic and statistical manual of mental disorders*, ed 4, Washington, DC, 1994, The Association.
†From North American Nursing Diagnosis Association: *NANDA nursing diagnoses: definitions and classifications, 1999-2000*, Philadelphia, 1999, The Association.

---

5. Identify barriers or problems that may precipitate exacerbation of the experience of fear, anxiety, and/or depression (e.g., perception of inadequate social support or perception of powerlessness over physical symptoms).
6. Verbalize clear, goal-directed, short-term plans that are achievable and problem-solution focused (see Collaborative Diagnoses box).

PLANNING

The nurse's awareness of the complexities of living with HIV disease is extremely critical in deriving an appropriate plan of care for the client and the client's family.

　　For clients who are diagnosed with adjustment disorders, the nurse considers a plan of action that will promote the following: prevent violence toward self; help clients address concerns in a coherent, goal-directed, problem-solving manner; increase social networking that will provide needed information and comfort; monitor adverse effects of stressors on clients' current level of adaptation; and use staff in an effective therapeutic alliance when social supports diminish or cannot provide the technical expertise the client requires.

IMPLEMENTATION

The challenges of working and intervening with clients are considerable and multiple. Families and caregivers also are greatly affected and often devastated by both the client's diagnosis and the functional and neuropsychiatric responses to the disease. Therefore it is important that families and significant others are considered and included in the interventions when appropriate and with the consent of the client.

　　For example, clients whose significant others are encouraged to engage in problem-solving coping methods (versus emotion-focused coping) may be more helpful to clients who are trying to minimize the emotional burden of their disease. Significant others need to be taught about the disease, its course, and what can be expected at various crisis points. Support groups for caregivers of persons with HIV/AIDS are available and appreciated by significant others dealing with issues of bereavement, fear of contagion, and the stress of caregiving. Support networks of a less formal design also exist to provide assistance for clients and their loved ones through newsletters and drop-in centers.

　　Clients with HIV/AIDS may have numerous symptoms; consequently, these clients require multiple interventions addressing various aspects of their spiritual, psychosocial, and physical well-being. The interventions discussed here are largely in the psychosocial domain, and they are directed toward altering maladaptive individual coping and treating impaired social interactions. Many nursing interventions for symptoms of HIV disease parallel

NURSING CARE PLAN

Steve, a 32-year-old Caucasian homosexual man, formerly a travel agent, has been retired for 2 years because of complications from AIDS. He has a history of depression since his early twenties for which he received outpatient counseling. He sees his physician regularly; currently he has esophageal candidiasis and wasting syndrome. He came to this clinic appointment expressing a great deal of hopelessness about his future. He stated that he didn't want to live anymore and that he was tired of fighting AIDS. When asked if he had a suicide plan, he stated that he could make it quick and fatal (e.g., jumping out a window of a 15-story building).

Nursing Diagnosis: Powerlessness related to responses to course of HIV disease and symptoms, as evidenced by verbalization of suicidal thoughts and plans, inability to forecast a positive future, verbalization of powerlessness as a result of physical decline, and decreased functioning.

Client Outcomes	Nursing Intervention	Evaluation
• Steve will verbalize absence of suicidal ideation and plans.	• Identify with Steve goals and aims relating to his life tasks, despite prognosis. Contract with Steve to avoid acting out with suicidal gestures or attempts *to facilitate the client's adaptive coping responses and decrease feelings of loss of control; to help support Steve's goal.*	• Steve progressively states optimism about achieving goals within his anticipated life span.
• Steve will verbalize increased feelings of personal competence and self-efficacy in relation to managing his symptoms.	• Identify with Steve options that he has in controlling his emotional and physical distress (e.g., stress management strategies and ways to cope with fatigue and diarrhea) *to counteract feelings of helplessness that, if not abated, result in hopelessness.*	• Steve identifies and begins to implement new strategies for coping with his symptoms. He verbalizes feelings of competence, as identified in the main outcome.
• Steve will develop a therapeutic alliance with staff.	• Engage Steve in an active problem-solving approach addressing each stressor and discussing appropriate coping options/strategies *to evaluate Steve's coping options/methods.*	• Steve regards the nurse as a facilitator and supportive resource. He initiates discussion of stressors and options.
• Steve will initiate social interactions with others with HIV to gain information and support.	• Offer referrals to Steve regarding support groups and particularly voluntary home care services *to help Steve gain information and support.*	• Steve attends support group of his choice or identifies at least one other person with AIDS whom he can talk to on a weekly basis.
• Steve will identify barriers or problems associated with exacerbation of his anxiety/depression.	• Assist Steve in reviewing what precipitating events and/or thoughts increase his anxiety/depression *to avoid such events, when possible, through increased awareness.*	• Steve expressed awareness of recurring stressors that worsen his anxiety and depression.
• Steve will verbalize goal-directed plans that are both achievable and problem-solution focused.	• Assist Steve in formulating goals that are realistic and achievable. These should be directed toward improving the quality of life and reducing stressors in day-to-day living *to decrease frustration and increase success through goal attainment.*	• Steve articulates two or three short-term goals he can realistically commit to with respect to his present condition.

interventions used with symptoms associated with other illnesses, particularly life-threatening cancers. People with HIV, however, experience other complications (e.g., dealing with stigma, estrangement from their family of origin, and inadequate medical intervention). These factors are related to emotional distress and negatively impact treatment. Successful coping with symptoms is a priority in maintaining these clients' quality of life.

The primary category of intervention in the psychosocial domain is facilitating adaptive coping to the multiple stressors the client will confront. Interventions for effective or adaptive coping to offer clients hope, increase self-worth, and reduce anxiety and feelings of powerlessness are the following:

Maintain or improve their quality of life.

Control or contain their feelings of fear, anxiety, grief, guilt, depression, and helplessness.

Maintain or enhance a sense of self-worth and positive self-esteem.

Avert a state of hopelessness and powerlessness.

Satisfactorily adapt their relationships as they are confronted with various stages of dependency on others.

Maintain physical functioning within capacity.

Along these lines nurses can also intervene to help clients cope adaptively to their phase of illness.

In terms of maintaining or improving clients' quality of life, nurses can intervene to alter the physical discomfort and psychosocial isolation clients experience. They can teach clients to handle pain and fatigue caused by their illness and/or treatment. In doing this, they are also helping the client to exert control and minimize feelings of helplessness.

Social support networks are important to the client with HIV/AIDS. Without them, social isolation and loneliness can occur. Also, disengagement is a normal process in adjusting to physical decline. The nurse needs to help the client preserve those relationships with friends and family who are capable of meeting the client's dependency needs. Loss of role functioning is usually very painful to a client but even more so when supportive relationships do not exist for the client.

Containing feelings of anxiety, helplessness, grief, guilt, depression, and fear is also important to maintaining the client's quality of life. Helping the client become informed about the illness and treatment will lessen the anxiety many clients experience because it relieves stress associated with uncertainty surrounding the disease. However, the nurse needs to consider that some clients are not comforted by instruction they are receiving because they do not understand the information and need further clarification.

Supporting clients when they are confronting the multiple losses concomitant with their disease is helpful in treating clients' feelings of grief and depression. These losses include deterioration of physical abilities and functions, as well as loss of roles, income, and social relationships. Loss of dignity related to declines in health and/or functional status may also occur. The client's distress may be reduced if nurses anticipate losses, prepare clients for coping, and supplement clients' resources by providing them with knowledge of financial and medical assistance.

Helping the client maintain or enhance a sense of self-worth and avert a state of powerlessness and hopelessness in the face of this serious disease requires thoughtful consideration about the ways that clients are affected by their

---

Nursing Care in the Community

Persons With HIV/AIDS

The continued epidemic of HIV/AIDS in the gay, heterosexual, and "people of color" communities presents challenges and opportunities for community mental health nurses. With health care becoming more of a managed system further constrained by capitation, the role of community mental health nurses is changing. Community mental health nurses are no longer bound to the traditions of the past. Instead, these nurses can become partners in community-based care for the majority of clients with HIV/AIDS.

The future of the long-term management of this chronic infection will see more and more home health care agencies providing home care in cooperation with major pharmaceutical companies and other community resource/support groups. Thus the high cost associated with acute hospitalization will be reduced. Already, more and more home health care agencies are providing direct care in the home. Pharmaceutical companies are providing a raft of services such as intravenous therapy, total parental nutrition, and the testing of newer drugs for the treatment of HIV/AIDS via established protocols. Many other agencies, along with community AIDS projects, are often involved in the care of these clients. Services such as social support, social services, peer support, and pet-assisted companionship are just a few of the growing services available in the community.

The community mental health nurse's role in working successfully with these clients must include confronting the self about personal attitudes, beliefs, and values about AIDS, gay lifestyles, and sexuality. Also, a thorough knowledge of AIDS and the biopsychosocial issues associated with the HIV-positive diagnosis, including its eventual progression to AIDS, its chronicity and sequelae, and death, is essential.

Nurses can offer much to these clients. Counseling, brief supportive therapy, and just being a caring presence can make a difference. Anxiety and depression must be addressed with these clients. The potential for suicide should be a concern. Social support, financial resources, housing needs, and possible job loss are other issues that need to be considered. Perhaps one of the most important interventions will be working with the client's partner, lover, and/or family.

The nurse must be prepared to work collaboratively with other health professionals. Teamwork for seamless coordination of all care services and referral to other appropriate community-based agencies will enhance the care and quality of life for these clients.

Newer drug therapies that suppress viral multiplication have promoted hope for improving the well-being of these clients. The recent announcement of the testing of an AIDS vaccine holds promise. Despite these advances, community mental health nurses still must emphasize safer sex practices, along with testing and education about engaging in high-risk behaviors. HIV/AIDS is still a major health and social problem because of the stigma attached to the diagnosis. These clients are often invisible in the community.

disease. Sometimes the nurse will teach the client how to respond to the curiosity of others. Hiding one's illness and minimizing its effects can be adaptive because it helps clients live as normally as possible despite their symptoms and effects of treatment.

Assisting the client in preserving relationships requires both direct and indirect intervention. Nurses can help clients understand reasons for reactions of family and friends. Less directly, they can assist these informal caregivers by teaching them how to respond to the client's illness and treatment. AIDS caregivers usually are concerned about contagion of the disease. Providing factual information to these caregivers may decrease any tendency of these supportive others to withdraw because of fear of becoming infected with HIV themselves. In cases where clients are sexually active with partners, nurses need to monitor, teach, and support them in adhering to safe sexual practices. The role of the nurse in dealing with persons with HIV/AIDS in the community is summarized in the Nursing Care in the Community box on p. 703.

A final important category of intervention is related to treatment of acute and subacute syndromes associated with cognitive impairment. The **AIDS Dementia Complex (ADC)** is a syndrome that includes cognitive, motor, and behavioral manifestations. Initial symptoms are usually memory impairment and concentration difficulties. These symptoms can be overlooked and are frequently confused with symptoms associated with depression. However, clients may complain of forgetfulness, "slowed thinking," and difficulty concentrating when engaged in conversations, watching TV programs, or reading. In some cases poor balance and coordination occur early on. As this syndrome progresses, with no chance of reversal, clients may become dependent on others for completion of activities of daily living. Clients' observation of declining functioning frequently causes emotional distress and social isolation. Early signs of inability to concentrate and lapses in short-term memory are within the client's awareness, although they may not always be described by the client.

Many clients and their caregivers fear the development of dementia. They may have observed friends who were exceedingly compromised by ADC in all areas—cognitive, motor, and behavior. In addition, AIDS dementia is not easily identified, and symptoms can wax and wane. This fact can cause a great deal of uncertainty and anxiety about one's diagnosis and evidence of decline. For this reason, early thorough assessment and teaching the client and caregivers about signs and symptoms are extremely important interventions leading to the client's ability to cope adaptively and avert severe states of helplessness and hopelessness.

With the advent of new therapies, researchers are hopeful that some clients with ADC will regain their lost faculties. **Antiretroviral therapy** is the use of certain drugs to treat the major opportunistic diseases associated with AIDS. **Opportunistic diseases** are diseases that commonly appear in clients with AIDS, especially when their T cell count drops. Whether these symptoms are reversible and what level of cognitive improvement can be made are the subjects of ongoing study.

Nurses working with clients with AIDS who also have dementia will participate in the neuropsychiatric assessment of their clients by recording problems related to memory, attention span, concentration, and motor deficits. They will provide support to the client, family, and friends who are assuming client care. Nurses may refer the client to day care. Caregivers or partners may welcome respite care or home care, depending on the client's functional status and needs. With clients such as these, it is important to help them and their families remember treatment and medication schedules. This may include checklists, bulletin boards, pillbox alarms, and other plans to promote self-care potential and ease the burden of care for significant others.

ADDITIONAL TREATMENT MODALITIES

Nursing interventions contribute significantly to the client's ability to cope effectively with HIV disease. But it is important to keep in mind that other disciplines and therapies play a critical role in the client's disease course. Currently accepted treatments of adjustment problems in clients with HIV/AIDS parallel those for other populations with adjustment disorders. However, there are important key differences addressed in this section that include particulars about pharmacologic intervention, the preferred format for individual counseling, psychosocial support networks specific to persons living with HIV/AIDS and their significant others, and the use of adjunct therapies (e.g., occupational and recreational therapies for stress reduction).

PHARMACOLOGIC INTERVENTION

Psychotropic medications can be useful in the treatment of clients with HIV disease. There are no medical reasons to avoid their use. The most commonly used psychotropic medications with clients with HIV/AIDS experiencing moderate to severe distress are antidepressants and anxiolytics.

Antidepressant medication can be prescribed if the client manifests a significant depressed or anxious condition. Sometimes an antidepressant is initiated prophylactically when new uncontrollable stressors are anticipated. Anxiolytics are prescribed in daily dosages or prn to curb the client's anxiety. The choice of antidepressant or anxiolytic and dosage of the medication will often depend on the client's neurovegetative symptoms and underlying physical illness. For example, for an agitated client with gastroenteritis who is also having difficulties with diarrhea because of the disease or complications from treatment, an antidepressant medication with more anticholinergic action may be the best choice. This medication will diminish diarrhea and provide a mild sedation. In addition to the individual's overall health status and specific emotional distress, the age of the client is important. Children and adolescents are generally treated with lower doses of psychotropic medications.

ALTERNATIVE THERAPIES

Alternative therapeutic programs for clients include many traditional and nontraditional therapies aimed at reducing stress and increasing chances of long-term survival. The stress of HIV infection is chronic and may persist over long periods of time with acute exacerbations. Dependency on psychotropic intervention alone is not the answer. Attention is drawn to recommended alternative actions.

There are well-documented techniques (e.g., stress reduction, relaxation, and cognitive restructuring techniques) that are extremely useful to many persons at various stages of HIV/AIDS. These include stress management strategies and progressive relaxation exercises that nurses can teach clients to help them cope more effectively. Manuals and self-help books, as well as short workshops, are available to teach clients these techniques. Some of these instructional aids are also on videotape.

Understanding & Applying Research

The purpose of this study was to describe the manner in which women cope with HIV infection by providing additional data about the prevalence of specific adaptive and maladaptive cognitive and behavioral coping responses and examining whether the prevalence of these responses varied across three ethnic groups (African-American, white, and Latina women). Women who were 18 years and older, HIV positive, and not currently pregnant were recruited; 53 women were interviewed, all of whom spoke English. In this sample of women, nearly 40% reported clinically significant levels of depressive symptomatology and anxiety on the Brief Symptom Inventory (BSI). Compared with normative samples, all infected women, regardless of ethnic group, reported distress levels. Prayer and rediscovery of what is important in life were their most frequent coping responses. Denial (refusal to believe one is HIV positive) and trying to feel better by eating, drinking, smoking, using drugs or medications, etc., were least often reported means of coping with HIV infection. The study suggests that clinicians should not overlook the importance of spiritual faith and practices in women adapting to HIV infection

Kaplan MS, Marks G, Mertens SB: Distress and coping among women with HIV infection: preliminary findings from a multiethnic sample, *Am J Orthopsychiatry* 67:80, 1997.

The individual's desire to control emotional distress through spiritual practices, diet, and exercise must be recognized. It is therefore important to recognize the role of prayer, in particular among women coping with HIV/AIDS (see Understanding & Applying Research box below). Proper exercise and healthy nutrition are important as general guidelines for addressing stress-related illnesses.

Clients must be cautioned that HIV-infected bodies are different from disease-free systems. Weight loss generated by diet changes and exercise is usually more of a problem than a desired goal. Unnecessary calorie depletion and calorie burning should be kept at a minimum. The recommendation for exercise should focus on moderation, with the major goal of exercise geared to strength building and resistance training. Adding muscle mass is a good thing; burning calories is not. Specific recommendations for diet therapy are not well established. What is known is that there is a relationship between nutritional status and survival. In a study by Guenter et al (1993), the nutritional status of persons with HIV infection who were treated with recent therapies (including antiretroviral agents) predicted their survival, even after adjusting for age and CD4 counts.

EVALUATION

If nursing interventions are successful, the client will show significant signs of improvement in coping ability. Nurses are expected to evaluate changes in client mood, behavior, and functional abilities. Clients' understanding of their illness and treatment should also be evident. A large part of the treatment of persons with HIV/AIDS is individualized teaching to help them regain or maintain a sense of control over their symptoms and disease.

Effective coping should be evidenced in the outcome criteria addressed in the treatment plan. That is, clients should demonstrate an ability to contain uncomfortable feelings of fear, anxiety, guilt, grief, and depression. Because their ability to manage their symptoms should have improved, their sense of self-worth and self-esteem should be enhanced. Relationships with others, especially those in caregiver roles, should have been strengthened by the added instruction and support of the nurse. The client should demonstrate a realistic level of hope as a result of the nurse's efforts to help the client find meaning in life and set small, realistic goals. Although clients may not experience a high level of wellness, they should experience a quality of life based on increased feelings of cognitive, behavioral, and decisional control. Helping clients achieve a sense of control helps the client avert high levels of fear, anxiety, and depression (psychologic health) and may also be vital to the client's ability to sustain physical health.

Summary of Key Concepts

1. HIV disease is considered a major public health problem around the world.
2. Persons may be infected with HIV but may be asymptomatic for long periods of time.
3. AIDS is the advanced stage of HIV disease.
4. AIDS may occur in both genders, in all age-groups, and in all ethnicities.
5. Although injection drug use and male homosexual activity are frequently reported risk behaviors for HIV infection, increasing rates of heterosexual transmission have been reported.
6. One principal DSM-IV diagnosis for emotional distress associated with HIV/AIDS is adjustment disorder.
7. Nursing assessment and interventions should be done in collaboration with the client and, in some cases, significant others.
8. Alternative therapy techniques such as stress reduction, relaxation, and cognitive restructuring, as well as customary coping responses (such as the use of prayer), have been found to be useful to many clients in various stages of HIV disease.

REFERENCES

American Psychiatric Association: *Diagnostic and statistical manual of mental disorders*, ed 4, Washington, DC, The Association.

Brown G, Rundell J: Suicidal tendencies in women with human immunodeficiency virus infection, *Am J Psychiatry* 146:556, 1989.

Buck B, Duffy VJ: The use of psychotropic medications in outpatient AIDS care, *AIDS Patient Care* 7(4):203, 1993.

Centers for Disease Control and Prevention: *HIV surveillance report, June 1997*, Atlanta, 1997, U.S. Department of Health and Human Services

Duffy VJ: Crisis points in HIV disease, *AIDS Patient Care* 8(1):28, 1994.

Frierson RL, Lippmann SB: Suicide and AIDS, *Psychosomatics* 29:226, 1988.

Gala C et al: The psychosocial impact of HIV infection in gay men, drug users and heterosexuals, *Br J Psychiatry* 163:651, 1993.

Glass RM: AIDS and suicide, *JAMA* 259:1369, 1988.

Guenter P et al: Relationships among nutritional status, disease progression and survival in HIV infection, *J Acquir Immune Defic Syndr* 6:1130, 1993.

Kaplan MS, Marks G, Mertens SB: Distress and coping among women with HIV infection: preliminary findings from a multiethnic sample, *Am J Orthopsychiatry* 67:80, 1997.

Kieger K et al: AIDS and suicide in California, *JAMA* 266:1881, 1988.

Mainous AG et al: Illustrations and implications of current models of HIV health service provision in rural areas, *AIDS Patient Care STDs* 11:25, 1997.

Marzuk PM et al: Increased risk of suicide in persons with AIDS, *JAMA* 259:1333, 1988.

McCain NL et al: The influence of stress management training in HIV disease, *Nurs Res* 45:246, 1996.

North American Nursing Diagnosis Association: *NANDA nursing diagnoses: definitions and classifications, 1999-2000*, Philadelphia, 1999, The Association.

Pergami A et al: The psychosocial impact of HIV infection in women, *J Psychosom Res* 37(7):687, 1993.

Perry S, Jacobsen P: Neuropsychiatric manifestations of AIDS-spectrum disorders, *Hosp Community Psychiatry* 37:135, 1986.

Perry S, Markowitz J: Psychiatric intervention for AIDS-spectrum disorders, *Hosp Community Psychiatr* 37:1001, 1986.

Plott RT et al: Suicide of AIDS patients in Texas: a preliminary report, *Tex Med* 85:40, 1989.

Rabkin JG et al: Effect of imipramine on mood and enumerative measures of immune status in depressed patients with HIV illness, *Am J Psychiatry* 151(4):516, 1994.

Shaffer HJ, Costikyan DS: Cocaine psychosis and AIDS: a contemporary diagnostic dilemma, *J Subst Abuse Treat* 5:9, 1988.

U.S. Department of Health and Human Services: Trends in AIDS among men who have sex with men—United States, 1989-1994, *MMWR* 44:401, 1995.

U.S. Department of Health and Human Services: Update: trends in AIDS incidence—United States, 1996, *MMWR* 46:861, 1997.

Notes

CHAPTER 31

Psychologic Aspects of Physiologic Illness

Ruth N. Grendell

OBJECTIVES

- Discuss the influence of mind-body interrelationships on wellness and health promotion.

- Describe the impact of mind-body interrelationships during physiologic illness or disease.

- Identify major physiologic and psychosocial stressors.

- Define the concepts of stress and adaptation.

- Describe the processes involved in mind-body response and adaptation to stress (cognitive appraisal, autonomic nervous system responses, and coping mechanisms).

- Describe the role and influence of social support in the adaptation to stress.

- Discuss examples of vulnerable groups at risk for psychologic-physiologic interactions to illness/disease.

- Design a plan of care that incorporates interventions for psychosocial and physiologic needs for an individual with a health care problem.

PSYCHOLOGIC ASPECTS OF PHYSIOLOGIC ILLNESS

HISTORICAL OVERVIEW

The mind-body-spirit connection has been a subject of interest for centuries. How human beings perceive and respond to environmental stimuli was as intriguing to early philosophers as it is to modern-day scientists. Aristotle believed that the heart was the center of thought, that the brain helped to cool the body, and that a heavy brain due to drowsiness forced the head to bend forward. Today these views seem naive, even humorous, but they were widely accepted truths as late as the nineteenth century (Swerdlow, 1995). Perhaps these concepts help to explain the use of common phrases such as "my heart is broken" to express deep sadness and "I cannot hold my head up any longer" to express extreme tiredness.

Traditionally the body, mind, and spirit have been considered as separate systems or units. In Western civilization, ancient healers of the body were "bleeders" or "bile examiners"; the mind was treated by magicians and alchemists; spiritual needs were the province of orthodox religions. Superstition, myths, and witchcraft were thought to be causes of disease, and rituals were used as remedies (Joseph, 1996; Swerdlow, 1995). Humans have been considered as puppets of the Gods and passive receptors to external environmental events. Rene Descartes, a French philosopher and mathematician (1596-1650), considered the body a machine that should be logically studied in the same manner as other machines. His premise was that the mind housed thoughts, consciousness, and soul but had no way to come directly in contact with reality;

therefore the mind was inaccessible to study. In contrast, he believed that a person's behavior was observable and could be interpreted. The separation of mind and body stayed in vogue until Sigmund Freud (1856-1939) reintroduced the connecting tie between them.

FACTORS CONTRIBUTING TO A CHANGE IN PHILOSOPHY
BIOMEDICAL MODEL

The biomedical model of traditional Western medicine has been based on a cause-and-effect relationship since the nineteenth century, when scientists discovered microbes as the origin of many physiologic diseases. This model was conducive to studying and explaining body functions; however, it did not explain functions or disease of the mind or interpret the interactions between mind, spirit, and body. The fact that some people survived tragic events, recovered from life-threatening illnesses, and were able to overcome disabilities while others did not, led scientists to examine the characteristics that differentiated survivors from those who succumbed.

EASTERN PHILOSOPHIC PERSPECTIVES

In contrast, Eastern philosophies view humans as capable of achieving a balance of mind-body-spirit through meditation, exercises, and self-discipline—practices that are intricately linked to Eastern religious philosophies. The use of acupuncture in Chinese medicine is based on the belief that the brain is controlled by the liver, heart, spleen, lungs, and kidneys, which communicate with the brain via energy channels (Swerdlow, 1995). Therapies such as meditation, self-hypnosis, biofeedback, acupuncture, and acupressure have been introduced to the Western world during the past several years. These therapies have been used in the pursuit of a healthy lifestyle, as alternatives to the use of drugs or surgery, and/or combined with traditional medicine as aides in coping with stress and illness. The blending of alternative and traditional therapies is central to the current holistic health care perspective (see Chapter 24).

HOLISTIC HEALTH CARE

Holistic health care emphasizes a person's self-responsibility in the promotion of psychologic, physiologic, and spiritual health and the prevention of illnesses that may disrupt that balance. Each person is perceived as unique and separate from others in experiencing and coping with life events. Past experiences and interactions with others influence the individual's current perceptions and interpretation of events. The selection and use of coping mechanisms can also be affected by genetic makeup, culture, and spiritual beliefs. This health care model integrates multiple disciplines in providing supportive measures to enable individuals to maintain health and to recover from an illness or manage long-term effects, when necessary. The model uses both traditional and alternative, or complementary, therapies to achieve its purposes. It is imperative that health care providers consider the dynamic interactions between mental and physical processes both in maintaining equilibrium and in contending with the disorders that may result from imbalances.

DISCOVERIES THROUGH ADVANCED TECHNOLOGY

Although scientific discovery about brain function has advanced impressively in the last decade, there remains a great deal to be learned. Current knowledge of brain-mind-body interactions has been gained primarily through the study of human psychologic and physiologic

responses to stress. Research pioneered by Hans Selye in the 1930s and supported with later studies by Lazarus, Folkman, and others has led to the development of several theories that correlate effects of stress and depressed immunity, illnesses, and depression and anxiety (Black and Matassarin-Jacobs, 1997; Monat and Lazarus, 1991). Although research supports these theories, the exact mechanism and effect at all cellular levels have remained unsolved. Stress as an etiologic factor in illness and human responses to stress are discussed later in this chapter.

The 1990s were declared by Congress to be the *"decade of the brain."* During this decade there has been an explosion of new discoveries about the complex interactions between the brain (mind) and body in both healthy and unhealthy conditions. Ninety percent of the knowledge of brain function has been learned within the last 10 years and has been greatly facilitated by the advanced technology in the fields of biochemistry and physics that has supported development of several new drugs and sophisticated imaging equipment. Diagnostic procedures are now enhanced by computer analytic models, and the use of biologic markers to monitor blood flow patterns, metabolic processes, and chemical reactions as they occur. Scientists have unlocked the genetic code and can frequently predict who is at greatest risk for specific physical and mental illnesses (Glod, 1998; Joseph, 1996; Swerdlow, 1995).

Before this time, scientists were primarily limited to indirect observation of brain function by comparing human behaviors with developmental standards or by correlating an individual's normal functional patterns with deficits subsequent to trauma or disease or as a result of genetic causes. Data derived from postmortem examination, via animal research, or through epidemiologic studies of disease patterns and results of pharmacotherapy and diagnostic procedures provided additional information.

BRAIN MAPPING

Earlier brain-mapping studies, conducted by electrically stimulating the brain during surgery, identified areas that control voluntary movement of a body part. Scientists discovered that large cortex sections of the brain are allocated to somatic areas that require the most dexterity, such as the muscles of the hands and those used for facial expression and speech. (Brain scans of Braille readers revealed that their "reading fingers" stimulated larger cortical areas than fingers of sighted persons.) The efficiency of each movement is dependent on input from various brain centers (e.g., the thalamus, the vestibular system, and sensory feedback from the involved muscles). The programmed movement is continuously corrected and adjusted until the process is completed (Porth, 1998; Swerdlow, 1995).

Three-dimensional computer images are currently used for more intricate plotting of the brain. For example, diagnostic electrodes inserted deep within the brain can

detect an exact area of highest seizure activity, and, subsequently, that portion of the cortex can be surgically removed to alleviate the problem. Scientists have also discovered that body movements, thoughts, recall of a memory, or expression of an emotion require involvement and coordination of several areas of the brain.

Almost all aspects of emotions, reasoning, processing of incoming sound, speech, and certain aspects of memory are negotiated in the right hemisphere of the brain, including dominant control over the autonomic nervous system. Expressive speech, math, and analytic reasoning are associated with the left hemisphere. Communication between the hemispheres permits crossover of information. Damage to one area of the brain can affect other areas involving behavior, emotion, and cognitive abilities. Damage to brain cells can also result in deficits in body function such as hemiparesis or paralysis following a cerebrovascular accident or head trauma.

COMMUNICATION PATHWAYS

Transfer of information from one hemisphere to the other is particularly noted in children before the age of 10 during periods of rapid neural dendrite growth. The flexibility, or plasticity, of the brain has been demonstrated in young children who have undergone hemispherectomies to alleviate brain-damaging seizures, often caused by Rasmussen's encephalitis. These children are often able to function at almost normal capacity. Transfer of information can also occur more slowly during adult years, as evidenced by the opposite hemisphere assuming control of functional ability when that function is lost in one hemisphere because of a cerebrovascular accident or head trauma (Glod, 1998; Joseph, 1996; Swerdlow, 1995).

BRAIN CELL GROWTH

A recent study has shown for the first time that the adult brain can generate new cells. These findings are contrary to previously held beliefs that the brain, unlike other organs, does not have regenerative capability. Five terminally ill study participants, ages 50 to 70, who had been diagnosed with throat cancer, were given a chemical tracer to monitor their tumor growth rates. Autopsy findings revealed that each of the patients had recently produced from 500 to 1000 new cells. This agent, which attaches to the DNA of dividing cells, was concentrated in the tumor cells and also in dividing cells in the hippocampus, which is involved in learning and memory. New evidence also indicates that the brain may contain "progenitor cells" that could grow into neurons in the presence of growth-stimulating hormones. Making new connections between neurons is possible even in older adults. These findings may offer tools for scientists to explore methods to treat brain injuries caused by diseases such as Alzheimer's disease and by cerebrovascular accidents (Graham, 1998; Swerdlow, 1995).

Biologists have isolated multipurpose embryonic stem cells in laboratory cultures that are capable of growing neurons, bone, muscle, or other body tissues. The researchers predicted that potential benefits from future engineering of stem cell growth could be (Goetinck, 1998):

Programming their development into nerve cells for testing drugs for Alzheimer's disease and to repair spinal cord injuries

Growing heart muscle cells to replace an area of scar tissue caused by myocardial damage

Evolving into brain cells to secrete dopamine for the treatment and control of Parkinson's disease

Growing bone marrow to replace damaged blood-forming tissues

Growing islet cells that would produce insulin

Evolving cells to decrease rejection of transplanted organs or tissue

BRAIN STRUCTURE AND MENTAL ILLNESS

Imaging procedures have revealed smaller brains and large ventricles in the brains of some people with schizophrenia. Studies have linked schizophrenia with neural chemical imbalances, genetic causes, and the mother's exposure to influenza during pregnancy. Other studies have suggested that depression, mania, and obsessive/compulsive disorders are associated with abnormalities in various regions of the brain. Positron emission tomography (PET) has identified specific areas of decreased brain activity in persons diagnosed with Alzheimer's disease. Advancing knowledge about the role of the brain's physical structure in mental illness should change our perceptions about mental illnesses. However, we still have much to learn about the brain functions that make us human, namely "the uniquely human 'consciousness,'" variously defined as language, introspection, self-awareness, and abstract thinking, which eludes scientific measurement (Black and Matassarin-Jacobs, 1997; Swerdlow, 1995).

APPLICATION OF SCIENTIFIC DISCIPLINES
PSYCHOBIOLOGY

Psychobiology is the melding of biology with the functions of the brain to describe the interplay between one's inherent biologic and genetic makeup and one's life experiences (Glod, 1998). Advances in this field moved slowly until the twentieth century, when scientists achieved a greater understanding of brain and body interactions. Current theory proposes that human experiences alter the structure and functions of the brain, especially during the first decade of life. These positive and negative experiences aid in defining who we are and how we think, and they affect our emotions and behavior. Key sensitive periods during exposure to an event are also influential in defining individuals and their behavior. Some studies have indicated that exposure to classical music in utero is associated with a higher IQ in infants; a mother's substance abuse during pregnancy is linked to a child's hyperactivity and inattention; and children exposed to sexual and physical abuse have less left brain development activity (Glod, 1998).

PSYCHONEUROIMMUNOLOGY

The branch of psychoneuroimmunology (formerly psychosomatic medicine) is concerned with the impact of emotional and psychologic disturbances on neural and immune systems, organic function and subsequent ailments such as cardiovascular disease, gastric ulcers, ulcerative colitis, asthma, migraine, dermatologic manifestations, arthritis, and cancer. The three processes of cognitive, neuroendocrine, and antibody formation by cellular and humeral (blood and plasma) immune systems are studied as a total network (Glod, 1998; Pender, 1996; Stuart and Laraia, 1998).

Dr. George Solomon at the University of California in Los Angeles first coined the term *psychoneuroimmunology* in 1964. In several studies conducted by Dr. Solomon and others, there were indications that immune response to disease was closely associated with emotions and attitudes toward stress (Glaser and Glaser, 1991; Groer, 1991). Prolonged exposure to stress and high anxiety levels has been linked to lowered immunity, whereas a greater resistance to illness has been associated with lower stress and anxiety. A possible explanation is that the immune and neuroendocrine cells share common signal pathways and receptor sites. There is evidence that endocrine hormones and neuropeptides can alter the function of immune cells, and products of the immune system can affect neuroendocrine function. Release of catecholamines by the sympathetic nervous system in response to stress can also have detrimental effects on the immune system. Research has also indicated a strong relationship between a series of losses experienced by elderly persons and illness episodes and death (Porth, 1998).

Much of the research has been concerned with immunodepression. Mental imagery is believed to aid in the release of chemicals in the brain and alter the immune system. Studies have been done on the beneficial effects of meditation and hypnosis on allergies and viral infections. Additional research is needed in other areas of the wellness/illness states (Dossey, 1998; Groer, 1991).

DISCOVERY OF ENDORPHINS

A major breakthrough in understanding the brain-mind-body connection resulted when molecular biologist Dr. Candace Pert and others isolated the opiate drug receptor in the brain in the mid-1980s (Monat and Lazarus, 1991;

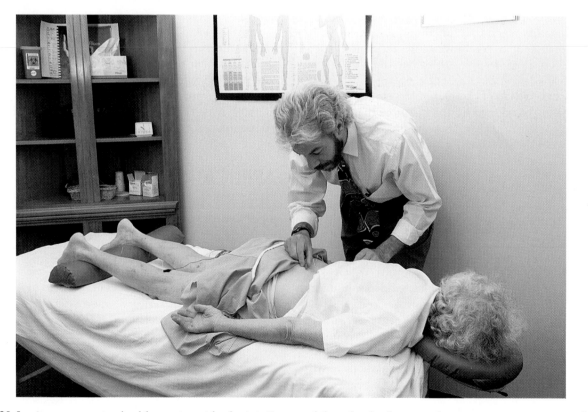

Figure 31-1   Acupuncture is a health practice with a basis in Eastern philosophy that has gained increasing acceptance in traditional health care. (Copyright Cathy Lander-Goldberg, Lander Photographics.)

Moyers, 1993; Porth, 1998; Swerdlow, 1995). This led to the discovery of endogenous morphines (endorphins) and other chemical communicators released by the brain, the immune and endocrine systems, and other parts of the body. It was discovered that the release of molecules from one part of the body, which provides instructions for action, are diffused to the surface of every body cell. Dr. Pert labeled these complex interactions a "psychosomatic communication network" and stated that all "emotions are (actually) neuropeptides attaching to receptors and stimulating an electrical charge on neurons" (Swerdlow, 1995). According to Pert, the residence of the mind is in the body, as well as the brain. At least 60 neuropeptides have been identified so far.

The peptides endorphin and enkephalin have been shown to relieve pain by the same mechanism as morphine and other narcotics. The use of placebos, acupuncture, and transcutaneous nerve stimulation are thought to release the endorphins and thus aid in pain relief (Figure 31-1). Mental imagery, music, and humor have been reported to serve as distractions from the person's focus on the pain and stress (Black and Massatarin-Jacobs, 1997; Selye, 1978; Smeltzer and Bare, 1996).

STRESS AS AN ETIOLOGIC FACTOR IN ILLNESS

A large body of literature exists concerning the relationship of **stress** (a nonspecific response of the body to any positive or negative demand placed on it), and the potential for illness. However, stress and its sources are often difficult to identify. Several research studies have been conducted across populations on the stressful effects of various life events (e.g., bereavement, divorce, clinical depression, chronic stressors, academic stress, and the incidence of mental and physical illnesses). Studies have also shown that persons do not always adapt positively to environmental disasters such as earthquakes, floods, and war. Stress can also be a result of positive life events (Glaser and Glaser, 1991; Glod, 1998; Monat and Lazarus, 1991). Box 31-1 depicts examples of many stress factors that are linked to physiologic, psychologic, and emotional responses or behaviors. Box 31-2 describes several indicators of stress.

A number of factors are now being considered as causes of illness and determinants of an individual's response, such as the number of stressors, intensity, and duration (Glod, 1998). The perception of control is also influenced by the person's cultural background, values, and beliefs. Other factors that may influence the response are the individual's past experience with the stressor or similar stressors and the capacity for **coping** with the life-

---

Box 31-1   Sources of Physiologic and Psychosocial Stressors

Physiologic Stressors
Infectious agents (viruses, bacteria, fungi)
Chemical agents (drugs, alcohol, poison)
Physical agents (heat/cold, radiation, electric shock, trauma)
Suppressed immune system
Genetic disorders
Illness processes
Aging processes

Psychosocial Stressors
Daily hassles (common frustrations)
Life events (birth/death, job change, role change, illness)
Major disasters (earthquake, flood)
War
Effects and response to the stressor are dependent on the individual's perception of the intensity of the stressor and:
   Acute/chronic duration of the stressor
   Cumulative effect of simultaneous stressors
   Sequence of stressors
   Severity of stressors
   Individual previous experience with stressors
   Amount of social support

Box 31-2   Indicators of Stress

Dryness of throat and mouth
Pounding of heart
Insomnia and/or nightmares
Increased urinary frequency
Muscle tension and migraine headaches
Pain in neck or lower back
Loss of or excessive appetite
Gastrointestinal signs and symptoms:
   "Butterflies" in stomach
   Cramping, constipation, or diarrhea
   Vomiting
   Change in menstrual cycle
   Body tics or twitches
   Flushing, sweating
   Nervous cough
General irritability, hyperexcitation, depression
Disturbed behavior
Feelings of unreality
Easily fatigued, weakness, dizziness
"Floating anxiety" without knowing exact cause
Overpowering urge to cry or run and hide
Easily startled, tension, heightened alertness
Inability to concentrate, loss of interest
Forgetfulness
Increased smoking
Increased use of drugs and/or alcohol
Accident proneness
Repetitive movements—picking at fingernails
Impulsive behavior, emotional instability
Nervous laughter
Stuttering or other speech difficulties
Hypermotility: pacing, restlessness

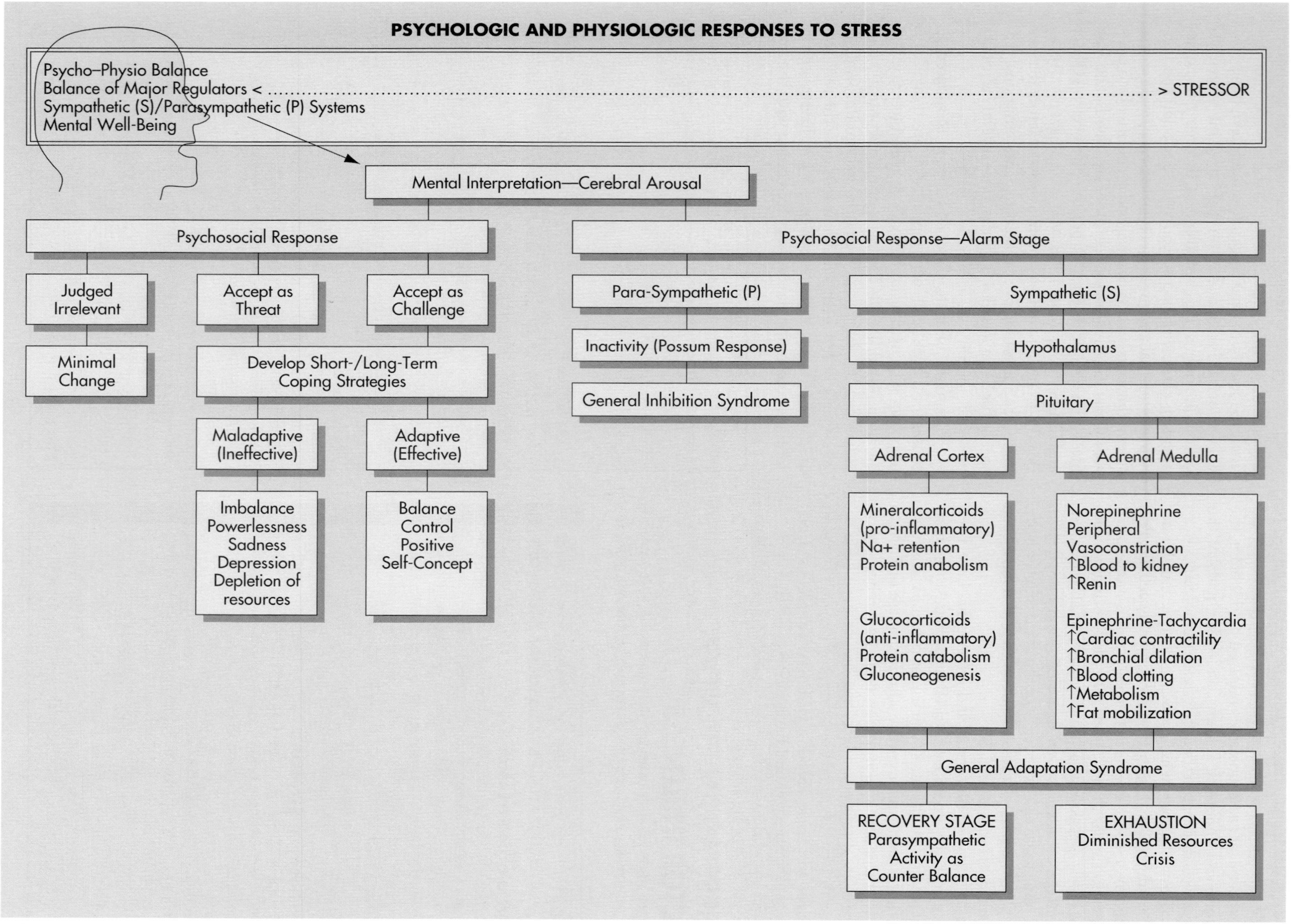

PSYCHOLOGIC AND PHYSIOLOGIC RESPONSES TO STRESS

Figure 31-2   Psychologic and physiologic responses to stress.   (Modified from Lewis S et al: *Medical-surgical nursing: assessment and management of clinical problems,* ed 5, St Louis, 1999, Mosby; and Kozier B, Erb G, Blais K: *Concepts and issues in nursing practice,* ed 2, Menlo Park, Calif, 1992, Addison-Wesley.)

style interruptions caused by stress or stressful events. Mind-body interaction is evident here.

THEORIES ON EFFECTS OF STRESS ON MIND AND BODY INTERACTIONS

Several theories have been developed to explain the impact of stress as a *response*, as a *stimulus*, or as a *transaction*. Some commonalities emerge through the examination of the various theories. (Figure 31-2 depicts an integration of three of the major theories.) Selye's theory (1978) demonstrates the nonspecific body response pattern to any form of stress; Lazarus and Folkman (1984, 1991) state that the individual's interpretation of the stress determines the degree and type of response; Nuernberger's theory proposes that the person "shuts down" and responses are suppressed.

Stress as a Response

Hans Selye's theory, first generated in 1936 during studies with laboratory animals, identified stress as a nonspecific stereotypically patterned biologic response to some environmental stressor—regardless of what the stressful stimulus might be. He defined the sequence of body responses to a stressor as the general adaptation syndrome (GAS). The three major phases are the alarm reaction, the stage of resistance, and the stage of exhaustion (Porth, 1998; Selye, 1978; Smeltzer and Bare, 1996).

The stimulation of the sympathetic nervous system is the primary response during the alarm reaction and is often referred to as the "flight or fight" mechanism. Increased activity of the hypothalamus-pituitary-adrenal axis (HPA) causes the release of endocrine hormones, particularly epinephrine, norepinephrine, and cortisol. During the stage of resistance the person continues to use sources of energy in order to adapt to the stressor. The stage of exhaustion is characterized by total expenditure of energy; the person usually becomes ill and may die without replenishment of resources. The condition may also be reversed by the use of internal and external resources such as stress reduction strategies (imagery, meditation), medication, nutrition, and psychotherapy. Adequate support systems and spiritual beliefs are also considered important resources.

In his many later studies, Selye and his associates also identified individual perception of a stressful event as a major influence on mind-body response. Recent studies have indicated that multiple bodily responses can occur because of a variety of stressors of different intensities. The characteristic patterned responses developed by each person can cross over from one stressful stimulus to another and are affected by the degree of emotional arousal (Black and Matassarin-Jacobs, 1997; Selye, 1978).

Selye's theory also proposes that there is a local adaptation syndrome (LAS) that involves the inflammatory response at a local site of injury that influences the subsequent repair process. The severity of the injury determines whether the systemic response is also initiated.

General Inhibition Syndrome Response to Stress

Nuernberger proposed an additional theory on adaptation to stress in 1981, which was labeled the general inhibition syndrome, or "possum response." This self-protective mechanism is due to the arousal of the parasympathetic system, the opposing branch to the sympathetic system. Stress is a reflection of an imbalance between these two systems, and prolonged or intense imbalances can lead to dysfunction. The imbalance is caused not by the external stressor, but by the individual's perception of threat, pain, or discomfort (Kozier, Erb, and Blais, 1992; Smeltzer and Bare, 1996) (Table 31-1).

Stress as a Stimulus

A stress stimulus may be positive or negative and may be endogenous (originate from within the body) or exogenous (originate from the surrounding environment). The stimulus elicits an adaptive response that requires an expenditure of energy and a change in the normal pattern of living (Porth, 1998; Selye, 1978). Several tools have been designed for use in research to determine the effect of previous events on illness.

The Holmes and Rahe Social Readjustment Scale developed in 1967 contains both positive and negative major life changes and has been used in numerous studies for identifying the impact of stress as a stimulus (Black and Matassarin-Jacobs, 1997; Monat and Lazarus, 1991; Smeltzer and Bare, 1996). The severity of impact for each life event is assigned a numerical value. The stress level is correlated with the total number and severity of life changes the person has encountered during the recent past and the amount of adjustment required. Such events could be loss of a job or retirement, marriage or divorce, a promotion or geographic change, the birth or adoption of a baby, or the death of a spouse. Studies have shown that people who experience a high level of stress are more prone toward illness and have lower coping ability with subsequent stress (see Understanding & Applying Research box on p. 717). However, caution should be used in the interpretation of this scale and similar stress scales because the potential influence of the individual's perception of a stressful event needs to be considered (Porth, 1998).

Several studies have indicated a relationship between minor daily life events, or hassles, and body system illnesses. Other studies have suggested a strong correlation between the clustering of previous life changes and the clusters of illnesses. The relationship between extended exposure to a stressful environment and changes in health status has also been shown (Monat and Lazarus, 1991; Pender, 1996; Porth, 1998).

Appraisal of the stressor can occur at both the conscious and unconscious levels. A generalized anxiety, or global response, is followed by a more specific response as the person has more time to mobilize coping resources. Thus the response pattern incorporates both physiologic and psychologic or emotional components. Maladaptive

Table 31-1	Examples of Physiologic Problems and Related Psychologic Effects	
Physiologic Problem	**Related Psychologic Effects**
Acute Problem	
Trauma	Anxiety
Surgery (disfigurement or alterations in body processes)	Fear of deformity, mutilation
Cardiovascular problems:	Lowered self-image and self-esteem
Myocardial infarction	Diminished self-confidence
Hypertension	Confusion
Cerebrovascular accident	Shock, inability to make decisions
Pain	Denial
Stressful event	
Major disaster (flood, earthquake)	
War	
Life-threatening diagnosis	
Chronic Problem	
Progressive effects of acute health problem	Powerlessness (uncertainty of future)
Epilepsy	Depression
Lupus erythematosus	Suicidal thoughts
Arthritis	Hopelessness
Renal/liver failure	Helplessness
Diabetes mellitus	Chronic fatigue
Posttraumatic stress syndrome	Insomnia
Terminal illness (cancer)	Worry over finances
Aging process/multiple health problems	Decisional conflict
Respiratory—chronic obstructive pulmonary disease (cystic fibrosis)	
Diminished immune response (AIDS)	

NOTE: A person may experience one or more psychologic effects with any of the above physiologic problems.

coping strategies can lead to increased vulnerability to other stressors or to one of the stress-related illnesses such as hypertension, gastric ulcers, or depression.

Examples of physiologic stressors that induce general and specific responses include traumatic accidents, chemicals, heat/cold, radiation or electrical shock, infectious agents, nutritional imbalances, faulty immune systems, and genetic disorders. Examples of psychologic stressors, or triggers, are victimization, unwanted controls, neglect, day-to-day stressors, major traumatic disasters, and life events. Stressors to the spiritual dimension are happenings that challenge one's values and beliefs, create a sense of abandonment, or are perceived as punishment (Black and Matassarin-Jacobs, 1997; Carson, 1989; Smeltzer and Bare, 1996).

Stress as a Transaction

Transactional, or process, theories of stress are based on the work of Lazarus, Folkman, and other associates, begun in 1966. They believed that neither the stimulus nor the response theories explained an individual's particular response to stress. The person who is confronted by a stressor makes a primary cognitive appraisal or judgment of its intensity. During primary appraisal, stressors can be classified as irrelevant, benign-positive, or stressful. Irrelevant demands often require minimal attention. Benign-positive stressors can be challenges and potential for growth.

Stressful demands are perceived as threats, as being harmful, or as losses. Secondary cognitive appraisal of the stressor judges which coping methods to use, whereas reappraisal evaluates whether coping methods have been effective. Stress is viewed as a dynamic state that requires effort in the process of adaptation or coping.

The sensitivity and vulnerability of an individual to the stressor are the determining factors of emotional and behavioral responses and may vary in intensity for an individual in different situations. Also, what may be an acutely stressful event to one person is not necessarily perceived as stressful by another. Coping mechanisms may also differ and can be effective or ineffective. The stress of daily hassles (minor life events) can be buffered by daily uplifts such as reading a good book, using prayer and meditation, or spending quality time with friends and family (Carson, 1989; Monat and Lazarus, 1991).

FRAMEWORK FOR STUDYING MIND/BODY RESPONSES TO STRESS

The mind-body connection is an important factor in the promotion of health and in the recuperative process from an illness. Mental and physical health are closely intertwined. Researchers have discovered several conditioning

Understanding & Applying Research

Panic disorder is associated with a variety of physical problems, including asthma, previous sexual and physical abuse, irritable bowel syndrome, and migraine headaches. It is widely misunderstood, and the individual may feel stigmatized. The DSM-IV (American Psychiatric Association, 1994) description of panic disorder states that it is "recurrent unexpected panic attacks followed by a least 1 month of persistent concern about having another attack." Symptoms include shortness of breath, chest pains, palpitations, fear of losing control, terror, and feeling a sense of impending doom, and 50% to 60% of affected persons have experienced depression. As symptoms escalate, there is increased use of emergency services and frequency of suicide attempts.

Postpartum panic episodes most often occur during the first 12 weeks after birth, with the average time being 7 weeks, and are often misdiagnosed as postpartum depression. This phenomenologic study, conducted over an 11-month period, investigated the symptoms experienced by six married women who had experienced a panic episode for the first time following the birth of a child. Five of the women were multiparas; one was a primipara. Five women had received medication therapy, and all had received psychiatric care. The study findings confirmed that the symptoms were similar to symptoms previously reported by individuals with other physiologic health problems.

Analysis of the interview transcripts resulted in 214 significant statements. After meanings of these statements were established, the statements were clustered into six main themes. The women felt paralyzed by the terrifying physical and emotional events and felt totally out of control; cognitive functioning was diminished during and between attacks; attempts to maintain composure and "hiding" their panic resulted in extreme exhaustion; they became consumed with trying "panic-prevention" methods; recurring attacks led to lowered self-esteem and feelings of disappointment in themselves for not being able to manage their lives; the mothers were haunted with the possibility of residual effects for themselves and their families.

Several nursing interventions were suggested, including providing information to new mothers regarding the possibility of panic attacks, reassurance that cognitive dysfunction is a natural consequence of the disorder, and establishing a trusting, supportive environment that allows women to admit their problem. Other suggested interventions were the use of diaries to aid in identifying panic trigger events and how to avoid them and the formation of a support group for women and their families. Information from mothers who have received treatment and conquered their panic and seeing how their children have developed may also be very beneficial for the recovery process.

Beck C: Postpartum onset of panic disorder, *Image J Nurs Sch* 30(2):131, 1998.

factors that determine the human response to stress. A person seeking medical help experiences a variety of emotions before the actual diagnosis, including anxiety, fear, grief, denial, and anger. Depression and helplessness often follow a diagnosis of a serious illness. Sometimes these individuals will try to hide their emotions, and health care providers must be alert to subtle cues.

Adaptation to illness involves several tasks such as managing the stress associated with threats to independence, control, self-concept, and body image; adjusting to potential limitations; dealing with an uncertain future; and dealing with the impact of illness on relationships with others. The complexity of individuals yields a variety of interpretations of the illness experience. People learn coping mechanisms that aid them in adapting to stress and apply them to similar situations (Black and Matassarin-Jacobs, 1997; Smeltzer and Bare, 1996).

Mental illness may go unrecognized when a person has a physical illness, and a physical illness and medications can exacerbate an existing psychiatric problem. Delirium, confusion, anxiety, sleep disorders, hallucinations, delusions, and personality changes can be a result of a physical problem. Stress, fluctuations in hormone levels such as hyperthyroidism, nutritional disorders, electrolyte imbalances, cancer, and vascular and neurologic conditions, including head injury and brain tumors, are the principal physical causes of changes in mental functioning. Additional risk factors include infections, hepatic encephalopathy, and surgical procedures. Exposure to anesthesia, nutritional imbalances, pain, and medications are particular high-risk factors for the elderly postoperative patient (Conrad, 1998).

STRESS AND PAIN RESPONSE

Some of the current psychologic research is focused on the relationship of stress and increased perception of pain. Studies have been conducted on the effects of biofeedback, meditation, and stress reduction techniques as distractions in lessening the perception of pain that has a physiologic base. Research has also explored the effects of social support on emotional and physical outcome and perception of pain (Black and Matassarin-Jacobs, 1997; Moyers, 1993; Smeltzer and Bare, 1996).

STRESS OF MEDICAL PROCEDURES

Additional studies have dealt with the stress people experience as they undergo medical tests, procedures, and surgery. Results have shown that people under stress are more depressed before and after surgery, require more anesthesia and analgesia, and have lower immune functioning than people who have lower stress levels (Dossey, 1991; Smeltzer and Bare, 1996).

COPING MEASURES/ADAPTATION TO STRESS

Several methods for coping with and reducing stress are derived from Eastern practices and have been introduced over the years. Exercise and recreation provide a variety of benefits, including increased oxygenation, changes in heart rate, and lowered blood pressure. Additional outcomes may be relaxation, peaceful sleep, distraction from concerns, increased appetite, and a feeling of general well-being. Music therapy and humor have also helped to relieve tension and anxiety and to reduce aggression. Use of saunas or massage helps individuals to relax and stimulates skin circulation. Pet therapy has been introduced as a means of social interaction to relieve tension and depression. Progressive relaxation, guided imagery, biofeedback, meditation, and yoga are used in both health and illness to induce calmness and to provide a sense of being in control of life events (see Chapter 24).

RESISTANCE AND COPING RESOURCES

Hardiness

The ability of some people to overcome diversity, to recover from a serious illness against all odds, or to survive severe tragedy has been an area of study by many scientists. The concept of **hardiness** has been used to describe a personality component that aids in mastering or controlling stressful events. Stress is often perceived as a challenge and opportunity for growth; the individual makes a commitment to meet that challenge. Studies have identified hardiness as a moderating factor in relation to stress and psychologic strain for both men and women in work situations, in survival rates for people with cancer, in lowering blood pressure, and in delaying conversion to AIDS in persons with AIDS-related complex.

Hardiness is not a unitary concept. Some components include self-confidence and an internal sense of control. Persons who exhibit hardiness usually take care of themselves and possess physical and mental health (Black and Matassarin-Jacobs, 1997; Pender, 1996; Pollack and Duffy, 1990; Smeltzer and Bare, 1996).

Resilience

Resilience is a similar character strength that refers to a kind of toughness, or the ability to bounce back and overcome adversity. **Resilience** is a dynamic process that involves protective factors such as effective problem-solving strategies and adaptability to situations that the person cannot control or change. Research has shown that resilient children can remain mentally healthy in spite of neglect and the mother's depressive symptoms (Conrad, 1998). The positive influence of an educational intervention on changing self-destructive behaviors of women who had suffered chaotic lives as victims of child or adult abuse and neglect was demonstrated in research by Myn-

att (1998). Resilience was also described as perseverance, having a balanced view of life, self-reliance, and feeling a sense of meaningfulness to life in elderly women in a study by Wagnild and Young (1990). Individuals often perceive themselves as "overcomers" rather than just "survivors." Enthusiasm, hardiness, resilience, buoyancy, emotional stability, optimism, and internal locus of control are descriptive terms of the "self-healing" personality according to Stuart and Laraia (1998).

An example of resilience is the perseverance of a sheriff's deputy in his recovery from a motorcycle accident that required the amputation of his left leg. Following several months of rehabilitation and adjustment to a prosthesis, he was able to pass the physical agility test for reinstatement on the force. He commented, "Being able to reach down inside yourself and overcome adversity will make you stronger . . . You'll find some strength you didn't know you had. The human spirit is greater than you think it is" (Associated Press, 1996).

Hope

Hope has been defined as a multidimensional construct that provides comfort while enduring life threats and personal challenges. Research was conducted on the coping strategies of four groups of individuals who were (1) facing heart transplants, (2) living with spinal cord injury, (3) surviving breast cancer, or (4) breast-feeding as working mothers. Findings from this study led to the following refined definition (Morse and Doberneck, 1995):

Hope is a response to a threat that results in the setting of a desired goal; the awareness of the cost of not achieving the goal; the planning to make the goal a reality, the assessment selection, and use of all internal and external resources and supports that will assist in achieving the goal; and the reevaluation and revision of the plan while enduring, working, and striving to reach the desired goal.

The human spirit has been defined as the unifying force that gives meaning and purpose to life and illness, as an important component of hope, and as an inner strength that allows the individual to transcend, or overcome, adverse circumstances. Several studies have demonstrated the significance of spiritual factors to an enhanced immunity and sense of well being (O'Neill and Kenny, 1998).

Internal Locus of Control

Individuals who have an **internal locus of control** believe in a personal responsibility in managing their lives and in minimizing risk factors that could affect mental and physical health. Choosing a healthy lifestyle, for example, involves appropriate diet, exercise, sufficient sleep, and use of stress reduction strategies to reduce the risks of heart disease and hypertension. When an illness does occur, these individuals call on inner strengths and participate in the recovery process. Higher levels of self-esteem, perception of a purpose in life, and lower levels of anxiety have been associated with a greater sense of control over one's life (Black and Matassarin-Jacobs, 1996; Kozier, Erb, and Blais, 1997).

A study of aging postpolio survivors indicated that individuals with a higher internal locus of control reported lower distress symptoms and more coping resources than persons who thought they had no control over the progressive symptoms of their disease. The individuals who perceived themselves in control were more active in the therapeutic treatment plan (Kuehn and Winters, 1994). Managing a chronic illness, however, often can be overwhelming, and these individuals wanted to decide when control could be assumed by caregivers (Thorne and Paterson, 1998).

Social Support

A sense of belonging and of being accepted, needed, loved, and valued as a human being are elements of social support. Affirmation of self-worth by others helps a person to recognize inner personal strengths and potential. Emotional support from significant others during a crisis event or a long-term difficult situation plays an important role in acceptance of an illness and in the selection of appropriate coping strategies.

The family is considered the primary social support group. The family that provides positive interactions among its own members may also relate to a wider social network within the community that can serve as additional resources in times of need. Organized support systems and self-help groups are also beneficial in promoting adaptation to a life change by creating a personal growth environment and buffering the negative effects of stressful events (Pender, 1996).

PERSONS AT RISK FOR PSYCHOLOGIC-PHYSIOLOGIC INTERACTIVE HEALTH PROBLEMS
PERSONS WITH ACUTE HEALTH PROBLEMS

Acute illnesses may suddenly interrupt or curtail a person's activities. There is usually a temporary loss of control over one's life and body. Fear, anxiety, powerlessness, helplessness, hostility, and anger are also common responses to illness. When an illness occurs, the person often questions, "Why me?" or "What did I do to deserve this?" Sometimes a person will deny being ill and attempt to continue with the usual roles or tasks. This may eventually contribute to complications and result in prolonged recuperation.

During recovery stages, the person who experiences lasting effects from an acute problem (e.g., a burn or spinal cord injury) must amend his or her self-identity and concept of self-worth that has previously been based on physical appearance. Often these persons believe that the traumatic experience has made them stronger and better persons. Empathy for others and a renewed religious faith often emerge after the traumatic event and become important facets of life (Black and Matassarin-Jacobs, 1997; Smeltzer and Bare, 1996).

PERSONS WITH CHRONIC HEALTH PROBLEMS

The long-term effects and unpredictability of chronic illness challenge the person's self-esteem, body image, and sexuality, as well as disrupt social relationships and usual role functions within the family, work, and community. The sense of autonomy is frequently lost (Eakes, Burke, and Hainsworth, 1998; Gorman, 1998; Thorne and Paterson, 1998).

Chronic illnesses have been identified as permanent or progressive health problems that require ongoing adaptation on the part of the individual and his or her social network. Depression is a common reaction accompanied by sleep disturbances, lack of appetite, neglect of personal appearance, and fatigue. Chronic conditions affect every aspect of the individual's life and require long-term monitoring by health professionals.

A sense of chronic sorrow is linked to an ongoing sadness regarding a situation that has no predictable end; it may be cyclic or recurrent; and it can be triggered internally or by external events that remind the person of actual or symbolic losses, disappointments, or fears. The sadness or sorrow can progress and intensify (Eakes and Burke, 1998). Chronic sorrow is unresolved when the current reality is markedly different from the idealized state, such as when a person with a chronic illness cannot meet the expectations of society. Bereaved individuals and family caregivers of persons with a chronic illness are also subject to chronic sorrow. A role change caused by the illness or death of a "significant other" is a reminder of the disparity between the present and the past.

Individuals with chronic illnesses sometimes take on a deviant **sick role.** They may use their illness for secondary gains of receiving attention or gaining control over other people, and as a means of avoiding responsibilities. These behaviors are frequently a result of anger, fear, or depression (Black and Matassarin-Jacobs, 1997). The "invalid" role can also be a result of self-pity. Rehabilitation from an illness occurs with the return to society and functioning at the individual's greatest potential. To achieve this goal, it is essential to involve family or significant others, and the client in instructions for recuperation and the activities that will promote recovery.

PERSONS WITH MULTIPLE HEALTH PROBLEMS

Multiple health problems are common occurrences as the person's physical and mental systems respond to chronic illness. The person with long-term diabetes mellitus is at risk for developing complications involving every physiologic system. The person who has chronic obstructive pulmonary disease (COPD) frequently has circulatory and cardiovascular problems as well. Complications of

COPD lead to respiratory failure, fluid and electrolyte imbalances, depression, and anxiety.

Endocrine imbalances can lead to a variety of disturbances of life-sustaining functions. Individuals with diminished immunity are at risk for a number of complications. Various degrees of psychologic distress accompany all of these conditions (Black and Matassarin-Jacobs, 1997). Many physical conditions are frequently accompanied by depression, anxiety, or full psychiatric disorders that are secondary to physical disorders.

ELDERLY PERSONS

The majority of our aging population in the United States live independently, and many older citizens are able to enjoy their retirement years. However, the aging process often brings multiple health problems and threatens independence. Aging produces a gradual decline in multisystem coordination. Changes are cumulative and progressive, and a healthy response to stress is diminished. An elderly person who has adequate cardiac function at rest may be unable to withstand extended exertion, and it may take longer for the heart rate to return to the baseline level. Other health problems include a lowered resistance to infection, and the decreased reserve capacity of hormonal and neural regulation often leads to slower reaction time (Black and Matassarin-Jacobs, 1997; Smeltzer and Bare, 1996).

Mental health disorders are a major problem for aging persons. Successful psychologic adjustment to aging is dependent on the person's ability to adapt to the multiple stressors, the severity of these stressors, and the person's ability to adapt to change. A positive self-image and finding a purpose or meaning in life are essential components.

PERSONS EXPERIENCING PAIN

There are several definitions of pain. McCaffery, Beebe, and Latham (1998) state that "pain is whatever the experiencing person says it is and exists whenever the person says it does." The experience of pain is dependent on many variables, such as the person's age, culture, gender, pain tolerance, perception, and the situation itself. Pain is a multidimensional phenomenon involving both physiologic and psychologic components. Physiologic responses to pain include tachycardia, diaphoresis, tachypnea, and fluctuations in blood pressure. Psychologic responses include a pattern of responses to protect oneself from harm. The pain becomes the major focus, and the individual often assumes a protective posture that will guard the painful part. High levels of anxiety are likely to increase the perception of pain, and the person will seek relief, such as through pacing back and forth, using restless hand movements, or using drugs or alcohol as distractions. Additional psychologic responses are impaired thought processes, changes in sleep patterns, fatigue, tension, restlessness, episodes of crying, and fearfulness of increased intensity or return of pain. Some may fear that the pain is an indication of a progression of the disease (Black and Matassarin-Jacobs, 1997; Porth, 1998).

PERSONS WITH TERMINAL ILLNESS

Spiritual distress is a common response of clients with life-threatening illness, since death becomes imminent. Grief, like pain, pervades every aspect of the person's existence. Grief is a normal response to loss. Physical alterations in heart rate and blood pressure, as well as changes in mood and affect, such as depression, are manifestations of grief. The dying process may extend over several months to a year or more and consist of many crises and plateaus. Each crisis results in increased anxiety; each plateau invokes a sense of hope.

ADDITIONAL POPULATIONS AT RISK FOR PSYCHOLOGIC-PHYSIOLOGIC INTERACTIONS

Additional populations at risk for psychologic-physiologic interactive stress-related effects include homeless persons, individuals who are in stressful occupations (e.g., policemen, health care workers) family caregivers for chronically ill persons or persons in crisis, and individuals exposed to abusive situations).

THE NURSING PROCESS

The six-step nursing process provides an efficient method for gathering the necessary information, for problem solving, for clinical decision making, and for delivering higher-quality, individualized client care. The cyclic nature of the nursing process minimizes errors and omission of important facets of client care through ongoing assessment and evaluation of client responses and reported perceptions, thoughts, and feelings.

The effective use of the nursing process also requires the nurse to have a thorough knowledge of science and theory related to nursing and other disciplines, particularly medicine and psychology (Doenges and Moorhouse, 1992; Smeltzer and Bare, 1996; Stuart and Laraia, 1998). The involvement of the client in the nursing process provides a sense of ownership and personal control while enhancing the client's responsibility and commitment to goal achievement.

ASSESSMENT

Assessment is one of the most essential components of the nursing process. A variety of resources are used by the nurse to collect data about the client's health status. Ideally, much of the information can be provided by the client. The health history should include questions pertaining to the client's current health problem and its impact on daily activities, social and family support systems, occupation, religion or belief, and ethnic-cultural background (see Chapter 7).

During the initial interview the nurse listens to the client's subjective report of symptoms and observes the person's verbal and nonverbal behaviors (see Understanding & Applying Research box below). When the client cannot provide an accurate report, another resource person can be used (Fortinash and Holoday-Worret, 1999).

The interviewing process continues during the physical assessment performed by the nurse. Often, the nurse is able to clarify previous comments regarding the client's perception of the current health problem. An important feature of the assessment is that it is mutually agreed on by the nurse and the individual client (Fortinash and Holoday-Worret, 1999). Information is also obtained from reports of diagnostic tests and procedures, from the client's record, and through consultation with other members on the health care team.

The final phase of assessment is the analysis of data. The information is categorized and organized into a logical format. The nursing diagnoses emerge from this framework and identify the existing needs.

NURSING DIAGNOSIS

When a conclusion has been made through data analysis, one or more diagnoses are made. The diagnostic statement serves as a method for describing a health problem or need that is responsive to nursing intervention. The statement is phrased to link the problem or need with its etiologic factors. For example, a person may be experiencing moderate to severe anxiety (diagnosis) related to the effects of a myocardial infarct or the possibility of open heart surgery (source or etiology). Nursing diagnoses can refer to actual or potential health problems and can also be used as etiologies for other nursing diagnoses.

More recently, the concept of wellness and the individual's strengths have been included on the North American Nursing Diagnosis Association (NANDA) list of approved diagnoses (NANDA, 1994). The diagnostic statement of coping, family: *potential for growth*, could indicate effective adaptation to change in the family structure due to illness of one member. A statement specific to health-seeking behaviors demonstrates an individual's desire to improve the level of wellness.

The diagnostic statement is further validated by coupling the diagnosis with a qualifying factor (e.g., anxiety [diagnosis], severe [qualifying factor]). Placing the diagnostic statement within the *Problem/need, Etiology,* and *Signs and symptoms or risk factors (PES) format provides a scientific basis and helps eliminate errors in judgment (Doenges and Moorhouse, 1992).

The client with severe anxiety related to a cardiac condition may be at high risk for further alteration in cardiac tissue perfusion, an increase in pain intensity, or impaired gas exchange, which can in turn lead to an overwhelming state of anxiety. The client's anxiety may trigger a fear about dying or helplessness and contribute to total unhealthy mind-body responses.

Understanding & Applying Research

The quality of the nurse's response may influence the outcome for people who experience distress, such as anxiety, anger, and depression related to variations in their state of health. The purpose of this study was to explore the relationship of the nurse's response, the client's perception that the nurse expressed empathy in responding to the client's need, and the influence on the client's distress level. Seventy medical-surgical nurses were asked to respond to a list of written statements of hypothetic situations; then each nurse was scheduled to view 13 videotapes of clients experiencing distress and state how he or she would respond in each situation. Responses were tabulated to obtain an empathy score. The researcher returned to the hospital unit and selected one of the clients cared for by the nurse on that day. The nurse then provided personal demographic data and information about the time spent with the client, including feelings about the client and the adequacy of the time spent with the client.

After obtaining consent, the client completed three questionnaires regarding the nurse-client interactions. The instruments were designed to measure (1) perceived empathy, (2) a self-report of feelings and moods, and (3) anxiety, depression, and anger. The findings revealed that nurses who had high scores on nurse-expressed empathy scales were also perceived by their clients as being highly empathic. These patients were less likely to have feelings of distress. Clients felt they were understood. "This study is one of the first to link behavioral measures of nurse empathy to patient outcomes."

Olson J: Relationships between nurse-expressed empathy, patient-perceived empathy and patient distress, *Image J Nurs Sch* 27(4):317, 1995.

OUTCOME IDENTIFICATION

"Outcomes are identified from the diagnoses" (McFarland and McFarlane, 1997). One or more expected client outcomes may be identified for each nursing diagnosis and can be physiologic, psychologic, cognitive, sociocultural, or spiritual. Expected outcomes should be stated as desirable client health states, be specific, and be in measurable terms. Outcomes are used to assist in the planning, intervention, and evaluation processes. For example, "The client will be able to express feelings about the effects of the recent myocardial infarction on future lifestyle" or "The client will recognize the relationship between feelings of anxiety and the occurrence and intensity of pain." Other examples of expected outcomes for the cardiac client would include the increase in the client's knowledge regarding the benefits of diet and exercise, and stress reduction techniques.

PLANNING

The planning phase includes establishing priority of needs, goals derived from the nursing diagnoses, and methods to achieve the stated objectives. The selection of appropriate nursing interventions to achieve the desired physiologic and psychologic outcomes is the next step of the planning phase. Interventions are based on scientific rationale and standards of care and are specific to the identified need.

Discharge planning and future needs are also components of the plan of care. Discharge planning begins when the person enters the health care setting. Continuity of care is essential as the person returns to the home environment.

IMPLEMENTATION

During the implementation phase the nurse carries out the identified interventions. A carefully constructed plan must also allow for some flexibility. Therefore the nurse is constantly monitoring the client's total response to the in-terventions. An analysis of these findings aids in making modifications or revisions to the plan of care.

Time constraints, interruptions, and other factors can limit the effectiveness of the nurse's intervention. Therefore to ensure continuity of care, the implementation phase requires a careful and concise documentation and appropriate reporting to other health care team members regarding progress in meeting the desired goals.

EVALUATION

The evaluation phase determines the appropriateness of the interventions and the client's progress or lack of progress in meeting the expected outcomes. The process requires a continual reassessment. Positive reinforcement and encouragement are also part of this phase, thus allowing modifications to the original plan if needed.

New problems may arise during the course of rehabilitation. Assessment, new or revised diagnoses, and expected outcomes may be necessary. There may be a need for referral to physical therapy, the home health nurse, social services, a support group, and so on. Priorities may need to be adjusted to meet the changing needs of care.

Planning for termination of nursing care is started when the desired outcomes have been achieved. Discharge planning for any unmet needs would ensure that continued services would be provided. Follow-through measures are taken, and the client and family caregivers

---

Nursing Care in the Community

Psychologic Aspects of Physiologic Illness

When a person who continues to be somewhat debilitated returns home from the hospital, family dynamics are affected in multiple ways. Even the return home of a woman and infant after childbirth may have disruptive effects on a functioning family, albeit it is generally a positive event in the long run. The client's perception of his or her level of functioning needs to be assessed for congruence with the family's perception of the client's needs. If too great a disparity exists, the client may deplete reserves of strength while trying to live up to expectations, or, conversely, the family may try to do too much and undermine the client's sense of autonomy. In either case the community mental health nurse must be able to facilitate communication among members to arrive at a realistic appraisal of the client's medical situation and mental health implications. Interventions may prevent the debilitating effects of depression, compounding a weakened condition.

Chronic physiologic illnesses are not only physically disabling, but they often provoke such frustration in the client that depression and suicidal behavior may result. This presents a challenging problem for the mental health nurse working in the community. Not only does the client require support, encouragement, and care as a result of physical symptoms, but the nurse must be constantly mindful of the state of the client's mental health and that of the family and support system. Emotional states are often labile, as physical symptoms fluctuate and vary. The client may present a positive affect to cover unacknowledged depression. Assessment requires direct questions if the client's mood seems incongruent with his or her physical condition. Therapeutic questions are often successfully interjected when offering information about the client's physical condition or about medication and potential side effects.

Factors that seem to be important in sustaining a relatively positive state of mind in the client are the client's perceived degree of autonomy, successful efforts to reduce stress, and minimal secondary gains from the maintenance of the helpless attitude. The client should always be allowed to do as much as possible independently, with frequent offers of assistance. The client should make decisions as a part of the treatment team and be given as much information as possible about available options. Stress reduction techniques such as visual or guided imagery or biofeedback can be taught to minimize anxiety. Physical contact such as massage may also be therapeutic. Pleasurable activities such as hobbies or reading should be explored and encouraged. To educate caregivers, the nurse should model the art of giving positive attention to clients and their families to encourage interactions, to reduce frustration, and to minimize demanding behavior.

Box 31-3   Woman With Terminal Illness

Anh Huynh, a 68-year-old Chinese/Vietnamese female with metastatic cancer of the cervix, is now in terminal stages after surgery 2 years ago and radium implant. She was admitted to the hospital for colostomy surgery and pain relief. She has been in the United States approximately 10 years but does not speak English. Her husband speaks little English; some family members are able to speak, write, and read English. Her religious beliefs are Buddhist, but she has no local affiliation. Her diet consists of typical Asian foods. The figure below depicts several stressors and the phases of the nursing process in outlining the plan of care.

*Nursing diagnoses include (but are not limited to):
Anxiety
Body image disturbance
Bowel incontinence
Communication, impaired verbal
Coping, ineffective individual
Family processes, altered
Fear
Grieving, anticipatory
Infection, risk for
Knowledge deficit related to diagnosis and treatment
Nutrition altered: less than body requirements
Pain
Powerlessness
Social interaction, impaired
Spiritual distress, risk for
Urinary elimination, altered, related to metastasis

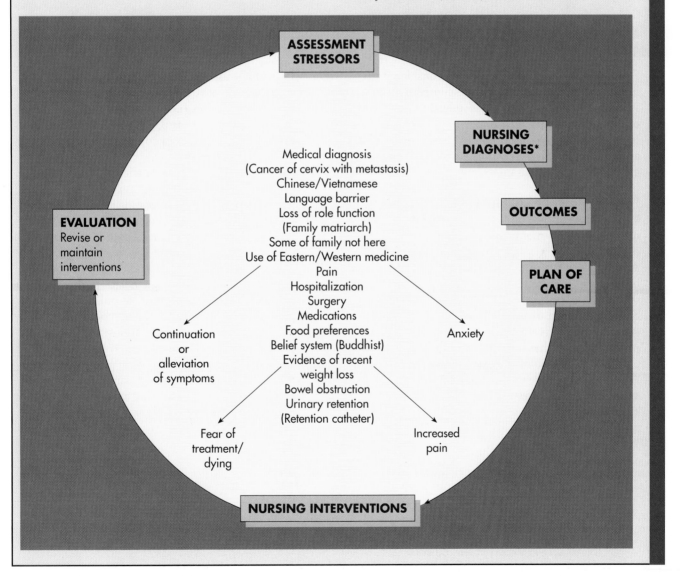

are given instructions in methods to enhance the recovery and health status in the future.

To meet this challenge of the evaluation phase, nurses must possess a comprehensive knowledge of the balance and imbalance of human biologic and behavioral responses to stress. In addition, nurses must consider the impact of life events and social, cultural, and value and belief systems on the individual in maintaining health and in adapting to stressful events and illness (McCloskey and Bulechek, 1996).

Choosing specific nursing interventions for a particular client is part of the clinical decision-making process. In addressing the psychologic needs of a physiologic illness, nurses must be able to:

> Understand the concept of stress.
> Recognize its manifestations on mind-body interactions.

Know which factors alter resistance to stress.
Formulate realistic plans to strengthen the positive influencing/coping factors.
Implement actions to reduce the individual's stress.
Educate the individual about how to control personal stressors (e.g., cognitive "reframing" of the stressful event, using diversional activities).
Include the client in decision making.
Provide positive reinforcement for effective coping measures.
Recognize own imbalances and incorporate stress reduction measures for self.
Promote a healthy lifestyle for self.

Box 31-3 presents the application of the steps in the nursing process to a woman with terminal illness.

Summary of Key Concepts

1. For centuries Western philosophers considered the mind, body, and spirit as separate components or systems. The human being was judged to be the sum of the individual parts.

2. In contrast, Eastern philosophies considered humans as part of their environment; past and present experiences played an important role in human behavior.

3. Holistic health care is a blend of Eastern and Western health care philosophies integrating alternative, or complementary, and traditional therapies.

4. A very strong relationship between stress and illness has been substantiated through theory and research.

5. Stress is referred to as a stimulus, a response; the stress may be perceived as a challenge or a threat; prolonged stress has been strongly associated with psychologic-physiologic illnesses.

6. A person's response to stress is varied and includes an integrated multisystem response of body, mind, and spirit.

7. Individuals use a variety of coping mechanisms in order to reduce stress and avoid discomfort.

8. Personal attributes (i.e., hardiness, resilience, hope, internal locus of control, and social support) are essential components in coping with stress, illness, or impending death.

9. Coping measures can be labeled as effective or ineffective; ineffective coping can result in illness.

10. The selection and use of coping mechanisms can be affected by genetic makeup, cultural and spiritual beliefs, past experiences, and interactions with others.

11. Certain individuals are at great risk for experiencing psychologic-physiologic health problems. These are related to acute, chronic, or multiple health problems; the elderly; the pain experience; terminal illnesses; stressful occupations; the homeless population; and advanced technologic procedures.

12. The effective use of the nursing process requires the nurse to have a thorough knowledge of science and theory related to nursing and other disciplines, particularly medicine and psychology.

REFERENCES

American Psychiatric Association: *Diagnostic and statistical manual of mental disorders*, ed 4, Washington, DC, 1994, The Association.

Associated Press: Deputy overcomes loss of limb: returns to duty, *San Diego Union-Tribune*, August 8, 1996.

Beck C: Postpartum onset of panic disorder, *Image J Nurs Sch* 30(2):131, 1998.

Black J, Matassarin-Jacobs E: *Medical-surgical nursing: a psychophysiological approach*, Philadelphia, 1997, WB Saunders.

Carson: *Spiritual dimensions of nursing practice*, Philadelphia, 1989, WB Saunders.

Conrad B: Maternal depressive symptoms and homeless children's mental health: risk and resiliency, *Arch Psychiatr Nurs* 12(1):50, 1998.

Doenges M, Moorhouse M: *Application of nursing process and nursing diagnosis*, Philadelphia, 1992, FA Davis.

Dossey B: Awakening the inner healer, *Am J Nurs* 91(8):31, 1991.

Dossey B: Using imagery to help your patient heal, *Am J Nurs* 98(1):41, 1998.

Dyer J, McGuinnes T: Resilience: analysis of the concept, *Arch Psychiatr Nurs* 10(5):276, 1996.

Eakes G, Burke M, Hainsworth M: Middle-range theory of chronic sorrow, *Image J Nurs Sch* 30(2):179, 1998.

Fortinash K, Holoday-Worret P: *Psychiatric nursing care plans*, ed 3, St Louis, 1999, Mosby.

Glaser, Glaser: Perspectives of psycho-immune response. In Adler R, Felton D, Cohen N, editors: *Psychoneuroimmunology*, San Diego, 1991, Academic Press.

Glod C: *Contemporary psychiatric mental health nursing: the brain-behavior connection*, Philadelphia, 1998, FA Davis.

Goetinck S: Key to repairing human tissue, *San Diego Union-Tribune*, p A-1, November 6, 1998.

Gorman L: Mental illness due to a general medical condition. In Glod C, editor: *Contemporary psychiatric mental health nursing: the brain-behavior connection*, Philadelphia, 1998, FA Davis.

Graham D: Brain can sprout new cells, researchers find, *San Diego Union-Tribune*, p A-1, October 30, 1998.

Groer M: Psychoneuroimmunology, *Am J Nurs* 91(8):33, 1991.

Jarrett M et al: The relationship between psychological distress and gastrointestinal symptoms in women with irritable bowel syndrome, *Nurs Res* 47(3):154, 1998.

Joseph R: *Neuropsychiatry, neuropsychology, and clinical neuroscience*, ed 2, Philadelphia, 1996, Williams & Wilkins.

Kozier B, Erb G, Blais K: *Concepts and issues in nursing practice*, ed 2, Park, Calif, 1992, Addison-Wesley.

Kozier B, Erb G, Blais K: *Professional nursing practice: concepts and perspectives*, Menlo Park, Calif, 1997, Addison-Wesley.

Kuehn A, Winters R: A study of symptom distress, health locus of control and coping resources of aging post-polio survivors, *Image J Nurs Sch* 26(4):325, 1994.

Lazarus R, Folkman S: *Stress, appraisal and coping*, New York, 1984, Springer.

Lazarus R, Folkman S: The concept of coping. In Monat A, Lazarus R, editors: *Stress and coping*, New York, 1991, Columbia University Press.

Lewis S et al: *Medical-surgical nursing: assessment and management of clinical problems*, ed 5, St Louis, 1999, Mosby.

Lindenberg C et al: Risk and resilience: building protective factors, *Matern Child Nurs J* 23(2):99, 1998.

McCaffery M, Beebe A, Latham J: *Pain: clinical manual for nursing practice*, ed 2, St Louis, 1998, Mosby.

McCloskey JC, Bulechek GM: *Nursing interventions classifications*, ed 2, St Louis, 1996, Mosby.

McFarland GK, McFarlane EA: *Nursing diagnosis and intervention*, ed 3, St Louis, 1997, Mosby.

Messner R, Lewis S: Double trouble: managing chronic illness and depression, *Nursing* 95(8):46, 1995.

Monat A, Lazarus R: *Stress and coping*, New York, 1991, Columbia University Press.

Morse J, Doberneck B: Delineating the concept of hope, *Image J Nurs Sch* 27(4):277, 1995.

Moyers B: *Healing of the mind*, New York, 1993, Doubleday.

Mynatt S: Increasing resiliency to substance abuse in recovering women with comorbid depression, *J Psychosoc Nurs* 36(1):28, 1998.

North American Nursing Diagnosis Association: *Nursing diagnoses: definitions and classification, 1999-2000*, Philadelphia, 1999, The Association.

Olson J: Relationships between nurse-expressed empathy, patient-perceived empathy and patient distress, *Image J Nurs Sch* 27(4):317, 1995.

O'Neill D, Kenny E: Spirituality and chronic illness, *Image J Nurs Sch* 30(3):275, 1998.

Pender N: Stress management. In *Health promotion in nursing practice*, ed 3, Stamford, Conn, 1996, Appleton & Lange.

Pollack, Duffy: The health-related hardiness scale: development and psychometric analysis, *Nurs Res* 39(4):218, 1990.

Porth C: *Pathophysiology: concepts of altered health states*, ed 5, Philadelphia, 1998, JB Lippincott.

Selye H: *Stress of life*, ed 2, New York, 1978, McGraw-Hill.

Smeltzer C, Bare B: Human response to illness. In Brunner, Sudarth: *Medical-surgical nursing*, ed 8, Philadelphia, 1996, Lippincott-Raven.

Stuart GW, Laraia MT: *Stuart and Sundeen's principles and practice of psychiatric nursing*, ed 6, St Louis, 1998, Mosby.

Swerdlow J: Quiet miracles of the mind, *National Geographic* 187(6):2, 1995.

Thorne S, Paterson B: Shifting images of chronic illness, *Image J Nurs Sch* 30(2):173, 1998.

Wagnild G, Young H: Resilience among older women, *Image J Nurs Sch* 22(4):252, 1990.

CHAPTER 32

Persons With Chronic Mental Illness

Alwilda Scholler-Joquish

OBJECTIVES

- Identify components of deinstitutionalization that have significantly affected persons with chronic mental illness.

- Discuss psychologic problems manifested by persons with chronic mental illness and the impact they have on the client and family.

- Describe several behavioral manifestations of chronic mental illness and how they affect a person's ability to function independently.

- Examine the relationship between poverty, chronic mental illness, and homelessness.

- Distinguish between the behavioral manifestations of chronic mental illness in persons who have been institutionalized and the behaviors of young people with chronic mental illness who have had few experiences with mental health treatment.

- Apply the nursing process to clients with chronic mental illness.

PERSONS WITH CHRONIC MENTAL ILLNESS

The impact of chronic mental illness on the individual, family members, health care providers, and the community is significant. Although any psychiatric diagnosis can result in a disabling condition, most references to **chronic mental illness** (a psychiatric disorder that persists over time with remissions and recurrence of severe and disabling symptoms) address the concerns of the most severely disabled individuals (Birren et al, 1992; Krauss and Slavinsky, 1982; Lipton and Cancro, 1995). Persons with chronic mental illness pose some of the most difficult social, medical, and political problems of our time. Each individual with a chronic mental illness will have a different life experience. However, each person lives in a world in which he or she is expected to have relationships with others and provide for shelter and the basic necessities of life. The impact of the degree and frequency of psychiatric symptoms will affect the ability to function effectively in the world in which the person lives. The general public is supportive of the person who recovers from a psychiatric illness and is able to resume normal functions. However, people with chronic mental illness are often shunned by society and isolated from the community (Kaplan and Sadock, 1998; Krauss and Slavinsky, 1982).

Nurses are the health care professionals who have the most frequent and most consistent involvement with the **chronically mentally ill** (persons who manifest the symptoms of chronic mental illness). Few people are so dependent on the compassionate and professional care provided by nurses as are persons with chronic mental illness and their families. Nurses help persons with chronic mental illness to develop

Chemical restraint The use of psychotropic drugs and sedatives to reduce or eliminate psychiatric symptoms. Symptom management through medication is another way to describe chemical restraint.

Chronic mental illness A psychiatric disorder that persists over time with remissions and recurrence of severe and disabling symptoms.

Chronically mentally ill Persons who manifest the symptoms of chronic mental illness.

Deinstitutionalization The process of returning psychiatric clients to the community, which includes limited admission and commitment policies.

Disaffiliated A person who does not associate with family, friends, or service providers.

Dual diagnosis A term used when the individual has two identified primary psychiatric diagnoses, most commonly used when one diagnosis is drug- or alcohol related. For example, the person may have both a substance-related disorder and a mood disorder.

Idea of influence A delusional belief that one's thought processes are being influenced by an external source, such as radar, space aliens, or another person.

Institutionalization Placing or confining persons with mental disorders in state-run facilities such as residential treatment programs designed to treat such disorders.

Parasitic One's total dependence on someone else for one's every need.

Restrictive admission policies A component of the deinstitutionalization process that limits the length of stay until symptoms are under control.

Restrictive commitment policies A component of the deinstitutionalization process that limits commitment to a psychiatric facility to cases where there is a threat to harm self and/or others.

Restrictive environment An environment that restricts the activity of a client to assist the client in regaining control of his or her behavior. The individual may be placed in open-door or closed-door seclusion during periods of extreme agitation, suicidal ideations, or threats of violence to self or others.

Sleep reversal A state in which normal sleeping patterns are reversed: the individual sleeps during the day and is active during the night.

Transinstitutionalization A process in which clients are transferred from one institution to another, such as from a psychiatric hospital to a nursing home.

strategies for coping with emotional and behavioral manifestations of their mental disorder. The individual is supported during times of crisis and encouraged during times of remission. Nurses also help family members cope with the challenges of living with a person with the behavioral and emotional manifestations of chronic mental illness.

DEVELOPMENT OF CHRONIC MENTAL ILLNESS

Chronic mental illness is diagnosed when it is believed that the person will have some manifestation of the disease process throughout his or her lifetime. The person with chronic mental illness may experience psychiatric transient and recurrent symptoms. Symptoms of chronic mental illness often are passed off as "odd" behaviors ("That's just her way") without recognition that these behaviors are clues to mental illness. Family members may tolerate a wide range of behaviors without clear understanding that an individual may have a psychiatric illness. Even treatment by mental health professionals in outpatient or inpatient facilities may not clearly identify the chronicity of the person's illness.

Chronic mental illness is often identified in retrospect. By the time symptoms have endured persistently enough for a major mental disorder to be confirmed, the individual may have had several episodes of symptomatic behavior. Looking back at the person's history of behavioral problems and symptoms, a pattern emerges that reveals the chronicity and impact of the mental disorder. Often the episodes were symptoms of a more comprehensive pattern of mental illness (Kaplan and Sadock, 1998; Lipton and Cancro, 1995; Rawnsley, 1991).

DIAGNOSTIC FEATURES

Persons with chronic mental illness have severe and persistent emotional disorders that interfere with their ability to live and function independently. The extent of disability has been defined by the National Plan for the Chronically Mentally Ill (U.S. Department of Health and Human Services, 1981). This definition includes disorders that interfere with the individual's ability to perform the activities of daily living, such as those related to personal hygiene and self-care, self-direction, interpersonal relationships, social interactions, learning, recreation, and economic self-sufficiency. The most common chronic mental illness medical diagnoses include schizophrenia, mood disorders, delusional disorders, delirium, dementia, amnestic and other cognitive disorders, and other psychotic disorders. In children the most common diagnoses include pervasive developmental disorders, childhood schizophrenia, conduct disorders, and mental retardation (American Psychiatric Association [APA], 1994; Kaplan and Sadock, 1998).

EFFECTS OF DEINSTITUTIONALIZATION

The Community Mental Health Act of 1965 was passed in response to many societal changes, including the advent of psychotropic drugs and the recognition of the effects of long-term **institutionalization** (placing or confining persons with mental disorders in state-run facilities such as residential treatment programs designed to treat such disorders). A combination of psycho-socio-political changes created the climate for change. From the psychologic perspective, it was clear that long-term institutionalization had negative effects on the client's mental status. New medications allowed for increased control of symptoms and more effective response to psychotherapy.

The federal law included the concept of mental health centers in the local communities. However, little funding was provided, and the number of centers was inadequate to meet the needs of the numbers of people who were discharged from the mental institutions. Persons with mental illness were sent home to live in the community without appropriate treatment programs, and there were many problems associated with the **deinstitutionalization** process (the process of returning psychiatric clients to the community, which includes limited admission and commitment policies). Families did not know how to cope, and many of the deinstitutionalized clients wandered away from their homes or residential treatment programs. Residents of local communities did not welcome the development of treatment programs in their neighborhoods for those with chronic mental illness. It has been almost 30 years since deinstitutionalization began, and there is strong evidence that persons with chronic mental illness still receive less care than they need (Aiken et al, 1986; Torrey, 1996).

YOUNG ADULTS WITH CHRONIC MENTAL ILLNESS

Some of the deinstitutionalization components included restriction of admissions to psychiatric facilities, as well as short-term hospital stays (Pepper and Ryglewicz, 1984; Torrey, 1988). These policies have probably contributed to the development of the new phenomenon known as the *young chronically mentally ill*. These adults, between ages 18 and 35, have the most severe, overt disorders. They lack internal controls, rarely take psychotropic medications, and exhibit excessive drug and alcohol abuse (Caton et al, 1989; Fischer and Breakey, 1986; Holcomb and Ahr, 1987).

It has been suggested that substance abuse is a form of self-medication for chronic mental illness. There is an indication that those with mood disorders are more likely to abuse cocaine, those with schizophrenia are more likely to use alcohol for symptom relief, and those with conduct disorders are more likely to abuse heroin and other drugs. Many of those with chronic mental illness are polysubstance abusers (Caton et al, 1989). A recent study suggested that reinforcement techniques may be effective in reducing cocaine use in persons with chronic mental illness (Shaner et al, 1997).

PSYCHOLOGIC MANIFESTATIONS OF CHRONIC MENTAL ILLNESS

The person with chronic mental illness will have numerous psychologic manifestations. The specific cognitive or behavioral manifestations may be associated with specific mental disorders, as well as with the individual's unique life history.

ALTERED THOUGHT PROCESSES

For the purposes of this chapter, altered thought processes will be defined as any disruption in the individual's ability to solve problems and think clearly. Alterations may include hallucinations, delusions, or confusion. (NOTE: NANDA [1999] describes hallucinations as sensory/perceptual alterations.) The alterations in thought processes may be transient, recurrent, or permanent. The recurrent and transient alterations in thought processes are a major difficulty that persons with chronic mental illness face in establishing independent living arrangements. One example is an **idea of influence,** in which the person believes that his or her thoughts are influenced by an external source.

Persons with chronic mental illness have limited skills in coping with the problems of day-to-day living. They may lack skills in communicating their thoughts and emotions to others. Additional stressors can precipitate major disruptions in their ability to cope (Kaplan and Sadock, 1998; Krauss and Slavinsky, 1982).

CHRONIC LOW SELF-ESTEEM

Chronic low self-esteem is a persistent problem for persons with chronic mental illness. Mental illness affects the self-perception and the ability to make sense out of life events. The delusions, hallucinations, and other negative symptoms of mental illness affect their memory, perception, and ability to think clearly. Persons with chronic mental illness are often excluded from social activities because they look and act different from others. They thus see themselves as ineffective and helpless; many are very much aware of their own deviance (Drew, 1991; Gerhart, 1990; Lefley, 1987; Mueser and Gingerich, 1994; Rawnsley, 1991). Persons with chronic mental illness who experience small successes resist making further attempts for fear of failure or expectations that they could do more (Bernheim and Lehman, 1985; Krauss and Slavinsky, 1982).

LONELINESS

Whether social isolation is self-imposed or results from avoidance of others, people with chronic mental illness are often lonely people. "Loneliness occurs when the need for intimacy is not met. It renders people emotionally paralyzed and helpless" (Copel, 1988). Some elements of loneliness include problems with social relationships, inability to make decisions, and a focus on weakness in self or others. Persons with chronic mental illness are often unable to express their feelings of loneliness and may withdraw further in fear of rejection. They experience a significant amount of distress in attempting to describe their feelings of loneliness. Loneliness is difficult for anyone, yet persons with a chronic mental illness are often unable to make the necessary changes in their lives or behaviors to break out of the experience of loneliness (Copel, 1988).

HOPELESSNESS

People who struggle with major mental illness can experience an overwhelming sense of worthlessness and hopelessness. Worthlessness is an awareness that one's efforts are ineffectual or insignificant. Feelings of worthlessness diminish the person's self-esteem and increase his or her risk of depression.

Hopelessness is a critical indicator of long-term suicidal risk (Kaplan and Sadock, 1998). It is a feeling that there are few alternatives or personal choices available. The individual is unable to mobilize energy to relieve feelings of futility and despair (Fortinash and Holoday-Worret, 1999).

DEPRESSION

Depressive episodes can accompany other mental disorders, making the life of the person with chronic mental illness much more difficult. Depression has been defined as "an emotional state, ranging in severity from mild to severe, characterized by discouragement, sadness, worthlessness, psychomotor retardation or agitation, and varying degrees of inability to care for self" (Kaplan and Sadock, 1998; McFarland et al, 1992).

> **⚠ CLINICAL ALERT**
>
> The possibility of suicide is an ever-present risk in schizophrenia, which may involve depression, delusions, and command hallucinations that may tell the person to attempt suicide (Torrey, 1995).

Depression may be related to the individual's awareness that he or she is unable to cope with the world. Persons who develop chronic mental illness as adults and who have experienced relationships and successes in life should be considered at high risk for suicide during depressive episodes. When depression accompanies schizophrenia or Alzheimer's disease, the risk of suicide increases significantly (see Chapter 12).

SUICIDE

Suicide has been defined as self-induced annihilation in a person who believes death is the best solution for his or her perceived problem. Suicide attempts in persons with chronic mental illness occur most often in persons with mood disorders or schizophrenia. Although persons with chronic mental illness may express suicidal ideations while in the hospital, they are more likely to commit suicide after they leave the nursing unit (Roy, 1995). However, any person with suicidal ideations or a past history of suicidal gestures should be considered at high risk for a suicide attempt. Chapter 28 discusses this topic in more depth.

It is important to explore the fantasies of suicidal patients about what the consequences would be if they were to commit suicide. Their fantasies may include wishes for revenge, power, control, punishment, sacrifice, reunion with the dead, or a new life. Persons most likely to act out suicidal fantasies may have lost a loved object, may have received an injury to their self-image, may experience overwhelming affects such as rage and guilt, or may identify with a suicide victim (Kaplan and Sadock, 1998).

BEHAVIORAL MANIFESTATIONS OF CHRONIC MENTAL ILLNESS

Persons with chronic mental illness often have difficulty in self-care, personal hygiene, independent living, interpersonal relations, and employment. Assaultive behaviors and criminal activity can alienate them from their family and professional mental health services. These behavioral manifestations may be present in young children, as well as adults and the elderly. The degree of disability will determine the extent and nature of the individual's behavioral manifestations. Persons with chronic mental illness who are receiving psychotropic medication in an inpatient setting may not exhibit the extent of disability demonstrated when they leave the hospital and resume living in the community. Persons who are noncompliant with their psychotropic medications may return to problematic behaviors once they return to their previous living situation. It is important to assess the extent and nature of the individual's behavior in the community, as described by the client and his or her family or caregivers.

> ## ⚠ CLINICAL ALERT
>
> It is estimated that 10% of all patients with schizophrenia kill themselves. They are most likely to commit suicide within the first 5 years of onset of symptoms. Persons at greatest risk are those with relapses and remission who have good insight into their illness, have poor response to medications, feel socially isolated, and feel hopeless about the future (Torrey, 1995).

ACTIVITIES OF DAILY LIVING

Activities of daily living are essential skills needed to live independently. Persons with chronic mental illness often lack basic self-maintenance skills such as personal grooming, table manners, and social interaction skills. Their careless behavior may result from impaired judgment, forgetfulness, or lack of motivation (Bellack and Mueser, 1986; Bernheim and Lehman, 1985).

> ## ⚠ CLINICAL ALERT
>
> Careless behaviors in handling cigarettes, sharp instruments, or hot liquids pose safety hazards to persons with chronic mental illness. These behaviors can be attributed to impaired judgment, forgetfulness, neglect of self, or lack of motivation (Bernheim and Lehman, 1985).

The lack of these essential skills interferes with the individual's ability to be accepted in community settings. The inability to function adequately in social settings is a major factor in the poor quality of life that many persons with chronic mental illness experience (Castle, 1997). Persons with schizophrenia often have poor social skills and are frequently asocial (Bachrach, 1996; Bellack and Mueser, 1986; Kouzis and Eaton, 1997; Torrey, 1995).

INDEPENDENT LIVING

During the deinstitutionalization process, it was believed that mental deterioration was caused by long-term hospitalization. It was not recognized that many persons with chronic mental illness are not fully capable of living in the community. More important, it was not recognized that such individuals would experience significant exacerbations during the course of their disease process (Belcher, 1991).

Personal survival depends on the person's ability to secure an income, locate a place to live, and maintain interpersonal relationships. Persons who live independently are responsible for obtaining food and clothing and for maintaining their living space. A large proportion of the people with chronic mental illness are living impoverished existences and rely heavily on others for financial and personal support (Hogstel, 1995; Lurigio and Lewis, 1989).

A recent study suggests that persons with chronic mental illness can successfully complete a daily activities check list, which serves as an assessment of the individual's ability to live independently (Brown, Hamera, and Long, 1996).

COMPLIANCE WITH MEDICATIONS

Persons with chronic mental illness may find it difficult to comply with a regular course of psychotropic medications. For some individuals this may be associated with attitudes about taking medications, whereas others may feel so much improvement that they believe they no longer need the medications (Ruscher, de Wit, and Mazmanian, 1997). The side effects of medications are one of the primary reasons these persons have for discontinuing their prescribed medical regimen (Piazza et al, 1997). The person's ability to remember his or her medications, the dosage, and the need for compliance needs to be assessed by the health care provider (So, Toglia, and Donohue, 1997). The longer a person is ill and the more educated the person is before the onset of mental illness, the more likely it is that the person will be well informed about his or her medications (Tempier, 1996). Educational programs designed for persons with chronic mental illness may enhance their ability to self-manage their own medications (Hornung et al, 1996; Ruscher, deWit, and Mazmanian, 1997).

MEDICAL ILLNESS IN THE CHRONICALLY MENTALLY ILL

Persons with chronic mental illness are subject to the same medical, surgical, obstetric, and physiologic conditions as the general population. It has been recognized that, as a group, the chronically mentally ill have a much higher rate of morbidity and mortality (Felker, Yazel, and Short, 1996). In some instances the increased number of illnesses may be associated with a lack of knowledge and awareness of the signs and symptoms of common health problems (Getty, Persese, and Knab, 1998). Some persons with chronic mental illness may not know how to access the health care system when they are ill, and their medical illness may not be recognized when they do present themselves for medical care. There is an indication that hospitalized psychiatric clients may not receive the same amount of pain medication as other clients (Wise and Mann, 1996). The assessment of the physical and psychiatric conditions of hospitalized clients is very important. Many medical conditions may exacerbate or mimic psychiatric disorders. Chronic mental illness results in a higher mortality rate than in the general population as a result of undiagnosed and untreated medical problems and self-destructive behaviors (Dembling, 1997; Felker, Yazel, and Short, 1996).

EMPLOYMENT

Work is a key factor in rehabilitation of persons with chronic mental illness because it provides meaning and organization in their lives. However, many skills are required to obtain a job, such as transportation to the place of employment, completing an application, and negotiating an interview. Persons with chronic mental illness may never have acquired job skills, or they may not be able to resume their former occupation. Once they secure a job, many are unable to retain it for a long period of time. The inability to obtain employment is a major difficulty for the psychiatric client and contributes significantly to the person's poor quality of living (Figure 32-1).

It has been suggested that persons who participate in supported employment that incorporates working and vo-

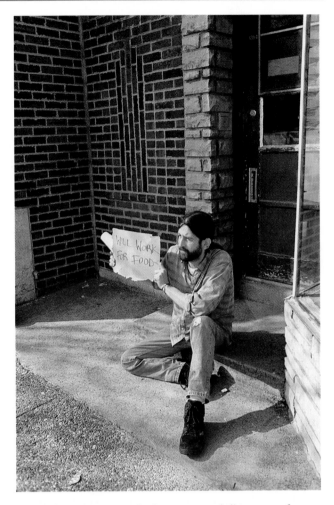

Figure 32-1 Persons with chronic mental illness are often unable to maintain regular employment and must rely on others for support. (Copyright Cathy Lander-Goldberg, Lander Photographics.)

cational services may be more successful in maintaining employment (Bond et al, 1997).

DEPENDENT LIVING WITH FAMILY

The majority of persons with chronic mental illness live with their families. Changes in the care of clients with chronic mental illness have shifted from a hospital-based program to a community-centered system, and families often serve as extensions of the mental health system (Saunders, 1997). Mental health professionals look to the family as primary support persons for individuals with chronic mental illness. Family members are expected to provide care management activities such as assessment, monitoring for compliance with the treatment regimen, and advocacy (Saunders, 1997). However, not all families are healthy enough to cope with the demands of the family member with chronic mental illness. The person's presence in the home drains financial, emotional, and personal resources. In some cases, the family is dysfunctional and may be unable to provide the necessary support for the person.

There are persons with chronic mental illness who are married and have had children before or during the onset of the severe psychiatric symptoms. A spouse may be repeatedly hospitalized or maintained primarily on an outpatient basis. A healthy spouse may be living with an adult whose behavior is unpredictable and even bizarre. During periods of exacerbation, the chronically mentally ill spouse may require frequent care and close supervision. The presence of children in the home can result in great stress for everyone concerned (Torrey, 1988).

Some persons with mood disorders are able to sustain minimal employment; however, they are unable to disguise their disorder from the family members, a dilemma that may be confusing for everyone concerned.

Children of persons with chronic mental illness are often at risk for mental illness themselves. The mental illness of a parent has a significant effect on the child's development (Powell, 1998). Unstable family life has been correlated with the subsequent development of chronic mental illness in the children. The children may also be at great risk for physical abuse. The home environment and the ability of family members to successfully cope should be evaluated by mental health professionals in any setting (Krauss and Slavinsky, 1982).

The behaviors of persons with chronic mental illness may be passive or hostile. Some individuals are **parasitic** (totally dependent on someone else for their every need), apathetic, and live in self-imposed isolation within the family unit. Others may refuse to take medication and reflect profound hopelessness and despair. Delusional thought processes, stereotyped bizarre behaviors, and eating disorders contribute to the disruption of the family living situation (Lipton and Cancro, 1995). Hostile, abusive, and assaultive behaviors may also be directed at family members. **Sleep reversal** (a state in which normal sleeping patterns are reversed and the individual sleeps during the day and is active during the night), running away, poor personal hygiene, and property damage are some of the most frustrating behaviors that disrupt the household (Bernheim and Lehman, 1985; Krauss and Slavinsky, 1982; Lefley, 1987; Steinglass and Horan, 1988). Families have reported that the highest burden in coping is with positive and negative symptoms of persons with bipolar disorders (Mueser et al, 1996).

SEXUALITY

There are numerous sexual and relationship problems associated with chronic mental illness (Bhui, Puffett, and Strathdee, 1997). These persons may have a normal sexual drive but may be unable to discern appropriate sexual responses. Individuals with chronic mental illness may be sexually promiscuous or could be exploited because of their desire for affection and acceptance. Persons with chronic mental illness are at an increased risk for HIV/AIDS and other sexually transmitted diseases (Carey et al, 1997).

Rape is not uncommon in women with chronic mental illness, who may be unable to discern inappropriate sexual advances. Pregnancies may occur during hospitalization, resulting in additional stressors for all concerned (News, 1997). Chronically mentally ill women are less likely to receive information about menstruation, birth control, or screening for breast or cervical cancer (Ritsher, Coursey, and Ferrell, 1997). They may be subject to unwanted pregnancies and poor prenatal care. These women are more likely to be exposed to violent behaviors and less likely to have a stable partner (Gold award, 1996; Miller and Finnerty, 1996; Ritsher, Coursey, and Ferrell, 1997).

There can also be inappropriate sexual acting-out behaviors by persons with chronic mental illness. Individuals may masturbate or expose themselves in ways that are offensive or threatening to others (Bernheim and Lehman, 1985; Issac and Armat, 1990). Efforts to control offensive sexual behavior have included punishment, stigmatization, and chemical castration. The use of medroxyprogesterone (Depo-Provera) can significantly reduce a man's sex drive and render him medically castrated.

VIOLENT AND CRIMINAL BEHAVIOR

Persons with chronic mental illness commit a disproportionate number of violent or criminal acts, which reveals lack of judgment and self-control (Isaac and Armat, 1990). These persons may respond with violence to perceived threats (Green, 1997). Violence by a person with chronic mental illness may pose a danger to family members or care providers. Children may be the targets of verbal and physical aggression. Violent behavior often makes community living difficult if not impossible. There is an even greater risk for violence in persons with a dual diagnosis (e.g., when drug and alcohol abuse coexist) (Bernheim and Lehman, 1985; Isaac and Armat, 1990; McFarland et al, 1989; Tardiff, 1984).

Many persons with chronic mental illness have had extensive contact with the criminal justice system (McFarland et al, 1989; Tardiff, 1984). People with mental illness commit crimes for a variety of reasons, such as poor impulse control and acting-out behaviors that include disorderly conduct, criminal trespass, disturbing the peace, and trespassing. Other persons with chronic mental illness tend to commit crimes such as shoplifting, petty theft, and prostitution as a means for survival (Lurigio and Lewis, 1989).

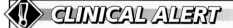 **CLINICAL ALERT**

Patients who were violent just before admission are more likely to attack the same person within 2 weeks after discharge (Tardiff et al, 1997).

There are also persons with chronic mental illness who commit violent crimes that pose a threat to public safety, such as residential burglary, assault, rape, and robbery. Young persons with chronic mental illness who have had little mental health treatment are more likely to be involved in criminal acts of violence. The three primary predictors of violence are a history of past violence, drug and alcohol abuse, and failure to take medication. It is estimated that as many as 1000 people in the United States are murdered each year by persons with chronic mental illness (Torrey, 1996).

Many mass murders have been committed by such people who experienced hallucinations or delusions caused by poor impulse control and substance abuse. With the restricted policies for hospitalization, many violent persons are treated for a brief period and then released. Persons with chronic mental illness who commit violent crimes are often delusional. These persons may commit crimes as a result of command hallucinations, whereby they believe they are told to perform certain acts. Others commit violent crimes because they are unable to control their impulsive urges (Kaplan and Sadock, 1998; Silva, Leong, and Weinstock, 1997).

Persons with chronic mental illness who commit criminal acts of violence are more likely to be placed in prison than in a psychiatric institution. Even in prison, persons with psychosis are legally allowed to choose whether they will take their medication. The rights of the individual and the goal of freedom of choice collide with the rights of family members to live without fear of harm to themselves or others (Isaac and Armat, 1990; Lurigio and Lewis, 1989; Tardiff, 1984).

PERSONS WITH CHRONIC MENTAL ILLNESS WHO HAVE SPECIAL PROBLEMS

Within the population of people with chronic mental illness there are subgroups with unique and special problems that affect their ability to respond to psychiatric interventions.

MENTALLY RETARDED PERSONS WITH CHRONIC MENTAL ILLNESS

Essential features of mental retardation are an IQ below 70 with impairments in adaptive functioning that began before the person was 18 years old. Behavioral patterns include cognitive deficits revealed in concreteness of thinking and neurologic dysfunction. Persons with mild to moderate retardation are believed to be more susceptible to mental illness. The conflict between the person's expectations and actual abilities may be a source of lifelong stress. In addition to a variety of personality disorders, the person with mental retardation and mental illness can experience affective, as well as psychotic, disorders. There are indica-

tions that at least 40% of individuals with mental retardation meet the criteria for at least one psychiatric disorder (Kaplan and Sadock, 1998). Depression and psychotic disorders are underreported in persons with mental retardation (Szymanski and Crocker, 1995). A breakdown of central nervous system processing is a common feature in persons with a dual diagnosis of mental retardation and mental illness. Self-stimulating and self-injurious behaviors are often associated with underlying neurologic dysfunction (Gorman, 1997). Treatment for this special population requires an interdisciplanary approach.

PERSONS WITH SENSORY AND COMMUNICATION IMPAIRMENTS

Individuals with sensory deprivations may experience many difficulties communicating with others when they are mentally healthy. The person with chronic mental illness who is sight or hearing impaired may be hospitalized much longer and receive less treatment (Dickert, 1988; Fitzgerald and Parkes, 1998). Cases have been reported in which hearing-impaired clients were institutionalized for many years before it became known that the individual's social deficits were not a result of mental illness. Any person with symptoms of chronic mental illness should receive a careful medical evaluation before a final diagnosis is made.

ELDERLY PERSONS WITH CHRONIC MENTAL ILLNESS

Elderly persons with chronic mental illness include those who have had mental illness for decades, as well as those whose mental disorder was diagnosed after the individual was over 50 years old. Elderly persons who develop chronic mental illness may have an insidious onset that is not immediately noted by their family members or care providers. Depression is a serious problem in the elderly and requires appropriate intervention to reduce the risk of suicide. Schizophrenia is usually manifested during the early years of a person's life, and there are many people who have grown old with this condition (Harvey et al, 1997). Nevertheless, schizophrenia may also manifest for the first time after age 45 (Harris and Jeste, 1995). Family members of elderly persons with chronic mental illness may find themselves becoming a primary caregiver in a most difficult situation (Krach and Yang, 1992; Post, 1995).

Alzheimer's disease and other dementias are the most common causes of mental illness in the elderly. As many as 20% of elderly persons over the age of 80 suffer from some form of dementia. The onset of dementia is insidious and requires careful evaluation and diagnosis (Kaplan and Sadock, 1998; McPherson, 1995.) The behavioral changes in the elderly with chronic mental illness are disturbing to spouses and adult children. Family members have concerns about the person's safety, as well as his or her memory loss and disorientation. Some elderly persons may become so agitated that they require intensive treatment (Mintzer et al, 1997). As the person with senile dementia continues to lose cognitive ability, he or she may strike out in fear at family members, who have become strangers. The mental deterioration of the elderly person may precipitate emotional disturbances in the spouse or adult children (Small, 1995).

The exploding population of people over the age of 65 was estimated to reach 35 million by the year 2000 and is expected to reach more than 64 million by the year 2030. It is anticipated that there will be 16 million mentally ill elderly persons by the year 2030. The combined effect of increased costs for extended care facilities and the limitations placed on services by insurance programs result in very limited care being provided for the aged chronically mentally ill. This places an increasingly large burden on the adult children. Most dependence needs of the elderly parents are being fulfilled by adult children, especially daughters. Not only is the burden of care very difficult, but it is often psychologically difficult for the caregiver who is now responsible for the dependent parent (Jarvik and Small, 1995) The awareness of the stress and psychologic strain for caregivers has resulted in a variety of educational programs designed to assist them in coping with unexpected life situations (Pruchno, Burant, and Peters, 1997; Seltzer and Li, 1996).

SUBSTANCE ABUSE

Persons with chronic mental illness who are also dependent on one or more substances are among the most difficult to treat in either psychiatric or substance abuse treatment programs. Persons with a **dual diagnosis** (i.e., they have two identified primary psychiatric diagnoses) have a high rate of hospitalization. There are many more persons with mental disorders who also abuse alcohol and drugs than in the general population. The coexistence of drug abuse and mental illness is associated with a more severe course of illness. Substance abuse can distort symptoms, as well as diminish impulse control. Persons with a dual diagnosis often have unstable living arrangements and may act out in violent and criminal behavior. They have more difficulty organizing their lives and are prone to homelessness. Persons with chronic mental illness who have a dual diagnosis are more difficult to treat than individuals with one primary psychiatric diagnosis (Caton et al, 1989; Osher and Kofoed, 1989).

CHILDREN AND ADOLESCENTS WITH CHRONIC MENTAL ILLNESS

Chronic mental illness is generally considered a diagnosis that occurs in a person's adult years. However, many chronic mental illnesses have their onset in childhood or adolescence. Schizophrenia can develop in children over 5 years of age. Bipolar disorders may be associated with other diagnoses such as conduct disorders. Although children in manic episodes engage in high-risk behaviors, they do so without intent to cause harm to anyone. Children of bipolar parents may not be identified until their symptoms become more severe (Cogan, 1998; Faedda et al, 1995).

For the most part, children who develop chronic mental illness at an early age will be severely affected throughout their lives. Many adolescents have manifestations of mental illness that may be recognized retrospectively. Chronic mental illnesses in children and youth have severe, long-lasting, and devastating effects on the children, their families, and society (Angold et al, 1998).

CHILDREN WITH CHRONIC MENTAL ILLNESS

It is difficult to consider the realities of children with chronic mental illness. The word *chronic* may refer to the anticipated length of treatment, a diagnostic category, or a set of behavioral patterns (Koret, 1981). Some of the symptoms of children with chronic mental illness include interpersonal problems, inability to learn or achieve at school, and behaviors that differ from the norm or are inconsistent with the child's age. These problems are generally long-standing and severe. It is often difficult to distinguish between behaviors of severely disturbed children and behaviors of those who are hearing impaired, sight impaired, or brain damaged (Kauffman, 1981; Koret, 1981; Silver, 1988; Szatmari, 1995).

Most children with chronic mental illness have no former level of optimal functioning to which they can return, because the basic components of personality functioning have never developed to a level approaching age-appropriate maturity. Unable to develop the prerequisites for growth, children with chronic mental illness tend to have deficits in every area of personality and social functioning (Kaplan and Sadock, 1998; Koret, 1981; Szatmari, 1995). Their lives may be filled with frightening thoughts, constant fear of failure, and overwhelming sadness. They may fear their own aggressiveness or that of others. Children with chronic mental illness may frighten other children or even adults, because they may be viewed as real physical threats. These children may be difficult to be

> ## ⚠ *CLINICAL ALERT*
>
> The characteristics of adolescents who attempt suicide and those who commit suicide are similar. The mental disorders that are most common in adolescents who attempt or complete suicide are bipolar disorder and schizophrenia. Adolescents with mood disorders, substance abuse, and a history of aggressive behavior are at very high risk. Depression is a more serious risk for girls, but boys may have a more severe psychopathology than girls who commit suicide (Kaplan and Sadock, 1998).

around because of their demanding, ungrateful, abusive, aggressive, or morose behaviors (Enzer, 1988).

Psychiatric disorders that occur in childhood include mood disorders, schizophrenia, conduct disorders, and autism (Caton et al, 1989; Kaplan and Sadock, 1998; Szatmari, 1995). It has been suggested that bipolar disorder can be diagnosed in young children (Faedda et al, 1995).

The self-concept of children with chronic mental illness is poor, since they often view themselves as bad or deficient, and many think of themselves as not entirely human. Their behavioral problems cover a wide range—from almost total withdrawal to acts of aggression toward self or others (Kaplan and Sadock, 1998; Kauffman, 1981).

ADOLESCENTS WITH CHRONIC MENTAL ILLNESS

Adolescence is a difficult and tumultuous time for many people. Young people in the midst of life transitions, hormonal changes, and relationship difficulties who also have a psychiatric illness can be challenging to their families and to mental health professionals. The onset of bipolar disorder in adolescence may be associated with conduct disorder. These adolescents may experience disruptions in their lives, including criminal activity, substance abuse, and aggressive and self-destructive behaviors (Hodgman, 1996).

Mental illnesses may not be recognized initially as family members attempt to make sense of the young person's behavior. Family members struggle with the burden of the adolescent's symptoms, the negative impact of the mental illness on the family members, and their own grief (Doornbas, 1997). Psychiatric disorders that may appear during adolescence include schizophrenia, mood disorders, bipolar disorder, conduct disorder, and substance abuse.

Vocational training can help these young persons with chronic mental illness to fulfill their need for meaningful activity (Lloyd and Bassett, 1997).

HOMELESS PERSONS WITH CHRONIC MENTAL ILLNESS

Many homeless persons with chronic mental illness have been institutionalized. However, an increasing number of the homeless are young persons with chronic mental illness with severe psychopathology who also have problems with drugs and alcohol. Social conditions such as poverty and unemployment, combined with persistent mental disorders, often result in homeless persons with chronic mental illness who are unable to maintain stable living arrangements. Homeless persons with chronic mental illness may also have a primary diagnosis of substance abuse. A significant number have a dual diagnosis, with one or more additional primary diagnoses (Cohen and Thompson, 1992; Fischer and Breakey, 1986).

Homelessness among people with chronic mental illness has multiple and often unrelated causes such as economic recession, unemployment, cutbacks in federal programs, **restrictive admission policies** (limiting the length of stay for inpatient psychiatric treatment), and a lack of adequate low-cost housing facilities (Baxter and Hopper, 1984; Bean et al, 1987; Belcher, 1991). A disproportionate number of homeless persons with chronic mental illness are members of racial minorities. The poor minority members with chronic mental illness have only their families or public institutions to provide care. Dependent adults can place such an enormous burden on their families that often the family must ask the person with chronic mental illness to leave. When forced out of their family home, these people often have no place to go except the street (Carter, 1991; Rossi and Wright, 1987; Torrey, 1988).

Homeless persons with chronic mental illness are among the hardest hit persons in society. Unable to think clearly, unable to make effective decisions, and unable to obtain medications, therapy, or shelter, they wander the streets of modern cities and rural communities.

With the increase in poverty and inadequate housing, the number of homeless women has increased. Homeless women tend to be young mothers with young children (Figure 32-2), single adults, or older women with overt psychopathology. Even though there has been an increase in homelessness among women, only 15% of all homeless people are female.

It is estimated that 25% of homeless women have a serious mental health problem. One study reported that 41% of these women had a major mental disorder such as schizophrenia or mood disorders, and that another 44% of the same group demonstrated severe anxiety disorders. Unmarried adult homeless women with chronic mental illness tend to have a history similar to the life experiences of men with chronic mental illness. These women have a high rate of alcoholism or substance abuse coexisting with personality disorders or other mental disorders. They may associate with one or more men for companionship and safety, or they may maintain a solitary existence, living in fear of assault and rape. The older homeless women with chronic mental illness are **disaffiliated** (they do not associate with family, friends, or service providers) (Strasser, 1978). These women tend to be the "bag ladies" who carry their personal possessions in plastic bags, shopping bags, or grocery carts (Figure 32-3). They are more likely to have psychotic disorders that may also be associated with alcoholism.

PROVIDERS OF CARE FOR PERSONS WITH CHRONIC MENTAL ILLNESS

Persons with chronic mental illness may live at home; in a community living arrangement with other persons with mental illness; or in an acute care hospital, psychiatric in-

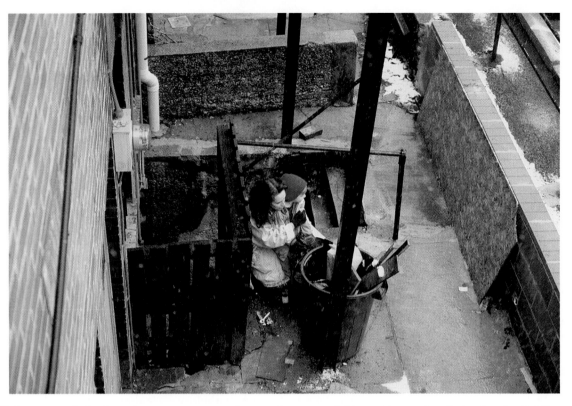

Figure 32-2 Many of the homeless are young mothers with young children. (Copyright Cathy Lander-Goldberg, Lander Photographics.)

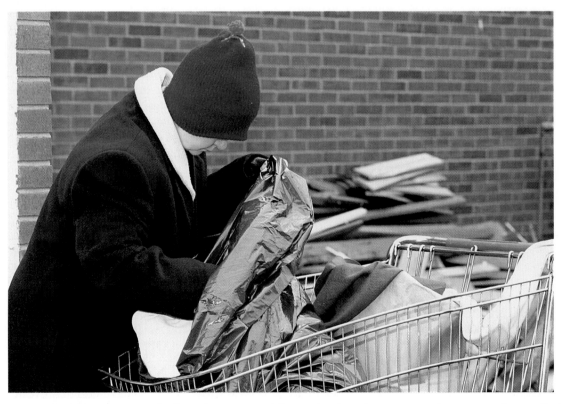

Figure 32-3 Many homeless persons suffer from chronic mental illness. They have few or no social supports and carry all of their personal belongings with them in bags or carts. (Copyright Cathy Lander-Goldberg, Lander Photographics.)

stitution, jail, or nursing home. In each case the nature of the care required and the care provided is different. It is important for nurses working with persons with chronic mental illness to be aware of the differences in care available in each of these settings.

PSYCHIATRIC INSTITUTIONS

Despite the impact of deinstitutionalization, state mental hospitals still provide more than 50% of all psychiatric inpatient care. The restrictive policies regarding admission criteria and length of stay result in short-term institutionalization. Managed care systems vigilantly restrict inpatient care for psychiatric clients. The urge to contain costs has resulted in minimizing the care for some of society's neediest persons (Sharfstein, Webb, and Stoline, 1995). However, short-term care may be stressful and disruptive to clients with schizophrenia, who account for the largest number (more than 70%) of hospital admissions in any year.

The psychiatric hospital maintains an important role in the treatment of severe mental illness. It provides a therapeutic, structured environment that is designed to meet the individual's need for care, protection, and control. It may also be an opportunity for the person with chronic mental illness to get away from a stressful situation. When persons with chronic mental illness are in crisis, the psychiatric hospital may be the most appropriate place in which to seek care. It also provides an opportunity for family members to work with the psychiatric treatment team in preparation for discharge (Menninger, 1995).

There is a "revolving door" effect with a significant number of clients who are admitted for short-term hospitalization and discharged when symptoms are under control. Thus persons with chronic mental illness may receive only episodic care aimed at controlling symptoms and are then discharged to family members, community programs, or their own care (Saunders, 1997).

GENERAL HOSPITALS

As the state mental hospitals reduced their bed capacity, general hospitals began to increase their number of psychiatric beds (Bellack and Mueser, 1986). Hospital units that had been unlocked began to receive young persons with chronic mental illness, as well as acutely ill psychiatric clients. Persons with chronic mental illness who were untreated or noncompliant in follow-up care were more likely to be psychotic and violent. They often required **restrictive environments** to protect them from harming themselves or others. A restrictive environment helps a client gain control of his or her behavior. The client may be placed in open-door or closed-door seclusion during periods of extreme agitation, suicidal ideation, or threats of violence to self or others.

Restrictive commitment policies limit commitment for admission to a psychiatric facility to persons who threaten to harm self or others. These policies have increased the number of persons with severe chronic mental illness who must rely on general community hospitals for care (Fenton et al, 1998). There are indications that changes in involuntary commitment laws have prevented people with severe mental illness from gaining access to appropriate psychiatric care. General hospital units have become locked wards to house people with chronic mental illness who were a threat to the safety of others (Fischer and Breakey, 1986; Pepper and Ryglewicz, 1984).

The restriction of mental health benefits by third-party payers has significantly reduced the amount of time a client may receive care. (Sharfstein, Webb, and Stoline, 1995).

AFTERCARE

Aftercare programs include a variety of community programs and services from partial hospitalization to sheltered living. The kind and type of programs available in a specific community will depend on the size and nature of the community, as well as the community's financial constraints. Outpatient clinics are often associated with acute care hospitals. The size of the outpatient programs and the extent of their services will depend on the availability of reimbursement for services (Surber et al, 1986). Insurance companies limit the number of days of therapy that they will pay for specific disorders.

A wide variety of community programs have been developed. Some include partial care services with day care provided in an acute care hospital and a return to the individual's place of residence at night. Partial care programs place their emphasis on improving the capabilities of persons with chronic mental illness (Marshall and Demmler, 1990; Menninger, 1995). Other living arrangements include lodgings for four or more people. In some situations a manager visits the residence once a day or at other periodic intervals. Some programs provide for a live-in manager who helps the residents resolve interpersonal or household issues. Assertive community programs have been associated with lower rates of rehospitalization (Gold award, 1997; Klinkenberg and Calsyn, 1996; Gater et al, 1997).

HOMELESS SHELTERS

Other types of community programs that provide services to persons with chronic mental illness include homeless shelters, soup kitchens, and substance abuse treatment programs. These individuals may consistently use the same program or go from place to place. Most service providers for the homeless have restrictions on serving individuals who are actively hallucinating, intoxicated, or displaying threatening acting-out behaviors. Persons who are noncompliant with the provider's rules are often refused admission or forced to leave the facility. Thus some of the most out-of-touch persons are turned away from the only places that remain available to them. Persons with chronic mental illness who become disaffiliated from family, health care services, and providers for the homeless often suffer the full ravages of untreated mental disorders. Shelters may provide an evening meal, a change of clothes, and a place to take a shower. However, they have no staff or facilities to deal with psychotic or violent homeless people with chronic mental illness.

FOSTER CARE

Foster care can be used as a temporary or permanent way of removing the child, adolescent, or adult with chronic mental illness from an unsafe environment. Children with chronic mental illness may be at risk of abusive behavior from parents or siblings. Therapeutic foster care must be carefully selected to ensure that the child is in a safe environment (Gross, 1995). Adults at risk in their own homes may be removed to foster care to receive appropriate physical care and interpersonal relationships (Green, 1995b).

NURSING HOMES

One of the results of deinstitutionalization has been the process of **transinstitutionalization** in which a person is transferred from one institution to another. Nursing homes were never designed to care for the client with chronic mental illness. They do not have psychiatrically trained staff to deal with active psychosis and must rely heavily on **chemical restraint** (the use of psychotropic drugs and sedatives to reduce or eliminate psychiatric symptoms). It is estimated that as many as 750,000 out of

2 million nursing home clients have chronic mental illness (Bellack and Mueser, 1986; Boyd and Luetje, 1992; Mosher-Ashley, 1991). Elderly persons with chronic mental illness who are admitted to or transferred to a nursing home may receive less care than those elders who are alert and aware of their surroundings. The former are at increased risk for behavioral manifestations related to inappropriate types or amounts of medications. Elders with chronic mental illness present the nursing home with the most behavioral problems and require specialized attention from geropsychiatric consultants such as nurses with advanced practice in geropsychiatry. Elders with chronic mental illness are also at risk for physical abuse or neglect from staff in nursing homes where staff members are not prepared or properly supervised.

PRISONS AND JAILS

Current reports suggest that from 6% to 15% of persons in city and county jails are chronically mentally ill and that up to 15% of the prison population have severe mental disorders. Many of these offenders have a history of mental illness and are unable to function well in society. A large number of these chronically mentally ill prisoners are also homeless (Jordan et al, 1996; Lamb and Weinberger, 1998; Teplin, Abram, and McClelland, 1996). Incarceration of chronically mentally ill persons poses serious problems for these individuals, as well as for the prison system.

 Client & Family **TEACHING GUIDELINES**

Tips for Managing a Crisis

1. It is important to attempt to reverse any escalation in psychotic symptoms and provide immediate protection and support for the person with chronic mental illness and for family members.
2. Warning signs of a crisis include sleeplessness, ritualistic behaviors, increased suspiciousness, and unpredictable outbursts.
3. Remember, things always go better if you speak softly and in simple sentences. It is uncommon for a person to lose total control of thoughts, feelings, and behaviors.
4. Accept the fact that the person with chronic mental illness is in an "altered state of reality" and may act out in response to hallucinations.
5. It is imperative to stay calm. Trust your feelings; if you are frightened, take immediate action. Do nothing to agitate the situation. If you are alone, call for someone to stay with you while professional help is on the way. If it is necessary to call the police, explain that your relative is mentally ill and that you need help during this crisis. (If police know that this is a psychiatric crisis, they are more likely to respond with strategies than if they think that criminal activity is in progress.)

6. Some simple tips include:
   Don't threaten. This may increase fear or increase the risk of assaultive behavior.
   Don't shout. If the person isn't listening to you, he or she is probably listening to other "voices."
   Don't criticize. It will only make things worse.
   Don't argue with other family members. This is not the time to fix blame or prove a point.
   Don't bait the person. This could lead to his or her acting out wild threats, and the consequences could be tragic.
   Don't stand over the mentally ill person. If the person is seated, seat yourself, since standing may pose a threat.
   Avoid continuous eye contact or touching. This may intimidate the person, especially if paranoia is present.
   Comply with requests that are not dangerous. This gives the individual a sense of control and may increase cooperation.
   Don't block the doorway. However, place yourself between the patient and an exit, in the event that you may need to leave the area.
   Evacuate. All family members should be evacuated in the event that the person appears to be out of control and there is risk for injury.

Some individuals are arrested for minor offenses and may be held in the local jail. When it is apparent that the offender has chronic mental illness, the person may be referred to a state psychiatric facility for treatment.

Family members may find it necessary to have a relative with chronic mental illness arrested for violent or threatening behavior. In some situations, emergency involuntary admissions require that the violent behavior be witnessed by the persons making the arrest or signing the commitment orders. If that does not happen, the individual may be jailed for his or her mental illness rather than admitted to a psychiatric facility. Many persons with severe mental illness serve long-term prison sentences with a minimal amount of psychiatric treatment. There is reason to be concerned that prison facilities are becoming like the asylums of the past.

FAMILY

The majority of people with chronic mental illness live with their families. The family members are key players in providing community mental health services. Family members are elected to assume responsibility for the client with little if any support, few resources, and no appreciation. The behaviors associated with chronic mental illness intrude on the lives of the family members and make extraordinary demands of them. The demands family members experience depend on their physical endurance and emotional health, as well as the nature and intensity of their relative's chronic mental illness.

Understanding & Applying Research

The purpose of this study was to examine the relationships among professional support, the caregiver's personal sense of control, and his or her sense of burden and well-being. A convenience (random) sample of primary caregivers of persons with chronic mental illness who were enrolled in a community-based rehabilitation program was used for this study. Ninety-four subjects were interviewed using a questionnaire that measured caregiver burden, depression, professional support, and the caregiver's personal sense of control.

The results suggest that most caregivers felt burdened by their responsibilities. There is an indication that caregiver burden is associated with depression. These data lend support to the importance of professional assistance and personal control in explaining differences in family members' burden experiences. The importance of practical advice in helping families manage their situations was consistent with other studies. This advice reduces the sense of burden by enhancing the family's sense of control. Nurses should counsel caregivers to include respite periods in their caregiving role and emphasize the need for support for the caregivers in all of their interactions with the family.

Reinhard SC: Living with mental illness: effects of professional support and personal control on caregiver burden, *Res Nurs Health* 17:79, 1994.

It is important to know that the family structure can provide the greatest support for adults with chronic mental illness. It is, however, a position of responsibility for the mentally healthy spouse and other family members. The family providers should be referred to self-help groups or for counseling to maintain their emotional stability. The Client and Family Teaching Guidelines box details information a nurse should provide to the family.

Under any circumstance, it is difficult to live with a family member who has a chronic mental illness, whether he or she is hospitalized, acting out, or in an interval between psychiatric symptoms. Nurses working with persons with chronic mental illness must be aware of the needs and concerns of the family members (Riebschleger, 1991) (see Understanding & Applying Research box).

HEALTH PROMOTION ACTIVITIES

Health promotion activities include many forms of health education programs and are often described in terms of illness prevention and a means of maintaining wellness. Health promotion activities for persons with chronic mental illness are planned to reduce the frequency of exacerbations, increase the individual's ability to live independently, improve medication compliance, improve health care practices, increase recognition of signs and symptoms indicating the need for interventions, and help families to function more effectively. Examples of health promotion activities include:

- Activities of daily living. These activities may be individually designed charts, plans developed with the family and client, or goals established with the individual and caregiver.
- Client and family education about medications, frequency, side effects, and the need for compliance. Individuals need to know about potential side effects and the appropriate action to take when they begin to be troubled by side effects or begin to think about discontinuing their medication.
- Family education, including the nature of chronic mental illness and the changes associated with long-term health problems. These educational programs should include signs and symptoms of exacerbation, as well as strategies about how to respond to positive and negative symptoms. Families should be instructed in developing methods for coping with individuals who may become psychotic and/or violent.
- Sexual education, including appropriate sexual behaviors and personal hygiene, as well as the importance of regular gynecologic examinations and recognition of abnormal signs and symptoms. Sexually active men must be taught about the use of condoms and avoiding unsafe sexual behaviors. Women need to know about the risks involved in pregnancy and how to protect themselves from unwanted pregnancy, sexually transmitted diseases, and the potential for violence.

- Support, encouragement, and assistance in coping with daily life events for families with chronically mentally ill persons. Spouses play a significant role in the quality of life for their partners. Exacerbations place additional strains on what may already be a difficult life situation. Children of chronically mentally ill parents need assurance that they are not responsible for their parents' illness. They may also need assistance in finding healthy adult role models.
- Health promotion programs for the community. These should consider the importance of reintegrating persons with chronic mental illness into the community. School programs could include signs and symptoms of mental illness in children and adolescents. Strategies for dealing with children and adolescents who talk about committing destructive acts against themselves or others should be developed.

Physicians and nurses providing medical care for clients with chronic mental illness should learn about the person's normal response to pain and discomfort. It is important that persons with chronic mental illness receive appropriate care when they become ill.

PUBLIC POLICY ISSUES

Nurses have opportunities to make an impact on public policies at the local, state, and national levels. National policies relating to persons with chronic mental illness must address the need for programs that are more flexible, comprehensive, and easier to access. There is a critical need for coordinated services with consistent financing at the city and state levels. Treatment programs in general, and psychiatric hospitals in particular, must be more creative in their approaches to treating clients with chronic mental illness. Individuals who are clearly unable to care for themselves must not be left to roam the streets without treatment and without access to psychiatric care. Persons who pose a threat to society because of their violent behavior require treatment in appropriate mental health facilities rather than criminal intervention that could worsen their condition.

One of the most acute problems facing persons with chronic mental illness is housing, because they vary in their need for supervised living arrangements. Provisions for housing in a variety of settings could be made available,

including adult foster care and residential treatment programs. Adequate low-income housing could be made available for persons with chronic mental illness who have low-paying jobs or those who subsist on entitlements alone. The lack of adequate housing is as severe a problem as the unavailability of adequate care (Belcher and DiBlasio, 1990; Lamb and Lamb, 1990).

Access to care is an increasingly important concern. The individual's ability to access the mental health system may be limited by his or her ability to seek assistance, as well as lack of knowledge. Nurses can play an important role in advocating for increased resources for mental health care. In addition, nurses can educate self-help groups and other community groups about the nature and impact of chronic mental illness. The quality of the available mental health care is also a concern for nurses. Short-term, episodic care is not sufficient to provide adequate care for persons with chronic mental illness. Walk-in mental health clinics could be made available for these clients and their families. The clinics could monitor medication compliance, as well as provide individual and/or group psychotherapy. Psychopharmacology alone is not sufficient treatment for persons with chronic mental illness. These individuals must also have access to psychotherapy to assist them with the complexity of their lives and their feelings.

Models for providing mental health services to persons with chronic mental illness vary according to regions of the country and resources available. Lehman (1989) has advocated a comprehensive health team approach to address the variety of problems these individuals experience. A treatment team of professionals can provide more and better coordinated services than mental health specialists working independently of one another.

Special programs can be developed for the care and treatment of homeless persons with chronic mental illness. There are strong indications that programs available at locations such as homeless shelters or soup kitchens can be effective means to reach homeless persons with chronic mental illness. Nurse-managed clinics in shelters and soup kitchens allow for easy access to health care professionals (Scholler-Joquish, 1993). These clinics could serve as a site for the distribution of psychotropic medications to help homeless persons with chronic mental illness increase their compliance with treatment and improve their ability to function in the world.

THE NURSING PROCESS

ASSESSMENT

When conducting an initial assessment interview with a person with chronic mental illness, it is important to be sensitive to the client's concerns. The establishment of a therapeutic relationship begins with the development of a sense of trust between the nurse and the client. The nurse should explain the nature and purpose of the interview and tell the client where the interview will take place and approximately how long it will last. The nurse must allow for as much privacy as possible. The nurse will use appropriate precautions when interviewing clients with chronic mental illness who have a history of poor impulse control or violent outbursts (see Nursing Assessment Questions). Effective assessment will provide the nurse with information about the nature of the client's problems. Clients with chronic mental illness often have unidentified medical problems or problems that have been neglected as a result of the individual's disordered lifestyle. Thus it is critical to conduct a thorough assessment of these clients, as each person will present a unique set of nursing problems (Box 32-1).

NURSING DIAGNOSIS

Nursing diagnosis is a process used to interpret the data collected during the assessment phase. Nursing diagnoses are statements that describe an individual's health state or alteration in a person's life processes (see Collaborative Diagnoses box on p. 745).

NURSING DIAGNOSIS FOR PERSONS WITH CHRONIC MENTAL ILLNESS

Safety and/or health risks:

Health maintenance, altered
Injury, risk for

Nutrition, altered: less than body requirements
Self-care deficit: bathing/hygiene
Self-care deficit: dressing/grooming
Self-mutilation, risk for
Violence, risk for: directed at others
Violence, risk for: self-directed

Perceptual/cognitive disturbances:

Anxiety
Fear
Hopelessness
Personal identity disturbance
Powerlessness
Self-esteem, chronic low
Sensory/perceptual alterations (hallucinations)
Thought processes, altered (delusions, impaired problem solving)

Problems in communicating and relating to others:

Communication, impaired verbal
Growth and development, altered
Sexuality patterns, altered
Social interaction, impaired
Social isolation

Disturbances in coping abilities (client and/or family):

Coping, defensive
Coping, ineffective family: compromised
Coping, ineffective family: disabling
Coping, ineffective individual
Denial, ineffective

NURSING ASSESSMENT QUESTIONS

Persons With Chronic Mental Illness

1. When did you first have trouble managing your own life?
   (To determine the duration of chronic mental illness disturbances)
2. What is the place like where you live?
   (To determine the person's current living situation)
3. Are there times when you hear voices talking to you?
   (To determine the presence of auditory hallucinations)
4. What are these voices telling you?
   (To determine if the voices are troubling or threatening)
5. Have there been times when you felt life wasn't worth living?
   (To determine the presence of hopelessness and depression)
6. Have there been times when you were so excited you could hardly contain yourself?
   (To determine the presence of mania)
7. Have there been times when you thought about hurting yourself or someone else?
   (To determine patterns of violence to self or others)

Box 32-1   Assessment of Clients With Chronic Mental Illness

Physiologic Disturbances

Physical integrity

The nurse will examine the client to determine if there is evidence of impaired skin integrity, such as abrasions, bruises, lacerations, scars, and needle puncture sites. Abrasions and bruises may indicate that the client with chronic mental illness was subjected to self-inflicted injury or trauma before admission. It is important to determine if the injuries are recent or nearly healed and the nature and source of the injuries. When examining abrasions and bruises, it is always important to determine if infection or inflammation is present. If there is a history suggestive of trauma or violence, it is important to carefully inspect the client's body surface for additional injuries.

Hormonal/metabolic patterns

Children with chronic mental illness may have inborn errors of metabolism. This information may be obtained through the client's history or from observing the child's physical characteristics. Does the client have a history of diabetes mellitus or kidney disease? Female clients should be assessed for their menstrual patterns. In each of these areas of concern, the nurse will want to know if the client is taking any medications for metabolic or hormonal disturbances.

Circulation

The nurse will assess the client's medical record for indications of neurologic changes and cardiac status.

Nutrition

Assessment of the client's nutritional history and present status is important, since many persons with chronic mental illness live a disorganized and confused lifestyle in which their nutritional intake may be significantly altered.

Physical regulation

Assessment of physical regulation will include the client's temperature and the potential for infection. The medication history for persons with chronic mental illness is important. It is necessary to know the nature and type of medications that the client has been prescribed and his or her compliance in taking the medications. Disturbances of the immune system should also be evaluated at this time.

Oxygenation

Assessment of the client's respiratory system will include evidence of dyspnea, cough, or labored breathing. It must be determined if the client smokes, how long he or she has been smoking, and the number of cigarettes smoked each day.

Elimination

It is essential to know if the client has normal elimination habits. The nurse will want to know if the client has difficulties in handling urine or stool, or ritualistic behaviors associated with elimination. The client's urine can also be screened for nonprescription drugs and psychotropic medications.

Mobility Disturbances

Activity

The nature and extent of the client's activity provide important information for the nurse. The presence of any physical disability such as paralysis or fractures will affect the development of the nursing care plan. The nurse will want to know if there are gait disturbances, tremors, or ritualistic behavior associated with moving from place to place. The client with chronic mental illness may demonstrate lethargic movements or may be hyperactive and move rapidly from place to place. Lethargy may be related to major depression or catatonic features of schizophrenia. Hyperactivity may be related to agitation associated with anxiety, hallucinations, paranoid delusions, or other mental or neurologic disorders.

Rest

The person with chronic mental illness may have developed sleeping patterns that differ from the norm. They may exhibit sleep reversal (sleeping during the daytime and being awake during the night). The nurse should assess the person's ability to fall asleep and remain asleep. Individuals who have difficulty falling asleep may have symptoms of depression or psychomotor agitation.

Recreation

Individuals with chronic mental illness may have a significant deficit in diversional activities. The person is often so preoccupied with symptoms of his or her mental disorder or the effort to get through each day that he or she leads a dull and uninteresting existence.

Environmental maintenance

The nurse's assessment of the client's ability to manage his or her living arrangement will provide important cues about the plan of care during treatment, as well as for discharge planning. If the person lives in a group situation, the nurse will want to know the extent to which he or she participates in maintaining individual and shared living space.

One of the very important components of this section includes assessing the individual's risk factor for injury, violence, and the possession of weapons. Persons with chronic mental illness may be at risk for harming themselves or others. Suicide rates are very high in persons with chronic mental illness, so the nurse will want to assess for suicidal ideations, gestures, or attempts. In assessing suicidal ideations or attempts, the nurse will want to know what method the individual used. It is also important to determine the person's availability of weapons and firearms.

Self-care

The ability of persons with chronic mental illness to perform activities of daily living such as personal hygiene and grooming may be significantly impaired. When these individuals have significant self-care deficits, they may not bathe or clean themselves appropriately.

Box 32-1   Assessment of Clients With Chronic Mental Illness—cont'd

Communication Disturbances

Verbal communication

In times of illness and stress, bilingual individuals often resort to their native language or may speak in a combined dialect that seems disordered and confused. The presence of speech impairments related to physical defects will provide the nurse with important cues. Verbal symptoms of psychiatric disorders include perseveration, circumstantiality, punning, rhyming, echolalia, mutism, word salad, cryptic language, symbolic references, neologisms, poverty of content, confabulation, and logorrhea.

Nonverbal communication

Nonverbal disturbances include posture, manner of dress, and gestures. Persons with chronic mental illness may crouch on the floor, pace back and forth, or retreat from others. Their ability to make and hold eye contact provides the nurse with important cues. Gestures may include ritualistic movements, striking themselves, or striking out at others. Inappropriate sexual behaviors are also important to note.

Cognitive Disturbances

Orientation

Assessment of the individual's orientation to time, place, and person is essential data for the plan of care. The person with chronic mental illness may be oriented to all three parameters or only one; for example, they may know who they are and where they are, but not the month or year. Mental confusion can be related to the individual's psychiatric disorder, side effects of medications, or physical disorders.

Memory

The nurse will assess the individual's memory to determine if he or she has intact recent and remote memory. The individual's ability to demonstrate abstract or concrete thinking affects his or her ability to understand and communicate effectively.

Perception

The person's understanding of the purpose and nature of treatment should also be assessed. Some persons with chronic mental illness may not be clear about why they have been admitted to an inpatient unit.

Thought processes

The person with chronic mental illness may exhibit one or more thinking disturbances. These may include dereistic and autistic thinking, delusions, thought withdrawal and insertion, thought blocking, thought broadcasting, magical thinking, looseness of association, ideas of reference, flight of ideas, ideas of influence, and tangentiality.

Persons with chronic mental illness may have well-defined delusions such as paranoid delusions in which they believe that a force is attempting to control their mind or to cause them harm. Obsessional thought patterns may take the form of ritualistic behaviors or may be manifested by an obsessive desire to control or possess another person.

Perceptual Disturbances

Sensory perception

The senses include vision, hearing, taste, touch, and smell. Any of these senses can be impaired by physical and mental disorders. Persons with chronic mental illness may have hallucinations involving one or more senses. The more common hallucinations involve the client hearing sounds or voices.

Attention

The nurse will assess the client's ability to follow directions, as well as verbal and visual cues. Evidence of psychiatric disturbance may include distractibility, hyperalertness, inattention, or selective inattention. The more manic the individual, the more likely it is that he or she will be easily distractible.

Self-concept

The person with chronic mental illness will, almost by definition, have significant disturbances in self-image, self-esteem, and personal identity. Assessment for these disturbances includes statements of negative self-concept and negative self-worth.

Meaningfulness

Persons with chronic mental illness may have difficulty finding meaning in a life that seems purposeless and hopeless. These individuals may express feelings of hopelessness that their life will ever get better. In addition, they may express powerlessness that they are able to effect any change in their life situation. When a person expresses feelings of hopelessness and meaninglessness, it is important to assess for suicidal ideations.

Relating Disturbances

Role

Each person has certain role expectations congruent with societal norms. The assessment of the person's marital status and relationship with parents, siblings, spouse, children, and others provides significant information about the individual's ability to function in society.

Sexual relationships may be difficult for the individual to maintain. There are wide variations in sexual expression among persons with chronic mental illness. Some may exhibit little interest, whereas others may have difficulty controlling their sexual behavior.

Socialization

Persons with chronic mental illness often have difficulties in maintaining social relationships with others. Their ability to develop a meaningful relationship with people outside their immediate family is often significantly impaired. The age of onset of the mental disorder will affect the individual's ability to socialize with others.

Continued

Box 32-1   Assessment of Clients With Chronic Mental Illness—cont'd

Feeling Disturbances

Comfort

The individual's awareness of pain or discomfort will be affected by his or her physical condition and the presence of any injuries before hospitalization. Some individuals with chronic mental illness may not be able to describe their sense of pain or discomfort and must rely on the nurse or others to be aware of changes that could affect their comfort level.

Emotional states

Persons with chronic mental illness may exhibit signs of mood disturbance such as major depression, anxiety, mania, agitation, and fear. The emotional disturbances will be related to the individual's mental disorder(s). Assessment includes evidence of the way the individual is coping with emotional disturbance. Anger and aggression may be expressed through sarcasm, fault finding, domineering behavior, and the threat or use of violence.

Problem-Solving Disturbances

Coping

The coping mechanisms of persons with chronic mental illness are often inadequate or inappropriate for the situation. Defense mechanisms that may be exhibited include rationalization, conversion, displacement, regression, introjection, projection, denial, disassociation, symbolization, fantasy, or splitting.

Participation

The individual's ability or willingness to participate in treatment is assessed on admission and on an ongoing basis. Persons with a history of noncompliance may exhibit compliance in a controlled environment. The degree of compliance with the therapeutic regimen can be assessed by nursing observations.

Judgment

Disturbances in judgment are common among persons with chronic mental illness. Impaired thought disorders and disorganized living experiences affect the individual's decision-making ability. These individuals may exhibit indecisiveness or may make poor judgments about themselves and others. The severity of the illness will affect the degree of difficulty the person experiences.

Client and family teaching needs:

Knowledge deficit (medication, treatment, symptoms)
Noncompliance (medication, therapy, aftercare)
Role performance, altered

OUTCOME IDENTIFICATION

Outcome criteria for persons with chronic mental illness include short-term and long-term client behaviors and responses to treatment. Outcomes will be stated in clear, measurable, and behavioral terms; can be identified as expected or anticipated; and, whenever possible, will include a time frame in which the client is expected to achieve them. Clients with chronic mental illness vary significantly in the extent and nature of their disorders. The following outcomes are not intended to be all-inclusive for clients with chronic mental illness.

Client will:

1. Verbalize absence of suicidal ideation or plan.
2. Display consistent, optimistic attitude.
3. List several reasons for wanting to live.
4. Demonstrate self-care appropriate for age.
5. Initiate conversation with staff.
6. Demonstrate effective problem-solving skills.
7. Express sense of self-worth.
8. Demonstrate absence of delusions.
9. Engage in positive relationships with significant others or identified support persons.
10. Verbalize feeling in control of self and situations.
11. Make choices regarding management of care.
12. Demonstrate absence of verbal intentions to harm self or others.
13. Demonstrate absence of violent or aggressive behaviors.
14. Communicate with others using appropriate language, tone, and speech pattern.
15. Participate in individual milieu and group activities without disruptions.
16. Demonstrate socially appropriate behavior.
17. Adhere to prescribed facility regimen.
18. Eat adequate amounts of different food groups.
19. Stop talking to self.
20. Seek staff when hallucinations begin.
21. Refrain from harming self or others.
22. Demonstrate reality-based thinking in verbal and nonverbal behavior.
23. Distinguish boundaries between self and others and the environment.
24. Use coping strategies in a functional, adaptive manner.
25. Demonstrate absence of overt confusion.
26. Demonstrate orientation to time, place, and person.
27. Sit through meals or other activities without agitation or restlessness.
28. Display control of angry, impulsive emotions.

COLLABORATIVE DIAGNOSES

DSM-IV Diagnoses*	NANDA Diagnoses†
Mood disorder:	Communication, impaired
Major depression,	verbal
recurrent	Coping, defensive
Bipolar disorder,	Coping, ineffective family:
depressed	disabling
Bipolar disorder, manic	Coping, ineffective individual
Bipolar disorder, mixed	Denial, ineffective
Psychoactive substance	Family processes, altered
abuse disorder	Hopelessness
(all types)	Injury, risk for
Schizophrenia,	Nutrition, altered: less than
catatonic type	body requirements
Schizophrenia,	Powerlessness
chronic,	Self-care deficit, bathing/
undifferentiated type	hygiene
Schizophrenia,	Self-care deficit, dressing/
paranoid type	grooming
Schizophrenia,	Self-esteem, chronic low
residual type	Sensory/perceptual alterations
Substance abuse	Social interaction, impaired
Substance	Social isolation
dependence	Thought processes, altered
	Violence, risk for: directed at
	others
	Violence, risk for: self-directed

*From American Psychiatric Association: *Diagnostic and statistical manual of mental disorders*, ed 4, Washington, DC, 1994, The Association.

†From North American Nursing Diagnosis Association: *NANDA nursing diagnoses: definitions and classifications, 1999-2000*, Philadelphia, 1999, The Association.

PLANNING

The nurse's knowledge and understanding of the complexities of providing care to persons with chronic mental illness are essential in the development of a comprehensive plan of care for the individual client. Each person with chronic mental illness will have his or her own history of mental disorders, previous treatment, coexisting medical illness, and current symptoms. Nursing care will address the acute and long-term needs of the individual and family members when appropriate.

It is important to remember that the individual's altered, disorganized thought process and/or mental deterioration may limit the extent to which he or she participates in the development of a plan of care. Many persons with chronic mental illness have been alienated from their families and live alone or live a homeless existence. For those persons, it may be necessary to include community mental health care providers in the development of the nursing care plan as described in the Nursing Care in the Community box.

IMPLEMENTATION

The plan of care for clients with chronic mental illness will vary depending on the nature of the person's mental disorder, age, and physical health status. Although the individual's mental disorder is long-term, the person with chronic mental illness will be admitted episodically for treatment of the disease process. General hospitals provide short-term care, whereas state psychiatric institutions provide longer-term care. Nursing interventions may be applied in either setting. However, achievement of the goals may take much longer for persons with severe mental illness.

Persons With Chronic Mental Illness

Nursing Care in the Community

The community mental health nurse assisting persons with chronic mental illness offers individualized and family support and monitors medication adherence and responses. Clients whose illnesses are in remission might have relatively smooth periods of functioning during which they need only minimal contact with the nurse. At these times their strengths should be assessed and encouraged. However, this period may be deceptive, not only for the nurse but also for the client. The client may begin to believe that the need for medication has passed and may discontinue prescriptions without consultation. Unfortunately, when medications are stopped, the person's thought processes often become progressively disorganized. Without a reality check from a supportive person, the mentally ill client may regress to the point of needing involuntary treatment. The nurse in the community must effectively monitor clients' behaviors so that, if possible, acute episodes are avoided. The community mental health nurse must to be able to distinguish between chronic low-level functioning and an acute psychotic state. An essential part of the nurse's role involves developing a relaxed and trusting relationship with the client and educating him or her to recognize and report antecedent symptoms of psychosis to facilitate early intervention.

Although it is critical to encourage continuity of the nurse-client relationship and promote attachment, it is equally important to connect the client to the outside world with meaningful employment, volunteer work, and constructive recreation. Many persons with mental illness live lives of fearful isolation and require immense amounts of encouragement to venture out of their restrictive environments. Clients need to have confidence in building a long-term relationship with a counselor or case manager, who can connect them with a group of peers for work, recreation, or education. These peer groups serve multiple functions of social support, corrective feedback, and integration of individuals into the community. The community mental health nurse will continue to monitor each client, as well as support group cohesiveness and community participation.

Persons with chronic mental illness experience impairment in their physical health, mental status, emotional responses, social status, and spiritual nature. The nurse providing care for the person with chronic mental illness will be challenged to prioritize a plan that addresses the client's most important needs. In addition to the manifestations of the disease process, these individuals need assistance with social interactions, self-esteem, knowledge of the disease process, compliance with the treatment regimen, and discharge planning. It is important to consider the individual's priorities when planning care away from the hospital. If the person's concerns are not addressed, it may affect his or her ability or willingness to remain compliant with the plan of care. Family members or community mental health care providers must be involved in the discharge planning process to maintain a functional status over a period of time.

NURSING INTERVENTIONS

1. Assess the risk of danger to self and others *to ensure safety and prevent violence.*
2. Encourage the client to alert the staff when self-destructive thoughts occur *to help manage destructive thoughts before acting on them.*
3. Orient the client to the milieu and modify the environment *to reduce situations that provoke anxiety.*
4. Provide positive feedback when the client demonstrates self-control *to ensure repetition of functional behaviors.*
5. Seclude the client during periods of high risk for harming self and others *to provide a safe environment.*
6. Educate family members about symptoms of non-compliance with psychotropic medications or exacerbation of the mental disorder *to promote knowledge, which may enhance compliance.*
7. Educate the family in self-protective actions in relation to the client *to ensure family safety.*
8. Provide nonthreatening reality orientation *to decrease the risk of upsetting the client and initiating harmful reactions.*
9. Instruct the client in recognizing harmful or inappropriate behaviors *to increase the client's self-awareness.*
10. Assess the client for delusions and hallucinations *to determine the level of psychosis.*
11. Interpret the meaning of the hallucination or delusion for the client *to determine the intent.*
12. Instruct the client to alert the staff when hallucinations begin *so that the staff can intervene and minimize their impact.*
13. Teach techniques to stop or reduce hallucinations, such as whistling, hand clapping, and loudly telling them to stop *to offer the client strategies to manage hallucinations.*
14. Praise efforts at controlling hallucinations *to reinforce the client's functional behavior.*
15. Work with clients to manage hygiene, grooming, and activities of daily living *to increase self-esteem by improving appearance and giving the client the satisfaction of self-help.*
16. Assist in selecting appropriate clothing *to reduce the incidence of ridicule by other clients.*
17. Monitor elimination and bathing patterns and establish a routine *to encourage proper hygiene and prevent injury to the bowel and bladder. Clients with psychosis often have trouble attending to activities of daily living.*
18. Set a regular eating schedule *to remind the client when it is time to eat. Clients with psychosis often forget or refuse to eat and could become physically ill.*
19. Supervise food preparation to ensure safety. *Persons with psychosis may be careless in food preparation.*
20. Assist with regulation of sleep-wake patterns *to promote healthy sleep patterns, because clients with chronic mental illness experience irregular sleep-wake patterns.*
    Provide activities to keep the client awake during the day.
    Encourage dressing before breakfast and staying awake all day.
    Promote relaxation at night.
21. Listen actively to the client's verbal and nonverbal communication *to elicit the client's style of communication and to better understand and anticipate the client's needs.*
22. Encourage the client to engage in conversations with others *to promote socialization and decrease isolation.*
23. Teach clients anxiety-reducing techniques when they are experiencing impaired communication *to reduce anxiety when clients are having difficulty expressing themselves.*

CASE STUDY

Joe was brought to the hospital by a psychiatric nurse who provides consultation to a homeless shelter. The shelter staff asked the nurse to see Joe, who was rocking back and forth on his cot. When the nurse spoke to Joe, he stated his name and date of birth. He said he had been homeless since he was 12 or 13 years of age, adding, "My family thought I was strange, and they sent me away. I found a place to stay in a junkyard. The old man who owned the junkyard let me stay there. He brought me food and let me sleep in a room behind his office. I stayed there until last month, when the old man died. I don't have anywhere to go. I can't stand the noise of the radio. The radio plays in my head all of the time. I just wish it would stop."

Critical Thinking—Diagnosis
1. Identify Joe's most immediate problems.
2. What might the hallucinations be saying to Joe?
3. What nursing diagnoses would be relevant for Joe?
4. What outcome criteria, based on the nursing diagnoses, might be established with Joe?

Bill was brought to the emergency department and admitted to the general hospital for psychiatric care. He had been treated in this hospital in the past and also had been committed to the state psychiatric institution three times in the past 10 years.

Bill was the fourth child and appeared to be normal in every respect until he had an onset of psychosis when he was 16 years old. He had lived at home until he was 28 years old and for the past 5 years had been living periodically in partial care facilities and supervised residential housing.

When Bill ran out of his antipsychotic medication 4 weeks ago, he began to be belligerent and threatened another resident, accusing him of stealing his food. When the resident manager tried to intervene, Bill became upset and ran away. His family was unable to locate him until they were notified that Bill was in the emergency department.

Bill had been living on the street and in missions since he ran away. The police had been called to a soup kitchen because Bill was assaultive, noncooperative, and belligerent to the staff and others. Bill fought with the police until they were able to restrain him and take him to the hospital. He had been without antipsychotic drugs for almost 1 month.

On admission to the unit, Bill was actively hallucinating. His affect was flat, and his movements were slow. When approached by the staff or other clients, Bill ignored them or spoke in a belligerent tone of voice. He has no history of drug or alcohol abuse. He was unkempt, and his clothing was soiled.

DSM-IV Diagnosis

Axis I	Schizophrenia, undifferentiated; chronic with acute exacerbation
Axis II	Deferred
Axis III	Deferred
Axis IV	Severity of psychosocial stressors = 5 Serious chronic illness in self
Axis V	GAF = 30 (current) GAF = 50 (past year)

Nursing Diagnosis: Sensory/perceptual alterations related to change in internal and external stimuli accompanied by impaired ability to respond to stimuli as evidenced by inattention to surroundings, misinterpretation of environment, hallucinations, and difficulty maintaining conversations.

Client Outcomes	Nursing Interventions	Evaluation
• Bill will seek staff when feeling anxious or when hallucinations begin.	• Continuously orient Bill to the nursing unit and to the events and activities that are going on *to present reality.* • Use clear, concrete statements and avoid abstract concepts *to help Bill understand the message.* • Reassure Bill that he is safe and will not be harmed *to help him begin to trust the environment.*	• Bill sought staff when he was feeling anxious and told them how he was feeling.
• Bill will be able to hold conversations without hallucinating.	• Focus on real events or activities *to reinforce reality and divert Bill's attention from his hallucinations.* • Describe Bill's hallucinatory behavior to him *to facilitate disclosure by reflecting on his behavior.* • Determine stressors that may trigger the hallucinations *to assist Bill in beginning to avoid or reduce his hallucinations.*	• Bill held conversations with staff, clients, and family without evidence of hallucinations.
• Bill will refrain from harming himself or others.	• Follow hospital's guidelines for chemical or mechanical restraint or seclusion when Bill is in danger of injuring himself or others *to prevent harm to Bill or others.* • Accept and support Bill's feelings underlying the hallucinations *to convey understanding and reduce anxiety.* • Set limits on Bill's behavior, when necessary, *to keep the environment safe for all clients.* • Encourage Bill to take medications *to control psychotic symptoms.*	• Bill did not harm himself and was not a threat to others.
• Bill will use techniques and activities to manage stress and anxiety.	• Praise Bill's efforts to use techniques to distract from or manage his hallucinations *to promote repetition of positive behavior.* • Provide a consistent, structured milieu *to promote trust, safety, and a sense of well-being.* • Provide group situations in which Bill can learn and practice activities of daily living *to increase feelings of adequacy.*	• Bill demonstrated effective use of techniques to manage his stress and feelings of anxiety before discharge.

Continued

Nursing Diagnosis: Social isolation related to negative experiences of aloneness or sensory/perceptual disturbances, as evidenced by running away from the partial care facility, withdrawal from the environment and others in the environment, noncommunicative manner, flat affect, and minimal or absent eye contact.

Client Outcomes	Nursing Interventions	Evaluation
• Bill will say that he is willing to engage in social interaction with others in the environment.	• Engage Bill in meaningful, nonthreatening individual and group interactions every day *to let him know that participation is expected and that he is a worthwhile member of the community.* • Act as a role model for social behaviors in one-to-one and in groups *to help Bill identify appropriate skills.*	• Bill said he was willing to participate in social interactions on the unit.
• Bill will participate in social activities with family and with others on the unit (e.g., meals, games, and crafts).	• Help Bill seek out other clients who have similar interests *to promote more enjoyable socialization.* • Praise Bill for attempts to seek out others with similar interests *to promote continued positive socialization.* • Encourage Bill's family to call him on the telephone and to visit him on the unit. *A strong family network will increase his social contacts and promote self-esteem.*	• Bill participated in social activities on the unit and had social contact with his family.
• Bill will express pleasure derived from social conversations with other clients, staff, and family.	• Provide Bill with graded activities according to his level of tolerance *to gradually expose him to more complex social interactions.* • Provide opportunities for Bill to go on outings *to encourage a variety of more complex social experiences.* • Encourage Bill to engage in social activities that are within his physical capabilities *to provide him with successful social experiences.*	• Bill expressed pleasure in participating in social activities before discharge.

24. Praise attempts to speak clearly and effectively *to encourage repetition of the client's clear, expressive behaviors.*
25. Enhance social skills, such as proper communication, eating/table manners, and social activities, *to promote the client's acceptability by others and increase self-esteem.*
26. Act as a role model for effective social interaction *to teach the client effective social skills.*
27. Praise successful social interactions or attempts *to reinforce positive social behavior.*
28. Teach the client and family about the disorder and symptom management *to promote knowledge, which may enhance compliance and reduce guilt.*
29. Arrange private meetings so that the family can express special concerns regarding the client *to clarify confusion about the illness and provide opportunities for expression of feelings.*
30. Teach the family to recognize early behavioral signs and symptoms of the client's failure to take medication *to be able to seek early intervention, promote medication compliance, and reduce recidivism.*

ADDITIONAL TREATMENT MODALITIES

Nurses working with persons with chronic mental illness will be involved in collaborative interventions with a variety of mental health specialists and disciplines. Clients with chronic mental illness require an interdisciplinary approach during hospitalization, for discharge planning, and for follow-up care after discharge.

Psychotropic Medications

Psychotropic medications are administered to reduce the client's psychotic behavior and help control anxiety. The most common medications used for clients with chronic mental illness are the antipsychotic drugs.

Medications such as haloperidol (Haldol) and loxapine (Loxitane) can be used for both acute episodes of psychosis and long-term management of the client with chronic mental illness. There is a high rate of extrapyramidal reactions with haloperidol. Nurses should note any evidence of side effects and report them to the practitioner. Antianxiety and antidepressant drugs are also used for clients with chronic mental illness (see Chapter 23 for further information about medications).

▲ NURSING CARE PLAN —cont'd

Nursing Diagnosis: Communication, impaired verbal, related to ineffective use of language in interacting with others, altered thought processes, or sensory/perceptual alterations, as evidenced by speaking minimally or not speaking for long periods.

Client Outcomes	Nursing Interventions	Evaluation
• Bill will communicate his thoughts in a coherent, goal-directed manner.	• Demonstrate a calm, quiet demeanor rather than attempting to force Bill to speak *to demonstrate acceptance of him.* • Actively listen and observe Bill's verbal and nonverbal cues during the communication process *to demonstrate an interest in meeting his needs.* • Anticipate Bill's needs until he is able to communicate effectively *to provide for his safety and comfort.*	• Bill communicated his thoughts and feelings in a goal-directed manner.
• Bill will demonstrate reality-based thought processes in verbal communication.	• Encourage Bill to approach other clients to engage in conversations *to allow him to practice communication skills in a safe setting.* • Help Bill to listen and engage in actual conversations with staff and other clients in individual and group activities *to encourage him to respond to reality rather than his own autistic thoughts.*	• Bill was able to maintain reality-based verbal communication with staff, peers, and family members before discharge.
• Bill will initiate strategies to decrease anxiety and promote meaningful and coherent verbal communication.	• Teach Bill strategies (e.g., deep breathing, replacing irrational or negative thoughts with realistic ones, seeking out a supportive person) to use when he initially experiences impaired verbal communication *to decrease anxiety and to promote more functional speech patterns.* • Praise Bill for his attempts to engage in coherent and meaningful conversations with others *to increase self-esteem and promote functional speech patterns.*	• Bill was able to identify and use effective strategies to control his anxiety and to promote effective verbal communication skills before discharge.

Nursing Diagnosis: Self-care deficit (bathing/hygiene, dressing/grooming) related to sensory/perceptual alterations or altered thought processes, as evidenced by withdrawal from reality and impaired ability to perform hygiene tasks, dress, or groom appropriately.

Client Outcomes	Nursing Interventions	Evaluation
• Bill will consistently perform personal hygiene and groom and dress appropriately.	• Assist Bill with personal hygiene, grooming, dressing, and laundry until he can function independently *to preserve his dignity and self-esteem.* • Establish routines for self-care, adding more complex tasks as Bill's condition improves *to organize his chaotic world and promote success.* • Praise Bill for attempts at self-care and each successfully completed task *to increase feelings of self-worth.*	• Bill performed all self-care activities of hygiene, dressing, and grooming in an appropriate manner before discharge.

Group, Occupational, and Other Therapies

The client with chronic mental illness will benefit from group therapy in which he or she has an opportunity to enhance communication skills. The group provides an opportunity to interact with others in a safe environment. Nurses and other therapists serve as role models for social interactions.

Occupational therapy can help the client with chronic mental illness to coordinate movements and express inner feelings through art forms. The client can also learn new dressing, grooming, and homemaking skills. The occupational therapist is an important adjunct to the psychiatric mental health nurse. Recreational therapy and movement or dance therapy can be an important asset in working with the client with chronic mental illness.

EVALUATION

The nurse is expected to evaluate changes in client behaviors and responses to treatment and interventions. Outcomes should be stated so that there is a specified time in which the desired behavior will be evaluated. At the time of evaluation, it is important to determine if the client has satisfactorily met the desired outcome or made progress toward achieving the outcome. The date that the outcome is achieved (and that outcome identification is no longer active) is noted. During evaluation, it may be decided that the original outcome identification is no longer applicable because of changes in the client's condition.

Summary of Key Concepts

1. Chronic mental illness is manifested by acute exacerbations and remissions.
2. Persons with chronic mental illness may have one or more mental disorders.
3. Chronic mental illness affects every aspect of an individual's life.
4. Persons with chronic mental illness may have difficulties with self-management of their medications.
5. Many chronic mental disorders are first evident during adolescence.
6. Persons with chronic mental illness do not die from their mental disorder and can have the same life span as any other adult.
7. Young adults with chronic mental illness are more likely to live chaotic lifestyles associated with undertreated mental disorders and substance abuse.
8. Persons with chronic mental illness generally live in impoverished conditions.
9. Persons with chronic mental illness have normal sexual drives and interests, although they may act them out in inappropriate ways.
10. There is a high rate of suicide among persons with chronic mental illness.
11. Family members of persons with chronic mental illness experience a significant amount of acute and chronic stress.
12. Persons with chronic mental illness can be helped to control hallucinations and delusions.
13. Family members of persons with chronic mental illness can learn how to prevent violence and intervene in sensory/perceptual disturbances.

REFERENCES

Aiken LH et al: Private foundations in health affairs: a case study of the development of a national initiative for the chronically mentally ill, *Am Psychol* 41(11):1290, 1986.

Akiskal HS, Weller EB: Child psychiatry: special areas of interest—mood disorders and suicide in children and adolescents. In Kaplan HI, Sadock BJ, editors: *Comprehensive textbook of psychiatry*, vol 2, ed 6, Baltimore, 1995, Williams & Wilkins.

American Psychiatric Association: *Diagnostic and statistical manual of mental disorders*, ed 4, Washington, DC, 1994, The Association.

Angold A et al: Perceived burden and service use for child and adolescent psychiatric disorders, *Am J Public Health* 88:75-80, 1998.

Bachrach LL: The chronic patient: patient's quality of life: a continuing concern in the literature, *Psychiatr Serv* 47:1305, 1996.

Bassuck E, Rosenberg L: Psychosocial characteristics of homeless children and children with homes, *Pediatrics* 85(3):257, 1990.

Bassuck E, Rubin L: Homeless children: a neglected population, *Am J Orthopsychiatry* 57(2):279, 1987.

Baxter E, Hopper K: Troubled on the streets: the mentally disabled homeless poor. In Talbott JA, editor: *The chronic mental patient: five years later*, Orlando, Fla., 1984, Grune & Stratton.

Bean GJ et al: Mental health and homelessness: issues and findings, *Soc Work* 32(5):411, 1987.

Belcher JR: Moving into homelessness after psychiatric hospitalization, *J Soc Serv Res* 14(3/4):63, 1991.

Belcher JR, DiBlasio FA: *Helping the homeless: where do we go from here?* Lexington, Mass, 1990, Lexington Books.

Bellack AS, Mueser KT: A comprehensive treatment program for schizophrenia and chronic mental illness, *Community Ment Health J* 22(3):174, 1986.

Benda BB: Crime, drug abuse and mental illness: a comparison of homeless men and women, *J Soc Serv Res* 13(30):39, 1990.

Bernheim KF, Lehman AF: *Working with families of the mentally ill*, New York, 1985, WW Norton.

Bhui K, Puffet A, Strathdee G: Sexual relationship problems amongst patients with severe chronic psychoses, *Soc Psychiatry Psychiatr Epidemiol* 32:459, 1997.

Birren JE et al: *Handbook of mental health and aging*, ed 2, San Diego, 1992, Academic Press.

Bond GR et al: An update on supported employment for people with severe mental illness, *Psychiatr Serv* 48:335, 1997.

Boyd MA, Luetje V: The individual who is severely and persistently mentally ill: directions for research and practice, *Issues Ment Health Nurs* 13:207, 1992.

Breakey WR et al: Health and mental health problems of homeless men and women in Baltimore, *JAMA* 262(1):1352, 1989.

Brooks GW: Vocational rehabilitation. In Talbott JA, editor: *The chronic mentally ill: treatment, programs, systems*, New York, 1981, Human Sciences Press.

Brown C, Hamera E, Long C: The daily activities check list: a functional assessment for consumers with mental illness living in the community, *Occup Ther Health Care* 10(3):33, 1996.

Carey MP et al: Behavioral risk for HIV infection among adults with a severe and persistent mental illness: patterns and psychological antecedents, *Community Ment Health J* 33(2):133, 1997.

Carter JH: Chronic mental illness and homelessness in black populations: prologue and prospects, *J Nat Med Assoc* 83(4):313, 1991.

Castle LN: Beyond medication: what else does the patient with schizophrenia need to reintegrate into the community? *J Psychosoc Nurs Ment Health Serv* 35(9):18, 1997.

Caton CLM et al: Young chronic clients and substance abuse, *Hosp Community Psychiatry* 40(10):1037, 1989.

Cogan MB: *Diagnosis and treatment*, (on-line), 1998.

Cohen CI, Thompson KS: Homeless mentally ill or mentally ill homeless? *Am J Psychiatry* 149(6):816, 1992.

Copel LC: Loneliness: a conceptual model, *Psychosoc Nurs* 26(1):14, 1988.

Dail PW: The psychosocial context of homeless mothers with young children: program and policy implications, *Child Welfare* 49(4):291, 1990.

Dembling B: Datapoints: mental disorders as contributing cause of death in the United States in 1992, *Psychiatr Serv* 48:45, 1997.

Dennis DL et al: A decade of research and services for homeless mentally ill persons: where do we stand? *Am Psychol* 46(11):1129, 1991.

Dickert J: Examination of bias in mental health evaluation of deaf patients, *Soc Work* 33(3):273, 1988.

Doornbas MM: The problems and coping methods of caregivers of young adults with mental illness, *J Psychol Nurs Ment Health Serv* 35(9):41, 1997.

Drake RE, Cotton PG: Depression, hopelessness and suicide in chronic schizophrenia, *Br J Psychiatry* 148:554, 1984.

Drake RE, Wallach MA: Substance abuse among the chronically mentally ill, *Hosp Community Psychiatry* 40(10):1041, 1989.

Drew N: Combating the social isolation of chronic mental illness, *J Psychosoc Nurs* 29(6):14, 1991.

Enzer NB: The real problem: human pain. In Looney JG, editor: *Chronic mental illness in children and adolescents*, Washington, DC, 1988, American Psychiatric Press.

Faedda GL et al: Pediatric-onset bipolar disorder: a neglected clinical and public health problem, *Harvard Rev Psychiatry* 3(4):171, 1995.

Felker B, Yazel JJ, Short D: Mortality and medical comorbidity amongst psychiatric patients: a review, *Psychiatr Serv* 47:1356, 1996.

Fenton WS et al: Randomized trial of general hospital and residential alternative care for patients with severe and persistent mental illness, *Am J Psychiatry* 155:516, 1998.

Ferguson MA: Psychiatric nursing in a shelter for the homeless, *Am J Nurs* 89:1060, 1989.

Fischer PJ, Breakey WR: Homelessness and mental health: an overview, *Int J Ment Health* 14(4):41, 1986.

Fitzgerald RG, Parkes CM: Blindness and loss of other sensory and cognitive functions, *Br MJ* 316(7138):1160, 1998.

Florenzano RU: Chronic mental illness in adolescence: a global overview, *Pediatrician* 18:142, 1991.

Forchuck C: Reconceptualizing the environment of the individual with a chronic mental illness, *Issues Ment Health Nurs* 12:159, 1991.

Forte JA: Operating a member-employing therapeutic business as part of an alternative mental health center, *Health Soc Work* 16(3):213, 1991.

Fortinash KM, Holoday-Worret PA: *Psychiatric nursing care plans*, ed 3, St. Louis, 1999, Mosby.

Foster GW et al: *Child care work with emotionally disturbed children*, Pittsburgh, 1972, University of Pittsburgh Press.

Gater R et al: The care of patients with chronic schizophrenia: a comparison between two services, *Psychol Med* 27:1325, 1997.

Gerhart UC: *Caring for the chronic mentally ill*, Itasca, Ill, 1990, FE Peacock.

Getty C, Perese E, Knab S: Capacity for self-care of persons with mental illnesses living in community residences and the ability of their surrogate families to perform health care functions, *Issues Ment Health Nurs* 19:53, 1998.

Goodman LA: The prevalence of abuse among homeless and housed poor mothers: a comparison study, *Am J Orthopsychiatry* 61(4):489, 1991.

Gold award: comprehensive prenatal and postpartum psychiatric care for women with severe mental illness, *Psychiatr Serv* 47:1108, 1996.

Gold award: linking mentally ill persons with services through crisis intervention, mobile outreach, and community education, *Psychiatr Serv* 48:1450, 1997.

Gorman PA: Sensory dysfunction in dual diagnosis: mental retardation/ mental illness and autism, *Occup Ther Ment Health* 13(1):3, 1997.

Green SA: Silence and violence, *Psychiatr Serv* 48:175, 1997.

Green WH: Child psychiatry: special areas of interest—schizophrenia with childhood onset. In Kaplan HI, Sadock BJ, editors: *Comprehensive textbook of psychiatry*, vol 2, ed 6, Baltimore, 1995a, Williams and Wilkins.

Green WH: Foster care. In Kaplan HI, Sadock BJ, editors: *Comprehensive textbook of psychiatry*, vol 2, ed 6, Baltimore, 1995b, Williams & Wilkins.

Gross RL: Foster care. In Kaplan HI, Sadock BJ, editors: *Comprehensive textbook of psychiatry*, vol 2, ed 6. Baltimore, 1995, Williams & Wilkins.

Harris M, Bachrach LL: Perspectives on homeless mentally ill women, *Hosp Community Psychiatry* 41(23):253, 1990.

Harris MJ, Jeste DP: Schizophrenia and delusional disorders. In Kaplan HI, Sadock BJ, editors: *Comprehensive textbook of psychiatry*, vol 2, ed 6, Baltimore, 1995, Williams & Wilkins.

Harvey PD et al: Cognitive impairment in geriatric chronic schizophrenic patients: a cross-national study in New York and London, *Int Geriatr Psychiatry* 12:1001, 1997.

Hellman RE: Issues in the treatment of lesbian women and gay men with chronic mental illness, *Psychiatr Serv* 47:1093, 1996.

Hier SJ et al: Social adjustment and symptomatology in two types of homeless adolescents: runaways and throwaways, *Adolescence* 25(100):761, 1990.

Hodgman CH: Adolescent psychiatric conditions, *Compr Ther* 22:796, 1996.

Hogstel MO: *Geropsychiatric nursing*, ed 2, St Louis, 1995, Mosby.

Holcomb WR, Ahr PR: Who really treats the severely impaired young adult client? A comparison of treatment settings, *Hosp Community Psychiatry* 38(6):625, 1987.

Hornung WP et al: Psychoeducational training for schizophrenic patients: background, procedure and empirical findings, *Patient Educ Counsel* 29:257, 1996.

Isaac RJ, Armat VC: *Madness in the streets*, New York, 1990, The Free Press.

Jarvik LF, Small GW: Introduction and overview. In Kaplan HI, Sadock BJ, editors: *Comprehensive textbook of psychiatry*, vol 2, ed 6, Baltimore, 1995, Williams & Wilkins.

Jordan BK et al: Prevalence of psychiatric disorders among incarcerated women: convicted felons entering prison, *Arch Gen Psychiatry*, 53:513, 1996.

Kaplan HI, Sadock BJ: *Kaplan and Sadock's synopsis of psychiatry: behavioral sciences/clinical psychiatry*, ed 8, Baltimore, 1998, Williams & Wilkins.

Kauffman JM: *Characteristics of children's behavior disorders*, ed 2, Columbus, Ohio, 1981, Charles E Merrill.

Klinkenberg WD, Calsyn RJ: Predictors of receipt of aftercare and recidivism among persons with chronic mental illness: a review, *Psychiatr Serv* 47:487, 1996.

Koret S: Specialized programs for the chronically mentally ill child. In Talbott JA, editor: *The chronic mentally ill: treatment, programs, systems*, New York, 1981, Human Science Press.

Kouzis AC, Eaton WW: Psychopathology and the development of disability, *Soc Psychiatry Psychiatr Epidemiol* 32:379, 1997.

Krach P, Yang J: Functional status of older persons with chronic mental illness living in a home setting, *Arch Psychiatr Nurs* 6(2):90, 1992.

Krauss JB, Slavinsky AT: *The chronically ill psychiatric patient and the community*, Boston, 1982, Blackwell Scientific Publications.

Lamb HR, Lamb DM: Factors contributing to homelessness among the chronically and severely mentally ill, *Hosp Community Psychiatry* 41(3):301, 1990.

Lamb HR, Weinberger LE: Persons with severe mental illness in jails and prisons: a review, *Psychiatr Serv* 49:483, 1998.

Lefley JP: Behavioral manifestations of mental illness. In Hatfield AB, Lefley HP, editors: *Families of the mentally ill: coping and adaptation*, New York, 1987, Guilford Press.

Lehman AF: Strategies for improving services for the chronic mentally ill, *Hosp Community Psychiatry* 40(9):916, 1989.

Lipton AA, Cancro R: Schizophrenia: clinical features. In Kaplan JI, Sadock BJ, editors: *Comprehensive textbook of psychiatry*, vol 1, ed 6, Baltimore, 1995, Williams & Wilkins.

Lloyd C, Bassett J: Life is for living: a pre-vocational programme for young people with psychosis, *Aust Occup Ther J* 44(2):82, 1997.

Lurigio AJ, Lewis DA: Worlds that fail: a longitudinal study of urban mental patients, *J Soc Issues* 45(3):79, 1989.

Marshall C, Demmler J: Psychosocial rehabilitation as treatment in partial care settings: service delivery for adults with chronic mental illness, *J Rehab* (2):27, 1990.

Martin J: The trauma of homelessness, *Int J Ment Health* 20(2):17, 1991.

McFarland BH et al: Chronic mental illness and the criminal justice system, *Hosp Community Psychiatry* 40(7):718, 1989.

McFarland GK et al: *Nursing diagnoses and process in psychiatric mental health nursing*, ed 2, Philadelphia, 1992, JB Lippincott.

McPherson S: Neurological evaluation. In Kaplan JI, Sadock BJ, editors: *Comprehensive textbook of psychiatry*, vol 2, ed 6, Baltimore, 1995, Williams & Wilkins.

Menninger WW: The chronically mentally ill. In Kaplan HI, Sadock BJ, editors: *Comprehensive textbook of psychiatry*, vol 2, ed 5, Baltimore, 1989, Williams & Wilkins.

Menninger WW: Role of the psychiatric hospital in the treatment of mental illness. In Kaplan JI, Sadock BJ, editors: *Comprehensive textbook of psychiatry*, vol 2, ed 6, Baltimore, 1995, Williams & Wilkins.

Miller LJ, Finnerty M: Sexuality, pregnancy, and childrearing among women with schizophrenia—spectrum disorders, *Psychiatr Serv* 47:502, 1996.

Mintzer, JE et al: The effectiveness of a continuum of care using brief and partial hospitalization for agitated dementia patients, *Psychiatr Serv* 48:1435, 1997.

Morrisey JP, Dennis DL: *NIMH-funded research concerning homeless mentally ill persons: implications for policy and practice*, Albany, 1986, New York State Office of Mental Health.

Mosher-Ashley PM: Attitudes of nursing and rest home administrators toward deinstitutionalized elders with psychiatric disorders, *Community Ment Health J* 27(4):241, 1991.

Mueser KT, Gingerich S: *Coping with schizophrenia: a guide for families*, Oakland, Calif, 1994, New Harbinger.

Mueser KT et al: Family burden of schizophrenia and bipolar disorder: perceptions of relatives and professionals, *Psychiatr Serv* 47:507, 1996.

News in mental health nursing: sex in the state hospital a continuing headache, *J Psychosoc Nurs* 35(6):6, 1997.

North American Nursing Diagnosis Association: *NANDA nursing diagnoses: definitions and classifications, 1999-2000*, Philadelphia, 1999, The Association.

Osher FC, Kofoed LL: Treatment of patients with psychiatric and psychoactive substance abuse disorders, *Hosp Community Psychiatry* 40(10):1025, 1989.

Pepper B: A public policy for the long-term mentally ill: a positive alternative to reinstitutionalization. *Am J Orthopsychiatry* 57(3):452, 1987.

Pepper B, Ryglewicz H: The young chronic patient: a new focus. In Talbott JA, editor: *The chronic mental patient*, 1984, Allyn & Bacon.

Piazza LA et al: Sexual functioning in chronically depressed patients treated with SSRI antidepressants: a pilot study, *Am J Psychiatry* 154:1757, 1997.

Post F: Geriatric psychiatry: schizophrenia and delusional disorders. In Kaplan HI, Sadock BJ, editors: *Comprehensive textbook of psychiatry*, vol 2, ed 6, Baltimore, 1995, Williams & Wilkins.

Powell J: First person account: paranoid schizophrenia—a daughter's story, *Schizophr Bull* 24:175, 1998.

Powers JL et al: Maltreatment among runaway and homeless youth, *Child Abuse Negl* 14(1):87, 1990.

Price V: Runaways and street youth. In Kneerin J, editor: *Homelessness: critical issues for policy and practice*, Boston, 1987, The Boston Foundation.

Pruchno RA, Burant CJ, Peters ND: Understanding the well-being of caregivers, *Gerontologist* 37:102, 1997.

Rawnsley MM: Chronic mental illness: the timeless trajectory, *Sch Inq Nurs Pract* 5(3):205, 1991.

Reinhard SC: Living with mental illness: effects of professional support and personal control on caregiver burden, *Res Nurs Health* 17:79, 1994.

Riebschleger JL: Families of chronically mentally ill people: siblings speak to social workers, *Health Soc Work* 16(2):94, 1991.

Ritsher JEB, Coursey RD, Ferrell EW: A survey on issues in the lives of women with severe mental illness, *Psychiatr Serv* 48:1273, 1997.

Rossi PH, Wright JD: The determinants of homelessness, *Health Affairs*, p 19, Spring 1987.

Rotherman-Borus MJ: Serving runaway and homeless youth, *Fam Community Health* 14(3):23, 1991.

Roy A: Emergency psychiatry. In Kaplan HI, Sadock BJ, editors: *Comprehensive textbook of psychiatry*, vol 2, ed 6, Baltimore, 1995, Williams & Wilkins.

Ruscher SM, de Wit R, Mazmanian D: Psychiatric patients' attitudes about medication and factors affecting noncompliance, *Psychiatr Serv* 48:82, 1997.

Saunders J: Walking a mile in their shoes . . . symbolic interaction for families living with severe mental illness, *J Psychosoc Nurs Ment Health Serv* 35(6):45, 1997.

Scholler-Jaquish A: Health care for the homeless: RN to BSN education, *Nurse Educ* 18(5):33, 1993.

Seltzer MM, Li LW: The transitions of caregiving: subjective and objective definitions, *Gerontologist* 36:614, 1996.

Shaner et al: Monetary reinforcement of abstinence from cocaine among mentally ill patients with cocaine dependence, *Psychiatr Serv* 48:807, 1997.

Sharfstein SS, Webb WL, Stoline AM: *Schizophrenia: questions and answers*, National Institute of Mental Health (on-line), 1995.

Sharfstein SS et al: *Schizophrenia: questions and answers*, National Institute of Mental Health (on-line), 1998.

Silva JA, Leong GB, Weinstock R: Violent behaviors associated with the antichrist delusion, *J Forensic Sci* 42:1058, 1997.

Silver LB: The scope of the problem in children and adolescents. In Looney JG, editor: *Chronic mental illness in children and adolescents*, Washington, DC, 1988, American Psychiatric Press.

Small GW: Alzheimer's disease and other dementing disorders. In Kaplan HI, Sadock BJ, editors: *Comprehensive textbook of psychiatry*, vol 2, ed 6, Baltimore, 1995, Williams & Wilkins.

So YP, Toglia J, Donohue MV: A study of memory functioning in chronic schizophrenic patients, *Occup Ther Ment Health* 13(1):1, 1997.

Steinglass P, Horan ME: Families and chronic medical illness. In Walsh F, Anderson C, editors: *Chronic disorders and the family*, New York, 1988, Haworth Press.

Strasser JA: Urban transient women, *Am J Nurs* 78(12):2076, 1978.

Surber RW et al: Effects of fiscal retrenchment on public mental health services for the chronic mentally ill, *Community Ment Health J* 22(3):215, 1986.

Szatmari P: Schizophrenia with childhood onset. In Kaplan JI, Sadock BS, editors: *Comprehensive textbook of psychiatry*, vol 2, ed 6, Baltimore, 1995, Williams & Wilkins.

Szymanski LS, Crocker AC: Mental retardation. In Kaplan HI, Sadock BJ, editors: *Comprehensive textbook of psychiatry*, vol 2, ed 6, Baltimore, 1995, Williams & Wilkins.

Tardiff K: Research on violence. In Talbott JA, editor: *The chronic mental patient: five years later*, New York, 1984, Grune & Stratton.

Tardiff, K et al: A prospective study of violence by psychiatric patients after hospital discharge, *Psychiatr Serv* 48:678, 1997.

Tempier R: Long-term psychiatric patients' knowledge about their medication, *Psychiatr Serv* 47:1385, 1996.

Teplin LA, Abram KM, McClelland GM: Prevalence of psychiatric disorders among incarcerated women. I. Pretrial jail detainees, *Arch Gen Psychiatry* 53:505, 1996.

Torrey EF: *Nowhere to go: the tragic odyssey of the homeless mentally ill*, New York, 1988, Harper.

Torrey EF: *Surviving schizophrenia*, ed 3, New York, 1995, Harper Perennial.

Torrey EF: *Out of the shadows: confronting America's mental illness*, New York, 1996, John Wiley & Sons.

U.S. Department of Health and Human Services: *National Plan for the Chronically Mentally Ill*, 1981, Washington, DC, The Department.

Wagner J, Menke E: The depression of homeless children: a focus for nursing intervention, *Issues Compr Pediatr Nurs* 14(1):17, 1991.

Wise TN, Mann LS: Utilization of pain medication in hospitalized psychiatric patients, *Gen Hosp Psychiatry* 18:422, 1996.

CHAPTER 33

Community Psychiatric Mental Health Nursing

Terry Patterson

OBJECTIVES

- Define deinstitutionalization.
- Discuss the factors that influenced the deinstitutionalization movement.
- Describe the components of community mental health nursing.
- Compare and contrast the community living arrangements available to psychiatric clients.
- List outpatient treatment options commonly available in community settings.
- Compare and contrast therapy and rehabilitation.
- Discuss the components of case management.
- Discuss the impact of managed care on community psychiatric rehabilitation.

Today, the emphasis in psychiatric treatment is on outpatient or community-based interventions. Community treatment of psychiatric clients occurs on a continuum of care that includes the community hospital, partial hospitalization programs, evaluation and treatment facilities, psychiatric rehabilitation programs, respite care, and a myriad of independent and semi-independent living arrangements. Community psychiatric mental health nursing encompasses a variety of treatment modalities and activity settings that address the treatment needs of psychiatric clients striving to maintain a position within the community.

ROLE OF THE NURSE

The role of the psychiatric nurse specializing in community mental health is to assist the client in maintaining the highest level of functioning and independence possible for that client, within the community. This role requires a sound understanding of human behavior and development, psychiatric disorders, and prevailing treatments. Keen assessment skills and insight based on experience and good judgment are necessary. Skill in group and family process is essential to the successful practice of community psychiatric mental health nursing. In addition, an extensive knowledge of the available community resources, the development and maintenance of community networks, the multidisciplinary treatment team process, and working with clients and families to facilitate community adjustment is required.

HISTORICAL PERSPECTIVE

Before the early 1960s all psychiatric care was administered and received in inpatient settings, primarily state hospitals. State hospitals have been in existence since the late eighteenth century, when the care of the men-

Activities of daily living The set of activities used in routine daily lives, such as personal hygiene, grooming, eating, and recreation.

Adult family home A living arrangement where a family takes in one or two boarders into their home to be a part of the family.

Adult residential rehabilitation program (ARRP) A 24-hour care facility; provides a mental health program and community living placements for persons who require more structure than is provided in group or board-and-care homes.

Capitation A system of reimbursement; a set amount of money is designated for each client regardless of the amount of services provided for the client.

Case management Clinical coordination of inpatient and outpatient treatments designed to support the client's highest level of functioning. Services include crisis intervention, supportive counseling, consultation/collaboration with multidisciplinary treatment providers, medication, and mental status monitoring.

Community mental health center An outpatient clinic that provides a myriad of mental health treatments for people in the community.

Congregate care facility A group home specializing in mental health clients. Group homes have 24-hour staffing and management, but not necessarily nursing staff. Also called board-and-care homes.

Deinstitutionalization Discharge from the psychiatric institution or hospital into the community. Specifically refers to the discharge of chronically mentally ill clients with long-term hospitalizations into less-structured care during the 1960s.

Independent living skills Activities required to maintain independent adult life (e.g., meal preparation, shopping, transportation, paying bills). Independent living skills are closely related to activities of daily living but require a higher level of skill and thinking.

Psychiatric rehabilitation/ skills training program Outpatient program designed to address cognitive, social, and functional deficits caused by mental illnesses.

tally ill was shifted from jails and poorhouses to a more humane setting. In the mid-1800s Dorothea Dix shaped hospital care for mentally ill persons by convincing legislators that caring for the mentally ill was a public responsibility.

In 1955, state hospitals reached a peak hospital census of 559,000 people. In the early 1960s the Joint Commission on Mental Illness and Health reported on the serious overcrowding of state hospitals, the ineffectiveness and debilitating nature of long-term hospitalization, and the high cost of institutional care. The result was the advent of the Mental Retardation Facilities and Community Mental Health Centers Construction Act in 1963 and Medicare and Medicaid programs in 1965. This began the deinstitutionalization movement that followed over the next 30 years.

DEINSTITUTIONALIZATION

During **deinstitutionalization**, federal dollars were distributed to communities to promote outpatient care of mental health needs on a local level. **Community mental health centers** were created to meet the perceived needs of the community with the intention of creating a system of preventive and follow-up care that would decrease the need for psychiatric hospitalization. Care for severely mentally ill persons was shifted from large state hospitals to communities. Between 1963 and 1980 the state hospital population decreased by 75%, from 504,000 to 138,000.

Psychotropic Medications

In addition to increased investments in community care, deinstitutionalization was highly influenced by two other factors. The introduction of phenothiazines and lithium carbonate in the late 1950s for the treatment of mental illnesses made possible the discharge of clients who previously were unremittingly psychotic. Today, further development of antipsychotic medications continues to greatly influence the prognosis of psychiatric treatment, leading to rapid and often premature discharge of clients from hospitals.

Legal Influences

The deinstitutionalization movement was also highly influenced by a civil rights movement that emphasized the rights of persons to self-determination. Legal decisions during this era made it difficult to commit people to mental institutions against their will. Litigation ensued for more treatment and less restrictive alternatives in the care of mentally ill persons. Treatment, rather than custodial care, became the focus of institutional settings. The U.S. Court of Appeals mandated the "least restrictive alternative to hospitalization" as the guide for the placement of clients, thus discouraging unnecessary hospitalization.

Social Acceptance

As with any social change process, the deinstitutionalization movement created a set of previously unseen problems. Often community acceptance lags behind legislative mandate. Communities were ill prepared to deal with chronically mentally ill individuals who had previously been treated in inpatient settings. Care in the community was poorly funded, poorly coordinated, and fragmented. The chronically mentally ill population shifted from the back wards of state hospitals to the back alleys of communities as many of the clients became homeless on discharge. Even with housing, many clients with mental disorders were poor, unemployed, and incapable of meeting basic needs of daily life. Community treatment lacked the continuity necessary for mentally ill persons to maintain function when discharged from the hospital. Many experts attribute the lack of community resources as the beginning of the "revolving door" syndrome for psychiatric clients—from the hospital to the community and back to the hospital.

CURRENT COMMUNITY PSYCHIATRIC TREATMENT SYSTEMS

To provide cogent care to clients and families, community psychiatric mental health nurses need to understand the context, diversity, and parameters of psychiatric treatment systems. Systems of care vary from state to state, county to county, and community to community. Community-based psychiatric treatment is often provided by public/private partnerships using grants and government funds, but it also may be provided by strictly private enterprises or strictly government agencies.

INTEGRATED SYSTEMS OF CARE

Integrated systems of care are designed to provide a full array of services along the continuum of mental health care. The continuum often begins with the state or community hospital, which is the most intensive treatment, and ends with medication management done by local general physicians or nurse practitioners who consult with psychiatrists. The array of services is intentionally and cooperatively designed to meet different levels of treatment intensity that are dictated by the clients' needs in the community.

In some communities, staff members from state and community hospitals, mental health centers, and county mental health facilities collaborate to track mental health needs and utilization. Some integrated systems are organized under an umbrella policy, with one agency assuming responsibility for overseeing mental health care within the designated service area. The umbrella or lead agency is responsible for providing or contracting with other agencies to provide the totality of mental health services within a designated geographic area. This agency is also responsible for providing data to funding sources about the numbers of persons served, as well as the service modalities and intensity of service provided to those numbers.

NONINTEGRATED SYSTEMS OF CARE

Nonintegrated systems of care do not have the overriding structure of integrated systems of care. Agencies within these systems contract directly with the funding source for services provided rather than through a local administrative system overseeing the structure of care. There are fewer formalized interagency agreements, and agencies may not communicate with each other about services that are provided. As a result, there is greater potential for duplication of services in nonintegrated systems. Many agencies within the system may provide the same types of services to the same clientele.

FUNDING

In most states, the state hospital system and the community treatment system are funded separately. In some states, mental health funding is distributed from the state directly to treatment providers. Other states distribute mental health dollars to each county government, which in turn distributes the money to treatment providers. Some states have developed a system of regional support networks (RSNs). A regional support network is an alliance or bonding together of a few counties to share the funding and the burden of mental health care. This approach is particularly advantageous in rural counties, where it is more difficult to secure treatment providers. As a general rule, when more layers of government are involved in the distribution of funding, more money is spent on administrative costs than on the clients. Local government or administrative offices, however, often have a clearer vision of the actual needs of the community being served, therefore avoiding waste on unnecessary programs.

PHILOSOPHY

Two separate philosophies currently dominate the organization of mental health care provider systems. These philosophies are sharply debated in urban areas and regional and state hospital catchment areas that have larger populations of persons with chronic mental illness. The central debate of the two philosophies is the issue of *freedom of choice* versus *continuity of care* for psychiatric clients.

Freedom of Choice

Freedom-of-choice advocates argue that all people, regardless of their disabilities, deserve a vast array of treatments from which to choose. In this mode, clients select from different modalities and treatment providers and may receive care at several different agencies. The client is empowered to design his or her own treatment. In the current trend of managed care, these systems operate on the idea of managed competition. An underlying assumption to this system approach is that agencies will compete to develop services that will best serve persons with mental disorders. In practice, freedom-of-choice systems have experienced some common problems with patient care. Persons with severe and persistent mental illness often have symptoms that affect their behavior, sometimes making them unpleasant or uncooperative and predisposing them to rejection. Many agencies will not choose to develop treatment options for severe mental disorders because of the nature of the work. Consequently, systems may actually have a dearth of services for the people within the system who need the most intervention. In addition, when a client has freedom of choice, so does the provider. Treatment providers in these systems can refuse to treat a person whose symptoms make him or her difficult to encounter, leaving a client who is difficult to treat without services. Combined with these problems is the fact that some severe mental disorders have a primary symptom of withdrawal. Often a client will withdraw from treatment as a result of impaired judgment due to worsening illness when in fact the treatment actually needs to increase. In a system built on a myriad of treatment options without a central contact, a client's withdrawal from treatment is less noticeable because of treatment fragmentation.

Continuity of Care

Continuity-of-care advocates argue that persons with severe and persistent mental illness need to have one stable treatment provider throughout all phases and episodes of their illness. The underlying assumption is that some symptoms of mental illness are the very processes that will disrupt a person's care and that need to be treated. Within these systems a central care provider or case manager is responsible for assessment, the securing of treatment, and referral to appropriate services. The majority of the services may or may not be provided by a central care coordinator, but the coordinator has the primary relationship with the client. A disadvantage of this system is that the client may be limited by the coordinator's view of the client's condition or situation, or of the system. A second disadvantage of this system is that when a case manager leaves, the client has a major disruption in a primary relationship and may feel the loss deeply. The advantages of this type of system are less treatment fragmentation and the fact that the client has someone to contact with whom he or she can interact and who will act on the client's behalf to coordinate care.

Many systems, whether offering freedom of choice or continuity of care, operate on the concept of *episodes of care*, following the medical model. Under this philosophy the client only encounters the system when his or her symptoms require care, much like the care an individual receives at the medical practitioner's office. The advantage of this model lies in its potential to serve increased numbers of clients because not all clients will require services at the same time. The disadvantage of this model is that primary prevention is not used. Often, clients will not encounter a provider until they need acute intervention. Acute and inpatient intervention is more costly, both to the system and to the client. Generally, the more severe the episode of illness, the longer and more difficult the recovery period, resulting in more disruption to the client's life.

MANAGED CARE

Managed care has emerged during this decade in an effort to stem the spiraling costs of health care. Although the economic rationale is clear, the clinical impact has not yet been established. Under managed health care plans, services at community mental health centers have been decreased. Mental health services remain stigmatized in the current health care system, with a disparity between allowable reimbursements for physical and mental illnesses.

Third-party payer systems hire nurses or case managers to review the effectiveness and cost-effectiveness of a client's treatment. This use of utilization review necessitates that nurses clearly articulate the needs and benefits of treatment for their clients. Goal-focused treatment, development of realistic and measurable treatment plans, and organization of care around accepted guidelines and preferred practices are the objectives of client advocacy under managed care (Schreter, 1997).

In some states the government now reimburses in a capitated system instead of the fee-for-service system used in previous years. In a fee-for-service system, treatment providers are reimbursed for each service rendered. In a capitated system **(capitation),** a flat fee is assigned for each client. The service provider is reimbursed the flat fee whether the client uses services minimally or maximally. Treatment providers changing to capitated systems must strategize to find cost-effective interventions to decrease the number of interventions needed or increase the numbers of persons served in order to survive at the same rate of pay. The implications for treatment in community mental health centers are enormous. Some treatment agencies deal with this new payment system by offering more group and less individual therapy. Other treatment agencies use the episodes-of-care model discussed previously.

COMPONENTS OF COMMUNITY PSYCHIATRIC CARE
COMMUNITY PSYCHIATRIC PROGRAMS
Research has clearly demonstrated that the combination of treatment programming and medication therapy is more effective for preventing relapse in psychiatric disorders than the use of medications alone (Janicak et al, 1998). Community psychiatric programs are outpatient programs offered by interdisciplinary teams that generally operate during work week hours. Because they operate during the day, in the past they have been termed day treatment programs. They generally operate in 3- to 6-hour time blocks and contain at least one of the basic treatment components of group therapy, which include psychoeducational classes, skills training, milieu therapy, and activities. Most clients attend voluntarily, although some clients may be mandated to the program as a least

restrictive alternative to inpatient treatment (see Understanding & Applying Research box).

In the field of psychiatric programming, a philosophic distinction is made between therapy and rehabilitation. Both therapy and rehabilitation are vital to the overall treatment of clients who are psychiatrically disturbed. Both have philosophic goals of preventing relapse or further deterioration. The distinction is in the focus of treatment. Therapy focuses on reducing the client's discomfort, liabilities, symptoms, and illness to aid community adjustment. Rehabilitation focuses on developing a person's strengths and assets and improving health by compensation to restore or increase community functioning (Anthony, 1978). There are four main models of community psychiatric programming: *partial hospitalization programs, traditional day treatment, psychiatric rehabilitation/skills training programs,* and *psychosocial clubhouse models.*

Partial Hospitalization Programs
Partial hospitalization programs are the most treatment intensive of the therapeutic models. These programs are one step away from the hospital on the treatment continuum of care and are specifically designed to avert client hospitalization. The program may reside in a hospital setting or at a mental health center. The actual location of the program will affect reimbursement with government and third-party payers. For example, Medicare will reimburse hospital-based partial hospitalization programs at a higher rate than nonhospital-based activities.

Clients enter partial hospitalization either when they are discharged from the hospital and are still in a fragile state or when they have become so symptomatic that they require intensive structure and intervention. This is a short-term intervention, and the average stay is 3 weeks to 3 months. Partial hospitalization programs are generally staffed with psychiatric mental health nurses, a psychiatrist, and bachelor-level psychology or social work staff. The package of treatment includes individual therapy, group therapy, psychoeducation classes, some structured activities, and medication monitoring. The goal of the program is to increase the client's functioning to a level that the client is able to maintain outside of the hospital. The focus is on reduction of symptoms that greatly inhibit or prohibit community living. A nurse working in a partial hospitalization program monitors symptoms and mental status, facilitates groups, teaches psychoeducation classes, plans and implements activities, and works with a psychiatrist in monitoring the effects and side effects of medications.

Traditional Day Treatment
Traditional day treatment is a therapeutic model similar to partial hospitalization. The client's stay is longer in this model, ranging from months to years, and the treatment is less intense. Many day treatment programs now include a component of skills training in addition to psychoeduca-

---

Understanding & Applying Research

Researchers compared the community functioning of 80 outpatients with persistent schizophrenia who had been treated either with psychosocial occupational therapy or with skills training by trained paraprofessionals. The subjects had been randomly assigned to receive occupational therapy or skills training 12 hours a week for 6 months and were then followed in the community for 18 months after the completion of the research treatment. Subjects receiving skills training demonstrated significantly greater independent living skills during the follow-up period. Skills training conducted by paraprofessionals can be effective in increasing a client's independent living skills. Based on this information, nurses can refer clients to other members of the treatment team for skills training, resulting in a cost savings to the client. Skills training is an effective way for the nurse to increase a patient's independent functioning in the community.

Liberman RP et al: Skills training versus psychosocial occupational therapy for persons with persistent schizophrenia, *Am J Psychiatry* 155(8), 1998.

tion classes and activities and list themselves as psychiatric rehabilitation programs. Basic program components may or may not include individual therapy, case management, or medication management but will include group therapy, psychoeducation classes, and activities. The nurse's role in this setting is to work with an interdisciplinary team as a program planner and facilitator to monitor the client's mental status and the effect of medications. A strong grasp of group therapy/process skills is required.

In the last decade, day treatment has been criticized as being nonhelpful to a client's recovery because the treatment encompasses leisure activities. The criticism is that a leisure activity is only something to do, not treatment. "Play" is an important part of the overall experience of all human beings and is often chosen deliberately as a strategy to assist in the rehabilitation of psychiatric clients. Play as a treatment addresses the neurocognitive and interpersonal deficits, such as the social withdrawal and lack of spontaneity experienced in severe mental disorders.

Psychiatric Rehabilitation/Skills Training Programs

Psychiatric rehabilitation/skills training programs distinguish themselves from other treatment programs by emphasizing different goals. The focus of these programs is for the client to acquire skills that will compensate for the neurocognitive and neuropsychiatric deficits caused by mental disorders. Although psychiatric rehabilitation has existed for decades, it is currently a highlighted treatment, with the recent increase in technology that clearly illuminates mental disorders as brain diseases. The primary assumption of the rehabilitation model is that the client has a deficit in a skilled performance or lacks the skills necessary for living, learning, or work (Anthony, 1978). The treatment goal is behavior-specific change, and the client, not the treatment provider, is responsible for implementing the treatment. A nurse working in this environment is responsible for helping the client to identify a specific area of need and then assisting the client in developing a realistic plan of intervention designated to induce behavioral change. The nurse is also responsible for creating and teaching psychoeducation/skill-building classes that address the neurocognitive needs of the clients (see Case Study box).

Psychosocial Clubhouse Models

Psychosocial clubhouse models are internationally prevalent, with 310 clubhouses in 21 countries today. The clubhouse model was begun in 1949 by a group of discharged psychiatric clients who met on the streets of New York City and banded together to start Fountain House. The underlying tenet of this model is that all people need a sense of belonging, a sense of being wanted and accepted, a sense of being needed, and a sense of generativity. The clubhouse provides a place for clients to fill important needs of food, clothing, shelter, social interac-

---

CASE STUDY

Merle is a 43-year-old man with a long history of chronic paranoid schizophrenia. He lives in a government-subsidized apartment and attends the local clubhouse model of treatment 5 days a week. At the clubhouse his primary job is washing dishes and serving food in the cafe. Within the clubhouse setting, Merle is socially appropriate and congenial. He exhibits no positive symptoms of his illness but has residual negative symptoms of blunted affect and compromised hygiene. He had expressed a desire to ride the bus, and the nurse offered to come to his apartment to teach him the bus route from his apartment to the club.

When the nurse arrives at Merle's apartment, she sees that it is a health hazard. Merle's kitchen counters are covered with moldy, dirty dishes adorned with cockroaches. Dirty laundry is piled throughout the house, and there is a strong odor of filth. Merle has hidden salami under the couch because he is afraid that the neighbors will steal it out of his refrigerator. There are cigarette burns on both the couch and the bed. There are no towels in the bathroom, about which Merle is unconcerned because, he says, he does not wash his hands after using the toilet, nor does he bathe.

Critical Thinking Questions

1. What is the nurse's primary concern? How will this affect Merle's treatment plan? Rank the concerns from highest to lowest priority.
2. What resources discussed in this chapter will be useful in Merle's treatment? How will the nurse discuss this with Merle?
3. Knowing the extent of Merle's compromised hygiene, what is the nurse's role in Merle's selection of clubhouse jobs? Does the nurse have an obligation to protect the health of other club members? What are some interventions that the nurse can develop that will help Merle work on this issue without embarrassing him within the club but still protect others?
4. What symptoms of schizophrenia in particular will interfere with Merle's ability to understand the connection between his apartment habits and his work at the clubhouse?

---

tion, and occupation for the members (Mastboom, 1992). Patients, or clubhouse members, come and work in some part of the club to keep the club functional. "In working side by side with [club] members, the staff become aware of the member's vocational and social potential and the . . . member begins to discover personal abilities and talents which can lead to greater social effectiveness and more meaningful work activities" (Fountain House, 1981). Most clubhouses have the following: a cafe where the members work to provide a daily meal and snacks; a maintenance unit where members do the cleaning and building upkeep; and a clerical or membership services unit where members answer phones, produce a daily paper, find locally available housing, and run a thrift shop. Some clubhouses have apartments that are rented to members. Most clubhouses have temporary employment positions that give members an opportunity to work at entry-level jobs in the community. A nurse employed in a clubhouse works alongside the members, facilitating the tasks and the processes of the clubhouse. This may mean helping a client clean the bathrooms or finding a suitable task for someone who is experiencing increased symptoms. It may mean talking to a prospective community employer or assisting members in organizing an annual clubhouse event. Whatever the actual daily task, it always includes the underlying nursing process of continual assessment of the client's mental status and facilitating group and program goals.

CLINICAL ALERT

The nurse must be constantly alert to suicidal ideation and intent. The period of highest risk is often the first month out of the hospital after the client has been discharged. Clients with schizophrenia who hear voices (auditory command hallucinations) instructing them to harm themselves are at equal or greater risk than those with depression. One predictor of suicidal risk is a history of previous attempts and the lethality of those attempts.

CASE MANAGEMENT

Psychiatric mental health nurses have been involved in the coordination of care for clients with mental illnesses for years. Because of the vast needs and the complex problems of persons with chronic mental illness, services are often provided in multiple sites by many different providers. This dramatically increases the potential for care fragmentation. Managing a mental illness requires careful coordination.

Case management is a strategy to coordinate care and reduce fragmentation. Psychiatric case management can be done by one case manager or an interdisciplinary team that incorporates nurses, physicians, and social workers who develop care for a specific patient population. Care coordination is the primary component of all case management models. The focus of case management is to advocate for individuals or families by integrating and coordinating care or multiple services (Bower, 1992). Goals for case management are multidimensional and include:

Enhancing client **activities of daily living**
Promoting appropriate use of resources
Preventing avoidable exacerbation of illness or inappropriate hospitalization
Delaying institutionalization
Improving the client's quality of life

The role of the nurse as case manager is to advocate for the client or the client's family by coordinating or providing services along the continuum of care throughout the entire illness. Effective case management has the potential to minimize health care costs to the client, to families, and to society (Box 33-1). The recommended minimum preparation for a nurse case manager is a baccalaureate degree in nursing with 3 years of appropriate clinical experience (American Nurses Association, 1994). Some case management programs exceed this recommendation, hiring only master's prepared nurses, whereas other case management programs hire bachelor-level psychology and social work majors.

LEVELS OF ASSISTED LIVING

Paramount to the client's adjustment is having a place to live within the community. Maslow's hierarchy of needs identifies food, shelter, and clothing as basic necessities that must be met before a person progresses to higher needs and levels of development (Maslow, 1954). During the era of deinstitutionalization a new class of mentally ill persons emerged—the homeless mentally ill. As people

---

Box 33-1   Why Case Management?

Case management addresses a wide variety of health care issues and needs. As a result, it is often implemented for multiple reasons, including the following:

1. Case management focuses on the full spectrum of needs presented by clients and their families; it is client focused. Client and family satisfaction within case management systems is generally high.
2. A strong component of case management is an outcome orientation to care. The goal is to move the client/family toward optimal care outcomes.
3. Case management facilitates and promotes coordination of client care, minimizing fragmentation.
4. Case management promotes cost-effective care by minimizing fragmentation, maximizing coordination, and facilitating client/family movement through the health care system.
5. Case management maximizes and coordinates the contributions of all disciplines within the health care team.
6. Case management responds to the needs of insurers and other third-party payers, specifically those related to outcome-based, cost-effective care.
7. The needs of clients, providers, and payers all receive attention within a case management system. Case management represents a merger of clinical and financial interests, systems, and outcomes.
8. Case management can be included in the marketing strategies of hospitals and other institutions to target clients/families, insurers, and employers.

Modified from American Nurses Association: *Case management by nurses,* Washington, DC, 1992, The Association.

were discharged from the hospital without follow-up care and with no place to go, they moved to the streets. People with psychiatric disorders are more likely than the average population to live in physically inadequate dwellings, in neighborhoods of high crime, and to pay a higher percentage of their income on housing (Owen et al, 1996). Over the last two decades communities have developed options along the continuum of community living arrangements that better suit the needs of persons with psychiatric disabilities. Persons with severe mental illness who live in an adult home experience lower rehospitalization rates (Rimmerman et al, 1992). Table 33-1 represents living arrangements along a continuum of care.

Adult residential rehabilitation programs (ARRPs), also known as intensive residential treatment facilities (IRTFs) or adult residential and treatment facilities (ARTFs), are designed for persons whose psychiatric disorders are so severe that they require continuous supervision. Until the advent of these programs, some persons with severe and persistent psychiatric disorders remained in the hospital indefinitely. ARRPs have 24-hour nursing staff and a consulting psychiatrist, living skills training, and rehabilitation programming all within the same facility. Residents in these programs often stay for 2 years while they systematically learn basic self-care skills they need to have in order to progress to the next level of community

Table 33-1	**Community Living Arrangements**				
Independent	**Semi-Independent**	**Adult Family Home**	**Structured Living Facilities**		**Intensive Residential Treatment Facility**
			Board-and-Care Homes, Congregate Care Facilities	Skilled Nursing Facilities	
Description of Function					
Lives on own or with others with no need for supervision	Shares responsibilities with two to four others	Family-type living situation	Structured living facility	Structured living facility	Need for highly structured, treatment-oriented residential living facility
Has freedom to do as he or she wishes	Has need for minimal structure and supervision	Does not require as much structure as structured living facilities and intensive residential care	Does not require as much structure as intensive residential care	Highly supervised 24-hour care	24-hour supervision
Exhibits responsible behavior	Works toward independent living, concentrating on needed skills	Requires 24-hour supervision	24-hour care		Different levels of need and care
Handles responsibilities, duties appropriately	Needs to live with others for ongoing support	Has some freedom and independence as appropriate to individual			
Client Criteria					
Stable	Able to demonstrate most skills to live independently satisfactorily	Demonstrates ability to get along with others	Able to cooperate with others	Functioning level warrants needed care	Poor history of compliance with treatment and community living
Able to demonstrate most skills needed to live independently satisfactorily	Able to cooperate with others	Follows house rules and treatment plan (if appropriate)	Follows house rules and structure	Unable to provide for self independently	Need for 24-hour supervision
Has good activities of daily living (ADL)	Has good ADL	Able to structure own time adequately		Follows facility rules and treatment plan	Able to follow rules of facility and treatment plan
Able to take medications on own responsibly	Able to take medications on own responsibly	Has good ADL			
Structures own time adequately	Structures own time adequately	Able to take own medications appropriately			

living. These skills include how to take medication as prescribed, how to describe medication side effects to their doctor, basic grooming and hygiene, and appropriate interpersonal behavior. Rehabilitation programming in these facilities follows the models of community psychiatric treatment programs described earlier in the chapter.

Congregate care facilities, or board-and-care homes, are group homes for persons with psychiatric illnesses that usually house 6 to 15 residents. Congregate care facilities provide food, housing, and supervision of medication regimens and daily living skills. Residents of these facilities often receive outpatient care at the local community mental health center. In some communities the community mental health centers provide free consultation to the congregate care facility. Most congregate care facilities require the resident to be involved in some kind of adjunct treatment.

Adult family homes provide a quieter, more personal living arrangement for clients needing supervision. Also called adult foster homes, these residential facilities are provided by families who agree to "adopt" one or two persons into their home. The client becomes a part of that family structure and is expected to fit into the normal routines of the household. The adult family home provider supervises medication regimens if necessary, expects the client to perform routine tasks of daily living, and assists the client in acquiring services and skills needed to live independently in the community. An adult family home is beneficial to the client who cannot tolerate the larger numbers of persons in congregate care facilities but is more difficult for clients who cannot tolerate the increased intimacy involved in being part of a family.

Semi-independent living is the designation for persons living with two to four other persons in the community with minimal supervision. Clients in these situations generally are assisted by **independent living skills** staff who systematically teach the residents the skills needed for adult independent life, such as cooking and budgeting.

HOME VISITS

Nurses in community psychiatric mental health nursing will see clients in a variety of living environments. As demonstrated by the previous section, there are many different living arrangements that people with psychiatric disorders may call home. "Home" may include a myriad of homeless shelters or the local park or nearest bridge.

Many home health agencies now have a subspecialty to provide psychiatric home health care, and case managers in community psychiatric care make home visits in certain circumstances. A broad range of psychiatric home visits are reimbursed by third-party payers, with each payer having specific criteria for reimbursement. For example, the requirement for reimbursement by Medicare is that the primary treating staff in the client's overall care is a psychiatrist.

SAFETY

Psychiatric home visits vary in focus, time spent, intensity, and outcome. It is crucial that the nurse planning a home visit evaluate the potential risks of that visit before the actual intervention. Risk evaluation always includes the cli-

---

CASE STUDY

Tom is a 20-year-old college student who was discharged from inpatient psychiatric services to independent living 2 weeks ago. He was originally brought to the hospital by four of his friends when he became drunk, belligerent, and threatening at a party. His friends reported that Tom's behavior had changed the previous month. Before he was hospitalized, Tom began staying up all night, consuming large quantities of alcohol, and fighting with other dorm residents, and he had gotten two speeding tickets in the previous week. In the hospital he was diagnosed with bipolar I disorder, single manic episode. He was treated with lithium carbonate 300 mg tid and clonazepam (Klonopin) 2 mg hs and discharged with a week's supply of medication. Today the nurse case manager received a call from Tom's apartment manager, who was concerned because Tom had sarcastically said he would just go kill himself when he was asked to turn his music down. The manager reports that other tenants are complaining that Tom makes noise at all hours of the night. The nurse has not seen Tom since his discharge 2 weeks ago and is unable to reach him by telephone.

Nursing Diagnoses
1. Injury, risk for, related to destructive behaviors and hyperactivity as evidenced by increased agitation and potentially injurious behavior (drinking alcohol, speeding, fighting)
2. Violence, risk for, self-directed, related to manic excitement as evidenced by increased motor activity and provocative behavior
3. Sleep pattern disturbance related to excessive hyperactivity
4. Social interaction, impaired, as evidenced by dysfunctional interaction with peers and others

Critical Thinking Questions
1. Should the nurse make a home visit? What factors will the nurse consider when making a decision about a home visit?
2. What assessments need to be done when Tom is seen? What other DSM-IV diagnoses need to be explored at this point? How will the nurse assess Tom's personal safety?
3. If Tom refuses to be seen or responds defensively or with denial, how will the nurse respond? How should the nurse proceed?
4. What other information is needed to complete the nursing assessment?

ent's history, the client's usual relationship with the nurse, the client's current or recent mental status, and the client's living situation. The nurse may decide to go alone or with another treatment provider or mental health professional.

CATEGORIES

The goals of community psychiatric mental health nursing home visits fall into three basic categories: client engagement, client assessment, and client teaching. Because many mental disorders exhibit primary symptoms of withdrawal or social isolation, it is sometimes necessary to first locate the person out in the community. Often the client is at home, having not been out of the house recently. These home visits are frequently not prearranged with the client because anticipation of a visit may increase the client's anxiety and lead to further exacerbation of symptoms. Also, some clients may avoid a visit, fearing that they might be involuntarily hospitalized. The goal of the visit is to reengage the client with the system of care by engaging the client with the primary case manager or nurse. Some clients are seen in their home for several months before they agree to engage in treatment at the local mental health center. Assertive outreach as a component of community psychiatric mental health care engages clients who generally resist traditional, office-based treatment (Herinckx et al, 1997).

A home visit is an illuminating part of treatment. Seeing the client within the context of his or her living situation expands the nurse's understanding of the client's overall functioning level. An outpatient clinic provides the location to assess how the client functions in a semipublic environment for a short period of time. A person's home gives the nurse a deeper sense of how he or she functions on more fundamental and enduring levels (e.g., with activities of daily living and independent living skills (see Client & Family Teaching Guidelines).

Neurocognitive deficits caused by mental illnesses frequently interfere with client learning and, more important, with the process of learning. Some clients are unable to perform a learned skill when the skill setting changes. A home visit is an effective approach for teaching basic independent living skills to clients who experience transfer-of-learning deficits. During home learning, clients have the opportunity to use their own equipment in their own setting, which increases the potential for task retention. The teaching process may need to be repeated if the client changes residences.

INCARCERATION

The incarceration of mentally ill persons is an urgent national problem. Estimates of the percent of the prison population with a diagnosable mental disorder range from 6% to 25%. Factors involved in the incarceration of mentally ill persons include homelessness, attitudes of com-

---

Client & Family TEACHING GUIDELINES

Schizophrenia

Teach the client:
1. Schizophrenia is a brain disorder that will require both chemotherapy and psychosocial therapy.
2. Withdrawal is a common symptom, and it is important to communicate with health care providers when beginning to feel more reluctant or afraid to interact with people.
3. It may take months for symptoms to get under control.
4. Increased involvement in therapy leads to a better outcome.

Teach the family:
1. Schizophrenia is a brain disease that affects 1% of the world's population. The brain disease has nothing to do with how the client was parented.
2. Chronic brain diseases put special stresses on the family. There are national organizations for education and support of family members, such as The National Alliance for the Mentally Ill (NAMI), that assist families with the emotional burden, decrease the isolation, and provide resource information on a local and national level.
3. High levels of expressed negative emotion within the family system may exacerbate symptoms of schizophrenia. It is important for all family members to find appropriate ways to express their grief and deal with conflict.
4. Prescribed medications for the client are important and may require supervision and monitoring by the family to ensure effectiveness and assess symptoms.
5. Local mental health centers and some school districts sometimes provide support groups to parents and to siblings of people with mental disorders.

---

munity and police force members, more rigid commitment criteria, and lack of adequate community supports. Nursing responsibilities in correctional institutions vary and may include the following:

Assessment of suicidality
Evaluation of mental status
Monitoring of effectiveness of medications
Liaison between the inmates and the community treatment providers
Provision of care when warranted

Providing general mental health treatment previously discussed in this chapter is necessary. Nurses working in this field may encounter a twofold stigma when working with the mentally ill and the incarcerated.

OTHER COMPONENTS OF COMMUNITY PSYCHIATRIC MENTAL HEALTH NURSING

Community psychiatric mental health nursing frequently involves crisis intervention both with individuals and with groups of people. Many communities have special multidisciplinary teams of mental health practitioners who provide mental health care as a component of disaster relief. Crisis intervention with groups and individuals is covered in Chapter 25.

Clients undergoing a severe exacerbation of psychiatric symptoms may need to be detained in a psychiatric hospital against their will for their own safety or for the safety of the community. Community psychiatric mental health nurses need a thorough understanding of the Involuntary Treatment Act covered in Chapter 5. Also, thorough knowledge of appropriate nursing interventions and other treatment modalities is essential.

Medication management is a fundamental role of the community psychiatric mental health nurse. Nurses may work in medication clinics or follow-up clinics where the primary identified role is to monitor the effects and side effects of the client's prescribed medication, or they may work in psychiatric rehabilitation programs where medication monitoring is one of many functions. Regardless of the nurse's vocational setting, a strong knowledge of psychopharmacology is required (see Chapter 23).

Summary of Key Concepts

1. Community psychiatric mental health services have greatly increased since the 1960s.
2. Community psychiatric mental health programming is an essential element in the treatment of persons with persistent mental illness.
3. Case management is a pivotal role for the community psychiatric mental health nurse.
4. Community psychiatric mental health nurses frequently collaborate with or participate in multidisciplinary teams.
5. A purpose of a psychiatric home visit is to engage the client in treatment, to assess the client, and/or to teach the client a community-based skill.
6. Managed care has a strong influence on the delivery of community psychiatric mental health care.

REFERENCES

American Nurses Association: *Statement on psychiatric mental health clinical nursing practice and standards of psychiatric mental health clinical nursing practice*, Washington, DC, 1994, The Association.

Anthony WA: *The principles of psychiatric rehabilitation*, Baltimore, 1978, University Park Press.

Bower KA: *Case management by nurses*, Washington, DC, 1992, American Nurses Association.

The Fountain House concept paper, New York, 1981, Fountain House.

Herinckx HA et al: Assertive community treatment versus usual care in engaging and retaining clients with severe mental illness, *Psychiatr Serv* 48(10):1297, 1997.

Janicak et al: *Treatment with antipsychotics: principles and practice of psychopharmacotherapy*, ed 2, Baltimore, 1998, Williams & Wilkens.

Liberman RP et al: Skills training versus psychosocial occupational therapy for persons with persistent schizophrenia, *Am J Psychiatry* 155(8), 1998.

Maslow AH: *Motivation and personality*, New York, 1954, Harper & Row.

Mastboom J: Forty clubhouses: models and practices, *Psychosoc Rehabil J*, 16(2), 1992.

Owen C et al: Housing accommodation preferences of people with psychiatric disabilities, *Psychiatr Serv* 47(6):628, 1996.

Rimmerman A et al: The rehabilitation of persons with severe mental illness in adult homes: the NYPCC study, *Psychosoc Rehabil J* 15(3):55, 1992.

Schreter RK: Essential skills for managed behavioral health care, *Psychiatr Serv* 48(5):653, 1997.

Notes

CHAPTER 34

Spirituality

Phillip R. Deming

OBJECTIVES

- Compare and contrast the meanings of spirituality, religion, and faith.

- Describe three reasons why a spiritual assessment is important and useful for clients experiencing mental or emotional illness.

- Explain the role of a chaplain or pastor as part of the interdisciplinary mental health care team.

- Develop a spiritual assessment that can be conducted by nurses when pastoral care is not available.

- Construct a nurse/client scenario, applying spiritual assessment and intervention strategies that are useful to the client's mental and emotional health.

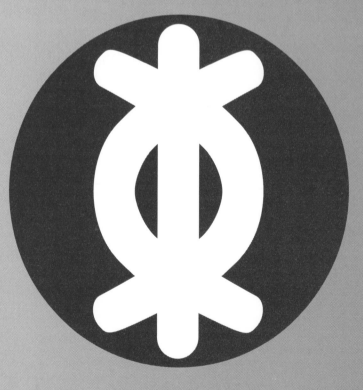

INTERRELATIONSHIP BETWEEN SPIRITUAL TRENDS AND MENTAL HEALTH ISSUES

The World Health Organization (1946) defined health as a state of complete physical, mental, and social well-being and not merely the absence of disease or infirmity. However, more recent definitions of health have included emotional and spiritual dimensions. In addition, health is no longer viewed as a passive state of being, but as a dynamic process of achieving higher levels of wellness within each dimension. According to Russell's model of well-being, spiritual health forms the overall umbrella under which all other dimensions are united. In this model, spirituality is not necessarily religious dogma, but rather, an individual's philosophy, value, and meaning of life. (Perrin and McDermott, 1997)

There is a growing belief that serious or chronic mental illness can be associated with increased feelings of loss and powerlessness. Mental illness, especially chronic mental illness, can lead to a cycle of loss: feelings of powerlessness, leading to hopelessness, leading to a sense of despair, which in turn feeds back into a deeper sense of loss. When quality spiritual care is provided in a consistent and effective manner as a key part of a multidisciplinary approach to treatment, both research (Perrin and McDermott, 1997) and anecdotal evidence indicate that there are significant benefits. These benefits can have both an impact on the client and an impact on other members of the health care team. One benefit is in the reduced length of inpatient stay for those clients who have had their spiritual concerns and questions addressed in an effective and helpful manner. Addressing client spiritual issues may also contribute to a decreased use of total system resources, in that client anxiety may be lessened, symptom control may be more effective, and there may be a reduced number of client complaints, all of which result in an increased level of client satisfaction (Perrin and McDermott, 1997).

The Joint Commission on Accreditation for Healthcare Organizations (JCAHO) the accrediting body for hospitals, provides the accreditation that is essential in order for a health care system to be eligible for Medicare, Medicaid, Social Security payments, and reimbursement from many third-party payers. Included in the JCAHO standards are requirements that a health care agency provide adequate spiritual care. The JCAHO provisions state that an organization must be able to provide for the spiritual care of patients, family, and staff, and that appropriate documentation should be available. So, in addition to treating the whole person, when one addresses the spirituality of a patient, one is also ensuring that the minimum standards of care are being met.

SPIRITUALITY AS A DIMENSION OF THE PERSON

As people, we have many facets. We are physical, cognitive, affective, relational, and spiritual. To ignore any of these components would omit a significant part of who we are, with equally significant consequences. Although everyone has a spiritual dimension, it may be expressed in many ways, both formal and informal. A person's spirituality addresses the core images regarding humanity, the divine, and the relationship between humanity and the divine. These images can be healing and sustaining, or they may be punitive and crippling. In the treatment of illness it is important to attend to the spiritual dimensions of a person.

SPIRITUALITY IN MENTAL HEALTH

Spirituality is an essential and integral part of who we are as individuals. Our spirituality is the thread that connects us with other people, with the world in which we live, and with the divine nature as we experience it. Through our spirituality we can make sense of powerful life experiences that would otherwise be confusing or devastating, and use them in ways that become life sustaining. Our spirituality allows us to make sense of the cycle of life and death. Spirituality gives us the hope and the strength to laugh and celebrate life while consciously acknowledging the reality of illness and tragedy.

Spirituality in mental health plays an important role. For many afflicted individuals, their spirituality gives them a powerful sense of hope in the face of an often devastating and chronic illness. For those who experience rejection by family and friends because of the illness's impact on their relationships, spirituality can help maintain a sense of connection and belonging. For those who may feel abandoned, a healthy spirituality can provide a sense of being loved and accepted for who they are as unique individuals, in spite of having a mental illness. Spirituality can also be a solid anchor for those individuals whose illnesses may create feelings of internal chaos. Left unattended, the same spirituality that helps an individual feel accepted and that provides hope can also become punitive or crippling in nature, rather than be a source of healing.

DEFINING THE TERMS

Spirituality is a search for the sacred, a need to have a conscious experience of the divine, however one conceives of it. Spirituality is that part of the person that deals with the transcendent and the universal. Spirituality recognizes one's relationship to the divine and sees how that relationship affects one's experience with people and all of creation. One's spirituality encompasses an understanding of the sacred, of the holy, of faith, and of all those things that are not physical. Spirituality may take expression in religion and ritual, but it is not limited to those things. Music, art, poetry, dance, and stories can all be spiritual expressions. Spirituality is the recognition that some connecting thread weaves through all creation; it is the search to more fully experience that connecting thread. The goals of spirituality are listed in Box 34-1.

Religion is a manner of expressing one's spirituality. It may be experienced through membership in a particular community that accepts a formal and organized system of beliefs, or it may be a less formal and more individual set of beliefs and practices. Religious expression may include ritual, ceremonies, music, art, and one's intentional participation in a community that has a specific understanding of history and the future. Christianity, Judaism, Buddhism, Hinduism, Taoism, and Islam are all formal systems of religious beliefs through which individual members are able to experience their spirituality. New Age spirituality is a collection of individual practices that are largely unconnected to formal communities.

Faith is the ability to draw on spiritual resources without having physical and empiric proof. It is an internal certainty that comes from one's own experience with the divine. Faith, although only a part of spirituality, is an essential component. It is through one's experience of faith that a deep individual spirituality can be mobilized to assist one in the challenges and celebrations of life.

STAGES OF FAITH IN SPIRITUAL PRACTICE AND INTERVENTIONS
STAGE I: IMPARTIAL INDIVIDUALS

Impartial individuals tend to do things in their own interest, are generally nominally or not involved in faith communities, and only have a casual acquaintance with faith community practices. They make up about 30% of the population.

Interventions for individuals in this stage usually include those things that are very well known in the general culture and may include formal readings such as the Twenty-Third Psalm, the poem "Footprints," the Serenity Prayer, the Lord's Prayer, or traditional hymns such as "Beautiful Savior" and "Amazing Grace." Alcoholics Anonymous (AA) and Narcotics Anonymous (NA) materials may be helpful as well.

STAGE II: INSTITUTIONAL INDIVIDUALS

Institutional individuals are regular church attendees who adhere to institutional rules and who largely adopt a "good person/bad person" concept; they make up about 40% of the population.

Interventions for individuals in this stage may include those in stage I, as well as visits from the minister and members of their local spiritual community; formal use of prayer, anointing, and laying on of hands; and use of prayer books and music that is specific to the denomination, congregation, or faith expression.

STAGE III: INDIVIDUAL SEEKERS

Individual seekers have left a formal religious community and often challenge many of their beliefs and tenants; they seek new answers or personal answers to questions, problems, or crises. On the surface they may appear to be in stage I, and they make up about 20% of the population.

Interventions for people in this stage are more individual, creative, and varied. They may encompass historic elements from various Eastern and Western spiritual traditions, including meditation, healing touch, devotional reading, communal prayer, and a variety of music. The individual is the best guide in selecting the spiritual re-

---

Box 34-1   **Goals of Spirituality**

Providing an image of the divine
Providing an image of humanity
Providing an understanding of the relationship between the divine and humanity
Helping to examine thoughts of divine punishment, reward, or neutrality
Helping to give belief and meaning to life
Helping to find a sense of duty, vocation, calling, or moral obligation
Helping to examine one's experience of the divine and sacred
Helping to cope with situations that conflict with spiritual understanding
Providing a format for spiritual rituals and practices
Providing a faith community
Providing authority and guidance for one's system of belief, meaning, and ritual

sources for this stage, and discussion and questions are equally important.

STAGE IV: INTEGRATED INDIVIDUALS

Integrated individuals have internalized their faith; they fully accept the rules they obey and believe that they are just and right. They may or may not belong to formal faith communities and are often seen as teachers or mystics. They make up about 10% of the population.

Interventions for individuals in this stage include many of the traditional rituals, rites, and expressions of formal spirituality that are found in stage II, but with an increased internal meaning. Individuals in this stage may have the need to leave a spiritual legacy.

MAJOR SPIRITUAL ISSUES

Some major spiritual issues include the fear of death and loss, both of self and others. Spirituality allows one to cope with these feelings by providing a sense of hope and meaning to experiences that would otherwise be crippling. Having a spiritual understanding that one's connection with creation is more than merely physical helps to ease the fear and pain of loss. Feeling connected to the divine eases feelings of abandonment, grief, and alienation, as well as promoting a sense of self-acceptance. Spirituality is thought to be a key component in the healing process and an integral part of the client's treatment plan.

The significant spiritual questions tend to remain constant, regardless of the health care need. Such issues as loss, fear, death, abandonment, and feelings of alienation may be present in clients with both physical and psychiatric illnesses. Responses to these feelings can range from finding new meanings and strength, to acceptance, to grief, to a sense of hopelessness. It is often a spiritual intervention to first acknowledge and validate these feelings, and then help the client to look at ways to rewrite their life story in such a manner as to encompass these experiences. One's spirituality can be a significant help during these times.

Before one can provide effective spiritual interventions, it is critical to identify those persons who are at significant spiritual risk. Individuals at spiritual risk are defined by Fitchett (1997) as those who have a high spiritual need, coupled with low spiritual resources to meet that need. These individuals have more risk for poor outcomes and should be the primary focus for outcome-based spiritual care.

INTERVENTION TOOLS

There are a variety of spiritual interventions that are possible. These interventions range from formal rituals and practices to informal types. Formal Christian rituals include sacraments, such as baptism, communion, and anointing. Additional formal practices include worship or memorial services, as well as formal confession and abso-

lution. On many of these occasions a chaplain will involve members of a local faith community, either in a leadership or a support role. Often a chaplain will be in contact with local worship communities to provide appropriate information for formal prayer services at a local church when requested by a client.

Informal rituals and practices include pastoral counseling, use of individual or group prayer at the hospital, reading of scripture, and the distribution of devotional books, cards, and other related materials. The use of rosaries or prayer beads, the playing of music, and the use of icons or pictures often allows the more experiential, noncognitive side of a patient's spirituality to be expressed. Verbal imagery is present in the telling of sacred stories from various traditions. Other forms of visual imagery are also used. Audiotapes and videotapes may be especially helpful. If the client has access to tapes of his or her own community worshipping, that can augment any mass media material that is available.

SPIRITUAL ASSESSMENT

Assessing an individual's spiritual need and what interventions are most helpful and appropriate in addressing that need is an essential component of a chaplain's role in a health care system. Approaching the client where he or she "is" in terms of spirituality requires the ability to acknowledge one's own biases and a willingness to put them aside during the interaction. To conduct the assessment in a systematic manner, Fitchett's 7 × 7 model of spiritual assessment (1993) is extremely helpful in that it views the client in a holistic manner, similar to a multidisciplinary approach. The first 7 in this multiaxis system describes seven identified key dimensions of an individual (Box 34-2).

Although all members of an interdisciplinary team may have some impact on and insight into each of these seven dimensions, there is usually a particular area of specialty that deals in more depth with each axis. Although the seventh dimension (spirituality) may be most commonly addressed by a pastor or chaplain, if there is no pastoral care department in the facility, and if the client has no specific faith community, these spiritual issues may

---

Box 34-2	**Seven Key Dimensions: Fitchett's Model of Spiritual Assessment**

1. Medical
2. Psychologic
3. Psychosocial
4. Family systems
5. Ethnic and cultural
6. Societal
7. Spiritual

Box 34-3   Spiritual Assessment Tool

The following reflective questions may assist you in assessing, evaluating, and increasing awareness of spirituality in yourself and others.

Meaning and Purpose

These questions assess a person's ability to seek meaning and fulfillment in life, manifest hope, and accept ambiguity and uncertainty:

What gives your life meaning?

Do you have a sense of purpose in life?

Does your illness interfere with your life goals?

Why do you want to get well?

How hopeful are you about obtaining a better degree of health?

Do you feel that you have a responsibility in maintaining your health?

Will you be able to make changes in your life to maintain your health?

Are you motivated to get well?

What is the most important or powerful thing in your life?

Inner Strengths

These questions assess a person's ability to manifest joy and recognize strengths, choices, goals, and faith:

What brings you joy and peace in your life?

What can you do to feel alive and full of spirit?

What traits do you like about yourself?

What are your personal strengths?

What choices are available to you to enhance your healing?

What life goals have you set for yourself?

Do you think that stress in any way caused your illness?

How aware were you of your body before you became sick?

What do you believe in?

Is faith important in your life?

How has your illness influenced your faith?

Does faith play a role in recognizing your health?

Interconnections

These questions assess a person's positive self-concept, self-esteem, and sense of self; sense of belonging in the world with others; capacity to pursue personal interests; and ability to demonstrate love of self and self-forgiveness:

How do you feel about yourself right now?

How do you feel when you have a true sense of yourself?

Do you pursue things of personal interest?

What do you do to show love for yourself?

Can you forgive yourself?

What do you do to heal your spirit?

These questions assess a person's ability to connect in life-giving ways with family, friends, and social groups and to engage in the forgiveness of others:

Who are the significant people in your life?

Do you have friends or family in town who are available to help you?

Who are the people to whom you are closest?

Do you belong to any groups?

Can you ask people for help when you need it?

Can you share your feelings with others?

What are some of the most loving things that others have done for you?

What are the loving things that you do for other people?

Are you able to forgive others?

These questions assess a person's capacity for finding meaning in worship or religious activities, and a connectedness with a divinity:

Is worship important to you?

What do you consider the most significant act of worship in your life?

Do you participate in any religious activities?

Do you believe in God or a higher power?

Do you think that prayer is powerful?

Have you ever tried to empty your mind of all thoughts to see what the experience might be?

Do you use relaxation or imagery skills?

Do you meditate?

Do you pray?

What is your prayer?

How are your prayers answered?

Do you have a sense of belonging in this world?

These questions assess a person's ability to experience a sense of connection with life and nature, an awareness of the effects of the environment on life and well-being, and a capacity for concern for the health of the environment:

Do you ever feel a connection with the world or universe?

How does your environment have an impact on your state of well-being?

What are your environmental stressors at work and at home?

What strategies reduce your environmental stressors?

Do you have any concerns for the state of your immediate environment?

Are you involved with environmental issues such as recycling environmental resources at home, work, or in your community?

Are you concerned about the survival of the planet?

From Dossey BM: Holistic modalities and healing moments, *Am J Nurs* 6:44, 1998.
Sources: Burkhardt MA: Spirituality: an analysis of the concept, *Holist Nurs Pract* 3(3):69, 1989; and Dossey BM et al, editors: *Holistic nursing: a handbook for practice*, ed 2, Gaithersburg, Md, 1995, Aspen.

never be addressed. Even in cases where one has a faith community, a client may be reluctant to delve too deeply into areas of spirituality that deal with mental illness; therefore interventions by the nurse addressing these issues may be crucial. Box 34-3 provides a spiritual assessment tool.

SPIRITUAL DIMENSION

The seventh dimension, the **spiritual dimension,** comprises the following seven axes.

Axis 1: Belief and Meaning

Belief and meaning form the central and foundational principle underlying this model. An individual views life in terms of what he or she perceives is life's meaning. In other words, whatever the individual believes in is important and gives meaning to life. This axis examines how a person makes sense of the world that he or she lives in, and what meanings are ascribed to people, relationships, events, thoughts, actions, and consequences. Some questions that may be included as one examines this axis include:

1. What are the beliefs a person has that give meaning and purpose to life, and what are the important symbols that reflect these?
2. How does a person's life story reflect or demonstrate these underlying themes?
3. Do any areas of the person's life story come into conflict with these underlying, foundational beliefs?
4. Do any current situations or problems come into direct conflict with these beliefs?
5. In what ways is the person able to consciously articulate these beliefs?
6. In what ways do these beliefs seem to be an unconscious part of the person's worldview?

Axis 2: Vocation and Obligation

Out of one's perception of belief and meaning flows a sense of what one needs to do with and in life. This axis is very closely linked to the first, in that one usually does what one considers important to do. If a task, action, or thought has no meaning, one is much less likely to do that action or to follow through on thoughts regarding that task. When life circumstances place one in a position in which actions come into conflict with core belief and meaning systems, crisis and significant stress may result. Questions that may be included in this axis are:

1. What sense of duty, vocation, calling, or moral obligation does this person have?
2. How actively has this client been able to express these in the past?
3. What impact does the client's current situation/illness have on these?

Axis 3: Experience and Emotion

In this axis, one examines questions that surround the emotional experience, both helpful and punitive, that one has encountered in experiencing one's own faith. Questions that may be examined in this axis include:

1. What experience of the divine or sacred has this person had?
2. What emotions or moods are associated with these contacts?
3. How does the client's current situation relate to these experiences?

Axis 4: Courage and Growth

This axis examines how one adapts to situations that may confront and conflict with the core beliefs and meanings that one holds. Questions in this axis examine how a client may deal with extremely stressful and challenging issues and include:

1. How spiritually adaptable is the client?
2. How has the client coped in the past with situations that were in conflict with his or her current spiritual understanding?
3. Must new experiences fit into existing belief systems, or can the person's beliefs adapt with new experiences?
4. How concrete is the person's spirituality?
5. How adaptable is the person currently?

Axis 5: Ritual and Practice

1. What are the spiritual rituals and practices of this individual?
2. Are they formal or informal?
3. Does the individual experience them on a regular basis?
4. How do they support the individual?
5. How does the client's current circumstances affect these rituals?

Axis 6: Community

1. Family of origin: How did the client's family of origin share spiritual experiences?
2. Current family structure: How does the client's current family share spiritual experiences?
3. How does the person view participation in a faith community?
   a. Faith community of origin
      (1) How formal was the client's faith community of origin?
      (2) How informal?
      (3) How active or inactive was the client?
   b. Current faith community
      (1) How formal was the patient's faith community of origin?

Spirituality and Well-Being

Spiritual well-being among our mentally ill clients is an unexplored area. It is the one aspect of care that we often neglect and/or overlook during our assessment. As an integral part of our assessment, do we even give any thought to the spiritual needs of our clients? Most likely we have a tendency to be caught up in the all-consuming task of trying to assist our clients in dealing with their multiple problems: behavioral, medication taking, money management, living arrangements, and possibly alcohol/drug usage. Unfortunately, we let these tasks of everyday living take precedence. Perhaps we ourselves are unable to deal with or be comfortable addressing our clients' religious needs. Or we just assume that spirituality is not important in their lives.

Assessment of the spiritual needs of our clients should include their religious and nonreligious beliefs and values. Their religious beliefs and values are going to be complex, personal, and private. For example, one client shared that her religious beliefs gave her a sense of space from a chaotic board-and-care environment, a sense of peace, and, more important for her, time for herself. Although a client's religious beliefs and values may not fit into what we consider accepted religious practices, they do serve a purpose by providing a tangible idea to hold onto. This client believed that the presence of a Higher Power outside herself could be guiding and supporting. Even for those clients who profess nonreligious beliefs in a mystical way—not delusional—these inner experiences of beliefs give them a sense of worth and promote self-esteem and self-confidence.

The available literature on spirituality and the mentally ill is sparse. However, the literature does point out that attending to our client's spiritual needs can serve as a buffer against the increased anxiety they confront in their daily lives. Despite this anxiety, affirmation of self is made easier through a spiritual presence. For many of our clients, their spiritual beliefs may be all they have, since family support, caring friends, and social networks may be nonexistent. Painfully aware of their losses, spirituality can serve to allay the angst associated with being mentally ill or perceived as different. Religion can help to improve the quality of life for our clients, who are often isolated, afraid, and lonely, and frequently ignored.

The use of prayer can serve as a source of strength in helping to overcome the uncertainty of living, managing, and surviving in what to them is a hostile, unfriendly world. We need to be able to facilitate and share in prayer with our clients as part of our therapeutic interventions.

In providing spiritual nursing interventions, we need to be comfortable in discussing religious beliefs and values, including our belief in God or a Higher Power, and be able to participate with our clients in their experiences. It is important for us to take the lead from our clients in order to determine from their perspective what it is that is needed at a particular moment. By bridging onto our client's expressed spiritual interests, we, as nurses, can foster a sense of hope and self-worth for giving meaning and purpose to their lives.

---

(2) How informal?

(3) How active or inactive was the client?

Axis 7: Authority and Guidance

1. What is the source of this client's system of belief, meaning, and ritual?
2. When faced with problems, tragedy, or doubt, where does the client look for guidance?
3. Does the client look for answers from internal or external sources?
4. Is this source fixed, or is it flexible?

STAGES OF FAITH

A key concept in understanding spiritual development is that one's faith tends to become internalized as one develops. As one develops, one's sense of faith, of meaning, of moral values, and of judgment moves from an external locus of control to an internal locus of control (Santrock, 1997). In assessing how best to assist a client in using his or her spirituality to address mental illness, it is essential to determine where the client is in his or her spiritual development. This is important in order to determine what interventions, if any, are appropriate. There are several significant models of both faith development and moral/

spiritual development that can help inform a chaplain of the relative foundations in which a patient is grounded.

The first model is James Fowler's stages of religious development theory (Box 34-4). In this theory, Fowler posits that an individual passes through various stages in a linear fashion, based on age. As such, this theory is much like many of the other individual development theories (Sandtrock, 1997).

STAGES OF MORAL DEVELOPMENT

A second important model that can help assess a client's spirituality and how illness or the current situation has challenged the client's spirituality is Kohlberg's six stages of moral development theory, in which Kohlberg posits that individuals move, in a linear fashion with age, through key areas of faith and spiritual reasoning. The theory indicates that individuals all move through one or more of the following stages:

Preconventional I. Avoid breaking rules in order to avoid punishment

II. Moral action based on satisfying needs

Box 34-4   **Fowler's Stages of Religious Development**

Stage 1: Intuitive-Projective Faith

A developmental stage that begins in early childhood
Intuitive images of good and evil.
Fantasy and reality are the same.

Stage 2: Mythical-Lyrical Faith

A developmental stage that can begin in middle to late childhood
More logical, concrete thought.
Literal interpretation of religious stories.
God is like a parent figure.

Stage 3: Synthetic-Conventional Faith

A developmental stage that can begin in early adolescence
More abstract thought.
Conformity to the religious beliefs of others.

Stage 4: Individuating-Reflexive Faith

A developmental stage that can begin in late adolescence to early adulthood
Individuals begin to take full responsibility for their religious beliefs.
In-depth exploration of one's values and religious beliefs.

Stage 5: Conjunctive Faith

A developmental stage that can begin in middle adulthood
Becoming more open to paradox and opposing viewpoints.
Stems from awareness of one's finiteness and limitations.

Stage 6: Universalizing Faith

A developmental stage that can begin in late adulthood
Transcending belief systems to achieve a sense of oneness with all beings.
Conflictual events are no longer viewed as paradoxes.

Conventional	I. Pleasing others and doing what is expected
	II. Maintaining order and following the law
Postconventional	I. Moral actions determined by individual rights and community standards
	II. Belief in universal ethical principles that can guide actions

Based on the work of Kohlberg and Fowler, the following model looks at four areas of spirituality, each having implications for effective pastoral interventions.

IMPARTIAL SPIRITUALITY

1. Individuals are considered to be "amoral."
2. They tend to do things in their own interest. ("What's in it for me?")
3. They are generally individuals who are not involved in faith communities or are only nominally involved.
4. They may have a casual, cultural acquaintance with a formal faith community.
5. They are a significant minority of the population.

INSTITUTIONAL SPIRITUALITY

1. Individuals are regular church attendees.
2. They adhere to outside, institutional rules.
3. They do things because they are told to do them.
4. They follow a good person/bad person concept.
5. They probably make up the largest percentage of the population.

INDIVIDUAL SPIRITUALITY

1. Individuals are seekers who have left a formal religious community.
2. They often challenge the tenants of formal religious communities.
3. They seek new answers or personal answers to questions, problems, or crises.
4. They can appear on the surface to be in the impartial stage of faith.
5. They are a smaller minority of the population.

INTEGRATED SPIRITUALITY

1. Individuals have internalized their faith.
2. These people obey "rules" because they fully accept them and feel that they are just and right.
3. They may or may not belong to formal faith communities.
4. They can be seen as teachers or mystics.
5. They make up a very small percentage of the population.

• • •

An accurate assessment of the client's stage of faith is extremely important in that it helps determine the nature of interventions that may be used. As in all models, these also have their limitations, and individuals tend to move along a continuum of spirituality and faith, rather than being locked into a particular stage. In some instances, a crisis may in fact be the initiator of a person's movement, in either direction, along the continuum. An individual in the first stage might likely be operating out of a "bargaining" position when dealing with a spiritual crisis that questions a core meaning held by the individual. An intervention that helped that individual become connected with a faith group, perhaps a return to a youthful experience of faith, may provide some additional spiritual tools that were not otherwise available to the person. It would probably be less effective to attempt to use interventions that encour-

CASE STUDY

This case illustrates the use of the assessment and intervention tools referred to in this chapter. It also reflects some of the significant aspects of spiritual care as they apply to both clients and nurses. The value of spiritual care as perceived by a client and a physician is also demonstrated.

Holistic Assessment

The client is a 66-year-old woman who has been hospitalized for an extensive period of time (approximately 6 weeks). The initial problems were major depression, anxiety, and a degenerative spinal condition that required several surgeries. The spinal condition is treatable, but the process will leave her with some permanent restrictions in movement and some possible residual pain. The client currently has significant chronic leg and lower back spasms and states that medication gives her little relief. Both the pain and the restrictions resulting from surgery have exacerbated her depression and anxiety.

    The client has been divorced for almost 40 years. Immediately after her divorce she and her four children moved 1500 miles away from her family and friends to seek employment in a manufacturing environment. Although two of her children live close by, only one child is in regular contact with the client. Although the client has a nominally Lutheran background, she has no local connection to a congregation and has not attended church regularly since leaving her home town. Both the client and her physician are extremely interested in her having regular visits for spiritual care, and both have stated that the visits provide the client with significant help and support.

The Client's Belief and Meaning

Being independent, stoic, and self-sufficient are important goals in life, which are to be valued and pursued.

The Client's Vocations and Obligations

The client's goal was to support, raise, and care for herself and her children without being dependent on others. She still seeks to care for her adult daughter—asking the spiritual caregiver to meet with her daughter to talk about performing a marriage ceremony.

The Client's Experience and Emotion

The client has had a life of struggle, which has been balanced against the rewards of accomplishing her goal to be independent and her pride in being self-sufficient.

The Client's Courage and Growth

The client is now struggling to find some meaning in her pain and suffering.

The Client's Ritual and Practice

The client has a strong, dependent need to have the poem "Footprints," the Twenty-Third Psalm, and the Lord's Prayer read to her; she requests few other institutional rituals.

The Client's Community

The client's community is a small one, consisting of her children, their spouses, and several grandchildren, mostly living some distance from the client.

---

aged and supported challenges to existing spiritual norms for a person in either the first or second stage, but it might be a very effective intervention to use when dealing with an individual in the third stage. For individuals who are in the fourth stage, often the elderly, the best possible pastoral intervention may be in learning from them, in being a student, and accepting their unique spiritual legacy.

SELECTED CASES OF CLINICAL SPIRITUAL INTERVENTIONS
PAIN

Patty, a patient with depression and anxiety, also had an extremely difficult case of pancreatitis, which required an inpatient stay of about 30 days. A few weeks after her discharge, she returned to talk. As she talked, she confessed that the ex-

perience had made a significant impact on her faith and spiritual viewpoint. When faced with agonizing pain for the first time in her life, this middle-age woman confided that the physical agony she felt connected her emotionally for the first time with the concept of "torment and damnation." Although her existing spiritual beliefs helped her to cope with the symptoms of her illnesses, the experience of excruciating pain caused her to question some of the fundamental spiritual principles that had guided her up to that point. Especially challenged during this illness was her understanding of the relationship between the divine and humanity, and her concept of ultimate punishment and reward.

SPIRITUAL TORMENT

Pete, a devout Mormon man in his mid-fifties, was in spiritual torment. His permanent developmental delay, coupled with his bipolar illness, had prevented him from marrying. His own

CASE STUDY—cont'd

The Client's Source of Authority and Guidance

The client's source of authority and guidance is largely external and is derived from her early Midwestern social norms and experiences with institutional religion. She grants pastors a great deal of power, authority, and control; the client also believes that common religious articles such as the Bible and prayer cards have an almost magical authority and power.

The Client's Stage of Faith Development

The client is basically in stage 1, the impartial stage of faith, and is now possibly seeking to move into the early phase of stage 2, the institutional religion stage.

Level of Spiritual Risk

This client is considered to be at significant spiritual risk. She has an extremely high need for spiritual care and has very limited-to-nonexistent resources with which to meet this need. In making a triage assessment of how to allocate scarce pastoral care resources, this client's particular situation would dictate that a significant amount of qualified pastoral care be provided.

Spiritual Care Plan

Using the assessment tools as previously described, the spiritual pastoral care plan was to see the patient often—daily if possible. During these visits the spiritual intervention tools of prayer, presence, and short scripture readings were used to help bolster the client's sense of God's care for her and to support her in the healing process. Another intervention strategy was to help the patient explore her stated desire to be connected to a local Lutheran church and to help identify ways in which she might do this. In addition, the spiritual caregiver helped the client explore, to the extent of her desire and ca-

pability, what meaning there might be for her in this illness and in her future physical limitations. The intent of this goal was to help the client find possible new meanings in her life as a result of this illness.

The benefit to the client in pursuing these spiritual care plan goals was the provision of help, support, and comfort. This spiritual support helped ease her sense of torment and pain, resulting in a reduced experience of suffering. The benefit to the hospital in pursuing these spiritual care plan goals was greater client satisfaction. As the client experienced significant relief in the periods following her spiritual care, her requests for nursing interventions decreased. The client was also more satisfied with her overall care and was less anxious about her prognosis. The client's physician reported that she was quite satisfied with the hospital's ability to address the client's spiritual needs and that in doing so the hospital helped the client to experience less pain and discomfort.

Critical Thinking—Assessment

1. Assess and prioritize the client's psychiatric, physical, and spiritual areas of concern, ensuring that all areas are addressed.
2. Describe the benefits of collaborating with the hospital chaplain in addressing the client's spiritual needs as part of a holistic assessment.
3. Given your knowledge of the stages of faith and the client's spiritual and religious background, which stage of faith best fits this client? What is the rationale for your choice?
4. How can your assessment of this client's family history of struggle, pride, and pain be used to guide you in your spiritual assessment? Consider the stages of the spiritual dimension as a guide.

---

understanding of his religious principles, whether they were completely accurate according to that faith tradition or not, led him to believe that he would never "be able to enter heaven." This statement was always made as part of a tearful, tormented lament. His own strong faith was "punishing" him. An appropriate intervention in this case was to listen to and acknowledge Pete's pain and help connect him with responsible members of his faith community, where he could address his concerns.

PUNISHMENT

Mary, a woman in her mid-fifties, was a devout Catholic. She believed that her lifelong bouts of major depression were an appropriate "punishment" for the sexual abuse she had experienced as a child. She clung to the belief that she was responsible for the abuse and that the enjoyment and attention she felt at the time only confirmed her worthlessness and lack of

capacity to be loved as an adult. In this case, where Mary was deeply entrenched in her denominational faith system, religious authority figures were seen to speak with much more authority than either physicians or other health care team members. Mary was introduced to a sympathetic priest who was also a trained psychotherapist. The interventions all centered around Mary's own belief system and included helping Mary to see herself as a survivor of abuse rather than as the responsible party. A sacramental ritual particular to her denomination was also included in order to eliminate Mary's deeply held "need" to be punished.

VOICES

Fred, a patient with schizophrenia and a member of a charismatic Protestant group, stated that he had the "gift of wisdom"; Fred's schizophrenic symptoms included auditory hallucinations. On further discussion with Fred, it was revealed that during worship services it was quite common for him and others to rise and to "speak in tongues," a regular occurrence within his denomination. He also revealed that the voices he heard were quite malevolent and frequently urged him to harm himself. In Fred's case the hospital chaplain provided the interventions. Without challenging the faith experience that Fred described having in worship services, the chaplain was able to help Fred see a distinction between the malevolent voices that urged him to harm himself and any prophetic experience that Fred might have within the understanding of his own religious concepts. Out of this distinction, Fred's reluctance to maintain his antipsychotic medication regimen diminished. This improved medication maintenance resulted in a better quality of life for Fred and fewer hospitalizations.

GUILT

Terry, a woman with bipolar disorder in her mid-forties, was riddled with guilt because of behaviors that she had demonstrated during previous manic phases of her illness. These actions had included both risky sexual acting out and behaving in ways that were financially irresponsible. Terry came from a mainstream, liturgical Protestant tradition whose culture had emphasized both "personal responsibility" and "spiritual consequences" for one's own actions. Terry believed that she was "condemned" and that there was nothing she could do to change that. In ongoing discussions Terry was provided with education about her illness and instructed on how her symptoms could be more effectively contained by correctly using and monitoring her medications. Terry was eventually able to view her illness in the same way she viewed a chronic physical illness, such as diabetes. This diminished her feelings of guilt. To help maintain her medication compliance, Terry also began to incorporate part of her faith tradition in her ongoing care by using the daily prayer rituals of her faith to help her take her medication.

HYPERRELIGIOSITY

Hank, a religiously preoccupied individual with schizoaffective disorder, would often respond in a tangential fashion when anyone engaged him in conversation. Any attempt to relate to Hank using the more traditional religious language of his own faith background would propel him into long, rambling, confused, and pressured ranting about his "special connection" to God "as a prophet." To engage Hank in spiritual discussions for either assessment or intervention purposes, it was necessary to use language that he did not identify as "religious." When Hank was engaged by staff in discussions about meaningful areas of spirituality that were couched in ordinary language rather than "spiritual language," the words that would usually trigger Hank's tangential responses were avoided, and he would enter into more meaningful dialogues with staff.

• • •

The role of spiritual caregiver, even in today's increasingly diverse and secular environment, still plays a significant part in the lives of individuals and health care organization. Chaplains, who most commonly hold these positions and who provide spiritual care on a variety of levels, have made an effective impact on the overall quality of client care. The various disciplines within the multidisciplinary health care team are usually seen by clients as having different levels of authority and "expertise" regarding spirituality and mental illness. For some clients, the physician is the "ultimate authority" when dealing with a health crisis and the subsequent challenges and interpretations of meaning that the crisis may hold. For others the "ultimate expertise" may be vested in a nurse, a social worker, or a therapist. For some individuals a chaplain may reflect an important image of "ultimate authority." To help clients with mental illness attempt to undertake a healing journey without addressing their spirituality and its authority in their lives may significantly impede the healing process.

Summary of Key Concepts

1. There is a growing belief that quality spiritual assessment can be significantly beneficial in reducing a client's feelings of powerlessness and despair.
2. Spirituality is an essential human dimension that helps connect people to each other, the community, and the world.
3. Spirituality, religion, and faith may be experienced and expressed in a variety of ways.
4. The Joint Commission on Accreditation for Health Care Organizations (JCAHO) includes the requirement for spiritual care in their standards.
5. Belief and meaning make up the central, foundational principle underlying an individual's spiritual dimension.
6. A person's spirituality can be influenced by culture, as well as life experiences.
7. For some individuals a chaplain may represent the "ultimate authority" for one's spiritual health, much as the nurse or physician is the authority for one's physical or mental health.

REFERENCES

Anderson H, Foley E: Experiences in need of ritual, *Christian Century,* 114(31):1002, 1997.

Appleby C: Integrated delivery: organized chaos, *Hosp Health Netw,* 71(14):50, 1997.

Becker V, editor: *Recovery devotional Bible, new international version,* Grand Rapids, Mich, 1993, Zondervan.

Culligan K: Spirituality and healing in medicine, *America* 175(5):17, 1996.

Episcopal Church: *The book of common prayer,* Philadelphia, 1979, Seabury Press.

Evans F: *New St. Joseph's people's prayer book,* New York, 1993, Catholic Book Publishing.

Fitchett G: *Assessing spiritual needs: a guide for caregivers,* Minn, 1993, Augsburg.

Fitchett G: *Developing outcome-focused spiritual care: facing the challenge of filling a new wineskin.* Unpublished monograph presented to the national meeting of the College of Chaplains, 1997.

Ford-Grabowsky M: *Prayers for all people,* New York, 1995, Doubleday.

Fowler JW: *Stages of faith,* San Francisco, 1981, Harper San Francisco.

Hall BA: Spirituality in terminal illness: an alternative view of theory, *J Holist Nurs* 15(1):82, 1997.

Holst L: *Hospital ministry,* New York, 1992, Crossroads.

Hunter RJ, editor: *Dictionary of pastoral care and counseling,* Nashville, 1996, Abingdon Press.

Job R, Shawchuck N: *A guide to prayer,* Nashville, Tenn, 1983, The Upper Room.

Kelly EW: *Spirituality and religion in counseling and psychotherapy,* 1995, American Counseling Association.

Moore T: *Care of the soul,* New York, 1992, HarperCollins.

Nichols JE: *The relationship between meaning in life and chronic illness,* master's thesis, San Diego, 1998, San Diego State University.

Nouwen H: *The wounded healer,* New York, 1990, Doubleday.

Oman M: *Prayers for healing,* Berkeley, Calif, 1997, Conari Press.

Perrin KM, McDermott RJ: The spiritual dimension of health: a review, *Am J Health Stud* 13(2):90, 1997.

Richards PS, Bergin AE: *A spiritual strategy for counseling and psychotherapy,* Washington, DC, 1997, American Psychological Association.

Roukema RW: *The soul in distress,* New York, 1997, Haworth Pastoral Press.

Santrock JW: *Life-span development,* Chicago, 1997, Brown & Benchmark.

Smith J: *The HarperCollins dictionary of religion,* New York, 1995, HarperCollins.

United Church Of Christ: *Book of worship,* New York, 1986, United Church Of Christ.

Warter C: *Recovery of the sacred,* Deerfield Beach, Fla, 1994, Health Communications.

DSM-IV Classification

NOS = Not Otherwise Specified.

An *x* appearing in a diagnostic code indicates that a specific code number is required.

An ellipsis (. . .) is used in the names of certain disorders to indicate that the name of a specific mental disorder or general medical condition should be inserted when recording the name (e.g., 293.0 Delirium Due to Hypothyroidism).

If criteria are currently met, one of the following severity specifiers may be noted after the diagnosis:
Mild
Moderate
Severe

If criteria are no longer met, one of the following specifiers may be noted:
In Partial Remission
In Full Remission
Prior History

DISORDERS USUALLY FIRST DIAGNOSED IN INFANCY, CHILDHOOD, OR ADOLESCENCE
Mental Retardation
NOTE: *These are coded on Axis II.*

317	Mild Mental Retardation
318.0	Moderate Mental Retardation
318.1	Severe Mental Retardation
318.2	Profound Mental Retardation
319	Mental Retardation, Severity Unspecified

Learning Disorders
315.00	Reading Disorder
315.1	Mathematics Disorder
315.2	Disorder of Written Expression
315.9	Learning Disorder NOS

Motor Skills Disorder
315.4	Developmental Coordination Disorder

Communication Disorders
315.31	Expressive Language Disorder
315.31	Mixed Receptive-Expressive Language Disorder

315.39	Phonologic Disorder
307.0	Stuttering
307.9	Communication Disorder NOS

Pervasive Developmental Disorders
299.00	Autistic Disorder
299.80	Rett's Disorder
299.10	Childhood Disintegrative Disorder
299.80	Asperger's Disorder
299.80	Pervasive Developmental Disorder NOS

Attention-Deficit and Disruptive Behavior Disorders
314.xx	Attention-Deficit/Hyperactivity Disorder
.01	Combined Type
.00	Predominantly Inattentive Type
.01	Predominantly Hyperactive-Impulsive Type
314.9	Attention-Deficit/Hyperactivity Disorder NOS
312.8	Conduct Disorder

Specify type: Childhood-Onset Type/Adolescent-Onset Type

313.81	Oppositional Defiant Disorder
312.9	Disruptive Behavior Disorder NOS

Feeding and Eating Disorders of Infancy or Early Childhood
307.52	Pica
307.53	Rumination Disorder
307.59	Feeding Disorder of Infancy or Early Childhood

Tic Disorders
307.23	Tourette's Disorder
307.22	Chronic Motor or Vocal Tic Disorder
307.21	Transient Tic Disorder

Specify if: Single Episode/Recurrent

307.20	Tic Disorder NOS

Elimination Disorders
___.__	Encopresis
787.6	With Constipation and Overflow Incontinence
307.7	Without Constipation and Overflow Incontinence
307.6	Enuresis (Not Due to a General Medical Condition)

Specify type: Nocturnal Only/Diurnal Only/Nocturnal and Diurnal

From American Psychiatric Association: *Diagnostic and statistical manual of mental disorders*, ed 4, Washington, DC, 1994, The Association.

Other Disorders of Infancy, Childhood, or Adolescence

309.21   Separation Anxiety Disorder

Specify if: Early Onset

313.23   Selective Mutism

313.89   Reactive Attachment Disorder of Infancy or Early Childhood

Specify type: Inhibited Type/Disinhibited Type

307.3   Stereotypic Movement Disorder

Specify if: With Self-Injurious Behavior

313.9   Disorder of Infancy, Childhood, or Adolescence NOS

DELIRIUM, DEMENTIA, AND AMNESTIC AND OTHER COGNITIVE DISORDERS
Delirium

293.0   Delirium Due to . . . *[Indicate the General Medical Condition]*

___.__   Substance Intoxication Delirium *(refer to Substance-Related Disorders for substance-specific codes)*

___.__   Substance Withdrawal Delirium *(refer to Substance-Related Disorders for substance-specific codes)*

___.__   Delirium Due to Multiple Etiologies *(code each of the specific etiologies)*

780.09   Delirium NOS

Dementia

290.xx   Dementia of the Alzheimer's Type, With Early Onset *(also code 331.0 Alzheimer's disease on Axis III)*
- .10   Uncomplicated
- .11   With Delirium
- .12   With Delusions
- .13   With Depressed Mood

Specify if: With Behavioral Disturbance

290.xx   Dementia of the Alzheimer's Type, With Late Onset *(also code 331.0 Alzheimer's disease on Axis III)*
- .0   Uncomplicated
- .3   With Delirium
- .20   With Delusions
- .21   With Depressed Mood

Specify if: With Behavioral Disturbance

290.xx   Vascular Dementia
- .40   Uncomplicated
- .41   With Delirium
- .42   With Delusions
- .43   With Depressed Mood

Specify if: With Behavioral Disturbance

294.9   Dementia Due to HIV Disease *(also code 043.1 HIV infection affecting central nervous system on Axis III)*

294.1   Dementia Due to Head Trauma *(also code 854.00 head injury on Axis III)*

294.1   Dementia Due to Parkinson's Disease *(also code 332.0 Parkinson's disease on Axis III)*

294.1   Dementia Due to Huntington's Disease *(also code 333.4 Huntington's disease on Axis III)*

290.10   Dementia Due to Pick's Disease *(also code 331.1 Pick's disease on Axis III)*

290.10   Dementia Due to Creutzfeldt-Jakob Disease *(also code 046.1 Creutzfeldt-Jakob disease on Axis III)*

294.1   Dementia Due to . . . *[Indicate the General Medical Condition not listed above] (also code the general medical condition on Axis III)*

___.__   Substance-Induced Persisting Dementia *(refer to Substance-Related Disorders for substance-specific codes)*

___.__   Dementia Due to Multiple Etiologies *(code each of the specific etiologies)*

294.8   Dementia NOS

Amnestic Disorders

294.0   Amnestic Disorder Due to . . . *[Indicate the General Medical Condition]*

Specify if: Transient/Chronic

___.__   Substance-Induced Persisting Amnestic Disorder *(refer to Substance-Related Disorders for substance-specific codes)*

294.8   Amnestic Disorder NOS

Other Cognitive Disorders

294.9   Cognitive Disorder NOS

MENTAL DISORDERS DUE TO A GENERAL MEDICAL CONDITION NOT ELSEWHERE CLASSIFIED

293.89   Catatonic Disorder Due to . . . *[Indicate the General Medical Condition]*

310.1   Personality Change Due to . . . *[Indicate the General Medical Condition]*

Specify type: Labile Type/Disinhibited Type/Aggressive Type/Apathetic Type/Paranoid Type/ Other Type/Combined Type/Unspecified Type

293.9   Mental Disorder NOS Due to . . . [Indicate the General Medical Condition]

SUBSTANCE-RELATED DISORDERS

[a]*The following specifiers may be applied to Substance Dependence:*

With Physiologic Dependence/Without Physiologic Dependence

Early Full Remission/Early Partial Remission

Sustained Full Remission/Sustained Partial Remission
On Agonist Therapy/In a Controlled Environment

The following specifiers apply to Substance-Induced Disorders as noted:

[I]With Onset During Intoxication/[W]With Onset During Withdrawal

Alcohol-Related Disorders
Alcohol Use Disorders

303.90	Alcohol Dependence[a]
305.00	Alcohol Abuse

Alcohol-Induced Disorders

303.00	Alcohol Intoxication
291.8	Alcohol Withdrawal

Specify if: With Perceptual Disturbances

291.0	Alcohol Intoxication Delirium
291.0	Alcohol Withdrawal Delirium
291.2	Alcohol-Induced Persisting Dementia
291.1	Alcohol-Induced Persisting Amnestic Disorder
291.x	Alcohol-Induced Psychotic Disorder
.5	With Delusions[I,W]
.3	With Hallucinations[I,W]
291.8	Alcohol-Induced Mood Disorder[I,W]
291.8	Alcohol-Induced Anxiety Disorder[I,W]
291.8	Alcohol-Induced Sexual Dysfunction[I]
291.8	Alcohol-Induced Sleep Disorder[I,W]
291.9	Alcohol-Related Disorder NOS

Amphetamine (or Amphetamine-Like)–Related Disorders
Amphetamine Use Disorders

304.40	Amphetamine Dependence[a]
305.70	Amphetamine Abuse

Amphetamine-Induced Disorders

292.89	Amphetamine Intoxication

Specify if: With Perceptual Disturbances

292.0	Amphetamine Withdrawal
292.81	Amphetamine Intoxication Delirium
292.xx	Amphetamine-Induced Psychotic Disorder
.11	With Delusions[I]
.12	With Hallucinations[I]
292.84	Amphetamine-Induced Mood Disorder[I,W]
292.89	Amphetamine-Induced Anxiety Disorder[I]
292.89	Amphetamine-Induced Sexual Dysfunction[I]
292.89	Amphetamine-Induced Sleep Disorder[I,W]
292.9	Amphetamine-Related Disorder NOS

Caffeine-Related Disorders
Caffeine-Induced Disorders

305.90	Caffeine Intoxication
292.89	Caffeine-Induced Anxiety Disorder[I]
292.89	Caffeine-Induced Sleep Disorder[I]
292.9	Caffeine-Related Disorder NOS

Cannabis-Related Disorders
Cannabis Use Disorders

304.30	Cannabis Dependence[a]
305.20	Cannabis Abuse

Cannabis-Induced Disorders

292.89	Cannabis Intoxication

Specify if: With Perceptual Disturbances

292.81	Cannabis Intoxication Delirium
292.xx	Cannabis-Induced Psychotic Disorder
.11	With Delusions[I]
.12	With Hallucinations[I]
292.89	Cannabis-Induced Anxiety Disorder[I]
292.9	Cannabis-Related Disorder NOS

Cocaine-Related Disorders
Cocaine Use Disorders

304.20	Cocaine Dependence[a]
305.60	Cocaine Abuse

Cocaine-Induced Disorders

292.89	Cocaine Intoxication

Specify if: With Perceptual Disturbances

292.0	Cocaine Withdrawal
292.81	Cocaine Intoxication Delirium
292.xx	Cocaine-Induced Psychotic Disorder
.11	With Delusions[I]
.12	With Hallucinations[I]
292.84	Cocaine-Induced Mood Disorder[I,W]
292.89	Cocaine-Induced Anxiety Disorder[I,W]
292.89	Cocaine-Induced Sexual Dysfunction[I]
292.89	Cocaine-Induced Sleep Disorder[I,W]
292.9	Cocaine-Related Disorder NOS

Hallucinogen-Related Disorders
Hallucinogen Use Disorders

304.50	Hallucinogen Dependence[a]
305.30	Hallucinogen Abuse

Hallucinogen-Induced Disorders

292.89   Hallucinogen Intoxication
292.89   Hallucinogen Persisting Perception Disorder (Flashbacks)
292.81   Hallucinogen Intoxication Delirium
292.xx   Hallucinogen-Induced Psychotic Disorder
   .11   With Delusions[I]
   .12   With Hallucinations[I]
292.84   Hallucinogen-Induced Mood Disorder[I]
292.89   Hallucinogen-Induced Anxiety Disorder[I]
292.9   Hallucinogen-Related Disorder NOS

Inhalant-Related Disorders
Inhalant Use Disorders

304.60   Inhalant Dependence[a]
305.90   Inhalant Abuse

Inhalant-Induced Disorders

292.89   Inhalant Intoxication
292.81   Inhalant Intoxication Delirium
292.82   Inhalant-Induced Persisting Dementia
292.xx   Inhalant-Induced Psychotic Disorder
   .11   With Delusions[I]
   .12   With Hallucinations[I]
292.84   Inhalant-Induced Mood Disorder[I]
292.89   Inhalant-Induced Anxiety Disorder[I]
292.9   Inhalant-Related Disorder NOS

Nicotine-Related Disorders
Nicotine Use Disorder

305.10   Nicotine Dependence[a]

Nicotine-Induced Disorder

292.0   Nicotine Withdrawal
292.9   Nicotine-Related Disorder NOS

Opioid-Related Disorders
Opioid Use Disorders

304.00   Opioid Dependence[a]
305.50   Opioid Abuse

Opioid-Induced Disorders

292.89   Opioid Intoxication

   Specify if: With Perceptual Disturbances

292.0   Opioid Withdrawal
292.81   Opioid Intoxication Delirium
292.xx   Opioid-Induced Psychotic Disorder
   .11   With Delusions[I]

   .12   With Hallucinations[I]
292.84   Opioid-Induced Mood Disorder[I]
292.89   Opioid-Induced Sexual Dysfunction[I]
292.89   Opioid-Induced Sleep Disorder[I,W]
292.9   Opioid-Related Disorder NOS

Phencyclidine (or Phencyclidine-Like)–Related Disorders
Phencyclidine Use Disorders

304.90   Phencyclidine Dependence[a]
305.90   Phencyclidine Abuse

Phencyclidine-Induced Disorders

292.89   Phencyclidine Intoxication

   Specify if: With Perceptual Disturbances

292.81   Phencyclidine Intoxication Delirium
292.xx   Phencyclidine-Induced Psychotic Disorder
   .11   With Delusions[I]
   .12   With Hallucinations[I]
292.84   Phencyclidine-Induced Mood Disorder[I]
292.89   Phencyclidine-Induced Anxiety Disorder[I]
292.9   Phencyclidine-Related Disorder NOS

Sedative-, Hypnotic-, or Anxiolytic-Related Disorders
Sedative, Hypnotic, or Anxiolytic Use Disorders

304.10   Sedative, Hypnotic, or Anxiolytic Dependence[a]
305.40   Sedative, Hypnotic, or Anxiolytic Abuse

Sedative-, Hypnotic-, or Anxiolytic-Induced Disorders

292.89   Sedative, Hypnotic, or Anxiolytic Intoxication
292.0   Sedative, Hypnotic, or Anxiolytic Withdrawal

   Specify if: With Perceptual Disturbances

292.81   Sedative, Hypnotic, or Anxiolytic Intoxication Delirium
292.81   Sedative, Hypnotic, or Anxiolytic Withdrawal Delirium
292.82   Sedative-, Hypnotic-, or Anxiolytic-Induced Persisting Dementia
292.83   Sedative-, Hypnotic-, or Anxiolytic-Induced Persisting Amnestic Disorder
292.xx   Sedative-, Hypnotic-, or Anxiolytic-Induced Psychotic Disorder
   .11   With Delusions[I,W]
   .12   With Hallucinations[I,W]
292.84   Sedative-, Hypnotic-, or Anxiolytic-Induced Mood Disorder[I,W]
292.89   Sedative-, Hypnotic-, or Anxiolytic-Induced Anxiety Disorder[W]

292.89   Sedative-, Hypnotic-, or Anxiolytic-Induced Sexual Dysfunction[I]

292.89   Sedative-, Hypnotic-, or Anxiolytic-Induced Sleep Disorder[I,W]

292.9   Sedative-, Hypnotic-, or Anxiolytic-Related Disorder NOS

Polysubstance-Related Disorder

304.80   Polysubstance Dependence[a]

Other (or Unknown) Substance–Related Disorders

Other (or Unknown) Substance Use Disorders

304.90   Other (or Unknown) Substance Dependence[a]

305.90   Other (or Unknown) Substance Abuse

Other (or Unknown) Substance–Induced Disorders

292.89   Other (or Unknown) Substance Intoxication

Specify if: With Perceptual Disturbances

292.0   Other (or Unknown) Substance Withdrawal

Specify if: With Perceptual Disturbances

292.81   Other (or Unknown) Substance–Induced Delirium

292.82   Other (or Unknown) Substance–Induced Persisting Dementia

292.83   Other (or Unknown) Substance–Induced Persisting Amnestic Disorder

292.xx   Other (or Unknown) Substance–Induced Psychotic Disorder

.11   With Delusions[I,W]

.12   With Hallucinations[I,W]

292.84   Other (or Unknown) Substance–Induced Mood Disorder[I,W]

292.89   Other (or Unknown) Substance–Induced Anxiety Disorder[I,W]

292.89   Other (or Unknown) Substance–Induced Sexual Dysfunction[I]

292.89   Other (or Unknown) Substance–Induced Sleep Disorder[I,W]

292.9   Other (or Unknown) Substance–Related Disorder NOS

SCHIZOPHRENIA AND OTHER PSYCHOTIC DISORDERS

295.xx   Schizophrenia

The following Classification of Longitudinal Course applies to all subtypes of Schizophrenia:

Episodic With Interepisode Residual Symptoms (specify if: With Prominent Negative Symptoms)/Episodic With No Interepisode Residual Symptoms/Continuous (specify if: With Prominent Negative Symptoms)

Single Episode in Partial Remission (specify if: With Prominent Negative Symptoms)/Single Episode on Full Remission Other or Unspecified Pattern

.30   Paranoid Type

.10   Disorganized Type

.20   Catatonic Type

.90   Undifferentiated Type

.60   Residual Type

295.40   Schizophreniform Disorder

Specify if: Without Good Prognostic Features/With Good Prognostic Features

295.70   Schizoaffective Disorder

Specify type: Bipolar Type/Depressive Type

297.1   Delusional Disorder

Specify type: Erotomanic Type/Grandiose Type/Jealous Type/Persecutory Type/Somatic Type/Mixed Type/Unspecified Type

298.8   Brief Psychotic Disorder

Specify if: With Marked Stressor(s)/Without Marked Stressor(s)/With Postpartum Onset

297.3   Shared Psychotic Disorder

293.xx   Psychotic Disorder Due to . . . [Indicate the General Medical Condition]

.81   With Delusions

.82   With Hallucinations

___.__   Substance-Induced Psychotic Disorder (refer to Substance-Related Disorders for substance-specific codes)

Specify if: With Onset During Intoxication/With Onset During Withdrawal

298.9   Psychotic Disorder NOS

MOOD DISORDERS

Code current state of Major Depressive Disorder or Bipolar I Disorder in fifth digit:

1 = Mild

2 = Moderate

3 = Severe Without Psychotic Features

4 = Severe With Psychotic Features

Specify: Mood-Congruent Psychotic Features/ Mood-Incongruent Psychotic Features

5 = In Partial Remission

6 = In Full Remission

0 = Unspecified

The following specifiers apply (for current or most recent episode) to Mood Disorders as noted:

[a]Severity/Psychotic/Remission Specifiers
[b]Chronic

[c]With Catatonic Features
[d]With Melancholic Features
[e]With Atypical Features
[f]With Postpartum Onset

The following specifiers apply to Mood Disorders as noted:

[g]With or Without Full Interepisode Recovery
[h]With Seasonal Pattern
[i]With Rapid Cycling

Depressive Disorders

296.xx Major Depressive Disorder
  .2x Single Episode[a,b,c,d,e,f]
  .3x Recurrent[a,b,c,d,e,f,g,h]
300.4 Dysthymic Disorder

    Specify if: Early Onset/Late Onset
    Specify: With Atypical Features

311 Depressive Disorder NOS

Bipolar Disorders

296.xx Bipolar I Disorder
  .0x Single Manic Episode[a,c,f]

    Specify if: Mixed

  .40 Most Recent Episode Hypomanic[g,h,i]
  .4x Most Recent Episode Manic[a,c,f,g,h,i]
  .6x Most Recent Episode Mixed[a,c,f,g,h,i]
  .5x Most Recent Episode Depressed[a,b,c,d,e,f,g,h,i]
  .7 Most Recent Episode Unspecified[g,h,i]
296.89 Bipolar II Disorder[a,b,c,d,e,f,g,h,i]

    Specify (current or most recent episode): Hypomanic/
    Depressed

301.13 Cyclothymic Disorder
296.80 Bipolar Disorder NOS
293.83 Mood Disorder Due to . . . *[Indicate the General
    Medical Condition]*

    Specify type: With Depressive Features/With Major
    Depressive-Like Episode/With Manic Features/With
    Mixed Features

___.__ Substance-Induced Mood Disorder *(refer to
    Substance-Related Disorders for substance-specific
    codes)*

    Specify type: With Depressive Features/With Manic
    Features/With Mixed Features
    Specify if: With Onset During Intoxication/With
    Onset During Withdrawal

296.90 Mood Disorder NOS

ANXIETY DISORDERS

300.01 Panic Disorder Without Agoraphobia
300.21 Panic Disorder With Agoraphobia
300.22 Agoraphobia Without History of Panic Disorder
300.29 Specific Phobia

    Specify type: Animal Type/Natural Environment
    Type/Blood-Injection-Injury Type/Situational Type/
    Other Type

300.23 Social Phobia

    Specify if: Generalized

300.3 Obsessive-Compulsive Disorder

    Specify if: With Poor Insight

309.81 Posttraumatic Stress Disorder

    Specify if: Acute/Chronic
    Specify if: With Delayed Onset

308.3 Acute Stress Disorder
300.02 Generalized Anxiety Disorder
293.89 Anxiety Disorder Due to . . . *[Indicate the General
    Medical Condition]*

    Specify if: With Generalized Anxiety/With Panic
    Attacks/With Obsessive-Compulsive Symptoms

___.__ Substance-Induced Anxiety Disorder *(refer to
    Substance-Related Disorders for substance-specific
    codes)*

    Specify if: With Generalized Anxiety/With Panic
    Attacks/With Obsessive-Compulsive Symptoms/
    With Phobic Symptoms
    Specify if: With Onset During Intoxication/With
    Onset During Withdrawal

300.00 Anxiety Disorder NOS

SOMATOFORM DISORDERS

300.81 Somatization Disorder
300.81 Undifferentiated Somatoform Disorder
300.11 Conversion Disorder

    Specify type: With Motor Symptom or Deficit/With
    Sensory Symptom or Deficit/With Seizures or
    Convulsions/With Mixed Presentation

307.xx Pain Disorder
  .80 Associated With Psychologic Factors
  .89 Associated With Both Psychologic Factors and a
    General Medical Condition

    Specify if: Acute/Chronic

300.7 Hypochondriasis

    Specify if: With Poor Insight

300.7 Body Dysmorphic Disorder
300.81 Somatoform Disorder NOS

FACTITIOUS DISORDERS

300.xx Factitious Disorder
  .16 With Predominantly Psychologic Signs and Symp-
    toms
  .19 With Predominantly Physical Signs and Symptoms

.19   With Combined Psychologic and Physical Signs and Symptoms
300.19 Factitious Disorder NOS

DISSOCIATIVE DISORDERS

300.12 Dissociative Amnesia
300.13 Dissociative Fugue
300.14 Dissociative Identity Disorder
300.6   Depersonalization Disorder
300.15 Dissociative Disorder NOS

SEXUAL AND GENDER IDENTITY DISORDERS
Sexual Dysfunctions

The following specifiers apply to all primary Sexual Dysfunctions:

Lifelong Type
Acquired Type
Generalized Type
Situational Type Due to Psychologic Factors
Due to Combined Factors

Sexual Desire Disorders

302.71 Hypoactive Sexual Desire Disorder
302.79 Sexual Aversion Disorder

Sexual Arousal Disorders

302.72 Female Sexual Arousal Disorder
302.72 Male Erectile Disorder

Orgasmic Disorders

302.73 Female Orgasmic Disorder
302.74 Male Orgasmic Disorder
302.75 Premature Ejaculation

Sexual Pain Disorders

302.76 Dyspareunia (Not Due to a General Medical Condition)
306.51 Vaginismus (Not Due to a General Medical Condition)

Sexual Dysfunction Due to a General Medical Condition

625.8   Female Hypoactive Sexual Desire Disorder Due to . . . *[Indicate the General Medical Condition]*
608.89 Male Hypoactive Sexual Desire Disorder Due to . . . *[Indicate the General Medical Condition]*
607.84 Male Erectile Disorder Due to . . . *[Indicate the General Medical Condition]*
625.0   Female Dyspareunia Due to . . . *[Indicate the General Medical Condition]*
608.89 Male Dyspareunia Due to . . . *[Indicate the General Medical Condition]*
625.8   Other Female Sexual Dysfunction Due to . . . *[Indicate the General Medical Condition]*
608.89 Other Male Sexual Dysfunction Due to . . . *[Indicate the General Medical Condition]*
___.__ Substance-Induced Sexual Dysfunction *(refer to Substance-Related Disorders for substance-specific codes)*

Specify if: With Impaired Desire/With Impaired Arousal/With Impaired Orgasm/With Sexual Pain
Specify if: With Onset During Intoxication

302.70 Sexual Dysfunction NOS

Paraphilias

302.4   Exhibitionism
302.81 Fetishism
302.89 Frotteurism
302.2   Pedophilia

Specify if: Sexually Attracted to Males/Sexually Attracted to Females/Sexually Attracted to Both
Specify if: Limited to Incest
Specify type: Exclusive Type/Nonexclusive Type

302.83 Sexual Masochism
302.84 Sexual Sadism
302.3   Transvestic Fetishism

Specify if: With Gender Dysphoria

302.82 Voyeurism
302.9   Paraphilia NOS

Gender Identity Disorders

302.xx Gender Identity Disorder
.6   In Children
.85   In Adolescents or Adults

Specify if: Sexually Attracted to Males/Sexually Attracted to Females/Sexually Attracted to Both/Sexually Attracted to Neither

302.6   Gender Identity Disorder NOS
302.9   Sexual Disorder NOS

EATING DISORDERS

307.1   Anorexia Nervosa

Specify type: Restricting Type; Binge-Eating/Purging Type

307.51 Bulimia Nervosa

Specify type: Purging Type/Nonpurging Type

307.50 Eating Disorder NOS

SLEEP DISORDERS
Primary Sleep Disorders
Dyssomnias

307.42 Primary Insomnia
307.44 Primary Hypersomnia

     Specify if: Recurrent

347   Narcolepsy
780.59 Breathing-Related Sleep Disorder
307.45 Circadian Rhythm Sleep Disorder

     Specify type: Delayed Sleep Phase Type/Jet Lag Type/Shift Work Type/Unspecified Type

307.47 Dyssomnia NOS

Parasomnias

307.47 Nightmare Disorder
307.46 Sleep Terror Disorder
307.46 Sleepwalking Disorder
307.47 Parasomnia NOS

Sleep Disorders Related to Another Mental Disorder

307.42 Insomnia Related to . . . *[Indicate the Axis I or Axis II Disorder]*
307.44 Hypersomnia Related to . . . *[Indicate the Axis I or Axis II Disorder]*

Other Sleep Disorders

780.xx Sleep Disorder Due to . . . *[Indicate the General Medical Condition]*
   .52   Insomnia Type
   .54   Hypersomnia Type
   .59   Parasomnia Type
   .59   Mixed Type
___.___ Substance-Induced Sleep Disorder *(refer to Substance-Related Disorders for substance-specific codes)*

     Specify type: Insomnia Type/Hypersomnia Type/Parasomnia Type/Mixed Type
     Specify if: With Onset During Intoxication/With Onset During Withdrawal

IMPULSE-CONTROL DISORDERS NOT ELSEWHERE CLASSIFIED

312.34 Intermittent Explosive Disorder
312.32 Kleptomania
312.33 Pyromania
312.31 Pathologic Gambling
312.39 Trichotillomania
312.30 Impulse-Control Disorder NOS

Adjustment Disorders

309.xx Adjustment Disorder
   .0   With Depressed Mood
   .24   With Anxiety
   .28   With Mixed Anxiety and Depressed Mood
   .3   With Disturbance of Conduct
   .4   With Mixed Disturbance of Emotions and Conduct
   .9   Unspecified

     Specify if: Acute/Chronic

PERSONALITY DISORDERS
Note: *These are coded on Axis II.*

301.0   Paranoid Personality Disorder
301.20 Schizoid Personality Disorder
301.22 Schizotypal Personality Disorder
301.7   Antisocial Personality Disorder
301.83 Borderline Personality Disorder
301.50 Histrionic Personality Disorder
301.81 Narcissistic Personality Disorder
301.82 Avoidant Personality Disorder
301.6   Dependent Personality Disorder
301.4   Obsessive-Compulsive Personality Disorder
301.9   Personality Disorder NOS

OTHER CONDITIONS THAT MAY BE A FOCUS OF CLINICAL ATTENTION
Psychologic Factors Affecting Medical Condition

316   . . . [Specified Psychologic Factor] Affecting . . . *[Indicate the General Medical Condition]*
     Choose name based on nature of factors:
     Mental Disorder Affecting Medical Condition
     Psychologic Symptoms Affecting Medical Condition
     Personality Traits or Coping Style Affecting Medical Condition
     Maladaptive Health Behaviors Affecting Medical Condition
     Stress-Related Physiologic Response Affecting Medical Condition
     Other or Unspecified Psychologic Factors Affecting Medical Condition

Medication-Induced Movement Disorders

332.1   Neuroleptic-Induced Parkinsonism
333.92 Neuroleptic Malignant Syndrome
333.7   Neuroleptic-Induced Acute Dystonia
333.99 Neuroleptic-Induced Acute Akathisia
333.82 Neuroleptic-Induced Tardive Dyskinesia
333.1   Medication-Induced Postural Tremor
333.90 Medication-Induced Movement Disorder NOS

Other Medication-Induced Disorder

995.2   Adverse Effects of Medication NOS

Relational Problems

V61.9   Relational Problem Related to a Mental Disorder or
        General Medical Condition
V61.20 Parent-Child Relational Problem
V61.1   Partner Relational Problem
V61.8   Sibling Relational Problem
V62.81 Relational Problem NOS

PROBLEMS RELATED TO ABUSE OR NEGLECT

V61.21 Physical Abuse of Child *(code 995.5 if focus of atten-
        tion is on victim)*
V61.21 Sexual Abuse of Child *(code 995.5 if focus of attention
        is on victim)*
V61.21 Neglect of Child *(code 995.5 if focus of attention is on
        victim)*
V61.1   Physical Abuse of Adult *(code 995.81 if focus of atten-
        tion is on victim)*
V61.1   Sexual Abuse of Adult *(code 995.81 if focus of atten-
        tion is on victim)*

Additional Conditions That May Be a Focus of Clinical Attention

V15.81 Noncompliance With Treatment
V65.2   Malingering
V71.01 Adult Antisocial Behavior
V71.02 Child or Adolescent Antisocial Behavior
V62.89 Borderline Intellectual Functioning
        Note: *This is coded on Axis II.*
780.9   Age-Related Cognitive Decline
V62.82 Bereavement
V62.3   Academic Problem
V62.2   Occupational Problem
313.82 Identity Problem
V62.89 Religious or Spiritual Problem
V62.4   Acculturation Problem
V62.89 Phase of Life Problem

ADDITIONAL CODES

300.9   Unspecified Mental Disorder (nonpsychotic)
V71.09 No Diagnosis or Condition on Axis I
799.9   Diagnosis or Condition Deferred on Axis I
V71.09 No Diagnosis on Axis II
799.9   Diagnosis Deferred on Axis II

MULTIAXIAL SYSTEM

Axis I   Clinical Disorders
          Other Conditions That May Be a Focus of Clinical
          Attention
Axis II   Personality Disorders
          Mental Retardation
Axis III General Medical Conditions
Axis IV   Psychosocial and Environmental Problems
Axis V   Global Assessment of Functioning

American Nurses Association (ANA) Standards of Psychiatric Mental Health Clinical Nursing Practice

STANDARDS OF CARE

Standard I. Assessment
The psychiatric mental health nurse collects client health data.

Standard II. Diagnosis
The psychiatric mental health nurse analyzes the assessment data in determining diagnoses.

Standard III. Outcome Identification
The psychiatric mental health nurse identifies expected outcomes individualized to the client.

Standard IV. Planning
The psychiatric mental health nurse develops a plan of care that prescribes interventions to attain expected outcomes.

Standard V. Implementation
The psychiatric mental health nurse implements the interventions identified in the plan of care.

Standard Va. Counseling
The psychiatric mental health nurse uses counseling interventions to assist clients in improving or regaining their previous coping abilities, fostering mental health, and preventing mental illness and disability.

Standard Vb. Milieu Therapy
The psychiatric mental health nurse provides, structures, and maintains a therapeutic environment in collaboration with the client and other health care providers.

Standard Vc. Self-Care Activities
The psychiatric mental health nurse structures interventions around the client's activities of daily living to foster self-care and mental and physical well-being.

Standard Vd. Psychobiological Interventions
The psychiatric mental health nurse uses knowledge of psychobiologic interventions and applies clinical skills to restore the client's health and prevent further disability.

From American Nurses Association: *A statement on psychiatric-mental health clinical nursing practice and standards of psychiatric-mental health clinical nursing practice*, Washington, DC, 1994, The Association.

Standard Ve. Health Teaching
The psychiatric mental health nurse, through health teaching, assists clients in achieving satisfying, productive, and healthy patterns of living.

Standard Vf. Case Management
The psychiatric mental health nurse provides case management to coordinate comprehensive health services and ensure continuity of care.

Standard Vg. Health Promotion and Health Maintenance
The psychiatric mental health nurse employs strategies and interventions to promote and maintain mental health and prevent mental illness.

ADVANCED PRACTICE INTERVENTIONS Vh to Vj
The following interventions (Vh to Vj) may be performed only by the certified specialist in psychiatric mental health nursing.

Standard Vh. Psychotherapy
The certified specialist in psychiatric mental health nursing uses individual, group, and family psychotherapy, child psychotherapy, and other therapeutic treatments to assist clients in fostering mental health, preventing mental illness and disability, and improving or regaining previous health status and functional abilities.

Standard Vi. Prescription of Pharmacologic Agents
The certified specialist uses prescription of pharmacologic agents in accordance with the state nursing practice act to treat symptoms of psychiatric illness and improve functional health status.

Standard Vj. Consultation
The certified specialist provides consultation to health care providers and others to influence the plans of care for clients, and to enhance the abilities of others to provide psychiatric and mental health care and effect change in systems.

Standard VI. Evaluation

The psychiatric mental health nurse evaluates the client's progress in attaining expected outcomes.

STANDARDS OF PROFESSIONAL PERFORMANCE

Standard I. Quality of Care

The psychiatric mental health nurse systematically evaluates the quality of care and effectiveness of psychiatric mental health nursing practice.

Standard II. Performance Appraisal

The psychiatric mental health nurse evaluates own psychiatric mental health nursing practice in relation to professional practice standards and relevant statutes and regulations.

Standard III. Education

The psychiatric mental health nurse acquires and maintains current knowledge in nursing practice.

Standard IV. Collegiality

The psychiatric mental health nurse contributes to the professional development of peers, colleagues, and others.

Standard V. Ethics

The psychiatric mental health nurse's decisions and actions on behalf of clients are determined in an ethical manner.

Standard VI. Collaboration

The psychiatric mental health nurse collaborates with the client, significant others, and health care providers in providing care.

Standard VII. Research

The psychiatric mental health nurse contributes to nursing and mental health through the use of research.

Standard VIII. Resource Utilization

The psychiatric mental health nurse considers factors related to safety, effectiveness, and cost in planning and delivering client care.

Mental Health Organizations

Chapter 1 Foundations of Psychiatric Mental Health Nursing

American Mental Health Foundation
2 East 86th Street
New York, NY 10028
(212) 737-9027

American Psychiatric Nurses Association (APNA)
1200 19th Street, NW, Suite 300
Washington, DC 20036-2401
http://www.apna.org

American Public Health Association
1015 15th Street, NW
Washington, DC 20005
(202) 789-5600
http://www.apha.org

Association of Child and Adolescent Psychiatric Nurses, Inc. (ACAPN)
1211 Locust Street
Philadelphia, PA 19107
(800) 826-2950

International Society of Psychiatric Consultation Liaison Nurses (ISPCLN)
7794 Grow Drive
Pensacola, FL 32514
(904) 474-4147

National Association for Mental Health, Inc.
1800 North Kent Street
Rosslyn Station
Arlington, VA 22209

National Institute of Mental Health
6001 Executive Boulevard
Rm. 8184, MSC 9663
Bethesda, MD 20892-9663
(301) 443-4513
http://www.nimh.nih.gov/

National Mental Health Association
1021 Prince Street
Alexandria, VA 22314
http://www.nmha.org

National Mental Health Consumers Association
P.O. Box 1166
Madison, WI 53701

Society for Education and Research in Psychiatric Mental Health Nursing (SERPN)
7794 Grow Drive
Pensacola, FL 32514
(904) 474-9024

World Federation for Mental Health
1021 Prince Street
Alexandria, VA 22314
(703) 684-7722
http://www.wfmh.com

Chapter 5 Legal-Ethical Issues

Bazelon Center for Mental Health Law
1101 15th Street NW, Suite 1212
Washington, DC 20005-5002

National Association for Protection and Advocacy Systems
900 2nd Street NE, Suite 211
Washington, DC 20002

Chapter 6 Cultural Issues

Office of Minority Health
Division of Information and Education
Rockwall II Building, Suite 1000
5600 Fishers Lane
Rockville, MD 20857
(301) 443-5224
http://www.omhrc.gov

Chapter 7 The Nursing Process

North American Nursing Diagnosis Association
1211 Locust St.
Philadelphia, PA 19107
(800) 647-9002

Chapter 9 Children and Adolescents

American Academy of Child and Adolescent Psychiatry
3615 Wisconsin Avenue NW
Washington, DC 20016

Child Welfare League of America
440 1st Street NW, Suite 310
Washington, DC 20001
http://www.cwla.org

National Association of Psychiatric Treatment Centers for Children
2920 Brandywine Street NW
Washington, DC 20008

National Organization of State Associations for Children
2219 California Street NW
Washington, DC 20008

Youth Suicide National Center
445 Virginia Avenue
San Mateo, CA 94402
(415) 342-5755

Youth Suicide Prevention
65 Essex Road
Chestnut Hill, MA 02167
(617) 738-0700

Chapter 11   The Elderly

American Association of Homes for the Aging
901 East Street NW, Suite 500
Washington, DC 20004-2037
(202) 783-2242
http://www.aahsa.org

American Association of Retired Persons
601 East Street NW
Washington, DC 20049
(202) 434-AARP
http://www.aarp.org

Foundation for Hospice and Homecare
519 C Street NE
Washington, DC 20002-5809
(202) 547-6586

International Federation on Aging
1909 K Street
Washington, DC 20049
(202) 662-4987
http://www.ifa-fiv.org

National Council on the Aging
409 3rd Street SW, Suite 200
Washington, DC 20024
(202) 479-1200
http://www.ncoa.org

Chapter 12   Anxiety and Related Disorders

Anxiety Disorders Association of America (ADAA)
6000 Executive Boulevard, Suite 513
Rockville, MD 20852
(301) 231-9350

Obsessive Compulsive Information Center
Dean Foundation
2711 Allen Boulevard
Middleton, WI 53562
(608) 827-2390

Chapter 13   Mood Disorders: Depression and Mania

Depression/Awareness, Recognition and Treatment (D/ART)
National Institute of Mental Health
5600 Fisher Lane, Room 7C-02
Rockville, MD 20857
(301) 443-4513
http://www.nimh.nih.gov

Depression and Related Affective Disorders Association
Johns Hopkins Hospital, Meyer 3-181
600 North Wolfe Street
Baltimore, MD 21205
(410) 955-4647

Depressives Anonymous: Recovery From Depression
329 East 62nd Street
New York, NY 10021
(212) 689-2600

Manic Depressive Association
53 West Jackson Boulevard, Suite 618
Chicago, IL 60654

National Depressive and Manic Depressive Association
730 North Franklin, Suite 501
Chicago, IL 60610
(312) 642-0049

National Foundation for Depressive Illness
P.O. Box 2257
New York City, NY 11016
(212) 268-4260
http://www.depression.org

Chapter 14   The Schizophrenias

American Schizophrenia Association
900 North Federal Highway, Suite 330
Boca Raton, FL 33432
(407) 393-6167

Schizophrenia.com
http://www.schizophrenia.com

Schizophrenics Anonymous
1209 California Road
Eastchester, NY 10709
(914) 337-2252

Chapter 15   Personality Disorders
Neurotics Anonymous International Liaison
11140 Bainbridge Drive
Little Rock, AR 72212
(501) 221-2809

Obsessive-Compulsives Anonymous
P.O. Box 215
New Hyde Park, NY 11040
(516) 741-4901

Chapter 16   Substance-Related Disorders
Adult Children of Alcoholics, Interim World Service Organization
P.O. Box 3216, 2522 West Sepulveda Boulevard
Torrance, CA 90505
(213) 534-1815

Al-Anon/Alateen Family Groups Headquarters
P.O. Box 862, Midtown Station
New York, NY 10018
http://www.al-anon-alateen.org

Alcoholics Anonymous (AA)
General Services Office
P.O. Box 450, Grand Central Station
New York, NY 10164
http://www.alcoholics-anonymous.org

American Council for Drug Education
204 Monroe Street
Rockville, MD 20850
(301) 294-0600
http://www.acde.org

Black Children of Alcoholic and Drug Addicted Persons
c/o National Black Alcoholism Council
417 Dearborn Street
Chicago, IL 60605
(312) 663-5780

Children of Alcoholics
23425 N.W. Highway
Southfield, MI 48075
(313) 353-3567

Children of Alcoholics Foundation, Inc.
200 Park Avenue, 31st Floor
New York, NY 10166
(212) 351-2680

Children Are People Too
493 Selby Avenue
St. Paul, MN 55102
(612) 227-4031

Cocaine Anonymous
3740 Overland Avenue, Suite G
Culver City, CA 90034
(213) 559-5833
http://www.ca.org

Hazelden Foundation
P.O. Box 11
Center City, MN 50012
(800) 328-9000
http://www.hazelden.org

Institute on Black Chemical Abuse
2614 Nicollet Avenue
Minneapolis, MN 55408
(612) 871-7878

International Commission for the Prevention of Alcoholism and Drug Dependency
12501 Old Columbia Pike
Silver Spring, MD 20904
(301) 680-6719

Narcotics Anonymous
P.O. Box 9999
Van Nuys, CA 91409
(818) 780-3951
http://www.na.org

National Association for Children of Alcoholics, Inc.
31582 Coast Highway, Suite B
South Laguna, CA 92677
(714) 499-3889

National Association for Native American Children of Alcoholics (NANACoA)
P.O. Box 18736
Seattle, WA 98114
(206) 322-5601
http://www.nanacoa.org

National Council on Alcoholism and Drug Dependence (NCADD)
12 West 21st Street
New York, NY 10010
(800) NCA-CALL or (212) 206-6770
http://www.ncadd.org

National Institute on Drug Abuse
Parklawn Building, 5600 Fishers Lane
Rockville, MD 20857
(301) 443-6480
http://www.nida.nih.gov

Smoker's Anonymous World Services
2118 Greenwich Street
San Francisco, CA 94123
(415) 922-8575

Chapter 17   Delirium, Dementia, and Amnestic and Other Cognitive Disorders

Alzheimer's Association
360 North Michigan Avenue, Suite 1102
Chicago, IL 60601
(800) 621-0379 (toll free)
(800) 572-6037 (toll free in Illinois)
http://www.alz.org

Alzheimer's Disease Education and Referral Center (A Division of the National Institute on Aging)
P.O. Box 8250
Silver Spring, MD 20907-8250
(800) 438-4380
http://www.alzheimers.org

Alzheimer's Disease International: The International Federation of Alzheimer's Disease and Related Disorders Society, Inc.
919 North Michigan Avenue, Suite 1000
Chicago IL 60611-1676
(312) 335-5777

Family Caregiver Alliance
1736 Divisadero Street
San Francisco, CA 94115
(415) 434-3388
http://www.caregiver.org

Chapter 18   Disorders of Childhood and Adolescence

Association for Children With Down Syndrome
2616 Martin Avenue
Bellmore, NY 11710
(516) 221-4700

Federation for Children With Special Needs
95 Berkeley Street, Suite 104
Boston, MA 02116
(617) 482-2915

Federation of Families for Children's Mental Health
1021 Prince Street
Alexandria, VA 22314-2971
(703) 684-7710
(703) 836-1040 (fax)
http://www.ffcmh.org

National Attention Deficit Disorder Association
42 Way to the River
West Newbury, MA 01985
(508) 462-0495
http://www.add.org

Chapter 19   Eating Disorders

American Anorexia/Bulimia Association (AA/BA)
165 West 46th Street, No. 1108
New York, NY 10036
(212) 575-6200
http://www.aabainc.org

Anorexia Bulimia Care, Inc.
545 Concord Avenue
Cambridge, MA 02138-1122
(617) 492-7670

Anorexia Nervosa and Related Eating Disorders (ANRED)
P.O. Box 5102
Eugene, OR 97405
(503) 344-1144
http://www.anred.com

Eating Disorders Awareness and Prevention (EDAP)
603 Stewart Street, No. 803
Seattle, WA 98101
(206) 382-3587
http://members.aol.com/edapinc/home.html

Massachusetts Eating Disorders Association, Inc. (MEDA)
92 Pearl Street
Newton, MA 02158
(617) 558-1881
http://www.medainc.org

National Anorexic Aid Society
1925 East Dublin-Granville Road
Columbus, OH 43229
(614) 436-1112

National Association of Anorexia Nervosa and Associated Disorders
P.O. Box 7
Highland Park, IL 60035
(847) 831-3438
http://members.aol.com/anad20/mdet.html

National Eating Disorders Screening Program
1 Washington Street, No. 304
Wellesley Hills, MA 02181
(781) 239-0071
http://www.nmisp.org

Overeaters Anonymous (OA)
P.O. Box 44020
Rio Rancho, NM 87174-4020
(505) 891-2664
http://www.overeatersanonymous.org

Additional Web sites:
http://www.laureate.com
http://www.gurze.com
http://www.eating-disorder.com

Chapter 27   Survivors of Violence

Batterers Anonymous
8485 Tamarind, Suite D
Fontana, CA 92335
(714) 355-1100

National Clearinghouse on Child Abuse and Neglect Information
330 C Street SW
Washington, DC 20447
(800) 394-3366 or (703) 385-7565
(703) 385-3206 (fax)
http://www.calib.com/nccanch

National Woman Abuse Prevention Project
1112 16th Street NW, Suite 920
Washington, DC 20036
(202) 857-0216

People Against Rape
P.O. Box 5318
River Forest, IL 60305
(708) 452-0737

Survivors of Incest Anonymous
P.O. Box 21817
Baltimore, MD 21222
(410) 433-2365

Women in Crisis
133 West 21st Street, 11th Floor
New York, NY 10011
(212) 242-4880

Chapter 30   Persons With AIDS

AIDS Action Council
729 8th Street SE, Suite 200
Washington, DC 20003
http://www.aidsaction.org

AIDS Prevention League
291 Crosby Street
Akron, OH 44303
(216) 476-4384

Chapter 32   Persons With Chronic Mental Illness

International Committee Against Mental Illness
P.O. Box 1921, Grand Central Station
New York, NY 10163
(914) 359-7387

National Alliance for the Mentally Ill (NAMI)
200 North Glebe Road
Suite 1015
Arlington, VA 22203
(800) 950-6264
http://www.nami.org

Chapter 33   Community Psychiatric Nursing Mental Health

Association of Community Health Nursing Educators
315 Con/HSLC Building
Lexington, KY
(606) 233-6534

Center for Family Support
386 Park Avenue South
New York, NY 10016
(212) 481-1082

Emotional Health Anonymous
P.O. Box 63236
Los Angeles, CA 90063-0236
(213) 268-7220
http://www.emotionsanonymous.org

National Association of Psychiatric Survivors
P.O. Box 618
Sioux Falls, SD 57101
(605) 334-4067

Cultural Competence in Clinical Practice/Implications for Nursing

Cultural competence refers to a set of practice standards developed and instituted by county health and county mental health departments in states across the country. They are required by specific managed care providers and other health care payers. The purpose of cultural competence is to ensure that clients of all cultures are given every opportunity to receive information about treatment in ways that they understand, considering their education, acculturation, and language.

SUMMARY OF CULTURAL COMPETENCE STANDARDS IN CLINICAL PRACTICE

Availability of professional interpreters who are capable of effectively communicating with the population they serve

A multicultural, multilingual staff who effectively represent the community they serve

Psychologic testing that is culturally sound and appropriate for the ethnically diverse population

Cultural components as part of the client admission interview, treatment plan, education plan, interventions, and discharge plan

Use of resources, including family and community, in helping clients meet cultural needs

Physician recognition of cultural factors that play a role in treatment compliance

Involvement in culturally competent community research and training

Provider involvement in ongoing cultural competence self-assessment

Agency/facility involvement in ongoing cultural competence self-assessment

Each cultural competence standard is accompanied by a series of objectives and outcomes for that standard. Methods of outcome and measurement include the following:

Submission of written protocols such as documentation in the medical record of how the language needs of the client were met.

Quarterly and annual reports, including an annual program review of the bilingual proficiency of staff and other agency support positions.

Periodic site reviews by designated county reviewers.

Client satisfaction survey reports in culturally sensitive areas.

Documentation in the medical record of client orientation, education, treatment goals, legal issues, program expectations of the client and provider, and confidentiality that meet cultural needs.

Availability of a clinic/hospital brochure describing treatment services in the preferred language of the client.

Minimum of 4 hours required for staff training per year, with submission of a report listing staff names and hours of cultural competence training. The staff training log must be kept on site.

A procedure/protocol for psychologists to access consultation when needed for assessment of ethnically diverse clients. This is to be documented in the client's medical record.

SUMMARY

In the current multilingual and ethnically diverse environment, the nurse and other health care providers are important advocates in helping clients and families understand and comply with treatment. This is particularly critical in the area of mental health, given the complex terminology and myriad behaviors and symptoms that require accurate interpretation by a culturally aware staff. Interpreters must be able to attach accurate meaning and purpose to a client's language so that nursing implications for effective treatment are clearly understood. Cultural diversity helps nurses and other health care disciplines recognize that people are more alike than different and that everyone deserves the best possible physical and psychologic treatment, regardless of language, culture, or ethnicity.

REFERENCE
Friedenberg J et al: *Cultural competence clinical practice standards*, San Diego, 1996-1997, San Diego County Department of Health Services.

Classification Systems

NURSING INTERVENTIONS CLASSIFICATION

Definition and Purpose

The Nursing Interventions Classification (NIC) is the first comprehensive standardized classification of treatments performed by nurses. The classification was researched and developed from 1987 through 1995 by the members of the Iowa Intervention Project Research Team, and its work was published in 1992 and again in 1996. The classification includes 433 interventions that nurses do for clients, whether collaborative or independent, or whether the care given is direct or indirect. The classification is used in all specialties and settings by both novice and seasoned practitioners. NIC interventions can be physiologic, such as airway suctioning and decubitus ulcer care, or psychosocial, such as anxiety reduction and assisting the client with coping skills. NIC interventions are effective in the treatment of physical or psychiatric illnesses, such as hypertension or cognitive disturbances, respectively. They are equally effective in preventing various types of illnesses, such as fall prevention or prevention of self-harm. NIC interventions are also used in health promotion, such as education about the health hazards of smoking, the value of good nutrition, and the importance of stress reduction. The purposed of NIC is to identify and refine nursing actions from groups of data found throughout current nursing texts and literature and to construct a taxonomy in which interventions can be systematically organized, with clear rules and principles for the interventions selected.

Research Methodology

Time-proven research methods were employed by the Iowa team to distinguish and refine the most relevant intervention labels from the myriad associated activities that accompanied the nursing problems or nursing diagnoses. Typically, most textbooks that were researched included several hundred of these "interventions," and quite often these actions were a combination of assessment and treatment activities, as well as a mixture of nurse-initiated and physician-initiated actions. During the analysis of content, the team discovered that each intervention label had anywhere from one to several hundred associated activities. Also, the lists of interventions for the same diagnosis varied enormously from one text to another. Research used in the expert surveys included a two-round Delphi questionnaire; responses from the first round of questions were used to modify the questionnaire during the second round. The process was such that groups of related intervention labels were ultimately selected as a result of an in-depth investigation process by nursing professionals. Lists of accompanying activities were computer generated, and participants were asked to create each activity according to the extent to which it was characteristic of the label. Fehring's research methodology was adapted for use with interventions and yielded intervention content validity (ICV) scores with critical and supporting activities. (Johnson and Maas, 1997).

Intervention Selection

NIC proposes that the following six factors be considered when selecting an intervention:

1. Desired client outcome
2. Characteristics of the nursing diagnosis
3. Research base for the intervention
4. Feasibility of performing the intervention
5. Acceptability of the intervention to the client
6. Capability of the nurse

Client Outcomes

Client outcomes should be identified before selecting an intervention, since effectiveness of nursing interventions is judged against outcome criteria. Outcomes describe the behaviors and feelings of the client in response to the care given. Many variables influence outcomes, which make it challenging for the nurse and other providers to determine a causal relationship between the nursing intervention and client outcomes. These variables include the following:

The clinical problem
The interventions prescribed
The health care providers
The environment in which care is received
The client's own motivation
The client's genetic structure and pathophysiology
The client's significant others

Pinkly (1991, cited in McCloskey and Bulechek, 1996) suggests that nurses should choose outcomes that apply to all of the identified nursing diagnoses, not just select outcomes aimed toward ameliorating the etiology of one diagnosis. Pinkly also states that the choosing of outcomes should be directed at maximizing health, as well as alleviating problems.

Summary

In conclusion, NIC represents a major effort to clearly define the treatments and activities performed by nurses, who make up the largest group of health care professionals in the world. Although nursing care is a critical component in client wellness and satisfaction, the specific impact of nursing care is often lost and difficult to measure. The following are a sampling of some critical questions that need to be addressed:

> What actions belong to the domain of nursing?
> How do these actions make a difference in the quality of care received?
> Are some nursing actions just as effective but less costly than care given by other disciplines?

Intervention Selection

The members of the Iowa Intervention Project Research Team continue to develop and refine the research of NIC in an effort to respond to these and other questions critical to the profession of nursing in the years ahead. For more information on NIC, refer to the work cited in McCloskey and Bulechek (1996) and other current literature.

NIC and NANDA Links

Like the North American Nursing Diagnosis Association (NANDA) taxonomy, NIC also serves to standardize language, which is a critical step toward validating a profession. Unlike NANDA, the phenomenon of concern with nursing interventions is nurse behavior or nurse activity (i.e., those things that nurses do to assist client status and client behavior to move toward an effective outcome), whereas the phenomenon of concern for nursing diagnoses or client outcomes sensitive to nursing care is the client behavior or client status. The widespread use of NANDA's nursing diagnosis language, which has been used throughout this text and others, has been instrumental in promoting an awareness of the need to standardize classifications in the areas of interventions and outcomes. Examples of major coded classifications include NANDA, NIC, ICD-10, and DSM-IV (see McCloskey and Bulechek, 1996, pp. 10-12).

NURSING OUTCOMES CLASSIFICATION

Definition and Purpose

The Nursing Outcomes Classification (NOC) presents the first comprehensive, standardized language used to describe client outcomes that are responsive to nursing interventions. The classification was developed by members of the Nursing-Sensitive Outcomes Classification team, which began its research in August 1991 and published its work in 1997. The classification currently contains 190 outcomes with indicators (e.g., observable client states, behaviors, or self-reported perceptions) that nurses can use to assess the effects of the interventions. Each outcome has a label (name); a definition; a set of indications; a measurement scale, which is in the process of being refined; and references. Indicators are selected based on the specific circumstance for an individual or client population. The nursing-sensitive outcomes are presented as neutral concepts that reflect a client's physical state, such as mobility or hydration, or psychologic state, such as coping or grieving. The team contends that neutral outcomes can be measured on a continuum, which differs from discrete goals, which are either met or unmet. The team believes that this neutral state helps nurses to identify and analyze outcomes recently achieved for specific client populations, as well as to identify realistic standards of care for specific populations. For example, clients can be aggregated in myriad ways, such as by nursing or medical diagnoses, or by service unit or illness acuity; and the difference in outcomes achievement can be analyzed by client characteristics, such as age, gender, or functional states. The NOC method of outcome selection is considered more effective than the usual practice, which is to set one standard or select a single goal for all clients, regardless of individual characteristics, which tends to produce ineffective outcomes attainment.

Research Methodology

The research team conducted two pilot studies to test content validity in measuring nursing-sensitive outcomes and indicators. Client satisfaction was included in the methodology. A literature review revealed client satisfaction with the following items:

> Safety
> Physical environment
> Availability of and access to care
> Providing client rights
> Caring
> Technical aspects of care
> Meeting physical needs
> Continuity of care
> Functional state
> Teaching/counseling
> Communication
> Symptom management
> Finances

Methodology and Conceptual Resolution

Following an in-depth literature search to identify and resolve methodology issues, the NOC team developed the following seven questions that provided the conceptual approach for NOC:

1. Who is the client?
2. What do client outcomes describe?

3. How abstract should outcomes be when developed?

4. How should outcomes be worded?

5. What are nursing-sensitive outcomes (e.g., outcomes that define the general client state, behavior, or self-reported perception resulting from nursing interventions?)

6. Are nursing-sensitive outcomes the resolution of nursing diagnoses?

7. When should client outcomes be measured?

Summary

The NOC was developed to fulfill the need to standardize and enhance the structure and language of nursing and its profession as a full participant in health care restructuring. For nurses to work effectively in the managed care environment and to improve quality and reduce costs, they must be able to accurately measure and document patient outcomes, which are influenced by nursing actions. Although it is widely accepted that nursing care is a strong driver in client satisfaction and wellness, the precise effect that nursing care has on client outcomes may remain lost and unmeasured if nurses continue to rely on physician-driven data only to meet client care needs. Nurses must persist in the effort to develop a common language or nomenclature that is used to organize the phenomena of nursing practice, while continuing to individualize the client.

Links to NIC and NANDA

The development of the NOC and NIC classification systems were clearly influenced by NANDA, whose standardization of a taxonomic structure for the classification of nursing diagnoses began in 1973, was formalized in 1982, and continues to develop and evolve. All three classifications strive to develop and refine a standard language that assists nurses in making decisions for health care practices and policies as managed competition in health care evolves. NOC, NIC, and NANDA are comprehensive companions that provide impetus in the teaching of diagnostic reasoning, critical thinking, and the continued development and refinement of nursing theory and knowledge.

REFERENCES

Johnson M, Maas ML, editors: *Nursing outcomes classification (NOC)*, St. Louis, 1997, Mosby.

McCloskey JC, Bulechek GM, editors: *Nursing interventions classification (NIC)*, ed 2, St. Louis, 1996, Mosby.

Managed Care

HISTORY AND DEVELOPMENT

Managed care is a generic term that refers to a wide variety of health care practices developed to regulate the rising costs of health care in the United States. An early model of managed care is known as the health maintenance organization (HMO). HMOs have been in existence since 1973, although by 1982 only 6% of the people in the United States were HMO members. However, since 1990, managed care practices have been used in a variety of ways across America, and most large companies have implemented managed care programs to provide health insurance coverage to their employees and often to their families.

KEY TERMS

1. *Managed care:* An oversight system of insurers or payers that monitors the delivery of health care, with the goal of controlling or reducing costs.

2. *Health Maintenance Organization (HMO):* An early model of managed care that provides or insures health care services for enrolled members under a prepaid sum or capitation arrangement.

3. *Capitation:* Payment given to a provider for a fixed fee per person that covers a defined range of health care services for a designated period of time, generally 1 year.

4. *Fee for service:* A commonly used health care reimbursement method based on services rendered, which is most likely a major factor in rising health care costs.

5. *Carve-out:* The separation of mental health from general medical benefits.

6. *Prospective payments:* A fixed fee that providers receive for delivery of health care during a defined illness episode. Diagnosis-related groups (DRGs) are the most common example of prospective payment for general health care. In mental health a typical example is the fixed target date per discharge that private hospitals receive for inpatient care for Medicare-insured clients, regardless of the client's length of stay or the amount of services rendered (Worley, 1997).

MANAGED CARE IN MENTAL HEALTH

The business sector has had a great influence on the effects of managed care in mental health. Twenty cents of every health care dollar is being spent on mental health services (Hilts, 1991, cited in Worley, 1997). Both public and private care sectors are working on ways to improve managed care as a cost-effective method of delivering mental health services. Managed care is more complicated in the mental health arena than in the general medical setting because of the need to establish relations between acute and long-term care, between medical and social services, and between services provided by physicians and those provided by the health care disciplines (Mechanic, 1993, cited in Worley, 1997). As a result of these differences in health care services, many insurance companies and other managed care companies have "carved out" the mental health benefit program and capitated it separately from other medical services. Therefore providers of mental health benefits are leery that these services will be overused; as a result, insurance policies tend to set different limits for psychiatric services than for other medical care. Psychiatric services tend to have higher deductibles, higher insurance rates (the percentage of the cost paid by the insured at the time of service), and lower utilization limits. Presently, managed care seems to afford greater access to health care than does fee-for-service case in the mental health sector, but it still limits critical services such as hospitalization, care given by a psychiatrist versus care given by other mental health professionals, and individual therapy versus group therapy (Mechanic, 1993, cited in Worley, 1997). A major crisis exists in the public sector that primarily serves a population of seriously and chronically mentally ill clients, whose needs include medical care, case management, housing, and rehabilitation. Many states are currently experimenting with more effective managed care methods for this chronically mentally ill population. Managed care has long been an agenda item for legislators in Washington, D.C., who have recently expressed the need for some reform in both the medical and the mental health sectors.

PSYCHIATRIC MENTAL HEALTH NURSING AND MANAGED CARE

The health care system's move from the hospital as the main service center of care to managed care regulations and provider oversights has had a major effect on psychiatry and psychiatric nursing. Immediate changes include the closing of psychiatric hospitals or units, the downsizing of staff, and the elimination of positions (Himali, 1995, cited in Worley, 1997). On the positive side, these changes are also forcing an expansion of the boundaries of practice and creating opportunities for practice along a broader health care continuum, which will benefit psychiatric mental health nurses in the long term. With the reduction in hospital days, there is a greater need for psychiatric home care, partial hospitalization, case management, and other supportive rehabilitative services. There are also opportunities for nurses to transfer education of patients and families from the hospital setting to the family and community environment. At the organizational level, medical record auditing and utilization review, as part of the clinical case management system, are critical elements of nursing skills needed to justify client acuity, inpatient treatment, length of stay, and reimbursement. At the clinical level, nurses will be motivated to develop innovative treatment programs and critical or clinical pathways that ensure managed care reimbursement. With the expansion of the nurse's role in mental health, there is an opportunity to focus on the actions and language of nursing, such as nursing diagnoses and client outcomes that are sensitive to nursing actions and interventions. As the population ages and the life span increases, nurses with a broad biopsychosocial background have greater opportunities in the expanding field of geropsychiatric nursing. Not to be ignored are the myriad opportunities for innovative nurses to manage wellness programs, stress reduction workshops, parenting classes, and illness prevention programs. The role of the school nurse now includes opportunities to work with a team of experts and parents, to help children diagnosed with attention-deficit disorder, dyslexia, and other problems that interfere with academic success and peer relations. Education involving diabetes mellitus, hypertension, smoking, and drugs and alcohol are fertile areas for community-based nursing.

SUMMARY

Managed care in the mental health environment provides a genuine challenge for psychiatry and psychiatric mental health nursing. During this juncture of managed care, it seems certain that the larger portion of mental health services will take place in the community versus the hospital setting. Psychiatric mental health nurses can respond by viewing these changes as opportunities to transfer their broad-based skills from the hospital to the home, the school, and the community. It is the comprehensive theory and practice of nursing, and not the environment of care, that defines nursing as a science and a profession. The broad background of biology, psychosocial knowledge, cultural competence, pharmacotherapy, and other treatment modalities allows nurses to flourish and succeed regardless of the type of health care services or setting. As psychiatric mental health nursing leaves the nineties and approaches the twenty-first century, opportunities in the managed care environment, no matter what shape it will take, appear limitless.

REFERENCE

Worley NK: *Mental health nursing in the community*, St. Louis, 1997, Mosby.

GLOSSARY

Abstinence   Voluntary refraining from a behavior or the use of a substance that has caused problems in psychosocial, biologic, cognitive/perceptual, or spiritual/belief dimensions of life, especially with regard to food, alcohol, or drugs.

Abuse   A maladaptive pattern of substance use leading to problems in psychosocial, biologic, cognitive/perceptual, or spiritual/belief dimensions of life.

Acculturation   The process of adapting to another culture.

Acting-out   The expression of internal affective states through external activities and behaviors, which are often destructive and/or maladaptive.

Activities of daily living (ADLs)   Categories of personal care (e.g., bathing, grooming, toileting).

Activity theory   Supports that maintaining an active lifestyle and social roles offsets the negative effects of aging.

Acute grief   The initial response to loss. Although it diminishes over time, acute grief may last for as long as several years, primarily depending on the meaning of the lost person/object for the survivor.

Adaptation   A constant, ongoing process that occurs along the time continuum and includes the dimensions of health and illness, beginning with birth and ending with death. It involves both cognitive and physiologic neural-chemical-endocrine processes.

Adjunct therapy   An action-oriented process with the primary intention of fostering adaptation and productivity for the purpose of minimizing pathology and promoting the maintenance of health.

Adjustment disorder   A short-term disturbance in mood or behavior with nonpsychotic manifestations resulting from identifiable stressors. The severity of the reaction is not predictable by the severity of the stressor.

Adult developmental theory   This theory suggests that although persons may complete developmental tasks of childhood, they continue to evolve as maturity progresses. Adulthood is divided into four age categories, and central themes of adult experience and development are articulated.

Adverse drug reaction   An unintended effect of a medication resulting in severe, unwanted symptoms or consequences.

Affect   Outward, bodily expression of emotions, ranging through joy, sorrow, anger, etc. **Blunted affect:** Restricted expression of emotions. **Flat affect:** Lack of outward expression of emotions. **Inappropriate affect:** Affect that is not congruent with the emotion being felt (e.g., laughing when sad). **Labile affect:** Rapid changes in emotional expression.

Affective instability   Rapidly fluctuating moods in which the individual is emotionally reactive to external events and lacks coping skills to manage feeling states.

Ageism   Systematic stereotyping and discrimination against the elderly.

Agnosia   The loss of comprehension of auditory, visual, or other sensations, although the senses are intact.

Agonist   A chemical that results in stimulation of activity of the target receptor.

Agranulocytosis   A drop in the production of leukocytes, specifically the neutrophil cell line, leaving the body defenseless against bacterial infection.

AIDS dementia complex (ADC)   A progressive neurologic syndrome caused by a subacute chronic HIV encephalitis. Cognitive impairment indicative of damage to the central nervous system is evidenced in these clients.

AIDS wasting syndrome (AWS)   During the later stages of AIDS, clients may experience a significant weight loss. A condition of an unexplained weight loss of 10%, along with chronic diarrhea, fatigue, or unexplained fever, and a loss of muscle mass, may occur during the later stages of AIDS.

Akathisia   Literally, "not sitting." A syndrome caused by dopamine-blocking drugs characterized by both motor restlessness and a subjective feeling of inner restlessness.

Alcoholism   A chronic, progressive, and potentially fatal biogenic and psychosocial disease characterized by impaired control over drinking, tolerance, and physical dependence that lead to loss of control, distorted thinking, and other social consequences.

Allopathic   The health beliefs and practices that are derived from the scientific models of the present time and involve the use of technology and other modalities of present-day health care, such as immunization, proper nutrition, and resuscitation.

Alpha$_1$ blockade   The process of inhibiting α_1-receptors that may result in orthostatic hypotension and reflex tachycardia.

Alter ego   A function of the therapist to reflect back the client's attitudes and feelings without including the client's negative connotations.

Alzheimer's disease A neurodegenerative disease characterized by progressive, irreversible, and lethal structural damage to the brain due to the presence of β-amyloid proteins and leading to loss of cognitive functions and symptoms of progressive dementia.

Analysis Taking apart collected data to examine and interpret each piece and identify variations from typical behaviors or responses. Discovering patterns or relationships in the data that may be cues or clues that require further investigation.

Anhedonia The loss of pleasure and interest in activities previously enjoyed or in life itself.

Anorexia nervosa An eating disorder classified in DSM-IV, characterized by self-starvation, weight loss below minimum normal weight, intense fear of being fat even when emaciated, distorted body image, and amenorrhea in females.

Antagonist A chemical that results in inhibition of activity of the target receptor.

Anticholinergic delirium Toxic effects of anticholinergic drugs characterized by confusion, perceptive disturbances, sleep disturbance, increased or decreased psychomotor activity, and change in level of consciousness. Also called atropine psychosis, this syndrome may present as a psychotic state.

Anticipatory grief Grief experienced before death or loss occurs (e.g., when a loved one has a terminal illness).

Antiretroviral therapy The use of drugs, such as AZT, ddI, and ddC. These drugs, often administered to clients via drug trials, treat the major opportunistic diseases associated with AIDS. Treatment with antiretroviral therapy can significantly affect the progression of AIDS by preventing opportunistic infections.

Anxiety A vague, subjective, nonspecific feeling of uneasiness, tension, apprehension, and sometimes dread or pending doom. Occurs as a result of a threat to one's biologic, physiologic, or social integrity arising from external influences. A universal experience and an integral part of human existence.

Aphasia *Expressive aphasia:* The inability to speak or write (also known as Broca's aphasia). **Global aphasia:** The complete loss of all motor and sensory uses of oral and written speech; expression and comprehension are severely impaired. **Receptive aphasia:** The inability to comprehend what is being said or written (also known as Wernicke's aphasia).

Appraisal As related to crisis, the ongoing perceptual process by which a potentially harmful event is distinguished from a potentially beneficial or irrelevant event.

Apraxia The loss of the ability to carry out purposeful, complex movements and to use objects properly.

Art medium Material or technical means of artistic expression.

Art therapy The use of artistic activities, such as painting and clay modeling, in psychotherapy and rehabilitation.

Assimilation To become absorbed into another culture and to adopt its characteristics.

Attending Demonstrating to a client attention to what he or she is saying.

Atypical depression Depression with features that include hypersomnia, weight gain, mood reactivity, and sensitivity in interpersonal relationships.

Autism A pervasive developmental disorder characterized by marked impairment of social and cognitive abilities.

Autodiagnosis Self-examination of one's own thoughts, feelings, perceptions, and attitudes about a particular client.

Autonomy versus shame and doubt Erikson's term for the second developmental crisis. Parental encouragement toward self-sufficiency in basic tasks of toileting, dressing, and feeding foster autonomy. Thwarted efforts by overcontrolling or undercontrolling parents result in the polar opposite, or shame and doubt. Shame is rage turned against the self. Doubt is an internal feeling of badness.

Battered women Women who are abused physically or mentally by their male intimates or those with whom they have been intimate.

Behavioral reorganization A new way of viewing development, emphasizing that new developmental capabilities are fit together and organized into previous capabilities in an orderly, patterned, and predictable fashion and build in a cumulative manner from earlier capabilities in a direction of greater complexity.

Bereavement The state of grieving.

Binge eating disorder (BED) A pattern of binge eating without the purging characteristic of bulimia nervosa. BED is commonly known as compulsive overeating. It is included in DSM-IV as a proposed diagnosis for further study.

Bioavailability The amount, usually described as a percentage, of a drug administered that reaches the blood.

Bipolar disorder A mood disorder characterized by episodes of mania and depression.

Blackout Acute anterograde amnesia without recognition formation of long-term memory (e.g., a period of memory loss during which there is no recall for activities, resulting from the ingestion of alcohol and/or other drugs).

Body image disturbance A perceptual disturbance in the way individuals subjectively perceive and experience their body shape, size, weight, and proportions. Typically, persons with anorexia complain of feeling "fat" or see their stomach/hips/thighs as fat when they are clearly underweight.

Body knowledge An "embodied" knowledge that allows a person to recognize familiar and unfamiliar mental, emotional, and body mechanisms—a sense of balance/imbalance changes.

Boundary The definition and separation of the self from others through the clarification of the limits and extent of responsibilities and duties of one's self in relationship to others.

Boundary violations Going beyond the established therapeutic relationship standards.

Bulimarexia An obsession with thinness, dieting, and a compulsive cycle of bingeing and purging. This syndrome is now labeled bulimia nervosa.

Bulimia nervosa An eating disorder classified in DSM-IV, characterized by recurrent episodes of binge eating subjectively experienced as out of control, followed by inappropriate compensatory behavior to prevent weight gain, such as self-induced vomiting; overuse of laxatives, diuretics, or diet pills; fasting; or excessive exercise. Also present is excessive preoccupation with body shape and weight.

Case finding The methodic and deliberate identification of people of any age who are ill and in need of care or who are at risk for incurring illness and injury.

Catastrophic reaction A sudden or gradual negative change in the behavior of dementia clients caused by their inability to understand and cope with stimuli in the environment.

CD4 count The CD4 lymphocyte count (T4 cell count) is the most commonly used marker to determine HIV progression. HIV attacks CD4 cells that help fight infections.

Chemical restraint The use of psychotropic drugs and sedatives to reduce or eliminate psychiatric symptoms.

Childhood incest Any type of exploitative sexual experience between relatives or surrogate relatives before the victim reaches the age of 18.

Child neglect Harm or threatened harm to a child's health or welfare by a parent, legal guardian, or any other person responsible for the child's health or welfare through either (1) failure to provide adequate food, clothing, shelter, or medical care, or (2) placing the child at unreasonable risk to health or welfare.

Child physical abuse Injury inflicted on a child that can range from minor bruises and lacerations to severe neurologic trauma and death. Psychologic abuse is also included.

Child psychologic abuse Rejection, degradation/devaluation, terrorization, isolation, corruption, exploitation, denying essential stimulation to a child, and unreliable and inconsistent parenting.

Chronic mental illness A psychiatric disorder that persists over time with remissions and recurrence of severe, disabling symptoms.

Chronic sorrow Grief in response to an ongoing loss, such as chronic illness in a loved one.

Chronically mentally ill Persons who have manifested the symptoms of chronic mental illness.

Clear and convincing evidence A burden of proof that requires more than the preponderance of evidence used in a civil proceeding and less than the "beyond a reasonable doubt" used in a criminal proceeding.

Clinical pathway A standardized format used to provide and monitor client care and progress by way of the case management, interdisciplinary health care delivery system. (Also known as critical pathway, care path, or Care Map.)

Closure Also called sharing. The last stage in a psychodrama or movement/dance therapy experience in which the experience is processed (verbally and nonverbally) and insight and a sense of completion are promoted.

Codependency An emotional, psychologic, and behavioral pattern of coping that an individual develops as a result of prolonged exposure to a dysfunctional pattern of behavior within the family of origin. The individual experiences difficulty with identity development and setting functional boundaries, which lead to taking care of others rather than self.

Cognition Awareness and subjective meaning of an event.

Cognitive rigidity The inability to adequately identify problems and corresponding solutions.

Cognitive triad A pattern of thinking noted in depressed people and characterized by (1) a negative self-assessment, (2) a negative view of the present, and (3) a negative view of the future.

Cohort A group united by one or more common factors.

Collegiality Working within a body of associates or colleagues (e.g., a team of home care providers).

Commitment A court order certifying that an individual is to be confined to a mental health facility for treatment.

Communication A reciprocal process of sending and receiving messages between two or more people and their environment; the vehicle for establishing a therapeutic relationship.

Community-linked health care Care provided by public and/or private partnerships using grant and government funds.

Comorbidity The co-occurrence of two or more psychiatric or other disorders. The simultaneous appearance of the disorders may be due to a causal relationship between the two or an underlying predisposition to both, or the disorders may be completely unrelated. For example, depression is a common comorbid disorder in clients with eating disorders. There are different theories about the association between eating disorders and mood disorders. Also known as dual diagnosis.

Compensatory developmental task Developmental tasks that deal with replacing losses with some other mechanism (e.g., developing new skills or hobbies after retirement).

Competency to stand trial The ability of the individual to understand the charges and the consequences, to understand the nature and object of the legal proceedings, and to advise an attorney and assist in the defense.

Compulsion An unremitting, repetitive impulse to perform a behavior (e.g., hand washing, ordering, checking) or mental acts (e.g., praying, counting, or repeating words silently), the goal of which is to prevent or reduce anxiety or distress and not to provide pleasure or gratification. In most cases the person feels driven to perform the compulsion to reduce the distress that accompanies an obsession or to prevent some dreaded event or situation.

Concentrated care Also called "intensive" care. Home care services delivered during a crisis, usually on a short-term basis, and designed to meet a specific, acute need.

Concrete operational period Piaget's term for the third stage of cognitive development whereby the child begins to think and reason in logical ways about the present and the past.

Confidentiality The right of the psychiatric client to keep information from people outside the health care team.

Congruence Consistency of agreement between verbal and nonverbal behavior.

Conscious suicidal intention A state of awareness characterized by a person's desire to accomplish death through self-means.

Continuity theory Promotes the premise that people become "more like themselves" as they age, maintaining continuity of habits, beliefs, and values.

Conventional morality Kohlberg's second stage of morality whereby moral decisions consider the perspective of the victim and are first based on a desire for approval from others to avoid guilt, and later based on defined rights, assigned duty, rules of the community, and respect for authority.

Conversion reaction A repression of an emotional problem by replacing it with a physical symptom. Most often involves the sensory organs or voluntary nervous system.

Coping Various strategies used, consciously or unconsciously, to deal with stress and tensions arising from perceived threats to psychologic integrity. It is the process of attempting to solve life problems.

Countertransference The nurse's irrational and inappropriate responses to a client because of a personal problem.

Creativity The ability to apply original ideas to the solution of problems; the development of theories, techniques, or devices; or the production of novel forms of art, literature, philosophy, or science.

Crisis A turning point marked by sharp improvement or sharp deterioration. A decision or event of great psychologic significance for an individual.

Crisis intervention Therapeutic techniques for helping individuals experiencing a crisis.

Crisis theory A theory that examines conscious coping abilities and unconscious defense mechanisms and how they help or inhibit interaction with the individual. Crises are separated into three categories: maturational, situational, and adventitious.

Cross-tolerance A condition in which tolerance to one drug often results in tolerance to chemically similar drugs. Tolerance is originally produced by long-term administration of one drug, which is manifested toward a second drug that has not been administered previously (e.g., tolerance to alcohol is accompanied by cross-tolerance to volatile anesthetics of barbiturates).

Decanoate Decanoic (10 carbon) acid ester, which is linked to the antipsychotics fluphenazine and haloperidol to create the long-acting antipsychotics. Dissolved in sesame oil and injected intramuscularly or subcutaneously, the rate-limiting pharmacokinetic step is the cleavage of the decanoate bond to release the active drug.

Defense   A means or method of protecting oneself; an unconscious mental activity or mental structure (e.g., a defense mechanism) that protects the ego from anxiety.

Defense mechanism   A structure of the psyche that protects the ego against unpleasant feelings or impulses. Defense mechanisms are unconscious and deny, falsify, or distort reality.

Deinstitutionalization   The process of returning psychiatric clients to the community, which includes limited admission and commitment policies.

Delayed grief   Grief that is not expressed or experienced until well after a loss, often as a result of circumstances such as being focused on survival (as among refugees).

Delirium   A disturbance of consciousness and a change in cognition that develop over a short period of time and tend to fluctuate during the course of the day, characterized by disorientation to time and place; reduced ability to focus, sustain, or shift attention; incoherent speech; and continual aimless physical activity.

Delusions   False beliefs that are fixed and resistant to reasoning.

Dementia   A global impairment of intellectual (cognitive) functions (e.g., thinking, remembering, reasoning) that usually is progressive and of sufficient severity to interfere with a person's normal social and occupational functioning.

Denial   A range of psychologic maneuvers designed to decrease awareness of the fact that substance use is the cause of an individual's problems rather than a solution to the problems.

Dependence, physical   A physiologic state of adaptation to a drug or alcohol, usually characterized by the development of tolerance to the drug's effects and the emergence of a withdrawal syndrome during prolonged abstinence.

Dependence, psychologic   The compulsive use of substances leading to a state of craving a drug or alcohol for its positive effect or to avoid negative effects associated with its absence, or the inability to exercise behavioral restraint.

Dependency ratio   The number of individuals below the age of 18 and over the age of 64 who are dependent on those persons ages 18 to 64.

Depo-Lupron Leuprolide   A synthetic analog of naturally occurring gonadotropin-releasing hormone. It inhibits gonadotropin secretion, thus suppressing testicular testosterone.

Depo-Lupron Medroxyprogesterone acetate   A medication used in the adjunctive treatment of sexual disorders; a sexual appetite suppressant; lowers testosterone level to a prepubescent level.

Derealization   The feeling that the surrounding world is not real or is distorted.

Dereism   A loss of connection with reality and logic that occurs just before autistic thinking. Thoughts become private and idiosyncratic. Dereism is seen in schizophrenia.

Detoxification   A treatment that helps the individual withdraw from the physical effects of alcohol and/or other addictive substances and helps eliminate severe withdrawal symptoms that can occur with abrupt withdrawal. It can be provided in a hospital setting, day treatment, or outpatient setting.

Devaluation   A method of coping whereby a person deals with emotional conflict or stressors by attributing exaggerated negative qualities to self or others.

Developmental contexts   The necessary circumstances that must exist for development to occur; some circumstances are related to nature (genes, inheritance), and others are related to nurture (environment).

Dichotomous thinking   A cognitive distortion common to people with eating disorders, in which an individual views a situation as all or nothing, black or white, all good or all bad. If a situation is less than perfect, it is perceived as a failure.

Disaffiliated   A person who does not associate with family, friends, or service providers.

Disengagement theory   The process of mutual withdrawal between the aging individual and society.

Dissociation   Occurs when an overwhelming event or experience is separated from an individual's conscious awareness.

Distress   A subjective response to internal or external stimuli that are threatening or perceived as threatening to the self.

Diurnal variation   Feeling worse or more depressed in the morning and better in the evening.

Double   The individual in psychodrama who operates as the "inner voice" of the protagonist to express repressed thoughts, feelings, and conflicts.

Double-bind   A situation in which contradictory messages are given to one person by another, demanding a response or choice between two opposing alternatives.

Dual diagnosis A term used when the individual has two identified primary psychiatric diagnoses, most commonly used when one diagnosis is drug or alcohol related. For example, the person may have both a psychoactive substance use disorder and a mood disorder.

Duty to warn The legal obligation of a mental health professional to warn an intended victim of potential harm from a client with mental illness.

Dysarthria Difficulty in articulating words: this is especially frustrating because the client knows what words to use but has trouble forming them (more commonly found in vascular dementias and strokes).

Dysfunctional grief Grief expressed to a significantly greater or lesser intensity over a significantly longer or shorter time than is culturally expected. It may manifest itself in serious physical and/or emotional disabilities.

Dysthymia A state of chronic, low-level depression lasting more than 2 years that may lead to more severe depression if untreated.

Dystonic Pertaining to unstable states or to some disorder.

Ego Freud's word for the self, whose major role is to find safe and appropriate ways for needs (instincts) to be met (gratified) in the external world. Lies mostly in the conscious.

Ego defenses Automatic psychologic processes that keep out the threat of internal and external stressors and dangers or deny awareness to protect the self. (Also known as defense mechanisms or mental mechanisms.)

Ego dissonance Inconsistency between attitudes and behaviors.

Ego dystonic pedophile A person who is cognitively aware that his or her behavior is inappropriate and is truly affected by this. This person might voluntarily seek treatment to deal with the disorder.

Ego state A coherent set of feelings developed by the child's organization of similar life experiences and accompanied by a related set of coherent and observable behavior patterns. There are three ego states defined in transactional analysis: parent, adult, and child.

Ego syntonic pedophile A person who is cognitively aware that his or her behavior is inappropriate; however, he or she is not troubled by this. This person will not voluntarily seek treatment because he or she sees no need to do so.

Elder abuse Includes psychologic or emotional neglect, psychologic or emotional abuse, violation of personal rights, financial abuse, physical neglect, and direct physical abuse to persons over age 65.

Empathy Projecting sensitivity and understanding of another's feelings and communicating the understanding in a way that the client understands.

Enactment The action portion in psychodrama in which a scene, or sequence of scenes, is portrayed.

Encopresis The repeated passage of feces into inappropriate places (e.g., clothing or floor), whether involuntary or intentional.

Endogenous agonist/antagonist A substance that occurs naturally in a cell or tissue that stimulates or inhibits a receptor (e.g., dopamine, GABA).

Enmeshed An individual's inability to differentiate or establish a personal identity. Enmeshed individuals have diffuse boundaries within the family and live solely for each other. Member roles are permeable, with a tendency to cut off outside interactions.

Enmeshed families A pattern of family relationships in which children are pressured to conform to parental expectations rather than express their individuality. Overinvolvement among family members, discouragement of outside relationships, and blurring of boundaries occur (e.g., a mother will "feel" her daughter's emotions).

Enuresis The repeated voiding of urine into bed or clothing, whether involuntary or intentional.

Epigenesis A developmental concept developed by Erikson that genetics and environmental experiences, which begin with conception and continue throughout life, determine the person's personality and the mentally healthy or destructive responses to the world.

Equilibrium A state of emotional balance.

Estradiol Endocrine testing for the female determines the level of estradiol in the bloodstream. Estradiol levels may reflect the level of sexual desire.

Ethnicity A cultural group's sense of identification associated with the group's common social and cultural heritage.

Ethnocentrism The tendency of members of one cultural group to view the members of other cultural groups in terms of the standards of behavior, attitudes, and values of their own group. Belief in the superiority of one's own group.

Ethnomethodology The study of people in context, through inductive, qualitative methods.

Eustress A nonspecific stress response associated with desirable events such as marriage, birth of a child, job promotion, etc., from the Greek word *eu* or "good."

Euthymia A mood that is normal and level.

Expert witness   Someone with education and experience on a specialized subject who is qualified as an expert and allowed to testify in order to assist the jury in understanding technical information.

External vacuum pump   A cylindric vacuum pump applied to the penis. When operated, it brings blood into the penis and traps it there, thus improving erection.

Extrapyramidal symptoms (EPS)   The collective term used to describe the motor side effect of dopamine-blocking medications. EPS includes acute dystonia, akathisia, parkinsonism, and tardive dyskinesia.

Faulty information processing   Fixed and rigid patterns of thinking that block the contextual aspects of a situation and are characteristic of depressed people.

Feedback   The measure by which the effectiveness of the message is gauged.

Feminist theory   Includes four major dimensions of wife abuse: (1) the explanatory utility of the constructs of gender and power, (2) the analysis of the family as a historically situated institution, (3) the crucial importance of understanding and validating women's experiences, and (4) the employment of scholarship for women.

Figure-background formation   The concept that an organism's foremost need or specific interest will define the reality of the moment.

First-pass effect   Refers to the process of orally administered drugs, when absorbed, first passing through the liver, where substantial percentages of the administered dose may be metabolized before the drug is distributed to the tissues.

Flight of ideas   The rapid shifting from one idea to another without completion of the preceding idea, commonly manifested in mania.

Forensic psychiatry   A branch of psychiatry that studies individuals who commit crimes and enter the court system, some of whom are incarcerated.

Formal operations period   Piaget's term for the fourth stage of cognitive development whereby the child learns to think in abstract and hypothetical ways about future events and learns to develop strategies for solving complex problems.

Generativity   In Erikson's personality theory, the positive outcome of one of the stages of adult personality development; the ability to do creative work or to contribute to the raising of one's children. The opposite of stagnation.

Generic approach   A method that focuses on the characteristic course of the particular kind of crisis rather than on the psychodynamics of each individual in crisis.

Genuineness   A quality of an effective nurse that encompasses openness, honesty, and sincerity.

Gerontology   The scientific study of the aging process involving multiple disciplines and settings.

Grief   The dynamic, natural psychologic and physiologic responses to loss. Grief affects physical, cognitive, behavioral, emotional, social, and spiritual aspects of the individual.

Grief work   The intense psychologic effort to (1) fully express the feelings associated with grief, (2) understand the relationship with the deceased, and paradoxically, (3) carry on with essential activities of daily living.

Half-life   The time required for the serum concentration of a drug to decrease by 50%. Drugs dosed at intervals less than their half-life will accumulate in the body, often to toxic levels.

Hallucination   A subjective disorder of perception in which one of the five senses is involved in the absence of external stimuli.

Hardiness   A sense of mastery or self-confidence needed to appropriately appraise and interpret health stressors.

Heritage consistency   The observance of the beliefs and practices of one's traditional cultural belief system.

Holism   A term with various interpretations and meanings. Holism in the broadest sense refers to a belief system in which persons are unified, complex, interdependent systems with interrelated physical, mental, emotional, spiritual, and social dimensions.

Homeopathic   Health beliefs and practices derived from traditional cultural knowledge to maintain health, prevent changes in health status, and restore health.

Humanistic nursing   A view of nursing as an interactive process that occurs between two people, one needing help and one willing to give help. Developed by Josephine Patterson and Loretta Zderad and based on existential theory and the phenomenologic method.

Hypochondriasis   A long-standing dependency. A preoccupation with the "sick role." A fear or belief that one has a serious illness, in spite of medical reassurances to the contrary.

Hypomania   The mood of elation with higher-than-usual activity and social interaction; not as expansive as full mania.

Id   The basic level of the personality that lies in the unconscious and consists of primitive drives and instincts aimed at self-preservation.

Ideas of influence   Delusional beliefs that one's thought processes are being influenced by an external source, such as radar, space aliens, or another person.

Ideas of reference   Incorrect interpretations of incidents and external events as having a particular or special meaning specific to the person.

Identified client   In family therapy, the member of the family (or group) whose behavior is seen as causing the problem for the family (or group).

Identity versus role confusion   Erikson's term for the fifth developmental crisis. Self-assurance of the previous stage leads to the adolescent's gaining a self-identity and the development of an ability to determine where the adolescent fits in society. Failure to develop a self-identity leads to role confusion, poor self-confidence, and alienation.

Imminence   The likelihood that an event will occur within a specific time period.

Incidence   The frequency of occurrences of a specific disorder within a designated time period; number of new cases.

Independent activities of daily living (IADLs)   Activities an individual requires in order to function in the community (e.g., shopping, preparing meals, and transportation).

Indifference   The manner in which the nurse interacts with the client that manifests disconnectedness and unconcern.

Individual approach   The individual approach differs from the generic approach in its emphasis on assessment, by a professional, of the interpersonal and intrapsychic processes of the person in crisis.

Industry versus inferiority   Erikson's term for the fourth developmental crisis. From the initiative achieved in the previous stage, the child develops an ability to master learning and develop peer relationships that lead to self-assurance or industry. Failure to master academic and social pursuits leads to inferiority and hinders attempts to try new things.

Inference   The interpretation of behavior, assumption of motive, and formation of a conclusion without having all the information.

Initiative versus guilt   Erikson's term for the third developmental crisis. Self-sufficiency allows the child to undertake and plan tasks and join with others in cooperative efforts resulting in increased initiative. If the child's desire to show initiative causes excessive conflict in the family, guilt results.

Insight   The ability to perceive oneself realistically and understand oneself.

Institutionalization   The act of placing or confining persons with mental disorders in state-run facilities, such as residential treatment programs designed to treat such disorders.

Interactive context of behaviors   Behavior is shaped and reinforced by interaction with one's social system while the social system is being shaped and reinforced by the same interaction.

Intermediate care   Short-term home care services designed to assist the client and family in achieving a planned, higher level of functioning.

Interoceptive deficits   The inability to correctly identify and respond to bodily sensations. Individuals with eating disorders are often out of touch with their bodies and either fail to recognize or mistrust physical sensations such as hunger, satiety, fatigue, or pain, as well as emotional states.

Interpersonal communication   Communication between two or more persons containing both verbal and nonverbal messages.

Intracorporal injections   Injections of various medications into the right and left corpus cavernosum to improve erection.

Intrapersonal communication   Communication occurring within oneself that can be functional or dysfunctional.

Intrapsychic   Pertaining to the mind or mental process.

Intuition   Insight into a situation without the benefit of critical analysis. (Also known as intuitive reasoning.)

Isolation   A feeling of aloneness with perceived social rejection or lack of support from others during a crisis.

Kindling   The creation of electrophysiologic sensitivity in the brain from stress that results in alteration of neural functioning.

Learned helplessness   The perception that events are uncontrollable, leading to apathy, helplessness, powerlessness, and depression.

Least restrictive alternative   Providing the least restrictive treatment in the least restrictive setting for a mental health client.

Legal duty   Something that an individual is required to do by law.

Lethality   The potential for causing death related to the level of danger associated with the suicidal plan, along a continuum from low to high probability (e.g., aspirin overdose versus a gunshot wound to the head). (A) **High** involves a precise suicide plan for the next 24 to 72 hours, with a lethal method, available means, intent to die, poor impulse control, and no rescue plan. (B) **Moderate** involves a less immediate or less lethal method and plan. (C) **Low** involves plans that are vague, imprecise, and sometimes include plans for rescue.

Libido   The energy of the instincts held in the id.

Life span   The maximum length of survival genetically fixed for each species.

Locus of control   An aspect of personality that deals with the degree of control one perceives over one's own destiny. **Internal locus of control** refers to the ability to actively control one's own destiny. **External locus of control** refers to the inability to control one's own destiny.

Loosening of associations   Thought disturbance in which the speaker rapidly shifts expression of ideas from one subject to another in an unrelated manner.

Loss   A process characterized by a series of overlapping stages that include common psychologic and behavioral manifestations of recognition, adjustment, and resolution.

Lovemap   A term coined by John Money that refers to an idiosyncratic image in the mind-brain that depicts the idealized lover and lovemaking activities.

Machismo   Compulsive masculinity characterized by a man's excessive need to control and dominate his wife at all costs.

Maintenance care   Home care services provided when the client has reached a stable, higher level of functioning, such as surveillance, client and family education, and emotional support. Concentrated and intermediate care is performed by skilled providers, and maintenance is performed by less skilled providers.

Mandatory outpatient treatment   The legal requirement that an individual undergo mental health treatment in an outpatient setting. The individual usually has been noncompliant and allegedly has a propensity for dangerous acts.

Mania   An elevated, expansive, or irritable mood accompanied by hyperactivity, grandiosity, and loss of reality.

Melancholic depression   Severe depression characterized by anhedonia, feeling worse in the morning, weight loss, and psychomotor retardation.

Message   The information (feelings or ideas) being sent and received.

Metabolism   The biotransformation of a drug molecule into a new molecule.

Metabolite   The result of biotransformation of a drug. Although most metabolites tend to be pharmacologically inactive and less toxic, there are important exceptions (e.g., fluoxetine is metabolized into the active metabolite norfluoxetine; ethanol is metabolized into the more toxic acetaldehyde).

Metamemory   One's self-perceptions of memory changes.

Metaneeds   As the physiologic and safety needs are met, the need for belonging and love emerges.

Milieu therapy   Re-creates a community atmosphere on an inpatient hospital unit, a partial hospitalization unit, or a day treatment setting to facilitate interaction between client peers to identify and problem solve issues that occur while relating to others.

Mirroring   A technique in psychodrama and movement/dance therapy in which one individual imitates the behavior patterns of another in order to show the person how other people perceive and react to him or her.

Mood   A feeling state reported by the client that can vary with external and internal changes.

Mourning   Feeling or expressing grief or sorrow.

Movement   Kinesthetic behavior in which individuals communicate by the use of body motions rather than formal language.

Movement/dance therapy   The use of movement to promote increased awareness of the body and changes in feeling states, cognition, and behavior.

Music   The science or art of assembling or performing intelligible combinations of tones in an organized, structured form.

Music therapy   The use of music to provide a variety of listening and participatory experiences adapted to the needs of the individual clients, such as an opportunity for nonverbal communication, shared experience, emotional expression, relaxation, and nonthreatening enjoyment.

Negative symptoms   A syndrome that includes flat affect, poverty of speech, poor grooming, withdrawal, and disturbance in volition.

Neuritic plaques   Maltese cross–appearing clumps composed of amyloid fibers found in the brains of clients with Alzheimer's disease.

Neurofibrillary tangle   The accumulation of twisted filaments inside brain cells, which is one of the characteristic structural abnormalities found on autopsy that confirms the diagnosis of Alzheimer's disease.

Neuroleptic   Literally, "to clasp the neuron"; the term used to describe antipsychotic medications.

Neuroleptic malignant syndrome   A rare but potentially lethal toxic reaction to dopamine-blocking drugs that presents with a constellation of symptoms, including fever, automatic instability, increased muscular rigidity, and altered mental status.

Neurotransmission   The process by which electrochemical signals are sent throughout the brain.

Neutrality   The manner in which the nurse interacts with the client that shows respect and acceptance regardless of the client's appearance or behavior.

Nihilism   Belief that existence is meaningless and useless.

Nocturnal penile tumescence   A test that uses a strain gauge around the penis to depict the pattern of arousal while the client sleeps.

Nonadrenergic   A neuronal system or neuron that manufactures and/or responds to norepinephrine.

Nonverbal communication   The nonverbal behaviors displayed by individuals during the process of an interaction.

Norms   The group's standards for behavior, attitudes and, at times, perceptions of their members; as such, they represent the shared expectations of appropriateness in behavior.

Nuclear family   A family made up of the parental dyad and the individual's siblings.

Object constancy   The ability to maintain a relationship regardless of frustration and changes in the relationship.

Object relations   The stability and depth of an individual's relations with significant others as manifested by warmth, dedication, concern, and tactfulness.

Objectivity   The state of remaining free from bias, prejudice, and personal identification in an interaction with another person.

Obsession   The persistent ideas, thoughts, impulses, or images about death, sexual matters, or religious matters that lead to efforts to resist them, are associated with marked distress or interference, and result in marked anxiety or distress.

Occupation   The goal-directed use of time, energy, interest, and attention to foster adaption and productivity, to minimize pathology, and to promote the maintenance of health.

Occupational therapy   The application of goal-directed, purposeful activity in the assessment and treatment of individuals with psychologic, physical, or developmental disabilities.

Opportunistic diseases   Diseases that commonly appear with AIDS clients, especially when their T cells drop; these diseases include cytomegalovirus and mycobacterium.

Organismic self-regulation   The concept that once the need is satisfied, it will recede and allow the emergence of the next need.

Overselect   A behavior commonly noted in children with psychiatric disorders. The child tends to be so specific about the stimuli that he or she selects to respond to that it appears as if there is no response at all.

Paradigm   A side-by-side example to show a clear pattern.

Paraphilia   A category of sexual deviations/disorders presenting with inappropriate sexual fantasies involving deviant sexual acts, inappropriate sexual urges, and acting-out of these fantasies and urges.

Parasitic   One's total dependence on someone else for one's every need.

Parasuicidal behavior   Suicidal gestures and attempts that are unsuccessful and of low lethality (e.g., superficial cutting of the wrists).

Penile-brachial index (PBI)   A test that determines the difference between the penile and brachial blood pressure that assesses vascularization to the penis.

Penile plethysmograph   A diagnostic test that determines a person's arousal pattern and level of arousal. This test may reveal the source of the client's arousal and the degree of its significance.

Performance inadequacy   The fear that beginning nurses may feel that they will not know what to say to help clients resolve their problems.

Perseveration   A disturbance in thought association in which there is a persistent repetition of the same idea in response to different questions.

Personality traits   Enduring patterns of perceiving, relating to, and thinking about the environment and oneself that are exhibited in a wide range of social and personal contexts.

Perturbation   A determination of an individual's level of distress, developed by Shneidman and rated on a scale of 19. Refers to how upset, disturbed, or perturbed the individual is.

Pervasive developmental disorder   A collection of disorders in which the child experiences deficits in a broad range of developmental areas.

Phobias   A group of disorders primarily characterized by avoidance of a specific situation or escape, if that situation is unexpectedly encountered.

Pleasure principle   The goal of experiencing pleasure while avoiding pain. This principle represents the id's goal in the personality to satisfy a person's innate needs and instincts.

Positive affirmation   A self-supporting message that reinforces confidence and enhances performance.

Positive cognitive set   The belief that success is possible and that one can achieve what one believes.

Positive regard   Acceptance of and respect for a client.

Positive symptoms   A syndrome that includes hallucinations, increased speech production with loose associations, and bizarre behavior.

Postconventional morality   Kohlberg's third stage of morality in which moral decisions reflect underlying ethical principles that consider societal needs and are first based on a sense of community respect and disrespect and later based on principles of justice, the reciprocity and quality of human rights, and respect for the dignity of human beings as individuals.

Postvention   Grief therapy after a death occurs but before pathology develops.

Poverty of thought   A psychopathologic thought disturbance in schizophrenia. The client's inability to think logically and sequentially is reflected in **poverty of content speech,** which is vague, repetitious, and disconnected.

Preconventional morality   Kohlberg's first stage of morality whereby moral decisions are self-centered and the child's behavior is first based on avoidance of punishment and later based on a desire to gain rewards or benefits.

Premorbid   The period just preceding the onset of a mental illness. Characteristics of the personality may indicate the type of disorder that may occur.

Preoperational period   Piaget's term for the second stage of cognitive development whereby the child remains egocentric, is oriented in the present, and only guesses about cause and effect.

Pressured speech   Rapid speech with an urgent quality.

Prevalence   The number of cases of a specific disorder in a normal population at a given point in time; the number of existing cases.

Primary prevention   Prevention efforts that focus on reduction of the incidence of mental disorders within the community. It is directed toward occurrence of mental health problems with emphasis on health promotion and prevention of disorders.

Primary process thinking   Prelogical thought that aims for wish fulfillment. It is associated with the pleasure principle characteristic of the id portion of the personality.

Privileged communication   Communication between a professional and a client that is confidential and protected from forced disclosure in court unless authorized by the client. The privilege is delegated by statutes in the various states.

Problem solving   The process involved in discovering the correct sequence of alternatives leading to a goal or to an ideational solution.

Prodromal symptoms   Early symptoms, such as a deterioration in functioning, that may mark the onset of a mental illness.

Projection   The process whereby a person deals with his or her emotional conflicts or stressors, both internal and external, by unconsciously and falsely attributing to another person his or her own unacceptable feelings, impulses, or thoughts.

Projective identification   The process whereby a person projects his or her emotional conflicts and stressors to another; however, this individual does not fully disavow what is projected. The individual remains aware of his or her own affects or impulses but misattributes them as justifiable reactions to the other person.

Protagonist   The individual, in psychodrama, who presents and acts out his or her emotional problems and interpersonal relationships.

Protein binding   The holding of a drug in the blood by circulating protein molecules. The percentage of a drug that is protein bound varies widely. The percentage of a drug that is protein bound is not pharmacologically active until released.

Psyche   The mind as the center of thought processes, emotions, and behavior.

Psychodrama   A form of psychotherapy in which an individual reenacts life situations in order to examine subjective experiences, promote insight, and alter specific behavior patterns.

Psychoeducation   A type of therapy that educates the client with a paraphilic disorder to identify situations/objects that may trigger inappropriate sexual activity, develop awareness of relapse prevention strategies, and acknowledge the importance of treatment compliance.

Psychologic morbidity   The prevalence of psychologic impairment in a specific population. With respect to AIDS, psychologic morbidity refers to the prevalence of emotional distress and syndromic conditions in persons with AIDS (PWAs).

Psychomotor agitation   Agitated motor activity.

Psychomotor retardation   The slowing of physiologic processes, resulting in slow movement, speech, and reaction time.

Psychosis   Having impaired ability to recognize reality and thus being unable to deal with life's demands.

Psychosocial stages   Theory by Erikson. A series of eight stages, distinct periods in a person's social development; each stage is marked by a particular type of crisis resulting from the ego's attempt to meet the demands of social reality.

Psychosomatic illness   Pertaining to a physical disorder that is notably influenced or caused by emotional or mental factors involving the mind and the body.

Psychotropic   Literally, "mind nutrition." The term used to describe drugs that affect the central nervous system.

Purging   The use of self-induced vomiting and/or the abuse of laxatives, diuretics, syrup of ipecac, diet pills, or enemas to avoid weight gain following a binge. One or more of these behaviors, as well as periods of fasting and excessive exercise during an episode of bulimia nervosa, may be used.

Reality principle   The goal of postponing immediate gratification until a suitable object for this satisfaction is found. The ego is ruled by this principle.

Receiver   The individual who both receives and interprets the message.

Receptors   Protein molecules located in the cell walls of tissues that receive chemical stimulation resulting in stimulation or inhibition of activity of the target cell.

Recreation   To create again by some form of play, amusement, or relaxation.

Recreational therapy   The use of recreational activities as an integral part of the rehabilitation or therapeutic process. The purpose is to increase enjoyment of life, stimulate activity and self-expression, enhance socialization, and counterbalance self-concern.

Reframing   A technique of changing the viewpoint of a situation and replacing it with another viewpoint that fits the facts equally well but changes the entire meaning.

Regressive developmental task   Developmental tasks that focus on adjustments to physical, psychologic, and functional changes due to aging.

Relapse/relapse prevention   The resumption of a pattern of substance use or dependency after a period of sobriety and/or the process in which indicators or warning signs appear before the individual's actual resumption of the substance. Relapse prevention is a means of helping the chemically dependent individual maintain behavioral changes over a prolonged period of time.

Repression   The involuntary exclusion of a painful, threatening experience. Begins in infancy and continues throughout life. Underlies all other defense mechanisms but also operates as its own defense mechanism.

Residual symptoms   Minor disturbances that may remain after an episode of schizophrenia but do not include delusions, hallucinations, incoherence, or gross disorganization.

Resistance   The inability, whether conscious or unconscious, to accept change; the denial of new problems.

Restrictive admission policies   A component of the deinstitutionalization process that limits the length of stay until symptoms are under control.

Restrictive commitment policies   A component of the deinstitutionalization process that limits commitment to a psychiatric facility to threat to harm self and/or others.

Restrictive environment   An environment that restricts the client's activity in order to help him or her regain control of his or her behavior. The individual may be placed in open-door or closed-door seclusion during periods of extreme agitation, suicidal ideations, or threats of violence to self or others.

Rites of passage   Rituals associated with life transitions that facilitate maturational development, such as puberty, marriage, birth, and death. These rites are commonly composed of three stages: separation, transition, and incorporation.

Roles   The socially expected behavior patterns usually determined by an individual's status in a particular group. Peplau identified four roles for the psychiatric nurse: (1) resource person, (2) counselor, (3) surrogate, and (4) technical expert.

Safeguards   Relapse prevention strategies employed to assist the individual in developing control over inappropriate sexual acting-out (reoffending) behaviors.

Safety   The sense of security developed within the therapeutic relationship when the responsibilities and expectations of each party are clearly defined. Safety develops from knowing the boundaries of a relationship and acting within them.

Schemata   The cognitive set of the self and world through which situations are perceived, coded, and interpreted.

Seasonal affective disorder (SAD) A mood disorder that occurs at a regular time each year.

Secondary gain Any benefit, such as personal attention, sympathy from others, or escape from unwanted responsibilities, as a result of illness. May be experienced when family or friends pay a great deal of attention to the client's eating behavior (e.g., preparing special meals or making special arrangements in an attempt to encourage him or her to eat).

Secondary prevention Prevention efforts directed toward reduction in the prevalence of mental disorders through early identification of problems and early treatment of those problems. This stage occurs after the problem arises and aims at shortening the course or duration of the episode.

Selective attention The ability to discriminate and focus on relevant information.

Self-actualization A concept developed by Maslow as an ongoing actualization of potentials, capacities, and talents as fulfillment of a mission, and as a greater knowledge and acceptance of one's own intrinsic nature.

Self-system Sullivan's term for the system that infants develop to cope with anxiety associated with the interpersonal process of need satisfaction and security. The individual develops self-appraisal as a result of significant others' responses to actions of the individual. Actions that cause anxiety result in "bad-me" self-appraisals. Actions that cause no anxiety result in "good-me" self-appraisals. Actions of disapproval cause severe anxiety, emotional withdrawal, and "not-me" self-appraisals.

Sender The individual who initiates the transmission of information.

Sensate focus A learned exercise developed by Masters and Johnson that involves concentrating on the sensations produced by touching.

Sensorimotor period Piaget's term for the first stage of cognitive development in which children use their senses and motor skills to manipulate the environment and develop the ability to differentiate self from objects.

Serostatus The presence or absence of HIV antibodies in the bloodstream. HIV status is determined through laboratory tests and is either seropositive or seronegative.

Seroconversion The term used to signify that HIV antibodies are discernible in the individual's laboratory blood tests. A person who was previously exposed to the HIV virus and showed no presence of the virus but subsequently tests positive for the virus has experienced seroconversion.

Serum level monitoring The process of obtaining blood samples to determine drug concentration.

Sick role A set of social expectations that an ill person meets, such as (1) being exempt from usual social role responsibilities, (2) not being morally responsible for being ill, (3) being obligated to "want to get well," and (4) being obligated to seek competent help.

Side effect An undesired nontherapeutic and often predictable consequence of medication. Frequently diminished with time. Contrast with adverse drug reaction.

Sleep reversal A state in which normal sleeping patterns are reversed; the individual sleeps during the day and is active during the night.

Sobriety The state of complete abstinence from alcohol and/or other drugs of abuse in conjunction with a satisfactory quality of life.

Social learning The process by which children acquire the behaviors they need to survive and function in society, which results from repeated interactions in their environments.

Social learning theory Bandura's theory that aggression is not instinctual but a learned behavior.

Social support The presence of other individuals who are able to give understanding, encouragement, and other assistance in life, especially during difficult times.

Socialization The process of being raised within a culture and acquiring the characteristics of the given group.

Somatization The conversion of mental states or experiences into bodily symptoms, associated with anxiety.

Splitting The process by which a person keeps the positive and negative aspects of self or others separate from each other. An individual who uses the unconscious defense mechanism of splitting cannot tolerate ambiguity; therefore people, events, or ideas are either good or bad, right or wrong, black or white, but not gray.

State disorders The diagnoses made on Axis I are considered state diagnoses. They constitute behavior patterns that are not as pervasive or long-lasting as trait disorders.

Stereotype To form an oversimplified, standardized opinion of a person or group of people that is often determined without adequate information.

Stress (1) A term that refers to both a stimulus and a response. It can denote a nonspecific response of the body to any demand placed on it, whether the causal event is negative (a painful experience) or positive (a happy occasion). (2) A state produced by a change in the environment that is perceived as challenging, threatening, or damaging to the person's dynamic equilibrium. (3) The wear and tear on the body over time. (4) Psychologic stress has been defined as all processes, whether originating in the external environment or within the person, that demand a mental appraisal of the event before the involvement or activation of any other system.

Subjectivity Emphasizing one's own moods, attitudes, and opinions in an interaction with another person.

Suicide The act of taking one's own life.

Suicide ideators Those persons who experience suicidal thinking on a consistent basis.

Suicidology The scientific and humane study of human self-destruction.

Sundowner's syndrome The confusion and irritation common in dementia clients at the end of the day, probably resulting from general tiredness and an inability to process any more information after a long day of struggling to interpret their environment correctly.

Superego The portion of the mind, differentiated from the ego, that contains the traditional values and taboos of society as interpreted by the child's parents and that becomes part of the self. Lies in the preconscious.

Sustained release Medications designed to provide slow, controlled dissolution, which allows longer dosing intervals.

Synthesis Combining several parts of relevant data into a single piece of information. Comparing behavioral patterns with learned theories or typical patterns of behavior in order to identify strengths and seek explanations for symptoms.

Syntonic Pertaining to a state of stability.

Tardive dyskinesia A syndrome of abnormal, involuntary movements occurring after months or years of treatment with drugs that block dopamine type 2 receptors. These movements, often described as oral, buccal, lingual, or masticatory, can occur throughout the body.

Taxonomy A classification of known phenomena under a hierarchical structure.

Teratogen A substance that causes developmental malformations in the fetus.

Tertiary prevention Prevention efforts that have the dual focus of reduction of residual effects of the disorder and rehabilitation of the individual who experienced the mental disorder.

Theme development The part of movement/dance therapy in which a specific issue or feeling is actively being explored.

Themes The recurring patterns of interactions the client experiences in relationships with self and/or others.

Therapeutic communication The interaction that takes place between the nurse and client. The content has meaning and focuses on the client's concerns.

Therapeutic milieu An environment designed to promote emotional health that is based on the assumption that the client is an active participant in his or her own life and therefore needs to be involved in the management of his or her behavior and environment.

Therapeutic play Age-appropriate play activities used purposefully by the nurse for assessment, intervention, and promotion of normal growth and development in children.

Therapeutic relationship A personal relationship convened to help one of the participants deal more effectively and maturely with some difficulty in life. It is a goal-directed, client-centered, and objective relationship.

Thought blocking The abrupt interruption in the flow of thoughts or ideas due to a disturbance in the speed of associations.

Tic A sudden, rapid, recurrent, nonrhythmic, stereotyped movement or vocalization that is considered irresistible but is often suppressible for short periods.

Tolerance Physiologic adaptation to the effect of drugs that diminishes effects with constant dosages or maintains the intensity and duration of effects through increased dosage.

Trait disorders Trait disorders are used to describe Axis II diagnoses. Axis II is used exclusively for the description of personality disorders and mental retardation, which are considered trait diagnoses. The symptoms of a personality disorder or mental retardation are not time limited, nor do they occur only in a time of crisis.

Transference The unconscious response whereby clients associate the nurse with someone significant in their lives.

Transgenerational violence When violence within the family is an accepted everyday occurrence, a natural, normal component of family living.

Transindividual perspective Looking beyond individuals to the family or community as the unit of care.

Transinstitutionalization A process in which clients are transferred from one institution to another, such as from a psychiatric hospital to a nursing home.

Transitional objects   Objects that remind one of a significant person. For example, a man keeps a picture of his wife on his desk, which reminds him of her during work hours.

Triggers   Stimuli that heighten unacceptable sexual cravings.

Trust   The reliance on the truthfulness or accuracy of the therapeutic relationship developed through a congruency between the therapist's words and actions.

Trust versus mistrust   Erikson's term for the first developmental crisis that the child tries to resolve. Consistent, predictable, and continuous care results in developing a sense of trust in oneself, others, and the world. Inconsistent, unpredictable, or discontinuous care results in the polar opposite, or mistrust of oneself, others, and the world.

Unconditional positive regard   The stance of the therapist modeling the unconditional acceptance of the client and based on the belief that the client is competent to direct himself or herself in his or her natural tendency to move forward toward integration.

Unconscious suicidal intention   A state outside of awareness during which persons engage in risk-taking behaviors that have a high likelihood of causing their deaths.

Underselect   The inability of children with psychiatric disorders to select which stimuli are most important; manifested by inappropriate responses to routine events.

Unipolar   A depressive disorder characterized by episodes of depression with no mania.

Vaginal dilators   A graduated series of cylindric dilators introduced into the vagina to decrease involuntary spasm.

Vaginal plethysmography   A test that uses a vaginal probe to assess blood flow to the female vagina. Blood flow is an indicator of arousal.

Verbal communication   Spoken or written words that compose the symbols of language.

Vicarious learning   Learning through imagining the experiences of others as if they are one's own.

Victimizer   Another term used to define a sex offender. This term may be used when discussing familial transmission of the paraphilia.

Vigilance   The ability to sustain attention over longer periods of time.

Violence   A term used to describe behavior that is physically or psychologically harmful, injurious, or assaultive (e.g., child abuse, domestic violence, elder abuse, family violence).

Warm-up   A stage of psychodrama and movement/dance therapy that focuses on introducing group members, increasing the comfort level, and determining the theme or issue to be addressed.

Xenophobia   A morbid fear of strangers and those who are not of one's own ethnic group.

Yohimbine   An α-adrenoreceptor blocker that may facilitate blood flow to the genitalia and therefore improve sexual arousal.

INDEX

GENERIC NAME; alprazolam
TRADE NAME; Xanax

CLASSIFICATION Antianxiety agent—benzodiazepine.

INDICATIONS & USES Anxiety, anxiety associated with depression, panic disorder.

USUAL ADULT DOSAGE RANGE 0.5-4 mg/day in anxiety; up to 10 mg/day in panic disorder in divided doses. Initial dosing is 0.25-0.5 mg bid to tid. Lower doses for geriatric clients.

AVAILABLE FORMS Tabs 0.25, 0.5, 1 mg.

PHARMACOKINETICS/DYNAMICS Rapidly absorbed. Average half-life is 12-15 hr. In some individuals, antianxiety effects may last <12 hr. Antianxiety effects may be rapidly apparent. Antipanic effects may be apparent in 1-2 wk.

SIDE EFFECTS Drowsiness, dizziness, ataxia. Rarely—nausea, vomiting, GI upset, blurred vision.

ADVERSE REACTIONS Rarely—increased aggression/irritability. **Oversedation and respiratory depression with other CNS depressants,** seizures on withdrawal.

INTERACTIONS Serum levels increased by cimetidine, oral contraceptives, disulfiram, nefazodone, erythromycin.

CONTRAINDICATIONS Coma, shock, alcohol intoxication, pregnancy. Use with caution in history of drug abuse/addiction. Use with caution in clients with liver or kidney disease.

NURSING CONSIDERATIONS Schedule IV controlled substance. Risk of respiratory depression when used with other CNS depressants. Abrupt discontinuation associated with anxiety, rebound insomnia, and seizures. Discontinuation titration may need to be as slow as 0.25 mg/day every week in some clients. Rapid absorption causing a "buzz" may reinforce drug-seeking behavior or may be perceived dysphorically in non-drug abuse population.

CLIENT TEACHING Avoid hazardous activities during initiation. Avoid alcohol. Drug should not be discontinued suddenly.

AVAILABLE IN CANADA Apo-Alpraz, Novo-Alprazol, Nu-Alpraz, Alti-Alprazolam, Gen-Alprazolam, Xanax, Xanax TS.

bold—Life-threatening reactions

GENERIC NAME; amantadine
TRADE NAME; Symmetrel

CLASSIFICATION Antiparkinsonian/antiviral.

INDICATIONS & USES Parkinsonism, prophylaxis and treatment of extrapyramidal symptoms, prophylaxis and treatment of influenza A.

USUAL ADULT DOSAGE RANGE For adults with normal renal function: 100 mg bid. Dosage must be reduced with decreasing renal function.

AVAILABLE FORMS Caps 100 mg; syr 50 mg/5 ml.

PHARMACOKINETICS/DYNAMICS Average half-life is 24 hr with normal renal function. Renal elimination. Full effects may be seen in 4-5 days. Amantadine may facilitate the release of dopamine in CNS neurons.

SIDE EFFECTS Dizziness, insomnia, impaired concentration, hypotension, irritability, depression, anxiety, ataxia, nausea, anorexia, livedo reticularis (blotchy spots on the skin) with chronic use.

ADVERSE REACTIONS Hallucinations and psychotic reactions, particularly in clients not taking antipsychotics or if doses are not reduced for impaired renal function. May exacerbate eczema.

INTERACTIONS May cause hypertension with MAOIs. May cause insomnia, irritability, seizures, irregular heartbeat with stimulants. May increase side effects of anticholinergic medications.

CONTRAINDICATIONS Uncontrolled psychosis, eczema, seizures.

NURSING CONSIDERATIONS Generally used for EPS when anticholinergics are contraindicated or ineffective. Monitor vital signs and for level of consciousness initially. Monitor for continued efficacy; may lose effectiveness over time. Abrupt discontinuation may result in acute worsening of symptoms.

CLIENT TEACHING Change body position slowly to prevent orthostatic hypotension. Report dyspnea, weight gain, dizziness, poor concentration, and behavioral changes. Abrupt discontinuation may cause parkinsonian crisis.

AVAILABLE IN CANADA Symmetrel, Endantadine, Gen-Amantadine.

bold—life-threatening reactions

GENERIC NAME; amitriptyline
TRADE NAME; Elavil

CLASSIFICATION Tricyclic antidepressant.

INDICATIONS & USES Major depression; anxiety, panic, eating disorders; chronic pain.

USUAL ADULT DOSAGE RANGE 50-300 mg/day. In major depression: 150-300 mg/day. Initial dosing is 50-75 mg/day in divided doses.

AVAILABLE FORMS Tabs 10, 25, 50, 75, 100, 150 mg/day in divided doses.

PHARMACOKINETICS/DYNAMICS Half-life varies from 10-46 hr in adults to 17-46 hr in the elderly. Partially metabolized to nortriptyline. Plasma therapeutic range (amitriptyline + nortriptyline): 120-250 mg/ml. Full therapeutic effects may not be apparent for 2-4 wk. Initial multiple daily dosing can often be consolidated to once or twice a day, once client is tolerant to side effects.

SIDE EFFECTS Sedation, dizziness, blurred vision, dry mouth, constipation, urinary retention, nausea, vomiting, tachycardia, orthostatic hypotension, tremor, cardiac conduction abnormalities, decreased libido, weight gain, allergic dermatitis, skin photosensitivity, reduced seizure threshold.

ADVERSE REACTIONS Exacerbation of untreated narrow-angle glaucoma, induction of mania, reduced seizure threshold, **potentially fatal in overdose.**

INTERACTIONS Increased levels—cimetidine, fluoxetine, antipsychotics, methylphenidate, propoxyphene. Decreased levels—barbiturates, phenytoin, chronic carbamazepine. Increased effects of epinephrine, norepinephrine, CNS depressants. **Severe hypertension with MAOIs.** Antacids reduce absorption.

CONTRAINDICATIONS Caution in clients with cardiovascular disease, arrhythmias, strokes, acute myocardial infarction, and thyroid disease/medications. May exacerbate signs and symptoms of glaucoma, benign prostatic hypertrophy, diabetes. Avoid in pregnant and lactating women.

NURSING CONSIDERATIONS Monitor level of sedation and vital signs carefully during dose titration. Suicide risk may be increased during initial improvement, particularly as psychomotor depression abates.

CLIENT TEACHING Therapeutic effects may take several weeks. May experience initial sedation and dizziness. Change positions slowly. Use hats and sunscreens to reduce risk with sun exposure.

AVAILABLE IN CANADA Apo-Amitriptyline, Elavil.

bold—Life-threatening reactions

GENERIC NAME; benztropine
TRADE NAME; Cogentin

CLASSIFICATION Antiparkinsonian, anticholinergic.

INDICATIONS & USES Parkinsonism, treatment and prevention of extrapyramidal symptoms caused by antipsychotic medications (excluding tardive dyskinesia).

USUAL ADULT DOSAGE RANGE 1-6 mg/day. Typical starting dose is 0.5-1 mg bid. Most clients have significant side effects at doses ≥6 mg/day.

AVAILABLE FORMS Tabs 0.5, 1, 2 mg; inj IM, IV 1 mg/ml.

PHARMACOKINETICS/DYNAMICS Rapidly absorbed. PO with effects in 1-2 hr. Very rapidly absorbed IM with effects in 10-30 min. The pharmacokinetics are not well characterized. Usually given bid, elimination is slow enough in some clients to allow qd dosing.

SIDE EFFECTS Dry mouth, blurred vision, tachycardia, urinary retention, constipation, nervousness, confusion.

ADVERSE REACTIONS **Paralytic ileus. Anticholinergic delirium (also called anticholinergic intoxication and atropine psychosis)**—confusion, disorientation, stupor. Flushing, hyperthermia, extreme agitation, hallucinations, hypotension, supraventricular tachycardia, markedly diminished or absent bowel sounds.

INTERACTIONS Additive anticholinergic effects with other medications, especially antipsychotics, tricyclic antidepressants, MAOIs, digoxin, furosemide (Lasix). Additive effects with CNS depressants.

CONTRAINDICATIONS Severe cardiac or GI disorders, benign prostatic hypertrophy, angle-closure glaucoma, neuroleptic malignant syndrome.

NURSING CONSIDERATIONS Increased risk of heat stroke. Evaluate for adequate hydration and constipation. May aggravate the movements of tardive dyskinesia. Elderly at increased risk for confusion and anticholinergic delirium.

CLIENT TEACHING Give with meals. May cause drowsiness, blurred vision, or dizziness. Avoid alcohol and other CNS depressants. Notify physician for rapid or pounding heartbeat. Use caution in hot weather.

AVAILABLE IN CANADA Apo-Benztropin, PMS-Benztropine, Cogentin.

bold—life-threatening reactions

GENERIC NAME; bupropion
TRADE NAME; Wellbutrin

CLASSIFICATION Aminoketone antidepressant.

INDICATIONS & USES Major depression. Often used in clients who have failed to respond to or cannot tolerate other antidepressant drugs. Seldom used as a first-choice drug.

USUAL ADULT DOSAGE RANGE 150-450 mg/day; initial dosing is 100 mg bid. Never administer more than 150 mg at one time, to minimize risk of seizure.

AVAILABLE FORMS Tabs 75, 100 mg.

AVAILABLE IN CANADA Wellbutrin SR.

PHARMACOKINETICS/DYNAMICS Half-life varies from 10-21 hr in adults. Full therapeutic effects may not be apparent for 2-4 wk.

SIDE EFFECTS Agitation, insomnia, headache, dizziness, slight weight loss, slight increases in blood pressure. Occasionally—mild, dry mouth, blurred vision, constipation, nausea, tremor.

ADVERSE REACTIONS Dose-related increased incidence of seizures, induction of mania, rarely—depersonalization and psychotic symptoms.

INTERACTIONS MAOIs increase side effects; l-dopa may increase side effects. Other drugs that reduce seizure threshold may increase seizure activity.

CONTRAINDICATIONS Preexisting seizure disorder, anorexia nervosa, bulimia (Clients with eating disorders may be at increased risk for seizures.)

NURSING CONSIDERATIONS Suicide risk may be increased during initial improvement, particularly as psychomotor depression abates. Low risk of fatality in overdose.

CLIENT TEACHING Therapeutic effects may take several weeks.

bold—Life-threatening reactions

GENERIC NAME; buspirone
TRADE NAME; BuSpar

CLASSIFICATION Antianxiety agent/azaspirone.

INDICATIONS & USES Anxiety disorders, adjunct in treatment of anxiety and aggression in developmentally disabled, adjunct in treatment of behavioral problems in brain-injured and elderly clients, adjunct in treatment of partial responders to SSRIs (e.g., fluoxetine) in depression and obsessive-compulsive disorder.

USUAL ADULT DOSAGE RANGE 15-60 mg/day. Typical starting dose is 5 mg tid. Because of the short half-life, tid dosing is usually required.

AVAILABLE FORMS Tabs 5, 10 mg.

AVAILABLE IN CANADA BuSpar, Apo-Buspirone, Buspirex, Bustab, Gen-Buspirone, Novo-Buspirone, Nu-Buspirone, PMS-Buspirone.

PHARMACOKINETICS/DYNAMICS Average half-life is 2.4 hr. Buspirone is a 5-HT₁ (serotonin) partial agonist. Efficacy in anxiety may not appear until second week of therapy. Full therapeutic effects may not be apparent for 2-4 wk.

SIDE EFFECTS Nausea, dizziness, headache, excitement, lightheadedness. Rarely—insomnia, drowsiness.

ADVERSE REACTIONS Rare reports of increased liver enzymes when used with trazodone.

INTERACTIONS Do not use with MAOIs. May increase haloperidol serum levels.

CONTRAINDICATIONS Severe hepatic or renal disease, pregnancy.

NURSING CONSIDERATIONS Many clients being treated for anxiety are accustomed to rapid antianxiety and sedative effects of benzodiazepines.

CLIENT TEACHING Educate client about potential side effects and delayed antianxiety effects of buspirone.

bold—Life-threatening reactions

GENERIC NAME; carbamazepine
TRADE NAME; Tegretol

CLASSIFICATION Anticonvulsant.

INDICATIONS & USES Generalized tonic-clonic and complex partial seizures, mixed seizure patterns, trigeminal neuralgia. Other uses: mood stabilizer in depression and bipolar disorder with and without lithium, aggression, rage, and impulse control disorders; adjunct in benzodiazepine withdrawal.

USUAL ADULT DOSAGE RANGE 200-1800 mg/day. Initial dosing is 200 mg bid.

AVAILABLE FORMS Tabs, chewable 100 mg, tabs 200 mg, oral susp 100 mg/5 ml.

PHARMACOKINETICS/DYNAMICS Initial half-life averages 36 hr in adults. Carbamazepine induces its own metabolism. After 4-6 wk the average half-life is 12-17 hr. **Once adequate serum levels are obtained, efficacy may be rapid in seizure disorders while taking 1-3 wk in mood disorders.** Plasma therapeutic range is 4-12 μg/ml. Persistent side effects can be serum level related and increase substantially in some clients at levels >7 μg/ml.

AVAILABLE IN CANADA Apo-Carbamazepine, Mazepine, Novo-Carbamaz, Nu-Carbamazepine, Taro-Carbamazepine, Tegretol.

PHARMACOKINETICS/DYNAMICS potentially the efficacy of oral contraceptives, warfarin, cyclic antidepressants, phenothiazines, haloperidol, clonazepam, thyroid hormone, theophylline, and doxycycline.

CONTRAINDICATIONS Bone marrow suppression, hypersensitivity to TCAs or carbamazepine. Use with caution in severe liver, renal, or cardiac disease and with increased intraocular pressure.

NURSING CONSIDERATIONS Monitor for decrease in WBC. Monitor for neurotoxicity in clients receiving lithium. Shake oral suspension well. Notify prescriber if symptoms of fever, sore throat, mouth ulcers, bleeding, or easy bruising occur. Take with food to minimize GI upset.

CLIENT TEACHING Risks of initial sedation, potential for failure of oral contraceptive. Report signs and symptoms of infection.

SIDE EFFECTS Blurred or double vision, drowsiness, hypotension, hypertension, urinary retention, rash, pruritus, nystagmus, paresthesia, nausea, vomiting, visual hallucinations, ataxia, photosensitivity, chills, confusion, leukocytosis, dizziness.

ADVERSE REACTIONS **Aplastic anemia, agranulocytosis**, thrombocytopenia, **Stevens-Johnson syndrome**, eosinophilia, antidiuretic effects leading to water intoxication, seizures on abrupt withdrawal.

INTERACTIONS Increases carbamazepine levels—erythromycin, fluoxetine, verapamil, propoxyphene, valproate, cimetidine, TCAs, diltiazem, INH, terfenadine. Carbamazepine decreases levels and

bold—Life-threatening reactions

GENERIC NAME; chlorpromazine
TRADE NAME; Thorazine

CLASSIFICATION Typical antipsychotic.

INDICATIONS & USES Symptomatic management of psychotic disorders, initial management of psychotic manic states, intractable hiccoughs.

USUAL ADULT DOSAGE RANGE 30-800 mg/day. Initial dosing is 20-75 mg every day in divided doses. Doses greater than 1000 mg/day are seldom required. Typical IM dose is 25-50 mg.

AVAILABLE FORMS Tabs 10, 25, 50, 100, 200 mg; time-rel caps 30, 75, 150, 200, 300 mg; syr 10 mg/5 ml; conc 30, 100 mg/ml; supp 25, 100 mg; inj IM, IV 25 mg/ml.

PHARMACOKINETICS/DYNAMICS Rapidly absorbed, half-life averages 10-30 hr. Onset of action: 30-60 min. Full therapeutic effects may not be apparent for 6-12 wk. Initial multiple daily dosing can often be consolidated to once or twice a day, once client is tolerant to side effects.

SIDE EFFECTS Sedation, dizziness, blurred vision, dry mouth, constipation, urinary retention, nausea, vomiting, **tachycardia, orthostatic hypotension,** acute dystonic reaction, stiffness, cogwheel rigidity, bradykinesia, akathisia, gynecomastia, galactorrhea, amenorrhea, decreased libido, retrograde ejaculation, weight gain, allergic dermatitis, skin photosensitivity, reduced seizure threshold.

ADVERSE REACTIONS Risk of tardive dyskinesia, **neuroleptic malignant syndrome.** Rarely—jaundice.

INTERACTIONS Additive effects with CNS depressants and anticholinergic drugs. Potentiates hypotensive effects of clonidine. Serum levels are increased by antidepressants and propranolol, reduced by carbamazepine and phenytoin. Epinephrine may result in reverse (hypotensive) effects. Antacids reduce absorption. Do not mix

liquid concentrate with apple juice, cranberry juice, grape juice, or Tang.

CONTRAINDICATIONS Contraindicated in coma, severe hypotension, acute subcortical brain damage. Relatively contraindicated in liver disease, renal insufficiency, blood dyscrasias, Parkinson's disease. May exacerbate signs and symptoms of glaucoma, benign prostatic hypertrophy, diabetes. Avoid in pregnant and lactating women.

NURSING CONSIDERATIONS Monitor level of sedation and vital signs carefully during dose titration. Topical contact with drug can lead to dermatitis. IM injections cause a burning pain. Rapid dose increases, IM injections, dehydration, and agitation are associated with increased incidence of neuroleptic malignant syndrome.

CLIENT TEACHING Rise from bed and change positions slowly to avoid dizziness. Use sugarless gums and candy for dry mouth. Use hats and sunscreens to reduce risk with sun exposure.

AVAILABLE IN CANADA Chlorpromanyl, Largactil.

bold—Life-threatening reactions

GENERIC NAME: citalopram hydrobromide
TRADE NAME: Celexa

CLASSIFICATION Atypical antidepressant.

INDICATIONS & USES Management of symptoms of depressive disorders.

USUAL ADULT DOSAGE RANGE Initially 20 mg/day; increased to 40 mg/day for treatment efficacy.

AVAILABLE FORMS Tabs 20, 40 mg.

PHARMACOKINETICS/DYNAMICS Potentiates serotonergic activity in the CNS by inhibiting neuronal uptake of serotonin (5HT). Highly selective SSRI with minimal effects on dopamine or norepinephrine. Steady-state plasma concentrations reached in 1 week with once-daily dosing.

SIDE EFFECTS Autonomic NS—diaphoresis, dry mouth; GI—nausea, diarrhea, dyspepsia; CNS—somnolence, insomnia, anxiety; GU—ejaculatory disorder, impotence (male), anorgasmy (female), tachycardia, postural hypotension.

ADVERSE REACTIONS Activation of mania, hypomania; suicide risk from overdose; severe dysfunction when used with MAOIs.

INTERACTIONS SSRIs and MAOI interaction have produced **serious, sometimes fatal results,** including hyperthermia, rigidity, myoclonus, vital sign fluctuations, mental changes (extreme agitation, delirium, coma).

CONTRAINDICATIONS No trials for use in clients with cardiovascular disorders. Not for use by breast-feeding women.

NURSING CONSIDERATIONS Monitor for extreme mood changes—potential suicide risk; monitor vital signs and other physical symptoms; be open to discussions of client's concerns over sexual dysfunction.

CLIENT TEACHING Drug may take 1 to 4 weeks before fully effective. Avoid use of alcohol and other mind/body-altering drugs. Notify physician before using OTC drugs, starting new prescription drugs, or intending to become pregnant. Stand up slowly to avoid dizziness. Do not operate hazardous machinery. Judgment and mental acuity may be compromised.

AVAILABLE IN CANADA Not available.

bold—Life-threatening reactions

GENERIC NAME: clomipramine
TRADE NAME: Anafranil

CLASSIFICATION Tricyclic antidepressant.

INDICATIONS & USES Obsessive-compulsive disorder, major depression, phobias, panic disorder, chronic pain.

USUAL ADULT DOSAGE RANGE 100-250 mg/day. Initial dosing is 25 mg/day at bedtime. Initial daytime doses should be given with meal to minimize GI upset.

AVAILABLE FORMS Caps 25, 50, 75 mg.

PHARMACOKINETICS/DYNAMICS In adults, half-life varies from 19-37 (mean, 32) hr for clomipramine and 54-77 (mean, 69) hr for desmethyl-clomipramine (active metabolite). Thus steady state may not be achieved for nearly 2 wk after dosage changes. Full therapeutic effects may not be apparent for several weeks. Initial multiple daily dosing can often be consolidated to once or twice a day, once client is tolerant to side effects.

SIDE EFFECTS Sedation, dizziness, blurred vision, dry mouth, constipation, urinary retention, nausea, vomiting, tachycardia, orthostatic hypotension, tremor, cardiac conduction abnormalities, decreased libido, weight gain, allergic dermatitis, skin photosensitivity, reduced seizure threshold, appetite disturbance, myoclonus, sweating.

ADVERSE REACTIONS Exacerbation of untreated narrow-angle glaucoma, induction of mania, reduced seizure threshold, **potentially fatal in overdose.**

INTERACTIONS Increased levels—cimetidine, fluoxetine, antipsychotics, methylphenidate, propoxyphene. Decreased levels—barbiturates, phenytoin, chronic carbamazepine. Increased effects of epinephrine, norepinephrine, CNS depressants. Severe **hypertension with MAOIs.** Antacids reduce absorption.

CONTRAINDICATIONS Caution in clients with cardiovascular disease, arrhythmias, strokes, acute myocardial infarction, and thyroid disease/medications. May exacerbate signs and symptoms of glaucoma, benign prostatic hypertrophy, diabetes. Avoid in pregnant and lactating women.

NURSING CONSIDERATIONS Monitor level of sedation and vital signs carefully during dose titration. Suicide risk may be increased during initial improvement, particularly as psychomotor depression abates.

CLIENT TEACHING Therapeutic effects may take several weeks. May experience initial sedation and dizziness. Change positions slowly. Use hats and sunscreens to reduce risk with sun exposure.

AVAILABLE IN CANADA Anafranil, Apo-Clomipramine, Gen-Clomipramine, Novo-Clopamine.

bold—Life-threatening reactions

GENERIC NAME: clonazepam
TRADE NAME: Klonopin

CLASSIFICATION Anticonvulsant—benzodiazepine.

INDICATIONS & USES Lennox-Gastaut syndrome (petit mal variant epilepsy), antianxiety, adjunctive treatment of bipolar disorder.

USUAL ADULT DOSAGE RANGE 0.5-10 mg/day in divided doses, bid or tid. Typical starting dose is 0.5 mg bid or tid.

AVAILABLE FORMS Tabs 0.5, 1, 2 mg.

PHARMACOKINETICS/DYNAMICS Rapidly absorbed. Half-life ranges from 18-50 hr.

SIDE EFFECTS Drowsiness, ataxia, hypotonia, hypersalivation. Rarely—nausea, vomiting, GI upset, blurred vision.

ADVERSE REACTIONS Rarely—euphoria followed by dysphoria, increased aggression/irritability. **Oversedation and respiratory depression with other CNS depressants,** seizures on withdrawal.

INTERACTIONS CNS depressants may increase levels of phenytoin, digoxin. Effects reduced by smoking, rifampin. Serum levels increased by cimetidine, valproate, disulfiram, oral contraceptives.

CONTRAINDICATIONS Coma, shock, alcohol intoxication, pregnancy, narrow-angle glaucoma. Use with caution in history of drug abuse/addiction.

NURSING CONSIDERATIONS Schedule IV controlled substance. Risk of respiratory depression when used with other CNS depressants. Abrupt discontinuation associated with anxiety, rebound insomnia, and seizures. Discontinuation titration may need to be as slow as 1 mg/day each week in some clients. Increased risk of ataxia and falls in the elderly.

CLIENT TEACHING Avoid hazardous activities during initiation. Avoid alcohol. Drug should not be discontinued suddenly.

AVAILABLE IN CANADA Rivotril, Alti-Clonazepam, Clonapam, Gen-Clonazepam, Nu-Clonazepam, PMS-Clonazepam, Rho-Clonazepam.

bold—Life-threatening reactions

GENERIC NAME: clozapine
TRADE NAME: Clozaril

CLASSIFICATION Atypical antipsychotic.

INDICATIONS & USES Treatment-refractory (failed to respond to typical antipsychotic medication) schizophrenia and schizoaffective disorders. Also used in treatment-refractory bipolar disorder, tardive dyskinesia, and emergent psychosis in treatment of Parkinson's disease.

USUAL ADULT DOSAGE RANGE 300-600 mg/day. Initial dosing is 12.5 mg once or twice a day. Total daily dose should not exceed 900 mg.

AVAILABLE FORMS Tabs 25, 100 mg.

PHARMACOKINETICS/DYNAMICS Rapidly absorbed; half-life averages 10-20 hr. PO onset of action: 30-60 min. Full therapeutic effects may not be apparent for 9-4 mo. Initial multiple daily dosing can often be consolidated to once or twice a day, once client is tolerant to side effects.

SIDE EFFECTS Sedation, fatigue, dizziness, blurred vision, dry mouth, constipation, diarrhea, urinary retention, nausea, vomiting, tachycardia, orthostatic hypotension, hypertension, weight gain, allergic dermatitis, skin photosensitivity, increased salivation, GI discomfort, diaphoresis, fever, neutropenia, eosinophilia.

ADVERSE REACTIONS **Agranulocytosis, seizures, possible neuroleptic malignant syndrome.**

INTERACTIONS Additive effects with CNS depressants (especially benzodiazepines). Epinephrine may result in reverse (hypotensive) effects. Serum levels are increased by antidepressants, cimetidine, and propranolol; reduced by carbamazepine and phenytoin. Antacids reduce absorption.

CONTRAINDICATIONS Contraindicated in coma, severe hypotension, acute subcortical brain damage, blood dyscrasia. Relatively contraindicated in liver disease, renal insufficiency. May exacerbate signs and symptoms of glaucoma, benign prostatic hypertrophy, diabetes. Avoid in pregnancy and lactating women.

NURSING CONSIDERATIONS Monitor level of sedation and vital signs carefully during dose titration. **Monitor WBC; do not start or give if WBC <3500/mm³.**

CLIENT TEACHING Use hats and sunscreens to reduce risk with sun exposure. Report lethargy, weakness, fever, sore throat, or other signs and symptoms of infection without delay. Weekly WBC monitoring required.

AVAILABLE IN CANADA Clozaril.

bold—Life-threatening reactions

GENERIC NAME; desipramine
TRADE NAME; Norpramin

CLASSIFICATION Tricyclic antidepressant.

INDICATIONS & USES Major depression, anxiety, panic, eating disorders, chronic pain.

USUAL ADULT DOSAGE RANGE 50-300 mg/day. In major depression, 150-300 mg/day; Initial dosing is 50-75 mg/day in divided doses.

AVAILABLE FORMS Tabs 10, 25, 50, 75, 100, 150 mg, caps 25, 50 mg.

PHARMACOKINETICS/DYNAMICS Half-life varies from 11-46 hr in adults. Plasma therapeutic range: 115-300 mg/ml. Full therapeutic effects may not be apparent for 2-4 wk. Initial multiple daily dosing can often be consolidated to once or twice a day, once client is tolerant to side effects.

SIDE EFFECTS Sedation, dizziness, blurred vision, dry mouth, constipation, urinary retention, nausea, vomiting, tachycardia, orthostatic hypotension, tremor, cardiac conduction abnormalities, decreased libido, weight gain, allergic dermatitis, skin photosensitivity, reduced seizure threshold.

ADVERSE REACTIONS Exacerbation of untreated narrow-angle glaucoma, induction of mania, reduced seizure threshold, **potentially fatal in overdose. Unexplained cardiac events resulting in sudden death have been reported in four children in the United States.**

INTERACTIONS Increased levels—cimetidine, fluoxetine, antipsychotics, methylphenidate, propoxyphene, quinidine. Decreased levels—barbiturates, phenytoin, chronic carbamazepine, chronic ethanol. Increased effects of epinephrine, norepinephrine, CNS depressants. **Severe hypertension with MAOIs.** Antacids reduce absorption.

CONTRAINDICATIONS Caution in clients with cardiovascular disease, arrhythmias, strokes, acute myocardial infarction, and thyroid disease/medications. May exacerbate signs and symptoms of glaucoma, benign prostatic hypertrophy, diabetes. Avoid in pregnant and lactating women.

NURSING CONSIDERATIONS Monitor level of sedation and vital signs carefully during dose titration. Suicide risk may be increased during initial improvement, particularly as psychomotor depression abates.

CLIENT TEACHING Therapeutic effects may take several weeks. May experience initial sedation and dizziness. Change positions slowly. Use hats and sunscreens to reduce risk with sun exposure.

AVAILABLE IN CANADA Norpramin, PMS-Desipramine, Alti-Desipramine, Novo-Desipramine, Nu-Desipramine.

bold—Life-threatening reactions

GENERIC NAME; diazepam
TRADE NAME; Valium

CLASSIFICATION Antianxiety agent, anticonvulsant—benzodiazepine.

INDICATIONS & USES Anxiety disorders, acute alcohol withdrawal, status epilepticus, adjunctive therapy in seizure disorders, skeletal muscle relaxant.

USUAL ADULT DOSAGE RANGE 2-40 mg/day.

AVAILABLE FORMS Tabs 2, 5, 10 mg, ext-rel caps 15 mg, IM/IV inj.

PHARMACOKINETICS/DYNAMICS Average half-life, including active metabolites, 100 hr. Very rapid PO absorption. IM absorption is erratic and unpredictable. Use in status epilepticus is IV.

SIDE EFFECTS Drowsiness, dizziness, ataxia. Rarely—nausea, vomiting, GI upset, blurred vision.

ADVERSE REACTIONS Anterograde amnesia. Rarely—increased aggression/irritability. Oversedation and **respiratory depression with other CNS depressants.**

INTERACTIONS CNS depressants, may increase levels of phenytoin, digoxin. Effects reduced by smoking, rifampin. Serum levels increased by cimetidine, valproate, oral contraceptives, disulfiram.

CONTRAINDICATIONS Coma, shock, alcohol intoxication, pregnancy. Use with caution in history of drug abuse/addiction.

NURSING CONSIDERATIONS Schedule IV controlled substance. Active metabolites with long half-life may result in accumulating effects over time. Risk of respiratory depression when used with other CNS depressants. Abrupt discontinuation associated with anxiety, rebound insomnia, and seizures. Rapid absorption causing a "buzz" may reinforce drug-seeking behavior or may be perceived dysphorically in non-drug abuse population.

CLIENT TEACHING Avoid hazardous activities during initiation. Avoid alcohol. Drug should not be discontinued suddenly.

AVAILABLE IN CANADA Vivol, Valium, Diazemuls, Apo-Diazepam.

bold—Life-threatening reactions

GENERIC NAME; diphenhydramine
TRADE NAME; Benadryl, Benalyn, various OTC products

CLASSIFICATION Antihistamine (H_1 blocker).

INDICATIONS & USES Acute and chronic treatment of drug-induced extrapyramidal reactions, hypnotic, sedation, allergy and cold symptoms; nausea, vomiting, vertigo, motion sickness.

USUAL ADULT DOSAGE RANGE 25-50 mg PO tid to qid. Acute dystonic reactions: 25-50 mg IM.

AVAILABLE FORMS Caps 25, 50 mg, tabs 25, 50 mg, elix 12.5 mg/5 ml, syr 12.5 mg/5 ml, inj IM, IV 10, 50 mg/ml.

PHARMACOKINETICS/DYNAMICS Rapidly absorbed, 50% bioavailable. Half-life varies considerably, between 3-9 hr in adults. IM effects begin in 15-30 min. Sedative effects after oral dosing are maximal at 1-3 hr. Nonspecific sedative effects are a result of histamine blockade. Substantial anticholinergic effects.

SIDE EFFECTS Drowsiness, sedation, fatigue, dry mouth, blurred vision, tachycardia, urinary retention, constipation, excitement, insomnia, confusion, nervousness.

ADVERSE REACTIONS With increased doses—risk of anticholinergic delirium.

INTERACTIONS Additive effects with CNS depressants, including alcohol. Severe cardiac or GI disorders, benign prostatic hypertrophy, angle-closure glaucoma.

CONTRAINDICATIONS Severe cardiac or GI disorders, benign prostatic hypertrophy, angle-closure glaucoma, stenosing peptic ulcer, asthma, nursing mother, infants.

NURSING CONSIDERATIONS/CLIENT TEACHING Increased risk of heat stroke. Evaluate for adequate hydration and constipation. May aggravate the movements of tardive dyskinesia. **Elderly at increased risk for confusion and anticholinergic delirium.** Injections should be deep IM, since superficial injections can be locally irritating.

AVAILABLE IN CANADA Benadryl, Allerdryl, AllerMax, Nytol, Nytol Extra Strength, PMS-Diphenhydramine.

bold—Life-threatening reactions

GENERIC NAME; fluoxetine
TRADE NAME; Prozac

CLASSIFICATION Antidepressant—serotonin selective reuptake inhibitor.

INDICATIONS & USES Major depression, obsessive-compulsive disorder.

USUAL ADULT DOSAGE RANGE 10-80 mg/day; Initial dosing is 20 mg qaw. Maximum dose is 80 mg/day.

AVAILABLE FORMS Pulvules 20 mg, caps 10 mg, liquid 20 mg/5 ml.

PHARMACOKINETICS/DYNAMICS In adults, half-life is 2-6 days for fluoxetine and 4-16 days for norfluoxetine (active metabolite). Thus steady state may not be achieved for a month or more after dosage changes. Full therapeutic effects may not be apparent for 2-4 wk.

SIDE EFFECTS Agitation, irritability, insomnia, headache, dizziness, GI upset, drowsiness, fatigue, diarrhea, tremor, sexual dysfunction, slight weight loss, akathisia, nervousness, sweating, occasionally—extrapyramidal symptoms, rarely—bradycardia.

ADVERSE REACTIONS Induction of mania, rash.

INTERACTIONS **Potentially fatal hypertensive crisis when MAOIs (including selegiline) are used within 5 wk of discontinuation.** Increased levels of haloperidol, tricyclic antidepressants, propranolol, benzodiazepines. Loss of therapeutic efficacy with cyproheptadine.

CONTRAINDICATIONS MAOI use within 5 wk. Avoid in pregnant and nursing mothers. May accumulate substantially in hepatic and renal disease and in debilitated clients.

NURSING CONSIDERATIONS Suicide risk may be increased during initial improvement, particularly as psychomotor depression abates.

CLIENT TEACHING Therapeutic effects may take several weeks. Low risk of fatality in overdose. Sexual dysfunction (loss of libido, delayed ejaculation, anorgasmy) may persist and interfere with compliance.

AVAILABLE IN CANADA Prozac, Apo-Fluoxetine, Novo-Fluoxetine, Nu-Fluoxetine, PMS-Fluoxetine.

bold—Life-threatening reactions

GENERIC NAME: fluphenazine
TRADE NAME: Prolixin, Permitil

CLASSIFICATION Typical antipsychotic.

INDICATIONS & USES Symptomatic management of psychotic disorders, initial management of psychotic manic states.

USUAL ADULT DOSAGE RANGE 1-20 mg/day. Initial dosing is 2.5-10 mg/day every day in divided doses. Fluphenazine decanoate 12.5-25 mg IM every 1-3 wk.

AVAILABLE FORMS HCl tabs 1, 2.5, 5, 10 mg; elix 2.5 mg/5 ml; conc 5 mg/ml; inj IM 10 mg/ml; enanthate, decanoate, inj SC, IM 25 mg/ml.

PHARMACOKINETICS/DYNAMICS Rapidly absorbed; half-life averages 10-20 hr. Onset of action: 30-60 min. Full therapeutic effects may not be apparent for 6-12 wk. Initial multiple daily dosing can often be consolidated to once or twice a day, once client is tolerant to side effects. The half-life of fluphenazine decanoate is approximately 14 days.

SIDE EFFECTS Sedation, nausea, vomiting, acute dystonic reaction, stiffness, cogwheel rigidity, bradykinesia, akathisia, synecomastia, galactorrhea, amenorrhea, decreased libido, weight gain, allergic dermatitis, skin photosensitivity, reduced seizure threshold.

ADVERSE REACTIONS Risk of tardive dyskinesia, **neuroleptic malignant syndrome**, seizures.

INTERACTIONS Additive effects with CNS depressants. Serum levels are increased by antidepressants and propranolol, reduced by carbamazepine and phenytoin. Antacids reduce absorption. Do not mix liquid concentrate with coffee, tea, cola, or apple juice.

CONTRAINDICATIONS Contraindicated in coma, severe hypotension, acute subcortical brain damage. Relatively contraindicated in liver

disease, renal insufficiency, blood dyscrasias, Parkinson's disease. May exacerbate signs and symptoms of glaucoma, benign prostatic hypertrophy, diabetes. Avoid in pregnant and lactating women.

NURSING CONSIDERATIONS Monitor level of sedation and vital signs carefully during dose titration. Rapid dose increases, dehydration, IM injections, and agitation are associated with increased incidence of neuroleptic malignant syndrome.

CLIENT TEACHING Use hats and sunscreen to reduce risk with sun exposure. Report fever and increasing stiffness immediately.

AVAILABLE IN CANADA Moditen, Apo-Fluphenazine.

bold—Life-threatening reactions

GENERIC NAME: haloperidol
TRADE NAME: Haldol

CLASSIFICATION Typical antipsychotic.

INDICATIONS & USES Symptomatic management of psychotic disorders, initial management of psychotic manic states.

USUAL ADULT DOSAGE RANGE 6-20 mg/day. Initial dosing is 0.5-10 mg/day every day in divided doses. Total daily doses as high as 100 mg/day may be required. Typical IM dose is 2-5 mg. Haloperidol decanoate, 25-100 mg IM q 4 wk.

AVAILABLE FORMS Tabs 0.5, 1, 2, 5, 10, 20 mg; conc 2 mg/ml; inj IM 5 mg/ml; Haldol Decanoate inj 50 mg/ml, 100 mg/ml.

PHARMACOKINETICS/DYNAMICS Rapidly absorbed; half-life averages 10-20 hr. Onset of action: 30-60 min. Full therapeutic effects may not be apparent for 6-12 wk. Initial multiple daily dosing can often be consolidated to once or twice a day, once client is tolerant to side effects. The half-life of haloperidol decanoate is approximately 21 days.

SIDE EFFECTS Sedation, nausea, vomiting, acute dystonic reaction, stiffness, cogwheel rigidity, bradykinesia, akathisia, synecomastia, galactorrhea, amenorrhea, decreased libido, weight gain, allergic dermatitis, skin photosensitivity, reduced seizure threshold.

ADVERSE REACTIONS Risk of tardive dyskinesia, **neuroleptic malignant syndrome**, seizures.

INTERACTIONS Additive effects with CNS depressants. Serum levels are increased by antidepressants and propranolol, reduced by carbamazepine and phenytoin. Antacids reduce absorption. Do not mix liquid concentrate with milk, coffee, tea, grape juice, or grapefruit juice.

CONTRAINDICATIONS Contraindicated in coma, severe hypotension, acute subcortical brain damage. Relatively contraindicated in liver disease, renal insufficiency, blood dyscrasias, Parkinson's disease. May exacerbate signs and symptoms of glaucoma, benign prostatic hypertrophy, diabetes. Avoid in pregnant and lactating women.

NURSING CONSIDERATIONS Monitor level of sedation and vital signs carefully during dose titration. Rapid dose increases, dehydration, IM injections, and agitation are associated with increased incidence of neuroleptic malignant syndrome.

CLIENT TEACHING Use hats and sunscreens to reduce risk with sun exposure. Report fever and increasing stiffness immediately.

AVAILABLE IN CANADA Apo-Haloperidol, Peridol, Haldol, Novo-Peridol, PMS-Haloperidol LA.

bold—Life-threatening reactions

GENERIC NAME: fluvoxamine
TRADE NAME: Luvox

CLASSIFICATION Antiobsessional—serotonin selective reuptake inhibitor.

INDICATIONS & USES Obsessive-compulsive disorder, major depression.

USUAL ADULT DOSAGE RANGE 100-300 mg/day. Initial dosing is 50 mg hs. Maximum dose is 300 mg/day; bid dosing is recommended for doses >100 mg/day. In unequal doses, larger dose should be at bedtime.

AVAILABLE FORMS Tabs 50, 100 mg.

PHARMACOKINETICS/DYNAMICS In adults, half-life is approximately 16 hr. Full therapeutic effects may not be apparent for 2-4 wk.

SIDE EFFECTS Somnolence, insomnia, nervousness, nausea, sexual dysfunction, weakness, dry mouth, dizziness, constipation, sweating, tremor, dyspepsia, anorexia, vomiting.

ADVERSE REACTIONS Induction of mania, rash, seizures.

INTERACTIONS **Potentially fatal hypertensive crisis when MAOIs (including selegiline) are used within 2 wk of discontinuation.** Diazepam should not be used. Alprazolam and triazolam doses should be halved. Increased astemizole and terfenadine levels may lead to cardiac arrhythmias. Theophylline dose should be decreased, and serum levels monitored closely. Warfarin may be increased by nearly 100%; monitor prothrombin times closely.

CONTRAINDICATIONS **MAOI use within 2 weeks.** Avoid in pregnant and nursing mothers. May accumulate substantially in hepatic and renal disease and in the debilitated. **Do not use with astemizole or terfenadine.**

bold—Life-threatening reactions

NURSING CONSIDERATIONS Suicide risk may be increased during initial improvement, particularly as psychomotor depression abates. Low risk of fatality in overdose. Sexual dysfunction (loss of libido, delayed ejaculation, anorgasmy) may persist and interfere with compliance.

CLIENT TEACHING Therapeutic effects may take several weeks.

AVAILABLE IN CANADA Luvox, Apo-Fluvoxamine, Alti-Fluvoxamine.

GENERIC NAME: imipramine
TRADE NAME: Tofranil

CLASSIFICATION Tricyclic antidepressant.

INDICATIONS & USES Major depression; anxiety, panic, eating disorders; chronic pain; childhood enuresis.

USUAL ADULT DOSAGE RANGE 50-300 mg/day. In major depression: 150-300 mg/day. Initial dosing is 50-75 mg/day in divided doses.

AVAILABLE FORMS Tabs 10, 25, 50 mg; inj IM 25 mg/2 ml.

PHARMACOKINETICS/DYNAMICS Half-life varies from 6-28 hr in adults to 21-35 hr in the elderly. Partially metabolized to desipramine. Plasma therapeutic range (imipramine + desipramine): 200-300 mg/ml. Full therapeutic effects may not be apparent for 2-4 wk. Initial multiple daily dosing can often be consolidated to once or twice a day, once client is tolerant to side effects.

SIDE EFFECTS Sedation, dizziness, blurred vision, dry mouth, constipation, urinary retention, nausea, vomiting, tachycardia, orthostatic hypotension, tremor, cardiac conduction abnormalities, decreased libido, weight gain, allergic dermatitis, skin photosensitivity, reduced seizure threshold.

ADVERSE REACTIONS Exacerbation of untreated narrow-angle glaucoma, induction of mania, reduced seizure threshold, **potentially fatal in overdose.**

INTERACTIONS Increased levels—cimetidine, fluoxetine, antipsychotics, methylphenidate, propoxyphene. Decreased levels—barbiturates, phenytoin, chronic carbamazepine. Increased effects of epinephrine, norepinephrine, CNS depressants. **Severe hypertension with MAOIs.** Antacids reduce absorption.

CONTRAINDICATIONS Caution in clients with cardiovascular disease, arrhythmias, strokes, acute myocardial infarction, and thyroid disease/medications. May exacerbate signs and symptoms of glaucoma, benign prostatic hypertrophy, diabetes. Avoid in pregnant and lactating women.

NURSING CONSIDERATIONS Monitor level of sedation and vital signs carefully during dose titration. Suicide risk may be increased during initial improvement, particularly as psychomotor depression abates.

CLIENT TEACHING Therapeutic effects may take several weeks. May experience initial sedation and dizziness. Change positions slowly. Use hats and sunscreens to reduce risk with sun exposure.

AVAILABLE IN CANADA Apo-Imipramine, Tofranil.

bold—Life-threatening reactions

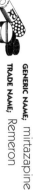

lithium

GENERIC NAME; lithium
TRADE NAME; Eskalith, Eskalith CR, Lithane, Lithobid, Cibalith-S

CLASSIFICATION Antimanic.

INDICATIONS & USES Bipolar disorder, adjunctive therapy in depression, adjunctive therapy in schizophrenia, adjunctive treatment in aggression.

USUAL ADULT DOSAGE RANGE 300-1800 mg/day in divided doses. Typical initial dosing—300 mg tid. Subsequent dosing is determined by serum level monitoring.

AVAILABLE FORMS Caps 150, 300, 600 mg; tabs 300, 450 mg; syrup 300 mg/5 ml.

PHARMACOKINETICS/DYNAMICS Average half-life in healthy adults is 18-27 hr. Half-life varies widely and is dependent on renal function. Maintenance therapeutic range in adults is 0.8-1.2 mEq/L.

SIDE EFFECTS Fine tremor, mild GI upset, diarrhea, polyuria, polydipsia, muscle weakness, lethargy, leukocytosis, hypothyroidism, exacerbation of psoriasis, acne, alopecia, weight gain.

ADVERSE REACTIONS (Including symptoms that may predict serious lithium toxicity)—coarsening of tremor, confusion, excessive sedation, ataxia, dysarthria, mental status deterioration, seizure, **coma, cardiovascular collapse.** Severe polyuria, polydipsia, and GI upset, goiter formation.

INTERACTIONS Increases lithium levels—hydrochlorothiazide, nonsteroidal antiinflammatory drugs (e.g., ibuprofen, indomethacin), angiotensin-converting enzyme inhibitors (e.g., captopril, enalapril). Decreases lithium levels—sodium bicarbonate, sodium chloride, theophylline, caffeine, urea. Potential for neurotoxicity when used with carbamazepine, calcium channel blockers. **Risk factor for neuroleptic malignant syndrome when used with typical anti-** psychotics. **Reductions in dietary sodium or excessive sweating result in increased or toxic lithium levels.**

CONTRAINDICATIONS Severe renal disease, cardiovascular disease, organic brain syndrome, dehydration. Use in pregnancy may increase risk of Ebstein's anomaly (cardiac valve formation).

NURSING CONSIDERATIONS Draw blood 12 hr after previous dose. Monitor for peripheral edema or sudden weight gain. May give with meals to reduce GI disturbance. GI disturbance common on initiation, but subsides. A return of GI symptoms may indicate lithium toxicity. Report excessive thirst or water consumption.

CLIENT TEACHING Report GI upset, sedation, ataxia, or increasing tremor immediately. It is important to **maintain stable salt intake in diet.**

AVAILABLE IN CANADA Carbolith, Lithane, Duralith, PMS-Lithium Carbonate, PMS-Lithium Citrate.

bold—Life-threatening reactions

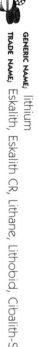

mirtazapine

GENERIC NAME; mirtazapine
TRADE NAME; Remeron

CLASSIFICATION Antidepressant.

INDICATIONS & USES Clinical depression.

USUAL ADULT DOSAGE RANGE 15-45 mg daily. Initial dosing is 15 mg PO hs.

AVAILABLE FORMS Tabs 15, 40 mg.

PHARMACOKINETICS/DYNAMICS Enhances central noradrenergic and serotonergic activity, ameliorating symptoms of depression.

SIDE EFFECTS CNS—somnolence, dizziness, asthenia, abnormal dreams, abnormal thinking, tremors, confusion; GI—nausea, increased appetite, dry mouth, constipation; GU—urinary frequency.

ADVERSE REACTIONS Agranulocytosis (rare), confusion.

INTERACTIONS Drug-drug; diazepam, other CNS depressants, possible additive CNS effects; MAOIs—sometimes **fatal** reaction. (Avoid concomitant use of CNS depressants of MAOIs.) Drug-lifestyle: alcohol use results in possible additive CNS effects (avoid use). May increase cholesterol, triglyceride, ALT (serum transaminase levels).

CONTRAINDICATIONS Clients with hypersensitivity to the drug. Drug should not be used with MAO inhibitor or within 14 days of initiating or discontinuing therapy with MAO inhibitor. At least 14 days should elapse after stopping mirtazapine before starting MAO inhibitor.

NURSING CONSIDERATIONS Use cautiously in clients with cardiovascular or cerebrovascular disease, seizure disorder, **suicidal ideations,** impaired hepatic or renal function, or history of mania or hypomania. Use cautiously in clients with conditions that predispose them to hypotension, such as dehydration, hypovolemia, or treatment with antihypertensive medication. Although **agranulocytosis** is rare, discontinue drug and monitor client closely if sore throat, fever, stomatitis or other signs of infection are present, along with a **low WBC count.** Monitor client closely for signs of dependence. It is not known whether mirtazapine causes physical or psychologic dependence.

CLIENT TEACHING Do not perform hazardous activities if somnolence occurs. Report signs and symptoms of infection, such as fever, chills, sore throat, mucous membrane ulceration, or flulike symptoms (may be agranulocytosis). Avoid alcohol and other CNS depressants while taking drug. Do not take concomitant medications without physician's approval. Clients should understand importance of therapy compliance. Female clients of childbearing age should report suspected pregnancy immediately and notify physician if breast-feeding.

AVAILABLE IN CANADA Not available.

---

lorazepam

GENERIC NAME; lorazepam
TRADE NAME; Ativan

CLASSIFICATION Antianxiety agent—benzodiazepine.

INDICATIONS & USES Anxiety, adjunct in treatment of agitation and irritability in other psychiatric disorders, sometimes used for insomnia.

USUAL ADULT DOSAGE RANGE 2-6 mg/day in divided doses (bid or tid); Acute use: 1-2 mg IM q4-6h.

AVAILABLE FORMS Tabs 0.5, 1, 2 mg; IM/IV inj 2,4 mg/ml.

PHARMACOKINETICS/DYNAMICS Average half-life is 10-20 hr. Absorption is considerably more rapid with PO concentrate and IM administration. Initial therapeutic effects may be observed within 15 min. Some clients require tid dosing to avoid breakthrough symptoms. No active metabolites.

SIDE EFFECTS Drowsiness, dizziness, ataxia. Rarely—nausea, vomiting, GI upset, blurred vision.

CONTRAINDICATIONS Coma, shock, alcohol intoxication, pregnancy. Use with caution in history of drug abuse/addiction.

ADVERSE REACTIONS Anterograde amnesia, rarely—increased aggression/irritability. Oversedation and respiratory depression with other CNS depressants.

INTERACTIONS CNS depressants, may increase levels of phenytoin, digoxin. Effects reduced by smoking, oral contraceptives.

NURSING CONSIDERATIONS Schedule IV controlled substance. Risk of respiratory depression when used with other CNS depressants. Abrupt discontinuation associated with anxiety, rebound insomnia, and seizures.

CLIENT TEACHING Avoid hazardous activities during initiation. Avoid alcohol. Drug should not be discontinued suddenly.

AVAILABLE IN CANADA Apo-Lorazepam, Novo-Lorazem, Ativan, Nu-Lorax.

bold—Life-threatening reactions

---

nefazodone

GENERIC NAME; nefazodone
TRADE NAME; Serzone

CLASSIFICATION Triazolopyridine antidepressant.

INDICATIONS & USES Major depression.

USUAL ADULT DOSAGE RANGE 300-600 mg/day. Initial dosing is 100 mg bid (50 mg bid in the elderly) for 1 wk, then increased to 150 mg bid. Maximum dose is 600 mg/day in divided doses.

AVAILABLE FORMS Tabs 100, 150, 200, 250 mg.

PHARMACOKINETICS/DYNAMICS In adults, half-life is approximately 2-4 hr. Full therapeutic effects may not be apparent for 2-4 wk.

SIDE EFFECTS Weakness, dry mouth, nausea, constipation, somnolence, dizziness, light-headedness, confusion, blurred vision, abnormal vision (visual flashes). The abnormal vision that may occur with initiation and/or dose increase is of short duration and not clinically significant.

ADVERSE REACTIONS Induction of mania.

INTERACTIONS **Potentially fatal cardiac arrhythmias with astemizole and terfenadine. Potentially fatal hypertensive crisis when MAOIs (including selegiline) are used within 2 wk of discontinuation.** May increase triazolam serum levels by 75% and alprazolam levels by 50%. May increase phenytoin levels by 10%.

CONTRAINDICATIONS **Never use with astemizole and terfenadine.** Avoid in pregnant and nursing mothers.

NURSING CONSIDERATIONS Suicide risk may be increased during initial improvement, particularly as psychomotor depression abates.

CLIENT TEACHING Therapeutic effects may take several weeks. May experience excessive sedation during initiation. Stand up slowly to avoid dizziness.

AVAILABLE IN CANADA Serzone.

bold—Life-threatening reactions

CLASSIFICATION Antipsychotic—thienbenzodiazepine.

INDICATIONS & USES Management of manifestations of psychotic disorders.

USUAL ADULT DOSAGE RANGE 5-10 mg/day. Do not exceed 20 mg/day.

AVAILABLE FORMS Tabs 5, 7.5, 10 mg.

PHARMACOKINETICS/DYNAMICS Basically unknown; binds to dopamine and serotonin receptors in the brain and may interfere with adrenergic, cholinergic, and histaminergic receptors.

SIDE EFFECTS CNS—somnolence, agitation, anxiety, hostility, Parkinsonian symptoms, euphoria; CV—orthostatic hypotension, chest pain, tachycardia, edema; EENT—amblyopia, corneal lesions; GI—nausea, vomiting, constipation, dry mouth, polydipsia; GU—premenstrual syndrome (PMS), metrorrhagia, hematuria, increased urinary tract infections.

ADVERSE REACTIONS Tardive dyskinesia, extrapyramidal symptoms, **neuroleptic malignant syndrome.**

INTERACTIONS Potentiates antihypertensives. Increased clearance of olanzapine when using carbamazepine. Diazepam and alcohol potentiate CNS effects.

CONTRAINDICATIONS Known hypersensitivity to the drug; client with liver impairment or cardiovascular dysfunction.

NURSING CONSIDERATIONS Monitor bilirubin, CBC, liver function studies; assess dizziness and tachycardia on rising; monitor constipation, urinary retention; increase bulk/fiber/water in diet. Use caution when dosing elderly clients.

CLIENT TEACHING Stand up slowly to avoid dizziness. Avoid overheating, driving, and alcohol intake. Use ice chips, sugarless gum, or candy for dry mouth. Notify physician of pregnancy. Teach client symptom recognition and to call physician with changes. Discuss dietary regulations to avoid constipation.

AVAILABLE IN CANADA Zyprexa.

bold—Life-threatening reactions

GENERIC NAME; paroxetine
TRADE NAME; Paxil

CLASSIFICATION Antidepressant—serotonin selective reuptake inhibitor.

INDICATIONS & USES Major depression, obsessive-compulsive disorder.

USUAL ADULT DOSAGE RANGE 10-50 mg/day. Initial dosing is 20 mg/day (10 mg/day in the elderly or debilitated). Maximum dose is 50 mg/day.

AVAILABLE FORMS Tabs 20, 30 mg.

PHARMACOKINETICS/DYNAMICS In adults, half-life is approximately 21 hr. Full therapeutic effects may not be apparent for 2-4 wk.

SIDE EFFECTS Agitation, irritability, insomnia, headache, dizziness, GI upset, dry mouth, constipation, sedation, sexual dysfunction, slight weight loss, tremor, akathisia, sweating, somnolence, nervousness, occasionally extrapyramidal symptoms.

ADVERSE REACTIONS Induction of mania, rash.

INTERACTIONS **Potentially fatal hypertensive crisis when MAOIs (including selegiline) are used within 2 wk of discontinuation.** Loss of therapeutic efficacy with cyproheptadine.

CONTRAINDICATIONS **MAOI use within 2 wk.** Avoid in pregnant and nursing mothers.

NURSING CONSIDERATIONS Suicide risk may be increased during initial improvement, particularly as psychomotor depression abates. Low risk of fatality in overdose. Sexual dysfunction (loss of libido, delayed ejaculation, anorgasmy) may persist and interfere with compliance.

CLIENT TEACHING Therapeutic effects may take several weeks.

bold—Life-threatening reactions

AVAILABLE IN CANADA Paxil.

GENERIC NAME; perphenazine
TRADE NAME; Trilafon

CLASSIFICATION Typical antipsychotic.

INDICATIONS & USES Symptomatic management of psychotic disorders, initial management of psychotic manic states.

USUAL ADULT DOSAGE RANGE 8-40 mg/day. Initial dosing is 4-8 mg/day. Typical IM dose is 5-10 mg.

AVAILABLE FORMS Tabs 2, 4, 8, 16 mg; sol 16 mg/5 ml; inj IM/IV 5 mg/ml; sus-rel tabs 8 mg.

PHARMACOKINETICS/DYNAMICS Rapidly absorbed, half-life averages 10-20 hr. Onset of action: 30-60 min. Full therapeutic effects may not be apparent for 6-12 wk. Initial multiple daily dosing can often be consolidated to once or twice a day, once client is tolerant to side effects.

ADVERSE REACTIONS Risk of tardive dyskinesia, **neuroleptic malignant syndrome.**

SIDE EFFECTS Sedation, dizziness, blurred vision, dry mouth, constipation, urinary retention, nausea, vomiting, tachycardia, orthostatic hypotension, acute dystonic reaction, stiffness, cogwheel rigidity, bradykinesia, akathisia, gynecomastia, galactorrhea, amenorrhea, decreased libido, retrograde ejaculation, weight gain, allergic dermatitis, skin photosensitivity, reduced seizure threshold.

INTERACTIONS Additive effects with CNS depressants and anticholinergic drugs. Serum levels are increased by antidepressants and propranolol, and reduced by carbamazepine and phenytoin. Epinephrine may result in reverse (hypotensive) effects. Antacids reduce absorption.

CONTRAINDICATIONS Contraindicated in coma, severe hypotension, acute subcortical brain damage. Relatively contraindicated in liver disease, renal insufficiency, blood dyscrasia, Parkinson's disease. May exacerbate signs and symptoms of glaucoma, benign prostatic hypertrophy, diabetes. Avoid in pregnant and lactating women.

NURSING CONSIDERATIONS Monitor level of sedation and vital signs carefully during dose titration. Rapid dose increases, dehydration, and agitation are associated with increased incidence of neuroleptic malignant syndrome.

CLIENT TEACHING Rise from bed and change positions slowly to avoid dizziness. Use sugarless gum and candy for dry mouth. Use hats and sunscreens to reduce risk with sun exposure.

AVAILABLE IN CANADA Apo-Perphenazine, Trilafon.

bold—Life-threatening reactions

GENERIC NAME; phenelzine
TRADE NAME; Nardil

CLASSIFICATION Antidepressant, monoamine oxidase inhibitor.

INDICATIONS & USES Atypical depression, treatment-refractory depression, panic disorder.

USUAL ADULT DOSAGE RANGE 45-90 mg/day. Can be given in divided doses. Thereafter may be increased 15 mg/day each week. Maximum dose is 90 mg/day.

AVAILABLE FORMS Tabs 15 mg.

PHARMACOKINETICS/DYNAMICS Well absorbed. Irreversibly inhibits monoamine oxidase (MAO). Maximal inhibition at a particular dose is complete in 5-10 days. After discontinuation, 2 weeks are required for resynthesis of baseline levels of MAO. Full therapeutic effects may not be apparent for 2-6 wk.

SIDE EFFECTS Orthostatic hypotension, dizziness, insomnia, paresthesia, sweating, flushing, edema, sexual dysfunction, weight gain.

ADVERSE REACTIONS **Hypertensive crisis secondary to tyramine-rich foods, stimulant drugs (e.g., nasal decongestants). Serotonin syndrome (autonomic instability, hyperthermia, rigidity, myoclonus, altered mental status—confusion, delirium, coma) with SSRIs.**

INTERACTIONS **Tyramine-rich foods, sympathomimetic drugs (e.g., phenylpropanolamine, ephedrine),** dextromethorphan, antihypertensives (reserpine, guanethidine), L-dopa, narcotics, antiasthmatics (epinephrine, isoproterenol), diuretics, general anesthetics.

CONTRAINDICATIONS Relatively contraindicated in renal disease, cardiovascular disease, hyperthyroidism, Parkinson's disease, asthma. May alter glucose treatment requirements in diabetes.

NURSING CONSIDERATIONS Monitor blood pressure closely. Assess for symptoms of hypertensive crisis reaction.

CLIENT TEACHING Teach client dietary restrictions, symptoms of hypertensive crisis reaction (pounding headache, neck stiffness, nausea, sweating), and drug interactions. Advise client not to take cough or cold preparation or weight loss pills without professional counsel.

AVAILABLE IN CANADA Nardil.

bold—Life-threatening reactions

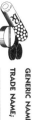

GENERIC NAME; propranolol
TRADE NAME; Inderal

CLASSIFICATION Antihypertensive—nonselective β-adrenergic blocking agent.

INDICATIONS & USES Hypertension, angina pectoris, cardiac arrhythmias, migraine headache, essential motor tremor, hypertrophic subaortic stenosis, pheochromocytoma, social phobias (including stage fright), adjunctive treatment of chronic aggression (including aggression in schizophrenia), drug-induced tremor (e.g., lithium tremor), akathisia.

USUAL ADULT DOSAGE RANGE 40-320 mg/day in divided doses. Required dose varies widely. Typical starting doses are 10-20 mg bid or tid. In general, treatment of cardiovascular disorders may require higher doses (up to 640 mg/day) than other indications. Performance anxiety may be treated with doses of 10-40 mg 30 min before event. Akathisia seldom requires doses >120 mg/day. Use of high doses (>640 mg/day) is controversial.

AVAILABLE FORMS Ext-rel caps 60, 80, 120, 160 mg; tabs 10, 20, 40, 60, 80, 90 mg; inj 1 mg/ml; oral sol 4 mg, 8 mg/ml; conc oral sol 80 mg/ml.

PHARMACOKINETICS/DYNAMICS Rapidly absorbed, average half-life is 3-6 hr. Onset of efficacy varies with the indication. Typical time to onset of therapeutic efficacy: social phobia—minutes; akathisia, tremor—1-2 days; full effects in chronic aggression may not be apparent for 2-4 mo.

SIDE EFFECTS Bradycardia, hypotension, dizziness, lethargy, fatigue, vivid dreams, epigastric distress, nausea, diarrhea, abdominal cramping, edema.

ADVERSE REACTIONS Wheezing, laryngospasm, pulmonary edema, depression.

INTERACTIONS Increased effects of insulin, oral hypoglycemics (e.g., glyburide), antihypertensives, calcium channel blockers. Increases plasma levels of chlorpromazine, thioridazine, haloperidol, theophylline. Monitor plasma levels of anticonvulsants.

CONTRAINDICATIONS **Cardiogenic shock, sinus bradycardia, heart block >1st degree, Wolff-Parkinson-White syndrome, bronchial asthma,** chronic obstructive pulmonary disease, Raynaud's syndrome. Relatively contraindicated in diabetes mellitus, hyperthyroidism, peripheral vascular disease, pregnancy, impaired hepatic or renal function.

NURSING CONSIDERATIONS Monitor pulse and orthostatic blood pressure, weight, closely at baseline and during drug regimen changes. Hold dose and notify prescriber for dizziness, ataxia, wheezing. CNS side effects and depression are more common at doses >240 mg/day. **Sudden discontinuation can result in profound tachycardia.**

CLIENT TEACHING Rise from bed and change positions slowly to avoid dizziness. Use sugarless gum and candy for dry mouth. Use hats and sunscreens to reduce risk with sun exposure.

AVAILABLE IN CANADA Apo-Propranolol, Inderal, Inderal LA, Nu-Propranolol.

bold—Life-threatening reactions

GENERIC NAME; risperidone
TRADE NAME; Risperdal

CLASSIFICATION Atypical antipsychotic.

INDICATIONS & USES Symptomatic management of psychotic disorders.

USUAL ADULT DOSAGE RANGE 4-8 mg/day; Initial dosing is 1 mg bid. Total daily doses as high as 16 mg/day may be required.

AVAILABLE FORMS Tabs 1, 2, 3, 4 mg

PHARMACOKINETICS/DYNAMICS Rapidly absorbed; half-life averages 10-20 hr. PO onset of action: 30-60 min. Full therapeutic effects may not be apparent for 6-12 wk.

SIDE EFFECTS Mild sedation, dizziness, nausea, vomiting, tachycardia, orthostatic hypotension, acute dystonic reaction, stiffness, cogwheel rigidity, bradykinesia, akathisia, gynecomastia, galactorrhea, amenorrhea, decreased libido, retrograde ejaculation, weight gain, allergic dermatitis, skin photosensitivity, reduced seizure threshold, anxiety, constipation, rhinitis, rash. Extrapyramidal symptoms are minimal at doses ≤6 mg/day, but increase with increasing dose.

ADVERSE REACTIONS Risk of tardive dyskinesia, **neuroleptic malignant syndrome.**

INTERACTIONS Additive effects with CNS depressants. Serum levels are increased by antidepressants and propranolol, reduced by carbamazepine and phenytoin. Antacids reduce absorption.

CONTRAINDICATIONS Contraindicated in coma, severe hypotension, acute subcortical brain damage. Relatively contraindicated in liver disease, renal insufficiency, blood dyscrasias, Parkinson's disease. May exacerbate signs and symptoms of glaucoma, benign prostatic hypertrophy, diabetes. Avoid in pregnant and lactating women.

NURSING CONSIDERATIONS Monitor level of sedation and vital signs carefully during dose titration.

CLIENT TEACHING Use hats and sunscreens to reduce risk with sun exposure. Report fever and increasing stiffness immediately.

AVAILABLE IN CANADA Risperdal.

bold—Life-threatening reactions

GENERIC NAME; quetiapine fumarate
TRADE NAME; Seroquel

CLASSIFICATION Antipsychotic drug—dibenzothiazepine derivative.

INDICATIONS & USES Management of manifestations of psychotic disorders.

USUAL ADULT DOSAGE RANGE 25 mg bid with increases in increments of 25-50 mg bid or tid on days 2 or 3, as tolerated. Antipsychotic efficacy at dose range of 150-750 mg/day. Expected steady-state concentration at 2 days.

AVAILABLE FORMS Tabs 25, 100, 200 mg

PHARMACOKINETICS/DYNAMICS Basically unknown. Proposed to act as antagonist at multiple neurotransmitter receptors in the brain: serotonin 5HT₁ and 5HT₂, dopamine, histamine, and adrenergic receptors. Eliminated mainly by liver metabolism; half-life about 6 hours.

SIDE EFFECTS CNS—dizziness, somnolence, cardiovascular—postural hypotension, tachycardia, peripheral edema; EENT—rhinitis, ear pain, GI—dry mouth, anorexia, constipation.

ADVERSE REACTIONS Leukopenia, seizures, hypothyroidism, extrapyramidal symptoms, neuroleptic malignant syndrome, suicide by overdose.

INTERACTIONS Use with caution when taking other centrally acting drugs. Potentiates cognitive and motor effects of alcohol. May enhance certain hypertensive agents and acts as antagonist with levodopa and dopamine agonists.

CONTRAINDICATIONS Avoid with pregnant or nursing women. Avoid if hepatic impairment or hypotensive problems.

NURSING CONSIDERATIONS **Caution with client history of seizures or hypotension. Monitor liver function values. Monitor for EPS and neuroleptic malignant syndrome symptoms.**

CLIENT TEACHING Avoid getting overheated or dehydrated. Avoid alcohol and using hazardous machinery or driving vehicle while taking medication. Stand up slowly (to avoid dizziness.) Contraindicated with breast-feeding. Teach client symptom recognition and to call physician about changes.

AVAILABLE IN CANADA Seroquel.

bold—Life-threatening reactions

GENERIC NAME; sertraline
TRADE NAME; Zoloft

CLASSIFICATION Antidepressant—serotonin selective reuptake inhibitor.

INDICATIONS & USES Major depression, obsessive-compulsive disorder.

USUAL ADULT DOSAGE RANGE 50-200 mg/day. Initial dosing is 50-100 mg/day. Maximum dose is 200 mg/day.

AVAILABLE FORMS Tabs 50, 100 mg

PHARMACOKINETICS/DYNAMICS In adults, half-life is approximately 25 hr. Full therapeutic effects may not be apparent for 2-4 wk.

SIDE EFFECTS Agitation, irritability, insomnia, headache, dizziness, GI upset, sexual dysfunction, slight weight loss, dry mouth, tremor, akathisia, increased side effects, diarrhea, occasionally—extrapyramidal symptoms, rarely—bradycardia.

ADVERSE REACTIONS Induction of mania, rash.

INTERACTIONS **Potentially fatal hypertensive crisis when MAOIs (including selegiline) are used within 2 wk of discontinuation.** Loss of therapeutic efficacy with cyproheptadine.

CONTRAINDICATIONS **MAOI use within 2 wk.** Avoid in pregnant and nursing mothers.

NURSING CONSIDERATIONS Suicide risk may be increased during initial improvement, particularly as psychomotor depression abates. Low risk of fatality in overdose. Sexual dysfunction (loss of libido, delayed ejaculation, anorgasmia) may persist and interfere with compliance.

CLIENT TEACHING Therapeutic effects may take several weeks.

AVAILABLE IN CANADA Zoloft.

bold—Life-threatening reactions

GENERIC NAME: tacrine hydrochloride
TRADE NAME: Cognex

CLASSIFICATION Centrally active, reversible anticholinesterase agent.

INDICATIONS & USES Palliative treatment of mild to moderate dementia of Alzheimer's type.

USUAL ADULT DOSAGE RANGE 10-40 mg. Initial dosing is 40 mg qid.

AVAILABLE FORMS Caps: 10, 20, 30, 40 mg.

PHARMACOKINETICS/DYNAMICS Reversibly inhibits the enzyme cholinesterase in the CNS, allowing buildup of acetylcholine and thereby improving cognitive functioning in patients with Alzheimer's disease.

SIDE EFFECTS CNS—agitation, ataxia, insomnia, abnormal thinking, somnolence, depression, anxiety, headache, fatigue, dizziness, confusion; GI—nausea, vomiting, diarrhea, dyspepsia, loose stools, anorexia, abdominal pain, constipation; respiratory—rhinitis, upper respiratory infection, cough; skin—rash, jaundice; other—myalgia, chest pain, weight loss.

ADVERSE REACTIONS Jaundice due to liver dysfunction, depression, confusion.

INTERACTIONS Drug-drug interactions: anticholinergics may decrease effectiveness of anticholinergics; cholinesterase inhibitors result in additive effects (toxicity); succinylcholine enhances neuromuscular blockade and prolongs duration of action; theophylline increases serum theophylline levels and prolongs theophylline half-life. Drug-food interactions: any food results in delayed absorption of the drug. Smoking decreases plasma concentration of the drug.

CONTRAINDICATIONS Clients with hypersensitivity to drug or acridine derivatives. Clients with elevated bilirubin. Clients with previously developed tacrine-related jaundice.

NURSING CONSIDERATIONS Use cautiously with clients with bradycardia or sick sinus syndrome; clients at risk for peptic ulcers, including clients taking NSAIDs; clients with a history of hepatic or renal disease; and clients with prostatic hyperplasia or urinary outflow impairment. Administer doses at regular intervals. Monitor serum ALT levels. If drug is discontinued for 4 wk or longer, a full dosage titration must be restarted and monitored.

CLIENT TEACHING Emphasize to client that the drug does not change the underlying degenerative disease and that positive effects are temporary. Abrupt discontinuation or large dose reduction may precipitate behavioral and cognitive dysfunction.

AVAILABLE IN CANADA Not available.

bold—Life-threatening reactions

GENERIC NAME: thioridazine
TRADE NAME: Mellaril

CLASSIFICATION Typical antipsychotic.

INDICATIONS & USES Symptomatic management of psychotic disorders; initial management of psychotic mania states; short-term management of depression, anxiety, and agitation.

USUAL ADULT DOSAGE RANGE 50-800 mg/day. Initial dosing is 50-100 mg bid or tid. Absolute maximum dose is 800 mg/day.

AVAILABLE FORMS Tabs 10, 15, 25, 50, 100, 150, 200, 300 mg; conc 30, 100 mg/ml; susp 25, 100 mg/5 ml; syrup 10 mg/15 ml.

PHARMACOKINETICS/DYNAMICS Rapidly absorbed; half-life averages 10-20 hr. Onset of action: 30-60 min. Full therapeutic effects may not be apparent for 6-12 wk. Initial multiple daily dosing can often be consolidated to once or twice a day, once client is tolerant to side effects.

SIDE EFFECTS Sedation, dizziness, blurred vision, dry mouth, constipation, urinary retention, nausea, vomiting, **tachycardia, orthostatic hypotension**, acute dystonic reaction, stiffness, cogwheel rigidity, bradykinesia, akathisia, gynecomastia, galactorrhea, amenorrhea, decreased libido, retrograde ejaculation, weight gain, allergic dermatitis, skin photosensitivity, reduced seizure threshold.

ADVERSE REACTIONS Risk of tardive dyskinesia, **neuroleptic malignant syndrome.** Doses >800 mg/day have been associated with pigmentary retinopathy and blindness.

INTERACTIONS Additive effects with CNS depressants and anticholinergic drugs. Serum levels are increased by antidepressants and propranolol, reduced by carbamazepine and phenytoin. Epinephrine may result in reverse (hypotensive) effects. Antacids reduce absorption.

CONTRAINDICATIONS Contraindicated in coma, severe hypotension, acute subcortical brain damage. Relatively contraindicated in liver disease, renal insufficiency, blood dyscrasias, Parkinson's disease. May exacerbate signs and symptoms of glaucoma, benign prostatic hypertrophy, diabetes. Avoid in pregnant and lactating women.

NURSING CONSIDERATIONS Monitor level of sedation and vital signs carefully during dose titration. Rapid dose increases, dehydration, and agitation are associated with increased incidence of neuroleptic malignant syndrome. Do not mix liquid concentrate with coffee, tea, or cola, apple, grape, pineapple, prune, or tomato juice; or Tang.

CLIENT TEACHING Rise from bed and change positions slowly to avoid dizziness. Use sugarless gum and candy for dry mouth. Use hats and sunscreens to reduce risk with sun exposure.

AVAILABLE IN CANADA Apo-Thioridazine, Mellaril.

bold—Life-threatening reactions

GENERIC NAME: thiothixene
TRADE NAME: Navane

CLASSIFICATION Typical antipsychotic.

INDICATIONS & USES Symptomatic management of psychotic disorders, initial management of psychotic manic states, acute agitation.

USUAL ADULT DOSAGE RANGE 6-30 mg/day. Initial dosing is 2-5 mg/day every day. Total daily doses as high as 60 mg/day may be required. Typical IM dose is 2-4 mg.

AVAILABLE FORMS Caps 1, 2, 5, 10, 20 mg; conc 5 mg/ml; inj IM 2 mg/ml; powder for inj 5 mg/ml.

PHARMACOKINETICS/DYNAMICS Rapidly absorbed; half-life averages 10-20 hr. PO onset of action: 1-2 hr. Full therapeutic effects may not be apparent for 6-12 wk. Initial multiple daily dosing can often be consolidated to once or twice a day, once client is tolerant to side effects.

SIDE EFFECTS Sedation, blurred vision, dry mouth, constipation, urinary retention, nausea, vomiting, tachycardia, orthostatic hypotension, acute dystonic reaction, stiffness, cogwheel rigidity, bradykinesia, akathisia, gynecomastia, galactorrhea, amenorrhea, decreased libido, retrograde ejaculation, weight gain, allergic dermatitis, skin photosensitivity, reduced seizure threshold.

ADVERSE REACTIONS Risk of tardive dyskinesia, **neuroleptic malignant syndrome,** seizures.

INTERACTIONS Additive effects with CNS depressants. Serum levels are increased by antidepressants and propranolol, reduced by carbamazepine and phenytoin. Antacids reduce absorption. Do not mix liquid concentrate with coffee, tea, apple juice, or cola.

CONTRAINDICATIONS Contraindicated in coma, severe hypotension, and acute subcortical brain damage. Relatively contraindicated in liver disease, renal insufficiency, blood dyscrasias, and Parkinson's disease. May exacerbate signs and symptoms of glaucoma, benign prostatic hypertrophy, and diabetes. Avoid in pregnant and lactating women.

NURSING CONSIDERATIONS Monitor level of sedation and vital signs carefully during dose titration. Rapid dose increases, dehydration, IM injections, and agitation are associated with increased incidence of neuroleptic malignant syndrome.

CLIENT TEACHING Use hats and sunscreens to reduce risk with sun exposure. Report fever and increasing stiffness immediately.

AVAILABLE IN CANADA Navane.

bold—Life-threatening reactions

GENERIC NAME: trazodone
TRADE NAME: Desyrel

CLASSIFICATION Triazolopyridine antidepressant.

INDICATIONS & USES Major depression, sleep disturbance, anxiety.

USUAL ADULT DOSAGE RANGE 50-600 mg/day. Initial dosing is 50-150 mg/day in divided doses.

AVAILABLE FORMS Tabs 50, 100, 150, 300 mg.

PHARMACOKINETICS/DYNAMICS In adults, half-life is approximately 6-11 hr. Full therapeutic effects may not be apparent for 2-4 wk.

SIDE EFFECTS Very sedating, dry mouth, blurred vision, constipation, urinary retention, somnolence, dizziness, orthostatic hypotension. Rarely—**priapism in males.**

ADVERSE REACTIONS Induction of mania, rarely—priapism.

INTERACTIONS Increased effects with CNS depressants, alcohol. Addition of fluoxetine may dramatically increase trazodone levels.

CONTRAINDICATIONS Avoid in pregnant and nursing mothers.

NURSING CONSIDERATIONS Suicide risk may be increased during initial improvement, particularly as psychomotor depression abates.

CLIENT TEACHING Therapeutic effects may take several weeks. May cause excessive sedation during initiation. Priapism is a medical emergency.

AVAILABLE IN CANADA Desyrel, Alti-Trazodone, Apo-Trazodone, PMS-Trazodone, Apo-Trazodone D, Alti-Trazodone Dividose, Novo-Trazodone, Nu-Trazodone D, Desyrel Dividose, Trazorel.

bold—Life-threatening reactions

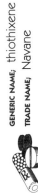

GENERIC NAME: triazolam
TRADE NAME: Halcion

CLASSIFICATION Hypnotic—benzodiazepine.

INDICATIONS & USES Short-term (7-10 days) treatment of insomnia.

USUAL ADULT DOSAGE RANGE Starting dose of 0.25 mg in adults, 0.125 mg in the elderly or debilitated; 0.5 mg should be reserved for exceptional cases and should not be exceeded.

AVAILABLE FORMS Tabs 0.125, 0.25, 0.5 mg.

PHARMACOKINETICS/DYNAMICS Rapidly absorbed. Half-life averages 2 hr. Rapid onset of sleep.

SIDE EFFECTS Sedation, fatigue, drowsiness, dizziness, ataxia.

ADVERSE REACTIONS Anterograde amnesia. Rarely—agitation, excitability, psychotic symptoms.

INTERACTIONS Addition of nefazodone, erythromycin may notably increase and prolong effects. CNS depressants; may increase levels of phenytoin, digoxin. Effects reduced by smoking, rifampin. Serum levels increased by cimetidine, valproate, oral contraceptives, disulfiram.

CONTRAINDICATIONS Coma, shock, alcohol intoxication, pregnancy. Use with caution in history of drug abuse/addiction.

NURSING CONSIDERATIONS Schedule IV controlled substance. Risk of respiratory depression when used with other CNS depressants. Monitor for next-morning sedation and reduced cognitive functioning. Abrupt discontinuation associated with anxiety, rebound insomnia.

CLIENT TEACHING Avoid hazardous activities during initiation. Avoid alcohol. Drug should not be discontinued suddenly.

AVAILABLE IN CANADA Apo-Triazo, Alti-Triazolam, Gen-Triazolam.

bold—Life-threatening reactions

GENERIC NAME: valproic acid, valproate sodium, divalproex sodium
TRADE NAME: Depakene, Depakene Syrup, Depakote, Depakote Sprinkle

CLASSIFICATION Anticonvulsant, antimanic.

INDICATIONS & USES Simple and complex absence seizures, tonic-clonic seizures, mixed seizures, bipolar disorder, episodic dyscontrol disorder.

PHARMACOKINETICS/DYNAMICS Average half-life is 8-20 hr in adults. Efficacy in seizures may occur several days after achieving therapeutic levels. Efficacy in mania may occur over 1-2 wk, but in as quickly as 3 days with aggressive dosing (e.g., starting at 500 mg tid). Therapeutic range for seizures is 50-120 µg/ml. Efficacy equivalent to lithium has been found when dosed to serum levels of 150 µg/ml. Therapeutic efficacy is seldom seen at levels <50 µg/ml.

USUAL ADULT DOSAGE RANGE Initially 15 mg/kg/day to a maximum of 60 mg/kg/day. Starting doses typically used vary from 250-500 mg bid. Some clinicians treat acute mania with starting doses of 500 mg tid.

AVAILABLE FORMS Caps 250 mg; tabs 125, 250, 500 mg; syr 250 mg/5 ml; 125 mg sprinkle capsules.

SIDE EFFECTS Drowsiness, nausea, vomiting, diarrhea, tremor, weight gain, transient hair loss, elevated serum ammonia, mild thrombocytopenia, pruritus.

ADVERSE REACTIONS Excess sedation, pancreatitis, liver enzymes >3 times normal. Rarely—**liver failure.** Teratogenic—associated with neural tube defects, most commonly spina bifida.

INTERACTIONS Decreases valproate levels—carbamazepine, phenobarbital, primidone, phenytoin. Increases valproate effect—salicylates, erythromycin.

CONTRAINDICATIONS Severe hepatic dysfunction, coma, pregnancy.

NURSING CONSIDERATIONS Monitor liver function tests.

CLIENT TEACHING May experience initial sedation. May take with food to reduce GI upset. Do not crush the coated (enteric) product Depakote.

AVAILABLE IN CANADA Epival, Depakene, Depakene Syrup, Deproic, Epiject IV, Gen-Valproic, Novo-Valproic, PMS-Valproic Acid, PMS-Valproic Acid EC.

bold—Life-threatening reactions

GENERIC NAME: trihexyphenidyl
TRADE NAME: Artane

CLASSIFICATION Antiparkinsonian, anticholinergic.

INDICATIONS & USES Parkinsonism, treatment and prevention of extrapyramidal symptoms caused by antipsychotic medications (excluding tardive dyskinesia).

USUAL ADULT DOSAGE RANGE 1-5 mg bid to qid. Typical starting dose 5 mg bid.

AVAILABLE FORMS Tabs 2, 5 mg, sus-rel caps 5 mg, elix 2 mg/5 ml.

PHARMACOKINETICS/DYNAMICS Rapidly absorbed. Peak effects in 1-2 hr. The pharmacokinetics are not well characterized. Usually given in 1-2 divided doses. Duration of efficacy varies from 6-12 hr.

SIDE EFFECTS Dry mouth, blurred vision, tachycardia, urinary retention, constipation, nervousness, confusion, excitation, euphoria.

ADVERSE REACTIONS **Paralytic ileus.** Anticholinergic delirium (also called anticholinergic intoxication and atropine psychosis)—confusion, disorientation, stupor, flushing, hyperthermia, extreme agitation, hallucinations, hypotension, supraventricular tachycardia, markedly diminished or absent bowel sounds.

INTERACTIONS Additive anticholinergic effects with other medications, especially antipsychotics, tricyclic antidepressants, MAOIs, digoxin, furosemide (Lasix).

CONTRAINDICATIONS Severe cardiac or GI disorders, benign prostatic hypertrophy, narrow angle-closure glaucoma, **neuroleptic malignant syndrome.**

NURSING CONSIDERATIONS Increased risk of heat stroke. Evaluate for adequate hydration and constipation. May aggravate the movements of tardive dyskinesia. **Elderly clients are at increased risk for confusion and anticholinergic delirium.** More stimulating than

benztropine. Euphoric side effect can result in drug-seeking behaviors by substance abusers.

CLIENT TEACHING Give with meals. May cause drowsiness, blurred vision, or dizziness. Avoid alcohol and other CNS depressants. Contact physician for rapid and pounding heartbeat. Use caution in hot weather.

AVAILABLE IN CANADA Apo-Trihex.

bold—Life-threatening reactions

GENERIC NAME: venlafaxine
TRADE NAME: Effexor

CLASSIFICATION Phenethylamine antidepressant, norepinephrine and serotonin reuptake inhibitor.

INDICATIONS & USES Major depression.

USUAL ADULT DOSAGE RANGE 150-350 mg/day. Initial dosing is 75 mg/day as 25 mg tid or 37.5 mg bid. Maximum dose is 375 mg/day in divided doses. Dose increases should be made at no less than 4-day intervals.

AVAILABLE FORMS Tabs 25, 37.5, 50, 75, 100 mg.

PHARMACOKINETICS/DYNAMICS In adults, venlafaxine's half-life is approximately 3-7 hr, and the active metabolite O-desmethylvenlafaxine's half-life is approximately 9-13 hr. Doses should be reduced in clients with severe hepatic or renal disease and in the elderly. Full therapeutic effects may not be apparent for 2-4 wk.

SIDE EFFECTS Asthenia, sweating, nausea, vomiting, constipation, anorexia, somnolence, dry mouth, dizziness, nervousness, anxiety, tremor, blurred vision, sexual dysfunction, insomnia.

ADVERSE REACTIONS Induction of mania, hypertension.

INTERACTIONS **Potentially fatal hypertensive crisis when MAOIs (including selegiline) are used within 2 wk of discontinuation.**

CONTRAINDICATIONS Avoid in pregnant and nursing mothers.

NURSING CONSIDERATIONS Suicide risk may be increased during initial improvement, particularly as psychomotor depression abates.

CLIENT TEACHING Therapeutic effects may take several weeks. May experience excessive sedation during initiation. Drug should not be discontinued suddenly.

AVAILABLE IN CANADA Effexor XR.

bold—Life-threatening reactions